汉英双解针灸大辞典

A CHINESE-ENGLISH DICTIONARY OF ACUPUNCTURE & MOXIBUSTION

中文主编 (Chinese Chief Editor)： 石学敏 (SHI, Xue-min)
英文主编 (English Chief Editor)： 张孟辰 (ZHANG, Meng-chen)

华夏出版社
Huaxia Publishing House

《汉英双解针灸大辞典》编纂委员会

主 任 委 员：石学敏
副主任委员：武连仲(中)　张孟辰(英)
编　　　委：刘嘉斌　李　力　郭宗仁　刘大勇　张文起
　　　　　　曹立娅　李　平　蒋戈利　王　舒　李志道
　　　　　　仇同庆　关启升　王荣武

中文　　　　　　　　　　　　　　英文

主　　编：石学敏　　　　　　　　主　　编：张孟辰
副 主 编：郭宗仁　武连仲　李志道　译　　者：李　力　曹立娅　李　平
编　　者：仇同庆　李桂兰　王　卫　　　　　　王　舒　蒋戈利　关启升
　　　　　孟　红　胡明海　尚秀葵　　　　　　张耀华　毛静远　白俊昆
　　　　　梁春雨　杨增瑞　袁洪霞　　　　　　高洪秀　李　华　张　培
　　　　　孟繁洁　　　　　　　　　　　　　　袁　杰　苗　菊　李菊菊
协　　编：陈秘水　李德元　李　锦　审　　译：刘嘉斌(主审)
　　　　　奚　阳　　　　　　　　　　　　　　刘大勇　张文起
绘　　图：房建国　　　　　　　　　　　　　　张坚(兼英文协译)

特约外籍专家：[美]Marnae C. Engil 博士

总 目 录

使用说明 …………………………………………………………… (1~2)
汉语拼音检字表 …………………………………………………… (3~7)
汉语拼音索引 ……………………………………………………… (8~56)
正文 ………………………………………………………………… (1~649)
附录 ………………………………………………………………… (1~81)
　一、中外针灸医家 ……………………………………………… (1~15)
　二、穴名索引 …………………………………………………… (16~22)
　三、插图索引 …………………………………………………… (23~25)
英文索引 …………………………………………………………… (26~81)

General Contents

Guide to the Use of this Dictionary ································· (1~2)
Word Index by the Phonetic Transcriptions of Chinese Characters ············· (3~7)
Syllable Index by the Phonetic Transcriptions of Chinese Characters ··········· (8~56)
The Main Body ·· (1~649)
Appendix ··· (1~81)
   I. Acupuncture-Moxibustion Famous Experts in China and the Other
      Countries ··· (1~15)
   II. Index of Acupoint Names ·· (16~22)
   III. Index of Illustrations ·· (23~25)
Index of English ··· (26~81)

使 用 说 明

一、本辞典收入有关中国针灸主要名词、术语4000余条,力求涵盖针灸学各主要领域的知识和操作要点,释文通俗、准确。

二、汉语条目按汉语拼音字母顺序排列。同音异声的,按四声顺序排列;同音同声的,按笔画多少排列。多字条目如第一个字相同,则按第二个字的汉语拼音字母顺序、四声以及笔画多少排列;第二个字相同,按第三个字排列,依此类推。

单字条目或多字条目首字字形相同而音或调不同者,分立条目。如:

  恶阻(è zǔ)   华盖(huá gài)
  恶食(wù shí)   华佗(huà tuó)

三、多义项条目,汉语均以①②③等数码排列。隶属同一汉语条目的各义项,如使用相同英译条目名,其英语仍按①②③等数码排列;如须各自使用不同的英译义项名,则以1、2、3等数码排列,不再另立条目。

四、汉语条目后均加注汉语拼音,置于圆括弧(　)内。穴位名称的英语采用汉语拼音(耳穴除外)。条目名和英语释义中的穴位名均不再标调。

声调只注原调,不注变调。

英语释义中的穴位名或经脉名有同音同声或同音异声的,均按汉语原序列出,同时在该英文后加注原汉字,以示区别。

五、与汉语书名对应的英语部分一律采用先汉语拼音(斜体)后英语音译的方法,汉语拼音不标调,英语意译置入圆括弧(　)内。

六、与汉语中草药名对应的英语部分,均采用先汉语拼音后拉丁字的方法,汉语拼音不标调,拉丁字置于圆括弧(　)内。

七、插图及其他符号的使用。

 1. 国际的经穴、奇穴以及耳穴均配有插图,标明其定位,该插图所在页码注在该穴位正名定位后的圆括弧(　)内。

 2. 汉语条目名均置于圆实点"●"之后。

 3. 穴位所属经脉或所在位置的英语缩写和代号,只在该穴位正名的对应英文后标出,置于圆括弧(　)内。

 4. 箭号"→"用于英语义项之后,指明相关或参见的条目及其所在页码。箭号后一般只有汉语条目名及页码。

 5. 书名条目名的汉语不加书名号,释义中的仍须加书名号。书名与章节名同时出现时,汉语部分用"·"隔开;其对应的英语中的汉语拼音仍用"·",英语意译部分中间用冒号。

八、汉、英释义中所含小标题,如"定位"、"层次解剖"等,均用〈　〉括注。

GUIDE TO THE USE OF THIS DICTIONARY

1. This dictionary includes more than 4000 main nouns and terms about the Chinese acupuncture-moxibustion, which involved the knowledge and operating essentials in the foundational fields of Chinese acupuncture-moxibustion study. And the explanations are simple and precise.

2. The entries in Chinese will be arranged by the order of the Chinese phonetic alphabet. The homonym nouns which are on different tones, will be arranged by the order of the four tones of modern standard Chinese pronunciation. The homonym nouns which are on the same tones, will be arranged by the order of numbers of Chinese charater strokes. If the first character is same, the multi-character entry will be arranged by the order of the second character's phonetic alphabet, four tones and stroke number; if the second same, it will be by the third; and so on and so forth.

The entries which are same character and different pronunciation or tones, will be put in different places, e.g.:

恶阻(è zǔ)   华盖(huá gài)

恶食(wù shí)   华佗(huà tuó)

3. The polysemant entries' Chinese characters are ordered on ①, ②, ③, and so on. The different meanings of the same Chinese entry, are ordered on ①, ②, ③, and so on, for English explantations; if necessary to use different English explantations, they are ordered on 1, 2, 3, and will not be put independently.

4. The Chinese entries will be all noted the Chinese phonetic transcriptions in the brackets. The names of acupoints in English will be on the Chinese phonetic transcription (except *ear-acupoints*). The names of the acupoints in the entries and English explantations, will be not signified the tones.

The tones will be only signified the original and not the tone sandi.

The names of the acupoints and the passages, the same pronunciation and the same tones, or the same pronunciation and the different tones, will be ordered on the Chinese originals, and will be signified the Chinese characters after the English explantations.

5. The English translations of the Chinese work titles will be signified their Chinese pronunciations, and after these, the English transliteration; the Chinese pronunciations will be not signified the tones. And their English free-translations will be in the brackets.

6. The English explantations of the names of herbs, are signified the Chinese pronunclations first and then the latin nouns; and the latin nouns are in the brackets.

7. The illustrations and the usage of the other signs:

   a. The passage, fractional and ear acupoints in the State Standard of China all will be concerted illustrations and signified their points. The illustration's pages are on the brackets of the referential acupoints.
   b. The Chinese entries will be following to the signs "●".
   c. The English abbreviations and codes of the acupoint passages and points will be only signified after the referential English explantations of the acupoints' original names, and in the brackets.
   d. The arrows "→" are after the English meanings, which are signified referential entries and their pages, After the arrows only are the names and the pages of the Chinese entries.
   e. The Chinese characters of the book titles are not signified punctuation marks "〈 〉". When the work titles and volume titles appear in the same places, the marks "·" will be put between the titles in the Chinese and also the English. And in the English free translations, it will be signified colons between them.

8. The headlines of Chinese and English explantations, for example "Location", "Regional anatomy", etc, will be all signified the marks "〈 〉".

汉语拼音检字表

A	暴 (15)	病 (25)	长 (39)	[chuāi]	攒 (58)	导 (76)	[dòu]
[ā]	[bèi]	[bó]	肠 (40)	揣 (51)	[cuàn]	捣 (77)	豆 (85)
阿 (1)	备 (16)	帛 (25)	[chè]	[chuān]	篡 (58)	[dé]	窦 (85)
[ài]	背 (16)	脖 (26)	彻 (41)	川 (51)	[cuī]	得 (77)	[dū]
艾 (1)	[běn]	膊 (26)	[chén]	穿 (51)	催 (58)	[dēng]	督 (85)
[ān]	本 (17)	[bò]	臣 (41)	[chuán]	[cuì]	灯 (77)	[dú]
安 (3)	[bēng]	擘 (26)	陈 (42)	传 (51)	焠 (58)	[dí]	独 (88)
[àn]	崩 (18)	[bǔ]	晨 (42)	[chuǎn]	[cún]	锝 (77)	犊 (88)
按 (3)	[bí]	补 (26)	[chēng]	喘 (51)	存 (59)	[dǐ]	[dù]
	鼻 (18)	[bù]	撑 (42)	[chuāng]	[cùn]	骶 (78)	妒 (88)
B	[bì]	不 (27)	[chéng]	窗 (51)	寸 (58)	[dì]	[duǎn]
[bā]	闭 (20)	步 (29)	成 (42)	[chuī]	[cuō]	地 (78)	短 (88)
八 (4)	痹 (20)		承 (42)	吹 (52)	搓 (59)	[diān]	[duàn]
巴 (8)	蔽 (20)	**C**	程 (45)	[chuí]		颠 (79)	断 (88)
[bá]	薛 (20)	[cǎi]	[chī]	垂 (52)	**D**	巅 (79)	[duì]
拔 (9)	臂 (20)	采 (30)	吃 (46)	[chún]	[dá]	癫 (79)	对 (89)
[bái]	髀 (22)	[cāng]	[chí]	唇 (52)	达 (59)	[diǎn]	兑 (89)
白 (10)	[biān]	苍 (30)	池 (46)	淳 (52)	[dǎ]	点 (80)	[dùn]
[bǎi]	砭 (22)	[cáng]	[chǐ]	[cī]	打 (59)	[diàn]	顿 (90)
百 (11)	[biǎn]	藏 (30)	尺 (46)	疵 (52)	[dà]	电 (80)	[duō]
[bān]	扁 (23)	[cáo]	齿 (47)	[cí]	大 (59)	雕 (82)	多 (91)
斑 (12)	[biàn]	曹 (31)	[chì]	慈 (52)	[dài]	[dīng]	[duó]
瘢 (12)	便 (24)	[cǎo]	豉 (47)	雌 (53)	代 (69)	丁 (82)	夺 (91)
[bàn]	辨 (24)	草 (31)	赤 (47)	磁 (53)	带 (70)	疔 (82)	
半 (12)	[biǎo]	[cè]	瘛 (48)	[cì]	[dān]	[dǐng]	**E**
[bàng]	表 (24)	侧 (31)	[chōng]	次 (53)	丹 (71)	顶 (83)	[é]
傍 (13)	[bié]	[chā]	冲 (48)	刺 (53)	单 (72)	[dìng]	蛾 (91)
[bāo]	别 (25)	插 (31)	[chóng]	[cōng]	担 (72)	定 (83)	额 (91)
包 (13)	[bīn]	[chán]	虫 (49)	葱 (56)	[dǎn]	[dōng]	[è]
胞 (13)	膑 (25)	缠 (31)	重 (50)	[cóng]	胆 (73)	东 (84)	呃 (92)
[bǎo]	[bīng]	镵 (31)	崇 (50)	从 (56)	[dàn]	[dòng]	恶 (92)
保 (15)	冰 (25)	[chǎn]	产 (32)	[cù]	亶 (75)	动 (84)	饿 (93)
[bào]	[bǐng]	产 (32)	[chāng]	卒 (57)	膻 (75)	[dǒu]	颔 (93)
报 (15)	秉 (25)	[cháng]	昌 (38)	猝 (58)	当 (76)	斗 (85)	[ér]
豹 (15)	[bìng]	昌 (38)	[chū]	[cuán]	[dǎo]		儿 (93)
			出 (51)	[cuán]			[ěr]

3

耳 (94)	扶 (118)	孤 (142)	含 (155)	[huá]	霍 (181)	量 (193)	[jiū]
[èr]	浮 (118)	[gǔ]	寒 (155)	华 (168)	**J**	[jiàng]	鸠 (219)
二 (100)	涪 (119)	谷 (142)	[hàn]	滑 (168)	[jī]	降 (193)	[jiǔ]
F	[fǔ]	骨 (142)	扞 (158)	[huà]	机 (181)	[jiāo]	九 (220)
[fā]	府 (119)	鼓 (146)	旱 (158)	化 (169)	鸡 (181)	交 (193)	灸 (222)
发 (103)	俯 (119)	臌 (146)	颔 (158)	华 (169)	积 (182)	椒 (199)	[jū]
[fān]	辅 (120)	[gù]	[háo]	[huái]	基 (182)	焦 (199)	居 (225)
翻 (103)	[fù]	固 (146)	毫 (159)	踝 (170)	箕 (182)	[jiǎo]	[jú]
[fán]	附 (120)	刮 (146)	[hé]	[huán]	激 (182)	角 (199)	局 (225)
樊 (103)	复 (120)	[guā]	禾 (160)	环 (170)	[jí]	脚 (200)	[jù]
燔 (104)	腹 (121)	[guān]	合 (160)	[huǎn]	极 (183)	[jiē]	巨 (225)
[fǎn]	**G**	关 (146)	何 (162)	缓 (172)	急 (183)	痎 (200)	聚 (228)
反 (104)	[gān]	[guàn]	和 (162)	[huàn]	疾 (184)	接 (200)	[juē]
返 (104)	干 (123)	罐 (149)	核 (162)	患 (172)	集 (185)	[jié]	撅 (228)
[fàn]	甘 (123)	[guāng]	颌 (162)	[huāng]	[jǐ]	节 (201)	[jué]
范 (105)	肝 (123)	光 (149)	颃 (162)	肓 (172)	脊 (185)	截 (201)	绝 (228)
[fàng]	疳 (130)	[guī]	颔 (162)	[huáng]	[jì]	解 (201)	厥 (229)
放 (105)	[gǎn]	归 (150)	鹘 (162)	皇 (173)	忌 (186)	[jiě]	橛 (230)
[fēi]	感 (131)	[guǐ]	鹤 (162)	黄 (173)	季 (186)	解 (201)	[jùn]
飞 (105)	[gāng]	鬼 (150)	[hēi]	癀 (176)	[jiā]	[jīn]	䐃 (230)
非 (106)	肛 (131)	[gǔn]	黑 (163)	[huī]	夹 (186)	巾 (202)	**K**
[fěi]	[gāo]	滚 (152)	[héng]	恢 (176)	颊 (187)	金 (202)	[kāi]
鲱 (107)	高 (131)	[guō]	横 (163)	[huí]	[jiǎ]	筋 (204)	开 (230)
[fèi]	膏 (132)	郭 (152)	衡 (164)	回 (177)	甲 (188)	[jǐn]	[kàn]
肺 (107)	[gē]	[guó]	[hóng]	迴 (177)	胛 (188)	紧 (204)	看 (231)
[fēn]	割 (133)	腘 (153)	红 (164)	蚘 (177)	[jiān]	[jìn]	[kāo]
分 (109)	[gé]	[guò]	[hóu]	[huì]	间 (188)	进 (204)	尻 (231)
[fēng]	阁 (133)	过 (153)	喉 (165)	会 (177)	肩 (188)	近 (206)	[kǎo]
丰 (109)	隔 (133)	**H**	[hòu]	绘 (179)	[jiǎn]	噤 (207)	考 (231)
风 (110)	膈 (139)	[há]	后 (165)	[hún]	睑 (192)	[jīng]	[kē]
锋 (116)	[gě]	虾 (154)	候 (166)	魂 (179)	[jiàn]	京 (207)	颗 (231)
[féng]	葛 (140)	蛤 (154)	[hū]	[hùn]	间 (192)	经 (208)	[ké]
冯 (116)	[gēn]	[hái]	呼 (167)	混 (179)	建 (192)	惊 (217)	咳 (231)
[fèng]	根 (140)	骸 (154)	[hú]	[huó]	剑 (192)	睛 (217)	[kè]
凤 (116)	跟 (141)	[hǎi]	狐 (167)	活 (179)	健 (193)	精 (218)	客 (232)
[fū]	[gōng]	海 (154)	胡 (167)	[huǒ]	箭 (193)	[jǐng]	[kǒng]
跗 (116)	公 (142)	[hài]	虎 (167)	火 (180)	姜 (193)	井 (218)	孔 (232)
[fú]	宫 (142)	害 (154)	[huā]	[huò]	[jiāng]	颈 (218)	[kòng]
伏 (117)	[gū]	[hán]	花 (168)	或 (181)	姜 (193)	痉 (219)	控 (232)

4

[kǒu]	蠡(242)	龙(253)	卵(264)	脑(276)	P	铺(299)	秦(319)
口(232)	[lǐ]	聋(255)	[méi]	[nào]	[pāi]	[pú]	[qǐn]
[kǔ]	李(242)	癃(255)	眉(265)	臑(277)	拍(288)	仆(299)	寝(319)
苦(234)	里(243)	[lóu]	梅(265)	[nèi]	[pái]	[pǔ]	[qīng]
[kù]	理(243)	楼(256)	[mén]	内(278)	排(288)	普(299)	青(320)
库(234)	[lì]	[lòu]	扪(266)	[néng]	[pán]	Q	清(321)
[kuài]	厉(243)	漏(256)	[mèng]	能(282)	盘(288)	[qī]	[qióng]
快(235)	利(243)	[lú]	梦(266)	[ní]	[páng]	七(300)	琼(321)
[kuān]	疠(244)	颅(257)	[miàn]	泥(282)	旁(288)	期(300)	[qiū]
髋(235)	痢(244)	[lù]	面(266)	[nì]	膀(289)	[qí]	丘(322)
[kuáng]	[lián]	鹭(257)	[miǎo]	逆(282)	[pèi]	齐(300)	[qiú]
狂(235)	廉(244)	[lǚ]	眇(268)	溺(283)	配(290)	岐(301)	球(322)
[kūn]	[liàn]	吕(257)	[míng]	[niǎn]	[pēn]	奇(301)	[qū]
昆(236)	练(244)	闾(258)	名(268)	捻(283)	贲(291)	脐(302)	曲(323)
L	炼(245)	膂(258)	明(268)	[niàn]	[pén]	骑(303)	屈(326)
[lā]	[liáng]	[lún]	[mìng]	念(284)	盆(291)	蛴(303)	胠(326)
拉(236)	梁(245)	轮(258)	命(269)	[niǎo]	[péng]	綦(303)	[qǔ]
[lá]	[liǎng]	[luǒ]	[miù]	尿(284)	彭(291)	[qǐ]	取(326)
喇(236)	两(246)	瘰(258)	缪(270)	[niè]	蓬(291)	起(303)	[qù]
[lán]	[liáo]	[luò]	[mó]	捏(285)	[pī]	[qì]	去(326)
兰(236)	髎(246)	络(259)	膜(270)	聂(285)	铍(291)	气(303)	[quán]
拦(237)	[liè]	M	[mǔ]	颞(285)	[pí]	[qiā]	权(327)
阑(237)	列(246)	[má]	拇(270)	[níng]	皮(291)	掐(315)	全(327)
[láo]	[lín]	麻(261)	踇(271)	凝(285)	琵(292)	[qiān]	泉(327)
劳(237)	邻(247)	[mǎ]	[mù]	[niú]	脾(292)	千(315)	拳(327)
[lǎo]	临(247)	马(261)	木(271)	牛(285)	[pǐ]	牵(316)	颧(327)
老(239)	[lìn]	[mái]	目(271)	[niǔ]	痞(296)	[qián]	[quē]
[lào]	淋(247)	埋(262)	募(274)	扭(286)	[piān]	前(316)	缺(328)
落(239)	[líng]	[mài]	N	[nǔ]	偏(296)	荨(318)	[què]
[léi]	灵(247)	麦(262)	[nà]	努(286)	[pián]	钱(318)	雀(328)
雷(239)	陵(250)	脉(262)	纳(275)	[nǚ]	骈(297)	[qiáng]	阙(328)
[lèi]	[liú]	[màn]	[nǎi]	女(286)	[píng]	强(318)	R
肋(240)	刘(250)	慢(263)	奶(276)	[nüè]	平(297)	[qiào]	[rán]
泪(240)	流(251)	[máng]	[nán]	疟(286)	屏(298)	窍(319)	然(329)
类(240)	留(251)	芒(263)	男(276)	O	[pò]	[qiē]	[ráng]
[lěng]	硫(252)	盲(264)	难(276)	[ōu]	迫(298)	切(319)	瀼(329)
冷(241)	[liù]	[máo]	[náng]	呕(287)	破(298)	[qié]	[rè]
[lí]	六(252)	毛(264)	囊(276)	[ǒu]	魄(298)	茄(319)	热(329)
离(241)	[lóng]	[mǎo]	[nǎo]	偶(287)	[pū]	[qín]	[rén]

5

人 (332)	疝 (348)	时 (386)	溲 (416)	替 (429)	团 (449)	[wū]	消 (493)
任 (334)	[shāng]	实 (386)	[sòu]	[tiān]	[tuī]	乌 (471)	哮 (495)
[rèn]	伤 (349)	食 (386)	嗽 (416)	天 (429)	推 (449)	屋 (472)	瘠 (495)
妊 (335)	商 (350)	[shǐ]	[sù]	[tiáo]	[tuì]	[wú]	[xiǎo]
[rì]	[shàng]	始 (388)	素 (416)	条 (437)	退 (450)	无 (472)	小 (495)
日 (337)	上 (351)	[shì]	[suàn]	调 (438)	[tún]	吴 (472)	[xiē]
[róng]	尚 (355)	视 (388)	蒜 (416)	[tiǎo]	臀 (450)	[wǔ]	歇 (505)
荣 (337)	[shāo]	势 (388)	[suí]	挑 (438)	[tuō]	五 (474)	[xié]
[ròu]	烧 (355)	是 (388)	随 (416)	[tiě]	托 (450)	舞 (481)	胁 (505)
肉 (337)	[shào]	释 (388)	髓 (417)	铁 (438)	脱 (450)	[wù]	斜 (505)
[rǔ]	少 (356)	[shǒu]	[sūn]	[tīng]		恶 (481)	[xiè]
乳 (338)	[shé]	手 (388)	孙 (417)	听 (438)	W		泻 (506)
[ruì]	舌 (358)	守 (405)	[suō]	[tíng]	[wài]	X	泄 (507)
锐 (339)	蛇 (359)	首 (405)	缩 (418)	葶 (439)	外 (452)	[xī]	解 (507)
[ruò]	[shè]	[shū]	[suǒ]	聤 (439)	[wán]	西 (482)	[xīn]
蒻 (340)	摄 (359)	枢 (405)	锁 (418)	[tǐng]	完 (456)	吸 (482)	心 (507)
	[shēn]	俞 (405)	所 (418)	艇 (440)	[wǎn]	息 (482)	辛 (510)
S	申 (359)	舒 (406)		[tōng]	碗 (457)	溪 (482)	新 (510)
[sāi]	身 (360)	输 (406)	T	通 (440)	[wàn]	膝 (482)	[xìn]
腮 (340)	[shén]	[shǔ]	[tā]	[tóng]	腕 (457)	蹊 (484)	囟 (510)
[sān]	神 (360)	属 (407)	他 (418)	同 (442)	[wáng]	[xí]	[xīng]
三 (340)	[shěn]	暑 (407)	[tāi]	铜 (442)	王 (458)	席 (484)	兴 (511)
[sǎn]	沈 (364)	鼠 (407)	胎 (418)	童 (443)	[wēi]	[xì]	惺 (511)
散 (346)	[shèn]	[shù]	[tài]	瞳 (443)	微 (460)	郄 (484)	[xíng]
[sāng]	肾 (364)	束 (407)	太 (419)	[tǒng]	[wéi]	细 (485)	行 (511)
桑 (347)	[shēng]	腧 (407)	[tán]	筒 (443)	维 (460)	[xiá]	[xiōng]
[sǎng]	生 (368)	[shuài]	弹 (423)	[tòng]	[wěi]	侠 (485)	胸 (512)
颡 (347)	[shèng]	率 (408)	痰 (423)	痛 (443)	尾 (460)	[xià]	[xiū]
[sè]	圣 (369)	[shuāng]	[táo]	[tōu]	委 (461)	下 (486)	休 (514)
色 (347)	胜 (369)	双 (408)	桃 (426)	偷 (444)	痿 (462)	夏 (491)	[xiù]
[sēng]	盛 (369)	[shuǐ]	陶 (426)	[tóu]	[wèi]	[xián]	绣 (514)
僧 (347)	[shī]	水 (408)	套 (427)	头 (444)	卫 (462)	痫 (491)	[xū]
[shā]	尸 (369)	[shuì]	[tè]	[tòu]	胃 (462)	[xiàn]	虚 (514)
莎 (347)	失 (369)	睡 (412)	特 (427)	透 (448)	[wēn]	陷 (492)	[xú]
砂 (348)	施 (370)	[sī]	[tí]	[tǔ]	温 (469)	[xiāng]	徐 (516)
[shān]	湿 (370)	丝 (412)	提 (427)	土 (449)	[wén]	香 (493)	[xǔ]
山 (348)	[shí]	[sì]	[tǐ]	[tù]	闻 (471)	[xiàng]	许 (517)
闪 (348)	十 (373)	四 (412)	体 (428)	吐 (449)	[wò]	项 (493)	[xù]
[shàn]	石 (384)	[sōu]	[tì]	[tuán]	卧 (471)	[xiāo]	絮 (518)

蓄 (518)	沿 (535)	[yí]	迎 (566)	原 (576)	掌 (585)	指 (603)	膪 (623)
[xuán]	研 (535)	胰 (551)	荥 (567)	缘 (577)	[zhàng]	趾 (604)	[zhuāng]
玄 (518)	盐 (535)	遗 (552)	营 (568)	[yuǎn]	胀 (585)	[zhì]	庄 (623)
旋 (518)	颜 (535)	颐 (552)	[yǐng]	远 (577)	瘴 (586)	至 (605)	[zhuàng]
悬 (518)	[yǎn]	[yǐ]	瘿 (568)	[yuē]	[zhǎo]	志 (605)	壮 (623)
璇 (520)	眼 (535)	以 (552)	[yōng]	约 (578)	爪 (586)	治 (606)	[zhuī]
[xuǎn]	[yàn]	[yì]	痈 (568)	[yuě]	[zhào]	秩 (606)	椎 (623)
选 (520)	燕 (535)	异 (552)	[yǒng]	哕 (578)	照 (586)	痔 (606)	[zhuō]
[xuàn]	[yáng]	疫 (552)	勇 (568)	[yuè]	[zhé]	滞 (607)	颛 (623)
眩 (521)	阳 (536)	意 (553)	涌 (568)	月 (578)	折 (587)	置 (608)	[zhuó]
[xuē]	扬 (542)	嗌 (553)	[yōu]	[yún]	辄 (587)	[zhōng]	着 (623)
薛 (521)	杨 (543)	谚 (553)	幽 (569)	云 (580)	[zhēn]	中 (608)	[zī]
[xué]	[yǎng]	翳 (553)	[yóu]	[yùn]	针 (587)	[zhǒng]	资 (624)
穴 (521)	仰 (544)	[yīn]	油 (569)	运 (580)	真 (598)	踵 (616)	[zǐ]
[xuè]	养 (544)	阴 (554)	[yǒu]	晕 (581)	甄 (598)	[zhòng]	子 (624)
血 (521)	[yāo]	殷 (563)	右 (570)	Z	箴 (598)	中 (616)	紫 (628)
[xūn]	腰 (544)	瘖 (563)	[yū]	[zā]	[zhěn]	[zhōu]	[zì]
熏 (531)	[yáo]	[yín]	瘀 (570)	匝 (582)	枕 (598)	周 (618)	自 (628)
[xún]	摇 (547)	寅 (564)	[yú]	[zá]	[zhèn]	[zhǒu]	[zōng]
循 (531)	[yào]	银 (564)	于 (571)	杂 (582)	振 (598)	肘 (619)	宗 (628)
Y	药 (547)	龈 (564)	鱼 (571)	[zàn]	震 (598)	[zhū]	综 (628)
[yā]	[yē]	断 (564)	鱼 (572)	赞 (582)	[zhēng]	珠 (620)	[zǒu]
丫 (532)	噎 (548)	[yǐn]	[yù]	[zàng]	怔 (598)	[zhǔ]	走 (628)
压 (532)	[yè]	引 (564)	玉 (572)	脏 (582)	蒸 (598)	主 (621)	[zú]
押 (533)	叶 (548)	饮 (565)	宛 (574)	藏 (583)	[zhèng]	煮 (621)	足 (628)
[yá]	夜 (549)	隐 (565)	郁 (574)	[zào]	正 (599)	[zhù]	[zǔ]
牙 (533)	液 (549)	瘾 (565)	彧 (575)	燥 (583)	政 (600)	注 (621)	阻 (648)
[yǎ]	掖 (549)	[yìn]	域 (575)	[zhà]	[zhī]	柱 (622)	组 (648)
哑 (533)	腋 (549)	印 (565)	[yuān]	炸 (583)	支 (600)	祝 (622)	[zuǎn]
[yān]	[yè]	[yīng]	渊 (575)	痄 (583)	知 (601)	疰 (622)	纂 (648)
咽 (534)	喂 (550)	应 (565)	[yuán]	[zhāng]	蜘 (601)	筑 (622)	[zuǒ]
[yán]	[yī]	缨 (566)	元 (576)	张 (584)	[zhí]	箸 (622)	左 (648)
言 (534)	一 (550)	膺 (566)	员 (576)	章 (585)	直 (601)	[zhuàn]	[zuò]
严 (534)	医 (550)	[yíng]	圆 (576)	[zhǎng]	[zhǐ]	转 (623)	坐 (649)

汉语拼音索引

A

ā shì xué	阿是穴	1
ài dǒu	艾斗	1
ài jiǔ	艾灸	1
ài jiǔ bǔ xiè	艾灸补泻	1
ài jiǔ tōng shuō	艾灸通说	1
ài juǎn	艾卷	2
ài juǎn jiǔ	艾卷灸	2
ài róng	艾茸	2
ài róng	艾绒	2
ài shī	艾师	2
ài tiáo	艾条	2
ài tiáo jiǔ	艾条灸	2
ài wán	艾丸	3
ài yuán	艾圆	3
ài zhù	艾炷	3
ài zhù jiǔ	艾炷灸	3
ān xié	安邪	3
àn fǎ	按法	3
àn jī qún qǔ xué	按肌群取穴	3
àn shén jīng qǔ xué	按神经取穴	4
àn zhěn	按诊	4

B

bā chōng	八冲	4
bā fǎ	八法	4
bā fēng	八风	4
bā guān	八关	5
bā guān dà cì	八关大刺	5
bā huá	八华	5
bā huì	八会	6
bā huì xué	八会穴	6
bā mài	八脉	6
bā mài bā xué	八脉八穴	6
bā mài bā xué pèi xué fǎ	八脉八穴配穴法	6
bā mài jiāo huì bā xué gē	八脉交会八穴歌	7
bā mài jiāo huì xué	八脉交会穴	7
bā mù huǒ	八木火	8
bā xié	八邪	8
bā zhèng	八正	8
bā zhuī xià	八椎下	8
bā dòu bǐng jiǔ	巴豆饼灸	8
bā dòu jiǔ zhēng qì jiǔ	巴豆酒蒸气灸	9
bā dòu shuāng jiǔ	巴豆霜灸	9
bá guàn fǎ	拔罐法	9
bá tǒng fǎ	拔筒法	9
bá yuán fǎ	拔原法	9
bá zhēn	拔针	9
bái fù zǐ jiǔ	白附子灸	10
bái hú jiāo jiǔ	白胡椒灸	10
bái hǔ yáo tóu	白虎摇头	10
bái huán shū	白环俞	10
bái jiè zǐ jiǔ	白芥子灸	10
bái rèn dīng	白刃疗	10
bái ròu jì	白肉际	10
bái zhēn	白针	11
bǎi chóng wō	百虫窝	11
bǎi fā shén zhēn	百发神针	11
bǎi huì	百会	11
bǎi láo	百劳	12
bǎi rì ké	百日咳	12
bǎi zhèng fù	百症赋	12
bān tū	斑秃	12
bān hén jiǔ	瘢痕灸	12
bàn cì	半刺	12
bàn xià jiǔ	半夏灸	13
bàng zhēn cì	傍针刺	13

拼音	词条	页码
bāo huāng	包肓	13
bāo bù zhèng	胞不正	13
bāo hán bù yùn	胞寒不孕	13
bāo huāng	胞肓	13
bāo lěng wú zǐ	胞冷无子	14
bāo mén	胞门	14
bāo mén zǐ hù	胞门、子户	14
bāo yī bù chū	胞衣不出	14
bāo yī bù xià	胞衣不下	14
bāo zhàng bù xià	胞胀不下	15
bāo zǔ	胞阻	15
bǎo jiàn jiǔ	保健灸	15
bào cì	报刺	15
bào jiǔ	报灸	15
bào tóu huǒ dān	报头火丹	15
bào wén cì	豹文刺	15
bào bìng zhě qǔ zhī tài yáng	暴病者取之太阳	15
bào máng	暴盲	16
bào tuō	暴脱	16
bèi jí jiǔ fǎ	备急灸法	16
bèi jiǎ zhōng jiān	背胛中间	16
bèi jiě	背解	16
bèi shù xué	背俞穴	16
bèi yáng guān	背阳关	17
běn chí	本池	17
běn jié	本节	17
běn jīng qǔ xué	本经取穴	18
běn shén	本神	18
bēng lòu	崩漏	18
bēng zhōng lòu xià	崩中漏下	18
bí chōng	鼻冲	18
bí chuān	鼻穿	18
bí dīng	鼻疔	18
bí hóng	鼻洪	19
bí huán	鼻环	19
bí jiāo	鼻交	19
bí jiāo è zhōng	鼻交頞中	19
bí liú	鼻流	19
bí nù	鼻衄	19
bí nù xuè	鼻衄血	19
bí tōng	鼻通	19
bí yuān	鼻渊	19
bí zhēn	鼻针	20
bí zhōng chū xuè	鼻中出血	20
bí zhǔn	鼻准	20
bì lóng	闭癃	20
bì zhèng	痹证	20
bì gǔ	蔽骨	20
bì xīn gǔ	蔽心骨	20
bì xī	薜息	20
bì gǔ	臂骨	20
bì jiān	臂间	20
bì jù yīn mài	臂巨（钜）阴脉	21
bì nǎo	臂脑	21
bì nào	臂臑	21
bì shào yáng mài	臂少阳脉	21
bì shào yīn mài	臂少阴脉	21
bì shí zǐ tóu	臂（臂）石子头	21
bì tài yáng mài	臂泰阳脉	21
bì tài yīn mài	臂泰阴脉	21
bì wǔ lǐ	臂五里	21
bì yáng míng mài	臂阳明脉	22
bì	髀	22
bì guān	髀关	22
bì shū	髀枢	22
bì yàn	髀厌	22
biān fǎ	砭法	22
biān jiǔ chù	砭灸处	22
biān lián fǎ	砭镰法	22
biān shí	砭石	22
biǎn gǔ	扁骨	23
biǎn píng yóu	扁平疣	23
biǎn què	扁鹊	23
biǎn què shén yīng zhēn jiǔ yù lóng jīng	扁鹊神应针灸玉龙经	23
biǎn què xīn shū	扁鹊心书	23
biǎn què zhēn chuán	扁鹊针传	23

biǎn táo tǐ	扁桃体 …… 23		**C**
biàn bì	便秘 …… 24		
biàn dú	便毒 …… 24	cǎi ài biān	采艾编 …… 30
biàn xuè	便血 …… 24	cǎi ài biān yì	采艾编翼 …… 30
biàn zhèng qǔ xué	辨证取穴 …… 24	cāng guī tàn xué	苍龟探穴 …… 30
biǎo lǐ pèi xué fǎ	表里配穴法 …… 24	cāng lóng bǎi wěi	苍龙摆尾 …… 30
bié yáng	别阳 …… 25	cāng zhú jiǔ	苍术灸 …… 30
bìn gǔ	膑骨 …… 25	cāng zhēn qì	藏针器 …… 30
bīng xiá yì	冰瑕翳 …… 25	cáo xī	曹溪 …… 31
bǐng fēng	秉风 …… 25	cǎo xié dài xué	草鞋带穴 …… 31
bìng ér	病儿 …… 25	cè fú zuò wèi	侧伏坐位 …… 31
bìng gé	病隔 …… 25	cè wò wèi	侧卧位 …… 31
bìng xiè chà	病蟹叉 …… 25	chā huā	插花 …… 31
bìng zǔ	病阻 …… 25	chán ěr	缠耳 …… 31
bó shū jīng mài	帛书经脉 …… 25	chán luò	缠络 …… 31
bó yāng	脖胦 …… 26	chán yāo huǒ dān	缠腰火丹 …… 31
bó jǐng	膊井 …… 26	chán shí	镵石 …… 31
bò xiè dú	擘蟹毒 …… 26	chán zhēn	镵针 …… 31
bǔ mǔ xiè zǐ fǎ	补母泻子法 …… 26	chǎn hòu bù yǔ	产后不语 …… 32
bǔ shēng xiè chéng	补生泻成 …… 26	chǎn hòu dà biàn nán	产后大便难 …… 32
bǔ xiè shǒu fǎ	补泻手法 …… 27	chǎn hòu ěr lóng	产后耳聋 …… 32
bǔ xiè xuě xīn gē	补泻雪心歌 …… 27	chǎn hòu fā jìng	产后发痉 …… 32
bǔ yuán	补元 …… 27	chǎn hòu fā rè	产后发热 …… 33
bǔ zhù tóng rén shù xué zhēn jiǔ tú jīng	补注铜人腧穴 针灸图经 …… 27	chǎn hòu fā zhì	产后发痓 …… 33
bù dé mián	不得眠 …… 27	chǎn hòu fù tòng	产后腹痛 …… 33
bù dé wò	不得卧 …… 28	chǎn hòu hàn yǔ bù zhǐ	产后汗雨不止 …… 34
bù dìng xué	不定穴 …… 28	chǎn hòu lì ji	产后痢疾 …… 34
bù mèi	不寐 …… 28	chǎn hòu mù tòng	产后目痛 …… 34
bù róng	不容 …… 28	chǎn hòu shāng fēng	产后伤风 …… 34
bù shèng bù xū yǐ jīng qǔ zhī	不盛不虚以经 取之 …… 28	chǎn hòu shāng hán	产后伤寒 …… 35
bù xiù gāng zhēn	不锈钢针 …… 28	chǎn hòu shāng shí	产后伤食 …… 35
bù yuè	不月 …… 29	chǎn hòu shuǐ zhǒng	产后水肿 …… 35
bù yuè shuǐ	不月水 …… 29	chǎn hòu tān huàn	产后瘫痪 …… 35
bù yùn	不孕 …… 29	chǎn hòu tóu tòng	产后头痛 …… 35
bù láng	步郎 …… 29	chǎn hòu xià lì	产后下利 …… 36
bù láng	步廊 …… 29	chǎn hòu xiǎo biàn bù tōng	产后小便不通 …… 36
		chǎn hòu xiǎo biàn shuò	产后小便数 …… 36

chǎn hòu xié tòng	产后胁痛 …… 37	chéng gǔ	成骨 …… 42
chǎn hòu xuàn yùn	产后眩晕 …… 37	chéng fú	承扶 …… 42
chǎn hòu xuè yùn	产后血晕 …… 37	chéng guāng	承光 …… 43
chǎn hòu yīn xià tuō	产后阴下脱 …… 38	chéng jiāng	承浆 …… 43
chǎn hòu zhòng shǔ	产后中暑 …… 38	chéng jīn	承筋 …… 43
chǎn hòu zǐ gōng bù shōu	产后子宫不收 … 38	chéng líng	承灵 …… 44
		chéng mǎn	承满 …… 44
chǎn hòu zǐ gōng tuō chū	产后子宫脱出 … 38	chéng mìng	承命 …… 44
chǎn nán	产难 …… 38	chéng qì	承泣 …… 44
chāng yáng	昌阳 …… 38	chéng shān	承山 …… 45
chāng yáng zhī mài	昌阳之脉 …… 38	chéng gāo	程高 …… 45
cháng gǔ	长谷 …… 39	chéng jiè	程玠 …… 46
cháng huì	长颊 …… 39	chéng tiān zuò	程天祚 …… 46
cháng jiá	长颊 …… 39	chéng yuē	程约 …… 46
cháng liáo	长髎 …… 39	chī nì	吃逆 …… 46
cháng pín	长频 …… 39	chí tóu	池头 …… 46
cháng píng	长平 …… 39	chǐ náo	尺桡 …… 46
cháng qiáng	长强 …… 39	chǐ zé	尺泽 …… 46
cháng sāng jūn	长桑君 …… 40	chǐ zhī wǔ lǐ	尺之五里 …… 47
chámg shé jiǔ	长蛇灸 …… 40	chǐ mài	齿脉 …… 47
cháng xī	长溪 …… 40	chǐ yá	齿牙 …… 47
cháng zhēn	长针 …… 40	chǐ bǐng jiǔ	豉饼灸 …… 47
cháng dào	肠道 …… 40	chì bái ròu jì	赤白肉际 …… 47
cháng fēng	肠风 …… 40	chì dài	赤带 …… 47
cháng jié	肠结 …… 40	chì fèng yíng yuán	赤凤迎源 …… 47
cháng kū	肠窟 …… 40	chì wū shén zhēn jīng	赤乌神针经 …… 47
cháng pì	肠澼 …… 40		
cháng rào	肠绕 …… 41	chì yóu dān	赤游丹 …… 48
cháng shān	肠山 …… 41	chì mài	瘈(瘦)脉 …… 48
cháng yí	肠遗 …… 41	chōng dào	冲道 …… 48
cháng yōng	肠痈 …… 41	chōng mài	冲脉 …… 48
chè yī	彻衣 …… 41	chōng mài bìng	冲脉病 …… 48
chén jué	臣觉 …… 41	chōng mén	冲门 …… 48
chén huì	陈会 …… 42	chōng yáng	冲阳 …… 49
chén shí róng	陈时荣 …… 42	chóng niè xīn tòng	虫啮心痛 …… 49
chén tíng quán	陈廷铨 …… 42	chóng tù	虫吐 …… 49
chén yán	陈言 …… 42	chóng xīn tòng	虫心痛 …… 50
chén xiè	晨泄 …… 42	chóng yǎo xīn tòng	虫咬心痛 …… 50
chēng kāi jìn zhēn	撑开进针 …… 42	chóng jiàn shí	重见时 …… 50

chóng gǔ	崇骨 …… 50	cì luò liáo fǎ	刺络疗法 …… 55
chōu qì bá guàn fǎ	抽气拔罐法 …… 50	cì shǒu	刺手 …… 55
chōu tiān fǎ	抽添法 …… 50	cì xuè bá guàn	刺血拔罐 …… 56
chū zhēn fǎ	出针法 …… 51	cì xuè liáo fǎ	刺血疗法 …… 56
chuǎi fǎ	揣法 …… 51	cōng bái jiǔ	葱白灸 …… 56
chuān jiāo bǐng jiǔ	川椒饼灸 …… 51	cōng chǐ hú jiǔ	葱豉糊灸 …… 56
chuān bí	穿鼻 …… 51	cóng róng zhì qì	从荣置气 …… 56
chuán rè jiǔ	传热灸 …… 51	cóng wèi qǔ qì	从卫取气 …… 56
chuán shī	传尸 …… 51	cóng yáng yǐn yīn	从阳引阴 …… 57
chuán shī jiǔ	传尸灸 …… 51	cóng yīn yǐn yáng	从阴引阳 …… 57
chuán shī láo	传尸痨 …… 51	cù diān	卒癫 …… 57
chuǎn xī xué	喘息穴 …… 51	cù zhòng	卒中 …… 57
chuāng lóng	窗笼 …… 51	cù zhòng fēng	卒中风 …… 57
chuī nǎi	吹奶 …… 52	cù zhòng	猝中 …… 58
chuī rǔ	吹乳 …… 52	cuán zhú	攒竹 …… 58
chuí jiāng	垂浆 …… 52	cuàn	篡 …… 58
chuí jǔ	垂矩 …… 52	cuī qì	催气 …… 58
chuí lián zhàng	垂帘障 …… 52	cuì cì	焠刺 …… 58
chuí qián	垂前 …… 52	cuì zhēn	焠针 …… 58
chuí shǒu	垂手 …… 52	cún zhēn tú	存真图 …… 58
chún lǐ	唇里 …… 52	cùn píng	寸平 …… 58
chún yú yì	淳于意 …… 52	cuō fǎ	搓法 …… 59
cī chuāng	疵疮 …… 52		
cí gōng	慈宫 …… 52		**D**
cí xióng pī lì huǒ	雌雄霹雳火 …… 53	dá	达 …… 59
cí zhēn	磁针 …… 53	dǎ è	打呃 …… 59
cì liáo	次髎 …… 53	dà bāo	大包 …… 59
cì mén	次门 …… 53	dà biàn bì jié	大便秘结 …… 59
cì fǎ	刺法 …… 53	dà biàn bù tōng	大便不通 …… 59
cì jī cān shù	刺激参数 …… 53	dà biàn nán	大便难 …… 59
cì jī diǎn	刺激点 …… 53	dà bó zi	大脖子 …… 59
cì jī qiáng dù	刺激强度 …… 54	dà bǔ dà xiè	大补大泻 …… 59
cì jī qū	刺激区 …… 54	dà cāng	大仓 …… 59
cì jìn	刺禁 …… 54	dà cháng	大肠 …… 60
cì jiǔ	刺灸 …… 54	dà cháng jīng	大肠经 …… 60
cì jiǔ fǎ	刺灸法 …… 54	dà cháng shǒu yáng míng zhī mài	大肠手阳明之脉 …… 61
cì jiǔ xīn fǎ yào jué	刺灸心法要诀 …… 55	dà cháng shù	大肠俞 …… 61
cì luò	刺络 …… 55	dà chōng	大冲 …… 61
cì luò bá guàn	刺络拔罐 …… 55		

拼音	词条	页码	拼音	词条	页码
dà chuí	大倾	61	dài mài bìng	带脉病	71
dà dū	大都	61	dài wǔ sè jù xià	带五色俱下	71
dà dūn	大敦	62	dài xià	带下	71
dà gǔ	大谷	62	dài xià bìng	带下病	71
dà gǔ	大骨	62	dài xià chì hòu	带下赤候	71
dà gǔ kōng	大骨空	62	dài xià hēi hòu	带下黑候	71
dà gǔ kǒng	大骨孔	62	dài xià huáng hòu	带下黄候	71
dà hè	大赫	62	dài xià qīng hòu	带下青候	71
dà héng	大横	63	dài xià wǔ sè	带下五色	71
dà jiē jīng fǎ	大接经法	63	dān biāo	丹熛	71
dà jù	大巨	64	dān dú	丹毒	71
dà líng	大陵	64	dān tián	丹田	72
dà mén	大门	64	dān fù zhàng	单腹胀	72
dà mǔ zhǐ tóu	大拇指头	64	dān gǔ	单鼓	72
dà quán	大泉	65	dān jié	担截	72
dà róng	大容	65	dǎn dào huí chóng bìng	胆道蛔虫病	73
dà shù	大腧	65	dǎn jīng	胆经	74
dà xī	大溪	65	dǎn náng	胆囊	74
dà xiè	大泻	65	dǎn shù	胆俞	75
dà xiè cì	大写刺	65	dǎn zú shào yáng zhī mài	胆足少阳之脉	75
dà yīn luò	大阴络	65			
dà yíng	大迎	65	dàn zhōng	亶中	75
dà yǔ	大羽	66	dàn zhōng	膻中	75
dà zhǐ(zhǐ) cì zhǐ(zhǐ)	大指(趾)次指(趾)	66	dāng róng	当容	76
dà zhǐ jié héng wén	大指节横纹	66	dāng yáng	当阳	76
dà zhǐ jié lǐ	大指节理	66	dǎo qì	导气	76
dà zhǐ jù máo	大趾聚毛	66	dǎo fǎ	捣法	77
dà zhēn	大针	66	dé qì	得气	77
dà zhōng	大钟	66	dēng cǎo jiǔ	灯草灸	77
dà zhōng jí	大中极	67	dēng huǒ jiǔ	灯火灸	77
dà zhǒu jiān	大肘尖	67	dēng xīn cǎo jiǔ	灯心草灸	77
dà zhù	大杼	68	dí zhēn	镝针	77
dà zhù jiǔ	大炷灸	69	dǐ duān	甑端	78
dà zhuàng jiǔ	大壮灸	69	dì cāng	地仓	78
dà zhuī	大椎	69	dì chōng	地冲	78
dài jiǔ gāo	代灸膏	69	dì fū zǐ zhēng qì jiǔ	地肤子蒸气灸	78
dài jiǔ tú qí gāo	代灸涂脐膏	70	dì hé	地合	78
dài mài	带脉	70	dì jī	地机	78

13

dì jī 地箕 …… 79
dì shén 地神 …… 79
dì wèi 地卫 …… 79
dì wǔ 地五 …… 79
dì wǔ huì 地五会 …… 79
diān 颠 …… 79
diān shàng 巅上 …… 79
diān kuáng 癫狂 …… 79
diān xián 癫痫 …… 80
diān zhèng 癫证 …… 80
diǎn cì 点刺 …… 80
diàn rè jiǔ 电热灸 …… 80
diàn zhēn fǎ 电针法 …… 80
diàn zhēn jī 电针机 …… 81
diàn zhēn má zuì 电针麻醉 …… 81
diàn zǐ wēn zhēn jiǔ 电子温针灸 …… 81
diāo mù 雕目 …… 82
dīng dé yòng 丁德用 …… 82
dīng yì 丁毅 …… 82
dīng chuāng 疔疮 …… 82
dīng chuāng zǒu huáng 疔疮走黄 …… 83
dīng dú 疔毒 …… 83
dǐng mén 顶门 …… 83
dǐng shàng huí máo 顶上回毛 …… 84
dìng chuǎn 定喘 …… 84
dìng xī cùn shù 定息寸数 …… 84
dōng yī bǎo jiàn 东医宝鉴 …… 84
dòng ěr shēn zhī 动而伸之 …… 84
dòng fǎ 动法 …… 85
dǒu zhǒu 斗肘 …… 85
dòu chǐ jiǔ 豆豉灸 …… 85
dòu cái 窦材 …… 85
dòu guì fāng 窦桂芳 …… 85
dòu hàn qīng 窦汉卿 …… 85
dòu shì bā xué 窦氏八穴 …… 85
dū jǐ 督脊 …… 85
dū mài 督脉 …… 86
dū mài bìng 督脉病 …… 86
dū mài luò 督脉络 …… 87
dū mài luò mài 督脉络脉 …… 87
dū mài luò mài bìng 督脉络脉病 …… 87
dū mài zhī bié 督脉之别 …… 87
dū shù 督俞 …… 87
dú yīn 独阴 …… 88
dú bí 犊鼻 …… 88
dù rǔ 妒乳 …… 88
duǎn cì 短刺 …… 88
duàn xù 断绪 …… 88
duàn zhēn 断针 …… 89
duì cè qǔ xué 对侧取穴 …… 89
duì ěr lún 对耳轮 …… 89
duì ěr lún hòu gōu 对耳轮后沟 …… 89
duì ěr lún shàng jiǎo 对耳轮上脚 …… 89
duì ěr lún xià jiǎo 对耳轮下脚 …… 89
duì ěr píng 对耳屏 …… 89
duì ěr píng hòu gōu 对耳屏后沟 …… 89
duì píng jiān 对屏尖 …… 89
duì yìng qǔ xué 对应取穴 …… 89
duì zhèng qǔ xué 对症取穴 …… 89
duì chōng 兑冲 …… 89
duì duān 兑端 …… 89
duì gǔ 兑骨 …… 90
dùn jiǔ 顿灸 …… 90
dùn ké 顿咳 …… 90
duō guàn 多罐 …… 91
duō suǒ wén 多所闻 …… 91
duó mìng 夺命 …… 91

E

é gēn 蛾根 …… 91
é zǐ 蛾子 …… 91
é 额 …… 91
é lú 额颅 …… 91
è nì 呃逆 …… 92
è lù bù jìn 恶露不尽 …… 92
è lù bù jué 恶露不绝 …… 92
è lù bù xià 恶露不下 …… 92
è lù bù zhǐ 恶露不止 …… 93

guǐ kū	鬼窟 …… 151	hán níng xuè zhì jīng bì	寒凝血滞经闭 … 155
guǐ lěi	鬼垒 …… 151	hán nüè	寒疟 …… 156
guǐ lù	鬼路 …… 151	hán qì huò luàn	寒气霍乱 …… 156
guǐ lù	鬼禄 …… 151	hán shàn	寒疝 …… 156
guǐ shì	鬼市 …… 151	hán shī lì	寒湿痢 …… 156
guǐ shì tóu	鬼舐头 …… 151	hán shī níng zhì tòng jīng	寒湿凝滞痛经 … 156
guǐ shòu	鬼受 …… 151		
guǐ táng	鬼堂 …… 151	hán shī xiè	寒湿泻 …… 157
guǐ tuǐ	鬼腿 …… 151	hán shī yāo tòng	寒湿腰痛 …… 157
guǐ xié	鬼邪 …… 151	hán tù	寒吐 …… 157
guǐ xīn	鬼心 …… 151	hán xié fù tòng	寒邪腹痛 …… 157
guǐ xìn	鬼信 …… 151	hán yǐn xiāo chuǎn	寒饮哮喘 …… 158
guǐ xué	鬼穴 …… 152	hán zé liú zhī	寒则留之 …… 158
guǐ yǎn	鬼眼 …… 152	hàn pí kāi còu lǐ	扞皮开腠理 …… 158
guǐ yíng	鬼营 …… 152	hàn lián cǎo jiǔ	旱莲草灸 …… 158
guǐ zhěn	鬼枕 …… 152	hàn	颔 …… 158
guǐ zhù	鬼注 …… 152	hàn yàn	颔厌 …… 158
gǔn cì tǒng	滚刺筒 …… 152	háo zhēn	毫针 …… 159
guō yù	郭玉 …… 152	háo zhēn cì	毫针刺 …… 160
guō zhōng	郭忠 …… 152	háo zhēn cì fǎ	毫针刺法 …… 160
guó	腘 …… 153	háo zhēn guī gé	毫针规格 …… 160
guò liáng zhēn	过梁针 …… 153	hé liáo	禾髎 …… 160
guò mén	过门 …… 153	hé gǔ	合谷 …… 160
guò mǐn qū	过敏区 …… 153	hé gǔ cì	合谷刺 …… 161
guò qī jīng xíng	过期经行 …… 154	hé gǔ dīng	合谷疔 …… 161
		hé gǔ jū	合谷疽 …… 161
H		hé gǔ	合骨 …… 161
há má	吓蟆 …… 154	hé lú	合颅 …… 161
há má wēn	蛤蟆瘟 …… 154	hé xué	合穴 …… 161
hái guān	骸关 …… 154	hé yáng	合阳 …… 161
hǎi dǐ	海底 …… 154	hé zhì nèi fǔ	合治内腑 …… 162
hǎi quán	海泉 …… 154	hé ruò yú	何若愚 …… 162
hài fēi	害蜚 …… 154	hé liáo	和髎 …… 162
hán sāi chuāng	含腮疮 …… 155	hé gǔ	核骨 …… 162
hán fǔ	寒府 …… 155	hé táo jiǔ	核桃灸 …… 162
hán huò luàn	寒霍乱 …… 155	hé	颌 …… 162
hán jī wèi tòng	寒积胃痛 …… 155	hé gàn	䯊骭 …… 162
hán jié	寒结 …… 155	hè dǐng	鹤顶 …… 162
hán jué	寒厥 …… 155		

拼音	词条	页码	拼音	词条	页码
hēi dài	黑带	163	huā yì bái xiàn	花翳白陷	168
héng cì	横刺	163	huá gài	华盖	168
héng gǔ	横骨	163	huá jīng	滑精	168
héng hù	横户	163	huá ròu mén	滑肉门	169
héng sān jiān cùn	横三间寸	164	huá shòu	滑寿	169
héng shé	横舌	164	huà nóng jiǔ	化脓灸	169
héng wén	横文	164	huà tuó	华佗	169
héng wén	横纹	164	huà tuó jiā jí	华佗夹脊	170
héng zhǐ tóng shēn cùn	横指同身寸	164	huà tuó xué	华佗穴	170
héng luò zhī mài	衡络之脉	164	huái	踝	170
hóng sī dīng	红丝疔	164	huái gǔ	踝骨	170
hóng wài xiàn jiǔ	红外线灸	165	huái jiān	踝尖	170
hóng wài xiàn xué wèi zhào shè fǎ	红外线穴位照射法	165	huán diào	环铫	170
			huán gǎng	环岗	170
hóng wài xiàn zhào shè fǎ	红外线照射法	165	huán gǔ	环谷	170
			huán tiào	环跳	170
hóng xiàn dīng	红线疔	165	huán tiào zhēn	环跳针	172
hóng yǎn	红眼	165	huán zhōng	环中	172
hóu bì	喉闭	165	huǎn fēng	缓风	172
hóu bì	喉痹	165	huàn mén	患门	172
hóu é	喉蛾	165	huāng mén	肓门	172
hòu dǐng	后顶	165	huāng mù	肓募	172
hòu guān	后关	166	huāng shū	肓俞	173
hòu qū	后曲	166	huáng fǔ mì	皇甫谧	173
hòu shén cōng	后神聪	166	huáng dài	黄带	173
hòu xī	后溪	166	huáng dǎn	黄疸	173
hòu yè	后腋	166	huáng dàn	黄瘅	174
hòu yè xià xué	后腋下穴	166	huáng dì	黄帝	174
hòu qì	候气	166	huáng dì jiǔ xū nèi jīng	黄帝九虚内经	174
hòu shí	候时	167			
hū xī bǔ xiè	呼吸补泻	167	huáng dì míng táng jiǔ jīng	黄帝明堂灸经	174
hú shàn	狐疝	167			
hú jiāo bǐng jiǔ	胡椒饼灸	167	huáng dì míng táng yǎn cè rén tú	黄帝明堂偃侧人图	174
hǔ kǒu	虎口	167			
hǔ kǒu bǎi yā	虎口百丫	168	huáng dì nèi jīng	黄帝内经	174
hǔ kǒu dīng	虎口疔	168	huáng dì nèi jīng míng táng	黄帝内经明堂	175
hǔ kǒu dú	虎口毒	168			
hǔ kǒu jū	虎口疽	168	huáng dì nèi jīng míng táng lèi chéng	黄帝内经明堂类成	175
hǔ yā dú	虎丫毒	168			

拼音	词条	页码	拼音	词条	页码
huáng dì nèi jīng tài sù	黄帝内经太素	175	huǒ chái tóu jiǔ	火柴头灸	180
			huǒ dài chuāng	火带疮	180
huáng dì qí bó lùn zhēn jiǔ yào jué	黄帝歧伯论针灸要诀	175	huǒ dān	火丹	180
			huǒ guàn fǎ	火罐法	180
huáng dì shí èr jīng mài míng táng wǔ zàng rén tú	黄帝十二经脉明堂五藏人图	175	huǒ guàn qì	火罐气	180
			huǒ nì	火逆	180
			huǒ yǎn	火眼	180
huáng dì zhēn jiǔ há má jì	黄帝针灸虾蟆忌	175	huǒ zhēn	火针	180
			huǒ zhēn liáo fǎ	火针疗法	180
huáng là jiǔ	黄蜡灸	176	huǒ zhū dīng	火珠疔	181
huáng shí píng	黄石屏	176	huò zhōng	彧中	181
huáng tǔ bǐng jiǔ	黄土饼灸	176	huò luàn	霍乱	181
huáng shì zhēn	黄士真	176			
huáng yè shàng chōng	黄液上冲	176	**J**		
huáng zhōng zǐ	黄中子	176			
huáng zǒu	癀走	176	jī guān	机关	181
huī cì	恢刺	176	jī guān chuāng	鸡冠疮	181
huí fā wǔ chù	回发五处	177	jī ké	鸡咳	181
huí gǔ	回骨	177	jī zǐ jiǔ	鸡子灸	181
huí qì	回气	177	jī zú zhēn fǎ	鸡足针法	181
huí xuán jiǔ	回旋灸	177	jī jù pǐ kuài xué	积聚痞块穴	182
huí qì	迴气	177	jī tù	积吐	182
huí jué	蚘厥	177	jī běn shǒu fǎ	基本手法	182
huì	会	177	jī mén	箕门	182
huì é	会额	177	jī zuò wèi	箕坐位	182
huì wéi	会维	177	jī guāng xué wèi zhào shè fǎ	激光穴位照射法	182
huì yáng	会阳	178	jī guāng zhēn	激光针	183
huì yīn	会阴	178	jí quán	极泉	183
huì yīn zhī mài	会阴之脉	178	jí jīng fēng	急惊风	183
huì yuán	会原	178	jí mài	急脉	184
huì zōng	会宗	178	jí ěr xú zé xū	疾而徐则虚	184
huì tú jīng luò tú shuō	绘图经络图说	179	jí hé cì	集合刺	185
hún hù	魂户	179	jǐ bèi wǔ xué	脊背五穴	185
hún mén	魂门	179	jǐ gǔ jiě zhōng	脊骨解中	185
hún shè	魂舍	179	jǐ nèi shù	脊内俞	185
hùn hé zhì	混合痔	179	jǐ sān xué	脊三穴	185
hùn jīng zhàng	混睛障	179	jǐ shū	脊俞	185
huó dòng biāo zhì	活动标志	179	jǐ suí yī	脊髓1	185
huó rén miào fǎ zhēn jīng	活人妙法针经	180	jǐ zhōng	脊中	185

jì xué	忌穴	186	jiàn	楗	193
jì xié	季胁	186	jiàn tóu zhēn	箭头针	193
jiā bái	夹白	186	jiāng jiāo zhēng qì jiǔ	姜椒蒸气灸	193
jiā chí jìn zhēn	夹持进针	186	jiāng wěi	畺尾	193
jiā chí yā shǒu	夹持押手	186	jiàng yā diǎn	降压点	193
jiā jí	夹脊	186	jiāo chā qǔ xué	交叉取穴	193
jiā jīng tù	夹惊吐	187	jiāo chōng	交冲	193
jiá	颊	187	jiāo gǎn	交感	193
jiá chē	颊车	187	jiāo huì xué	交会穴	193
jiá lǐ	颊里	188	jiāo jīng bā xué	交经八穴	198
jiǎ gēn	甲根	188	jiāo jīng miù cì	交经缪刺	198
jiǎ fèng	胛缝	188	jiāo xìn	交信	198
jiān gǔ	间谷	188	jiāo yí	交仪	199
jiān shǐ	间使	188	jiāo bǐng jiǔ	椒饼灸	199
jiān	肩	188	jiāo yùn wěn	焦蕴稳	199
jiān jiǎ	肩胛	188	jiǎo	角	199
jiān jiān	肩尖	189	jiǎo fǎ	角法	199
jiān jiě	肩解	189	jiǎo sūn	角孙	199
jiān jǐng	肩井	189	jiǎo wō shàng	角窝上	199
jiān liáo	肩聊	189	jiǎo wō zhōng	角窝中	199
jiān liáo	肩髎	189	jiǎo zhēn	角针	199
jiān mài	肩脉	190	jiǎo qì	脚气	200
jiān nèi shù	肩内俞	190	jiǎo qì bā chù jiǔ	脚气八处灸	200
jiān nèi yú	肩内髃	190	jiǎo qì chōng xīn	脚气冲心	200
jiān níng zhèng	肩凝症	190	jiǎo qì gōng xīn	脚气攻心	200
jiān shù	肩俞	190	jiǎo qì rù xīn	脚气入心	200
jiān tóu	肩头	190	jiǎo ruò	脚弱	200
jiān wài shù	肩外俞	190	jiē nüè	痎疟	200
jiān yú	肩髃	191	jiē gǔ	接骨	200
jiān zhēn	肩贞	191	jiē jǐ	接脊	200
jiān zhōng shù	肩中俞	191	jiē jīng qǔ xué	接经取穴	201
jiān zhù	肩柱	192	jiē qì tōng jīng	接气通经	201
jiān zhù gǔ	肩柱骨	192	jié	节	201
jiǎn fèi	睑废	192	jié cháng	截肠	201
jiàn gé jiǔ	间隔灸	192	jié gēn liáo fǎ	截根疗法	201
jiàn jiē jiǔ	间接灸	192	jié nüè	截疟	201
jiàn lǐ	建里	192	jiě huò	解惑	201
jiàn jù	剑巨	192	jiě mài	解脉	202
jiàn zhēn	剑针	193	jiě xī	解溪	202

拼音	词条	页码	拼音	词条	页码
jīn zhēn	巾针	202	jīng hòu bù tiáo	经候不调	208
jīn chuāng jìng	金疮痉	202	jīng hòu bù xíng	经候不行	208
jīn jīn	金津	202	jīng hòu bù yún	经候不匀	208
jīn jīn yù yè	金津玉液	202	jīng hòu fù tòng	经后腹痛	209
jīn kǒng xián	金孔贤	203	jīng jīn	经筋	209
jīn lán xún jīng	金兰循经	203	jīng luàn	经乱	209
jīn lán xún jīng qǔ xué tú jiě	金兰循经取穴图解	203	jīng luò	经络	209
jīn mén	金门	203	jīng luò gǎn chuán xiàn xiàng	经络感传现象	209
jīn téng yù guì zhēn jīng	金滕玉匮针经	203	jīng luò huì biān	经络汇编	210
jīn yě tián	金冶田	203	jīng luò jiān zhù	经络笺注	210
jīn zhēn	金针	203	jīng luò jīng xué bō lí rén	经络经穴玻璃人	210
jīn zhēn fù	金针赋	203	jīng luò kǎo	经络考	210
jīn sù	筋束	204	jīng luò mǐn gǎn xiàn xiàng	经络敏感现象	210
jīn suō	筋缩	204			
jīn zhī fǔ	筋之府	204	jīng luò quán shū	经络全书	210
jǐn àn màn tí	紧按慢提	204	jīng luò shū yào	经络枢要	210
jǐn tí màn àn	紧提慢按	204	jīng luò xiàn xiàng	经络现象	211
jìn	进	204	jīng luò xué qū dài	经络穴区带	211
jìn fǎ	进法	206	jīng mài	经脉	211
jìn zhēn	进针	206	jīng mài bù tiáo	经脉不调	211
jìn zhēn fǎ	进针法	206	jīng mài bù tōng	经脉不通	211
jìn zhēn guǎn	进针管	206	jīng mài bù xíng	经脉不行	211
jìn zhēn qì	进针器	206	jīng mài fēn tú	经脉分图	211
jìn bù qǔ xué	近部取穴	206	jīng mài fēn yě	经脉分野	211
jìn dào qǔ xué	近道取穴	206	jīng mài tú kǎo	经脉图考	211
jìn jié duàn qǔ xué	近节段取穴	207	jīng mài zhī hǎi	经脉之海	212
jìn qǔ	近取	207	jīng mén sì huā	经门四花	212
jìn shì	近视	207	jīng qì	经气	212
jìn kǒu lì	噤口痢	207	jīng qì bù tiáo	经气不调	212
jīng gǔ	京骨	207	jīng qián biàn xuè	经前便血	212
jīng mén	京门	207	jīng qián fù tòng	经前腹痛	212
jīng bì	经闭	208	jīng qián qí xià tòng	经前脐下痛	212
jīng bì bù lì	经闭不利	208	jīng qú	经渠	213
jīng bié	经别	208	jīng shǐ	经始	213
jīng bù tiáo	经不调	208	jīng shuǐ	经水	213
jīng chí	经迟	208	jīng shuǐ bù dìng	经水不定	213
jīng duàn qián hòu zhū zhèng	经断前后诸症	208	jīng shuǐ bù tiáo	经水不调	213

jīng shuǐ bù tōng	经水不通	213	jīng huá	精滑	218
jīng shuǐ bù xíng	经水不行	213	jīng lù	精露	218
jīng shuǐ hòu qī	经水后期	213	jīng míng	精明	218
jīng shuǐ pǐ sè	经水否涩	213	jǐng xué	井穴	218
jīng shuǐ sè shǎo	经水涩少	213	jǐng	颈	218
jīng shuǐ wú cháng	经水无常	213	jǐng bǎi láo	颈百劳	218
jīng shuǐ xiān hòu wú dìng qī	经水先后无定期	213	jǐng bì	颈臂	219
			jǐng chōng	颈冲	219
jīng shuǐ xiān qī	经水先期	213	jǐng zhōng	颈中	219
jīng suì	经隧	213	jǐng zhuī	颈椎	219
jīng wài qí xué	经外奇穴	214	jìng	痉	219
jīng wài xué	经外穴	214	jìng zhèng	痉证	219
jīng xíng fù tòng	经行腹痛	214	jiū wěi	鸠尾	219
jīng xíng hòu qī	经行后期	214	jiū wěi gǔ duān	鸠尾骨端	220
jīng xíng huò qián huò hòu	经行或前或后	214	jiǔ bù zhēn jīng	九部针经	220
			jiǔ cì	九刺	220
jīng xíng xiān hòu wú dìng qī	经行先后无定期	214	jiǔ gōng kāo shén	九宫尻神	220
			jiǔ juàn	九卷	221
jīng xíng xiān qī	经行先期	214	jiǔ líng	九灵	221
jīng xué	经穴	215	jiǔ liù bǔ xiè	九六补泻	221
jīng xué cè dìng	经穴测定	215	jiǔ liù shù	九六数	221
jīng xué fā míng	经穴发明	215	jiǔ qū	九曲	221
jīng xué huì jiě	经穴汇解	215	jiǔ qū zhōng fǔ	九曲中府	221
jīng xué zhěn duàn fǎ	经穴诊断法	215	jiǔ xū	九虚	221
jīng xué zuǎn yào	经穴纂要	216	jiǔ yí	九宜	221
jīng xuè bù dìng	经血不定	216	jiǔ zhēn	九针	221
jīng yàn qǔ xué	经验取穴	216	jiǔ bān	灸瘢	222
jīng zǎo	经早	216	jiǔ bǎn	灸板	222
jīng zhà lái zhà duō	经乍来乍多	217	jiǔ chuāng	灸疮	222
jīng zhà lái zhà shǎo	经乍来乍少	217	jiǔ chuāng gāo yào	灸疮膏药	223
jīng zhōng	经中	217	jiǔ cì	灸刺	223
jīng fēng	惊风	217	jiǔ diàn fēng	灸癜风	223
jīng gé tù	惊膈吐	217	jiǔ fǎ	灸法	223
jīng jì	惊悸	217	jiǔ fǎ mì chuán	灸法秘传	223
jīng jué	惊厥	217	jiǔ gǎn	灸感	223
jīng tù	惊吐	217	jiǔ huā	灸花	224
jīng míng	睛明	217	jiǔ huǒ mù	灸火木	224
jīng zhōng	睛中	218	jiǔ láo	灸痨	224
jīng gōng	精宫	218	jiǔ liáo qì	灸疗器	224

pinyin	词	页
jiǔ qì jiǔ	灸器灸	224
jiǔ ruò	灸焫	224
jiǔ shī	灸师	224
jiǔ xiāo	灸哮	224
jiǔ xuè bìng	灸血病	225
jiǔ zhǎn	灸盏	225
jiǔ zhào	灸罩	225
jū liáo	居髎	225
jú bù qǔ xué	局部取穴	225
jù chù	巨处	225
jù cì	巨刺	225
jù gǔ	巨骨	226
jù jiǎo	巨搅	226
jù jiào	巨窌	226
jù jué	巨觉	226
jù liáo	巨髎	226
jù què	巨阙	226
jù què shù	巨阙俞	227
jù xū	巨虚	227
jù xū shàng lián	巨虚上廉	227
jù xū xià lián	巨虚下廉	227
jù yáng	巨阳	227
jù zhēn	巨针	227
jù máo	聚毛	228
jù quán	聚泉	228
juē	撅	228
jué chǎn	绝产	228
jué gǔ	绝骨	228
jué jīng qián hòu zhū zhèng	绝经前后诸证	228
jué yáng	绝阳	229
jué yùn xué	绝孕穴	229
jué zǐ	绝子	229
jué	厥	229
jué shū	厥俞	229
jué yáng	厥阳	229
jué yīn shū	厥阴俞	230
jué zhèng	厥证	230
jué gǔ	橛骨	230
jùn ròu	䐃肉	230

K

pinyin	词	页
kāi hé bǔ xiè	开阖补泻	230
kāi hé shū	开阖枢	231
kàn bù qǔ xué	看部取穴	231
kāo	尻	231
kāo shén	尻神	231
kǎo zhèng zhōu shēn xué fǎ gē	考正周身穴法歌	231
kē lì shì pí nèi zhēn	颗粒式皮内针	231
ké sòu	咳嗽	231
ké sòu xuè	咳嗽血	231
ké xuè	咳血	232
kè zhǔ rén	客主人	232
kǒng guǎng péi	孔广培	232
kǒng xué	孔穴	232
kǒng zuì	孔最	232
kòng nǎo shā	控脑砂	232
kǒu	口	232
kǒu cùn	口寸	232
kǒu hé liáo	口禾髎	232
kǒu wēn	口温	234
kǒu yǎn wāi xié	口眼㖞斜	234
kǔ hú jiǔ	苦瓠灸	234
kù fáng	库房	234
kuài chā jìn zhēn	快插进针	235
kuān	髋	235
kuān gǔ	髋骨	235
kuáng zhèng	狂证	235
kūn lún	昆仑	236

L

pinyin	词	页
lā guàn fǎ	拉罐法	236
lǎ ma xué	喇嘛穴	236
lán mén	兰门	236
lán jiāng fù	拦江赋	237
lán wěi	阑尾	237
láo gōng	劳宫	237
láo lìn	劳淋	238

láo nüè	劳疟 ………… 238	liáng guān	梁关 ………… 245	
láo shāng yuè jīng guò duō	劳伤月经过多 … 238	liáng mén	梁门 ………… 245	
láo sǔn yāo tòng	劳损腰痛 …… 238	liáng qiū	梁丘 ………… 246	
láo zhài	劳瘵 ………… 239	liǎng chà gǔ	两叉骨 ……… 246	
lǎo shǔ chuāng	老鼠疮 ……… 239	liǎng shǒu yán zǐ gǔ	两手研子骨 … 246	
lào zhěn	落枕 ………… 239	liáo liáo	髎髎 ………… 246	
léi fēng	雷丰 ………… 239	liè quē	列缺 ………… 246	
léi huǒ shén zhēn	雷火神针 …… 239	lín jìn qǔ xué	邻近取穴 …… 247	
léi huǒ zhēn fǎ	雷火针法 …… 239	lín qì	临泣 ………… 247	
lèi tóu	肋头 ………… 240	lìn quán	淋泉 ………… 247	
lèi xià	肋䏚 ………… 240	lìn zhèng	淋证 ………… 247	
lèi kōng	泪空 ………… 240	líng dào	灵道 ………… 247	
lèi kǒng	泪孔 ………… 240	líng guāng fù	灵光赋 ……… 248	
lèi jīng	类经 ………… 240	líng guī bā fǎ	灵龟八法 …… 248	
lèi jīng fù yì	类经附翼 …… 240	líng guī fēi téng	灵龟飞腾 …… 249	
lèi jīng tú yì	类经图翼 …… 240	líng qiáng	灵墙 ………… 249	
lěng bì	冷秘 ………… 241	líng shū	灵枢 ………… 249	
lěng jiǔ	冷灸 ………… 241	líng shū jīng	灵枢经 ……… 249	
lěng jué	冷厥 ………… 241	líng shū jīng mài yì	灵枢经脉翼 … 249	
lěng zhàng	冷瘴 ………… 241	líng tái	灵台 ………… 249	
lěng zhēn	冷针 ………… 241	líng xū	灵墟 ………… 250	
lí zuǒ yòu nán	离左右南 …… 241	líng hòu	陵后 ………… 250	
lí gōu	蠡沟 ………… 242	liú dǎng	刘党 ………… 250	
lǐ hào	李浩 ………… 242	liú jǐn	刘瑾 ………… 250	
lǐ mèng zhōu	李梦周 ……… 242	liú wán sù	刘完素 ……… 250	
lǐ shǒu dào	李守道 ……… 242	liú yuán bīn	刘元宾 ……… 251	
lǐ shǒu xiān	李守先 ……… 242	liú huǒ	流火 ………… 251	
lǐ xué chuān	李学川 ……… 242	liú qì fǎ	流气法 ……… 251	
lǐ yù	李玉 ………… 243	liú zhù bā xué	流注八穴 …… 251	
lǐ yuán	李源 ………… 243	liú zhù zhǐ wēi fù	流注指微赋 … 251	
lǐ nèi tíng	里内庭 ……… 243	liú	留 …………… 251	
lǐ yuè pián wén	理瀹骈文 …… 243	liú qì fǎ	留气法 ……… 251	
lì duì	厉兑 ………… 243	liú zhēn	留针 ………… 251	
lì jī	利机 ………… 243	liú huáng jiǔ	硫磺灸 ……… 252	
lì zǐ jǐng	疠子颈 ……… 244	liú zhū jiǔ	硫朱灸 ……… 252	
lì jí	痢疾 ………… 244	liù fèng	六缝 ………… 252	
lián quán	廉泉 ………… 244	liù fǔ xià hé xué	六腑下合穴 … 252	
liàn zhēn fǎ	练针法 ……… 244	liù hé	六合 ………… 253	
liàn qí fǎ	炼脐法 ……… 245	liù huá	六华 ………… 253	

liù jīng	六经 ……………… 253	luò què	络却 ……………… 259
liù jīng biāo běn	六经标本 …………… 253	luò xì	络郄 ……………… 260
liù jīng pí bù	六经皮部 …………… 253	luò xué	络穴 ……………… 260
lóng hàn	龙颔 ……………… 253		
lóng hǔ guī fèng	龙虎龟凤 ………… 254		# M
lóng hǔ jiāo téng	龙虎交腾 ………… 254	má yè jiǔ	麻叶灸 …………… 261
lóng hǔ jiāo zhàn	龙虎交战 ………… 254	mǎ dān yáng	马丹阳 …………… 261
lóng hǔ shēng jiàng	龙虎升降 ………… 254	mǎ dān yáng shí èr xué	马丹阳十二穴 …… 261
lóng hǔ shēng téng	龙虎升腾 ………… 254		
lóng quán	龙泉 ……………… 255	mǎ sì míng	马嗣明 …………… 261
lóng quán dīng	龙泉疔 …………… 255	mǎ wáng duī hàn mù bó shū	马王堆汉墓帛书 … 261
lóng xián sù	龙衔素 …………… 255		
lóng xuán	龙玄 ……………… 255	mǎ xián tiě zhēn	马衔铁针 ………… 262
lóng yuān	龙渊 ……………… 255	mái xiàn liáo fǎ	埋线疗法 ………… 262
lóng kuì	聋聩 ……………… 255	mái zhēn liáo fǎ	埋针疗法 ………… 262
lóng yǎ	聋哑 ……………… 255	mài lì jiǔ	麦粒灸 …………… 262
lóng	癃 ………………… 255	mài lì zhǒng	麦粒肿 …………… 262
lóng bì	癃闭 ……………… 255	mài	脉 ………………… 262
lóng bì shí zhèng	癃闭实证 ………… 256	mài dù	脉度 ……………… 263
lóng bì xū zhèng	癃闭虚证 ………… 256	mài qì	脉气 ……………… 263
lóu yīng	楼英 ……………… 256	màn jīng fēng	慢惊风 …………… 263
lòu gǔ	漏谷 ……………… 256	máng zhēn	芒针 ……………… 263
lòu jiān fēng	漏肩风 …………… 257	máng zhēn liáo fǎ	芒针疗法 ………… 264
lòu yīn	漏阴 ……………… 257	máng cháng xué	盲肠穴 …………… 264
lú xī	颅息 ……………… 257	máo cì	毛刺 ……………… 264
lú xìn	颅囟 ……………… 257	máo gèn jiǔ	毛茛灸 …………… 264
lù sī ké	鹭鸶咳 …………… 257	máo jì	毛际 ……………… 264
lǚ guǎng	吕广 ……………… 257	mǎo nán mǎo běi	卯南卯北 ………… 264
lǚ kuí	吕夔 ……………… 258	mǎo nán yǒu běi	卯南酉北 ………… 265
lǚ xì	吕细 ……………… 258	méi běn	眉本 ……………… 265
lǚ shàng	闾上 ……………… 258	méi chōng	眉冲 ……………… 265
lǚ	膂 ………………… 258	méi tóu	眉头 ……………… 265
lúnyī lúnèr lúnsān lúnsì lúnwǔ lúnliù	轮1 轮2 轮3 轮4 轮5 轮6 …… 258	méi zhěn xiàn	眉枕线 …………… 265
		méi hé qì	梅核气 …………… 265
luǒ lì	瘰疬 ……………… 258	méi huā zhēn	梅花针 …………… 266
luò	络 ………………… 259	mén fǎ	扪法 ……………… 266
luò cì	络刺 ……………… 259	mèng shī jīng	梦失精 …………… 266
luò mài	络脉 ……………… 259	mèng yí	梦遗 ……………… 266
luò qì	络气 ……………… 259	miàn jiāo	面窌 ……………… 266

27

miàn tān	面瘫	266	mù lín qì	目临泣	272
miàn tòng	面痛	267	mù nèi zì	目内眦	272
miàn wáng	面王	267	mù ruì zì	目锐眦	272
miàn yán	面岩	267	mù shàng gāng	目上纲	272
miàn yù	面玉	267	mù shàng wǎng	目上网	273
miàn zhēn	面针	267	mù wài zì	目外眦	273
miàn zhèng	面正	267	mù wài wéi	目外维	273
miǎo	眇	268	mù xì	目系	273
míng jiā jiǔ xuǎn	名家灸选	268	mù yī	目1	273
míng guāng	明光	268	mù yì	目瞖	273
míng jiǔ	明灸	268	mù shù jīng	募腧经	274
míng táng	明堂	268	mù xué	募穴	274
míng táng jīng	明堂经	268	mù yuán	募原	274
míng táng jīng luò tú cè	明堂经络图册	268			

N

míng táng jīng tú	明堂经图	268	nà gān fǎ	纳干法	275
míng táng kǒng xué	明堂孔穴	268	nà jiǎ fǎ	纳甲法	275
míng táng kǒng xué tú	明堂孔穴图	268	nà qì fǎ	纳气法	275
míng táng kǒng xué zhēn jiǔ zhì yào	明堂孔穴针灸治要	269	nà zhī fǎ	纳支法	275
			nà zǐ fǎ	纳子法	275
míng táng rén xíng tú	明堂人形图	269	nǎi jī	奶积	276
míng táng tú	明堂图	269	nǎi pí	奶脾	276
míng táng xuán zhēn jīng jué	明堂玄真经诀	269	nǎi xuǎn	奶癣	276
			nán yīn fèng	男阴缝	276
míng táng zhēn jiǔ tú	明堂针灸图	269	nán chǎ	难产	276
mìng guān	命关	269	náng dǐ	囊底	276
mìng mén	命门	270	náng ěr	囊耳	276
miù cì	缪刺	270	náng xià fèng	囊下缝	276
mó yuán	膜原	270	nǎo bēng	脑崩	276
mǔ zhǐ tóng shēn cùn	拇指同身寸	270	nǎo diǎn	脑点	276
mǔ zhǐ lǐ héng wén	蹈趾里横纹	271	nǎo gài	脑盖	276
mù xiāng bǐng	木香饼	271	nǎo hán	脑寒	276
mù bāo	目胞	271	nǎo hù	脑户	276
mù běn	目本	271	nǎo kōng	脑空	277
mù chì zhǒng tòng	目赤肿痛	271	nǎo lòu	脑漏	277
mù chuāng	目窗	272	nǎo shèn	脑渗	277
mù èr	目2	272	nào	臑	277
mù gāng	目纲	272	nào huì	臑会	277
mù jiào	目窌	272	nào jiāo	臑交	277

拼音	词条	页码	拼音	词条	页码	拼音	词条	页码
nào jiāo	臑窌	277	niǎn zhuǎn bǔ xiè	捻转补泻	283
nào shū	臑俞	277	niǎn zhuǎn fǎ	捻转法	283
nèi bí	内鼻	278	niǎn zhuǎn jìn zhēn	捻转进针	284
nèi cè	内侧	278	niǎn yíng yào tiáo	念盈药条	284
nèi chuī rǔ yōng	内吹乳痈	278	niào bāo	尿胞	284
nèi ěr	内耳	278	niào chuáng	尿床	284
nèi fēn mì	内分泌	278	niào dào	尿道	284
nèi guān	内关	278	niào lái	尿来	284
nèi huái	内踝	279	niào xuè	尿血	284
nèi huái jiān	内踝尖	279	niē qǐ jìn zhēn	捏起进针	285
nèi huái qián xià	内踝前下	279	niè yíng	聂莹	285
nèi jīn	内筋	279	niè	颞	285
nèi jīng	内经	279	niè rú	颞颥	285
nèi jīng míng	内睛明	279	níng zhǐ yì	凝脂翳	285
nèi jiǔ	内灸	279	niú pí xuǎn	牛皮癣	285
nèi kūn lún	内昆仑	280	niǔ shāng	扭伤	286
nèi lìn	内淋	280	nǔ fǎ	努法	286
nèi lóng yǎn	内龙眼	280	nǚ xī	女膝	286
nèi shēng zhí qì	内生殖器	280	nǚ xū	女须	286
nèi tài chōng	内太冲	280	nǚ yīn fèng	女阴缝	286
nèi tíng	内庭	280	nuè	疟	286
nèi wài èr jǐng tú	内外二景图	280	nuè bìng	疟病	286
nèi wài zhì	内外痔	280	nuè jí	疟疾	287
nèi xī yǎn	内膝眼	281
nèi yáng chí	内阳池	281	**O**
nèi yíng xiāng	内迎香	281	ǒu tù	呕吐	287
nèi zhì yīn	内至阴	282	ǒu xuè	呕血	287
nèi zhì	内痔	282	ǒu cì	偶刺	287
néng jìn qiè yuǎn zhèng	能近怯远症	282	ǒu jīng qǔ xué	偶经取穴	288
ní qián	泥钱	282
ní tǔ jiǔ	泥土灸	282	**P**
ní wán gōng	泥丸宫	282	pāi xiè dú	拍蟹毒	288
nì ér duó zhī	逆而夺之	282	pái guàn fǎ	排罐法	288
nì jiǔ	逆灸	282	pái zhēn	排针	288
nì zhēn jiǔ	逆针灸	283	pán fǎ	盘法	288
nì zhù	逆注	283	páng tíng	旁廷	288
nì xuè	溺血	283	páng guāng	膀胱	289
niǎn	捻	283	páng guāng jīng	膀胱经	289
niǎn fǎ	捻法	283	páng guāng shū	膀胱俞	290

páng guāng zú tài yáng zhī mài	膀胱足太阳之脉 …… 290	píng jiān qiē jì hòu wō		屏间切迹后窝 …… 298
pèi xué fǎ	配穴法 …… 290	píng lún qiē jì	屏轮切迹 …… 298
pēn mén	贲门 …… 291	píng shàng qiē jì	屏上切迹 …… 298
pén qiāng	盆腔 …… 291	píng yì	屏翳 …… 298
péng jiǔ sī	彭九思 …… 291	pò ké	迫咳 …… 298
péng yòng guāng	彭用光 …… 291	pò shāng fēng	破伤风 …… 298
péng lái huǒ	蓬莱火 …… 291	pò hù	魄户 …… 298
pī zhēng	铍针 …… 291	pū jiǔ	铺灸 …… 299
pí bù	皮部 …… 291	pú cān	仆参 …… 299
pí fū zhēn	皮肤针 …… 292	pǔ jì fāng	**普济方** …… 299
pí nèi zhēn	皮内针 …… 292		
pí zhì xià	皮质下 …… 292		# Q
pí pá	琵琶 …… 292	qī cì mài	七次脉 …… 300
pí	脾 …… 292	qī xīng zhēn	七星针 …… 300
pí héng	脾横 …… 293	qī mén	期门 …… 300
pí jīng	脾经 …… 293	qí cì	齐刺 …… 300
pí shè	脾舍 …… 293	qí bó	岐伯 …… 301
pí shū	脾俞 …… 293	qí bó jiǔ	岐伯灸 …… 301
pí wèi xū ruò jīng bì	脾胃虚弱经闭 …… 295	qí bó jiǔ jīng	岐伯灸经 …… 301
pí xū biàn xuè	脾虚便血 …… 295	qí bó zhēn jīng	岐伯针经 …… 301
pí xū dài xià	脾虚带下 …… 295	qí gǔ	岐骨 …… 301
pí xū tù xuè	脾虚吐血 …… 295	qí jīng	奇经 …… 301
pí xū xiāo chuǎn	脾虚哮喘 …… 295	qí jīng bā mài	奇经八脉 …… 301
pí xū xiè	脾虚泻 …… 296	qí jīng bā mài kǎo	奇经八脉考 …… 302
pí zhī dà luò	脾之大络 …… 296	qí jīng nà guà fǎ	奇经纳卦法 …… 302
pí zhī dà luò bìng	脾之大络病 …… 296	qí jīng nà jiǎ fǎ	奇经纳甲法 …… 302
pí zú tài yīn zhī mài	脾足太阴之脉 …… 296	qí shū	奇输 …… 302
pǐ gēn	痞根 …… 296	qí xué	奇穴 …… 302
piān gǔ	偏骨 …… 296	qí	脐 …… 302
piān jiān	偏肩 …… 297	qí páng xué	脐旁穴 …… 302
piān lì	偏历 …… 297	qí shàng xià wǔ fēn xué	脐上下五分穴 …… 302
pián zhǐ yā shǒu	骈指押手 …… 297	qí xià liù yī	脐下六一 …… 303
píng bǔ píng xiè fǎ	平补平泻法 …… 297	qí zhōng	脐中 …… 303
píng chuǎn	平喘 …… 297	qí zhōng sì biān xué	脐中四边穴 …… 303
píng héng qū	平衡区 …… 297	qí zhú mǎ xué	骑竹马穴 …… 303
píng yì	平翳 …… 297	qí cáo jiǔ	蛴螬灸 …… 303
píng zhēn fǎ	平针法 …… 298	qí zhēn	綦针 …… 303
píng jiān	屏尖 …… 298	qì bì	气秘 …… 303

qì chōng	气冲 …… 303
qì duān	气端 …… 304
qì fǎn	气反 …… 304
qì fǔ	气府 …… 304
qì gǔ	气鼓 …… 305
qì guǎn	气管 …… 305
qì hǎi	气海 …… 305
qì hǎi shū	气海俞 …… 305
qì hé	气合 …… 307
qì hù	气户 …… 307
qì jiē	气街 …… 308
qì jué	气厥 …… 308
qì lìn	气淋 …… 308
qì lóng	气癃 …… 309
qì mén	气门 …… 309
qì nà sān jiāo	气纳三焦 …… 309
qì shè	气舍 …… 309
qì shū	气俞 …… 310
qì táng	气堂 …… 310
qì xū bēng lòu	气虚崩漏 …… 310
qì xū jīng xíng xiān qī	气虚经行先期 … 310
qì xū xīn jì	气虚心悸 …… 310
qì xū yuè jīng guò duō	气虚月经过多 … 310
qì xū zhì chuāng	气虚痔疮 …… 311
qì xū zǐ gōng tuō chuí	气虚子宫脱垂 … 311
qì xué	气穴 …… 311
qì xuè bù zú wěi zhèng	气血不足痿证 … 312
qì xuè xū ruò rǔ shǎo	气血虚弱乳少 … 312
qì xuè xū ruò tòng jīng	气血虚弱痛经 … 312
qì yīn liǎng shāng tuō jū	气阴两伤脱疽 … 312
qì yǐng	气瘿 …… 313
qì yù bēng lòu	气郁崩漏 …… 313
qì yù è nì	气郁呃逆 …… 313
qì yù wèi tòng	气郁胃痛 …… 313
qì yuán	气原 …… 314
qì zhēn	气针 …… 314
qì zhī yīn xī	气之阴郄 …… 314
qì zhì bìng suǒ	气至病所 …… 314
qì zhì jīng xíng hòu qī	气滞经行后期 … 314
qì zhì tòng jīng	气滞痛经 …… 314
qì zhì xuè yū jīng bì	气滞血瘀经闭 … 315
qì zhì xuè yū tuō jū	气滞血瘀脱疽 … 315
qì zhōng	气中 …… 315
qiā fǎ	掐法 …… 315
qiān jīn fāng	千金方 …… 315
qiān jīn shí xué gē	千金十穴歌 …… 315
qiān jīn yào fāng	千金要方 …… 316
qiān jīn yì fāng	千金翼方 …… 316
qiān zhèng	牵正 …… 316
qián dǐng	前顶 …… 316
qián fà jì xué	前发际穴 …… 317
qián gǔ	前谷 …… 317
qián guān	前关 …… 317
qián hòu pèi xué fǎ	前后配穴法 …… 317
qián hòu zhèng zhōng xiàn	前后正中线 …… 318
qián liè xiàn	前列腺 …… 318
qián shén cōng	前神聪 …… 318
qián má zhěn	荨麻疹 …… 318
qián má zhěn diǎn	荨麻疹点 …… 318
qián jìng hú	钱镜湖 …… 318
qiáng cì jī	强刺激 …… 318
qiáng jiān	强间 …… 318
qiáng yáng	强阳 …… 319
qiào yīn	窍阴 …… 319
qiē fǎ	切法 …… 319
qié bìng	茄病 …… 319
qín chéng zǔ	秦承祖 …… 319
qín yuè rén	秦越人 …… 319
qīn zhēn shì pí nèi zhēn	揿针式皮内针 … 319
qīng dài	青带 …… 320
qīng hào	青昊 …… 320
qīng líng	青灵 …… 320
qīng líng quán	青灵泉 …… 320
qīng lóng bǎi wěi	青龙摆尾 …… 320
qīng máng	青盲 …… 320
qīng lěng quán	清冷泉 …… 321
qīng lěng yuān	清冷渊 …… 321

拼音	词条	页码
qióng yáo fā míng shén shū	琼瑶发明神书	321
qióng yáo zhēn rén bā fǎ shén zhēn	琼瑶真人八法神针	322
qiū jīng lì	丘经历	322
qiū jué	丘珏	322
qiū xū	丘虚	322
qiū xū	丘墟	322
qiú hòu	球后	322
qū bìn	曲鬓	323
qū chā	曲差	323
qū chí	曲池	323
qū chǐ	曲尺	324
qū fà	曲发	324
qū gǔ	曲骨	324
qū jiá	曲颊	324
qū jiǎ	曲甲	324
qū jiǎo	曲角	324
qū jié	曲节	325
qū quán	曲泉	325
qū yá	曲牙	325
qū yuán	曲垣	325
qū zé	曲泽	326
qū gǔ	屈骨	326
qū gǔ duān	屈骨端	326
qū	胠	326
qǔ xué fǎ	取穴法	326
qù zhǎo	去爪	326
quán liáo	权髎	327
quán bù chǎn	全不产	327
quán xún yì	全循义	327
quán mén	泉门	327
quán yè	泉液	327
quán yīn	泉阴	327
quán jiān xué	拳尖穴	327
quán	颧	327
quán liáo	颧髎	327
quē pén	缺盆	328
quē rǔ	缺乳	328
què zhuó fǎ	雀啄法	328
què zhuó jiǔ	雀啄灸	328
què shù	阙俞	328

R

rán gǔ	然谷	329
rán gǔ	然骨	329
rán hòu	然后	329
ráng xiè	瀼泄	329
rè bì	热秘	329
rè bì	热痹	330
rè bìng wǔ shí jiǔ shū	热病五十九俞	330
rè fǔ	热府	330
rè huò luàn	热霍乱	330
rè jiǔ	热灸	330
rè jué	热厥	331
rè lìn	热淋	331
rè qì huò luàn	热气霍乱	331
rè rù yíng xuè jìng zhèng	热入营血痉证	331
rè shàn	热疝	331
rè tù	热吐	332
rè zé jí zhī	热则疾之	332
rè zhàng	热瘴	332
rén bù	人部	332
rén cái	人才	332
rén héng	人横	332
rén jìng jīng	人镜经	332
rén shén	人神	333
rén tǐ jīng xué mó xíng	人体经穴模型	333
rén yíng	人迎	333
rén zhōng dīng	人中疔	333
rén mài	任脉	334
rén mài bìng	任脉病	334
rén mài luò mài	任脉络脉	335
rén mài luò mài bìng	任脉络脉病	335
rén mài zhī bié	任脉之别	335
rèn shēn ěr míng	妊娠耳鸣	335
rèn shēn fēng jìng	妊娠风痉	335
rèn shēn fù tòng	妊娠腹痛	335

拼音	词条	页码
rèn shēn jìng	妊娠痉	336
rèn shēn ǒu tù	妊娠呕吐	336
rèn shēn shāng shí	妊娠伤食	336
rèn shēn xián zhèng	妊娠痫证	336
rèn shēn xiǎo fù tòng	妊娠小腹痛	336
rèn shēn zhòng fēng	妊娠中风	336
rì gān chóng jiàn	日干重见	337
rì guāng jiǔ	日光灸	337
rì yuè	日月	337
róng bèi huí bì bā fǎ	荣备回避八法	337
ròu lǐ zhī mài	肉里之脉	337
ròu xì	肉郄	338
ròu zhù	肉柱	338
rǔ chuī	乳吹	338
rǔ é	乳蛾	338
rǔ é	乳鹅	338
rǔ gēn	乳根	338
rǔ pǐ	乳癖	338
rǔ shàng	乳上	338
rǔ shǎo	乳少	339
rǔ xià	乳下	339
rǔ xuǎn	乳癣	339
rǔ yōng	乳痈	339
rǔ zhōng	乳中	339
ruì zhēn	锐针	339
ruì zhōng	锐中	340
ruò	爇	340

S

拼音	词条	页码
sāi xiàn	腮腺	340
sān bǎi liù shí wǔ huì	三百六十五会	340
sān bǎi liù shí wǔ jié	三百六十五节	340
sān bǎi liù shí wǔ luò	三百六十五络	340
sān bǎi liù shí wǔ xué	三百六十五穴	340
sān biàn cì	三变刺	340
sān bù	三部	341
sān cái	三才	341
sān cái jiě	三才解	341
sān chí	三池	341
sān cì	三刺	341
sān guǎn	三管	341
sān jiān	三间	341
sān jiāo	三焦	342
sān jiāo jīng	三焦经	342
sān jiāo shǒu shào yáng zhī mài	三焦手少阳之脉	342
sān jiāo shū	三焦俞	343
sān jiǎo jiǔ	三角灸	343
sān jiǎo wō	三角窝	343
sān jiǎo wō hòu lóng qǐ	三角窝后隆起	343
sān jié jiāo	三结交	343
sān jìn yī tuì	三进一退	344
sān léng zhēn	三棱针	344
sān lǐ	三里	344
sān máo	三毛	344
sān qí liù yí zhēn yào jīng	三奇六仪针要经	344
sān shāng	三商	344
sān shuǐ	三水	344
sān tuì yī jìn	三退一进	344
sān xiāo	三消	345
sān yáng	三阳	345
sān yáng luò	三阳络	345
sān yáng sān yīn	三阳三阴	345
sān yáng wǔ huì	三阳五会	345
sān yīn	三阴	346
sān yīn jiāo	三阴交	346
sān yīn sān yáng	三阴三阳	346
sǎn cì	散刺	346
sǎn mài	散脉	347
sǎn xiào	散笑	347
sǎn zhēn fǎ	散针法	347
sāng mù jiǔ	桑木灸	347
sāng zhī jiǔ	桑枝灸	347
sǎng dà	颡大	347
sè máng	色盲	347
sēng tǎn rán	僧坦然	347
shā dāo	莎刀	347

拼音	词条	页码	拼音	词条	页码
shā lìn	砂淋	348	shàng sān lǐ	上三里	353
shā shí lìn	砂石淋	348	shàng wǎn	上脘	353
shān gēn	山根	348	shàng xià pèi xué fǎ	上下配穴法	354
shān tiào zhēn jiǔ jīng	山眺针灸经	348	shàng xiāo	上消	354
shān zhī shēng jiāng jiǔ	山栀生姜灸	348	shàng xīng	上星	354
shǎn guàn	闪罐	348	shàng yín lǐ	上龈里	354
shǎn guàn fǎ	闪罐法	348	shàng yíng xiāng	上迎香	355
shǎn huǒ fǎ	闪火法	348	shàng zhù	上杼	355
shàn	疝	348	shàng gǔ	尚骨	355
shàn qì	疝气	348	shāo shān huǒ	烧山火	355
shàn qì xué	疝气穴	349	shāo zhēn	烧针	355
shāng jìng	伤痉	349	shāo zhēn wěi	烧针尾	355
shāng rǔ tù	伤乳吐	349	shāo zhuó jiǔ	烧灼灸	356
shāng shí ǒu tù	伤食呕吐	349	shào chōng	少冲	356
shāng shí tù	伤食吐	349	shào fǔ	少府	356
shāng shí xiè	伤食泻	349	shào gǔ	少谷	357
shāng gài	商盖	350	shào guān	少关	357
shāng lù bǐng jiǔ	商陆饼灸	350	shào hǎi	少海	357
shāng qiū	商丘	350	shào jí	少吉	357
shāng qū	商曲	350	shào shāng	少商	357
shāng yáng	商阳	350	shào yáng mài	少阳脉	357
shàng bāo xià chuí	上胞下垂	351	shào yáng wéi	少阳维	358
shàng bìng xià qǔ	上病下取	351	shào yīn mài	少阴脉	358
shàng cí gōng	上慈宫	351	shào yīn shù	少阴俞	358
shàng dū	上都	351	shào yīn xì	少阴郄	358
shàng è xué	上腭穴	351	shào zé	少泽	358
shàng ěr gēn	上耳根	351	shé	舌	358
shàng gǔ	上骨	351	shé běn	舌本	358
shàng guān	上关	352	shé héng	舌横	358
shàng guǎn	上管	352	shé xià xué	舌下穴	358
shàng jì	上纪	352	shé yàn	舌厌	359
shàng jù xū	上巨虚	352	shé chuàn chuāng	蛇串疮	359
shàng kūn lún	上昆仑	352	shé dān	蛇丹	359
shàng lián	上廉	352	shé tóu	蛇头	359
shàng liáo	上髎	353	shé tóu dīng	蛇头疔	359
shàng lín	上林	353	shè fǎ	摄法	359
shàng mén	上门	353	shè lǐng chuāng	摄领疮	359
shàng qì hǎi	上气海	353	shēn mài	申脉	359
shàng qǔ	上取	353	shēn jiāo	身交	360

拼音	词条	页码	拼音	词条	页码
shēn zhù	身柱	360	shèn zú shào yīn zhī mài	肾足少阴之脉	368
shén cáng	神藏	360	shēng chéng shù	生成数	368
shén cōng	神聪	360	shēng chéng xī shù	生成息数	368
shén dào	神道	360	shēng jiāng jiǔ	生姜灸	368
shén dēng huǒ	神灯火	361	shēng shú	生熟	368
shén dēng zhào fǎ	神灯照法	361	shēng zhí qū	生殖区	369
shén fēng	神封	361	shèng bǐng zǐ	圣饼子	369
shén fǔ	神府	361	shèng jì zǒng lù	圣济总录	369
shén guāng	神光	362	shèng yù gē	胜玉歌	369
shén jīng shuāi ruò diǎn	神经衰弱点	362	shèng zé xiè zhī	盛则泻之	369
shén jiǔ jīng lún	神灸经纶	362	shī zhù	尸注	369
shén mén	神门	362	shī jīng	失精	369
shén nóng jīng	神农经	362	shī mián	失眠	370
shén què	神阙	363	shī mián xué	失眠穴	370
shén táng	神堂	363	shī qì	失气	370
shén tíng	神庭	363	shī xìn	失信	370
shén yìng jīng	神应经	364	shī zhěn	失枕	370
shén zhēn huǒ	神针火	364	shī guā shù	施刮术	370
shén zōng	神宗	364	shī dú dài xià	湿毒带下	370
shěn hào wèn	沈好问	364	shī jiǎo qì	湿脚气	370
shèn	肾	364	shī rè bēng lòu	湿热崩漏	371
shèn gān zhī bù	肾肝之部	364	shī rè biàn xuè	湿热便血	371
shèn jīng	肾经	364	shī rè dān dú	湿热丹毒	371
shèn náng fēng	肾囊风	365	shī rè jìn yīn wěi zhèng	湿热浸淫痿证	371
shèn qì	肾气	365	shī rè lì	湿热痢	371
shèn shàng xiàn	肾上腺	365	shī rè shé dān	湿热蛇丹	372
shèn shū	肾俞	365	shī rè shī zhěn	湿热湿疹	372
shèn xì	肾系	365	shī rè xié tòng	湿热胁痛	372
shèn xū bù yùn	肾虚不孕	365	shī rè xiè	湿热泻	372
shèn xū dài xià	肾虚带下	366	shī rè zhì chuāng	湿热痔疮	373
shèn xū jīng luàn	肾虚经乱	366	shī zhěn	湿疹	373
shèn xū jīng xíng hòu qī	肾虚经行后期	366	shí biàn	十变	373
shèn xū jīng xíng xiān hòu wú dìng qī	肾虚经行先后无定期	366	shí èr cì	十二刺	373
shèn xū xiāo chuǎn	肾虚哮喘	367	shí èr cóng	十二从	373
shèn xū xiè	肾虚泻	367	shí èr jié	十二节	374
shèn xū yāo tòng	肾虚腰痛	367	shí èr jié cì	十二节刺	374
shèn xū yuè jīng guò shǎo	肾虚月经过少	367	shí èr jìn	十二禁	374
shèn xū zǐ gōng tuō chuí	肾虚子宫脱垂	368	shí èr jīng biāo běn	十二经标本	375
			shí èr jīng bié	十二经别	376

拼音	词条	页码
shí èr jīng dòng mài	十二经动脉	376
shí èr jīng jīn	十二经筋	377
shí èr jīng mài	十二经脉	377
shí èr jīng mài gē	十二经脉歌	377
shí èr jīng shuǐ	十二经水	378
shí èr jīng zhī hǎi	十二经之海	378
shí èr jīng zǐ mǔ bǔ xiè gē	十二经子母补泻歌	378
shí èr pí bù	十二皮部	378
shí èr rén tú	十二人图	378
shí èr shǒu fǎ	十二手法	378
shí èr zhèng jīng	十二正经	379
shí èr zhǐ cháng	十二指肠	379
shí èr zì fēn cì dì shǒu fǎ	十二字分次第手法	379
shí liù luò mài	十六络脉	379
shí qī zhuī	十七椎	379
shí sān guǐ xué	十三鬼穴	379
shí sān xué	十三穴	380
shí sì fǎ	十四法	380
shí sì jīng	十四经	380
shí sì jīng fā huī	十四经发挥	380
shí sì jīng fā huī hé zuǎn	十四经发挥合纂	380
shí sì jīng xué	十四经穴	380
shí wáng	十王	382
shí wǔ bié luò	十五别络	382
shí wǔ luò	十五络	382
shí wǔ luò mài	十五络脉	382
shí wǔ zhuī	十五椎	383
shí xuān	十宣	383
shí yī mài	十一脉	384
shí yī mài jiǔ jīng	十一脉灸经	384
shí gōng	石宫	384
shí guān	石关	384
shí lìn	石淋	385
shí lóng ruì	石龙芮	385
shí mén	石门	385
shí què	石阙	385
shí zàng yòng	石藏用	386
shí zhēn	石针	386
shí xíng dùn ké	时行顿咳	386
shí àn jiǔ	实按灸	386
shí rè yá tòng	实热牙痛	386
shí rè yān hóu zhǒng tòng	实热咽喉肿痛	386
shí dào	食道	386
shí dòu	食窦	386
shí gōng	食宫	387
shí guān	食关	387
shí jī wèi tòng	食积胃痛	387
shí yán jiǔ	食盐灸	387
shí zhǐ	食指	387
shí zhì fù tòng	食滞腹痛	387
shǐ guāng	始光	388
shǐ sù	始素	388
shì chì rú bái	视赤如白	388
shì qū	视区	388
shì wù yì sè	视物易色	388
shì tóu	势头	388
shì dòng bìng	是动病	388
shì dòng suǒ shēng bìng	是动、所生病	388
shì sēng kuàng	释僧匡	388
shì sēng kuàng zhēn jiǔ jīng	释僧匡针灸经	388
shì zhàn chí	释湛池	388
shǒu chà fā	手叉发	388
shǒu dà zhǐ jiǎ hòu	手大指甲后	389
shǒu fū	手夫	389
shǒu huái	手踝	389
shǒu jué yīn biāo běn	手厥阴标本	389
shǒu jué yīn jīng bié	手厥阴经别	389
shǒu jué yīn jīng jīn	手厥阴经筋	389
shǒu jué yīn jīng jīn bìng	手厥阴经筋病	389
shǒu jué yīn luò mài	手厥阴络脉	389
shǒu jué yīn luò mài bìng	手厥阴络脉病	390
shǒu jué yīn xīn bāo jīng	手厥阴心包经	390
shǒu jué yīn xīn bāo jīng bìng	手厥阴心包经病	390
shǒu nì zhù	手逆注	390

拼音	词条	页码
shǒu sān lǐ	手三里	390
shǒu sān yáng jīng	手三阳经	391
shǒu sān yīn jīng	手三阴经	391
shǒu shàng lián	手上廉	391
shǒu shào yáng biāo běn	手少阳标本	392
shǒu shào yáng jīng bié	手少阳经别	392
shǒu shào yáng jīng jīn	手少阳经筋	392
shǒu shào yáng jīng jīn bìng	手少阳经筋病	392
shǒu shào yáng luò mài	手少阳络脉	393
shǒu shào yáng luò mài bìng	手少阳络脉病	393
shǒu shào yáng sān jiāo jīng	手少阳三焦经	393
shǒu shào yáng sān jiāo jīng bìng	手少阳三焦经病	393
shǒu shào yáng shǒu jué yīn jīng bié	手少阳、手厥阴经别	394
shǒu shào yáng zhī zhèng	手少阳之正	394
shǒu shào yīn biāo běn	手少阴标本	394
shǒu shào yīn jīng bié	手少阴经别	394
shǒu shào yīn jīng jīn	手少阴经筋	395
shǒu shào yīn jīng jīn bìng	手少阴经筋病	395
shǒu shào yīn luò mài	手少阴络脉	395
shǒu shào yīn luò mài bìng	手少阴络脉病	395
shǒu shào yīn xì	手少阴郄	395
shǒu shào yīn xīn jīng	手少阴心经	395
shǒu shào yīn xīn jīng bìng	手少阴心经病	396
shǒu shào yīn zhī bié	手少阴之别	396
shǒu shào yīn zhī zhèng	手少阴之正	396
shǒu suí kǒng	手髓孔	396
shǒu tài yáng biāo běn	手太阳标本	396
shǒu tài yáng jīng bié	手太阳经别	396
shǒu tài yáng jīng jīn	手太阳经筋	397
shǒu tài yáng jīng jīn bìng	手太阳经筋病	397
shǒu tài yáng luò mài	手太阳络脉	397
shǒu tài yáng luò mài bìng	手太阳络脉病	397
shǒu tài yáng shǒu shào yīn jīng bié	手太阳、手少阴经别	397
shǒu tài yáng xiǎo cháng jīng	手太阳小肠经	398
shǒu tài yáng xiǎo cháng jīng bìng	手太阳小肠经病	398
shǒu tài yáng xué	手太阳穴	398
shǒu tài yáng zhī bié	手太阳之别	398
shǒu tài yáng zhī zhèng	手太阳之正	398
shǒu tài yīn biāo běn	手太阴标本	398
shǒu tài yīn fèi jīng	手太阴肺经	398
shǒu tài yīn fèi jīng bìng	手太阴肺经病	399
shǒu tài yīn jīng bié	手太阴经别	400
shǒu tài yīn jīng jīn	手太阴经筋	400
shǒu tài yīn jīng jīn bìng	手太阴经筋病	400
shǒu tài yīn luò mài	手太阴络脉	400
shǒu tài yīn luò mài bìng	手太阴络脉病	400
shǒu tài yīn zhī bié	手太阴之别	401
shǒu tài yīn zhī zhèng	手太阴之正	401
shǒu wǔ lǐ	手五里	401
shǒu xià lián	手下廉	401
shǒu xīn	手心	401
shǒu xīn zhǔ zhī bié	手心主之别	401
shǒu xīn zhǔ zhī zhèng	手心主之正	401
shǒu yáng míng biāo běn	手阳明标本	401
shǒu yáng míng dà cháng jīng	手阳明大肠经	401
shǒu yáng míng dà cháng jīng bìng	手阳明大肠经病	403
shǒu yáng míng jīng bié	手阳明经别	403
shǒu yáng míng jīng jīn	手阳明经筋	403
shǒu yáng míng jīng jīn bìng	手阳明经筋病	403
shǒu yáng míng luò mài	手阳明络脉	403
shǒu yáng míng luò mài bìng	手阳明络脉病	404
shǒu yáng míng shǒu tài yīn	手阳明、手太阴	

拼音	词条	页码
yīn jīng bié	经别	404
shǒu yáng míng zhī bié	手阳明之别	404
shǒu yáng míng zhī zhèng	手阳明之正	404
shǒu yú	手鱼	404
shǒu zhǎng hòu bái ròu jì xué	手掌后白肉际穴	404
shǒu zhǎng hòu bì jiān xué	手掌后臂间穴	404
shǒu zhēn	手针	404
shǒu zhǐ bǔ xiè fǎ	手指补泻法	404
shǒu zhōng zhǐ dì yī jié xué	手中指第一节穴	405
shǒu zú dà zhǐ zhǎo jiǎ	手足大指爪甲	405
shǒu zú suǐ kǒng	手足髓孔	405
shǒu qì	守气	405
shǒu qiào yīn	首窍阴	405
shū chí	枢持	405
shū rú	枢儒	405
shū fǔ	俞府	405
shū mù pèi xué fǎ	俞募配穴法	406
shū zhāng yā shǒu	舒张押手	406
shū	输	406
shū cì	输刺	406
shū mài	输脉	406
shū niào guǎn	输尿管	406
shū xué	输穴	406
shū zhī mài	输之脉	406
shǔ lèi	属累	407
shǔ shī gǎn mào	暑湿感冒	407
shǔ fèn jiǔ	鼠粪灸	407
shǔ lòu	鼠瘘	407
shǔ wěi	鼠尾	407
shù gǔ	束骨	407
shù xué	腧穴	407
shù xué zhé zhōng	腧穴折衷	408
shuài gǔ	率谷	408
shuāng mù tōng jīng	双目通睛	408
shuǐ	水	408
shuǐ bìng	水病	408
shuǐ dào	水道	408
shuǐ fēn	水分	409
shuǐ gōu	水沟	409
shuǐ gǔ	水鼓	409
shuǐ guàn fǎ	水罐法	410
shuǐ jiǔ	水灸	410
shuǐ mén	水门	410
shuǐ qì	水气	410
shuǐ quán	水泉	410
shuǐ tù	水突	411
shuǐ xué	水穴	411
shuǐ yuán	水原	411
shuǐ zhēn	水针	411
shuǐ zhǒng	水肿	411
shuì shèng sǎn	睡圣散	412
sī luò	丝络	412
sī zhú	丝竹	412
sī zhú kōng	丝竹空	412
sì bái	四白	412
sì dú	四渎	412
sì fèng	四缝	413
sì gēn sān jié	四根三结	413
sì hǎi	四海	414
sì hé	四合	414
sì héng wén	四横纹	414
sì huā	四花	414
sì huá	四华	414
sì jiē	四街	414
sì jīng	四经	414
sì mǎn	四满	414
sì qì jiē	四气街	415
sì shén cōng	四神聪	415
sì wān fēng	四弯风	415
sì zhōu qǔ xué	四周取穴	415
sì zǒng xué gē	四总穴歌	415
sōu xuè	溲血	416
sòu xuè	嗽血	416
sù liáo	素髎	416
sù wèn	素问	416
suàn qián jiǔ	蒜钱灸	416

suí biàn ěr tiáo qì	随变而调气…… 416	tài yǐ shén zhēn jí jiě	太乙神针集解 … 422
suí ěr jì zhī	随而济之……… 416	tài yǐ shén zhēn xīn fǎ	太乙神针心法 … 422
suí nián zhuàng	随年壮………… 416	tài yīn	太阴…………… 422
suí zhèng qǔ xué	随症取穴……… 417	tài yīn luò	太阴络………… 422
suǐ fǔ	髓府…………… 417	tài yīn mài	太阴脉………… 422
suǐ hǎi	髓海…………… 417	tài yīn qiāo	太阴跷………… 423
suǐ kōng	髓空…………… 417	tài yuān	太渊…………… 423
suǐ kǒng	髓孔…………… 417	tài zhōng	太钟…………… 423
suǐ shù	髓俞…………… 417	tài zǔ	太祖…………… 423
suǐ zhōng	髓中…………… 417	tán fǎ	弹法…………… 423
sūn dǐng yí	孙鼎宜………… 417	tán huǒ xīn jì	痰火心悸……… 423
sūn luò	孙络…………… 417	tán jué	痰厥…………… 424
sūn mài	孙脉…………… 417	tán rè xiāo chuǎn	痰热哮喘……… 424
sūn sī miǎo	孙思邈………… 417	tán shī bù yùn	痰湿不孕……… 424
sūn sī miǎo zhēn jīng	孙思邈针经…… 418	tán shī ké sòu	痰湿咳嗽……… 424
sūn zhuō sān	孙卓三………… 418	tán shī yuè jīng guò shǎo	痰湿月经过少 … 424
suō jiǎo cháng yōng	缩脚肠痈……… 418	tán shī zǔ zhì jīng bì	痰湿阻滞经闭 … 425
suǒ gǔ	锁骨…………… 418	tán yǐn ǒu tù	痰饮呕吐……… 425
suǒ shēng bìng	所生病………… 418	tán zhì è zǔ	痰滞恶阻……… 425
		tán zhuó rǔ pǐ	痰浊乳癖……… 425
		tán zhuó tóu tòng	痰浊头痛……… 425

T

		tán zhuó xiōng bì	痰浊胸痹……… 426
tā jīng qǔ xué	他经取穴……… 418	táo zhī jiǔ	桃枝灸………… 426
tāi fēng	胎风…………… 418	táo cí zhēn	陶瓷针………… 426
tāi wèi bù zhèng	胎位不正……… 418	táo dào	陶道…………… 426
tāi xuǎn	胎癣…………… 418	táo zhēn	陶针…………… 426
tāi yī bù chū	胎衣不出……… 419	tào guǎn jìn zhēn	套管进针……… 427
tāi yī bù xià	胎衣不下……… 419	tào guǎn shì pí fū zhēn	套管式皮肤针 … 427
tài bái	太白…………… 419	tè dìng xué	特定穴………… 427
tài cāng	太仓…………… 419	tí chā bǔ xiè	提插补泻……… 427
tài chōng	太冲…………… 419	tí chā fǎ	提插法………… 428
tài chōng mài	太冲脉………… 420	tí fǎ	提法…………… 428
tài líng	太陵…………… 420	tí niē jìn zhēn	提捏进针……… 428
tài quán	太泉…………… 420	tí qì fǎ	提气法………… 428
tài xī	太溪…………… 420	tí zhēn fǎ	提针法………… 428
tài yáng	太阳…………… 420	tǐ biāo biāo zhì	体表标志……… 428
tài yī	太一…………… 421	tǐ biāo jiě pāo biāo zhì	体表解剖标志 … 428
tài yǐ	太乙…………… 421	tǐ biāo jiě pāo biāo zhì dìng wèi fǎ	体表解剖标志定位法 …………… 428
tài yǐ shén zhēn	太乙神针……… 421		
tài yǐ shén zhēn fāng	太乙神针方…… 422		

tǐ wèi	体位	429	tiān xíng chì yǎn	天行赤眼 …… 436
tǐ zhēn	体针	429	tiān xīng shí èr xué	天星十二穴 …… 436
tì jiǔ gāo	替灸膏	429	tiān xīng shí yī xué	天星十一穴 …… 436
tiān bù	天部	429	tiān yī	天医 …… 436
tiān cái	天才	429	tiān yìng xué	天应穴 …… 436
tiān chí	天池	429	tiān yǒu	天牖 …… 436
tiān chōng	天冲	430	tiān yuán tài yǐ gē	天元太乙歌 …… 436
tiān chuāng	天窗	430	tiān zhù	天柱 …… 437
tiān cōng	天聪	430	tiān zhù gǔ	天柱骨 …… 437
tiān diào fēng	天吊风	430	tiān zōng	天宗 …… 437
tiān dǐng	天顶	430	tiáo kǒu	条口 …… 437
tiān dǐng	天鼎	431	tiáo qì	调气 …… 438
tiān fǔ	天府	431	tiáo qì fǎ	调气法 …… 438
tiān gài	天盖	431	tiǎo cǎo zī	挑草子 …… 438
tiān guǐ	天癸	431	tiǎo cì	挑刺 …… 438
tiān huì	天会	431	tiǎo zhēn liáo fǎ	挑针疗法 …… 438
tiān huǒ	天火	431	tiǎo zhì fǎ	挑治法 …… 438
tiān jīng	天泾	431	tiǎo zhì fǎ	挑痔法 …… 438
tiān jǐng	天井	431	tiě zhēn	铁针 …… 438
tiān jiǔ	天灸	432	tīng hē	听呵 …… 438
tiān jiù	天臼	432	tīng hé	听河 …… 438
tiān liáo	天髎	432	tīng gōng	听宫 …… 439
tiān lóng	天笼	433	tīng huì	听会 …… 439
tiān mǎn	天满	433	tíng lì bǐng jiǔ	葶苈饼灸 …… 439
tiān nán xīng jiǔ	天南星灸	433	tíng ěr	聤耳 …… 439
tiān qú	天瞿	433	tíng ěr shí zhèng	聤耳实证 …… 439
tiān qú	天衢	433	tíng ěr xū zhèng	聤耳虚证 …… 440
tiān quán	天泉	433	tǐng jiǎo	艇角 …… 440
tiān róng	天容	433	tǐng zhōng	艇中 …… 440
tiān shèng zhēn jīng	天圣针经	434	tōng gǔ	通谷 …… 440
tiān shī	天湿	434	tōng guān	通关 …… 440
tiān shū	天枢	434	tōng jiān	通间 …… 440
tiān tū	天突	434	tōng jīng jiē qì	通经接气 …… 440
tiān wēn	天温	435	tōng lǐ	通里 …… 440
tiān wǔ huì	天五会	435	tōng lǐ	通理 …… 441
tiān xī	天溪	435	tōng mén	通门 …… 441
tiān xiāo	天哮	435	tōng tiān	通天 …… 441
tiān xiāo qiàng	天哮呛	436	tōng xuán zhǐ yào fù	通玄指要赋 …… 441
tiān xíng chì rè	天行赤热	436	tóng míng jīng pèi xué fǎ	同名经配穴法 …… 442

tóng míng jīng qǔ xué	同名经取穴 …… 442	tuō yí wèi	托颐位 …………… 450
tóng shēn cùn	同身寸 ………… 442	tuō gāng	脱肛 …………… 450
tóng yīn zhī mài	同阴之脉 ……… 442	tuō gāng shí zhèng	脱肛实证 ……… 451
tóng rén	铜人 …………… 442	tuō gāng xū zhèng	脱肛虚证 ……… 451
tóng rén shù xué zhēn jiǔ tú jīng	铜人腧穴针灸图经 ……… 442	tuō gǔ dīng	脱骨疔 ………… 451
		tuō gǔ jū	脱骨疽 ………… 451
tóng rén zhēn jiǔ fāng	铜人针灸方 …… 443	tuō jū	脱疽 …………… 451
tóng rén zhǐ yào fù	铜人指要赋 …… 443	tuō yōng	脱痈 …………… 451
tóng xuán	童玄 …………… 443	tuō zhèng	脱证 …………… 452
tóng zǐ liáo	瞳子髎 ………… 443		
tǒng jiǔ	筒灸 …………… 443		

W

tòng bì	痛痹 …………… 443	wài bí	外鼻 …………… 452
tòng jīng	痛经 …………… 444	wài cè	外侧 …………… 452
tōu zhēn	偷针 …………… 444	wài chuī rǔ yōng	外吹乳痈 ……… 452
tóu chōng	头冲 …………… 444	wài ěr	外耳 …………… 452
tóu fèng	头缝 …………… 444	wài ěr dào kǒu	外耳道口 ……… 453
tóu héng gǔ	头横骨 ………… 444	wài gǎn fēng zhěn	外感风疹 ……… 453
tóu lín qì	头临泣 ………… 444	wài gǎn ǒu tù	外感呕吐 ……… 453
tóu pí zhēn	头皮针 ………… 444	wài gōu	外勾 …………… 453
tóu qiào yīn	头窍阴 ………… 444	wài guān	外关 …………… 453
tóu téng	头疼 …………… 445	wài huái	外踝 …………… 454
tóu tòng	头痛 …………… 445	wài huái jiān	外踝尖 ………… 454
tóu wéi	头维 …………… 445	wài huái qián jiāo mài	外踝前交脉 …… 454
tóu xuàn	头眩 …………… 445	wài huái shàng	外踝上 ………… 454
tóu zhēn	头针 …………… 446	wài jīn jīn yù yè	外金津玉液 …… 454
tóu zhēn liáo fǎ	头针疗法 ……… 446	wài jīng	外经 …………… 454
tòu cì	透刺 …………… 448	wài jiǔ gāo	外灸膏 ………… 454
tòu tiān liáng	透天凉 ………… 448	wài kē jiǔ fǎ lùn cuì xīn shū	外科灸法论粹新书 ……… 455
tǔ gān	土疳 …………… 449		
tù xuè	吐血 …………… 449	wài láo gōng	外劳宫 ………… 455
tuán gǎng	团岗 …………… 449	wài líng	外陵 …………… 455
tuī ěr nà zhī	推而纳之 ……… 449	wài qiū	外丘 …………… 455
tuī guàn fǎ	推罐法 ………… 449	wài shēng zhí qì	外生殖器 ……… 456
tuī yǐn	推引 …………… 449	wài shū	外枢 …………… 456
tuī zhēn	推针 …………… 450	wài tái mì yào	外台秘要 ……… 456
tuì	退 ……………… 450	wài xī yǎn	外膝眼 ………… 456
tuì fǎ	退法 …………… 450	wài zhì	外痔 …………… 456
tún	臀 ……………… 450	wán gǔ	完骨 …………… 456
tún zhōng	臀中 …………… 450		

拼音	词条	页码
wǎn jiǔ	碗灸	457
wàn	腕	457
wàn gǔ	腕骨	457
wàn huái zhēn	腕踝针	457
wàn láo	腕劳	457
wàn zhǎng bèi cè héng wén	腕掌、背侧横纹	458
wàn	踠	458
wáng bīng	王冰	458
wáng chù míng	王处明	458
wáng guó ruì	王国瑞	458
wáng hào gǔ	王好古	458
wáng huái yǐn	王怀隐	458
wáng kāi	王开	458
wáng kè míng	王克明	458
wáng tāo	王焘	459
wáng wéi yī	王惟一	459
wáng yǔ	王禹	459
wáng zhí zhōng	王执中	459
wáng zōng quán	王宗泉	459
wáng zuǎn	王纂	459
wēi zhēn	微针	460
wéi bāo	维胞	460
wéi dào	维道	460
wéi gōng	维宫	460
wéi huì	维会	460
wěi cuì	尾翠	460
wěi lú	尾闾	461
wěi qióng gǔ	尾穷骨	461
wěi yì	尾翳	461
wěi yáng	委阳	461
wěi zhōng	委中	461
wěi zhōng yāng	委中央	462
wěi bì	痿躄	462
wěi zhèng	痿证	462
wèi shēng zhēn jiǔ xuán jī mì yào	卫生针灸玄机秘要	462
wèi shì jié	卫世杰	462
wèi	胃	462
wèi cāng	胃仓	462
wèi fǎn	胃反	463
wèi fǔ bù hé bù mèi	胃腑不和不寐	463
wèi guǎn	胃管	463
wèi hán è nì	胃寒呃逆	463
wèi hán è zǔ	胃寒恶阻	463
wèi jīng	胃经	463
wèi qū	胃区	463
wèi rè bí nǜ	胃热鼻衄	464
wèi rè è nì	胃热呃逆	464
wèi rè è zǔ	胃热恶阻	466
wèi rè fēng zhěn	胃热风疹	466
wèi rè ǒu tù	胃热呕吐	466
wèi rè rǔ yōng	胃热乳痈	466
wèi rè tù xuè	胃热吐血	467
wèi shū	胃俞	467
wèi tòng	胃痛	467
wèi wǎn	胃脘	468
wèi wǎn tòng	胃脘痛	468
wèi wǎn xià shū	胃脘下俞	468
wèi wéi	胃维	469
wèi xīn tòng	胃心痛	469
wèi xū è zǔ	胃虚恶阻	469
wèi zhī dà luò	胃之大络	469
wèi zú yáng míng zhī mài	胃足阳明之脉	469
wēn hé jiǔ	温和灸	469
wēn liū	温溜	470
wēn jiǔ	温灸	470
wēn jiǔ qì	温灸器	470
wēn nüè	温疟	470
wēn qí fǎ	温脐法	470
wēn tǒng jiǔ	温筒灸	471
wēn zhēn	温针	471
wēn zhēn jiǔ	温针灸	471
wén rén qí nián	闻人耆年	471
wò wèi	卧位	471
wò zhēn	卧针	471
wū méi jiǔ	乌梅灸	471
wū méi zhēng qì jiǔ	乌梅蒸汽灸	472

拼音	词条	页码
wū yì	屋翳	472
wú bān hén jiǔ	无瘢痕灸	472
wú míng	无名	472
wú míng zhǐ	无名指	472
wú rè jiǔ	无热灸	472
wú zǐ	无子	472
wú fù guì	吴复桂	472
wú jiā yán	吴嘉言	473
wú kūn	吴昆	473
wú qiān	吴谦	473
wú wén bǐng	吴文炳	473
wú yì dǐng	吴亦鼎	473
wú zhī yīng	吴之英	474
wǔ bèi zǐ jiǔ	五倍子灸	474
wǔ bèi zǐ zhēng qì jiǔ	五倍子蒸气灸	474
wǔ biàn	五变	474
wǔ biàn cì	五变刺	474
wǔ chù	五处	475
wǔ cì	五刺	475
wǔ duó jìn cì	五夺禁刺	475
wǔ gēng xiè	五更泄	475
wǔ guò	五过	475
wǔ hǔ	五虎	475
wǔ huì	五会	475
wǔ jié cì	五节刺	476
wǔ jìn	五禁	476
wǔ jīng	五经	476
wǔ jué	五决	476
wǔ lǐ	五里	476
wǔ mén	五门	476
wǔ mén shí biàn	五门十变	477
wǔ nì	五逆	477
wǔ qū shù	五胠俞	477
wǔ sè dài xià	五色带下	477
wǔ shí jiǔ cì	五十九刺	478
wǔ shū	五枢	478
wǔ shù pèi xué fǎ	五腧配穴法	478
wǔ shù xué	五腧穴	479
wǔ tài zhī rén	五态之人	479
wǔ xié cì	五邪刺	480
wǔ xíng	五行	480
wǔ zàng cì	五脏刺	481
wǔ zàng liù fǔ zhī hǎi	五脏六腑之海	481
wǔ dǎo zhèn chàn kòng zhì qū	舞蹈震颤控制区	481
wù shí	恶食	481
wù zǐ	恶子	481
wù zì	恶字	481

X

拼音	词条	页码
xī fāng zǐ míng táng jiǔ jīng	西方子明堂灸经	482
xī bēi fǎ	吸杯法	482
xī tǒng	吸筒	482
xī bāo	息胞	482
xī tāi	息胎	482
xī gǔ	溪谷	482
xī xué	溪穴	482
xī	膝	482
xī dǐng	膝顶	482
xī guān	膝关	482
xī mù	膝目	483
xī páng	膝旁	483
xī shàng	膝上	483
xī wài	膝外	483
xī xià	膝下	483
xī yǎn	膝眼	483
xī yáng guān	膝阳关	484
xī xué	膝穴	484
xí hóng	席弘	484
xí hóng fù	席弘赋	484
xì luò	系络	484
xì mén	郄门	484
xì xué	郄穴	485
xì yáng	郄阳	485
xì zhōng	郄中	485
xì xīn jiǔ	细辛灸	485

xiá bái	侠白 …… 485	xià yīng	夏英 …… 491	
xiá chéng jiāng	侠承浆 …… 486	xián zhèng	痫证 …… 491	
xiá shàng xīng	侠上星 …… 486	xián zhèng shí zhèng	痫证实证 …… 492	
xiá xī	侠溪 …… 486	xián zhèng xū zhèng	痫证虚证 …… 492	
xiá yù quán	侠玉泉 …… 486	xiàn gǔ	陷谷 …… 492	
xià bìng shàng qǔ	下病上取 …… 486	xiàn gǔ	陷骨 …… 493	
xià bù bīng lěng bù yùn	下部冰冷不孕 …… 487	xiàn xià zé jiǔ zhī	陷下则灸之 …… 493	
xià chún dīng	下唇疔 …… 487	xiāng fù bǐng	香附饼 …… 493	
xià dū	下都 …… 487	xiāng liú bǐng	香硫饼 …… 493	
xià dú	下渎 …… 487	xiāng shā jiǔ	香砂灸 …… 493	
xià ěr gēn	下耳根 …… 487	xiàng qiáng xué	项强穴 …… 493	
xià fān	下瘢 …… 487	xiāo dàn	消瘅 …… 493	
xià guān	下关 …… 487	xiāo kě	消渴 …… 494	
xià guǎn	下管 …… 487	xiāo lì	消疬 …… 494	
xià hé xué	下合穴 …… 487	xiāo luò	消泺 …… 494	
xià héng	下横 …… 488	xiāo pǐ shén huǒ zhēn	消癖神火针 …… 494	
xià huāng	下肓 …… 488	xiāo chuǎn	哮喘 …… 495	
xià jí	下极 …… 488	xiāo kě	痟渴 …… 495	
xià jí shū	下极俞 …… 488	xiǎo cháng	小肠 …… 495	
xià jí zhī shū	下极之俞 …… 488	xiǎo cháng jīng	小肠经 …… 495	
xià jì	下纪 …… 488	xiǎo cháng qì	小肠气 …… 495	
xià jù xū	下巨虚 …… 489	xiǎo cháng shǒu tài yáng zhī mài	小肠手太阳之脉 …… 495	
xià kūn lún	下昆仑 …… 489			
xià lì	下利 …… 489	xiǎo cháng shū	小肠俞 …… 496	
xià lián	下廉 …… 489	xiǎo ér bàn shēn bù suí	小儿半身不遂 …… 496	
xià liáo	下髎 …… 489	xiǎo ér è nì	小儿呃逆 …… 496	
xià lín	下林 …… 490	xiǎo ér gān lì	小儿疳痢 …… 496	
xià líng	下陵 …… 490	xiǎo ér gān shòu	小儿疳瘦 …… 496	
xià líng sān lǐ	下陵三里 …… 490	xiǎo ér gāng yǎng	小儿肛痒 …… 496	
xià qì hǎi	下气海 …… 490	xiǎo ér guī xiōng xué	小儿龟胸穴 …… 497	
xià qǔ	下取 …… 490	xiǎo ér hán jué	小儿寒厥 …… 497	
xià sān lǐ	下三里 …… 490	xiǎo ér hūn mí	小儿昏迷 …… 497	
xià shǒu bā fǎ	下手八法 …… 490	xiǎo ér jī xiōng xué	小儿鸡胸穴 …… 497	
xià sì fèng	下四缝 …… 490	xiǎo ér jué zhèng	小儿厥证 …… 497	
xià wǎn	下脘 …… 490	xiǎo ér ké sòu	小儿咳嗽 …… 497	
xià xiāo	下消 …… 491	xiǎo ér má bì zhèng	小儿麻痹证 …… 498	
xià xuè	下血 …… 491	xiǎo ér míng táng zhēn jiǔ jīng	小儿明堂针灸经 …… 498	
xià yāo	下腰 …… 491			
xià zhēn shí sì fǎ	下针十四法 …… 491	xiǎo ér ǒu tù	小儿呕吐 …… 498	

xiǎo ér rè jué	小儿热厥 …… 498	xié táng	胁堂 …… 505
xiǎo ér rè xiè	小儿热泻 …… 499	xié tòng	胁痛 …… 505
xiǎo ér shēn rè tù xiè	小儿身热吐泻 …… 499	xié cì	斜刺 …… 505
xiǎo ér shí xián	小儿食痫 …… 499	xié shì	斜视 …… 506
xiǎo ér shuǐ jīng	小儿睡惊 …… 499	xiè fāng bǔ yuán	泻方补圆 …… 506
xiǎo ér tán xiè	小儿痰泻 …… 499	xiè nán bǔ běi	泻南补北 …… 506
xiǎo ér tóu tòng	小儿头痛 …… 500	xiè yuán bǔ fāng	泻圆补方 …… 507
xiǎo ér tuō gāng	小儿脱肛 …… 500	xiè zǐ suí mǔ	泻子随母 …… 507
xiǎo ér wěi zhèng	小儿痿证 …… 500	xiè	泄 …… 507
xiǎo ér xiè xiè	小儿泄泻 …… 501	xiè xiè	泄泻 …… 507
xiǎo ér yáng jué	小儿阳厥 …… 502	xiè mài	解脉 …… 507
xiǎo ér yí niào	小儿遗尿 …… 502	xīn	心 …… 507
xiǎo ér yīn jué	小儿阴厥 …… 502	xīn bāo jīng	心包经 …… 508
xiǎo ér yuě	小儿哕 …… 502	xīn huǒ kàng shèng niào xuè	心火亢盛尿血 …… 509
xiǎo ér zhēn	小儿针 …… 503	xīn jì	心悸 …… 509
xiǎo gǔ kōng	小骨空 …… 503	xīn jīng	心经 …… 509
xiǎo gǔ kǒng	小骨孔 …… 503	xīn pí liǎng xū bù mèi	心脾两虚不寐 …… 509
xiǎo gǔ	小谷 …… 503	xīn shǒu shào yīn zhī mài	心手少阴之脉 …… 509
xiǎo hǎi	小海 …… 503	xīn shū	心俞 …… 509
xiǎo huí xiāng jiǔ	小茴香灸 …… 503	xīn tòng	心痛 …… 510
xiǎo jí	小吉 …… 504	xīn xì	心系 …… 510
xiǎo méi dāo	小眉刀 …… 504	xīn xià tòng	心下痛 …… 510
xiǎo tiān xīn	小天心 …… 504	xīn zhǔ	心主 …… 510
xiǎo xī	小溪 …… 504	xīn zhǔ shǒu jué yīn xīn bāo luò zhī mài	心主手厥阴心包络之脉 …… 510
xiǎo zhēn	小针 …… 504		
xiǎo zhǐ(zhǐ)cì zhǐ(zhǐ)	小指(趾)次指(趾) …… 504	xīn è bí yuān	辛頞鼻渊 …… 510
xiǎo zhǐ jiān	小指尖 …… 504	xīn jí míng táng jiǔ fǎ	新集明堂灸法 …… 510
xiǎo zhǐ jiān	小趾尖 …… 504	xīn jiàn	新建 …… 510
xiǎo zhǐ tóu	小指头 …… 504	xīn shè	新设 …… 510
xiǎo zhǐ zhǎo wén	小指爪纹 …… 504	xìn huì	囟会 …… 510
xiǎo zhú	小竹 …… 505	xìn zhōng	囟中 …… 511
xiǎo zhù jiǔ	小炷灸 …… 505	xīng lóng	兴隆 …… 511
xiǎo zhuàng jiǔ	小壮灸 …… 505	xīng xīng	惺惺 …… 511
xiǎo zhǒu jiān	小肘尖 …… 505	xíng bì	行痹 …… 511
xiē	歇 …… 505	xíng jiān	行间 …… 511
xiē jīng	歇经 …… 505	xíng qì fǎ	行气法 …… 512
xié	胁 …… 505	xíng zhēn	行针 …… 512
xié jiào	胁窌 …… 505	xíng zhēn zhǐ yào fù	行针指要赋 …… 512

拼音	词条	页码	拼音	词条	页码
xíng zhēn zǒng yào gē	行针总要歌	512	xuán lí	悬厘	518
xiōng	胸	512	xuán lú	悬颅	519
xiōng bì	胸痹	513	xuán mìng	悬命	519
xiōng bì	胸薜	513	xuán qǐ jiǔ	悬起灸	519
xiōng qiāng qū	胸腔区	513	xuán quán	悬泉	519
xiōng táng	胸堂	513	xuán shū	悬枢	519
xiōng tōng gǔ	胸通谷	513	xuán zhōng	悬钟	519
xiōng xiāng	胸乡	513	xuán zhù	悬柱	520
xiōng zhī yīn shū	胸之阴俞	514	xuán jī	璇玑	520
xiōng zhuī	胸椎	514	xuǎn fàn	选饭	520
xiū xī lì	休息痢	514	xuǎn xué fǎ	选穴法	520
xiù qiú fēng	绣球风	514	xuàn yùn	眩晕	520
xū bì	虚秘	514	xuàn yùn shí zhèng	眩晕实证	520
xū hán ǒu tù	虚寒呕吐	514	xuàn yùn xū zhèng	眩晕虚证	521
xū hán xiōng bì	虚寒胸痹	515	xuē jǐ	薛己	521
xū hán wèi tòng	虚寒胃痛	515	xuē lì zhāi	薛立斋	521
xū huǒ yá tòng	虚火牙痛	515	xué	穴	521
xū lǐ	虚里	515	xué dào	穴道	521
xū rè yān hóu zhǒng tòng	虚热咽喉肿痛	515	xué wèi	穴位	521
xū rè jīng xíng xiān qī	虚热经行先期	516	xué wèi chāo shēng cì jī fǎ	穴位超声刺激法	521
xū zé bǔ zhī	虚则补之	516	xué wèi cí liáo fǎ	穴位磁疗法	522
xú chūn fǔ	徐春甫	516	xué wèi fēng bì liáo fǎ	穴位封闭疗法	522
xú ér jí zé shí	徐而疾则实	516	xué wèi jī guāng liáo fǎ	穴位激光疗法	522
xú fèng	徐凤	517	xué wèi lěng fū fǎ	穴位冷敷法	523
xú jí bǔ xiè	徐疾补泻	517	xué wèi mái xiàn fǎ	穴位埋线法	523
xú tíng zhāng	徐廷璋	517	xué wèi xī yǐn qì	穴位吸引器	523
xú wén zhōng	徐文中	517	xué wèi zhào shè fǎ	穴位照射法	523
xú yuè	徐悦	517	xué wèi zhù shè fǎ	穴位注射法	523
xǔ xī	许希	517	xuè bì	血闭	524
xǔ yù qīng	许裕卿	517	xuè gǔ	血鼓	524
xù zhēn	絮针	518	xuè hǎi	血海	524
xù xuè chéng zhàng	蓄血成胀	518	xuè hán jīng chí	血寒经迟	524
xuán wù huì yào zhēn jīng	玄悟会要针经	518	xuè hán jīng xíng hòu qī	血寒经行后期	525
xuán wù sì shén zhēn fǎ	玄悟四神针法	518	xuè hán yuè jīng guò shǎo	血寒月经过少	525
xuán ěr chuāng	旋耳疮	518	xuè jué	血厥	525
xuán jī	旋机	518	xuè kuī jīng bì	血亏经闭	525
xuán jī	旋玑	518	xuè lìn	血淋	526
xuán jiāng	悬浆	518	xuè luò	血络	526

xuè mài	血脉	526		yā zhěn	压诊	532
xuè mén	血门	526		yā shǒu fǎ	押手法	533
xuè nà bāo luò	血纳包络	526		yá	牙	533
xuè rè bēng lòu	血热崩漏	527		yá tòng	牙痛	533
xuè rè jīng xíng xiān qī	血热经行先期	527		yǎ mén	哑门	533
xuè rè jīng zǎo	血热经早	527		yān hóu	咽喉	534
xuè rè yuè jīng guò duō	血热月经过多	527		yān hóu zhǒng tòng	咽喉肿痛	534
xuè shǎo bù yùn	血少不孕	528		yán yǔ èr qū	言语二区	534
xuè sī dīng	血丝疔	528		yán yǔ sān qū	言语三区	534
xuè xì	血郄	528		yán zhèn	严振	534
xuè xū bù yùn	血虚不孕	528		yán pí cì	沿皮刺	535
xuè xū chǎn hòu tóu tòng	血虚产后头痛	528		yán zǐ	研子	535
xuè xū fēng zào niú pí xuǎn	血虚风燥牛皮癣	528		yán xiāo	盐哮	535
xuè xū jīng xíng hòu qī	血虚经行后期	528		yán	颜	535
xuè xū shī zhěn	血虚湿疹	529		yǎn	眼	535
xuè xū tóu tòng	血虚头痛	529		yǎn jiǎn xià chuí	眼睑下垂	535
xuè xū xīn jì	血虚心悸	529		yǎn xì	眼系	535
xuè xū yuè jīng guò shǎo	血虚月经过少	530		yàn kǒu	燕口	535
xuè yū bēng lòu	血瘀崩漏	530		yáng bái	阳白	536
xuè yū bù yùn	血瘀不孕	530		yáng chí	阳池	536
xuè yū chǎn hòu tóu tòng	血瘀产后头痛	530		yáng cì	阳刺	536
xuè yū jīng xíng hòu qī	血瘀经行后期	530		yáng fǔ	阳辅	536
xuè yū tòng jīng	血瘀痛经	531		yáng gāng	阳刚	537
xuè yū yuè jīng guò shǎo	血瘀月经过少	531		yáng gāng	阳纲	537
xūn jiǔ	熏灸	531		yáng gǔ	阳谷	537
xūn qí fǎ	熏脐法	531		yáng guān	阳关	537
xún fǎ	循法	531		yáng huáng	阳黄	538
xún jǐ	循脊	532		yáng jiāo	阳交	538
xún jì	循际	532		yáng kū	阳窟	538
xún jīng kǎo xué biān	循经考穴编	532		yáng líng	阳陵	538
xún jīng gǎn chuán xiàn xiàng	循经感传现象	532		yáng líng quán	阳陵泉	538
xún yuán	循元	532		yáng luò	阳络	539
				yáng míng mài	阳明脉	539
				yáng qiāo	阳跷	539
				yáng qiāo bìng	阳跷病	539
				yáng qiāo mài	阳跷脉	539

Y

yā chā dú	丫叉毒	532		yáng shuǐ	阳水	539
yā zhǐ	丫指	532		yáng suì dìng jiǔ	阳燧锭灸	540
yā tòng diǎn	压痛点	532		yáng wéi bìng	阳维病	540

拼音	词条	页码	拼音	词条	页码
yáng wéi mài	阳维脉	540	yáo fǎ	摇法	547
yáng wéi xué	阳维穴	540	yào bǐng jiǔ	药饼灸	547
yáng wěi	阳萎	540	yào dìng jiǔ	药锭灸	547
yáng wěi shí zhèng	阳萎实证	541	yào niǎn jiǔ	药捻灸	547
yáng wěi xū zhèng	阳萎虚证	541	yào tǒng fǎ	药筒法	547
yáng xī	阳溪	541	yào wù ài juǎn	药物艾卷	548
yáng xū bēng lòu	阳虚崩漏	541	yào wù fā pào jiǔ	药物发泡灸	548
yáng xū è nì	阳虚呃逆	542	yào wù fā pào liáo fǎ	药物发泡疗法	548
yáng xū fù tòng	阳虚腹痛	542	yào xūn zhēng qì jiǔ	药熏蒸气灸	548
yáng zé	阳泽	542	yē gé	噎膈	548
yáng zhī líng quán	阳之陵泉	542	yē sè	噎塞	548
yáng zhōng yǐn yīn	阳中隐阴	542	yè chá shān	叶茶山	548
yáng cì	扬刺	542	yè guǎng zuò	叶广祚	549
yáng jì zhōu	杨继洲	543	yè guāng	夜光	549
yáng jiè	杨介	543	yè mén	液门	549
yáng jìng zhāi zhēn jiǔ quán shū	杨敬斋针灸全书	543	yè jiān	掖间	549
yáng shàng shàn	杨上善	543	yè mén	掖门	549
yáng xún	杨珣	543	yè	腋	549
yáng yán qí	杨颜齐	544	yè mén	腋门	549
yǎng kào zuò wèi	仰靠坐位	544	yè qì	腋气	550
yǎng wò wèi	仰卧位	544	yè xià xué	腋下穴	550
yǎng lǎo	养老	544	yè	䏲	550
yāo dǐ zhuī	腰骶椎	544	yī fū fǎ	一夫法	550
yāo hù	腰户	544	yī jìn sān tuì	一进三退	550
yāo jǐ tòng	腰脊痛	544	yī yáng	一阳	550
yāo mù	腰目	545	yī yuè jīng zài xíng	一月经再行	550
yāo mù jiào	腰目窌	545	yī gōng zhēn	医工针	550
yāo qí	腰奇	545	yī huǎn	医缓	550
yāo shū	腰俞	545	yī jīng xiǎo xué	医经小学	551
yāo tòng	腰痛	545	yī xué gāng mù	医学纲目	551
yāo tòng diǎn	腰痛点	546	yī xué rù mén	医学入门	551
yāo tòng xué	腰痛穴	546	yī zōng jīn jiàn	医宗金鉴	551
yāo yǎn	腰眼	546	yí dǎn	胰胆	551
yāo yáng guān	腰阳关	546	yí shū	胰俞	551
yāo yí	腰宜	547	yí dào	遗道	552
yāo zhù	腰注	547	yí jīng	遗精	552
yāo zhù	腰柱	547	yí xiè	遗泄	552
yáo bǐng fǎ	摇柄法	547	yí	颐	552
			yǐ tòng wéi shū	以痛为输	552

拼音	词条	页码	拼音	词条	页码
yì jīng qǔ xué	异经取穴	552	yīn tuō	阴脱	559
yì dú lì	疫毒痢	552	yīn wéi bìng	阴维病	559
yì ké	疫咳	553	yīn wéi mài	阴维脉	559
yì shè	意舍	553	yīn wéi xué	阴维穴	559
yì rǔ	嗌乳	553	yīn wěi	阴萎	559
yì xǐ	谚谞	553	yīn xì	阴郄	559
yì fēng	翳风	553	yīn xū bēng lòu	阴虚崩漏	560
yì míng	翳明	554	yīn xū è nì	阴虚呃逆	560
yīn bāo	阴包	554	yīn xū huǒ wàng bù mèi	阴虚火旺不寐	560
yīn bāo	阴胞	554	yīn xū huǒ wàng ké xuè	阴虚火旺咳血	560
yīn bù sāo yǎng	阴部瘙痒	554	yīn xū huǒ wàng niào xuè	阴虚火旺尿血	561
yīn cì	阴刺	554	yīn xū ké sòu	阴虚咳嗽	561
yīn dǐng	阴鼎	554	yīn xū luǒ lì	阴虚瘰疬	561
yīn dū	阴都	554	yīn xū ǒu tù	阴虚呕吐	561
yīn dú bā xué	阴独八穴	555	yīn xū rǔ pǐ	阴虚乳癖	561
yīn gǔ	阴谷	555	yīn xū wèi tòng	阴虚胃痛	562
yīn guān	阴关	555	yīn xū xié tòng	阴虚胁痛	562
yīn hú shàn	阴狐疝	555	yīn yáng pèi xué fǎ	阴阳配穴法	562
yīn huáng	阴黄	555	yīn yáng xué	阴阳穴	562
yīn jiāo	阴交	556	yīn yǎng	阴痒	562
yīn jié	阴结	556	yīn zhī líng quán	阴之陵泉	563
yīn jìng xué	阴茎穴	556	yīn zhōng yǐn yáng	阴中隐阳	563
yīn lián	阴廉	556	yīn jǔ	殷榘	563
yīn líng	阴陵	557	yīn mén	殷门	563
yīn líng quán	阴陵泉	557	yīn mén	瘖门	563
yīn luò	阴络	557	yín mén	寅门	564
yīn mén sāo yǎng	阴门瘙痒	557	yín zhēn	银针	564
yīn mén yǎng	阴门痒	557	yín jiāo	龂交	564
yīn náng fèng	阴囊缝	557	yín jiāo	龈交	564
yīn náng xià héng wén	阴囊下横纹	557	yǐn huǒ fǎ	引火法	564
yīn qiāo bìng	阴跷病	558	yǐn zhēn	引针	564
yīn qiāo mài	阴跷脉	558	yǐn xì	饮郄	565
yīn qiāo xué	阴跷穴	558	yǐn bái	隐白	565
yīn qié	阴茄	558	yǐn zhěn	瘾疹	565
yīn shì	阴市	558	yìn táng	印堂	565
yīn shuǐ	阴水	558	yīng tū	应突	565
yīn tǐng	阴挺	559	yīng mài	缨脉	566
yīn tǐng xià tuō	阴挺下脱	559	yīng	膺	566
yīn tù	阴突	559	yīng chuāng	膺窗	566

yīng shū	膺俞……566	yù hù	玉户……572
yīng zhōng	膺中……566	yù huán shū	玉环俞……573
yīng zhōng shū	膺中俞……566	yù lóng fù	玉龙赋……573
yíng ér duó zhī	迎而夺之……566	yù mén tóu	玉门头……573
yíng fēng lěng lèi	迎风冷泪……566	yù quán	玉泉……573
yíng fēng liú lèi	迎风流泪……567	yù táng	玉堂……573
yíng fēng rè lèi	迎风热泪……567	yù tián	玉田……573
yíng suí	迎随……567	yù yè	玉液……574
yíng suí bǔ xiè	迎随补泻……567	yù yīng	玉英……574
yíng xiāng	迎香……567	yù zhěn	玉枕……574
yíng shù zhì wài jīng	荥输治外经……567	yù zhěn gǔ	玉枕骨……574
yíng xué	荥穴……568	yù zhù	玉柱……574
yíng chí	营池……568	yù chén zé chú zhī	宛陈则除之……574
yǐng qì	瘿气……568	yù mào	郁冒……574
yōng jū shén mì jiǔ jīng	痈疽神秘灸经……568	yù zhèng	郁证……574
yōng jū shén miào jiǔ jīng	痈疽神妙灸经……568	yù zhōng	郁中……575
yǒng quán	勇泉……568	yù zhōng	彧中……575
yǒng quán	涌泉……568	yù zhōng	域中……575
yōu mén	幽门……569	yuān yè	渊液……575
yóu fēng	油风……569	yuān yè	渊腋……575
yóu niǎn jiǔ	油捻灸……569	yuán ér	元儿……576
yòu guān	右关……570	yuán jiàn	元见……576
yòu yù yè	右玉液……570	yuán zài	员在……576
yū xuè tóu tòng	瘀血头痛……570	yuán zhēn	员针……576
yū xuè wèi tòng	瘀血胃痛……570	yuán zhù	员柱……576
yū xuè xié tòng	瘀血胁痛……570	yuán lì zhēn	圆利针……576
yū xuè xīn jì	瘀血心悸……570	yuán zhēn	圆针……576
yū xuè xiōng bì	瘀血胸痹……571	yuán zhù	圆柱……576
yú fǎ kāi	于法开……571	yuán luò pèi xué fǎ	原络配穴法……576
yú	鱼……571	yuán xué	原穴……577
yú cháng	鱼肠……571	yuán zhōng	缘中……577
yú fù	鱼腹……571	yuǎn dào qǔ xué	远道取穴……577
yú jì	鱼际……571	yuǎn gé qǔ xué	远隔取穴……577
yú luò	鱼络……571	yuǎn jié duàn qǔ xué	远节段取穴……577
yú wěi	鱼尾……572	yuǎn jìn pèi xué fǎ	远近配穴法……578
yú yāo	鱼腰……572	yuǎn qǔ	远取……578
yú gǔ	髃骨……572	yuē wén	约纹……578
yù fáng shū	玉房俞……572	yuě	哕……578
yù guì zhēn jīng	玉匮针经……572	yuè bì	月闭……578

拼音	词条	页码	拼音	词条	页码
yuè bù tōng	月不通	578	zàng shū	藏输	583
yuè hòu bù tiáo	月候不调	578	zào rè ké sòu	燥热咳嗽	583
yuè hòu guò duō	月候过多	578	zhà sāi	炸腮	583
yuè jì	月忌	578	zhà sāi	痄腮	583
yuè jīng bù tiáo	月经不调	578	zhāng jiè bīn	张介宾	584
yuè jīng bù tōng	月经不通	579	zhāng quán	张权	584
yuè jīng bù xíng	月经不行	579	zhāng yuán sù	张元素	584
yuè jīng bù yún	月经不匀	579	zhāng zhì cōng	张志聪	584
yuè jīng guò duō	月经过多	579	zhāng zhòng jǐng	张仲景	584
yuè jīng guò shǎo	月经过少	579	zhāng dí	章迪	585
yuè jīng luò hòu	月经落后	579	zhāng mén	章门	585
yuè jīng sè shǎo	月经涩少	579	zhǎng zhōng	掌中	585
yuè jīng xiān qī	月经先期	579	zhàng	胀	585
yuè jīng zhì sè	月经滞涩	579	zhàng bìng	胀病	586
yuè shǐ bù tiáo	月使不调	579	zhàng nüè	瘴疟	586
yuè shǐ bù lái	月使不来	579	zhǎo fǎ	爪法	586
yuè shì bù lái	月事不来	579	zhǎo qiē	爪切	586
yuè shì bù tōng	月事不通	579	zhǎo qiē jìn zhēn	爪切进针	586
yuè shuǐ lái fù tòng	月水来腹痛	579	zhǎo qiē yā shǒu	爪切押手	586
yuè shuǐ bù lái	月水不来	579	zhǎo shè	爪摄	586
yuè shuǐ bù tiáo	月水不调	579	zhào hǎi	照海	586
yuè shuǐ bù tōng	月水不通	580	zhé zhēn	折针	587
yún mén	云门	580	zhé jīn	辄筋	587
yún qí zǐ	云岐子	580	zhēn	针	587
yùn dòng qū	运动区	580	zhēn ài	针艾	588
yùn qì fǎ	运气法	581	zhēn bǐng jiǔ	针柄灸	588
yùn yòng qū	运用区	581	zhēn bó shì	针博士	588
yùn zhēn	运针	581	zhēn cì bǔ xiè fǎ	针刺补泻法	588
yùn jiǔ	晕灸	581	zhēn cì gǎn yīng	针刺感应	588
yùn tīng qū	晕听区	581	zhēn cì jiǎo dù	针刺角度	588
yùn zhēn	晕针	581	zhēn cì má zuì	针刺麻醉	588
			zhēn cì shǒu fǎ	针刺手法	589

Z

拼音	词条	页码	拼音	词条	页码
zā fēng	匝风	582	zhēn fǎ	针法	589
zá bìng shí yī zhèng gē	杂病十一证歌	582	zhēn fāng	针方	589
zàn cì	赞刺	582	zhēn fāng liù jí	针方六集	589
zàng bìng qǔ yuán	脏病取原	582	zhēn gǎn	针感	590
zàng zào	脏燥	582	zhēn gōng	针工	590
zàng shū	藏俞	583	zhēn hé	针盒	590
			zhēn jiě fǎ	针解法	590

51

zhēn jīng	针经 …… 590	zhēn tóu bǔ xiè	针头补泻 …… 597
zhēn jīng jié yào	针经节要 …… 590	zhēn tuì	针退 …… 597
zhēn jīng zhāi yīng jí	针经摘英集 …… 591	zhēn xiàng bǔ xiè	针向补泻 …… 597
zhēn jīng zhǐ nán	针经指南 …… 591	zhēn yǎn	针眼 …… 597
zhēn jiǔ	针灸 …… 591	zhēn yáo	针摇 …… 597
zhēn jiǔ dà chéng	针灸大成 …… 591	zhēn cháng	真肠 …… 598
zhēn jiǔ dà quán	针灸大全 …… 591	zhēn quán	甄权 …… 598
zhēn jiǔ liáo fǎ	针灸疗法 …… 592	zhēn shí	箴石 …… 598
zhēn jiǔ gǎn yīng xiàn xiàng	针灸感应现象 …… 592	zhěn	枕 …… 598
zhēn jiǔ gē fù	针灸歌赋 …… 592	zhěn gǔ	枕骨 …… 598
zhēn jiǔ jī chéng	针灸集成 …… 592	zhèn ái	振埃 …… 598
zhēn jiǔ jiǎ yǐ jīng	针灸甲乙经 …… 592	zhèn chàn fǎ	震颤法 …… 598
zhēn jiǔ jīng xué tú kǎo	针灸经穴图考 …… 593	zhēng chōng	怔忡 …… 598
zhēn jiǔ jié yào	针灸节要 …… 593	zhēng qí fǎ	蒸脐法 …… 598
zhēn jiǔ jù yīng	针灸聚英 …… 593	zhēng qí zhì bìng fǎ	蒸脐治病法 …… 599
zhēn jiǔ jù yīng fā huī	针灸聚英发挥 …… 593	zhèng jīng	正经 …… 599
zhēn jiǔ quán shēng	针灸全生 …… 593	zhèng nüè	正疟 …… 600
zhēn jiǔ sì shū	针灸四书 …… 593	zhèng yíng	正营 …… 600
zhēn jiǔ sù nàn yào zhǐ	针灸素难要旨 …… 593	zhèng hé shèng jì zǒng lù	政和圣济总录 …… 600
zhēn jiǔ tǐ wèi	针灸体位 …… 594	zhī gōu	支沟 …… 600
zhēn jiǔ tú jīng	针灸图经 …… 594	zhī jié	支节 …… 600
zhēn jiǔ tú yào jué	针灸图要诀 …… 594	zhī zhèng	支正 …… 601
zhēn jiǔ wèn dá	针灸问答 …… 594	zhī rè gǎn dù cè dìng fǎ	知热感度测定法 …… 601
zhēn jiǔ wèn duì	针灸问对 …… 594	zhī zhū gǔ	蜘蛛鼓 …… 601
zhēn jiǔ xué	针灸学 …… 594	zhí cháng	直肠 …… 601
zhēn jiǔ yào zhǐ	针灸要旨 …… 595	zhí cháng xià duàn	直肠下段 …… 602
zhēn jiǔ yì xué	针灸易学 …… 595	zhí cì	直刺 …… 602
zhēn jiǔ zá shuō	针灸杂说 …… 595	zhí ěr	直耳 …… 602
zhēn jiǔ zé rì biān jí	针灸择日编集 …… 595	zhí gǔ	直骨 …… 602
zhēn jiǔ zhì liáo cì jī diǎn	针灸治疗刺激点 …… 595	zhí jiē jiǔ	直接灸 …… 602
		zhí lǔ gǔ	直鲁古 …… 602
zhēn jiǔ zī shēng jīng	针灸资生经 …… 595	zhí zhēn cì	直针刺 …… 602
zhēn jiǔ zuǎn yào	针灸纂要 …… 596	zhǐ	指 …… 603
zhēn má	针麻 …… 596	zhǐ bá	指拔 …… 603
zhēn má dìng liàng	针麻定量 …… 596	zhǐ bō fǎ	指拨法 …… 603
zhēn má yòu dǎo qī	针麻诱导期 …… 596	zhǐ chí	指持 …… 603
zhēn shī	针师 …… 596	zhǐ cuō	指搓 …… 603
zhēn shí	针石 …… 596	zhǐ cùn dìng wèi fǎ	指寸定位法 …… 603
		zhǐ dīng	指疔 …… 603

拼音	词条	页码
zhǐ gēn	指根	604
zhǐ liú	指留	604
zhǐ mí fù	指迷赋	604
zhǐ niǎn	指捻	604
zhǐ qiē jìn zhēn	指切进针	604
zhǐ xún	指循	604
zhǐ yā jìn zhēn fǎ	指压进针法	604
zhǐ zhēn	指针	604
zhǐ	趾	604
zhì gōng	至宫	605
zhì róng	至荣	605
zhì yáng	至阳	605
zhì yīn	至阴	605
zhì yíng	至营	605
zhì shì	志室	605
zhì chuǎn	治喘	606
zhì fǔ zhě zhì qí hé	治腑者治其合	606
zhì wěi dú qǔ yáng míng	治痿独取阳明	606
zhì zàng zhě zhì qí shù	治脏者治其俞	606
zhì biān	秩边	606
zhì chuāng	痔疮	606
zhì hé diǎn	痔核点	607
zhì chǎn	滞产	607
zhì xià	滞下	607
zhì zhēn	滞针	607
zhì zhēn	置针	608
zhōng bìng páng qǔ	中病旁取	608
zhōng chōng	中冲	608
zhōng cì jī	中刺激	608
zhōng dū	中都	608
zhōng dú	中渎	609
zhōng dú	中犊	609
zhōng fēng	中封	609
zhōng fǔ	中府	609
zhōng gào kǒng xué tú jīng	中诰孔穴图经	610
zhōng guǎn	中管	610
zhōng guó zhēn jiǔ xué	中国针灸学	610
zhōng guó zhēn jiǔ zhì liáo xué	中国针灸治疗学	610
zhōng huá zhēn jiǔ xué	中华针灸学	610
zhōng jí	中极	611
zhōng jiān jǐng	中肩井	611
zhōng jǔ	中矩	611
zhōng kōng	中空	611
zhōng kuí	中魁	611
zhōng liáo	中髎	612
zhōng lǚ	中膂	612
zhōng lǚ nèi shū	中膂内俞	612
zhōng lǚ shū	中䐃输	612
zhōng lǚ shū	中膂俞	612
zhōng píng	中平	612
zhōng qì fǎ	中气法	613
zhōng quán	中泉	613
zhōng shǒu	中守	613
zhōng shū	中枢	613
zhōng tíng	中庭	614
zhōng wǎn	中脘	614
zhōng wù	中恶	614
zhōng xì	中郄	614
zhōng xiāo	中消	615
zhōng zhǐ jié	中指节	615
zhōng zhǐ tóng shēn cùn	中指同身寸	615
zhōng zhǔ	中渚	615
zhōng zhù	中注	616
zhōng zhù	中柱	616
zhǒng	踵	616
zhòng fēng	中风	616
zhòng fēng bù yǔ xué	中风不语穴	616
zhòng fēng qī xué	中风七穴	616
zhòng jīng luò	中经络	617
zhòng shǔ	中暑	617
zhòng shǔ qīng zhèng	中暑轻证	617
zhòng shǔ zhòng zhèng	中暑重证	617
zhòng yè	中暍	618
zhòng zàng fǔ	中脏腑	618
zhòng zàng fǔ bì zhèng	中脏腑闭证	618
zhòng zàng fǔ tuō zhèng	中脏腑脱证	618

拼音	词条	页码
zhōu gǔ	周谷	618
zhōu hàn qīng	周汉卿	618
zhōu róng	周荣	618
zhōu yíng	周营	619
zhǒu	肘	619
zhǒu hòu bèi jí fāng	肘后备急方	619
zhǒu hòu gē	肘后歌	619
zhǒu jiān	肘尖	619
zhǒu liáo	肘聊	620
zhǒu liáo	肘髎	620
zhǒu shū	肘俞	620
zhǒu zhuī	肘椎	620
zhū dǐng	珠顶	620
zhū xíng lóng qǐ	珠形隆起	620
zhǔ kè	主客	621
zhǔ kè pèi xué fǎ	主客配穴法	621
zhǔ kè yuán luò pèi xué fǎ	主客原络配穴法	621
zhǔ bá tǒng	煮拔筒	621
zhǔ yào bá guàn fǎ	煮药拔罐法	621
zhǔ zhēn fǎ	煮针法	621
zhù shè shì jìn zhēn	注射式进针	621
zhù shì	注市	621
zhù xià	注夏	622
zhù gǔ	柱骨	622
zhù dìng	祝定	622
zhù bù	疰布	622
zhù bīn	筑宾	622
zhù bīn	筑滨	622
zhù zhēn	箸针	622
zhuǎn gǔ	转谷	623
zhuàn	腨	623
zhuàn cháng	腨肠	623
zhuāng shū	庄俞	623
zhuàng	壮	623
zhuī dǐng	椎顶	623
zhuō	颜	623
zhuó bì	着痹	623
zhuó fū jiǔ	着肤灸	624
zhuó ròu jiǔ	着肉灸	624
zī mài	资脉	624
zǐ bào	子豹	624
zǐ bìng	子病	624
zǐ gōng	子宫	624
zǐ gōng bù shōu	子宫不收	624
zǐ gōng tuō chū	子宫脱出	624
zǐ gōng tuō chuí	子宫脱垂	625
zǐ hù	子户	625
zǐ mào	子冒	625
zǐ mǔ bǔ xiè fǎ	子母补泻法	625
zǐ tòng	子痛	626
zǐ wǔ bā fǎ	子午八法	626
zǐ wǔ bǔ xiè	子午补泻	626
zǐ wǔ dǎo jiù	子午捣白	626
zǐ wǔ fǎ	子午法	626
zǐ wǔ jīng	子午经	626
zǐ wǔ liú zhù	子午流注	626
zǐ wǔ liú zhù zhēn fǎ	子午流注针法	626
zǐ wǔ liú zhù zhēn jīng	子午流注针经	627
zǐ wǔ liú zhù zhú rì àn shí dìng xué gē	子午流注逐日按时定穴歌	627
zǐ xián	子痫	627
zǐ zàng léng wú zǐ	子脏冷无子	628
zǐ gōng	紫宫	628
zì jiǔ	自灸	628
zōng jīn	宗筋	628
zōng mài	宗脉	628
zōng hé shǒu fǎ	综合手法	628
zǒu guàn fǎ	走罐法	628
zú dà zhǐ cóng máo	足大趾丛毛	628
zú dì èr zhǐ shàng	足第二指上	628
zú jiào	足窍	629
zú jù yáng mài	足巨(钜)阳脉	629
zú juǎn yīn mài	足卷阴脉	629
zú jué yīn biāo běn	足厥阴标本	629
zú jué yīn gān jīng	足厥阴肝经	629
zú jué yīn gān jīng bìng	足厥阴肝经病	630
zú jué yīn jīng bié	足厥阴经别	630

zú jué yīn jīng jīn	足厥阴经筋 …… 630		bìng	…………… 639
zú jué yīn jīng jīn bìng	足厥阴经筋病 …… 630		zú shào yīn zhī bié	足少阴之别 …… 639
zú jué yīn luò mài	足厥阴络脉 …… 630		zú shào yīn zhī zhèng	足少阴之正 …… 639
zú jué yīn luò mài bìng	足厥阴络脉病 …… 631		zú tài yáng biāo běn	足太阳标本 …… 639
zú jué yīn mài	足厥阴脉 …… 631		zú tài yáng jīng bié	足太阳经别 …… 639
zú jué yīn zhī bié	足厥阴之别 …… 631		zú tài yáng jīng jīn	足太阳经筋 …… 640
zú jué yīn zhī zhèng	足厥阴之正 …… 631		zú tài yáng jīng jīn bìng	足太阳经筋病 …… 640
zú lín qì	足临泣 …… 631		zú tài yáng luò mài	足太阳络脉 …… 640
zú qiào yīn	足窍阴 …… 631		zú tài yáng luò mài bìng	足太阳络脉病 …… 640
zú sān lǐ	足三里 …… 632		zú tài yáng páng guāng jīng	足太阳膀胱经 …… 640
zú sān yáng jīng	足三阳经 …… 632			
zú sān yīn jīng	足三阴经 …… 632		zú tài yáng páng guāng jīng bìng	足太阳膀胱经病 …… 641
zú shàng lián	足上廉 …… 632			
zú shào yáng biāo běn	足少阳标本 …… 632		zú tài yáng xué	足太阳穴 …… 641
zú shào yáng dǎn jīng	足少阳胆经 …… 633		zú tài yáng zhī bié	足太阳之别 …… 641
zú shào yáng dǎn jīng bìng	足少阳胆经病 …… 635		zú tài yáng zhī zhèng	足太阳之正 …… 642
			zú tài yáng zú shào yīn jīng bié	足太阳、足少阴经别 …… 642
zú shào yáng jīng bié	足少阳经别 …… 635			
zú shào yáng jīng jīn	足少阳经筋 …… 635		zú tài yīn biāo běn	足太阴标本 …… 642
zú shào yáng jīng jīn bìng	足少阳经筋病 …… 636		zú tài yīn jīng bié	足太阴经别 …… 642
			zú tài yīn jīng jīn	足太阴经筋 …… 642
zú shào yáng luò mài	足少阳络脉 …… 636		zú tài yīn jīng jīn bìng	足太阴经筋病 …… 642
zú shào yáng luò mài bìng	足少阳络脉病 …… 636		zú tài yīn luò	足太阴络 …… 642
			zú tài yīn luò mài	足太阴络脉 …… 643
zú shào yáng mài	足少阳脉 …… 636		zú tài yīn luò mài bìng	足太阴络脉病 …… 643
zú shào yáng xué	足少阳穴 …… 636		zú tài yīn mài	足泰阴脉 …… 643
zú shào yáng zhī bié	足少阳之别 …… 637		zú tài yīn pí jīng	足太阴脾经 …… 643
zú shào yáng zhī zhèng	足少阳之正 …… 637		zú tài yīn pí jīng bìng	足太阴脾经病 …… 644
zú shào yáng zú jué yīn jīng bié	足少阳、足厥阴经别 …… 637		zú tài yīn zhī bié	足太阴之别 …… 644
			zú tài yīn zhī zhèng	足太阴之正 …… 644
zú shào yīn biāo běn	足少阴标本 …… 637		zú tài yáng mài	足泰阳脉 …… 644
zú shào yīn jīng bié	足少阴经别 …… 637		zú tōng gǔ	足通谷 …… 644
zú shào yīn jīng jīn	足少阴经筋 …… 637		zú wǔ lǐ	足五里 …… 644
zú shào yīn jīng jīn bìng	足少阴经筋病 …… 638		zú xià lián	足下廉 …… 645
zú shào yīn luò mài	足少阴络脉 …… 638		zú xīn	足心 …… 645
zú shào yīn luò mài bìng	足少阴络脉病 …… 638		zú yáng guān	足阳关 …… 645
zú shào yīn mài	足少阴脉 …… 638		zú yáng míng biāo běn	足阳明标本 …… 645
zú shào yīn shèn jīng	足少阴肾经 …… 638		zú yáng míng jīng bié	足阳明经别 …… 645
zú shào yīn shèn jīng	足少阴肾经病		zú yáng míng jīng jīn	足阳明经筋 …… 645

zú yáng míng jīng jīn bìng	足阳明经筋病 …… 646	zú yáng míng、zú tài yīn jīng bié	足阳明、足太阴经别 …… 648
zú yáng míng luò mài	足阳明络脉 …… 646	zú yùn gǎn qū	足运感区 …… 648
zú yáng míng luò mài bìng	足阳明络脉病 …… 646	zǔ bìng	阻病 …… 648
zú yáng míng mài	足阳明脉 …… 647	zǔ xué	组穴 …… 648
zú yáng míng wèi jīng	足阳明胃经 …… 647	zuǎn	纂 …… 648
zú yáng míng wèi jīng bìng	足阳明胃经病 …… 648	zuǒ yòu pèi xué fǎ	左右配穴法 …… 648
zú yáng míng zhī bié	足阳明之别 …… 648	zuǒ yòu zhuàn	左右转 …… 649
zú yáng míng zhī zhèng	足阳明之正 …… 648	zuò gǔ shén jīng	坐骨神经 …… 649
		zuò wèi	坐位 …… 649

A

●阿是穴[ā shì xué]　①腧穴分类名。见"腧穴"条。②指按压痛点取穴。见《千金方》。又名压痛点、天应穴、不定穴等。这一类腧穴既无具体名称，又无固定位置，而是以压痛点或其它反应点作为针灸部位。

Ashi Point　①A category of acupoints. →腧穴(p.407)②Referring to point selection in accordance with tenderness, seen in *Qianjin Fang* (*Prescriptions Worth a Thousand Gold*), also named pressing point, touch point, non-fixed point, etc. Points of this kind have neither specific term nor fixed location, but are selected as acupoints according to tenderness or pain at the site of sensitivity.

●艾斗[ài dǒu]　灸具名。结构分上下两部：上部用金属丝绕成弹簧斗；下部用人造革或石棉衬垫制成。垫旁各一条丝带固定艾斗，将艾装于斗中点燃后供温灸用。

Moxibustion Dipper　A moxibustion apparatus, composed of two parts. The upper part is a spring dipper wound up with metal wire, and the lower part is a leatherette or asbestos pad. On either side of the pad, there is a silk ribbon for fixing the dipper. The moxa wool is placed inside the dipper and lit for moxibustion.

●艾灸[ài jiǔ]　灸法的一种。即以艾绒为主要施灸材料，直接或间接地放置在穴位上施灸。艾绒中还可掺入少量的香燥类药末，以加强作用。因其制成的形状及运用方法的不同，又可分艾炷灸、艾条灸、灸器灸等。详见各条。

Moxa Wool Moxibustion　A moxibustion method which uses moxa wool as the main material, the moxa wool is put directly or indirectly on or over the points for moxibustion. Sometimes, fragrant herbal powder may be mixed with the moxa wool to enhance the effect. Becaus of the diversified shapes and applications of moxa wool, moxa wool moxibustion can be divided into moxa cone moxibustion, moxa stick moxibustion and moxibustion with a moxibustion apparatus. →艾炷灸(p.3)、艾条灸(p.2)、灸器灸(p.224)

●艾灸补泻[ài jiǔ bǔ xiè]　出《灵枢·背输》。艾灸时，以其火力的大小区分补泻。施行补法时，不要吹旺艾火，让它徐燃自灭。灸毕后，用手轻轻地揉按，使真气聚而不散，达到补其正气的目的。施行泻法时，宜吹旺艾火，使其快燃快灭，火力较旺。灸毕，不以手揉按，使邪气得以宣散。

Reinforcing and Reducing of Moxibustion　Originally from *Lingshu*:*Beishu* (*Miraculous Pivot*:*Back-Shu Points*). In moxibustion, the reinforcing and reducing methods are differentiated according to different fires. When performing the reinforcing method, do not blow on the fire, let it burn slowly and go out by itself. After moxibustion, give gentle massage with the hand to make the genuine-qi gather and not disperse for the purpose of strengthening the body resistance qi. When performing the reducing method, blow on the fire and let it burn and go out quickly. After moxibustion, do not give massage so as to dispel the evil qi.

●艾灸通说[ài jiǔ tōng shuō]　书名。日本后滕省(仲介)著，内容专论灸法。分制法精粗、艾炷大小、灸数多少、灸法异同、脊骨长短、点位狭阔、灸疮要发、艾火非燥、不选时日、火无良毒等篇。于公元1762年(日宝历壬午年)刊行。

Aijiu Tongshuo (*A General Exposition of Moxibustion*)　A book written by a Japanese, Sho Goto(Chukai), dealing specially with moxibustion therapy. Contents：Refined and coarse preparation of moxa wool, size of moxa cones, the number of cones used in each treatment, similarities and differences of moxibustion methods, length of the spinal column, broadness of the points, formation of the moxibustion sores, strength of moxa fire, no selections of time, moxa fire without poisons, etc.

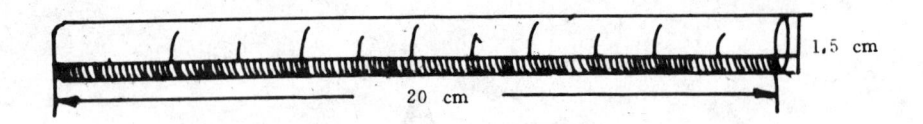

图1 艾条

Fig 1　Moxa stick

The book was published in 1762 (the year of Renwu, Japanese Baoli period).

●艾卷[ài juǎn] 灸具名。为艾条之别称。见该条。

Moxa Roll　A moxibustion appliance, another name for moxa stick. →艾条(p.2)

●艾卷灸[ài juǎn jiǔ] 灸法的一种。为艾条灸之别称。见该条。

Moxa Roll Moxibustion　One of the moxibustion methods, another name for moxa stick moxibustion. →艾条灸(p.2)

●艾茸[ài róng] 施灸材料。出《外科正宗》卷二。即艾绒。见该条。

Moxa Down　A moxibustion material. The term is from Vol. 2 of *Waike Zhengzong* (*Orthodox Manual of External Diseases*). →艾绒(p.2)

●艾绒[ài róng] 施灸材料。又称艾茸。灸法所用的主要材料,由艾叶加工制成。于夏季艾叶茂盛时割取,晒干捣碎,除去枝梗、杂质,即成细软的绒状物。根据加工程度不同而有粗细之分。细艾绒杂质少,纤维短,可塑性强,多用于直接灸,粗艾绒杂质稍多,纤维长,多用于间接灸。

Moxa Wool　A moxibustion material, also named moxa down. The main material for moxibustion which is processed from moxa leaves. Collect the leaves in summer while the plant is exuberant, dry and grind them, remove the stalks and impurities, making a fine, soft wool-like substance. According to the extent prepared, there is refined wool and coarse wool. The refined moxa wool, with less impurities, shorter fibres, and a good plasticity is mostly used in direct moxibustion, while the coarse moxa wool, with more impurities and longer fibres, is mainly used in indirect moxibustion.

●艾师[ài shī] 出《铁崖先生古乐府》。指专门施行灸法的医师。

Moxibustion Doctor　A term originally from *Tieya Xiansheng Guyue Fu* (*Mr. Tieya's Ancient Folk-Songs*), referring to doctors who specialized in moxibustion therapy.

●艾条[ài tiáo] 灸具名。又称艾卷。用艾绒制成的条状物,一般分纯艾卷和药艾卷两种。后者是在艾绒中掺入一定的药物制成。制作时,取纯净的艾绒20克(如制药艾条,则加入药末6～8克,与艾绒拌匀),平铺在长28厘米、宽15厘米的棉纸上,折叠棉纸两端,然后将其卷紧,并用白芨液或鸡蛋清封口,晒干收藏备用。参见"艾灸"条。

Moxa Stick　A moxibustion appliance, also called moxa roll, a stick made of moxa wool, divided into pure moxa stick and herbal moxa stick. The latter is made of moxa wool mixed with certain herbs. Preparation of the stick: Put 20g of pure moxa wool (for the making of herbal moxa stick, mix 6～8g of herbal powder into the wool) evenly spread out a piece of cotton paper 28 cm in length and 15 cm in width. Fold the two edges of the paper and then roll up tightly. Seal up with the fluid of Bai Ji or with egg white. Dry and store for use. →艾灸(p.1)

●艾条灸[ài tiáo jiǔ] 艾灸法的一种。是用特制的艾条在穴位上熏灸或灼烫的方法,有悬起灸和实按灸二种。悬起灸,一般每处灸3～5分钟,以皮肤温热而起红晕为度。根据施术方法的不同,又分为温和灸、雀啄灸、回旋灸等;实按灸,主要是指太乙神针、雷火神针的应用。详见各条。

Moxa Stick Moxibustion　A moxibustion method with a specially-made moxa stick to smoke and cauterize the point. There is suspended moxibustion and push-down moxibus-

tion. Suspended moxibustion does not stop until, after 3～5 minutes, the skin becomes red and the patient feels warm. According to the manipulations, it is further divided into mild moxibustion, sparrow-pecking moxibustion, revolving moxibustion, etc. Push-down moxibustion mainly refers to the applications of great monad herbal moxa stick and thunder-fire herbal moxa stick. →**悬起灸**(p. 519)、**实按灸**(p. 386)、**温和灸**(p. 469)、**回旋灸**(p. 177)、**太乙神针**(p. 421)、**雷火神针**(p. 239)

●**艾丸**[ài wán] 施灸材料。又称艾圆。将艾绒团聚成丸,作灸用,施灸方法与艾炷同。每个艾丸,亦称一壮。参见"艾炷"、"艾炷灸"条。

Moxa Ball A moxibustion material, also called moxa sphere. Roll the moxa wool into a ball for moxibustion, its manipulation is similar to that of moxa cones. Each moxa ball is also called one "zhuang". →**艾炷**(p. 3)、**艾炷灸**(p. 3)

●**艾圆**[ài yuán] 施灸材料。出《普济方》卷四百二十三。为艾丸之别称。详见该条。

Moxa Sphere Another name for a moxa ball, a moxibustion material, originally from Vol. 423 of *Puji Fang*(*Prescriptions for Universal Relief*). →**艾丸**(p. 3)

●**艾炷**[ài zhù] 施灸材料。用艾绒制做成的上尖下平的圆锥形小体。可依灸治的需要,分为大艾炷、中艾炷、小艾炷三种。

Moxa Cone A moxibustion material, tapered with the tip of the cone at the top and the flat at the bottom made of moxa wool. According to the needs of moxibustion, moxa cones vary in size—large, medium and small.

●**艾炷灸**[ài zhù jiǔ] 灸法的一种。将艾炷直接或间接地置于穴位上施灸的方法。可分为直接灸、间接灸二种。详见各条。

Moxa Cone Moxibustion A moxibustion method of putting a moxa cone directly or indirectly on the point, divided further into direct moxibustion and indirect moxibustion. →**直接灸**(p. 602)、**间接灸**(p. 192)

●**安邪**[ān xié] 经穴别名。出《针灸甲乙经》。即仆参。详见该条。

Anxie Another name for Pucan(BL 61), a meridian point originally from *Zhenjiu Jiayi Jing*(*A-B Classic of Acupuncture and Moxibustion*). →**仆参**(p. 299)

●**按法**[àn fǎ] 针刺手法名。十四法之一。①指针刺前用手指按压穴位。②指针刺时将针向下按入。又称插法。

Pressing One of the 14 methods referring to ① pressing the point with fingers before acupuncture, or ② pushing the needle downward during acupuncture, also called thrusting.

●**按肌群取穴**[àn jī qún qǔ xué] 取穴法之一。在病

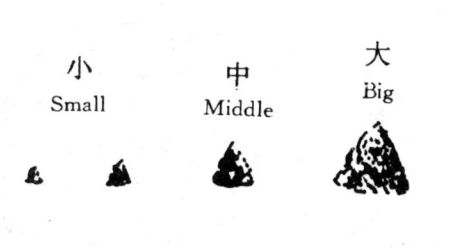

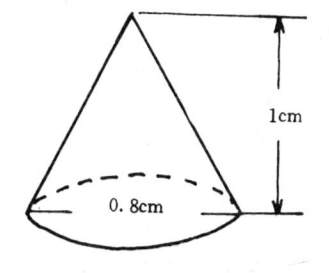

图2 艾 炷

Fig 2 Moxa cones

变所在的肌肉或肌群处选取穴位。常用于肌肉瘫痪、萎缩等症。如股直肌麻痹取伏兔,胫前肌麻痹取足三里等。

Selection of Points According to Muscle Groups   A method of point-selection. Select the point on the muscle or muscle group where the disease lies. It is often used for myoparalysis and muscular atrophy, etc., e. g. Futu (ST 32) for paralysis of musculus rectus femoris, and Zusanli (ST 36) for paralysis of musculus tibialis anterior, etc.

●按神经取穴[àn shén jīng qǔ xué]   取穴法之一。指按照神经的分布选取有关的穴位,多数选用与脊神经相应的夹脊穴和某些分布在神经丛或神经干通路上的穴位。如手指麻木,取正中神经上的内关、桡神经上的曲池。小腿疼痛,取腓神经上的阳陵泉、胫神经上的委中。

Selection of Points According to the Distribution of Nerves   A method of point-selection referring to selecting points according to the distribution of nerves. In most of the cases Jiaji (EX — B2) points related to the spinal nerves, and the points distributed on the neuro-plexus or nerve-trunk are selected, e. g., select Neiguan (PC 6) at the nervus medianus and Quchi (LI 11) at the nervus radialis to treat numbness of fingers; select Yanglingquan (GB 34) at the nervus peroneus and Weizhong (BL 40) at the tibial nerve to treat leg pain, etc.

●按诊[àn zhěn]   诊法之一。又称触诊。用手对病人体表进行触摸按压,以获得诊断印象的一种诊察方法。包括按肌表、按手足、按胸腹、按颈部、按经脉、按腧穴等。参见"压诊"条。

Pressing for Diagnosis   One of the diagnostic methods, also called palpation. A way of getting a diagnostic impression of the disease by palpating the body surface of the patient with the hand. It includes palpation of the muscle and skin, hands and feet, chest and abdomen, neck, meridians, acupoints, etc. →压诊(p. 532)

B

●八冲[bā chōng]   经外穴别名。出《千金要方》。即八风。详见该条。

Bachong   Another name for Bafeng (EX-LE 10), a set of eight extra points, originally from *Qianjin Yaofang* (*Essential Prescriptions Worth a Thousand Gold*). →八风(p. 4)

●八法[bā fǎ]   ①配穴法。出《针灸大全》。指八脉交会八穴的用法,主要指灵龟八法及飞腾八法。详见该条。②针刺手法。为下手八法的别称。详见该条。

Eight Methods   ① Methods for point prescription originally from *Zhenjiu Daquan* (*A Complete Work of Acupuncture and Moxibustion*), referring to the applications of the eight confluent points, mainly the application of Eight Methods of Intelligent Turtle and Eight Methods of Soaring. →灵龟八法(p. 243)、飞腾八法(p. 105) ② Needling techniques, another name for the eight methods for needling manipulations. →下手八法(p. 490)

●八风[bā fēng]   ①经外穴名。出《奇效良方》。又名八冲、阴独八穴。〈定位〉在足背侧第一至五趾间,趾蹼缘后方赤白肉际处,一足四穴,左右共八穴(图3)。〈层次解剖〉踇趾与第二趾之间的八风穴,层次解剖同行间穴(足厥阴肝经)。第二趾与第三趾之间者,层次解剖同内庭穴(足阳明胃经)。第四趾与小趾之间者,层次解剖同侠溪穴(足少阳胆经)。第三趾与第四趾之间的八风穴的层次解剖是:皮肤→皮下组织→第三与第四趾的趾长、短伸肌腱之间→第三、四跖骨头之间。浅层布有足背中间皮神经的趾背神经和足背浅静脉网。深层有跖背动脉的分支趾背动脉,跖背静脉的属支趾背静脉。〈主治〉头痛、牙痛、毒蛇咬伤、脚背红肿、足趾麻木等。向上斜刺0.5~1寸。或点刺出血。②出《灵枢·九宫八风》。指八方的来风。

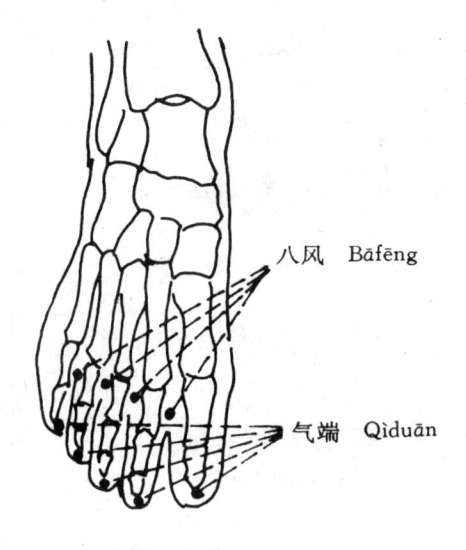

风。

图3 八风、气端穴
Fig 3 Bafeng and Qiduan points

1. **Bafeng**(EX-LE 10) A set of extra points, originally from *Qixiao Liangfang* (*Prescriptions of Wonderful Efficacy*), also named Bachong, Yindubaxue. 〈Location〉eight points on the instep of both feet, at the junction of the red and white skin proximal to the margin of the webs between each two neighboring toes. (Fig. 3.) 〈Regional anatomy〉 The layer anatomy of Bafeng(EX-LE 10) between the great and 2nd toes is the same as that in Xingjian(LR 2). The layer anatomy of Bafeng(EX-LE 10) between the 2nd and 3rd toes is the same as that in Neiting(ST 44). The layer anatomy of Bafeng(EX-LE 10) between the 4th and little toes is the same as that in Xiaxi(GB 43). The layer anatomy of Bafeng(EX-LE 10) between the 3rd and 4th toes is: skin → subcutaneous tissue → between tendons of long and short extensor muscles of 3rd and 4th toes → between heads of 3rd and 4th metatarsal bones. In the superficial layer, there are the dorsal digital nerve of the intermediate dorsal cutaneous nerve of the foot and the superficial venous network of the foot. In the deep layer, there are the dorsal digital artery from the dorsal metatarsal artery, and the dorsal digital vein to the dorsal metatarsal vein. 〈Indications〉 headache, toothache, snakebite, redness and swelling at the dorsum of foot, numbness of toes, etc. 〈Method〉Puncture 1 cun obliquely upwards or prick to cause bleeding.

2. **Eight Winds** Oringnally from *Lingshu*: *Jiu Gong Ba Feng* (*Miraculous Pivot*: *Nine Palaces and Eight Winds*), referring to the winds from the eight directions.

●八关[bā guān] 经外穴别名。即八邪。详见该条。

Baguan Another name for the extra point Baxie(EX-UE 9). →八邪(p. 8)

●八关大刺[bā guān dà cì] 针刺方法。出《素问病机气宜保命集》卷下。指针刺八邪出血的方法。用于治疗烦热甚者，或用于目疾睛痛欲出者。

Big Puncture at Baguan A needling technique originally from *Suwen*: *Bingji Qiyi Baoming Ji* (*Plain Questions*: *Collection of Pathology, Five Motions, Six Climatic changes and Health Preserving*), referring to the method of bleeding Baxie(EX-UE 9) by puncturing it, used for treating severe dysphoria with a smothering sensation or eye pain with a prolapsing feeling.

●八华[bā huá] 经外穴名。见《经外奇穴治疗诀》。位于背部，以两乳头间距离的1/4为边长，作一等边三角形，一角顶置大椎穴上，底边呈水平，下端两角是穴。再以此三角形之一角顶置于上两角之中点，其下端两角亦是穴。如此再量两次，共得八穴，称八华。上六穴称六华。灸治虚弱羸瘦、骨节疼痛、盗汗咳嗽等。

Bahua(EX-B) A set of extra points, seen in *Jingwai Qixue Zhiliao Jue* (*Pithy Formulas for Treatment with Extra Points*). 〈Location〉 on the back, take 1/4 of the distance between the two nipples as the side of an equilateral triangle, place the vertex angle on Dazhui(DU 14) point, and the base is horizontal. Two points are at the tips of the two basal angles. Move the triangle down and place the vertex angle on the midpoint between the above two points, another two points are at the basal angles of this triangle. Move the triangle downward another two times, and you will get four

表1 八 会 穴

Table 1 The Eight Influential Points

八会 Organs or Tissues	穴名 Influential Point	经属 Specialties of the Points
脏会 Zang organs	章门 Zhangmen(LR 13)	肝经穴 the Point of the Liver Meridian
腑会 Fu organs	中脘 Zhongwan(RN 12)	任脉穴 the Point of the Ren Meridian
气会 Qi	膻中 Danzhong(RN 17)	任脉穴 the Point of the Ren Meridian
血会 Blood	膈俞 Geshu(BL 17)	膀胱经穴 the Point of the Bladder Meridian
筋会 Tendons	阳陵泉 Yanglingquan (GB 34)	胆经合穴 the He(sea)Point of the Gallbladder Meridian
脉会 Vessels	太渊 Taiyuan(LU 9)	肺经输穴 the Shu(stream) Point of the Lung Meridian
骨会 Bones	大杼 Dazhu(BL 11)	膀胱经穴 the Point of the Bladder Meridian
髓会 Marrow	绝骨(悬钟) Juegu(Xuanzhong)(GB 39)	胆经穴 the Point of the Gallbladder Meridian

more points. All eight points are called Bahua, the upper six are called Liuhua (Ex-B). 〈Indications〉 general weakness, emaciation, painful joints, night sweating, cough, etc. 〈Method〉moxibustion.

●**八会**[bā huì] 即八会穴,见该条③。

Bahui →**八会穴**3. (p. 6)

●**八会穴**[bā huì xué] ①经穴分类名。指脏、腑、气、血、筋、脉、骨、髓等精气所会聚的腧穴。八会穴与其所属的八种脏器组织的生理功能有密切关系。故在治疗方面,凡与此八者相关的病证均可选用相关的八会穴来治疗。见表1。②指八脉交会穴。详见该条。③经外穴名。见《千金要方》。位于阳溪穴下0.5寸。灸治癫狂,白内障,近视,高血压,中风,卵巢疾患等。

1. **Eight Influential Points** Name of a point category, referring to the eight points at which the essence qi of zang-organs, fu-organs, qi, blood, tendons, vessels, bones and marrow respectively gathers. These 8 points have close relations with the physiological functions of the above eight organs or tissues, therefore, the diseases concerning the above organs or tissues could be treated by the relevant ones of the eight points. See Table 1.

2. **Eight Confluence Points** →**八脉交会穴** (p. 7)

3. **Bahuixue(EX-UE)** An extra point, originally from *Qianjin Yaofang* (*Essential Prescriptions Worth a Thousand Gold*). 〈Location〉 0.5 cun below Yangxi(LI 5). 〈Indications〉 manic-depressive psychosis, cataract, myopia, hypertension, windstroke, ovarian diseases, etc. 〈Method〉moxibustion.

●**八脉**[bā mài] 经脉名。出《难经·二十七难》。奇经八脉之简称。详见该条。

Eight Merdians Originally from *Nanjing: Ershiqi Nan* (*The Classic of Questions: Question 27*). Short for the Eight Extra Meridians. →**奇经八脉**(p. 301)

●**八脉八穴**[bā mài bā xué] 八脉交会穴的别名。详见该条。

Eight Points of the Eight Extra Meridians Another name for the Eight Confluence Points. →**八脉交会穴**(p. 7)

●**八脉八穴配穴法**[bā mài bā xué pài xué fǎ] 即八脉交会穴的配穴法。详见八脉交会穴。

The Combination of Eight Confluence

Points. →八脉交会穴(p. 7)

●八脉交会穴歌 [bā mài jiāo huì bā xué gē] 针灸歌赋名。出《医经小学》。内容概括八脉八穴的配伍关系。歌曰：公孙冲脉胃心胸，内关阴维下总同。临泣胆经连带脉，阳维目锐外关逢。后溪督脉内眦颈，申脉阳跷络亦通。列缺任脉行肺系，阴跷照海膈喉咙。参见"八脉交会穴"条。

Ba Mai Jiaohui Baxue Ge（Verses on the Eight Confluence Points） A title of the verses on acupuncture and moxibustion, originally from *Yijing Xiaoxue* (*Collection of Elementary Medical Classics*). The verses summarized the cooperative relationships among the eight confluence points. The verses read: Gongsun (SP 4) connects with Chong Meridian for treating diseases of the stomach, the heart and the chest. and Neiguan (PC 6) meets the Yinwei Meridian and has the same effects as Gongsun (SP 4). Zulinqi (GB 41), a point of the Gallbladder Meridian, is related to Dai Meridian for treating the disease of Dai Meridian, while Waiguan (SJ 5) meets Yangwei Meridian for treating the outer canthus disease. Houxi (SI 3) joins the Du Meridian to treat the inner canthus and neck disease. and Shenmai (BL 62) connects with Yangqiao Meridian to obtain the same effects as Houxi (SI 3). Lieque (LU 7), with the Ren Meridian, regulates the lung system, Zhaohai (KI 6) connects with Yinqiao Meridian to treat diaphragm and throat diseases. →八脉交会穴(p. 7)

●八脉交会穴 [bā mài jiāo huì xué] 经穴分类名。原名八脉交会八穴，出《针经指南》。又名流注八穴，交经八穴、八脉八穴、窦氏八穴。指奇经八脉与十二经脉气相通的八个腧穴。八穴即公孙、内关、后溪、申脉、足临泣、外关、列缺、照海。这些穴能主治头身各部的多种病症，其作用是从本经通向奇经八脉。见表2。

Eight Confluence points A Category of points, of which the original name was the eight confluence points of the eight extra meridians, from *Zhenjing Zhinan* (*Guide to the Classics of Acupuncture*), also called eight ebb-flow points, eight points of crossed meridians, eight points of the eight meridians or Dou's eight points. Referring to the points at which the qi of the eight extra meridians and the qi of the 12 regular meridians are connected, including Gongsun (SP 4), Neiguan (PC 6), Houxi (SI 3), Shenmai (BL 62), Zulinqi

表2　　　　　　　　八脉交会穴表
Table 2　　　　　　　The Eight Confluence Points

经属 Meridian the Point Pertains to	八穴 8 Confluence Points	通八脉 Extra Meridian	会合部位 Connected Parts
足太阴 Foot-Taiyin	公孙 Gongsun (SP 4)	冲脉 Chong Meridian	胃 stomach 心 heart 胸 chest
手厥阴 Hand-Jueyin	内关 Neiguan (PC 6)	阴维 Yinwei Meridian	
手少阳 Hand—Shaoyany	外关 Waiguan (SJ 5)	阳维 Yangwei Meridian	目外眦 outer canthus 颊、颈 cheek, neck, 耳后 anricular back 肩 gion, shoulder
足少阳 Foot—Shaoyany	足临泣 Zulinqi (GB 41)	带脉 Dai Meridian	
手太阳 Hand-Taiyang	后溪 Houxi (SI 3)	督脉 Du Meridian	目内眦 inner canthus 项、耳 nape, ear 肩胛 scapula
足太阳 Foot-Taiyang	申脉 Shenmai (BL 62)	阳跷 Yangqiao Meridian	
手太阴 Hand-Taiyin	列缺 Lieque (LU 7)	任脉 Ren Meridian	胸、肺 chest, lung, 膈 diaphragm, 喉咙 throat
足少阴 Foot-Shaoyin	照海 Zhaohai (KI 6)	阴跷 Yingiao Meridian	

(GB 41) Waiguan (SJ 5), Lieque (LU 7), Zhaohai (KI 6). These points whose effects may lead to their connected extra meridians from their own meridians, can be used for treating various diseases of the head and body. See Table 2.

●八木火[bā mù huǒ] 施灸材料。指松、柏、竹、橘、榆、枳、桑、枣八种木材燃烧的火。《黄帝虾蟆经》辨灸火木法、《小品方》、《外台秘要》、《医宗金鉴》和《刺灸心法要诀》等书均论及八木火，意为用八木之火施灸，易伤血脉、肌肉、骨髓，故当忌用。

Eight-Wood Fires Moxibustion materials, referring to the fires of burning pine, cypress, bamboo, tangerine, elm, trifoliate orange, mulberry, and jujube. Discrimination of the Wood for Moxibustion in *Huangdi Hama Jing* (*The Yellow Emperor's Frog Classic*), *Xiaopin Fang* (*Prescriptions in Brief*), *Waitai Miyao* (*Clandestine Essentials from the Imperial Library*) and *Experiential Knacks on Needling Techniques*, in *Yizong Jinjian* (*Gold Mirror of Orthodox Medical Lineage*), all discussed the eight-wood fires. Since moxibustion by the eight-wood fires may damage blood vessels, muscles and marrow, their use should be avoided.

●八邪[bā xié] 经外穴名。出《医经小学》。又名八关。〈定位〉在手背侧，微握拳，第1～5指间，指蹼缘后方赤白肉际处，左右共八穴（图76）。〈层次解剖〉皮肤→皮下组织→骨间背侧肌→骨间掌侧肌→蚓状肌。浅层布有掌背动、静脉或指动、静脉和指背神经。深层有指掌侧总动、静脉或指掌侧固有动、静脉和指掌侧固有神经。〈主治〉手指关节麻木和疼痛、头痛、项强、咽痛、牙痛、目疾、疟疾、毒蛇咬伤等。向上斜刺0.5～1寸，或点刺出血。

Baxie (EX-UE 9) Set of extra points, originally from *Yijing Xiaoxue* (*Collection of Elementary Medical Classics*), also named Baguan. 〈Location〉Four points on the dorsum of each hand, at the junction of the red and white skin proximal to the margin of the webs between each two of the five fingers of each hand when a loose fist is made. (Fig. 76)〈Regional anatomy〉skin→subcutaneous tissue→dorsal interosseous muscle→palmar interosseous muscle→lumbrical muscle. In the superficial layer, there are the dorsal metacarpal artery and vein or the dorsal digital artery and vein and the dorsal disital nerve. In the deep layer, there are the common digital palmar artery and vein or the proper palmar digital artery and vein and the proper palmar digital nerve. 〈Indications〉numbness and pain of fingers, headache, stiff neck, sore throat, toothache, eye diseases, malaria, snakebite, etc. 〈Method〉Puncture obliquely 0.5～1 cun or prick to cause bleeding.

●八正[bā zhèng] 指八方之正位。出《素问·八正神明论》即东、南、西、北、东南、西南、东北、西北。又释作四时八节的正气。春、夏、秋、冬，八方各有正常的风，又有致病的虚邪。在针刺时，要顺天时而行，此为后世"子午流注针法"所本。

Eight Directions A general name for the eight due directions, originally from *Suwen: Bazheng Shenming Lun* (*Plain Questions: On Eight Natural Qi and Divinity*), i.e., the east, south, west, north, southeast, southwest, northeast and northwest. The term is also interpreted as the natural qi of the four seasons and the 8 directions. When acupuncture is given, we should follow natural qi and seasonal qi, which was the basis of the later "midnight-noon circulation acupuncture".

●八椎下[bā zhuī xià] 经外穴名。见《针灸孔穴及其疗法便览》。位于后正中线，第8胸椎棘突下陷中。主治疟疾。斜刺0.5～1寸；可灸。

Bazhuixia (EX-B) An extra point, seen in *Zhenjiu Kongxue Jiqi Liaofa Bianlan* (*Guide to Acupoints and Acupuncture Therapeutics*). 〈Location〉on the posterior midling, in the depression below the spinous process of the 8th thoracic vertebra. 〈Indication〉malaria. 〈Method〉Puncture obliquely 0.5～1 cun. Moxibustion is applicable.

●巴豆饼灸[bā dòu bǐng jiǔ] 间接灸的一种。是用巴豆作间隔物而施灸的一种灸法。其法有二：①取巴豆10粒，捣碎研细，加入白面3克，成膏状，捏作饼，放于脐中，上置艾炷施灸。也可与隔葱灸合用，疗效更著。②取黄连末适量，用巴豆10粒，二药混合制成膏状，放入脐中，上置艾炷灸之。临床上适用于食积、腹痛、泄泻、胸痛、小便不通诸症。

Ba Dou (Croton Tiglium)-Cake-Separated Moxibustion A form of indirect moxibustion, i.e., a method of using *Ba Dou (Croton Tiglium)* cake as the intercalating material for indirect moxibustion. ⟨Methods⟩ ①Grind 10 grains of *Ba Dou (Semen Crotonis)* into fine powder and mix it with 3 g of flour and some water, making a medicinal extract. Mould the cake and place it in the umbilicus with a moxa cone on it. Ignite the moxa for moxibustion. If this method is used together with garlic-separated moxibustion, the therapeutic effect will be better. ②Mix some powder of *Huang Lian (Rhizoma Coptidis)* and the powder of 10 grains of *Ba Dou (Semen Crotonis)* into a paste, and put it in the umbilicus, place a moxa cone on it, thus to perform moxibustion. Clinically, this moxibustion method is applied to treat retention of food, abdominal pain, diarrhea, thoracic pain and retention of urine, etc.

●巴豆酒蒸气灸[bā dòu jiǔ zhēng qì jiǔ] 灸法的一种。取50~60度白酒250毫升，将巴豆(去壳)5~10粒投入酒中，置火上煮沸后，再将酒倒入瓶中或小杯中，乘热用蒸气熏灸劳宫穴，用治颜面神经麻痹。

Moxibustion with the Vapor from Ba Dou (Croton Tiglium) Spirit A moxibustion method. Take 250 ml of white spirit of 50~60 degrees and put 5~10 grains of *Ba Dou (Semen Crotonis)* (peeled) in it. Boil the spirit and then pour it into a bottle or a small cup to vaporize Laogong (PC 8) for facial paralysis.

●巴豆霜灸[bā dòu shuāng jiǔ] 天灸的一种。取巴豆霜、雄黄各等分，研细混匀，收贮瓶中备用。于疟疾发作前5~6小时，取药面如绿豆大放在1.5×1.5厘米胶布中央，敷贴于病人两耳后的乳突部(相当于完骨处)，敷灸7~8小时取下。用于治疗疟疾。

Moxibustion with Ba Dou Shuang (Pulvis Crotonis Tiglium) One form of crude herb moxibustion. Take equal amount of *Ba Dou Shuang (Pulvis Crotonis Tiglium)* and *Xiong Huang (Realgar)*, grind them into fine powder and mix them, store them in a bottle, ready for use. 5~6 hours before an attack of malaria, take some prepared powder, of which a volume is just like that of a mung bean and put it in the center of a plaster which is 1.5× 1.5 cm² in size. Stick the plasters on the mastoid processes behind the ears (i.e. Wangu, GB 12). Remove the plasters after 7 to 8 hours. The therapy is used for the treatment of malaria.

●拔罐法[bá guàn fǎ] 治病方法之一。见《五十二病方》。又称吸杯法、吸筒、角法、拔筒法。系应用各种方法排除杯罐内空气形成负压，使其紧吸在体表上来治疗疾病。通过吸拔，引起局部充血或瘀血，能起到活血、行气、止痛、消肿等作用。临床又分火罐法、水罐法、抽气拔罐法等多种。用于治疗咳嗽、肺炎、哮喘、头痛、胸胁痛、风湿痹痛、扭伤、腰痛、胃痛、疮疖痈肿及毒蛇咬伤等。

Cupping. A therapy seen in *Wushier Bingfang (Prescription for Fifty-Two Diseases)*, i.e., to expel the air in the cup by various means to create a negative pressure inside and produce suction of the cup to the skin; also named "sucking cup", "sucking tube", "horn cupping", or "bamboo cupping". This therapy causes local hyperemia or passive congestion so as to promote the circulation of blood and the flow of qi, alleviate pain and relieve swelling, etc. It is clinically divided into fire cupping, cupping with boiled cup and cupping by extracting air, etc. ⟨Indications⟩ cough, pneumonia, asthma, headache, pain in chest and hypochondrium, wind-dampness, Bi-syndrome, sprain, lumbago, stomachache, carbuncle, furuncle, sores, and snake-bite, etc.

●拔筒法[bá tǒng fǎ] 见《外科正宗》卷二。为拔罐法之别称。详见该条。

Bamboo Cupping Another name for cupping, from Vol. 2 of *Waike Zhengzong (Orthodox Manual of External Diseases)*. →拔罐法 (p. 9)

●拔原法[bá yuán fǎ] 取穴法之一。王海藏所倡用。指各经之病选用其原穴进行治疗。

Selection of Yuan (Primary) Points A principle of selecting points in acupuncture, advocated by Wang Haizang, i.e. to select the Yuan (primary) point of a certain meridian to treat diseases related to it.

●拔针[bá zhēn] 针刺手法名。为出针法之别称。详见该条。

Pulling Out the Needle A term used in acupuncture, another name for withdrawing the needle. →出针法(p. 51)

●白附子灸[bái fù zǐ jiǔ] 天灸的一种。取白附子适量,研为细末,加水调如膏状,敷于穴位上,胶布固定。如敷涌泉穴治疗牙痛等。

Moxibustion with Bai Fu Zi (Rhizoma Typhonii) A kind of medicinal vesication. Grind an appropriate amount of a dried tuber of *Bai Fu Zi* (*Typhonium giganteum*) into a fine powder, mix it with water and stir them into a paste. Apply the paste to certain acupoints and fix it with adhesive plasters, e. g., apply it to Yongquan (KI 1) to treat toothache.

●白胡椒灸[bái hú jiāo jiǔ] 天灸的一种。取白胡椒适量,研为细末,敷于穴位上,胶布固定。如敷大椎穴能治疗疟疾。

White Pepper Moxibustion A kind of medicinal vesication. Grind an appropriate amount of white pepper into a fine powder, then apply it to certain acupoints and fix it with adhesive plasters, e. g., apply it to Dazhui (DU 14) to treat malaria.

●白虎摇头[bái hǔ yáo tóu] 针刺手法名。出《金针赋》。针法是:将针捻入,并用中指拨动针体,使针左右摇动,再予上提,同时进行摇振,有如用手摇铃一般,可以推动经气。

White Tiger Shaking Its Head A needling technique, from *Jinzhen Fu* (*Ode to Gold Needle*). ⟨Method⟩ Insert the needle with rotation, pluck the body of the needle to make it move left and right, then lift the needle up while shaking it, as if ringing a bell, to promote the circulation of meridian qi.

●白环俞[bái huán shū] 经穴名。出《针灸甲乙经》。属足太阳膀胱经。又名玉环俞、玉房俞。⟨定位⟩在骶部,当骶正中嵴旁1.5寸,平第四骶后孔(图7)。⟨层次解剖⟩皮肤→皮下组织→臀大肌→骶结节韧带→梨状肌。浅层布有臀中和臀下皮神经。深层布有臀上、下动、静脉的分支或属支,骶神经丛和骶静脉丛。主治白带、疝气、遗精、月经不调、腰腿痛。直刺0.8～1寸;可灸。

Baihuanshu (BL 30) A meridian point, originally from *Zhenjiu Jia-Yi Jing* (*A-B Classic of Acupuncture and Moxibustion*), a point on the Bladder Meridian of Foot-Taiyang, also named Yuhuanshu and Yufangshu. ⟨Location⟩ on the sacrum and on the level of the 4th posterior sacral foramen, 1.5 cun lateral to the median sacral crest. (Fig. 7) ⟨Regional anatomy⟩ skin→subcutaneous tissue→greatest gluteal muscle→sacrotuberous ligament→piriform muscle. In the superficial layer, there are the middle and inferior clunial nerves. In the deep layer, there are the branches or tributaries of the superior and inferior gluteal arteries and veins and the sacral nervous plexus and sacral venous plexus. ⟨Indication⟩ leucorrhea, hernia, emission, irregular menstruation, lumbocrural pain. ⟨Method⟩ Puncture perpendicularly 0.8～1 cun. Moxibustion is applicable.

●白芥子灸[bái jiè zǐ jiǔ] 天灸的一种。白芥子研末,醋调为糊膏状,每次用5～10克贴敷穴位上,油纸敷盖,橡皮膏固定;或将白芥子细末10克,放置在3厘米直径的圆形胶布中央,直接贴敷在穴位上。敷灸时间约为2～4小时,以局部充血潮红,或皮肤起泡为度。该法主治风寒湿痹、肺结核、哮喘、口眼㖞斜等症。

Bai Jie Zi (Semen Sinapis Albae) Moxibustion A form of medicinal vesication with *Bai Jie Zi* (*Semen Sinapis Albae*) ground to a powder, and then mixed with vinegar to form a paste, apply 5～10 g to the acupoint, cover it with oilpaper and fix it with an adhesive plaster. Or, put 10 g of the powder in the centre of a piece of round adhesive plaster, 3 cm in diameter, and apply it directly to the acupoint. Keep it on for 2～4 hours until a local flush or blister appears. ⟨Indications⟩ arthralgia due to wind-cold-dampness, tuberculosis, asthma, and other disorders such as facial hemiparalysis, etc..

●白刃疔[bái rèn dīng] 即鼻疔中白者。详见该条。

Naked-Sword-Like Furuncle Synonymous with furuncle with white head in the vestibule of the nose. →鼻疔(p. 18)

●白肉际[bái ròu jì] 部位名。出《灵枢·经脉》。指手足掌(蹠)面与背面的交界处。因掌面肤色较白,故名。

Border of White Skin A term used for the location of points, from *Lingshu: Jingmai* (*Miraculous Pivot: Meridians*), referring to the border line between the palm (or sole) and the dorsum of the hand (or foot). The skin of the palm or sole is whitish, hence the name.

●白针[bái zhēn] 针刺术语。见《千金要方》卷三十。又称冷针。指单纯的针刺方法, 与温针等对举。

Ordinary Needling An acupuncture terminology, from Vol. 30 of *Qianjin Yaofang* (*Essential Prescriptions Worth a Thousand Gold*) also named cold needling, referring to ordinary acupuncture in comparison with warm needling, etc.

●百虫窝[bǎi chóng wō] ①经外穴名。见《针灸大成》。又名血郄、百虫窠。〈定位〉屈膝, 在大腿内侧, 髌底内侧端上3寸, 即血海上1寸(图33)。〈层次解剖〉皮肤→皮下组织→股内侧肌。浅层布有股神经的前皮支, 大隐静脉的属支。〈主治〉风疹、湿疹、皮肤瘙痒症、下部生疮等。直刺1～1.5寸；可灸。②经穴别名。出《针灸大全》。即血海。详见该条。

1. **Baichongwo** (EX-LE 3) An extra point seen in *Zhenjiu Dacheng* (*A Great Compendium of Acupuncture and Moxibustion*), also named Xuexi or Baichongke. 〈Location〉 3 cun above the medial superior corner of the patella of the thigh with the knee flexed, i.e. 1 cun above Xuehai (SP 10) (Fig. 33) 〈Regional anatomy〉 skin → subcutaneous tissue → medial intermuscle of thigh. In the superficial layer, there are the anterior cutaneous branch of the femoral nerve and great saphenous vein. In the deep layer, there are the muscular branch of the femoral artery and vein and the femoral nerve. 〈Indications〉 ruhella, eczema, cutaneous pruritus, sores on the lower body. 〈Method〉 Puncture perpendicularly 1～1.5 cun. Moxibustion is applicable.

2. **Baichongwo** Another name for Xuehai (SP 10), a meridian point from *Zhenjiu Daquan* (*A Complete Work of Acupuncture and Moxibustion*). →血海(p.524)

●百发神针[bǎi fā shén zhēn] 艾条灸的一种。见《种福堂公选良方》卷二。以乳香、没药、生川附子、血竭、川乌、草乌、檀香末、降香末、大贝母、麝香各12克, 母丁香49粒, 净蕲艾绒30克, 卷制如雷火针。治偏正头风、腰痛、小肠疝气、痈疽、发背、痰核初起不破烂等, 各按穴灸之。

Baifa Magic Needling A form of moxa-stick moxibustion, seen in Vol. 2 of *Zhong futang Gongxuan Liangfang* (*Zhongfutang Effective Prescriptions*). Preparation of herbal moxa stick: *Ru Xiang* (*Frankincense*) 12 g, *Mo Yao* (*Myrrh*) 12 g, raw *Chuan Fu Zi* (*Radix Aconiti Carmichaeli*) 12 g, *Xue Jie* (*Resina Draconis*) 12 g, *Chuan Wu* (*Radix Aconiti*) 12 g, *Cao Wu* (*Radix Aconiti Kusnezoffii*) 12 g, *Tan Xiang* (*Lignum Santali*) 12 g, *Da Bei Mu* (*Bulbus Fritillariae Cirhosae*) 12 g, *She Xiang* (*Moschus*) 12 g, 49 grains of *Mu Ding Xiang* (*Semen Syzigii Aromatici*) and *Ai Rong* (Moxa Wool) 30 g. Grind all of the above herbs into a powder to make a moxa stick like the thunder-fire herbal moxa stick. 〈Indications〉 migraine, headache, lumbago, hernia, carbuncle, cellutitis, lumbodorsal cellutitis, subcutaneous module in an early stage without ulceration. 〈Method〉 Apply moxibustion to the selected acupoints with this herbal moxa stick.

●百会[bǎi huì] 经穴名。出《针灸甲乙经》。属督脉, 为督脉、手足三阳之会。又名三阳五会、天满、巅上、泥丸宫、维会、三阳五会。〈定位〉在头部, 当前发际正中直上5寸, 或两耳尖连线的中点处(图28)。〈层次解剖〉皮肤→皮下组织→帽状腱膜→腱膜下疏松组织。布有枕大神经、额神经的分支和左、右颞浅动、静脉及枕动、静脉吻合网。〈主治〉头痛、眩晕、惊悸、健忘、尸厥、中风不语、癫狂、痫证、癔病、瘈疭、耳鸣、鼻塞、脱肛、痔疾、阴挺、泄泻。平刺0.5～0.8寸；可灸。

Baihui (DU 20) A meridian point of the Du Meridian, and the meeting point of the Du Meridian, the three Yang Meridians of the hand and the three Yang Meridians of the foot, from *Zhenjiu Jia-Yi Jing* (*A-B Classic of Acupuncture and Moxibustion*), also named Sanyangwuhui, Tianman, Dianshang, Niwangong, Weihui, Sanyang or Wuhui. 〈Location〉 on the head, 5 cun directly above the midpoint of the anterior hairline, or at the midpoint of the line connecting the apexes of both ears. (Fig. 28) 〈Regional anatomy〉 skin → subcutaneous tissue → epicranialaponeurosis → sub-

aponeurotic loose tissue. There are the branches of the greater occipital and frontal nerves, and the anastomotic network of the left and right superficial temporal arteries and veins with the left and right occipital arteries and veins in this area. 〈Indications〉 headache, dizziness, palpitation due to fright, amnesia, corpse-like syncope, aphasia from apoplexy, manic-depressive psychosis, epilepsy, hysteria, colic convulsion, tinnitus, stuffy nose, proctoptosis, hemorrhoid, prolape of the uterus, diarrhea. 〈Method〉Puncture 0.5~0.8 cun horizontally. Moxibustion is applicable.

● 百劳[bǎi láo] ①经穴别名。见《针灸大全》。即大椎。详见该条。②指随痛处取穴。所指与"阿是穴"相同。③经外穴名。位于大椎上2寸,旁开各1寸处。灸治瘰疬。

1. **Bailao** Another name for Dazhui (DU 14), a meridian point from *Zhenjiu Daquan* (*A Complete Work of Acupuncture and Moxibustion*). → 大椎(p.69)
2. Referring to the method of selecting tender or sensitive points synonymous with Ashi points.
3. **Bailao**(EX−B) An extra point. 〈Location〉 2 cun above Dazhui (DU 14) and 1 cun lateral to the posterior midline. 〈Indication〉 scrofula. 〈Method〉 moxibustion.

● 百日咳[bǎi rì ké] 即顿咳的别名。详见该条。

Wooping Cough another name for paroxymal cough. → 顿咳(p.90)

● 百症赋[bǎi zhèng fù] 针灸歌赋名。见《针灸聚英》。撰人不详。其内容列举多种病证的针灸配穴,便于诵读,影响很广。

Baizheng Fu(A Verse on 100 Diseases) One of the verses on acupuncture and moxibustion, from *Zhenjiu Juying* (*Essentials of Acupunture and Moxibustion*). The verse, whose writer is unknown, lists point prescriptions for many diseases. Since it is convenient for reading and reciting, it has a wide influence.

● 斑秃[bān tū] 病名。指头皮部突然发生斑状脱发,又称油风。患者头发迅速成片脱落,呈圆形或不规则形,小如指甲,大如钱币,一至数个不等,皮肤平滑而有光泽。多由肝肾不足,风邪外袭,风盛血燥所致;或由气滞血瘀,发失所养所致。血虚者,伴有头晕失眠,舌淡红,苔薄,脉细弱,血瘀者,病程较长,面色晦黯,舌边有紫色瘀点,脉涩。治宜养血祛风,活血化瘀。取阿是穴、百会、风池、膈俞、足三里、三阴交。局部可用梅花针叩刺。还可用艾条在患部熏灸,至皮肤呈微红时为止。

Alopecia Areata A disease also named alopecia areata due to pathogenic wind referring to a sudden occurrence of loss of hair in circular patches, resulting in spots of smooth, glossy, bald scalp of various sizes, mostly due to deficiency of the liver and kidney, exterior attack of wind, dryness in blood with domination of pathogenic wind; or, qi stagnation and blood stasis, hair lacking nourishment. In cases of blood deficiency, hair loss is accompanied by dizziness, insomnia, a pink tongue with thin coating, and a thready, weak pulse. In cases of blood stasis over a prolonged period of time, it is accompanied by a dim complexion, petechia on the sides of the tongue and a choppy pulse. 〈Theatment principle〉 Nourish the blood to expel wind and promote blood circulation to remove stasis. 〈Points selection〉Ashi points, Baihui(DU 20), Fengchi(GB 20), Geshu(BL 17), Zusanli(ST 36) and Sanyinjiao(SP 6). 〈Method〉 Tap with plum-blossom needle locally, or fumigate the affected parts with a moxa-stick until the skin turns reddish.

● 瘢痕灸[bān hén jiǔ] 为化脓灸的别称。详见该条。

Scarring Moxibustion Another name for festering moxibuston. → 化脓灸(p.169)

● 半刺[bàn cì] 《内经》刺法名。出《灵枢·官针》。是五刺之一。指浅刺皮肤,快速出针的刺法。与九刺中的毛刺相仿。近代应用的皮肤针即由此发展而来。参见"毛刺"条。

Extremely Shallow Puncture Name of a needling method in *Neijing* (*The Inner Canon of Huangdi*), originally from *Lingshu: Guanzhen* (*Miraculous Pivot: Official Needles*). One of the five needling techniques, in which the needle is punctured very superficially and withdrawn swiftly. It is similar to the shallow needling of the nine needling meth-

● 半夏灸[bàn xià jiǔ]　天灸的一种。取生半夏、葱白各等份,共捣料如膏状,贴于穴位或患处。适于治疗急性乳腺炎。也可将药膏揉成栓状,塞于一侧鼻孔。每次30分钟,每日二次。用以治疗鼻渊。

Ban Xia（Rhizoma Pinelliae）Moxibustion　A form of medicinal versiculation.〈Manipulation〉Take equal amounts of dried tuber of Ban Xia(Pinellia Ternata) and scallion stalk, pound them into a paste, and apply it to acupoints or affected parts to treat acute mastadenitis. The paste can also be kneaded into an embolus, and placed in one nostril for 30 minutes, twice a day, to treat rhinorrhea with turbid discharge.

● 傍针刺[bàng zhēn cì]　《内经》刺法名。出《灵枢·官针》。先直刺一针,再在近旁斜向加刺一针。因其正旁配合而刺,故称傍针刺。多用于压痛比较明显,且固定不移,久久不愈的痹证。

Adjacent Puncture　One of the needling methods in Neijing（The Inner Canon of Huangdi）, originally from Ling shu: Guanzhen（Miraculous Pivot: Official Needles）. Insert a needle perpendicularly into the affected parts, and then another needle obliquely toward the first needle at a nearby point. It's so named because the two needles are punctured at nearby points.〈Indication〉lingering arthralgia-syndrome with obvious and fixed tenderness.

● 包肓[bāo huāng]　经穴别名。出《备急千金要方》。即胞肓。详见该条。

Baohuang　Another name for Baohuang（BL 53）, a meridian point from Beiji Qianjin Yaofang（Essential Prescriptions Worth a Thousand Gold for Emergencies）. →胞肓(p.13)

● 胞不正[bāo bù zhèng]　病证名。见《产家要诀》。又称胎位不正。正常胎位中,绝大多数为枕前位。如果妊娠30周后,经产前检查发现枕后位、臀位、横位等异常胎位,谓之胞不正。多因经产妇腹壁松弛而引起,或因气滞、惊恐,影响胎胞转运所致。治宜舒气导滞,矫正胎位。用艾条灸两侧至阴穴15分钟。每天1～2次,至胎位转正为止。

Abnormal Position of Fetus　A disease from Chanjia Yaojue（Pithy Formulas for Childbirth）, also named malposition of fetus. The usual position of a fetus is on occipitoanterior position; but, after 30 weeks of pregnancy, if the fetus is found in an occipitoposterior position, breech presentation, or transverse position, etc., this means that the fetus is malpositioned.〈Causes〉plurigravida with abdominal muscular relaxation, or stagnation of qi, panic, etc. affecting fetal movement.〈Treatment principle〉Promote the flow of qi, remove stagnancy and correct the position of the fetus.〈Method〉Apply moxa-stick moxibustion to bilateral Zhiyin（BL 67）point for 15 minutes, once or twice a day until the position of the fetus is normal.

● 胞寒不孕[bāo hán bù yùn]　不孕证型之一。又称宫冷不孕、胞冷无子、子脏冷无子、下部冰冷不孕。多因肾阳不足,寒自内生,胞宫失于温煦;或经期调摄不慎,风寒客于胞中,以致胞宫寒冷,难以摄精所致。证见经行愆后,质稀色黯,小腹冷痛,形寒肢冷,或兼见腰酸腿软,小便清长,舌淡苔薄,脉沉迟。治宜暖宫散寒。取阴交、曲骨、命门、气海。

Sterility due to Retention of Cold in the Uterus　A form of sterility, also named sterility due to cold uterus, childlessness due to cold in the uterus, childlessness due to cold uterus, and sterility due to the ice-coldness lower abdomen.〈Etiology and pathology〉insufficiency of kidney-yang leading to a production of cold in the interior, and a failure of kidney-yang to warm the uterus; or improper nursing during the menstrual period and wind-cold invading the uterus leading to a cold uterus in which sperm cannot be kept.〈Manifestations〉delayed menstrua period, dilute and dark menstrual blood, cold-pain in lower abdomen, cold body and limbs, often accompanied by lumbar soreness and lassitude in the legs, clear and excessive urine, a pale tongue with little coating, a deep and slow pulse.〈Treatment principle〉Warm the womb and dispel cold.〈Point selection〉Yinjiao（RN 7）, Qugu（RN 2）, Mingmen（Du 4）and Qihai（RN 6）.

● 胞肓[bāo huāng]　经穴名。出《针灸甲乙经》。属足太阳膀胱经。又名包肓。〈定位〉在臀部,平第二骶后

孔,骶正中嵴旁开3寸(图7)。〈层次解剖〉皮肤→皮下组织→臀大肌→臀中肌。浅层布有臀上皮神经和臀中皮神经。深层有臀上动、静脉,臀上神经。〈主治〉肠鸣、腹胀、腰脊痛、大小便不利、阴肿。直刺0.8～1寸;可灸。

Baohuang(BL 53) A meridian point on the Bladder Meridian of Foot-Taiyang, from *Zhenjiu Jia-Yi Jing*(*A-B Classic of Acupuncture and Moxibustion*), also named Baohuang (包肓). 〈Location〉 on the buttocks, and on the level of the 2nd posterior sacral foramen, 3 cun lateral to the median sacral crest. (Fig. 7) 〈Regional anatomy〉skin→subcutaneous tissue → greatest gluteal muscle → middle gluteal muscle. In the superficial layer, there are the superior and middle clunial nerves. In the deep layer, there are the superior gluteal artery and vein and the superior gluteal nerve. 〈Indications〉 borborygmus, abdominal distention, pain along spinal column, dysuria and constipation, pudental swelling. 〈Method〉 Puncture 0.8～1 cun perpendicularly. Moxibustion is applicable.

●胞冷无子[bāo lěng wú zǐ] 即胞寒不孕的别名。详见该条。

Childlessness due to Cold in the Uterus Another name for sterility due to retention of cold in the uterus. →胞寒不孕(p. 13)

●胞门[bāo mén] ①经穴别名。出《针灸甲乙经》。即气穴。详见该条。②经外穴名。详见"胞门、子户"条。

1. **Baomen** Another name for Qixue (KI 13), a meridian point from *Zhenjiu Jia-Yi Jing*(*A-B Classic of Acupuncture and Moxibustion*). →气穴(p. 311)

2. **Baomen** An extra point → 胞门、子户(p. 14)

●胞门、子户[bāo mén zǐ hù] 经穴名。见《千金要方》。关元穴左侧,旁开2寸为胞门穴;关元穴右侧,旁开2寸为子户穴。与今之"水道"穴同位。〈主治〉妇女不孕、漏胎下血、腹痛、难产、白带多、腹中积聚等。直刺1～1.5寸;可灸。孕妇禁针。参见"气穴"条。

Baomen and Zihu(EX-CA) Two extra points seen in *Qianjin Yaofang*(*Essential Prescriptions Worth a Thousand Gold*). 〈Location〉 Baomen and Zihu are located 2 cun to the right of Guanyuan(RN 4), in the same place as Shuidao(ST 28). 〈Indications〉 female sterility, vaginal bleeding during pregnancy, abdominal pain, dystocia, leukorrhea, abdominal masses, etc. 〈Method〉 Puncture perpendicularly 1～1.5 cun. Moxibustion is applicable. Contraindicated in pregnancy. →气穴(p. 311)

●胞衣不出[bāo yī bù chū] 即胞衣不下的别名。详见该条。

Lingering placenta Another name for retention of placenta. →胞衣不下(p. 14)

●胞衣不下[bāo yī bù xià] 病证名。出《经效产宝》。又名胞衣不出、息胞、息胎、胞胀不下、儿衣不出。分娩之后,胎盘经过较长时间不能娩出者,称为胞衣不下。可分为两种证型。①气虚者,多由于产妇体质虚弱,元气不足;或产程过长,用力过多,耗伤气血,无力送出胞衣所致。症见产后胞衣不下、少腹微胀、按之不痛、有块不坚、阴道流血量多、色淡、并伴有面色㿠白、脉虚弱。治宜补气养血。取关元、三阴交、独阴。②血瘀者,多由于产时调摄失宜,感受寒邪,至令气血凝滞,或败血瘀滞胞中所致。症见产后胞衣不下、小腹冷痛、拒按、按之有块且硬、恶露甚少、色黯红、舌质微紫、脉沉弦而涩。治宜行气活血、温经祛瘀。取中极、气海、合谷、三阴交、肩井、独阴。

Retention of Placenta A disease from *Jingxiao Chanbao*(*Treasury of Effective Prescriptions in Obsterics*), also named lingering placenta, resting placenta, delayed delivery of placenta, retained placenta, retardative fetus, lingering afterbirth, or retardative delivery of afterbirth, referring to the case in which the placenta cannot be delivered long after childbirth. There are two types: ①The qi deficiency type is due to weak constitution of parturient, deficiency of yuan (primary)-qi or too much strength used during a long delivery leading to the consumption and damage of qi and blood, the parturient then has no strength to deliver the placenta. 〈Manifestations〉retention of placenta, mild distension in the lower abdomen, no pain while with pressure, soft mass in the lower abdomen, excessive light-coloured blood from the vagina, a pale complexion, spiritlessness and tiredness, intolerance to cold, a preference for warmth, a pale

tongue with a thin, whitish coating, and a feeble and weak pulse. 〈Treatment principle〉 Invigorate qi and nourish the blood. 〈Point selection〉Guanyuan(RN 4), Sanyinjiao(SP 6), and Duyin(EX-LE 11). ②Blood stasis due to improper care during delivery and invasion of cold leading to the stagnation of qi and blood or, retention of lochioschesis. 〈Manifestations〉 retention of placenta, cold-pain in the lower abdomen and refusal to be pressed, gelosis found by pressing, less lochia with dark-red color, purplish tongue, deep, wiry and choppy pulse. 〈Treatment principle〉Promote the flow of qi and blood, remove blood stasis by warming the meridians. 〈Point selection〉 Zhongji (RN 3), Qihai(RN 6), Hegu(LI 4), Sanyinjiao(SP 6), Jianjing(GB 21), and Duyin(EX-LE 11).

●胞胀不下[bāo zhàng bù xià] 胞衣不下的别名。详见该条。

Retained Placenta Another name for retention of placenta. →胞衣不下(p. 14)

●胞阻[bāo zǔ] 妊娠腹痛的别名。详见该条。

Embarrassment of the Fetus Another name for abdominal pain during pregnancy. →妊娠腹痛(p. 335)

●保健灸[bǎo jiàn jiǔ] 指以增强人体抗病能力而达到强身保健为目的的灸法。保健灸常用穴有足三里、关元、气海、膏肓等。多用连续的化脓灸来预防疾病。

Moxibustion for Health Protection A moxibustion method used to keep fit by improving the body resistance. Commonly used points are Zusanli(ST 36), Guanyuan(RN 4), Qihai (RN 6), Gaohuang(BL 43), etc. Successive festering moxibustions are usually applied at those points to prevent diseases.

●报刺[bào cì] 《内经》刺法名。出《灵枢·官针》。为十二刺之一。本法为治游走性疼痛的刺法,可当其痛处下针,再按到痛处后,将前刺之针拔出重刺。报作复解,即当针复刺之意。

Trigger Puncture A needling method of Neijing(The Inner Canon of Huangdi) from Lingshu: Guanzhen (Miraculous Pivot: Official Needles). One of the twelve needlings; used to treat wandering pain by puncturing a painful trigger point directly, retaining the needle there in until another painful trigger point is found, then withdrawing the needle and puncturing the second painful trigger point. This is a repeated needling at the trigger points(Ashi points).

●报灸[bào jiǔ] 灸法用语。见《针灸资生经》。即分次重复灸治,指多壮灸或反复多次施灸治疗疾病。

Repeated Moxibustion A method of moxibustion from Zhenjiu Zisheng Jing(Acupuncture-Moxibustion Classic for Saving Life) i.e., to apply moxibustion repeatedly, referring to multi-moxa-cone moxibustion or repeated moxibustion treatments for some diseases that cannot be cured with one time moxibustion.

●报头火丹[bào tóu huǒ dān] 发于头部的丹毒。详见该条。

Erysipelas Overhead Erysipelas occurring on the head. →丹毒(p. 71)

●豹文刺[bào wén cì] 刺法名。见《灵枢·官针》。是五刺之一。指用散刺络脉出血的方法,以刺到血脉为目的,出血点多,因其前后左右均刺,形如豹文,故名。本法与九刺中的络刺、十二刺中的赞刺,都是指刺络出血法。参见各条。

Leopard-Spot Puncture One of the five ancient needling techniques from Lingshu: Guanzhen (Miraculous Pivot: Official Needles), i.e. to give scattered collateral pricking, reaching the blood vessel so as to cause bleeding. So many bleeding spots appear that they look like leopard spots, hence the name. This method, together with the collateral pricking in the nine needling methods and the repeated shallow puncture in the twelve needlings, belongs to the blood-letting method. →络刺(p. 259)、赞刺(p. 582)

●暴病者取之太阳[bào bìng zhě qǔ zhī tài yáng] 《内经》治则之一。对急性病症的治疗可取太阳经腧穴。

Selecting Taiyang Meridian for Fulminating Diseases One of the principles of treatment from Neijing (The Canon of Internal Medicine). i.e., points of Taiyang meridians can be used to treat acute diseases.

●**暴盲**[bào máng] 病证名。见《证治准绳》。多因暴怒,肝阳上亢,精明失用;或气滞血瘀,气血不能运精于目所致。其证发病急骤,病人视力突然丧失。肝阳上亢者,症见头目眩晕,心烦易怒,胁肋胀痛,颜赤舌绛,脉弦。治宜清肝明目。取睛明、瞳子髎、太冲、光明。气滞血瘀者,症见头痛且胀,烦躁口渴,舌有紫斑,脉涩。治宜行气活血明目。取睛明、瞳子髎、内关、膈俞。

Sudden Loss of Vision A disease from the *Zhengzhi Zhunsheng*(*Standards of Diagnosis and Treatment*). Primarily due to rage and hyperactivity of the liver-yang leading to failure of the eye functions, or to qi stagnation and blood stasis leading to the qi and blood being unable to transfer essence to the eyes. The disease progresses rapidly, causing patients to have a sudden loss of eyesight. In the case of liver-yang rising, vision loss is accompanied by dizziness and vertigo, vexation, irritability, pain in the hypochondrium and a flushed face. Treat by puncturing Jingming (BL 1), Togziliao(GB 1), Taichong (LR 3) and Guangming (GB 37) to remove intensive heat from the liver and improve eyesight. Stgnation of qi and blood is accompanied by a distending pain in the head, dysphoria, thirst, petechia of the tongue and a choppy pulse. Treat by puncturing Jingming (BL 1), Tongziliao (GB 1), Neiguan(PC 6), and Geshu(BL 17) to promote the circulation of qi and blood and thus improve activity of vision.

●**暴脱**[bào tuō] 病证名。指因中风,大汗,剧泻,大失血等逆变为阴阳离决者。参见"脱证"条。

Sudden Collapse A disease referring to dissociation of yin and yang due to transformative changes such as apoplexy, profuse sweating, severe diarrhea, profuse loss of blood. → 脱证(p. 452)

●**备急灸法**[bèi jí jiǔ fǎ] 书名。南宋闻人耆年撰,一卷,成书于1226年。书中载痈疽、腹痛、吐泻等二十余种急性病的灸法,并附简明图说。1245年,孙炬卿将此书与《竹阁经验备急药方》合刊,仍称《备急灸法》。后附的《骑竹马灸法》记载了治发背的灸法。

Beiji Jiufa(*Moxibustion Methods for Emergencies*) A single-volume book, completed by Wenren Qinian in 1226 during the Southern Song Dynasty. It recorded methods of moxibustion for treating over 20 acute diseases such as boils, abdominal pain, vomiting and diarrhea, etc. There are also brief illustrations with a set of simple pictures attached to the book. In 1245, Sun Juqing combined this book and *Zhuge Jingyan Beiji Yaofang*(*Experienced Prescriptions for Emergencies from a Bamboo Pavilion*)into one, which retained the original name of *Beiji Jiufa*(*Moxibustion Methods for Emergencies*). Its appendix, *Qi Zhuma Jiufa* (*Moxibustion while on a Bamboo Horse*), recorded the moxibustion methods for lumbodorsal cellalitis.

●**肩胛中间**[bèi jiǎ zhōng jiān] 经外穴名。见《肘后备急方》。在肩胛骨冈下窝,当肩胛骨外、上、下三角之中点。灸治癫狂。

Beijiazhongjian(EX-B) An extra point from *Zhouhou Beiji Fang*(*A Handbook of Prescriptions for Emergencies*).〈Location〉in the infraspinous fossa of the scapula, at the central point of a triangle formed by connecting the lateral, superior and inferior points of the scapula. 〈Indications〉manic-depressive disorders. Method moxibustion.

●**背解**[bèi jiě] 经穴别名。出《针灸甲乙经》。即腰俞。详见该条。

Beijie Another name for Yaoshu(DU 2), a meridian point from *Zhenjiu Jia-Yi Jing*(*A-B Classic of Acupuncture and Moxibustion*). → 腰俞(p. 545)

●**背俞穴**[bèi shū xué] ①经穴分类名。出《灵枢·背腧》。指脏腑经气输注于背腰部的腧穴。背俞穴位于背腰部足太阳膀胱经的第一侧线上,大体依脏腑位置而上下排列,分别冠以脏腑之名,共十二穴。各脏腑疾病,常在相关的背俞穴出现压痛或敏感等异常反应,从而进行诊断和治疗。见表3。②泛指背部各经穴。见《资生经》。

Back-Shu Points 1. Name of a group of classified meridian points from *Lingshu*:*Beishu* (*Miraculous Pivot*:*Back-Shu Points*), referring to the points into which the meridian qi of zang and fu organs infuse at the back. They are all on the first side line of the Bladder Meridian of Foot-Taiyang in the dorsolumbar

region, and are named after zang or fu organs respesctively. These points are located in positions near their related organs. Disases related to zang or fu organs frequently lead to abnormal reactions such as tenderness or sensitivity at those points. These points therefore help in diagnosis and treatment(See Table 3).
2. A general term for all the meridian points on the back, originally from *Zhenjiu Zisheng Jing* (*Acupuncture and Moxibustion Classic for Saving Life*).

● 背阳关[bèi yáng guān] 经穴别名。出《针灸大全》。即腰阳关。详见该条。

Beiyangguan Another name for Yaoyangguan (DU 3), a meridian point from *Zhenjiu Daquan* (*A Complete Work of Acupunction and Moxibustion*). →腰阳关(p.546)

● 本池[běn chí] 经穴别名。出《针灸甲乙经》。即廉泉。详见该条。

Benchi Another name for Lianquan (RN 23), a meridian point from *Zhenjiu Jia-Yi Jing* (*A-B Classic of Acupuncture and Moxibustion*). →廉泉(p.244)

● 本节[běn jié] 部位名。指掌指关节或跖趾关节。以关节两端的圆形突起(包括关节囊所覆盖处)为准,区分为"本节前"和"本节后"。即以远端为前,近端为后。

Basic Joints of Extremities Joints of the body, referring to the metacarpaphalangeal and metatarsophalangeal joints (including both the joints and the parts covered by the joint capsules). "Anterior to the basic joints of extremities" means distal to these joints and "posterior to the basic joints of extremities" means proximal to these joints.

表3 十二背俞穴
Table 3 The 12 Back-Shu Points

六脏 Six Zang Organs	背俞 Back-Shu Points	六腑 Six Fu Organs	背俞 Back-Shu Points
肺 Lung	肺俞 Feishu(BL 13) Lung-shu	大肠 Large Intestine	大肠俞 Dachangshu(BL 25) Large-intestine-shu
肾 Kidney	肾俞 Shenshu(BL 23) Kidney-shu	膀胱 Bladder	膀胱俞 Pangguangshu(BL 28) Bladder-shu
肝 Liver	肝俞 Ganshu(BL 18) Liver-shu	胆 Gallbladder	胆俞 Danshu(BL 19) Gallbladder-shu
心 Heart	心俞 Xinshu(BL 15) Heart-shu	小肠 Small Intestine	小肠俞 Xiaochangshu(BL 27) Small-intestine-shu
脾 Spleen	脾俞 Pishu(BL 20) Spleen-shu	胃 Stomach	胃俞 Weishu(BL 21) Stomach-shu
心包 Pericardium	厥阴俞 Jueyinshu(BL 14) Pericardium-shu	三焦 Sanjiao	三焦俞 Sanjiaoshu(BL 22) Sanjiao-shu

● 本经取穴[běn jīng qǔ xué]　取穴法之一。指在疾病所属的经脉上选取穴位。如肺病取太渊、鱼际。脾病取太白、三阴交。急性腰痛针水沟等。

Acupoint Selection along the Affected Meridian　One of the principles of point selection, i. e. selecting acupoints along the diseased meridian, e. g, puncturing Taiyuan(LU 9), and Yuji(LU 10)for lung diseases, Taibai(SP 3)and Sanyinjiao(SP 6)for spleen diseases; and Shuigou(DU 26)for acute lumbar muscle sprain, etc.

● 本神[běn shén]　经穴名。出《针灸甲乙经》。属足少阳胆经, 为足少阳、阳维之会。又名直耳。〈定位〉在头部, 当前发际上0.5寸, 神庭旁开3寸, 神庭与头维连线的内2/3与外1/3的交点处。(图28)〈层次解剖〉皮肤→皮下组织→额肌。布有眶上动、静脉和眶上神经以及颞浅动、静脉额支。〈主治〉头痛、目眩、癫痫、小儿惊风、颈项强痛、胸胁痛、半身不遂。平刺0.5～0.8寸; 可灸。

Benshen(GB 13)　A Meridian point from *Zhenjiu Jia-Yi Jing*(*A-B Classic of Acupuncture and Moxibustion*), a point on the Gallbladder Meridian of Foot-Shaoyang and Yangwei Meridians, also named Zhier. 〈Location〉on the head, 0.5 cun within the anterior hair line, 3 cun lateral to Shenting(DU 24), at the juncture of the lateral 1/3 and medial 2/3 of the distance between Shenting(DU 24)and Touwei(ST 8). (Fig. 28)〈Regional anatomy〉skin → subcutaneous tissue → frontal muscle. There are frontal branches of superficial temporal artery and vein lateral branches of frontal artery and vein, and lateral branches of frontal nerve. 〈Indications〉headache, dizziness and vertigo, epilepsy, infantile convulsion, stiffness and pain of the neck, pain in the chest and hypochondrium, hemiplegia. 〈Method〉Puncture horizontally 0.5～0.8 cun. Moxibustion is applicable.

● 崩漏[bēng lòu]　病证名。见《济生方》。又称崩中漏下。崩, 指不在经期突然阴道大量出血, 来势急骤, 出血如注; 漏, 是出血量少, 淋沥不止。或经期血来, 量少而持续日久不止者。前人以其出血淋沥不断, 如器之漏而故名。在发病过程中, 两者常易互相转化。如崩血渐少, 可能致漏, 漏势发展又可转变为崩, 因此, 不易截然分开, 故多以崩漏并称。本病主要由于冲任损伤, 不能固摄所致。临床分血热崩漏、湿热崩漏、气郁崩漏、血瘀崩漏、气虚崩漏、阳虚崩漏、阴虚崩漏。详见各条。

Metrorrhagia and Metrostaxis　A disease from *Jisheng Fang*(*Recipes for Saving Lives*), also termed as bursting and leaking. Bursting means sudden massive bleeding prior to or beyond the menstrual period. Leaking means incessant dripping of blood from the uterus. It also refers to light but lingering menstrual blood during menstruation. In the process of the disease, bursting and leaking are often interconvertible, i. e. bursting may turn into leaking and vice versa, therefore, the two can not be divided and are often termed together as bursting-leaking, i. e. metrorrhagia and metrostaxis. It is mainly due to impairment and debility of the Chong and Ren Meridians, which therefore fail to control the blood. Clinically, it is divided into many types according to causes: metrorrhagia and metrostaxis due to blood-heat, damp-heat, qi stagnation, blood stasis, qi deficiency, yang insufficiency, and yin deficiency. → 血热崩漏(p. 527)、气郁崩漏(p. 313)、血瘀崩漏(p. 530)、气虚崩漏(p. 310)、阳虚崩漏(p. 541)、阴虚崩漏(p. 560)

● 崩中漏下[bēng zhōng lòu xià]　崩漏的别名。详见该条。

Bursting and Leaking　Another name for metrorrhagia and metrostaxis. → 崩漏(p. 18)

● 鼻冲[bí chōng]　经穴别名。出《针灸甲乙经》。即曲差。详见该条。

Bichong　Another name for Qucha(BL 4), a meridian point from *Zhenjiu Jia-Yi Jing*(*A-B Classic of Acupuncture and Moxibustion*). → 曲差(p. 323)

● 鼻穿[bí chuān]　经外穴别名。见《针灸经外奇穴治疗诀》。即上迎香。详见该条。

Bichuan　Another name for Shangyingxiang(EX-HN 8), an extra point seen in *Zhenjiu Jingwei Qixue Zhiliao Jue*(*Pithy Acupuncture Formulas for Treatment with Extra Points*). → 上迎香(p. 355)

● 鼻疔[bí dīng]　病证名。见《外科正宗》。红者, 又

名火珠疔；白者，又名白刃疔。由肺经火毒凝聚而成。生鼻孔内，自觉麻痒，红肿胀痛，或生小白泡，顶硬根突，堵塞鼻窍，甚则痛引脑门，腮唇俱肿，破流脓水，易引起疔毒内攻。治宜清热解毒。详见"疔疮"条。

Furuncle of Nose A disease, from *Waike Zhengzong* (*Orthodox Manual of External Diseases*), referring to a furuncle inside the nose. Red ones are known as fire-bead-like furuncles and white ones as naked-sword-like furuncles. They are usually due to accumulation of fire-toxin in the Lung Meridian. It is marked by itching redness, swelling, distending pain, or a small white vesicle with a hard tip and protruding root blocking the nasal cavity. Severe cases may induce pain in the forehead, swelling of the checks and lips, pus on breakage, and an internal attack of furunculosis. It should be treated by clearing heat and toxic materials. →疔疮(p. 82)

● 鼻洪[bí hóng] 指鼻中出血不止。参见"鼻衄"条。

Serious Case of Epistaxis Endless bleeding from inside the nose. →鼻衄(p. 19)

● 鼻环[bí huán] 经外穴名。出《刺疔捷法》。在面部，当鼻翼向外隆突最高点与面相接处。〈主治〉疔疮、酒齇鼻等。沿皮刺0.3～0.5寸。或点刺出血。

Bihuan(EX-HN) An extra point from *Ciliao Jiefa* (*Simple Acupuncture Methods for Boils*) 〈Location〉on the border between the highest point on the lateral protuberance of alanasi and cheek. 〈Indications〉 furuncle, brandy nose, etc. 〈Method〉Puncture subcutaneously 0.3～0.5 cun or bleed by pricking.

● 鼻交[bí jiāo] 鼻交頞中穴的简称。详见该条。

Bijiao Shortened name for Bijiaoezhong (EX-HN). →鼻交頞中(p. 19)

● 鼻交頞中[bí jiāo è zhōng] 经外穴名。见《千金翼方》。又名鼻交。在鼻骨最高处凹陷中。〈主治〉癫风、角弓反张、羊鸣、大风、青风、面如虫行、卒风、多眠健忘、心中愦愦、口噤不识人、黄疸、八种大风。沿皮刺0.3～0.5寸；可灸。

Bijiaoezhong（EX-HN） An extra point, from *Qianjin Yifang* (*Supplement to Essential Prescriptions Worth a Thousand Gold*), also called Bijiao.〈Location〉in the depression slightly above the highest part of the nasal bone.〈Indications〉depressive psychosis, opisthotonus, bleating, leprosy, bluish glaucoma, facial windstroke, drowsiness, amnesia, vexation, lockjaw, failure to recognize others, jaundice, and eight kinds of leprosy.〈Method〉Puncture Subcutaneously 0.3-0.5 cun. Moxibustion is applicable.

● 鼻流[bí liú] 经外穴名。见《千金要方》。在鼻孔口，禾髎穴上方，正鼻孔口之中间处。〈主治〉中风、面瘫、鼻塞、鼻炎、流涕，以及嗅觉减退、三叉神经痛、咀嚼肌痉挛等。斜刺0.3～0.5寸。

Biliu(EX-HN) An extra point, from *Qianjin Yaofang* (*Essential Prescriptions Worth a Thousand Gold*),〈Location〉above Heliao (LI 19), on the midpoint of the lower border of the nostril.〈Indications〉facial paralysis, stuffy nose, running nose hyposmia, rhinitis, prosopalgia, masticatory spasm, etc..〈Method〉Puncture obliquely 0.3～0.5 cun.

● 鼻衄[bí nù] 病证名。见《素问玄机原病式》。又名鼻中出血、鼻衄血。若鼻中出血不止，名为鼻洪。多由肝火、肺热，胃热所致。临床分为肺热鼻衄和肝火鼻衄。详见该条。

Epistaxis A disease from *Suwen Xuan Jiyuan Bing shi* (*Exploration of Mysterious Etiology in Plain Questions*), also called bleeding from inside the nose or nasal bleeding. Endless bleeding from inside the nose is named "serious case of epistaxis". This pathologic state is usually due to liver fire, retention of pathogenic heat in the lung or stomach-heat, and is clinically divided into epistaxis due to lung-heat, epistaxis due to stomach-heat, and epistaxis due to liver-fire. →肺热鼻衄(p. 108)胃热鼻衄(p. 464)肝火鼻衄(p. 124)

● 鼻衄血[bí nù xuè] 即鼻衄。详见该条。

Nasal Bleeding. →鼻衄(p. 19)

● 鼻通[bí tōng] 经外穴别名。见《常用新医疗法手册》。即上迎香。详见该条。

Bitong Another name for Shangyingxiang (EX-HN 8), an extra point from *Changyong Xingyi Liaofa Shouce* (*A Manual of New Therapies in Frequent Use*). →上迎香(p. 355)

● 鼻渊[bí yuān] 病证名。出《素问·气厥论》。又名辛頞鼻渊。重症名脑漏、脑渗。又名脑寒、脑崩、控脑

砂。以鼻流腥臭脓涕，鼻塞，嗅觉减退为主症。临床分为风寒化热鼻渊和肝胆火旺鼻渊。详见各条。

Thick Discharge from Nose A disease from *Suwen: Qijue Lun* (*Plain Questions: On Reversed Flow of Qi of Zang-Fu Organs*), referring to rhinorrhea and sinusitis, also called tingling in the roof of the nose and rhinorrhea. The serious case is called leaking of the brain or oozing of the brain. Also called brain coldness, brain collapse or uncotrolled brain. 〈Main manifestations〉 copious foul, purulent discharge from the nose accompanied by stuffy nose, hyposmia. Clinically it is divided into: thick discharge from nose due to heat resulting from wind-cold; thick discharge from nose due to fire in the liver and the gallbladder. →风寒化热鼻渊(p. 111)、肝胆火旺鼻渊(p. 124)

●鼻针[bí zhēn] 治病方法之一。指针刺鼻部特定穴位以治病的方法。其选用穴位以《灵枢·五色》的记载为依据，但临床应用不广泛。

Nasal Acupuncture An acupuncture therapy, i.e., to treat diseases by needling particular points on the nose, the points are selected according to what is recorded in *Lingshu: Wuse* (*Miraculous Pivot: Five Colors*), but this therapy is not extensively used in clinic.

●鼻中出血[bí zhōng chū xuè] 即鼻血。详见该条。

Bleeding from Inside the Nose. →鼻衄(p. 19)

●鼻准[bí zhǔn] ①部位名。指鼻端。②经穴别名。见《奇效良方》。即素髎。详见该条。

1. **Apex Nasi** A body part, referring to the apex of the nose.
2. **Bizhun** Another name for Suliao (DU 25), a meridian point from *Qixiao Liangfang* (*Prescriptions of Wonderful Efficacy*). →素髎(p. 416)

●闭癃[bì lóng] 即癃闭。详见该条。

Dysuria Synonymous with uroschesis, referring to retention of urine. →癃闭(p. 255)

●痹证(bì zhèng) 病证名。见《证治汇补》。指外邪侵入肢体经络、肌肉、关节，气血流行不畅，引起疼痛、肿大、重胀或麻木等症，甚则动转困难，总称痹证。多因卫气不固，腠理疏松，或感受风、寒、湿、热之邪，痹阻经络所致。临床分为行痹、痛痹、着痹、热痹

四种。详见各条。

Arthralgia Syndrome A disease, from *Zheng zhi Huibu* (*A Supplement to Diagnosis and Treatment*), generally referring to pain, swelling pressure, distention or numbness, even stiffness, in serious cases, of muscles or joints due to an invasion of exogenous pathogenic factors upon the extremity meridians and collaterals, muscles and joints and the failure of qi and blood to flow freely. It is mostly induced by instability of the defensive energy, loose striae of the skin, or by the patient's suffering from pathogenic wind-cold dampness or heat, thus causing the stagnation of meridians and collaterals. It is clinically divided into 4 kinds: migratory arthralgia, pain arthralgia (cold arthralgia), lingering arthralgia (damp arthralgia) and heat arthralgia. →行痹(p. 511)、痛痹、(p. 443)着痹(p. 623)、热痹(p. 330)

●蔽骨[bì gǔ] 部位名。见《针灸甲乙经》。指胸骨剑突。因其包埋于腹直肌鞘内较为隐蔽，不易触及而得名。

Hidden Bone A body part from *Zhenjiu Jia-Yi Jing* (*A-B Classic of Acupuncture and Moxibustion*), referring to the xiphoid process of the sternum. It is so named because it stays inside the vagina musculi recti abdominis and is hard to feel.

●蔽心骨[bì xīn gǔ] 部位名。见《类经图翼》。即蔽骨。详见该条。

Xiphoid A body part from *Leijing Tuyi* (*Supplements to Illustrated Classified Canon of Internal Medicine of the Yellow Emperor*), also named hidden bone. →蔽骨(p. 20)

●薜息[bì xī] 经穴别名。出《备急千金要方》。即乳根。详见该条。

Bixi Another name for Rugen (ST 18), a meridian point from *Beiji Qianjin Yaofang* (*Essential Prescriptions Worth a Thousand Gold for Emergencies*). →乳根(p. 338)

●臂骨[bì gǔ] 骨骼名。指尺骨和桡骨。

Forearm Bones Bones of the body, referring to the ulna and radius.

●臂间[bì jiān] 经外穴名。见《千金要方》。在前臂掌侧，当掌后横纹正中直上五横指，掌长肌腱与桡侧

腕屈肌腱之间。〈主治〉疔肿。直刺0.5～1寸;可灸。

Bijian(EX-UE)　An extra point from *Qianjin Yaofang*(*Essential Prescriptions Worth a Thousand Gold*).〈Location〉on the palmar side of the forearm, 5 fingers' breadth above the middle point of the crease of wrist, and between the long palmar muscle and radial carpal flexer muscle.〈Indications〉furuncle and sores.〈Method〉Puncture perpendicularly 0.5～1 cun. Moxibustion is applicable.

●臂巨(钜)阴脉[bì jù yīn mài]　早期经脉名。出《帛书》。与手太阴经类似。

Meridian of Arm-Juyin　An earlier name of a meridian, originally from *Bo Shu* (*Silk Book*), similar to the Meridian of Hand-Taiyin.

●臂脑[bì nǎo]　经穴别名。出《太平圣惠方》。即臂臑。详见该条。

Binao　Another name for Binao(LI 14), a meridian point, seen in *Taiping Shenghuifang* (*Imperial Benevolent Prescriptions*).→臂臑(p. 21)

●臂臑[bì nào]　经穴名。出《针灸甲乙经》。属手阳明大肠经,为手足太阳、阳维交会穴。又名头冲、颈冲、颈中、臂脑。〈定位〉在臂外侧,三角肌止点处,当曲池与肩髃连线上,曲池上7寸。(图48和图6)〈层次解剖〉皮肤→皮下组织→三角肌。浅层有臂外侧上、下皮神经等分布。深层有肱动脉的肌支。主治瘰疬、颈项拘急、肩臂疼痛、目疾。直刺0.5～1寸,或斜刺0.8～1.2寸;可灸。

Binao(LI 14)　A meridian point seen in *Zhenjiu Jia-Yi Jing*(*A-B Classic of Acupuncture and Moxibustion*), a point of the Large Intestine Meridian of Hand Taiyang and the crossing point of the Hand- and Foot-Taiyang Meridians and the Yingwei Meridian, also named Touchong, Jingchong, Jingzhong and Binao(臂脑).〈Location〉on the lateral side of the arm, at the insertion of the deltoid muscle, on the line connecting Quchi(LI 11)and Jianyu(LI 15), 7 cun above Quchi(LI 11). (Figs. 48 & 6)〈Regional anatomy〉skin → subcutaneous tissue → deltoid muscle. In the superficial layer, there are the inferior and superior lateral cutaneous nerves of the arm. In the deep layer, there are the muscular branches of the brachial artery.〈Indications〉scrofula, spasmodic rigidity of the neck, pain in the shoulder and arm and eye diseases.〈Method〉Puncture perpendicularly 0.5～1 cun, or puncture obliquely 0.8～1.2 cun. Moxibustion is applicable.

●臂少阳脉[bì shào yáng mài]　早期经脉名。出《帛书》。与手少阳经类似。

Meridian of Arm-Shaoyang　An earlier name of a meridian, originally from *Boshu*(*Silk Book*), similar to the Meridian of Hand-Shaoyang.

●臂少阴脉[bì shào yīn mài]　早期经脉名。出《帛书》。与手少阴经类似。

Meridian of Arm-Shaoyin　An earlier name of a meridian, originally from *Bo Shu* (*Silk Book*), similar to the Meridian of Hand-Shaoyin.

●臂(臂)石子头[bì shí zǐ tóu]　经外穴名。出《千金要方》。在前臂掌侧桡侧缘,腕横纹上3寸处。〈主治〉马黄黄疸。可灸。

Bishizitou(EX-UE)　An extra point, originally from *Qianjin Yaofang* (*Essential Prescriptions Worth a Thousand Gold*)〈Location〉in the palmar aspect, on the radial border of the forearm, 3 cun above the transverse wrist crease.〈Indications〉jaundice.〈Method〉Moxibustion is applicable.

●臂泰阳脉[bì tài yáng mài]　早期经脉名。出《帛书》。与手太阳经类似。

Meridian of Arm-Taiyang　An earlier name of a meridian, originally from *Bo Shu*(*Silk Book*), similar to the Meridian of Hand-Taiyang.

●臂泰阴脉[bì tài yīn mài]　早期经脉名。出《帛书》。与手太阴经类似。

Meridian of Arm-Taiyin　An earlier name of a meridian, originally from *Bo Shu*(*Silk Book*), similar to the Meridian of Hand-Taiyin.

●臂五里[bì wǔ lǐ]　经穴别名。出《圣济总录》。即手五里。详见该条。

Biwuli　Another name for Shouwuli(LI

13), a meridian point originally from *Sheng Ji Zonglu*(*Imperial Medical Encyclopaedia*). → 手五里(p. 401)

● 臂阳明脉[bì yáng míng mài] 早期经脉名。出《帛书》。与手阳明经类似。

Meridian of Arm-Yangming An earlier name of a meridian, originally from *Bo Shu* (*Silk Book*), similar to the Meridian of Hand-Yangming.

● 髀[bì] 部位名,一说指股之上端;一说膝上通称髀。即大腿部。

Bone of the Thigh A body part, referring to ①the upper part of the thigh, or ②the whole part above the knee i. e., the thigh.

● 髀关[bì guān] ①经穴名。出《灵枢·经脉》。属足阳明胃经。〈定位〉在大腿前面,当髂前上棘与髌底外侧端的连线上,屈股时,平会阴,居缝匠肌外侧凹陷处(图86)。〈层次解剖〉皮肤→皮下组织→阔筋膜张肌与缝匠肌之间→股直肌→股外侧肌。浅层布有股外侧皮神经。深层有旋股外侧动、静脉的升支,股神经的肌支等。〈主治〉髀阴痿痹,足麻不仁,腰肌疼痛,筋急不得屈伸。直刺0.6～1.2寸;可灸。②部位名。指大腿前上方的弯曲处。

1. Biguan (ST 31) A meridian point, from *Lingshu: Jingmai* (*Miraculous Pivot: Meridians*), on the Stomach Meridian of Foot-Yangming. 〈Location〉on the anterior side of the thigh and on the line connecting the anteriosuperior iliac spine and the superiolateral corner of the patella, on the level of the perineum when the thigh is flexed, in the depression lateral to the sartorius muscle(Fig. 86). 〈Regional anatomy〉 skin→subcutaneous tissue→ between tensor muscle of fascia lata and sartorius muscle→rectus muscle of thigh→lateral vastus muscle of thigh. In the superficial layer, there is the lateral cutaneous nerve of the thigh. In the deep layer, there are the ascending branches of tje lateral circumfles femoral artery and vein and the muscular branches of the femoral nerve. 〈Indications〉 paralysis of lower extremities, numbness of foot, pain in the lumbar muscles, muscular contraction leading to the failure of the muscle to flex and extend. 〈Method〉 Puncture perpendicularly 0.6～1.2 cun. Moxibustion is applicable.

2. Thigh Pass A body part, i. e. the anterior upper bending spot of the thigh.

● 髀枢[bì shū] 部位名。出《灵枢·骨度》。指髋关节。

Thigh Pivot A body part, from *Lingshu: Gudu* (*Miraculous Pivot: Bone Measurement*), referring to the hip joint.

● 髀厌[bì yàn] ①指髋关节部,与髀枢义同。②指环跳穴。详见该条。

1. Epiglottis of Thigh Synonymous with thigh pivot.

2. Biyan →环跳(p. 170)

● 砭法[biān fǎ] 古针法。出《帛书》。又名砭镰法、飞针。用尖石、石片或陶瓷碎片在疮疡、红肿处割刺,以排除脓血,使热毒外泄,肿消痛减。

Stone Needling An ancient acupuncture method, originally from *Bo Shu*(*Silk Book*), also called stone needling therapy or flying needle. A method of using pointed stones, pieces of stone or fragments of ceramics to cut and prick at sores and ulcers or red-swollen areas for pus drainage and blood letting, thus expelling noxious heat and relieving pain and swelling.

● 砭灸处[biān jiǔ chù] 腧穴别名。详见该条。

Applicable Places for Stone Needling and Moxibustion Another name for acupoints. →腧穴(p. 407)

● 砭镰法[biān lián fǎ] 古针法。即砭法。详见该条。

Stone Needle Therapy An ancient acupuncture method. →砭法(p. 22)

● 砭石[biān shí] 古针具名。出《素问·宝命全形论》等篇。中国古代的一种石制医疗工具,又称石针。其形状或者有锋,或者有刃,所以又称针石或镵石。因此,砭石是各种不同石针的总称。而一边磨锐的刀形石块也称为砭石,主要用于切割脓肿以排脓放血。参见"石针"、"针石"、"镵石"条。

Sharp Stone A term for ancient needles, originally from *Suwen: Bao Ming Quan Xing Lun*(*Plain Questions: On Mainteinance of Life and Body*) and other chapters. A primary medical instrument made of stone in ancient China, also called stone needle. With a sharp point or cutting edge it is also called needling stone or sagital stone. Therefore, "stones used

for needling" is a general term for a diversity of stone needles. A knife-like stone with one edge sharpened is also called sharp stone, mainly used to cut abscesses for pus drainage and blood letting. →石针(p. 386)、针石(p. 596)、镵石(p. 31)

●扁骨[biǎn gǔ] ①经穴别名。出《太平圣惠方》。即肩髃穴。见该条。②骨骼名。指颅盖、肩胛等形如板，无髓腔的骨。

1. **Biangu**   Another name for Jianyu (LI 15), a meridian point originally from *Taiping Shenghui Fang* (*Imperial Benevolent Prescriptions*). →肩髃(p. 191)

2. **Flat Bone**   Name of skeleton, referring to bones which resemble flat boards in shape and have no medullary cavity, such as the skullcap, scapula, etc.

●扁平疣[biǎn píng yóu] 病证名。是发生于皮肤的小赘物。表面光滑的扁平小疣，如半粒或黄豆大小，呈浓褐色或正常肤色，一般无痛痒。本病多由风热之邪搏于肌肤，或因肝气郁结，气血凝滞，发于肌肤而成。根据扁平疣所发部位，按循经取穴同局部取穴相结合的原则，取阳明经穴为主治疗。取中渚、丘墟、曲池、鱼际、阿是穴。风热所致者，加风池、商阳；肝郁所致者，加行间、侠溪。

Flat Wart   A disease referring to a small flat vegetation occurring on the skin with a smooth surface and deep brown or normal color. The spot can be as small as a soybean or a grain of rice, it usually occurs without pain or itching. It is generally caused by conjoint invasion of pathogenic wind and heat in muscles and skin or, liver-qi stagnation causing the stagnation of qi and blood and affecting muscles and skin. According to the location of the flat wart and the principle of combining the selection of points along the course with that of local points, select the points on the yangming meridians as a principle treatment, e. g., Zhongzhu (SJ 3), Qiuxu (GB 40), Quchi (LI 11), Yuji (LU 10) and Ashi point. For cases due to pathogenic wind-heat, add Fengchi (GB 20) and Shangyang (LI 11); for cases due to the stagnation of the liver qi, Xingjian (LR 2), Xiaxi (GB 43).

●扁鹊[biǎn què] 人名。即战国时医学家秦越人，秦氏号扁鹊。参见"秦越人"条。

Bian Que   A medical expert in the period of the Warring States (475-421 B. C.). →秦越人 (p. 319)

●扁鹊神应针灸玉龙经[biǎn què shén yīng zhēn jiǔ yù lóng jīng] 书名。元代王国瑞著，一卷。成书于1329年。内载玉龙歌等多首针灸歌诀，对于针灸临床治疗有很多宝贵经验。该书现存于《四库全书》中。

Bian Que Shenying Zhenjiu Yulong Jing (**Bian Que's Jade Dragon Classics of Acupuncture and Moxibustion**)   A one volume book written by Wang Guorui of the Yuan Dynasty, finished in 1329, recorded in the book were the Jade Dragon Verse and many other verses on acupuncture and moxibustion which contain valuable experience for clinical treatment of acupuncture and moxibustion. This book is now included in *Siku Quanshu* (*Complete Works of Four Treasuries*).

●扁鹊心书[biǎn què xīn shū] 书名。宋代窦材著，三卷，撰于1146年。作者以《内经》为指导，上卷论施治原则、经络、灸法；中、下卷述及各病证的治疗。其中较为重视灸治。

Bian Que Xin Shu (**Bian Que's Medical Experiences**)   A book written by Dou Cai of the Song Dynasty, with the *Huangdi Neijing* (*Inner Canon of Huangdi*) as its guide, which has three volumes in all. The first volume deals with treatment principles, meridians, collaterals and moxibustion, and the second and third volumes deal with the treatment of various diseases. In addition, more emphasis is laid on moxibustion in the book.

●扁鹊针传[biǎn què zhēn chuá] 书名。撰人不详，已佚。见宋人《崇文总目》。

Bian Que Zhen Chuan (**Bian Que's Bequeathed Acupuncture Techniques**)   Title of a lost book from the Song Dynasty, the author unknown. Recorded in *Chongwen Zongmu* (*Chong Wen Complete Catalogue*).

●扁桃体[biǎn táo tǐ] ①耳穴名。位于八区，参见牙条。用于治疗急性扁桃体炎、咽炎。②耳穴名。为轮1、轮2、轮3、轮4、轮5之别称。详见各条。

Tonsil (MA)   ① An auricular point, located

in the 8th section. →牙(MA)(p. 533)〈Indications〉 acute tonsillitis and phanynitis. ② A set of auricular points. →轮1(p. 258)轮2(p. 258)轮3(p. 258)轮4(p. 258)轮5(p. 258)

●便秘[biàn bì] 病证名。又名大便难、大便不通、大便秘结。指大便干燥坚硬,排出困难。或排便次数少,通常二、三天以上不大便者。有正虚与邪实的不同。临床上分为热秘、气秘、虚秘、冷秘四种。详见各条。

Constipation A disease, also called dyschesia, difficult bowel movement or dry stool, referring to difficulty in defecation with discharge of dry and impacted feces or infrequent defecation, e. g. having a bowel movement only once every 2~3 days or less. Constipation can be classified as deficient or excess type. Clinically, it is also divided into constipation due to heat, constipation due to disorder of qi, constipation of insufficient type, and constipation of cold type. →热秘(p. 329)气秘(p. 303)虚秘(p. 514)冷秘(p. 241)

●便毒[biàn dú] 经外穴名。见《外科大成》。在前臂屈侧,当掌长肌腱与桡侧腕屈肌腱之间,腕横纹上约4寸处。施灸可治肿痛。

Biandu (EX-UE) An extra point, originally from *Waike Dacheng* (*A Great Compendium of External Diseases*).〈Location〉on the flexor side of the forearm, between the tendons of the long palmar muscle and radial flexor muscle of the wrist, appoximately 4 cun above the crease of the wrist.〈Indication〉swelling and pain due to passing stools with poisonous materials.〈Method〉moxibustion.

●便血[biàn xuè] 病证名。出《素问·阴阳别论》。又称下血。指血从肛门而出。多由脾气虚弱,不能统血;或由大肠湿热所致。临床分为脾虚便血和湿热便血。详见各条。

Hemafecia A disease, originally from *Suwen:Yin Yang Bielun* (*Plain Questions:Supplementary Exposition of Yin and Yang*), also called passing blood, referring to the discharge of blood through the anus, mainly caused by the failure of the spleen to keep the flow of blood within the vessels resulting from insufficiency of the spleen or large intestinal damp-heat. Clinically it is divided into hemafecia due to hypofunction of the spleen and that due to damp-heat pathogen. →脾虚便血(p. 295)、湿热便血(p. 371)

●辨证取穴[biàn zhèng qǔ xé] 取穴法之一。根据辨证施治的原则,分析病证与脏腑、经络之间的关系,选取有关穴位。如失眠症属心脾两虚的,可选神门、三阴交。属肝胆火旺的,可选阳陵泉、太冲。属心肾不交的,可选神门、太溪。又如目视昏花,取肝俞以养肝明目。阴虚火旺的齿痛,取太溪以滋阴降火,均是。

Point Selection in Accordance with Differentiation of Syndrome One of the point-selecting principles relevant points are selected according to the principles of determining treatment on the basis of the differentiation of syndromes and through analyses of the relation between manifestations of a disease and zang-fu organs, meridians and collaterals, e. g., select Shenmen(HT 7) and Sanyinjiao(SP 6) for insomnia due to deficiency of qi and blood in the heart and spleen; Taichong (LR 3) and Yanglingquan (GB 34) for insomnia due to excess of fire in the liver and the gallbladder;Shenmen(HT 7)and Taixi (KI 3)for insomnia due to breakdown of the normal physiological coordination between the heart and the kidney. Select Ganshu (BL 18) for blurred vision to nourish the liver and improve visual acuity;select Taixi(KI 3)to nourish yin and reduce pathogenic fire for toothache caused by hyperactivity of fire due to yin deficiency, etc.

●表里配穴法[biǎo lǐ pèi xué fǎ] 配穴法之一。指按照十二经脉阳经与阴经的表里关系来配穴。如胃病取足阳明胃经的足三里和足太阴脾经的公孙;喉痛取手阳明大肠经的合谷和手太阴肺经的鱼际。古代文献中记载的原络配穴法,亦属此法范围。参见该条。

Exterior-Interior Point Prescription A method of the selection of related points, based on the exterior-interior relationship of the twelve Yin and Yang meridians, e. g., to select Zusanli(ST 36)and Gongsun(SP 4)for the treatment of stomach diseases;select Hegu (LI 4)and Yuji(LU 10)for sore-throat, etc. The combined selection of the Yuan(primary) point and Luo(connecting)point recorded in

ancient works belongs to this method. →原络配穴法(p. 576)

●**别阳**[bié yáng] ①经穴别名。出《针灸甲乙经》。即阳池。详见该条。②经穴别名。出《针灸甲乙经》。即阳交。详见该条。

Bieyang Another name for ① Yangchi(SJ 4), a meridian point, originally from *Zhenjiu Jia-yi Jing*(*A-B Classic of Acupuncture and Moxibustion*). →阳池(p. 536) ② Yangjiao (GB 35), a meridian point, originally from *Zhenjiu Jia-Yi Jing*(*A-B Classic of Acupuncture and Moxibustion*). →阳交(p. 538)

●**膑骨**[bìn gǔ] 经穴别名。见《针灸大全》。即环跳。详见该条。

Bingu Another name for Huantiao (GB 30), a meridian point originally from *Zhenjiu Dacheng* (*A Great Compendium of Acupuncture and Moxibustion*). i. e. →环跳(p. 170)

●**冰瑕翳**[bīng xiá yì] 目翳的别名。详见该条。

Thin Nebula→目翳(p. 273)

●**秉风**[bǐng fēng] 经穴名。出《针灸甲乙经》。属手太阳小肠经。为手阳明、太阳、手、足少阳之会。〈定位〉在肩胛部，冈上窝中央，天宗直上，举臂有凹陷处（图48和图65）。〈层次解剖〉皮肤→皮下组织→斜方肌→冈上肌。浅层布有第二胸神经后支的皮支和伴行的动、静脉。深层有肩胛上神经的分支和肩胛上动、静脉的分支或属支分布。主治肩胛疼痛、上肢酸麻。直刺0.5～0.7寸，可灸。不宜向锁骨上窝上方刺，以免损伤肺脏。

Bingfeng (SI 12) A meridian point, originally from *Zhenjiu Jia-Yi Jing* (*A-B Classic of Acupuncture and Moxibustion*), a point of the Small Intestine Meridian of Hand-Taiyang and the crossing point of the Yangming Meridian of Hand, the Taiyang Meridian of Hand and the Shaoyang Meridians of Hand and Foot. 〈Location〉 on the scapula, at the centre of the suprascapular fossa, directly above Tianzong (SI 11), in the depression found when the arm is raised. (Figs. 48 & 65) 〈Regional anatomy〉 skin→subcutaneous tissue→trapezius muscle→suprasinous muscle. In the superficial layer, there are the cutaneous branches of the posterior branches of the 2nd thoracic nerve and their accompanying arteries and veins. In the deep layer, there are the branches of the suprascapular nerve and the branches or tributares of the suprascapular artery and vein. 〈Indications〉 pain in scapular region, aching and numbness of the upper limb. 〈Method〉 Puncture perpendicularly 0.5～0.7 cun. Moxibustion is applicable. 〈Caution〉 Do not puncture the needle towards the region above the supraclavicular fossa to avoid hurting the lung.

●**病儿**[bìng ér] 即恶阻。详见该条。

Sickness in Pregnancy→恶阻(p. 93)

●**病隔**[bìng gé] 即恶阻。详见该条。

Affected Diaphragm Causing Sickness →恶阻 (p. 93)

●**病蟹叉**[bìng xiè chà] 即虎口疔。详见该条。

Fore-Legs of a Diseased Crab →虎口疔(p. 168)

●**病阻**[bìng zǔ] 即恶阻。详见该条。

Sickness due to Gravidity →恶阻(p. 93)

●**帛书经脉**[bó shū jīng mài] 医学文献名。长沙马王堆汉墓出土帛书之一。因其原无篇名，故据所载十一脉名为《帛书经脉》，名《十一脉灸经》。又分为《足臂十一脉灸经》和《阴阳十一脉灸经》。所论经脉与《内经》主要不同点：①只有十一脉而无十二经；②手脉称臂不称手，无臂厥阴；《阴阳十一脉经》不称臂三阳，而称为肩脉、耳脉、齿脉；③十一脉起止点、走行方向与《内经》的十二经不同，未提经络，亦未形成"如环无端"的循环概念；④十一脉中只有口条脉提到和脏腑联系，且多与《内经》不同；⑤所载各脉的病候，比《内经》简略。

Bo Shu Jingmai(Meridians of the Silk Book)

A medical work, one of the silk books unearthed in the Tomb of Han Dynasty at Ma Wang Mound in Changsha. Because no title was seen on the original, the title of *Bo Shu Jingmai*(*Meridians of the Silk Book*)was given to it later in accordance with the eleven meridians recorded in it. It was also entitled *Shiyimai Jiujing* (*Moxibustion Classic of the Eleven Meridians*), which is divided into *Zubi Shiyi Mai Jiujing*(*Moxibustion Classic of the Eleven Meridians of Foot and Arm*)and *Yin-Yang Shiyi Mai Jiujing* (*Moxibustion Classic of the Eleven Yin and Yang Meridians*). The main difference between the meridians dis-

cussed in this book and those discussed in *Huangdi Neijing* (*The Yellow Emperor's Inner Canon*) are as follows: ① Only eleven meridians are mentioned in the former rather than the twelve regular meridians mentioned in the latter. ② The meridians of the hand are referred to as those of the arm in the former with the absence of the Meridian of Arm-Jueyin; the three Yang Meridians of Arm are referred to as the shoulder meridian; the ear meridian and the tooth meridian in *Yin-Yang Shiyi Mai Jiujing* (*Moxibustion Classic of the Eleven Yin and Yang Meridians*). ③ The starting and ending points and the course directions of the eleven meridians are different from those in *Neijing* (*The Canon of Internal Medicine*). The concept of the meridian and collateral is not mentioned and the circulative concept of the meridians (like a circle without end) is also not formulated. ④ Only 4 out of the 11 meridians mentioned are related to zang-fu organs, and the relationship differs greatly from that in *Neijing* (*The Canon of Internal Medicine*). ⑤ Manifestations of diseases of separate meridians recorded in this book are simpler than those in *Neijing* (*The Inner Canon of Huangdi*).

●膊胦 [bó yāng] 经穴别名。出《针灸甲乙经》。即气海。详见该条。

Boyang Another name for Qihai (RN 6), a meridian point originally from *Zhenjiu Jia-Yi Jing* (*A-B Classic of Acupuncture and Moxibustion*). i.e. →气海 (p. 305)

●膊井 [bó jǐng] 经穴别名。出《太平圣惠方》。即肩井。详见该条。

Bojing Another name for Jianjing (GB21), a meridian point originating from *Taiping Shenghui Fang* (*Imperial Benevolent Prescriptions*). →肩井 (p. 189)

●擘蟹毒 [bò xiè dú] 即虎口疔。详见该条。

Thumb-Crad Poison →虎口疔 (p. 168)

●补母泻子法 [bǔ mǔ xiè zǐ fǎ] 针刺补泻手法之一。为子母补泻法之别称。详见该条。

The Combination of Reinforcing Mother Point and Reducing Son Point A kind of reinforcing and reducing method of acupuncture, another name for mother-child reinforcing-reducing. →子母补泻法 (p. 625)

●补生泻成 [bǔ shēng xiè chéng] 针刺补泻法之一。以针刺深浅结合生成数分补泻：补法从1～5分，即用一、二、三、四、五"生数"；泻法从6～10分，即用六、七、八、九、十"成数"。由于阳经的经浅、络深；阴

表4　　　　　　　　补　生　泻　成
Table 4　　　　　Reinforcing the growing and reducing the grown

经　脉 Meridians	络　脉 Collaterals	针刺浅深 Needling Depth (cun)	
		补 (生数) Reinforcement (Growing Number)	泻 (成数) Reduction (Grown Number)
膀胱、肾、三焦 bladder, kidney, sanjiao	胃、心、心包 stomach, heart, pericardium	1分 0.1(1)	6分 0.6(6)
小肠、心、心包 small intestine, heart, pericardium	膀胱、肺、三焦 bladder, lung, sanjiao	2分 0.2(2)	7分 0.7(7)
胆、肝 gallbladder, liver	大肠、脾 large intestine, spleen	3分 0.3(3)	8分 0.8(8)
大肠、肺 large intestine, lung	小肠、肝 small intestine, liver	4分 0.4(4)	9分 0.9(9)
胃、脾 stomach, spleen	胆、肾 gallbladder, kidney	5分 0.5(5)	1寸 1(10)

经的经深、络浅,所用补泻浅的标准各不同。各经规定的数字见表4。

Reinforcing the Growing and Reducing the Grown A kind of reinforcing and reducing methods of acupuncture, differentiating the reinforcing method and the reducing method according to the needling depth in combination with the growing and grown numbers. The needling depth of the reinforcing method is from 0.1～0.5 cun, namely, one, two, three, four and five, which are the so-called growing numbers; the needling depth of the reducing method is from 0.6 to 1 cun, namely, six, seven, eight, nine and ten, which are the so-called grown numbers. Because of the shallow meridians and deep collaterals of the Yang meridians the deep meridians and shallow collaterals of the Yin meridians, the standard of the needling depth varies from one to the other. The needling depth stipulated for each meridian is listed in Table 4.

●补泻手法[bǔ xiè shǒu fǎ]　针刺术语。指针刺补泻的操作手法。如捻转补泻法、提插补泻法等多种。补泻法中有的不属于手法操作则不宜称手法,如子母补泻等。但一般统称为针刺补泻法。参见该条。

Reinforcing and Reducing Manipulations An acupuncture term, referring to the manipulations of reinforcing and reducing during acupuncture. e.g. twirling reinforcing-reducing manipulation, reinforcing and reducing by lifting and thrusting the needle, and so on. Of the reinforcing and reducing methods, some do not belong to manipulations, so it is not appropriate to call them manipulations. e.g., mother-child reinforcing-reducing method, etc. But, they can generally be called reinforcing and reducing methods in acupuncture therapy. →针刺补泻法(p.588)

●补泻雪心歌[bǔ xiè xuě xīn gē]　针灸歌赋名。撰人不详,疑为席弘撰。

Bu Xie Xue Xin Ge（Verse for Clear Understanding of Reinforcing and Reducing） One of the verses on acupuncture. No details are known about its compiler. Xi Hong is hearsaid to be compiler.

●补元[bǔ yuán]　经穴别名。出《医学纲目》。即天枢。详见该条。

Buyuan Another name for Tianshu(ST 25), a meridian point from *Yixue Ganmu* (*An Outline of Medicine*). →天枢(p.434)

●补注铜人腧穴针灸图经[bǔ zhù tóng rén shū xué zhēn jiǔ tú jīng]　书名。无名氏补注。其在宋代王惟一《铜人腧穴针灸图经》三卷本的基础上,加入金大定丙午(1186年)闲邪聩叟的《针灸避忌太乙图序》而成五卷本。书中卷一、二载十二经穴和任、督脉穴;卷三、四、五分十二部,介绍各穴的主治和针灸方法。对经络、腧穴进行整理,并有增益。

Buzhu Tongren Shuxue Zhenjiu Tujing（Supplementary Annotation for the Illustrated Manual of Points Acupuncture and Moxibustion on a Bronze Statue with Acupoints） Title of a book of which the notes were supplemented by an anonymous author. Based on the three-volume version of *Tongren Shuxue Zhenjiu Tujing* (*The Illustrated Manual of Points for Acupuncture and Moxibustion on a Bronze Statue with Acupoints*) written by Wang Weiyi in the Song Dynasty, a five-volume edition came into being with the edition of *Zhenjiu Biji Taiyi Tuxu* (*Preface of Taiyi Diagram of Cautions in Acupunture*), Compiled by Xian Xie Kui Sou in the year of Bing Wu(1186)in the regime of Dading of the Jin Dnasty. The first two volumes deal with the points of the twelve regular meridians and the Ren and Du meridians. Volume 3～5 include twelve parts, in which the indications and the techniques of acupuncture and moxibustion of separate points are introduced. The meridians and points are systematically arranged and supplemented.

●不得眠[bù dé mián]　病证名。出《金匮要略·惊悸吐衄下血胸满瘀血病脉证治》。又名不得卧、不寐。即失眠症。详见"不寐"条。

Inability to Sleep A disease from *Jingui Yaolüe: Jingji Tuniü Xiaxue Xiongman Yuxue Bingmai Zhengzhi* (*Synopsis of the Golden Chamber: Pulse Conditions, Symptoms and Treatments of Fright, Palpitation, Bleeding, Fullness in Chest and Blood Stasis*), also named difficult sleep or insomnia. →不寐(p.

28)

● 不得卧 [bù dé wò]　见《素问·逆调论》。即失眠、不寐。详见"不寐"条。

Difficult Sleep　Insomnia, seen in *Suwen*: *Nitiao Lun* (*Plain Questions*: *On Disharmony*). →不寐(p. 28)

● 不定穴 [bù dìng xué]　与阿是穴同义。见《扁鹊神应针灸玉龙经》。又名天应穴。详见"阿是穴"条。

Unfixed Points　Synonymous with Ashi points, from *Bian Que Shen-Ying Zhenjiu Yulong Jing* (*Bianque's Jade Dragon Classics of Acupuncture and Moxibustion*), also named Tianying points. →阿是穴(p. 1)

● 不寐 [bù mèi]　病证名。出《难经·四十六难》。又名不得眠、不得卧、失眠。指以经常性入睡困难、睡眠不足为特征的病证。其轻者经常入寐迟缓，或寐而时醒；其重者彻夜不眠。由气血失调，脏腑失和，阴阳逆乱，使神不安宁所致。临床可分为心脾两虚不寐、阴虚火旺不寐、胃腑失和不寐、肝火上扰不寐。详见各条。

Insomnia　A disease, from *Nanjing*: *Sishiliu Nan* (*The Classic of Questions*: *Question* 46), also called inability to sleep, or difficult sleep. 〈Manifestations〉 frequent difficulty in going to sleep, or lack of sleep. In mild cases, the patient often falls asleep slowly or wakes up frequently during sleep; in severe cases, he has no sleep at all through the night. 〈Pathology〉 disorder of qi and blood, disharmony between Zang and Fu organs and imbalance between Yin and Yang, which leads to instability of the spirit (mind). Clinically, this disease is divided into the following types: insomnia due to heart and spleen deficiency, insomnia due to yin deficiency and fire preponderance, insomnia due to derangement of the stomach and insomnia due to upward disturbance of the liver fire. → **心脾两虚不寐** (p. 509) **阴虚火旺不寐** (p. 560) **胃腑不和不寐** (p. 463) **肝火上扰不寐** (p. 124)

● 不容 [bù róng]　经穴名。出《针灸甲乙经》。属足阳明胃经。〈定位〉在上腹部，当脐中上6寸，距前正中线2寸(图60.4和图40)。〈层次解剖〉皮肤→皮下组织→腹直肌鞘前壁→腹直肌。浅层布有第六、七、八胸神经前支的外侧皮支和前皮支及腹壁浅静脉。深层有腹壁上动、静脉的分支或属支，第六、七胸神经前支的肌支。〈主治〉腹胀、呕吐、胃痛、食欲不振、喘咳、呕血、心痛、胸背胁痛。直刺0.5～1寸；可灸。

Burong (ST 19)　A meridian point, from *Zhenjiu Jia-Yi Jing* (*A-B Classic of Acupuncture and Moxibustion*), a point on the Stomach Meridian of Foot-Yangming. 〈Location〉 on the upper abdomen, 6 cun above the centre of the umbilicus and 2 cun lateral to the anterior midline. (Figs. 60.4 & 40) 〈Regional anatomy〉 skin→subcutaneous tissue→anterior sheath of rectus muscle of abdomen→rectus muscle of abdomen. In the superficial layer, there are the lateral and anterior cutaneous branches of the anterior branches of the 6th to 8th thoracic nerves and the superficial epigastric vein. In the deep layer, there are the branches or tributaries of the superior epigastric artery and vein and muscular branches of the anterior branches of the 6th and 7th thoracic nerves. 〈Indications〉 abdominal distension, vomiting, stomachache, poor, appetite, cough, asthma, haemate-mesis, precordial pain, chest, back and hypochondriac pains. 〈Method〉 Puncture perpendiculary 0.5～1 cun. Moxibustion is applicable.

● 不盛不虚以经取之 [bù shèng bù xū yǐ jīng qǔ zhī]　针灸治疗原则之一。出《灵枢·经脉》和《禁服》等篇。对虚实不明显的病症，只须按经取穴治疗，而不必分补泻，与"盛则泻之，虚则补之"的原则并列。

Selecting Points on the Affected Meridian Where a Neither-Excess-Nor-Deficiency Syndrome Lies　One of the principles of acupuncture treatment, from *Lingshu*: *Jingmai* (*Miraculous Pivot*: *Meridians*) and *Lingshu*: *Jin Fu* (*Miraculous Pivot*: *Disciplines and Submission*). A syndrome without obvious symptoms and signs of deficiency and excess will be treated with points according to the affected meridian instead of being treated by means of reinforcing or reducing. This principle of treatment is juxtaposed with the principles of "reducing for excess syndromes" and "reinforcing for deficiency syndromes".

● 不锈钢针 [bù xiù gāng zhēn]　针具名。近代以不锈钢为原料制成医用针具，一般多采用铬镍合成的不

锈钢制造。具有硬度强、质地韧、富有弹性和不易锈蚀等优点,为临床所常用。

Stainless Steel Needle A kind of needle, developed in modern times, made of stainless steel. The stainless steel in common use is chrome-nickel steel. This type of needle is tough, pliable, resilient, rustless and corrosion-resistant, therefore, it is commonly used in the clinic.

●**不月**[bù yuè] 经闭的别名。详见该条。

No Menses Another name for amenorrhea. →经闭(p. 208)

●**不月水**[bù yuè shuǐ] 经闭的别名。详见该条。

No Mensual Blood Another name for amenorrhea. →经闭(p. 208)

●**不孕**[bù yùn] 病证名。出《素问·骨空论》。又称无子、绝子、全不产、绝产、断绪。指夫妇同居三年以上,配偶健康,而不受孕;或曾孕育,但间隔三年以上未再受孕者,称为不孕。多因先天不足,肾气虚弱;或精血亏损,冲任虚衰,胞脉失养;或命门火衰,寒邪客于胞中;或气滞血瘀,胞络不通;或痰湿内生,闭塞胞宫所致。临床可分为肾虚不孕、血虚不孕、胞寒不孕、血瘀不孕、痰湿不孕等,详见各条。

Sterility A disease from *Suwen*: *Gukong Lun* (*Plain Questions*: *On Apertures of Bones*), also named childlessness, no offspring, no issue, no delivery or no posterity. Referring to cases where, three or more years after a couple begin living together, even though the man is healthy, the woman does not become pregnant; or to cases where, an interval of more than three years after an impregnation passes, and the woman no longer becomes pregnant. ⟨Etiology and pathology⟩ congenital insufficiency, deficiency of kidney-qi; loss and damage of essence and blood, asthenia and deficiency of Chong and Ren meridians, the loss of nourishment in the uterine; the decline of fire of the life gate, attack by pathogenic cold upon the uterus; stagnation of qi and blood leading to the obstruction of the uterine collaterals, or internal phlegm-dampness obstructing the uterus clinically. It is divided into sterility due to kidney deficiency, due to blood deficiency, due to retention of cold in the uterus, due to blood stasis and due to phlegm-dampness. →**肾虚不孕**(p. 365)、**血虚不孕**(p. 528)、**胞寒不孕**(p. 13)、**血瘀不孕**(p. 530)、**痰湿不孕**(p. 424)

●**步郎**[bù láng] 经穴别名。出《备急千金要方》。即步廊。详见该条。

Bulang Another name for Bulang(KI 22), a meridian point from *Beiji Qianjin Yaofang* (*Essential Prescriptions Worth a Thousand Gold for Emergencies*). →**步廊**(p. 29)

●**步廊**[bù láng] 经穴名。出《针灸甲乙经》。属足少阴肾经。⟨定位⟩在胸部,当第五肋间隙,前正中线旁开2寸(图40)。⟨层次解剖⟩皮肤→皮下组织→胸大肌。浅层布有第五肋间神经的前皮支,胸廓内动、静脉的穿支。深层有胸内、外侧神经的分支。⟨主治⟩胸痛、咳嗽、气喘、呕吐、不嗜食、乳痈。斜刺或平刺0.5～0.8寸;可灸。不可深刺,以免伤及内脏。

Bulang (KI 22) A point on the Kidney Meridian of Foot-Shaoyin, from *Zhenjiu Jia-Yi Jing* (*A-B Classic of Acupuncture and Moxioustion*). ⟨Location⟩ on the chest, in the 5th intercostal space, 2 cun lateral to the anterior midline. (Fig. 40) ⟨Regional anatomy⟩ skin → subcutaneous tissue → greater pectoral muscle. In the superficial layer, there are the anterior cutaneous branches of the 5th intercostal nerve and the perforating branches of the internal thoracic artery and vein. In the deep layer, there are the branches of the medial and lateral pectoral nerves. ⟨Indications⟩ chest pain, cough, asthma, vomiting, anorexia, acute martitis. ⟨Method⟩ Puncture obliquely or along the skin 0.5～0.8 cun. Moxibustion is applicable. Deep insertion should be avoided in case the internal organs are injured.

C

●采艾编[cǎi ài biān] 书名。为灸法专书,清叶广祚撰,四卷,刊于1668年。该书讨论了经脉经穴的部位、名称、主治、诊法及内、外、妇、儿各科疾病的灸法。

Cai Ai Bian (A Book on Adoption of Moxibustion) A book in four volumes, compiled by Ye Guangzuo of the Qing Dynasty, published in 1668. It discusses the locations, names, indications, diagnostic methods and of meridian points, and the treatment with moxibustion for internal, external, gynaecological and paediatrical diseases.

●采艾编翼[cǎi ài biān yì] 书名。清叶茶山撰,三卷,刊于1805年。其于灸法之外兼及药物,是《采艾编》的补充。卷一为经络、腧穴及灸法总论;卷二介绍各种疾病的灸法并配合药物;卷三介绍治疗外科病的方药。

Cai Ai Bianyi (Supplement to the Book on Adoption of Moxibustion) A book in three volumes, compiled by Ye Chashan, published in 1805, including the application of herbs, in addition to moxibustion methods, a supplement to *Cai Ai Bian* (*A Book on Adoption of Moxibustion*). Vol. 1 deals with meridians, points and an introduction to moxibustion, Vol. 2 introduces moxibustion methods with the combination of herbs for treating various diseases, and Vol. 3 the prescriptions and herbs for external diseases.

●苍龟探穴[cāng guī tàn xué] 针刺手法名。出《金针赋》。为飞经走气四法之一,与赤凤迎源对称。其法当将针刺入穴位后,退至浅层,然后依次斜向上、下、左、右,分别用三进一退的钻剔动作。如龟入土,探穴四方。有通行经气的作用。

Green Turtle Probing Its Cave A needling technique, from *Jinzhen Fu* (*Ode to Gold Needle*). One of the four methods of accelerating the flow of meridian-qi, corresponding to the method of "red phonix encountering the source" ⟨Manipulation⟩ After the insertion of the needle, lift it to the shallow layer, then, successively move the needle upwards, downwards, leftwards and rightwards; thrusting three times and lifting one time, as if a turtle were digging into the earth in four directions to find its cave. ⟨Function⟩ Promote the circulation of meridian qi.

●苍龙摆尾[cāng lóng bǎi wěi] 青龙摆尾之别称。详见该条。

Blue Dragon Wagging Its Tail Another name for green dragon wagging its tail. →青龙摆尾(p. 320)

●苍术灸[cāng zhú jiǔ] 间接灸的一种。见《医学入门》。又称隔苍术灸。是用苍术作间隔物而施灸的一种灸法。将苍术削成圆锥形,底面要切平,并用细针穿刺数个小孔,然后将尖头插进外耳道,于底面上置艾炷,点燃施灸。一般每次灸5—14壮,用于治疗耳暴聋、耳鸣等症。孕妇不宜使用。

Cang Zhu (Rhizoma Atractylodis) Moxibustion A kind of indirect moxibustion seen in *Yixue Rumen* (*An Introduction to Medicine*), also named Cang Zhu (*Rhizoma Atractylodis*)-separated moxibustion. ⟨Method⟩ Shape this herb into a circular cone, whose bottom is cut flat with several holes bored in it. Put the tip of the cone of atractylodes rhizome into the external auditory canal with a moxa cone on the bottom of it, then light the moxa cone. Generally 5-14 moxa-cones will be burnt at a time. ⟨Indications⟩ sudden deafness and tinnitus, etc. This method is not suitable for pregnant women.

●藏针器[cáng zhēn qì] 针刺用具。储藏针刺用品以便携带,古代多用布帛包裹,称针包。又有以金属制成的针筒。近代有以皮革或塑料制成的藏针夹以及笔管式的藏针管等。

Needle Container A container used to keep the articles for acupuncture in order to carry conveniently. In ancient times, acupuncture appliances were wrapped in cloth and silk, which was called a needle bag. Some were tubes made of metal and were called needle tubes. In recent times, needle cases and pen-like tubes made of leather or plastics have come into being.

●曹溪[cáo xī] 经穴别名。出《普济方》。即风府。详见该条。

Caoxi Another name for Fengfu(DU 16), a meridian point from *Puji Fang* (*Prescriptions for Universal Relief*). →风府(p.111)

●草鞋带穴[cǎo xié dài xué] 经穴别名。出《玉龙经·五龙歌》。即解溪。详见该条。

Caoxiedaixue Another name for Jiexi (ST 41), a meridian point from *Yulong Jing: Yulong Ge* (*Jade Dragon Classic: Jade Dragon Verses*). →解溪(p.202)

●侧伏坐位[cè fú zuò wèi] 针灸体位名。患者身体正坐，两臂侧屈伏于案上，头侧伏于臂，面部朝向一侧的体位。适用于取头部一侧、面颊及耳前后部位的腧穴。

Sitting with Head Turning Aside A body position. Have the patient take a sitting position with both arms leaning on a table, then turn the face to the side so that the head may rest on the arms. The position is suitable for selecting points on the side of head and cheeks and points around the auricle.

●侧卧位[cè wò wèi] 针灸体位名。患者身体一侧着床，头面、胸腹朝向一侧的体位。适用于取身体侧面少阳经腧穴，和上、下肢的部分腧穴。

Lateral Recumbent Position A body position. Have the patient lie on his/her side. This is suitable for selecting points on Shaoyang Meridians which distribute on the side of the body and some of the points of the upper and lower limbs.

●插花[chā huā] 经外穴名。出《刺疔捷法》。在头部，当额角（头维）直上1.5寸处。主治头面疔疮、偏头痛等。沿皮刺0.3～0.5寸；可灸。

Chahua (EX-HN) An extra point from *Ci Ding Jiefa* (*Simple Acupuncture Method for Boils*). 〈Location〉on the head, 1.5 cun directly above Equ (Touwei ST 8).〈Indications〉furuncles on head and face, migraine. etc.〈Method〉Puncture along the skin 0.3-0.5 cun. Moxibustion is applicable.

●缠耳[chán ěr] 即聤耳。详见该条。

Troublesome Ear→聤耳(p.439)

●缠络[chán luò] 络脉名。出《经络汇编》。指从系络分出的更细小络脉。

Twining Collaterals A kind of collateral, from *Jingluo Huibian* (*An Expository Manual of Meridians and Collaterals*), referring to the smaller and thinner collaterals branching from the large ones.

●缠腰火丹[chán yāo huǒ dān] 病证名。见《疡科选粹》，又名火带疮、蛇串疮。指生于胸胁及腹部一侧的疱疹疾病。详见"蛇丹"条。

Burning Sores Around Waist A disease seen in *Yangke Xuancui* (*Essence in Treatment of Sores*), also named "burning sores along the waist" or "snake-like blisters", referring to herpletic lesions on the chest and the side of the trunk. →蛇丹(p.359)

●镵石[chán shí]古针具名。见《素问·宝命全形论》。砭石的一种，即一端锥形，形象如箭头的石块。参见"砭石"条。

Sagital Stone An ancient needle seen in *Suwen: Baoming Quanxing Lun* (*Plain Questions: On Mainteinance of Life and Body*); a kind of stone used for needling i.e. a stone with one cone-shaped end like an arrow head. →砭石(p.22)

●镵针[chán zhēn] 针具名。见《灵枢·九针十二原》。又称箭头针，为古代九针之一。其长一寸六分，形似箭头，头大末锐，当末端一分处收小，形成尖端。用于浅刺皮肤泻血，治头身热证等。后人在此基础上发展为皮肤针。

Shear Needle A needle seen in *Lingshu: Jiu Zhen Shier Yuan* [*Miraclous Pivot: Nine Needles and Twelve Yuan (Primary) Points*], also named arrowhead needle or sagital needle. One of the nine classical needles with a length of 1.6 cun, shaped like an arrowhead. The head is big and the tip is sharp. At 0.1 cun far from the tip, it begins to taper and forms a

sharp end. The needle is used to let out blood and treat heat syndromes. Later, on the basis of this, it developed into the dermal needle.

●产后不语[chǎn hòu bù yǔ] 病证名。出《经效产宝·续篇》。多因产后败血不去,停积于心;或产后气血两虚,心气虚不能上通于舌;或痰热乘心,心气闭塞所致。败血停心者,证见面色紫黑、胸闷。治宜活血开郁。取神门、通里、膻中、印堂、太冲。心气虚者,证见心悸、气短、自汗。治宜补益气血。取神门、通里、内关、足三里。痰热乘心者,证见喉间有痰声、面热胸闷。治宜清痰热。取神门、通里、印堂、丰隆、内关。

Postpartum Aphasia A disease from *Jingxiao Chanbao*: *Xupian* (*Treasury of Effective Prescriptions in Obstetrics*: *Continuation*). 〈Etiology and pathology〉 ochioschesis upward which disturbs the heart; or the deficiency of qi and blood leading to a failure of heart qi in reaching the tongue, or heart qi obstruction due to the invasion of phlegm and heat into the heart. 〈Manifestations〉 those with syndromes of lochia disturbing the heart: dark purple comlexion, oppressive feeling in the chest. 〈Treatment principle〉 Activate blood cirulation and release stagnation. 〈Point selection〉 Shenmen (HT 7), Tongli (HT 5), Danzhong (RN 7), Yintang (EX-HN 3) and Taichong (LR 3). 〈Manifestations〉 those with a syndrome of heart-qi deficiency: palpitation, shortness of breath, and spontaneous perspiration. 〈Treatment principle〉 Invigorate qi and nourish blood. 〈Point selection〉 Shenmen (HT 7), Tongli (HT 5), Neiguan (PC 6) and Zusanli (ST 36). 〈Manifestations〉 those with a syndrome of heart attacked by phlegm and heat: wheezing sound in the throat, flushed face, and oppressive feeling in the chest. 〈Treatment principle〉 Clear phlegm and heat. 〈Point selection〉 Shenmen (HT 7), Tongli (HT 5), Yintang (EX-HN 3), Fenglong (ST 40) and Neiguan (PC 6).

●产后大便难[chǎn hòu dà biàn nán] 病证名。出《金匮要略·妇人产后病脉证并治》。多因产后失血,伤津,阴液不能润肠所致。证见产后饮食如常、大便不畅、或数日不解、或便时干燥疼痛、艰涩难下、面色萎黄、皮肤不润、舌淡苔薄、脉虚弦而涩。治宜养血润燥。取脾俞、胃俞、大肠俞、天枢、支沟、足三里。

Postpartum Constipation A disease from *Jingui Yaolüe*: *Furen Chanhoubing Maizheng Bingzhi* (*Synopsis of the Golden Chamber*: *Pulse Conditions, Syndromes and Treatment of Postpartum Diseases*). 〈Etiology and pathology〉 loss of blood, impairment of body fluids, and the inability of yin fluid to moisten the intestine. 〈Manifestations〉 normal diet, difficult bowel movements, or no bowel movements for several days, or painful and difficult defecation with dry stool, sallow complexion, dry skin, pale tongue with thin coating, feeble, wiry and choppy pulse. 〈Treatment principle〉 Enrich the blood and moisten the dryness. 〈Point selection〉 Pishu (BL 20), Weishu (BL 21), Dachangshu (BL 25), Tianshu (ST 25), Zhigou (SJ 6) and Zusanli (ST 36).

●产后耳聋[chǎn hòu ěr lóng] 病证名。见《诸病源候论》。多因产后气血损伤,肾虚气弱,精气不能上述于耳所致。证见产后突然耳聋、头晕、腰膝疲软乏力、舌淡、脉虚细。治宜补益肾气。取肾俞、关元、翳风、听会、侠溪、中渚。

Postpartum Deafness A disease seen in *Zhubing Yuanhou Lun* (*General Treatise on the Etiology and Symptomatology of Diseases*), caused by impairment of qi and blood, deficiency of kidney qi, and inability of essence qi to reach the ears. 〈Manifestations〉 sudden deafness, dizziness, lassitude and debility in the loins and knees, pale tongue, feeble and thready pulse. 〈Treatment principle〉 Tonify the kidney qi. 〈Point selection〉 Shenshu (BL 23), Guanyuan (RN 4), Yifeng (SJ 17), Tinghui (GB 2), Xiaxi (GB 43) and Zhongzhu (SJ 3).

●产后发痉[chǎn hòu fā jìng] 病证名。出《金匮要略·妇人产后病脉证并治》。又称产后发痓。指产后突然颈项强直,四肢抽搐,甚至口噤不开,角弓反张。多因产后阴血大亏,筋失所养,复为风邪所袭,引动肝风;或产后汗出过多,亡血伤津,虚极生风所致。临床有两种证型。复感风邪者,兼见发热恶寒、头项强痛、舌苔薄、脉浮而弦。治宜疏肝祛风,开窍醒神。取百会、风府、大椎、曲池、阳陵泉、太冲、十二井穴。虚极生风者,兼见面色苍白或萎黄、目瞑、神昏、舌淡红无苔、脉虚细。治宜育阴熄风。取劳宫、百会、水沟、行间、涌泉、太溪。

Postpartum Convulsion A disease from *Jingui Yaolüe: Furen Chanhoubing Maizheng Bingzhi* (*Synopsis of the Golden Chamber: Pulse Conditions, Syndromes and Treatment of Postpartum Diseases*), also named postpartum spasm, referring to a sudden stiff neck, convulsions of the four limbs, even opisthotonos and lockjaw appearing after delivery. 〈Etiology and pathology〉heavy loss of yin-blood, lack of nourishment of tendons, wind-evil attack resulting in the stir of liver-wind, or oversweating, leading to the impairment of blood and body fluids and extreme deficiency resulting in the stir of internal wind. Clinically, there are two kinds of syndromes: ① Syndrome with simultaneous invasion of wind. 〈Manifestations〉 fever and chills, headache, stiff neck, thin tongue coating, floating and wiry pulse. 〈Treatment principle〉 Disperse the depressed liver-qi and dispel wind; induce resuscitation and restore consciousness. 〈Point selection〉Baihui(DU 20), Fengfu(DU 16), Dazhui (DU 14), Quchi(LI 11), Yanglingquan (GB 34), Taichong(LR 3) and the Twelve Jing (Well) points. ② Syndrome of internal wind due to extreme deficiency. 〈Manifestations〉 pale or sallow complexion, heavy eyes, unconsciousness, pink tongue without fur, feeble and thready pulse. 〈Treatment principle〉 Nourish yin and calm the endopatnic wind. 〈Point selection〉Laogong (PC 8), Baihui(DU 20), Shuigou (DU 26), Xingjian (LR 2), Yongquan (KI 1) and Taixi(KI 3).

● 产后发热[chǎn hòu fā rè]　病证名。见《医学纲目》。指分娩后,因各种原因引起的发热。常见的有血虚、血瘀、外感等。血虚者,多因产时失血,阴不敛阳,虚热内生。证见身热、头晕、心悸或腹痛绵绵,舌淡红、脉细数。治宜补气血,清虚热。取百会、关元、足三里、内关、大椎、曲池、合谷。血瘀者,多因产后恶露不下,瘀血停滞,以致气机不利,营卫失调。证见寒热时作、恶露不下或下亦甚少、血色紫黯,挟有血块、少腹胀痛拒按、舌略紫、脉弦涩。治宜活血散瘀清热。取中极、气冲、地机、大椎、曲池、曲泽、十二井穴。外感者,多因产后气血骤虚,卫外不固,外邪乘虚袭入。证见恶寒发热、头痛身痛、腰背酸楚、无汗、苔白、脉浮。治宜养血祛风。取足三里、大椎、曲池、外关、合谷、委中。

Postpartum Fever A disease seen in *Yixue Gangmu* (*An Outline of Medicine*), referring to various kinds of fevers after delivery, generally caused by deficiency of blood, stagnation of blood and invasion of external evils. Deficiency of blood resulting from hemorrhage during delivery will lead to a failure of yin in restraining yang, and then deficient heat will be produced inside. 〈Manifestations〉fever, dizziness, palpitation, continuous mild abdominal pain, pink tongue, thready and rapid pulse. 〈Treatment principle〉 Nourish qi and blood, clear deficient heat. 〈Point selection〉 Baihui(DU 20), Guanyuan(RN 4), Zusanli (ST 36), Neiguan(PC 6), Dazhui (DU 14), Quchi(LI 11) and Hegu(LI 4). Stagnation of blood resulting from retention of lochia will cause disturbances of qi movements, and then imbalance of ying(nutrient qi)and wei (defensive qi). 〈Manifestations〉 chills and fever, lochioschesis or less lochia, dark purple blood with clots, lower abdominal distending pain and refusal to be pressed, purplish tongue, wiry and choppy pulse. 〈Treatment principle〉 Promote blood circulation by removing blood stasis and clearing beat. 〈Point selection〉 Zhongji (RN 3), Qichong(ST 30), Diji (SP 8), Dazhui(DU 14), Quchi (LI 11), Quze (PC 3) and Twelve Jing(Well)Points. Cases of external evil result from deficiency of qi and blood and failure of defensive qi in protecting the body against evils. 〈Manifestations〉chills and fever, headache, general aching, soreness in back and loins, no sweat, whitish tongue coating and floating pulse. 〈Treatement principle〉 Nourish blood and expel wind. 〈Point selection〉Zusanli(ST 36), Dazhui (DU 14), Quchi(LI 11), Waiguan(SJ 5), Hegu(LI 4) and Weizhong(BL 40).

● 产后发痓[chǎn hòu fā zhì]　即产后发痉。详见该条。

Postpartum Spasm→产后发痉(p. 32)

● 产后腹痛[chǎn hòu fù tòng]　病证名。见《古今医鉴》。又称儿枕痛。产妇分娩之后,小腹疼痛,称为产

后腹痛。多因血虚、血瘀、寒凝等所致。血虚者，证见小腹隐痛、腹软喜按、恶露量少色淡、头晕耳鸣、大便燥结、舌淡苔薄、脉虚细。治宜补血益气，调理冲任。取关元、气海、膈俞、足三里、三阴交。血瘀者，证见小腹胀痛、痛连胸胁、或小腹可摸到硬块、恶露量少、涩滞不畅、其色紫黯夹有瘀块、舌质微紫、脉弦涩。治宜行气化瘀，通络止痛。取中极、归来、膈俞、血海、太冲。寒凝者，证见小腹冷痛拒按、得热稍减、面色青白、四肢不温、舌质黯淡、苔白滑、**脉沉迟**。治宜助阳散寒，温通胞脉。取关元、气海、肾俞、三阴交。

Postpartum Abdominal Pain A disease seen in *Gujin Yijian* (*A Medical Reference of the Past and Present*), also named abdominal pain after delivery. The lower abdominal pain following childbirth is called postpartum abdominal pain. Mostly due to deficiency of blood, blood stasis and accumulation of cold. The syndrome of deficiency of blood is accompanied by dull lower adominal pain, relieved by soft pressure on the abdomen, less lochia with light red color, dizziness, tinnitus constipation, pale tongue with thin coating, feeble and thready pulse. 〈Treatment principle〉 Enrich the blood and nourish qi; regulate the Chong and Ren meridians. 〈Point selection〉 Guanyuan(RN 4), Qihai(RN 6), Geshu(BL 17), Zusanli(ST 36) and Sanyinjiao(SP 6). The syndrome of blood stasis is accompanied by lower abdominal distending pain rediating to the chest and hypochondrium, or a palpable mass in the lower abdomen, lochiorrhea with light flow, dark purple blood and clots, purplish tongue, wiry and choppy pulse. 〈Treatment principle〉 Activate qi and remove blood stasis; resolve obstruction in the meridians to relieve pain. 〈Point selection〉 Zhongji(RN 3), Guilai (ST 29), Geshu(BL 17), Xuehai(SP 10) and Taichong (LR 3). The syndrome of cold accumulation is accompanied by cold pain in the lower abdomen refusing to be pressed, but slightly relieved by heat, pale green face, cold limbs, dark grey tongue, whitish coating with fluid, deep and slon pulse. 〈Treatment principle〉 Strengthen yang and dispel cold; warm the uterine collaterals. 〈Point selection〉 Guanyuan (RN 4), Qihai (RN 6), Shenshu (BL 23) and Sanyinjiao(SP 6).

●**产后汗雨不止**[chǎn hòu hàn yǔ bù zhǐ] 病证名。出《女科指要》。多因产后心肾气虚，身体大虚，不能统摄津液所致。证见汗出如雨、头晕、心悸气短。治宜养心益肾。取心俞、肾俞、神门、太溪、合谷、三阴交。

Dripping with Sweat after Delivery A disease originally from *Nüke Zhiyao* (*Essential of Obstetrics and Gynecology*), mostly caused by qi-deficiency of the kidney and heart after delivery, severe deficiency of the body and failure to control body fluids. 〈Manifestations〉 dripping with sweat, dizziness, palpitation and shortness of breath. 〈Treatment principle〉 Nourish the heart and invigorate the kidney. 〈Point Selection〉 Xinshu (BL 15), Shenshu (BL 23), Shenmen (HT 7), Taixi (KI 3), Hegu (LI 4), Sanyinjiao(SP 6).

●**产后痢疾**[chǎn hòu lì jí] 即产后下利。详见该条。

Postpartum Dysentery →产后下利(p. 36)

●**产后目痛**[chǎn hòu mù tòng] 病证名。见《胎产证治录》。多因产后出血过多所致。证见眼痛不能视、羞明隐涩、眼睑无力。治宜补血养营。取睛明、太阳、鱼腰、肾俞、关元、太溪。

Postpartum Ophthalmodynia A disease, originally from *Taichan Zhengzhi Lu* (*Diagnosis and Treatment of Obstetrical Diseases*), mostly caused by overbleeding after childbirth. 〈Manifestations〉 unable to see due to pain of the eye, photophobia with xerophthalmia, inert eye-lashes. 〈Treatment principle〉 Enrich blood and nourish ying (nutrient). 〈Point selection〉 Jingming (BL 1), Taiyang (EX-HN 5), Yuyao (EX-HN 4), Shenshu (BL 23), Guanyuan(RN 4), and Taixi(KI 3).

●**产后伤风**[chǎn hòu shāng fēng] 病证名。多因产后气血两虚，风邪外乘所致。证见鼻塞声重、流清涕、自汗、恶风、舌淡苔白、脉浮无力。治宜扶正祛邪。取风门、百会、列缺、风池、肺俞、合谷。

Invasion by Wind after Delivery A disease mostly caused by invasion from wind evil, due to deficiency of qi and blood after delivery. 〈Manifestations〉 stuffy nose, low voice, running nose with clear nasal discharge, spontaneous perspiration, aversion to wind, pale tongue with white coating, superficial and

weak pulse. ⟨Treatment principle⟩ Support body energy to eliminate evils. ⟨Point selection⟩ Fengmen (BL 12), Baihui (DU 20), Lieque (LU 7), Fengchi (GB 20), Feishu (BL 13), and Hegu (LI 4).

● 产后伤寒[chǎn hòu shāng hán] 病证名。见《诸病源候论》。多因产后气血大虚，卫外不固，寒邪乘虚侵肌表所致。证见产后恶寒发热、头痛、无汗或有汗，脉浮。治宜补虚为主，佐以祛邪。取百会、风池、风门、肺俞、关元、血海、列缺、合谷。

Invasion by Cold after Dlivery A disease, originally from *Zhubing Yuanhou Lun* (*General Treatise on the Etiology and Smptomatology of Diseases*). Generally due to a severe deficiency of qi and blood leading to the failure of superficial qi to protect the body and allowing an invasion of cold evils. ⟨Manifestations⟩ chills with fever, headache, anhidropsis or sweating, superficial pulse. ⟨Treatment principle⟩ Strengthen the body energy and clear the pathogenic factors. ⟨Point selection⟩ Baihui (DU 20), Fengchi (GB 20), Fengmen (BL 12), Feishu (BL 13), Guanyuan (RN 4), Xuehai (SP 10), Lieque (LU 7), Hegu (LI 4).

● 产后伤食[chǎn hòu shāng shí] 病证名。见《傅青主女科》。多因产后饮食不节，损伤脾胃所致。证见脘腹满闷、嗳腐吞酸、大便酸臭、舌苔腻、脉滑。治宜健脾和胃。取脾俞、胃俞、建里、中脘、足三里、商丘。

Postpartum Dyspepsia A disease originally from *Fu Qingzhu's Nüke* (*Fu Qingzhu's Obstetrics and Gynecology*), mostly caused by improper diet after delivery leading to injury of the spleen and the stomach. ⟨Manifestations⟩ fullness and distention in the epigastrium and abdomen, eructation with fetid odor and reguritation, sour, foul stool, greasy tongue coating and slippery pulse. ⟨Treatment principle⟩ Strengthen the spleen and stomach. ⟨Point selection⟩ Pishu (BL 20), Weishu (BL 21), Jianli (RN 11), Zhongwan (RN 12), Zusanli (ST 25) and Shangqiu (SP 5).

● 产后水肿[chǎn hòu shuǐ zhǒng] 病证名。见《绛血丹书》。多因产后脾肾之阳虚损，水湿不得敷布，溢于肌肤四肢所致。证见手足浮肿渐及周身、小便短少、神疲、脘痞、舌淡苔白、脉沉细弱。治宜健脾温肾，助阳利水。取脾俞、肾俞、水分、气海、太溪、足三里。

Postpartum Edema A disease originally from *Jiang Xue Dan Shu* (*A Precious Book on the Treatment of Bleeding*). Generally caused by yang deficiency of the spleen and kidney after delivery, which leads to failure to transfer body fluids, resulting in the retention of body fluids in superficial muscles and skin and the four limbs. ⟨Manifestations⟩ gradual spread of edema, first to the limbs, then to the whole body, oliguria, fatigue, fullness in the epigastrium, pale tongue with white coating, deep thin and weak pulse. ⟨Treatment principle⟩ Strenghten the spleen and warm the kidney; induce diuresis by restoring yang. ⟨Point selection⟩ Pishu (BL 20), Shenshu (BL 23), Shuifen (RN 9), Qihai (RN 6), Taixi (KI 3), and Zusanli (ST 36).

● 产后瘫痪[chǎn hòu tān huàn] 病证名。见《胎产方案》。多因生产时失血过多，经脉空虚所致。证见产后半身不遂、手足麻木不仁、拘挛不知痛痒。治宜补气养血。取肩髃、曲池、手三里、外关、环跳、阳陵泉、足三里、三阴交、阳溪、昆仑。

Postpartum Paralysis A disease originally from *Taichan Fangan* (*Treatment Plans in Obstetrics*). Generally caused by severe blood loss during delivery which leads to deficiency of the meridians. ⟨Manifestations⟩ postpartum hemiplegia, numbness and spasm with bradyesthesia of the extremities. ⟨Treatment principle⟩ Invigorate qi and nourish blood. ⟨Point selection⟩ Jianyu (LI 15), Quchi (LI 11), Shousanli (LI 10), Waiguan (SJ 5), Huantiao (GB 30), Yanglingquan (GB 34), Zusanli (SP 36), Sanyinjiao (SP 6), Yangxi (LI 5) and Kunlun (BL 60).

● 产后头痛[chǎn hòu tóu tòng] 病证名。见《妇人良方大全》。多因产后失血过多，不能上荣于脑；或恶露停留胞宫，循经冲于脑所致。可分产后血虚头痛，产后血瘀头痛。

Postpartum Headache A disease seen in *Furen Liangfang Daquan* (*A Complete Work of Effective Prescriptions for Women*). Generally caused by severe blood loss after delivery leading to failure to nourish the brain; or, due to lochia remaining in the uterus. It can be divided into postpartum headache due to blood

deficiency and postpartum headache due to bloodstasis.

●产后下利[chǎn hòu xià lì] 病证名。出《金匮要略·妇人产后病脉证并治》。又称产后痢疾。多因产后饮食伤及脾胃,饮食停积于内;产后气血虚少更兼热邪伤阴,或恶露不下,败血渗入大肠所致。伤食者,证见下利兼腹胀痛、里急窘迫、舌苔厚腻、脉滑。治宜导滞攻下。取天枢、上巨虚、合谷、中脘。热邪伤者,取天枢、上巨虚、合谷、中脘。热邪伤阴者,证见下利脓血、兼发热腹痛、里急后重、身体困倦、虚烦不眠、唇干口渴、舌红、脉数。治宜养血清利湿热。取天枢、上巨虚、合谷、三阴交。

Postpartum Diarrhea A disease, originally from *Jingui Yaolüe: Furen Chanhoubing Maizheng Bingzhi* (*Synopsis of the Golden Chamber: Pulse Conditions, Symptoms and Treatment of Postpartum Diseases*), also termed as postpartum dysentery. Generally caused by improper diet after delivery which injures the spleen and the stomach, leading to food remaining inside the body;or to postpartum qi and blood deficiency accompanied by the injury of yin due o heat evil;or to postpartum lochioschesis which causes the lochioschesis to seep into the large intestine. Cases due to improper diet are manifested as dysentery with abdominal pain and distention, tenesmus, thick and greasy tongue coating, slippery pulse. ⟨Treatment principle⟩ Remove stagnancy and purge obstruction of the fu organs. ⟨Point selection⟩Tianshu (ST 25), Shangjuxu (ST 37),Hegu(LI 4), and Zhongwan (RN 12). Cases due to the injury of yin by pathogenic heat are manifested as dysentery with pus and blood , accompanied by fever and abdominal pain, tenesmus, fatigue, insomnia due to deficiency vexation, dry lips and thirst, red tongue and rapid pulse. ⟨Treatment principle⟩ Nourish blood and eliminate damp and heat. ⟨Point selection⟩ Tianshu (ST 25),Shangjuxu(ST 37),Hegu(LI 4)and Sanyinjiao (SP 6).

●产后小便不通[chǎn hòu xiǎo biàn bù tōng] 病证名。指产后尿闭,小腹胀急疼痛,甚则坐卧不安。多因素体虚弱,产时劳力伤气;或失血过多,气随血耗,脾肺气虚,不能通调水道,下输膀胱;或损伤肾气,以及肾阳不足,不能化气行水,或产后情志不畅,肝气郁结,气机阻滞,清浊升降失调,膀胱不利所致。临床分虚、实两证,兼见小腹胀满而痛,精神萎靡、言语无力。治宜温肾补气利水。取阴谷、肾俞、三焦俞、气海、脾俞、委阳。实证者,兼见小腹胀痛、精神抑郁,甚则两胁胀痛,舌红苔黄、脉数。治宜理气行滞利尿。取膀胱俞、中极、三阴交、阴陵泉、太冲。

Postpartum Retention of Urine A disease referring to the retention of urine with hypogastric distention and pain, and restless after delivery. Generally due to the weakness of the patient and over consumption of qi resulting from overstrain during delivery ;or ,from over bleeding leading to qi deficiency of the spleen and lung, failure to clear and regulate water passage to transfer the urine into the urinary bladder; or , the injury of the kidney leading to deficiency of the kidney yang, failure to dispel dampness and promote diuresis; or ,to the stagnation of liver qi and the disorder of qi caused by postpartum depressed emotions, leading to disturbance in ascending and descending the clear turbid qi, and the dysfunction of the urinary bladder. The disease is clinically divided into two types: deficiency and excess. Cases of deficiency are manifested as hypogastric distention, fullness and pain, listlessness, and inertia of speech. ⟨Treatment principle⟩ Warm the kidney, invigorate genuine qi, and promote diuresis. ⟨ Point selection⟩ Yingu (KI 10),Shenshu (BL 23), Sanjiaoshu(BL 22),Qihai(RN 6),Pishu(BL 20),and Weiyang(BL 39). Cases of excess are manifested as hypogastric distention and pain, mental depression, distention and pain in both sides of the hypochondriac region, red tongue with yellow coating, rapid pulse. ⟨Treatment principle⟩Regulate and promote the flow of qi, and induce diuresis. ⟨ Point selection ⟩ Pangguangshu (BL 28), Zhongji (RN 3), Sanyinjiao (SP 6), Yinlingquan (SP 9), and Taichong (LR 3).

●产后小便数[chǎn hòu xiǎo biàn shuò] 病证名。出《诸病源候论》。多因气虚不固,冷气乘虚侵入膀胱,膀胱失约,或因产后肾气虚弱,虚热移于膀胱所致。

可分虚寒、虚热两种证型。虚寒者,证见产后小便频数、色白、神气怯弱、畏寒肢冷、舌质淡、脉沉细。治宜温补下焦。取肾俞、三焦俞、气海、委阳、百会、中极。虚热者,证见产后小便频数涩痛、小腹坠胀、口苦、舌红苔黄、脉数。治宜疏利膀胱,清热。取三阴交、阴陵泉、膀胱俞、中极、行间。

Postpartum Frequency of Urination A disease seen in *Zhubing Yuanhou Lun(General Treatise on the Etiology and Symptomatology of Diseases)*. Generally due to cold evil invading the urinary bladder, resulting from failure of asthenic superficial qi to protect the body, causing the urinary bladder to be unable to control urination; or, due to the shift of heat into the urinary bladder resulting from puerperal deficiency of kidney qi. The disease can be divided into cold due to dificiency and heat due to deficiency. The former is manifested as postpartum frequent urination with whitish urine, listlessness, intolerance of cold and cold limbs, pale tongue and deep and thin pulse. ⟨Treatment principle⟩ Warm and strengthen the lower-Jiao. ⟨Point selection⟩ Shenshu(BL 23). Sanjiaoshu (BL 22), Qihai (RN 6), Weiyang(BL 39), Baihui(DU 20), Zhongji (RN 3). The latter is manifested as postpartum frequent urination with difficulty and pain, distention of the lower abdomen with a dropping feeling, bitter taste, red tongue with yellow coating, rapid pulse. ⟨Treatment principle⟩ Remove heat and regulate the function of the urinary bladder. ⟨Point selection⟩ Sanyinjiao (SP 6), Yinlingquan (SP 9), Pangguangshu (BL 28), Zhongji (RN 3), and Xingjian(LR 22).

●产后胁痛[chǎn hòu xié tòng] 病证名。出《达生保赤编》。多因气血瘀滞,或产后失血过多,肝脉失养所致,证见产后出现一侧或两侧胁肋部疼痛。治宜活血祛瘀,理气止痛。取期门、支沟、阳陵泉、足三里、太冲、行间。

Postpartum Hypochondriac Pain A disease originally from *Dasheng Baochi Bian(A Collection of Works on Successful Delivery and Care of Children)*. Generally due to the stagnation of qi and blood stasis, or puerpareal severe blood loss, which leads to the failure to nourish the liver meridian. ⟨Manifestations⟩ pain in either one or both sides of the hypochondriac region. ⟨Treatment principle⟩ Remove blood stasis by promoting blood circulation and alleviate pain by regulating the flow of qi. ⟨Point selection⟩ Qimen (LR 14), Zhigou (SJ 6), Yanglingquan(GB 34), Zusanli(ST 36), Taichong(LR 3), and Xingjian(LR 2).

●产后眩晕[chǎn hòu xuàn yùn] 即产后血晕。详见该条。

Postpartum Dizziness →产后血晕(p. 37)

●产后血晕[chǎn hòu xuè yùn] 病证名。出《经效产宝》。又称郁冒、产后眩晕。产妇分娩后,突然发生头晕、目眩眼花、不能起坐;或心下满闷、恶心呕吐、或痰涌气急、甚则神昏口噤、不省人事,称为产后血晕。是产后危证之一。临床分两种证型。血虚气脱者,多因产妇平素气血虚弱,复因产后失血过多,气随血脱,心神失养所致。证见突然昏晕、不醒人事、面色苍白、甚则四肢厥冷、冷汗淋漓、脉微细或浮大而虚。治宜回阳救逆,补气益血。取关元、气海、三阴交、足三里。寒凝血瘀者,多因产时感寒,恶露不下,血瘀气逆,并走于上,心神受扰所致。证见产后恶露不下,或下亦很少,少腹阵痛拒按、心下急满、气息喘促、神昏不省人事、两手握拳、牙关紧闭、面色紫黯、口唇舌质发紫、脉涩。治宜温经散寒,行血祛瘀。取中极、阴交、三阴交、支沟、公孙。

Postpartum Dizziness due to Blood Problems

A disease, originally from *Jing Xiao Chan Bao(Treasury of Effective Prescriptions in Obsterics)*, also named oppressive feeling and dizziness or postpartum dizziness. It is so named due to blood problems after delivery marked by a sudden onset of dizziness, blurred vision and inability to sit up; or by epigastric distention and fullness, nausea and vomiting; or by dyspnea with copious sputum, even mental confusion, lockjaw and unconscionsness. It is one of the dangerous diseases seen after delivery. It is clinically divided into two types. Cases of blood-deficiency and qi-exhaustion are mostly due to puerperant-constitutional weakness in qi and blood, followed by severe blood loss after childbirth, which causes blood-exhaustion, leading to

malnutrition of the heart and mind. ⟨Manifestations⟩ a sudden onset of dizziness, unconsciousness, pale complexion, numb cold limbs, dripping with cold sweat, weak, slightly pulse or weak and floating pulse. ⟨Treatment principle⟩ Recuperate depleted yang, rescue the patient from collapse and invigotate qi and blood. ⟨Point selection⟩ Guanyuan (RN 4), Qihai (RN 6), Sanyinjiao (SP 6), Zusanli (ST 36). Cases of blood stasis and cold accumulation are mostly due to the invasion of cold evil during delivery and the retention of lochia leading to blood stasis and qi counterflow, qi and blood gathering and moving upwards, interfering with the heart and mind. ⟨Manifestations⟩ lochiostasis or little lochia after delivery, pain and tenderness in the lower abdomen, epigastric distress, dyspnea, unconsciousness, clenched fists, lockjaw, dark purple complexion dark, purple lips and tongue, choppy pulse. ⟨Treatemnt principle⟩ Dispel cold by warming the meridians; remove blood stasis by promoting circulation of blood. ⟨Point selection⟩ Zhongji (RN 3), Yinjiao (RN 7), Sanyinjiao(SP 6), Zhigou(SJ 6) and Gongsun (SP 4).

●产后阴下脱[chǎn hòu yīn xià tuō] 病证名。出《诸病源候论》。又名产后子宫脱出、产后子宫不收，即产后子宫脱垂。多因宿有虚冷，产时用力过度，其气下冲所致，证见子宫脱出或伴有阴道壁下垂。参见"子宫脱垂"条。

Postpartum Prolapse of Genital Structure A disease originally from *Zhubing Yuanhou Lun* (*General Treatise on the Eticology and Symtomatology of Diseases*), also named posrpartum prolapse of uterus, postpartum relaxation of uterus, postpartum hysteroptosis. Generally due to the patient originally manifesting cold due to deficiency, and overstrain during delivery, leading to the sinking of qi. ⟨Manifestations⟩ hysteroptosis or the prolapse of the vaginal wall. →子宫脱垂(p. 625)

●产后中暑[chǎn hòu zhòng shǔ] 病证名。见《石室秘录》。多因产后气血未复，盛夏炎热，暑邪乘虚侵袭肌体，阴气卒绝，阳气暴壅，经络不通所致。证见产后1～3天内，高热、头晕、头痛、心烦口渴、胸闷呕吐，甚则烦躁不安、神志不清、四肢抽搐。治宜清泄暑热，宁心开窍。取大椎、百会、水沟、曲池、内关、合谷、足三里、太冲、委中、陷谷。

Postpartum Heat-Stroke A disease originally from *Shishi Milu* (*Secret Records in the Stone House*). Generally due to the attack of summer heat evil on the patient with deficiency of qi and blood after delivery in midsummer, leading to the sudden obsruction of yinqi, the severe accumulation of yang-qi and the blockage of meridians. ⟨Manifestations⟩ high fever, dizziness, headache, irritability, thirst, oppressive feeling in the chest, vomiting, and even dysphoria, unconciousness and convulsion of the four limbs within 1～3 days after delivery. ⟨Treatment principle⟩ Remove summer heat, relieve mental stress and regain consciousness. ⟨Point selection⟩ Dazhui (DU 14), Baihui (DU 20), Shuigou (DU 26), Quchi (LI 11), Neiguan (PC 6), Hegu (LI 4), Taichong (LR 3), Zusanli (ST 36), Weizhong (BL 40), and Xiangu (ST 43).

●产后子宫不收[chǎn hòu zǐ gōng bù shōu] 即产后阴下脱，详见该条及"子宫脱垂"条。

Postpartum Relaxation of Uterus i.e. postpartum prolapse of genital structure. →产后阴下脱(p. 38)、子宫脱垂(p. 625)

●产后子宫脱出[chǎn hòu zǐ gōng tuō chū] 即产后阴下脱。详见该条及"子宫脱垂"条。

Postpartum Prolapse of Uterus i.e. postpartum prolapse of genital structure. →产后阴下脱(p. 38)、子宫脱垂(p. 625)

●产难[chǎn nán] 即滞产。详见该条。

Delivery with Difficulty →滞产(p. 607)

●昌阳[chāng yáng] 经穴别名。出《针灸甲乙经》。即复溜。详见该条。

Changyang Another name for Fuliu(KI 7), a meridian point seen in *Zhenjiu Jia-Yi Jing* (*A-B Classic of Acupuncture and Moxibustion*). →复溜(p. 121)

●昌阳之脉[chāng yáng zhī mài] 经脉名。出《素问·刺腰痛篇》。指足少阴经在小腿部的支脉。王冰认为指阴跷脉，其穴为交信。张介宾等解释作"复溜"，《针灸甲乙经》复溜，别名昌阳。

Chanyang Meridian A meridian originally

from *Suwen*: *Ci Yaotong Pian* (*Plain Questions*: *On Treatment of Lumbago with Acupuncture*), referring to the branch of the Meridian of Foot-Shaoyang in the medial shank, which is called the Yinqiao Meridian by Wang Bing, and its point is Jiaoxin (KI 8). Also explained by Zhang Jiebin, etc. as Fuliu (KI 7), another name for which is Changyang in *Zhenjiu Jia-Yi Jing* (*A-B Classic of Acupuncture and Moxibustion*).

●长谷[cháng gǔ] 经外穴名。见《千金要方》。又名循际、长平、循脊、循元。在神阙旁开2.5寸。主治泄痢、不嗜食、食不消。直刺1.0～1.5寸；可灸。

Changgu (EX-CA) An extra point seen in *Qianjin Yaofang* (*Essential Prescriptions Worth a Thousand Gold*), also called Xunji, Changping, Xunji Xunyuan. 〈Location〉2.5 cun lateral to Shenque (RN 8). 〈Indications〉Diarrhea and dysentery, lack of appetite and indigestion. 〈Method〉Puncture perpendicularly 1.0～1.5 cun. Moxibustion is applicable.

●长频[cháng huì] 经穴别名。出《针灸大成》。即口禾髎。详见该条。

Changhui Another name for Kouheliao (LI 19), a merdidan point originally from *Zhenjiu Dacheng* (*A Great Compendium of Acupuncture and Moxibustion*). →口禾髎(p. 232)

●长颊[cháng jiá] 经穴别名。出《针灸聚英》。即口禾髎。详见该条。

Changjia Another name for Kouheliao (LI 19), a meridian point originally from *Zhenjiu Juying* (*Essentials of Acupuncture and Moxibustion*). →口禾髎(p. 232)

●长髎[cháng liáo] 经穴别名。出《针灸大全》。即口禾髎。详见该条。

Changliao Another name for Kouheliao (LI 19), a meridian point originally from *Zhenjiu Daquan* (*A Complete Work of Acupuncture and Moxibustion*). →口禾髎(p. 232)

●长频[cháng pín] 经穴别名。出《铜人腧穴针灸图经》。即口禾髎。详见该条。

Changpin Another name for Kouheliao (LI 19), a meridian point originally from *Tongren Shuxue Zhenjiu Tujing* (*Illustrated Manual of Points for Acupuncture and Moxibustion on a Bronze Statue with Acupoints*). →口禾髎(p. 232)

●长平[cháng píng] ①经穴别名。出《针灸甲乙经》。即章门。详见该条。②经外穴别名。出《千金翼方》。即长谷。详见该条。

Changping Another name for ① Zhangmen (LR 13), a meridian point originally from *Zhenjiu Jia-Yi Jing* (*A-B Classic of Acupuncture and Moxibustion*). →章门(p. 585) ② Changgu (EX-CA), an extra point originally from *Qianjin Yifang* (*Supplement to the Essential Prescriptions Worth a Thousand Gold*). →长谷(p. 39)

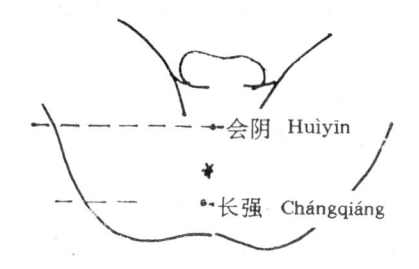

图 4 长强和会阴穴

Fig 4 Changqiang and Huiyin Points

●长强[cháng qiáng] 经穴名。出《灵枢·经脉》属督脉，《针灸甲乙经》为督脉络穴。又名气之阴郄、橛骨、尾闾、鸠尾、下极之俞、胸之阴俞。〈定位〉在尾骨端下，当尾骨端与肛门连线的中点处（图12）。〈层次解剖〉皮肤→皮下组织→肛尾韧带。浅层主要布有尾神经的后支。深层有阴部神经的分支，肛神经，阴部内动静脉的分支或属支，肛动、静脉。主治泄泻、痢疾、便秘、便血、痔疾、癫狂、痫证、瘈疭、脊强反折、癃淋、阴部湿痒、腰脊、尾骶部疼痛。斜刺，针尖向上与骶骨平行刺入 0.5～1.0寸。可灸。不得刺穿直肠，以防感染。

Changqiang (DU 1) A meridian point, orginally from *Lingshu*: *Jingmai* (*Miraculous Pivot*: *Merdians*), a point on the Du Meridian, taken as the Luo (Connecting) point of the Du Meridian in *Zhenjiu Jia-Yi Jing* (*A-B Classic of Acupuncture and Moxibustion*), also named Qizhiyinxi, Juegu, Weilü, Jiuwei, Xiajizhishu Xiongzhiyinshu. 〈Locaion〉below the

tip of the coccyx midway between the tip of the coccyx and the anus. (Fig. 12) 〈Regional anatomy〉 skin→subcutaneous tissue→anococcygeal ligament. In the superficial layer, there are the posterior branches of the coccygeal nerve. In the deep layer, there are the end nerve of the pudendal nerve and the artery and vein of the internal pudendal artery and vein. 〈Indications〉 diarrhea, dysentery, constipation, bloody stool, hemorrhoids, manic-depressive psychosis, epilepsy, clonic convulsion, back rigidity, opisthotonus, dysuria and stranguria, pruritis vulvae due to damp. heat, pain in the spinal column and coccyx. 〈Method〉 Puncture obliquely 0.5～1.0 cun upward toward the coccys. Moxibustion is applicable. Do not puncture through the rectal tube in case of infection.

●长桑君[cháng sāng jūn]　人名。战国时代医家,熟谙禁方,擅长针灸。名医秦越人(扁鹊)曾师事之而尽得其传。

Changsang Jun　A medical expert in the Warring States period (475 B. C.). He was good at applying secret recipes and acupuncture and moxibustion. The well-known doctor Qin Yueren(Bian Que) once learned medicine and obtained much from him.

●长蛇灸[cháng shé jiǔ]　灸法的一种。又称铺灸。用大蒜适量,去皮捣泥,平铺于脊柱(自大椎穴至腰俞穴)上,宽厚各约6毫米,周围用桑皮纸封固,然后用黄豆大的艾炷分别在大椎穴及腰俞穴上施灸,至患者口鼻内觉有蒜味时止。民间用以治疗虚痨。

Long Snake Moxibustion　One of the moxibustion methods, also named spreading moxibustion. Take some garlic, peel and pound it, spread the pounded garlic on the spinal column from Dazhui (DU 14) to Yaoshu(DU 2) about 6 mm both in thickness and width. Cover the skin with mulberry paper, then apply respectively to Dazhui (DU 14) and Yaoshu (DU 2), burning cones of moxa, as big as soybeans, until the patient has the smell of garlic both in his mouth and nose. It is used for the treatment of consumptive diseases.

●长溪[cháng xī]　经穴别名。出《针灸甲乙经》。即天枢。详见该条。

Changxi　Another name for Tianshu (ST 25), a meridian point orginally from *Zhenjiu Jia-Yi Jing* (*A-B Classic of Acupuncture and Moxibustion*). →天枢(p. 434)

●长针[cháng zhēn]　针具名。出《灵枢·九针论》。又称环跳针。其针长七寸,针身细长而锋利。可用于深刺,为治疗病邪较深的病证。近代发展为芒针。

Long Needle　An acupuncture instrument, originally form *Lingshu: Jiu Zheng Lun* (*Miraculous Pivot: On Nine Needles*), also calld Huantiao (GB 30) needle. The needle, which is 7 cun long and has a long thin boby with a sharp tip, is used for deep puncture to treat diseases due to pathogenic factors in the deep layers. Today the long needle has developed into the elongated needle.

●肠道[cháng dào]　经外穴别名。出《腧穴学概论》。即肠遗。详见该条。

Changdao　Another name for Changyi (EX-CA), an extra point originally from *Shuxuexue Gailum* (*An Outline of Acupoints*). →肠遗(p. 41)

●肠风[cháng fēng]　经外穴别名。见《中国针灸》。即阳刚。详见该条。

Changfeng　Another name for Yanggang (EX), an extra point seen in *Zhongguo Zhenjiu*(*Chinese Acupuncture and Moxibustion*). →阳刚(p. 537)

●肠结[cháng jié]　经穴别名。出《千金翼方》。即腹结。详见该条。

Chanjie　Another name for Fujie (SP 14), a meridian point orignally from *Qianjin Yifang* (*A Supplement to Essential Prescriptions Worth a Thousand Gold*). →腹结(p. 121)

●肠窟[cháng kū]　经穴别名。出《外台秘要》。即腹结。详见该条。

Changku　Another name for Fujie (SP 14), a meridian point originally from *Waitai Miyao* (*Clandestine Essentials form the Imperial Library*). →腹结(p. 121)

●肠澼[cháng pì]　病证名。出《素问·通评虚实论》等篇。痢疾的古称。详见"痢疾"条。

Changpi　A disease, seen in *Suwen: Tong Ping Xushi Lun* (*Plain Questions : A Thor-

ough Discssion of Deficiency and Excess), etc., the archaic name for dysentery. →痢疾 (p. 244)

●肠绕[cháng rào] 经外穴名。见《针灸集成》。在中极两旁相去各2寸处,位同归来穴。灸治大便闭塞。

Changrao(EX-CA) An extra point seen in *Zhenjiu Jicheng* (*A Collection of Acupuncture and Moxibustion*).〈Location〉2 cun lateral to Zhongji (RN 3), in the same position as of Guilai (ST 29).〈Indication〉constipation.〈Method〉moxibustion.

●肠山[cháng shān] 经穴别名。见《铜人腧穴针灸图经》。即承山。详见该条。

Changshan Another name for Chengshan (BL 57), a meridian point seen in *Tongren Shuxue Zhenjiu Tujing* (*Illustrated Manual of Points Acupuncture and Moxibustion on a Bronze Statue with Acupoints*). →承山 (p. 45)

●肠遗[cháng yí] 经外穴名。见《千金要方》。又名肠道。在下腹部,当中极穴旁开2.5寸处。灸治大便不通。

Changyi(EX-CA) An extra point, seen in *Qianjin Yaofang* (*Essential Prescriptions Worth a Thousand Gold*), also named Changdao.〈Location〉in the lower abdomen, 2.5 cun lateral to Zhongji (RN 3).〈Indication〉constipation.〈Method〉moxibustion.

●肠痈[cháng yōng] 病证名。出《素问·厥论》。以右少腹疼痛为主症。因本病有右腿不能伸直的体征,故有缩脚肠痈之称。本病多因恣食膏粱厚味,温热蕴于肠间;或饱食后剧烈运动,肠络受损;或感受寒邪,郁而化热,导致脏腑气血壅滞,酿成肠痈。证见初起先觉绕脐作痛,继则疼痛转移至右下腹部,以手按之其痛加剧,痛处固定不移,腹皮微急,右腿屈而难伸,伴有发热恶寒、恶心呕吐、便秘溲赤、舌苔黄腻、脉洪数。治宜清热导滞、活血散结。取曲池、天枢、上巨虚、地机。

Acute Appendicitis A disease originally from *Suwen*: *Jue Lun* [*Plain Questions*: *On Jue-Syndromes* (*Syncope, Reverse of Qi, Extreme Cold and Heat*)], charaterized by pain in the lower right abdomen, also named acute appendicitis with foot shrinking because of the symptom of the patient's inability to stretch the right leg. Mostly due to the accumulation of damp-heat in the intestine caused by overeating or rich fatty diet; or due to impairment of the intestine collaterals caused by an attack of cold evil, leading to stagnated heat, stagnation of qi and blood of zang-fu, and finally resulting in acute appendicitis.〈Manifestations〉At first, pain appears around the umbilicus, then moves to lower right abdomen and fixes there with severe pain under pressure, slight tension of the abdominal wall, and a shrunken right leg which is difficult to stretch out. Accompanied by fever, aversion to cold, nausea and vomiting, constipation, deep colored urine, a yellowish and greasy tongue coating with a surging and rapid pulse.〈Treatment principle〉Clear away heat and resolve stagnation, activate blood and remove obstruction.〈Point selection〉Quchi(LI 11), Tianshu(ST 25), Shangjuxu(ST 37), and Diji(SP 8).

●彻衣[chè yī] 《内经》刺法名。出《灵枢·刺节真邪》。为刺法五节之一。指对阳气有余之外热,阴气不足之内热,两热搏结,热甚如怀抱炭火一样病证,取天府、大杼、中膂俞以泻热,然后补手、足太阴经,使其出汗,其热退汗液减少时,病就痊愈。其效验有如脱除衣服。

Taking Off Clothes One of the five acupuncture techinques from *Neijing* (*The Canon of Internal Medicine*), found in *Lingshu: Cijie Zhenxie* (*Miraculous Pivot: Acupuncture Principles and Diseases*), referring to a technique which induces sweat. Used to relieve two kinds of excess heat syndromes; exterior heat due to excess yang qi, and internal heat caused by deficeient yin qi, both of which cause the patient to feel as if they were carrying charcoal fire in their arms. To treat, puncture Tianfu(LU 3), Dazhu(BL 11), and Zhonglüshu(BL 29) to reduce heat. Then, puncture points on the Hand and Foot-Taiyin Meridians with the reinforcing method. The disease is cured when heat is relieved and sweat decreased. The intended effect resembles removing clothes, hence the name.

●臣觉[chén jué] 经外穴名。出《千金要方》。又名巨搅、巨觉。在背部,肩胛骨内上角边际,当两手相抱

时,中指端尽处是穴。主治狂走、喜怒悲泣、肩胛痛等。斜刺0.5～0.8寸;可灸。

Chenjue(EX-B) An extra point, originally from *Qianjin Yaofang* (*Essential Prescriptions Worth a Thousand Gold*), also named Jujiao or Jujue. ⟨Location⟩ on the back, at the margin of the superior-medial angle of the scapula, at the place touched by the extremity of the middle finger when the arms embrace the body. ⟨Indications⟩ walking in madness, abnormal emotions of joy, anger, sorrow and weeping, pain in the scapula, etc.. ⟨Method⟩ Puncture 0.5～0.8 cun obliquely. Moxibustion is applicable.

●陈会[chén huì] 人名。明针灸家,字善同,号宏纲,丰城横江里(今属江西)人。精于针灸,著《广爱书》十卷。后其弟子重新校正、增补,为《神应经》。

Chen Hui An expert in acupuncture and moxibustion during the Ming Dynasty, who styled himself Shantong and was called Honggang. He came from Hengjianli, Feng Cheng (in today's Jiangxi Province). Proficient in acupuncture and moxbustion, he wrote *Guang'aishu* (*A Book on Fraternity*), in ten volumes. The book was later rectified and supplemented by his disciples, and entitled *Shenying Jing* (*Classic of God Merit*).

●陈时荣[chén shí róng] 人名。明针灸家,字颐春,华亭(今上海松江)人,精于针灸。事见《松江府志》。

Chen Shirong An expert in acupuncture and moxibustion during the Ming Dynasty, who styled himself Yichun, came from Huating (today's Songjiang, Shanghai). Further details about him can be seen in *Songjianfu Zhi* (*Annals of Songjiangfu*).

●陈廷铨[chén tíng quán] 人名。清针灸家,字隐荟,清泉(属湖南衡阳)人。撰《罗遗编》三卷,成书于1763年。

Chen Tingquan An expert in acupunture and moxibustion during the Qing Dynasty, who styled himself Yinyan, a native of Qingquan (today's Hengyang, Hunan Province), compiler of *Luoyi Bian* (*A Collection of the Lost*) in three volumes, which was completed in 1763.

●陈言[chén yán] 人名。明针灸家,建阳人。撰《杨敬斋针灸全书》。参见该条。

Chen Yan An expert in acupuncture and moxibustion during the Ming Dynasty, a native of Jianyang. He compiled *Yang Jingzhai Zhenjiu Quanshu* (*Yang Jingzhai's Complete Work of Acupuncture and Moxibustion*)→《杨敬斋针灸全书》(p. 543)

●晨泄[chén xiè] 见《杂病源流犀烛·泄泻源流》。即五更泄。详见该条。

Early Morning Diarrhea Seen in *Zabing Yuanliu Xizhu*: *Xiexie Yuanliu* (*Bright Candle to Pathology of Miscellaneous Diseases*: *Pathology of Diarrhea*).→五更泄(p. 427)

●撑开进针[chēng kāi jìn zhēn] 进针方法之一。又称舒张押手。其法用左拇指、食指将穴位附近的皮肤向两侧撑开绷紧后,右手持针刺入穴位。适用于皮肤松驰而需直刺的部位,如腹部各穴。

Inserting the Needle While Unfolding the Skin One of the methods of inserting the needle, also named hand-pressing for unfolding the skin. ⟨Method⟩ After unfolding and tightening the skin adjacent to the acupoint on both sides with the left thumb and index finger, puncture the acupoint with the needle held in the right hand. Applicable where the skin is flaccid and perpendicular needling is required, such as the acupoints on the abdomen.

●成骨[chéng gǔ] 经外穴名。见《针灸经外奇穴图谱》。位于膝关节腓侧,股骨外上髁最高点处。⟨主治⟩腰痛、鹳口疽、坐马痈等。浅刺出血。

Chengu(EX-LE) An extra point seen in *Zhenjiu Jingwai Qixue Tupu* (*An Atlas of Extra Points for Acupuncture and Moxibustion*). ⟨Location⟩ on the fibular side of the knee joint, the highest point of the external epicondyle of femur. ⟨Indications⟩ lumbago, carbuncle on the coccygeal region, carbuncle adjacent to the anus, etc. ⟨Method⟩ Puncture shallowly and cause bleeding.

●承扶[chéng fú] 经穴名。出《针灸甲乙经》。属足太阳膀胱经,又名扶承、肉郄、阴关。⟨定位⟩在大腿后面,臀下横纹的中点(图83)。⟨层次解剖⟩皮肤→皮下组织→臀大肌→股二头肌长头及半腱肌。浅层布有

股后皮神经及臀下皮神经的分支。深层有股后皮神经本干,坐骨神经及其并行动、静脉。〈主治〉痔疾、腰、骶、臀、股部痛。直刺1.5～2.5寸;可灸。

Chengfu(BL 36) A meridian point originally from *Zhenjiu Jia-Yi Jing*(*A-B Classic of Acupuncture and Moxibustion*),a point on the Bladder Meridian of Foot-Taiyang,also named Fucheng, Rouxi, Yinguan. 〈Location〉on the posterior side of the thigh,at the midpoint of the inferior gluteal crease. (Fig. 83)〈Regional anatomy〉skin→subcutaneous tissue→greatest gluteal muscle→long head of biceps muscle of thigh and semitendinous muscle. In the superficial layer,there are the branches of the posterior femoral cutaneous nerve and the inferior clunial nerve. In the deep layer,there are the trunk of the posterior femoral cutaneous nerve,the sciatic nerve and the accompanying arteries and veins. 〈Indications〉Hemorrhoids, pain in the lumber, sacral, gluteal and femoral regions. 〈Method〉Puncture perpendicularly 1.5～2.5 cun. Moxibustion is applicable.

● 承光[chéng guāng] 经穴名。出《针灸甲乙经》。属足太阳膀胱经。〈定位〉在头部,当前发际正中直上2.5寸,旁开1.5(图28)。〈层次解剖〉皮肤→皮下组织→帽状腱膜。浅层布有眶上神经和眶上动、静脉。深层为腱膜下疏松组织和颅骨外膜。〈主治〉头痛、目眩、呕吐、烦心、目视不明、鼻塞多涕、热病无汗。平刺0.3～0.5寸;可灸。

Chengguang (BL 6) A meridian point, origially from *Zhenjiu Jia-Yi Jing*(*A-B Classic of Acupuncture and Moxibustion*), a point on the Bladder Meridian of Foot-Taiyang. 〈Location〉on the head, 2.5 cun directly above the midpoint of the anterior hairline and 1.5 cun lateral to the midline. (Fig. 28)〈Regional natomy〉skin→subcutaneous tissue epicraniala poneurosis. In the superficial layer, there are the supraorbital nerve and the supraorbital artery and vein. In the deep layer, there are the subaponeurotic loose connective tissue and the pericranium. 〈Indications〉headache, blurred vision, vomiting, irritability, blindness, stuffy nose with nasal discharge, fever without sweat. 〈Method〉Puncture subcutaneously 0.3～0.5 cun. Moxibustion is applicable.

● 承浆[chéng jiāng] ①经穴名。出《针灸甲乙经》,属任脉,为足阳明、任脉之会。又名天池、悬浆、垂浆、鬼市。〈定位〉在面部,当颏唇沟的正中凹陷处。(见图5和图28)〈层次解剖〉皮肤→皮下组织→口轮匝肌→降下唇肌→颏肌。布有下牙槽神经的终支颏神经和颏动、静脉。〈主治〉口眼㖞斜、唇紧、面肿、齿痛、齿衄、龈肿、流涎、口舌生疮、暴喑不言、消渴嗜饮、小便不禁、癫痫。斜刺0.3～0.5寸;可灸。②部位名。唇下颏上中央凹陷处。

1. **Chengjiang**(RN 24) A meridian point originally from *Zhenjiu Jia-Yi Jing* (*A-B Classic of Acupuncture and Moxibustion*) a point on the Ren Meridian, the converging point of the Stomach Meridian of Foot-Yangming and the Ren Meridian, also named Tianchi, Xuanjiang, Chuijiang or Guishi.〈Location〉on the face, in the depression at the midpoint of the mentolabial sulcus. (Figs. 5 & 28)〈Regional anatomy〉skin→subcutaneous tissue→orbicular muscle of mouth → depressor muscle of lower lip→mental muscle. There are the mental nerve of the inferior alveolar nerve and the mental artery and vein in this area. 〈Indications〉deviation of the eye and mouth, tight lip, facial swelling, toothache, bleeding from the gum, swelling of the gums, salivation, ulcer in the mouth, sudden loss of voice, diabetes with thirst relieved by dribbling urination, epilepsy. 〈Method〉Puncture obliquely 0.3～0.5 cun. Moxibustion is applicable.

2. **Chengjiang** A part of the body, located in the depression at the centre below the lip and above the mentum.

● 承筋[chéng jīn] 经穴名。出《针灸甲乙经》。属足太阳膀胱经。又名腨肠、直肠、真肠。〈定位〉在小腿后面,当委中与承山的连线上,腓肠肌肌腹中央,委中下5寸(图83)。〈层次解剖〉皮肤→皮下组织→腓肠肌→比目鱼肌。浅层布有小隐静脉,腓肠内侧皮神经。深层有胫后动、静脉,腓动、静脉和胫神经。〈主治〉小腿痛、膝痠重、腰背拘急、痔疾、霍乱转筋。直刺0.5～1.0寸;可灸。

Chengjin(BL 56) A meridian point, originally from *Zhenjiu Jia-Yi Jing* (*A-B Classic*

of Acupuncture and Moxibustion), a point on the Bladder Meridian of Foot-Taiyang, also named Zhuanchang, Zhichang, Zhenchang. ⟨Location⟩ on the back, below the spinous process of the 2nd thoracic vertebra, 3 cun lateral to Chengshan (BL 57), at the centre of the gastrocnemius muscle belly, 5 cun below Weizhong (BL 40). (Fig. 83) ⟨Regional anatomy⟩ skin→subcutaneous tissue→gastrocnemius musele→seleus muscle. In the superficial layer, there are the small saphenous vein and the medial cutaneous nerve of the calf. In the deep layer, there are the posterior tibial artery and vein, the peroneal artery and vein and the tibial nerve. ⟨Indications⟩ pain in the leg, soreness and heavy sensation in the knee, contraction of the lumbar area and back, hemorrhoids, cholera morbus and spasm. ⟨Method⟩ Puncture perpendicularly 0.5～1.0 cun. Moxibustion is applicable.

●承灵[chéng líng] 经穴名。出《针灸甲乙经》。属足少阳胆经,为足少阳、阳维之会。〈定位〉在头部,当前发际上4.0寸,头正中线旁开2.25寸(图28)。〈层次解剖〉皮肤→皮下组织→帽状腱膜→腱膜下疏松结缔组织。布有枕大神经和枕动、静脉的分支。〈主治〉头痛、目眩、目痛、鼻渊、鼻衄、鼻窒、多涕。平刺0.5～0.8寸;可灸。

Chengling(GB 18) A meridian point, originally from *Zhenjiu Jia-Yijing* (*A-B Classic of Acupuncture and Moxibustion*), a point on the Gallbladder Meridian of Foot-Shaoyang, the converging point of the Gallbladder Meridian of Foot-Shaoyang and the Yangwei Meridian. ⟨Location⟩ on the head, 4 cun above the anterior hairline and 2.25 cun lateral to the midline of the head. (Fig. 28) ⟨Regional anatomy⟩ skin→subcutaneous tissue→epicranial aponeurosis→loose connective tissue below aponeurosis. There are the greater occipital nerve and the branches of the occipital artery and vein in this area. ⟨Indications⟩ headache, dizziness, pain in the eye, rhinorrhea, epistaxis, stuffy nose with much nasal discharge. ⟨Method⟩ Puncture subcutaneously 0.5～0.8 cun. Moxibustion is applicable.

●承满[chéng mǎn] 经穴名。出《针灸甲乙经》。属足阳明胃经。〈定位〉在上腹部,当脐中上5寸,距前正中线2寸(图86和图40)。〈层次解剖〉皮肤→皮下组织→腹直肌鞘前壁→腹直肌。浅层布有第六、七、八胸神经前支的外侧皮支和前皮支及腹壁浅静脉,深层有腹壁上动、静脉的分支或属支,第六、七、八胸神经前支的肌支。〈主治〉胃痛、呕吐、腹胀、肠鸣、食欲不振、喘逆、吐血、胁下坚痛。直刺0.5～1.0寸;可灸。

Chengman(ST 20) A meridian point, originally from *Zhenjiu Jia-Yi Jing* (*A-B Classic of Acupuncture and Moxibustion*), a point of the Stomach Meridian of Foot-Yangming. ⟨Location⟩ in the upper abdomen, 5 cun above the centre of the umbilicus and 2 cun lateral to the anterior midline. (Figs. 86 & 40) ⟨Regional anatomy⟩ skin→subcutaneous tissue→anterior sheath of rectus musde of abdomen→rectus muscel of abdomen. In the superficial layer, there are the lateral and anterior cutaneous branches of the anterior branches of the 6th to 8th thoracic nerves and the superficial epigastric vein. In the deep layer, there are the branches or tributaries of the superior epigastric vein. In the deep layer, there are the branches or tributaries of the superior epigastric artery and vein and the muscular branches of the anterior branches of the 6th to 8th thoracic nerves. ⟨Indications⟩ astric pain, vomiting, abdominal distension, borborygmus, anorexia, dyspnea, hemoptysis, sharp pain in the hypochondrium. ⟨Method⟩ Puncture perpendicularly 0.5～1.0 cun. Moxibustion is applicable.

●承命[chéng mìng] 经外穴名。出《千金要方》。在小腿内侧,当太溪穴直上3寸处。〈主治〉癫痫、下肢浮肿。直刺0.5-1.0寸;可灸。

Chengming(EX-LE) An extra point, originally from *Qianjin Yaofang* (*Essential Prescriptions Worth a Thousand Gold*). ⟨Location⟩ on the medial side of the leg, 3 cun straight above Taixi (KI 3). ⟨Indications⟩ epilepsy and edema of the lower extremities. ⟨Method⟩ Puncture perpendicularly 0.5～1.0 cun. Moxibustion is applicable.

●承泣[chéng qì] 经穴名。出《针灸甲乙经》。属足阳明胃经,为阳蹻、任脉、足阳明之会。又名鼷穴,面髎。〈定位〉在面部,瞳孔直下,当眼球与眶下缘之间

(图28)。〈层次解剖〉皮肤→皮下组织→眼轮匝肌→眶脂体→下斜肌。浅层布有眶下神经的分支,面神经的颧支。深层有动眼神经的分支,眼动、静脉的分支或属支等结构。〈主治〉眼睑瞤动、目赤肿痛、迎风流泪、夜盲、口眼歪斜。紧靠眶下缘缓慢直刺0.3～0.7寸,不宜提插及大幅度捻转,以防刺破血管引起血肿;禁灸。

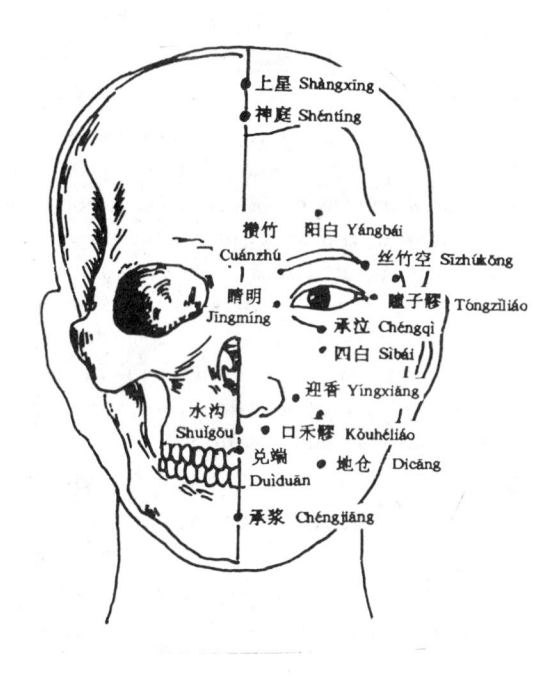

图5 承泣等前头部穴

Fig 5 Chengqi and other points of head

(Anterior view)

Chengqi (ST 1) A meridian point, originally from *Zhenjiu Jia-Yi Jing* (*A-B Classic of Acupuncture and Moxibustion*), a point on the Stomach Meridian of Foot-Yangming, the converging point of the Yangqiao Meridian, the Ren Meridian and the Meridian of Foot-Yangming, also named Xixue or Mianliao. 〈Location〉on the face, directly below the pupil, in the depression of the infraorbital ridge. (Fig. 28)〈Regional anatomy〉skin→subcutaneous tissue→orbicular muscle of eye →adipose body of orbit→inferior oblique muscle. In the superficial layer, there are the branches of the infraordital nerve and the zygomatic branches of the facial nerve. In the deep layer, there are the branches of the oculomotor nerve and the branches or tributaries of the ophthalmic artery and vein. 〈Indications〉twitching of eyelids, redness with swelling and pain of the eye, lacrimation when attacked by wind, night blindness, deviation of the eye and mouth. 〈Method〉Puncture perpendicularly 0.3～0.7 cun along the infraorbital ridge. Lift and thrust the needle slowly, and twirl the needle with a large amplitude, taking care not to prick the blood vessels and cause hemotoma. Moxibustion is forbidden.

●承山 [chéng shān] 经穴名。出《灵枢·卫气》。属足太阳膀胱经。又名鱼腹、肉柱、玉柱、肠山、鱼肠。〈定位〉在小腿后面正中,委中与昆仑之间,当伸直小腿或足跟上提时腓肠肌肌腹下出现尖角凹陷处(图83)。〈层次解剖〉皮肤→皮下组织→腓肠肌→比目鱼肌。浅层布有小隐静脉和腓肠肌内侧皮神经。深层有胫神经和胫后动、静脉。〈主治〉腰背病、腿痛转筋、痔疾、便秘、脚气、鼻衄、癫疾、疝气、腹痛。直刺0.7～1寸;可灸。

Chengshan (BL 57) A meridian point, originally from *Lingshu:Wei Qi* (*Miraculous Pivot:Defensive Qi*), a point on the Bladder Meridian of Foot-Taiyang, also named Yufu, Rouzhu, Yuzhu, Changshan or Yuchang. 〈Location〉on the posterior midline of the leg, between Weizhong (BL 40) and Kunlun (BL 60), in a pointed depression formed below the gestrocnemius muscle belly when the leg is stretched or the heel is lifted. (Fig. 83)〈Regional anatomy〉skin→subcutaneous tissue→gastrocnemius muscle→soleus muscle. In the superficial layer, there are the small saphenous vein and the medial cutaneous nerve of the calf. In the deep layer, there are the tibial nerve and the posterior tibial artery and vein. 〈Indications〉pain in the lumbar area and the back, spasm with pain in the leg, hemorrhoids, constipation, beriberi, epistaxis, disorder or the head or epilepsy, hernia pain. 〈Method〉Puncture perpendicularly 0.7～1.0 cun. Moxibustion is applicable.

●程高 [chéng gāo] 人名。东汉针灸家,涪翁的弟

子,郭玉的老师。见《后汉书·郭玉传》。

Cheng Gao An expert in acupuncture and moxibustion during the Eastern Han Dynasty, a disciple of Fu Weng, teacher of Guo Yu. Cf. *Hou Han Shu: Guo Yu Zhuan* (*History of the Later Han Dynasty: Biography of Guo Yu*).

●程玠[chéng jiè] 人名。明代医家,字文玉,号松崖,歙县(今属安徽)人。精于医,善针灸,著《松崖医经》等。见《安徽通志》。

Cheng Jie A doctor during the Ming Dynasty, who styled himself Wen Yu and was called Song Ya, a native of Shexian County (in today's Anhui Province). Proficient in medicine and good at acupuncture and moxibustion, he compiled *Song Ya Yijing* (*Song Ya's Medical Classic*), etc. Cf. *Anhui Tongzhi* (*General Annals of Anhui Province*).

●程天祚[chéng tiān zuò] 人名。南北朝以前针灸家,里籍不详。撰《程天祚针经》。六卷。见《隋书·经籍志》。书佚。

Cheng Tianzuo An expert in acupuncture and moxibustion prior to the North and South Dynasties, whose personal background is unknown. Author of the six-volume *Cheng Tianzuo Zhenjing* (*Cheng Tianzuo's Moxibustion Classic*) which is no longer extant. Cf. *Suishu: Jing Ji Zi* (*History of the Sui Dynasty: Records of Classics and Books*).

●程约[chéng yuē] 人名。宋针灸家,字孟博,婺源(今属江西)人。世代为医,善针灸,著《医方图说》。见《婺源县志》。

Cheng Yue An expert in acupuncture and moxibustion during the Song Dynasty, who styled himself Mengbo, a native of Wuyuan (in today's Jianxi Province). He came from a long line of doctors and was therefore well trained in acupuncture and moxibustion. He wrote *Yifang Tushuo* (*Illustration of Prescriptions*). Cf. *Wuyuan Xianzhi* (*Annals of Wuyuan County*).

●吃逆[chī nì] 病证名。见《医经溯洄集》。即呃逆。详见该条。

Hiccup While Eating A disease seen in *Yijing Suhui Ji* (*A Discourse on the Tracing Back of Medical Classics*), i. e. hiccup. →呃逆 (p.)

●池头[chí tóu] 经穴别名。出《针灸资生经》。即温溜。详见该条。

Chitou Another name for Wenliu (LI 7), a meridian point originally from *Zhenjiu Zisheng Jing* (*Acupuncture-Moxibustion Classic for Saving Life*). →温溜 (p. 470)

●尺桡[chǐ náo] 经外穴名。见《中医杂志》(1957.4)位于前臂伸正中线上,腕背横纹中点上6寸处。〈主治〉精神病、上肢麻痹或瘫痪等。直刺1.0～1.5寸,或透向对侧皮下。

Chinao (EX-UE) An extra point seen in *Zhongyi Zazhi* (*Journal of Traditional Chinese Medicine*) (April, 1957). 〈Location〉 on the midline of the back side of the forearm, 6 cun above the midpoint of the dorsal transverse crease of the wrist. 〈Indications〉 mental disorder, numbness of the upper limbs or paralysis, etc. 〈Method〉 Puncture perpendicularly 1.0～1.5 cun or through to the subcutaneous region of the opposite side.

●尺泽[chǐ zé] 经穴名。出《灵枢·本输》。属于手太阴肺经,为本经合穴。又名鬼受、鬼堂。〈定位〉在肘横纹中,肱二头肌腱桡侧凹陷处(图52和图16)。〈层次解剖〉皮肤→皮下组织→肱桡肌→桡神经→肱肌。浅层有头静脉,前臂钱侧皮神经等。深层有桡神经,桡侧副动、静脉前支,桡侧返动、静脉等。〈主治〉咳嗽、气喘、咯血、潮热、咽喉肿痛、舌干、胸部胀满、吐泻、小儿惊风、肘臂挛痛、乳痈。直刺0.5～0.8寸,或点刺出血;可灸。

Chize (LU 5) A meridian point, originally from *Lingshu: Benshu* (*Miraculous Pivot: Meridian Points*), the He (Sea) point of the Lung Meridian of Hand-Taiyin, also named Guishou or Guitang. 〈Location〉 In the cubital crease, in the depression of the radial side of the tendon of the bicepsmuscle of the arm. (Figs. 52 & 16) 〈Regional anatomy〉 skin → subcutaneous tissue → brachioradial muscle → radial nerve → brachial muscle. In the superficial layer, there are the cephalic vein and the lateral cutaneous nerve of the forearm and so on. In the deep layer, there are the radial nerve, the anterior branches of the radial col-

lateral artery and vein and the radial recurrent artery and vein. 〈Indications〉 cough, dyspenea, hemoptysis, afternoon fever, sore throat, dryness of the tongue, distension and fullness in the chest, vomiting and diarrhea, infantile convulsion, spasmodic pain of the elbow and arm, acute mastitis. 〈Method〉 Puncture perpendicualarly 0.5～0.8 cun, or prick to cause bleeding. Moxibustion is applicable.

●尺之五里[chǐ zhī wǔ lǐ] 经穴别名。出《灵枢·小针解》,即手五里。详见该条。

Chizhiwuli Another name for Shouwuli (LI 13), a meridian point originally from *Lingshu: Xiaozhen Jie* (*Miraculous Pivot: Explanation of Delicate Needling*). →手五里(p.401)

●齿脉[chǐ mài] 经脉名,出《阴阳十一脉灸经甲本》。即手阳明大肠经。详见该条。

Tooth Meridian A meridian, originally from *Yinyang Shiyi Mai Jiujing Jiaben* (*Moxibustion Classic of the Eleven Yin-Yang Meridians*). →手阳明大肠经(p.401)

●齿牙[chǐ yá] 经穴别名。出《针灸经纶》。即颊车。详见该条。

Chiya Another name for Jiache (ST 6), a meridian point originally from *Zhenjiu Jinglun* (*Treatise on Acupuncture Classic*). →颊车(p.187)

●豉饼灸[chǐ bǐng jiǔ] 间接灸的一种。见《千金要方》。即隔豉饼灸。详见该条。

Fermented Soybean-Cake Moxibustion One type of indirect moxibustion seen in *Qianjin Yaofang* (*Essential Prescriptions Worth a Thousand Gold*). →隔豉饼灸(p.134)

●赤白肉际[chì bái ròu jì] 部位名。指手足部掌面(白肉)与背面(赤肉)皮肤的移行处。

Junction of the Red and White Skin A part of the body, referring to the line between the palm (the whitish skin) and dorsum (the reddish skin) on the hand or foot.

●赤带[chì dài] 病证名。见《千金要方》。又称带下赤候。指从阴道流出淡红似血非血的粘液,淋沥连绵不断。多因忧思伤脾,肝郁火炽,灼伤冲任带脉所致。治宜扶脾气,清肝火。取脾俞、肝俞、三阴交、足三里、带脉、间使、行间。

Leukorrhea with Bloody Discharge A disease seen in *Qianjin Yaofang* (*Essential Prescriptions Worth a Thousand Gold*), also named leukorrhagia with reddish discharge, referring to light colored bloody mucous discharged continuously of the spleen, and the stagnation of liver-qi, leading to excessive pathogenic fire, thus resulting in the impairment of the Chong, Ren, and Dai Meridians. 〈Treatment principle〉 Strengthen spleen-qi and clear away liver-fire. 〈Point selection〉 Pishu (BL 20), Ganshu (BL 18), Sanyinjiao (SP 6), Zusanli (ST 36), Daimai (GB 26), Jianshi (PC 5) and Xingjian (LR 2).

●赤凤迎源[chì fēng yéng yuán] 针刺手法名。出《金针赋》。为飞经走气四法之一,与苍龟探穴相对,又称凤凰展翅。其法当先将针刺入深层,得气后再上提至浅层,候针自摇,再插入中层,进行上下、左右的提插、捻转动作,手指一捻一放,形如赤凤展翅飞旋,有通行经气的作用。

Red Phoenix Encountering the Source A needing technique originally from *Jinzhen Fu* (*Ode to the Gold Needle*), one of the four methods of quick needling over the meridians, the opposite of the green turtle probing point method, also termed "spreading of the phoenix's wings". 〈Method〉 Insert the needle to the deep layer, then lift it to the superficial tissue. After getting a needling response, wait until the needle shakes itself before thrusting it back to the middle layer. Manipulate it by lifting it left and right. The fingers twirl and spread the needle repeatedly as if a red phoenix were spreading her wings while hovering in the sky. The method has the function of promoting the circulation of meridian-qi.

●赤乌神针经[chì wū shén zhēn jīng] 书名。张子存撰。原见于《隋书·经籍志》,不著撰人姓名。后由《唐书·经籍志》订补。书佚。

Chi Wu Shen Zhen Jing (***Classic on Red-Black Miraculous Acupuncture***) A book written by Zhang Zicun, originally from *Suishu: Jing Ji Zhi* (*The History of the Sui Dynasty: Records of Classics and Books*). Whose author is unknown. Later it was revised and supplemented into *Tangshu: Jing Ji*

Zhi (*The History of the Tang Dynasry: Records of Classics and Books*). It is no longer extant.

● 赤游丹 [chì yóu dān] 即丹毒。以其色赤，发无定处，故名。详见"丹毒"条。

Unfixed Red Erysipelas Also erysipelas, so named because of its reddish color and unfixed pathogenic site. →丹毒(p.71)

● 瘈(瘛)脉 [chì mài] 经穴名。出《针灸甲乙经》。属手少阳三焦经，又名资脉。在头部，耳后乳突中央，当角孙至翳风之间，沿耳轮连线的中、下三分之一的交点处(图28)。在耳后肌上；有耳后动、静脉；布有耳大神经耳后支。主治头痛、耳聋、耳鸣、小儿惊痫、呕吐、泄痢。平刺0.3～0.5寸，或点刺出血；可灸。

Chimai (SJ 18) A meridian point, originally from *Zhenjiu Jia-Yi Jing* (*A-B Classic of Acupuncture and Moxibustion*), a point on the Sanjiao Meridian of Hand-Shaoyang, also named Zimai. ⟨Location⟩ on the head, at the centre of the mastoid process, and at the junction of the middle third and lower third of the line connecting Jiaosun (SJ 20) and Yifeng (SJ 17) along the curve of the ear helix. (Fig. 28) ⟨Regional anatomy⟩ skin→subcutaneous tissue→posterior auricular muscle. There are the great auricular nerve, the posterior auricular branches of the facial nerve and the posterior auricular artery and vein in this area. ⟨Indications⟩ headache, deafness, tinnitus, infantile convulsion, vomiting, diarrhea and dysentery. ⟨Method⟩ Puncture subcutaneously 0.3～0.5 cun or prick to cause bleeding. Moxibustion is applicable.

● 冲道 [chōng dào] 经穴别名。见《循经考穴编》。即神道。详见该条。

Chongdao Another name for Shendao (DU 11), a meridian point seen in *Xunjing Kaoxue Bian* (*Studies on Acupoints along Meridians*). →神道(p.360)

● 冲脉 [chōng mài] 奇经八脉之一。又名太冲脉。出《灵枢·逆顺肥瘦》。其循行，起于小腹内，浅出气街部，与足少阴经并行，夹脐旁直上，至胸中散开，上行的一支至咽喉，上行至鼻之内窍，分别散络唇口。下行者，注入肾之大络，出于气街部。沿大腿内侧，斜入腘中，经过胫骨内廉，到内踝后又分两支。一支向下并于足少阴肾达足底，一支向前至足跗上行于足大趾。另一支，从小腹分出，向内贯脊，行于背部。

Chong Meridian One of the Eight Extra Meridians, also named the Great Chong Meridian, originally from *Lingshu: Nishun Feishou* (*Miraculous Pivot: Circulatory Direction of Meridians and Body Constitution*). ⟨Course of the meridian⟩ It begins at the lower abdomen, emerges at the groin and runs abreast the Foot-Shaoyin Meridian, ascends along both sides of the umbilicus and splits when reaching the chest. The ascending branch reaches the throat, goes up to the nostril, and distributes around the lips. The descending branch enters the major collateral of the kidney, comes out from the groin, goes along the medial side of the thigh, obliquely reaches the popliteal fossa, passes through the medial side of the tibia and divides into ramifications when reaching the medial malleolous, of which one goes downwards, meets with the Kidney Meridian of Foot-Shaoyin at the sole of the foot while the other runs forwards to the dorsum of the foot and then to the big toe; yet another branch divides from inside the lower abdomen, runs to the spinal column and travels along the back.

● 冲脉病 [chōng mài bìng] 奇经八脉病候之一。见《素问·骨空论》。证见气急上冲、心胸腹痛、月经不调、崩漏、不育等。

Diseases of Chong Meridian One of the diseases of the Eight Extra Meridians, seen in *Suwen: Gu Kong Lun* (*Plain Questions: On the Apertures of Bones*), manifested with upwards reverse of qi, pain in heart, chest and abdomen, irregular menstruation, metrorrhagia, metrostaxis and sterility.

● 冲门 [chōng mén] 经穴名。出《针灸甲乙经》。属足太阴脾经，为足太阴、厥阴之会。又名慈宫、上慈宫。⟨定位⟩在腹股沟外侧，距耻骨联合上缘中点3.5寸，当髂外动脉搏动处的外侧(图84和图40)。⟨层次解剖⟩皮肤→皮下组织→腹外斜肌腱膜→腹内斜肌→腹横腰肌→髂腰肌。浅层有旋髂浅动、静脉的分支或属支，第十一、十二胸神经前支和第一腰神经前支的外侧皮支。深层有股神经，第十一、十二胸神经前支和第一腰神经前支的肌支，旋髂深动、静脉。⟨主治⟩腹痛、疝气、痔痛、小便不利、缺乳、胎气上冲。直

刺0.5~0.7寸,可灸。

Chongmen (SP 12)　A meridian point, originally from *Zhenjiu Jia-Yi Jing* (*A-B Classic of Acupuncture and Moxibustion*), a point on the Spleen Meridian of Foot-Taiyin, the converging point of the Meridians of Foot-Taiyin and Foot Jueyin, also named Cigong or Shangcigong. 〈Location〉 at the lateral and of the inguinal groove, 3.5 cun lateral to the midpoint of the inguinal groove, 3.5 cun lateral to the midpoint of the upper border of the symphysis pubis, lateral to the midpoint of the upper border of the symphysis pubis, lateral to the pulsating external iliacartery (Figs. 84 & 40). 〈Regional anatomy〉 skin → subcutaneous tissue → aponeurosis of external oblique of abdomen → internal oblique muscle of the abdomen → transverse muscle abdomen → iliopsoas muscle. In the superficial layer, there are the branches or tributaries of the superficial circumflex iliac artery and vein, the lateral cutaneous branches of the anterior branches of the 11th and 12th thoracic nerves and the lst lumbar nerve. In the deep layer, there are the muscular branches of the anterior branches of the 11th and 12th thoracic nerve and the lst lumbar nerve, the femoral nerve, and the deep circumflex iliac artery and vein. 〈Indications〉 abdominal pain, hernia. hemorrhoid with pain, difficulty in urination, lack of lactation, reversed excessive qi due to fetus. 〈Method〉 Puncture perpendicularly 0.5~0.7 cun. Moxibustion is applicable.

●冲阳[chōng yáng]　①经穴名。出《灵枢·本输》。属足阳明胃经,为本经原穴,又名会原。〈定位〉在足背最高处,当拇长伸肌腱与趾长伸肌腱之间,足背动脉搏动处(图86)。〈层次解剖〉皮肤→皮下组织→拇长伸肌腱与趾长伸肌腱之间→短伸肌→中间楔骨。浅层布有足背内侧皮神经,足背静脉网,深层有足背动、静脉和腓深神经。〈主治〉胃痛、腹胀、不嗜食、口眼㖞斜、面肿齿痛、足痿无力、脚背红肿、善惊、癫狂。避开动脉,直刺0.2~0.5寸,禁灸。②经穴别名。出《针灸甲乙经》。即迎香,详见该条。

1. **Chongyang** (ST 42)　A meridian point, originally from *Lingshu: Benshu* (*Miraculous Pivot: Meridian Points*), the Yuan (Primary) Point of the Stomach Meridian of Foot-Yangming, also named Huiyuan. 〈Location〉 on the dome of the instep of the foot, between the tendons of the long extensor muscle of the great toe and the long extensor muscle of the toes, where the pulsation of the dorsal artery of the foot is palpable (Fig. 86). 〈Regional anatomy〉 skin → subcutaneous tissue → between tendons of long extensor muscle of great toe and long extensor muscle of toes → short extensor muscle of great toe → intermediate cuneiform bone. In the superficial layer, there are the medial dorsal cutaneous nerve and dorsal venous network of the foot. In the deep layer, there are the dorsal pedal artery and vein and the deep peroneal nerve. 〈Indications〉 astralgia, abdominal distention, poor appetite, deviation of the mouth and eye, edema of the face, toothache, muscular atrophy and weakness of the foot, redness and swelling of the dorsum of the foot, susceptibility to fright, manic-depressive psychosis. 〈Method〉 Avoiding (puncturing) the artery, puncture perpendicularly 0.2~0.5 cun. Moxibustion is forbidden.

2. **Chongyang**　Another name of Yingxiang (LI 20), a meridian point originally from *Zhenjiu Jia-Yi Jing* (*A-B Classic of Acupuncture and Moxibustion*). → 迎香 (p. 567)

●虫啮心痛[chóng niè xīn tòng]　病证名。见《丹溪心法附余》卷十五。即虫心痛。详见该条。

Epigastric Pain due to Bit by Parasites　A disease seen in Vol. 15 of *Danxi Xinfa Fuyu* (*Supplement to Danxi's Experience*). → 虫心痛 (p. 50)

●虫吐[chóng tù]　病证名。因肠道蛔虫上扰于胃而致的呕吐,可分寒、热两种证型。寒证者,多因胃经受寒,迫虫扰胃上逆所致。证见呕吐清稀、腹部时痛时止、面色青白。治宜温胃安蛔,取中脘、关元、足三里。温针灸。热证者,多因胃经火逆,以致虫动不安扰胃上逆所致,证见呕吐清稀涎沫、腹部时痛时止、面色口唇红赤。治宜清胃安蛔。取中脘、曲池、内庭、梁门。

Vomiting Caused by Intestinal Parasitosis　A disease referring to vomiting due to intestinal parasites interfering with the stomach. It can be divided into two types: cold and heat.

The cold type is mostly due to cold pathogens affecting the meridian of the stomch, forcing the parasites upwards and interfering with the stomach. 〈Manifestations〉 vomiting with thin discharge, intermittent abdominal pain, pale and green complexion. 〈Treatment principle〉 Warm the stomach to quiet the parasites. 〈Point selection〉 Zhongwan (RN 12), Guanyuan (RN 4) and Zusanli (ST 36). 〈Method〉 Warm stomach to quiet the parasites. The heat type is mostly due to excess fire of the stomach, leading to irritated parasites interfering the stomach. 〈Manifestations〉 vomiting with thin saliva, intermittent abdominal pain, flushed face and red lips. 〈Treatment principle〉 Clear heat from the stomach to quiet the parasites. 〈Point selection〉 Zhongwan (RN 12), Quchi (LI 11), Neiting (ST 44) and Liangmen (ST 21).

●虫心痛[chóng xīn tòng] 病证名。出《千金要方》。又名啮心痛、虫咬心痛。即胆道蛔虫病。详见该条。

Epigastric Pain due to Enterositosis A disease originally from *Qianjin Yaofang* (*Essential Prescriptions Worth a Thousand Gold*), also named epigastric pain due to a parasite bite or epigastric pain due to snapping by parasites. →胆道蛔虫病(p.73)

●虫咬心痛[chóng yǎo xīn tòng] 病证名。见《丹溪心法附余》卷十五。即虫心痛。详见该条。

Epigastric Pain due to Snap by Parasites A disease seen in Vol. 15 of *Danxi Xinfa Fuyu* (*Supplement to Danxi's Experience*). →虫心痛(p.50)

●重见时[chóng jiàn shí] 子午流注针法用语。又称日干重见。按干支记时,每个时辰又重复见到同一天干。如甲日于甲戌时开穴,后第十个时辰为甲申,重见甲。乙日于乙酉时开穴,后第十个时辰为乙未,重见乙。本法规定,阳日重见时,取三焦经的五输穴,称为气纳三焦;阴日重见时,取心包经的五输穴。称为血纳包络。

The Meeting-Once-Again Period A term for midnight-noon ebb flow needling method, also termed "day and stem meet once again". According to the method of calculating the time by stems matching branches, the same heavenly stems meet again every 10 two-hour period. For instance, an acupoint is selected at the period of Jiawu in the day of Jia, the next 10 two-hour period is Jiashen, when the Jias meet again; an acupoint is selected in the period of Yiyou in the day of Yi, the next 10 two-hour period is Yiwei, when the Yis meet again. The rules of the method are : select the five shu points of the Sanjiao Meridian when Yang days meet again, which is called "qi being brought into the Sanjiao"; select the five Shu points of the Pericardium Meridian when Yin days meet again, which is termed as "blood being brought into the pericardium".

●崇骨[chóng gǔ] 经外穴名。出《针灸集成》。又名椎顶、太祖,在项部且正中线上,当第六颈椎棘突下缘。〈主治〉感冒、咳嗽、疟疾、项强、支气管炎、癫痫等,直刺0.5～1寸;可灸。

Chonggu (EX-HN) An extra point, orginally from *Zhenjiu Jicheng* (*A Collection of Acupuncture and Moxibustion*), also named *Zhuiding* or *Taizu*. 〈Location〉on the posterior midline of the nape, at the inferior edge of the spinous process of the 6th cervical vertebra. 〈Indications〉common cold, cough, malaria, rigidity of the neck, bronchitis, epilepsy. 〈Method〉Puncture perpendicularly 0.5～1.0 cun. Moxibustion is applicable.

●抽气拔罐法[chōu qì bá guàn fǎ] 拔罐法的一种。用特制的罐,罐底有橡皮活塞,接通吸引器抽成负压,使罐吸着于皮肤上以治疗病痛,吸附力较强,并可随时调节或测量负压大小。

Cupping by Extracting Air A cupping method. Use a specially made cup with a rubber piston fixed at the bottom of the cup, connect it to the air extractor, extract the air to form a negative pressure inside, making the cup absorbent on the skin for treating diseases. The absorption is fairly strong, and the negative pressure of the cup can be regulated and measured at any time.

●抽添法[chōu tiān fǎ] 针刺手法名。出《金针赋》。抽,意为上提;添,意为按纳。其法与纳气法类似。先紧按慢提九数,得气后,阳阳转换针向,多用提按(或当呼气时按纳,吸气时上提),使气到病痛部位,再直起针向下按纳。用于瘫痪、半身不遂。

Lifting-Pushing Method A term for a

needling technique, originally from *Jinzhen Fu* (*Ode to the Gold Needle*). Lifting means lifting up the needle, whereas pushing means thrusting it. This therapy is similar to the qi-accepting method. 〈Method〉Thrust quickly and lift slowly nine times first. After the arrival of qi, change the insertion direction of the needle slowly. Adopt mostly the method of lifting and thrusting the needle (push and thrust the needle while the patient expires and lift the needle while the patient inspires) to make the qi reach the affected region, then straighten the needle and thrust and push it downwards. 〈Indications〉paralysis and hemiplegia.

●出针法[chū zhēn fǎ] 针法术语。又称起针、拔针、排针、发针、引针。指行针已毕，将针从穴内退出的方法。即先以左手拇、食指或中、食指，固定被刺腧穴周围皮肤，右手持针轻微捻退至皮下，然后迅速拔出；或将针轻捷地直接向外拔出。出针的快慢，必须结合病情和各种补泻手法的需要，切不可妄用强力，粗心大意。

Needle-Withdrawing A term for a needling technique, also named needle-taking-out, needle-pulling, needle-removing, needle-releasing, or needle-getting-up. It refers to the method of withdrawing the needle from the acupoint, when the needling is done. Press and tighten the skin around the inserted point with the thumb and index finger or the middle and index fingers of the left hand, rotate the needle gently and lift it to the subcutaneous layer, then withdraw it quickly; or directly withdraw the needle quickly and gently. To withdraw the needle quickly or slowly depend on the patient's condition and the requirements of the different methods of reinforcing and reducing. Too powerful and casual withdrawal of the needle should be avoided.

●揣法[chuǎi fǎ] 针刺辅助手法名。见《针灸大成》。为下手八法之一。指在针刺之前，先用手指揣摸病人肢体以探索穴位，随后下针。

Seeking A term in auxiliary acupuncture manipulations, seen in *Zhenjiu Dacheng* (*A Great Compendium of Acupuncture and Moxibustion*), one of the eight manipulations of acupuncture, referring to the seeking of the points on the patient's body with the fingers before inserting the needle.

●川椒饼灸[chuān jiāo bǐng jiǔ] 间接灸法之一。出《肘后方》。即隔川椒灸。详见该条。

Chuan Jiao (Pericarpium Zanthoxyli)-Cake Moxibustion One of the indirect moxibustion methods, originally from *Zhou Hou Fang* (*A Handbook of Prescriptions*). →隔川椒灸(p.134)

●穿鼻[chuān bí] 经外穴别名。出《刺疗捷法》。即上迎香。详见该条。

Chuanbi Another name for Shangyingxiang (EX-HN 8), an extra point originally from *Ci Ding Jiefa* (*Simple Acupuncture Method for Boils*). →上迎香(p.355)

●传热灸[chuán rè jiǔ] 为温针之别称。详见该条。

Heat-Conducting Moxibustion Another name for warming the needle. →温针(p.471)

●传尸[chuán shī] 古病证名。见《外台秘要》卷十三。即肺痨。详见该条。

Walking Corpse An archaic name for pulmonary tuberculosis, seen in Vol. 13 of *Waitai Miyao* (*Clandestine Essentials from the Imperial Library*). →肺痨(p.107)

●传尸灸[chuán shī jiǔ] 经外穴名。见《外台秘要》。位于小腿伸侧胫骨前嵴，当内外踝连线中点直上3寸，灸治肺痨。

Chuanshijiu (EX-LE) An extra point, seen in *Waitai Miyao* (*Clandestine Essentials from the Imperial Library*). 〈Location〉on the anterior side of the leg, lateral to the spine of the tibia, 3 cun above the midpoint of the line connecting the medial and external malleolus. 〈Indication〉pulmonary tuberculosis. 〈Method〉moxibustion.

●传尸痨[chuán shī láo] 古病证名。即肺痨。详见该条。

Corpse-Walking Tuberculosis An archaic name for pulmonary tuberculosis. →肺痨(p.107)

●喘息穴[chuán xī xué] 经外穴别名。即定喘。详见该条。

Chuanxixue →定喘(p.84)

●窗笼[chuāng lóng] ①部位名。指耳部。②经外别

名。出《针灸甲乙经》。即天窗。详见该条。

Chuanglong ① A part of the body, referring to the ear. ② Another name for Tianchuang(SI 16), a meridian point originally from *Zheniu Jia-Yi Jing*(*A-B Classic of Acupuncture and Moxibustion*). →天窗(p. 430)

●吹奶[chuī nǎi] 即乳痈。详见该条。

Mammary Abscess →乳痈(p. 339)

●吹乳[chuī rǔ] 病证名。出《儒门事亲》。又名乳吹,即乳痈。分内吹乳痈和外吹乳痈两种。详见各条。

Acute Mastitis Another name for breast abscess, originally from *Rumen Shiqin*(*Confucians' Duties to Their Parents*), also named mammary abscess, divided into two types: acute mastitis during pregnancy and postpartum mastitis. →乳痈(p. 339). 内吹乳痈(p. 278). 外吹乳痈(p. 452)

●垂浆[chuí jiāng] 经穴别名。出《圣济总录》。即承浆。详见该条。

Chuijiang Another name for Chengjiang (RN 24), a meridian point from *Shengji Zonglu*(*Imperial Medical Encyclopaedia*). →承浆(p. 43)

●垂矩[chuí jù] 经外穴别名。即中矩。详见该条。

Chuiju →中矩(p. 611)

●垂帘障[chuí lián zhàng] 病证名。即目翳别名。详见该条。

Trachomatous Pannus Another name for eye macula. →目翳(p. 273)

●垂前[chuí qián] 耳穴名。又名神经衰弱点,位于4区,参见牙条。用于治疗神经衰弱、牙痛。

Anterior Ear Lobe(MA) An ear point, also named neuresthenic point, located in the 4th area of the ear, used to treat neurasthenia and toothache. →牙(p. 533)

●垂手[chuí shǒu] 经穴别名。出《医学原始》。即风市。详见该条。

Chuishou Another name for Fengshi (GB 31), a meridian point from *Yixue Yuanshi*(*Origin of Medicine*). →风市(p. 115)

●唇里[chún lǐ] 经外穴名。出《千金要方》。在口腔内,下唇粘膜上,与承浆穴相对处。〈主治〉黄疸、瘟疫、口噤、口臭、面颊肿、齿龈炎、口腔炎等,点刺出血.

Chunli(EX-HN) An extra point, originally from *Qianjin Yaofang*(*Essential Prescriptions Worth a Thousand Gold*). 〈Location〉in the mouth, on the mucous membrane of the lower lip, opposite to Chengjiang (RN 24). 〈Indications〉 jaundice, pestilence, trismus, foul breath, edema of face, gingivitis, stomatitis, etc. 〈Method〉Prick to cause bleeding.

●淳于意[chún yú yì] 人名。西汉著名医家,齐临菑(今山东临淄)人。曾任齐太仓长,故又称仓公。曾先后随公孙光、公乘阳庆等人学医,医术高明,亦善针灸。现存其临证实录25例。见《史记·扁鹊仓公列传》。

Chunyu Yi A famous physician during the Western Han Dynasty, a native of Linzi in the area of Qi (today's Linzi, Shandong Province). He was once in charge of the storehouse of grain in the area of Qi, and so was also named Canggong (Storehouseman). He once learned medicine from Gongsun Guang and Gongsheng Yangqing, etc.. His medical skill was excellent, and he also specialized in acupuncture and moxibustion. The concrete records on 25 cases of his clinical practice exist today. Cf. *Shi Ji*: *Bian Que Canggong Liezhuan*(*Historical Records*: *Biographies of Bian Que and Canggong*.)

●疵疮[cī chuāng] 即疔疮。详见该条。

Ci Chuang →疔疮(p. 82)

●慈宫[cí gōng] ①经穴别名。出《针灸甲乙经》。即冲门。详见该条。②经外穴名。见《千金要方》。当耻骨联合中点(横骨)旁开2.5寸。〈主治〉泄泻、痢疾、月经不调。直刺0.5～1寸;可灸。

1. **Cigong** Another name for Chongmen (SP 12), a meridian point originally from *Zhenjiu Jia-Yi Jing*(*A-B Classic of Acupuncture and Moxibustion*). →冲门(p. 48)

2. **Cigong**(EX) An extra point originally from *Qianjin Yaofang*(*Essential Prescriptions Worth a Thousand Gold*). 〈Location〉2.5 cun lateral to the midpoint of the symphysis pubis. 〈Indications〉diarrhea, dysentery, irregular menstruation. 〈Method〉Puncture perpendicularly 0.5～1.0 cun. Moxibustion is applica-

●**雌雄霹雳火**[cí xióng pī lì huǒ] 直接灸法的一种。见《外科正宗》卷二。用麝香3克、丁香、雌黄、雄黄各少许，研为细末，搓入艾绒内，作小艾炷，放于患处施灸。灸至局部肉焦为度，或知痛灸至知痒，知痒灸至知痛，可用于治疗阴毒、阴疽、阴发背。

Male-Female Thunderbolt Fire A kind of direct moxibustion, from Vol. 2 of *Waike Zhengzong* (*Orthodox Manual of External Diseases*). Grind 3g of musk and a small amount of cloves, orpiment and realgar into a fine powder, mix it with moxa wool, make small moxa cones, and put the cones directly on the affected part of the body for moxibustion. Stop moxibustion when local skin is burnt, or when the patient itches if he feels pain, or *vice versa*. The method is used to treat yin-pathogens, yin-cellulitis and yin-lumbodorsal cellulitis.

●**磁针**[cí zhēn] 针具名。用带有磁性的铁针或钢针进行针刺。

Magnetic Needle A needling instrument, puncturing with a magnetic needle made of iron or steel.

●**次髎**[cì liáo] 经穴名。出《针灸甲乙经》。属足太阳膀胱经。〈定位〉在骶部，当髂后上棘内下方，适对第2骶后孔处(图7)。〈层次解剖〉皮肤→皮下组织→竖脊肌→第二骶后孔。浅层布有臀中皮神经。深层有第二骶神经和骶外侧动、静脉的后支。〈主治〉腰痛、月经不调、赤白带下、痛经、疝气、小便赤淋、腰以下至足不仁。直刺0.8～1寸；可灸。

Ciliao (BL 32) A meridian point originally from *Zheniu Jia-Yi Jing* (*A-B Classic of Acupuncture and Moxibustion*), a point on the Blader Meridian of Foot-Taiyang. 〈Location〉 on the sacral region, medial and inferior to the posterior superior iliac spine, in the 2nd posterior sacral foramen (Fig. 7). 〈Regional Anatomy〉 skin → subcutaneous tissue → erector spinal muscle → 2nd posterior sacral foramen. In the superficial layer, there is the middle clunial nerve. In the deep layer, there are the posterior branches of the 2nd sacral nerve and the lateral sacral artery and vein. 〈Indications〉 lower back pain, irregular menstruation, leukorrhea with reddish discharge, dysmenorrhea, hernia, scanty dark urine, numbness from the loin to the foot. 〈Method〉 Puncture perpendicularly 0.8～1.0cun. Moxibustion is applicable.

●**次门**[cì mén] 经穴别名。出《针灸甲乙经》。即关元。详见该条。

Cimen Another name for Guanyuan (RN 4), a meridian point, originally from *Zhenjiu Jia-Yi Jing* (*A-B Classic of Acupuncture and Moxibustion*). →关元(p. 148)

●**刺法**[cì fǎ] 针刺术语。即针法的别称，详见该条。

Acupuncture Technique An acupuncture term, i.e. needling technique. →针法(p. 589)

●**刺激参数**[cì jī cān chù] 针刺术语。指针刺时对穴位施加刺激条件及刺激量等方面的各项数据。手法运针的刺激参数，包括手法操作过程中提插、捻转的幅度、频率及持续时间。电针刺激参数，一般包括脉冲电流的强度、频率、波形、波宽及刺激时间等。因刺激参数的不同，临床所产生的效果也不同，各项之间还存在着交互作用，与刺激时间长短也有一定关系。记录和积累参数，并加以分析，对研究针刺原理，提高临床疗效和交流经验等都有着重要意义。

Stimulation Parameter An acupuncture term, denoting various datum of the stimulation condition and intensity applied to the point during acupuncture. The stimulation parameters of acunpuncture manipulation include the amplitude, frequency and the sustained time of lifting, thrusting and twirling. The stimulation of parameters of electrical acupuncture generally include the intensity, frequency, wave form, wave width and stimulating time of the pulse current. Different stimulation parameters may cause different clinical effects, and interaction exists among them. However, the effects are related to the stimulation time. Recording, accumulating and analysing the stimulation parameters are very significant to the researches of acupuncture mechanism, improvement of clinical effects, and exchange of experience.

●**刺激点**[cì jī diǎn] 近代对针灸腧穴的一种称谓，或称为针灸治疗刺激点。因穴位都具有治疗疾病的作用，故名。

Stimulation Point   A modern name for acupoint, also called stimulation point for acupuncture and moxibustion therapy. This name exists because all the points have the function of treating diseases.

●刺激强度[cì jī qiáng dù]   刺法术语。指针灸刺激的强弱程度,分强刺激、中刺激、弱刺激三种。大致由手法的轻重,针刺的深浅,针的粗细,针数的多少,刺激频率的快慢和持续时间的久暂等方面所构成。重、深、粗、多、快、久等构成了强刺激;轻、浅、细、少、慢、暂等构成了弱刺激;介于强、弱刺激之间的,为中刺激。不同刺激强度对机体可产生不同的效应,不同病人对同样刺激强度的针灸刺激的反应也有所差异。所以,针灸治疗时,要根据辨证论治的原则,灵活地掌握好适当的刺激强度。

Stimulation Intensity   A term for acupuncture techniques, referring to how strong the acupuncture stimulation is. It divided into three levels: strong, medium and weak. The intensity is related to the force of manipulation, the depth of insertion, the thickness of needles, the number of needles used, the stimulating frequency, and the stimulation time. Strong stimulation is to manipulate the needle forcefully, insert the needle deeply, use many and thick needles, apply a high frequency and for a long time, etc.. Weak stimulation is to manipulate the needle gently, insert the needle shallowly, use thin and few needles, apply low frequency and for a short time, etc. Medium stimulation is between the strong and the weak. Different stimulation intensities may cause different effects and the same stimulation intensities may also vary in intensity. Therefore, during treatment with acupuncture and moxibustion, proper stimulation intensities should be adopted flexibly on the basis of differentiation of syndromes.

●刺激区[cì jī qū]   与刺激点比较而言,其刺激的部位是一个面或一条线,而不是一个点。如皮肤针、头针等刺法,即将人体划分为若干刺激区。

Areas for Stimulation   In comparison with the stimulation points, the areas for stimulation are not points, but a surface or a line. For example, dermal needling or scalp acupuncture is just to stimulate certain areas on the body surface.

●刺禁[cì jìn]   针刺术语。指针刺的禁忌,包括禁刺部位(重要脏器、大血管、脑脊髓)和禁刺时机(如过饥、过饱、过度疲劳、情绪激烈变动等)。《灵枢·终始》等篇提出十二禁、五禁、五过、五夺禁刺、五逆等内容。参见各条。

Contraindications of Needling   An acupuncture term, referring to the cautions to be observed during acupuncture, including forbidden areas (e. g. important organs, great blood vessels, brain and spinal cord) and forbidden times (e. g. when patient is starving, has overeaten, is overstrained, or has violent mood changes) for acupuncture. The following contraindications were stated in *Lingshu: Zhongshi* (*Miraculous Pivot: End and Beginning*) and other chapters: twelve contraindications, five contraindications, acupuncture contraindications of five kinds of exhaustion; five excesses and five deteriorations. →十二禁(p. 374)五禁(p. 476)五过(p. 475)五夺禁刺(p. 475)五逆(p. 477)。

●刺灸[cì jiǔ]   针灸术语。又称灸刺,指针刺和艾灸。

Acupuncture and Moxibustion   A term of acupunsture and moxibustion, also called moxibustion and acupuncture, referring to acupuncture and moxibustion therapies.

●刺灸法[cì jiǔ fǎ]   中医治疗方法之一。指各种针刺和灸治方法。早在《黄帝内经》中就有五刺、九刺、十二刺和艾灸方法的记载,后世又续有发展,为针灸学术重要组成部分,使用适当与否,对临床疗效有很大影响。参见"针法"、"刺法"、"针刺手法"和"灸法"各条。

Techniques of Acupuncture and Moxibustion
  A therapy of traditional Chinese medicine, referring to various techniques used in acupuncture and moxibustion. When *Huangdi Neijing* (*The Yellow Emperor's Inner Canon*) came into being, five needling techniques, nine needling methods, twelve needlings and the techniques of moxibustion were recorded in it. They were further developed by later generations, thus constituting an important component of the science of

acupuncture and moxibustion. Whether these techinques are applied suitably or not will bear greatly on the clinical effects. →针法(p. 589). 刺法(p. 53)针刺手法(p. 589)灸法(p. 223)

●**刺灸心法要诀**[cì jiǔ xīn fǎ yào jué] 书名。针灸著作，八卷(即清·吴谦等编纂《医宗金鉴》卷七十九～八十六)。全书以七言歌诀为主，歌诀之后加注，并附插图一百三十四幅，易于习诵掌握。卷七十九为九针、十二经井、荥、输、经、合、原、络穴、八会穴及经脉流注；卷八十为周身骨度及各部诸穴；卷八十一～八十四为十二经及奇经的循行和经穴部位。卷八十五为头、胸腹背及手足各部的要穴及主治病证；卷八十六为各种灸法及针灸禁忌等。

Cijiu Xinfa Yaojue (Essentials of Acupuncture and Moxibustion in Verse) A book on acupuncture and moxibustion in 8 volumes, i.e. Vols. 79~86 of *Yizong Jinjian(Gold Mirror of Orthodox Medical Lineage)* by Wu Qian of the Qing Dynasty. The book was written mainly in the form of verses with 7 characters to each line and with annotations and 134 diagrams attached, which makes it easy to read, recite and master. Vol. 79 of the book deals with the nine needles, the point of Jing (Well), Ying (Spring), Shu (Stream), Jing (River), He (Sea), Yuan (Primary) and Luo(Connecting) points, the eight influential points and the cyclical flow of the twelve regular meridians; Vol. 80 involves proportional measurements of the whole body and the points in different areas; Vols. 81~84 explain the distribution and circulation of the twelve regular meridians and the extra meridians, also the locations of meridian points; Vol. 85 introduces the main points on the head, chest, abdomen, back, hand and foot and the indications of these points as well; Vol. 86 elaborates different moxibustion methods and the contraindications of acupuncture and moxibustion.

●**刺络**[cì luò] 针刺方法名。出《灵枢·血络论》。用三棱针或皮肤针等在浅表络脉上点刺或散刺，以放出适量血液。可用于治疗急性扁桃体炎、急性结膜炎、急性扭伤、中暑、中风昏迷、丹毒、急性胃肠炎、头痛、高血压、肺水肿等。须避免伤及动脉。体质虚弱，低血糖、低血压、血液病者，以及妊娠妇女，均不宜应用此法。

Collateral Pricking A needling method, originally from *Lingshu: Xueluo Lun (Miraculous Pivot: On Superficial Venules)*, referring to pricking and clumpy pricking on the superficial collateral with a three-edged needle or cutaneous needle to let out the proper amount of blood. 〈Indications〉acute tonsillitis, acute conjunctivitis, acute sprain, heat stroke, apoplexy coma, acute gastroenteritis, headache, hypertension, pulmonary edema, etc.. Try to avoid injurying arteries. The method is unadvisable for patients with weak constitution, hypoglycemia, hypotension or hematopathy, and pregnant women.

●**刺络拔罐**[cì luò bá guàn] 拔罐法之一。又称刺血拔罐。用三棱针、皮肤针等刺出血后再拔罐，以吸出少量血液。多用于软组织劳损扭伤、肩、背或腰腿风湿痛等症。对贫血、有出血倾向的病证，大血管所在部位，均不宜使用。

Bleeding before Cupping One of the cupping methods, also named blood-letting cupping, referring to blood-letting with a three-edged or cutaneous needle, followed by cupping, so as to draw out a small amount of blood. It is mainly used to treat soft tissue injury, sprain, pain of the shoulder and back, or lumbago due to pathogenic wind-dampness, etc. It is advisable to apply the method to patients with anemia or those susceptible to bleeding, or where big blood vessels lie.

●**刺络疗法**[cì luò liáo fǎ] 即刺血疗法。详见该条。
Collateral Pricking Therapy →刺血疗法(p. 56)

●**刺手**[cì shǒu] 针刺用语。毫针进针时，两手同时操作，一般将持针的手(右手)称为刺手。其作用主要是掌握针具，进针时使针尖迅速刺透皮肤进入身体，然后施行适当的捻转、提插等各种手法。

Needle-Holding Hand An acupuncture term. Both hands work together when inserting the filiform needle. The one (right hand) which holds the needle is usually called the acupuncturing hand. The main function of this hand is to control the needle and insert the needle rapidly through the skin into the body so as to apply various proper manipulation

techniques, such as lifting and thrusting, twirling or rotating.

●刺血拔罐[cì xuè bá guàn] 为刺络拔罐之别称。详见该条。

Blood-Letting Cupping Another name for bleeding cupping. →刺络拔罐(p. 55)

●刺血疗法[cì xuè liáo fǎ] 又称放血疗法、刺络疗法。是用三棱针、小眉刀、皮肤针等器具刺破人体上的一些浅表血管，放出适量血液以治疗疾病的一种方法。适用治疗扁桃体炎、神经性皮炎、过敏性皮炎、急性扭伤、中暑、痈疖、发热、头痛、鼻炎、急性结膜炎、急性角膜炎、丹毒、湿疹、淋巴管炎、静脉炎、痔疮等。凡体弱、贫血、低血压、妇女妊娠或产后等慎用，对有出血倾向及血管瘤患者，不宜使用。

Blood-letting Therapy Also named bleeding therapy or collateral pricking therapy, a therapeutic technique to prick the superficial blood vessels and draw out a proper amount of blood with a three-edged needle, a small eyebrowlike knife or a cutaneous needle. 〈Indications〉 tonsillitis, neurodermatitis, allergic dermatitis, acute sprain, heatstroke, carbuncle and furuncle, fever, headache, rhinitis, acute conjunctivitis, acute keratitis, erysipelas, exzeme, lymphangitis, phlebitis, hemorrhoid, etc. Careful consideration should be given to patients with a weak constitution, anemia, or hypotension, and patients who are pregnant or have just given birth, when this therapy is applied. The method should not be used for patients with a tendency to bleed or patients with angioma.

●葱白灸[cōng bái jiǔ] 天灸的一种。取葱白适量，洗净后捣如泥膏状，敷于穴位或患部。如敷于患部可治疗急性乳腺炎。也可与生姜、鲜疳积草合用，共捣如膏状，于晚上睡前敷于涌泉穴，翌日晨起取去之，治疗小儿养营不良。

Moxibustion with Scallion Stalk One of the medicinal vesiculation therapies. Take a proper amount of the stalk of Chinese green onion and after washing it, pound it into a mash or paste, then apply it to acupoints or affected area. For instance, apply the mash to the surface of the breast to treat acute mastitis. The scallion stalk can also be used together with fresh ginger and fresh Gan Ji herb. Pound them into a paste; apply it to the point Yongquan(KI 1) before sleeping, and remove it the next morning for treating malnutrition of children.

●葱豉糊灸[cōng chǐ hú jiǔ] 天灸的一种。取豆豉30克，生姜60克，食盐30克，葱白适量，上药共捣如糊膏状，敷于脐上(神阙穴)，油纸覆盖，胶布固定。并以热水袋敷其上，每日2次。适于治疗流行性感冒。

Moxibustion with Scallion Stalk and Fermented Soybean One of the medicinal vesiculation therapies. Take 30g of fermented soybean, 60g of fresh ginger, 30g of salt, and the proper amount of Chinese green onion stalk, and pound them into a paste. Apply it to the navel(Shenque, RN 8), then cover the area with oil paper and fix the paper with adhesive tape. Finally, place a bag of hot water on the area. The therapy is given twice a day to treat epidemic influenza.

●从荣置气[cóng róng zhì qì] 刺法用语。出《难经·七十六难》。与"从卫取气"相对，为针刺泻法的要领。荣，通营。指营气所行的部分，即深部。意指泻法操作要于深部候气并向浅部引提。后世刺法中的泻法，用先深后浅，即以此为理论依据。参见"从卫取气"条。

Directing Qi from Rong A term used to describe an acupuncture technique, from *Nanjing*: *Qishiliu Nan* (*Classic of Questions*: *Question* 76). This technique is the opposite of "taking qi from wei". It is the essential principle of reducing for using acupuncture. Rong is a general term for Ying, referring to the deep part, where ying qi (nutrient qi) travels. The term refers to the manipulation technique of reducing, or waiting for qi in the deep area and then lifting it to the superficial area. Later reducing methods, i. e., first needling deeply and then shallowly are based on this theory. →从卫取气(p. 56)

●从卫取气[cóng wèi qǔ qì] 刺法用语。出《难经·七十六难》。与"从荣置气"相对，为针刺补法的要领。卫，指卫气所行的部位，即浅部；取是候气之意。指补法的操作须于浅部候气，并往下按纳。后世刺法中的补法用先浅后深，即以此为理论依据。参'从荣置气'

条。

Taking Qi from Wei A term used to describe an acupuncture technique, from *Nan Jing*: *Qishiliu Nan* (*Classic of Questions*: *Question* 76). This technique is the opposite of "directing qi from Rong". It is the essential principle of reinforcing for using acupuncture. Wei refers to the superficial area where wei qi (Defensive qi) travels. This term refers to the manipulation technique of reinforcing, or waiting for qi in the superficial area and then pressing it down to the deep area. Later reinforcing methods, i.e. first needling shallowly and then deeply, are based on this theory. → 从荣置气(p. 56)

●从阳引阴[cóng yáng yǐn yīn] 《内经》取穴法则之一。出《素问·阴阳应象大论》。指病在阴经则先刺阳经以引导之。《卫生宝鉴》卷七引云歧子《医学新说》:治中风偏枯,取十二经井穴,先从足太阳经井穴至阴开始,依十二经流注次序至手太阳小肠经井穴少泽为止。称此为大接经从阳引阴。详见"大接经法"条。

Guiding Yin from Yang A principle for selecting acupoints, recorded in *Neijing* (*The Inner Canon of Huangdi*), originally from *Suwen*: *Yin-Yang Yingxiang Dalun* (*Plain Qestions*: *On Correspondence of Yin-Yang with Nature*). When yin-meridians are attacked by pathogenic factors, yang-meridians are to be punctured first to guide the factors. Vol. 7 of *Weisheng Baojian* (*A Treasured Mirror of Health Protection*) quoted *Yixue Xinshuo* (*New Theories in Medicine*) written by Yun Qizi: Select the Jing (Well) points of the Twelve Regular Meridians to treat apoplexy in the order of the cyclical flow of the Twelve Regular Meridians. Begin with Zhiyin (BL 67), the Jing (Well) point of the Meridian of Foot-Taiyang and end at Shaoze (SI 1), the Jing (Well) point of the Small Intestine Meridian of Hand-Taiyang. This is called great joined meridians of guiding yin from yang. → 大接经法(p. 63)

●从阴引阳[cóng yīn yǐn yáng] 《内经》取穴法则之一。出《素问·阴阳应象大论》。指病在阳经,当先刺阴经以引导之。《卫生宝鉴》卷七引云歧子《医学新说》:治中风偏枯,取用十二经井穴,先从手太阴肺经井穴少商开始,顺序刺至足厥阴肝经井穴大敦为止,称此为大接经从阴引阳。详见"大接经法"。

Guiding Yang from Yin A principle for selecting acupoints, recorded in *Neijing* (*The Canon of Internal Medicine*), originally from *Suwen*: *Yin-Yang Yingxiang Dalun* (*Plain Questions*: *On correspondence of Yin-Yang with Nature*). When yang meridians are attacked by pathogenic factors, yin meridians are to be punctured first to guide the factors. Vol. 7 of *Weisheng Baojian* (*A Treasured Mirror of Health Protection*) quoted *Yixue Xinshuo* (*New Theories in Medicine*) written by Yun Qizi: Selecting the Jing (Well) points of the Twelve Regular Meridians to treat apoplexy, in the order of the cyclical flow of the Twelve Regular Meridians. Begin with Shaoshang (LU 11) the Jing (Well) point of the Lung Meridian of Hand-Taiyin and end at Dadun (LR 1), the Jing (Well) point of the Liver Meridian of Foot-Jueyin. This is called great joined meridians of guiding yang from yin. → 大接经法(p. 63)

●卒癫[cù diān] 经外穴名。见《千金要方》。在阴茎根部上方凹陷处。〈主治〉卒癫。用灸法。

Cudian (EX) An extra point from *Qianjin Yaofang* (*Essential Prescriptions Worth a Thousand Gold*). 〈Location〉in the depression above the root of penis. 〈Indications〉sudden onset of depressive psychosis. 〈Method〉moxibustion.

●卒中[cù zhòng] 即中风。见《三因极一病证方论·中风治法》。一作猝中,又称卒中风。详见"中风"条。

Wind-stroke Another name for Apoplexy, from *Sanyin Jiyi Bingzheng Fanglun*: *Zhongfeng Zhifa* (*Treatise on the Three Categories of Pathogenic Factors of Diseases and the Prescriptions*: *Therapy for Apoplexy*). Also termed sudden stroke or sudden windstroke. → 中风(p. 616)

●卒中风[cù zhòng fēng] 见《千金要方》卷八。即卒中。详见该条。

Sudden Windstroke Another name for apoplexy, from Vol. 8 of *Qianjin Yaofang*(*Es*

sential Prescriptions Worth a Thousand Gold).
→卒中(p. 57)

●猝中[cù zhòng] 即卒中。见该条。

Sudden Stroke →卒中(p. 57)

●攒竹[cuán zhú] 经穴名。出《针灸甲乙经》。属足太阳膀胱经。又名始光、夜光、明光、光明、员在、员柱、眉头、眉本。〈定位〉在面部,当眉头陷中,眶上切迹处(图5和图28)。〈层次解剖〉皮肤→皮下组织→眼轮匝肌。浅层布有额神经的滑车上神经、眶上动、静脉的分支或属支。深面有面神经的颞支和颧支。〈主治〉头痛、眉棱骨痛、目眩、目视不明、目赤肿痛、迎风流泪、近视、眼睑瞤动、面瘫。治疗眼病,可向下斜刺0.3~0.5寸治疗头痛、面瘫,可平刺透鱼腰;禁灸。

Cuanzhu (BL 2) A meridian point, from *Zhenjiu Jia-Yi Jing (A-B Classic of Acupuncture and Moxibustion)*. It belongs to the Bladder Meridian of Foot-Taiyang. Also named Shiguang, Yeguang, Mingguang, Guangming, Yuanzai, Yuanzhu, Meitou or Meiben. 〈Location〉 on the face, in the depression of the medial and of the eyebrow, at the supraorbital notch (Figs. 5&28). 〈Regional anatomy〉 skin → subcutaneous tissue → orbicular muscle of eye. In the superficial layer, there are the supratrochlear nerve of the frontal nerve, and the branches or tributaries of the superior orbital artery and vein. In the deep layer, there are the temporal and zygomatic branches of the facial nerve. 〈Indications〉 headache, supraorbital pain, dizziness, poor vision, redness, swelling and pain of the eye, lacrimation when exposed to wind, myopia, twitching of eyelids, and facial paralysis, etc. 〈Method〉 Puncture obliquely downwards 0.3~0.5 cun for ophthalmopathy; puncture to Yuyao (EX-HN 4) for headache and facial paralysis. Moxibustion is forbidden.

●篡[cuàn] 部位名。指肛门部。

Cuan A part of the body, referring to the anal region.

●催气[cuī qì] 针刺术语。指针刺未得气时应用各种行针手法,以取得感应。如应用循法、弹法等。

Promoting Qi A term used in acupuncture, referring to promoting the arrival of qi (needling sensation) by using various kinds of manipulation techniques such as pressing or plucking methods, etc., when the patient has a delayed needling reaction.

●焠刺[cuì cì] 《内经》刺法名。出《灵枢·官针》。为九刺之一。是将针烧红后,刺入机体,治疗寒痹、瘰疬、阴疽等病证的一种针刺方法。

Heat Needling (Red-Hot Needling) A needling technique recorded in *Neijing (The Canon of Internal Medicine)*, originally from *Lingshu: Guanzhen (Miraculous Pivot: Official Needles)*, one of the nine needling methods. After the needle is heated to red-hot, insert it into the body. 〈Indications〉 arthralgia due to cold, scrofula, and yin type cellulitis, etc..

●焠针[cuì zhēn] 为火针之别称。详见该条。

Red-Hot Needle (or Heated Needle) Another name for the fire needle. →火针(p. 180)

●存真图[cún zhēn tú] 古代脏腑图。又名《存真环中图》,一卷,宋代杨介编。见《郡斋读书后志》。"存真"指脏腑,"环中"指经络。这是十二世纪初,北宋统治者利用被处决人的尸体,遣医并画工绘图,又经杨介考订而成,是我国较早的人体解剖图谱。已佚。

Cunzhen Tu (Pictures of Reserving the True) Ancient drawings of zang-fu organs, also named *Cunzhen Huanzhong Tu (Pictures of Circulatory Courses and Reserving the True)*, a single volume, compiled by Yang Jie in the Song Dynasty, seen in *Junzhai Dushu Houzhi (Records After Reading in the County Study)*, *Cunzhen (Reserving the True)* refers to the zang-fu organs and *Huan-zhong (Circulatory courses)* refers to the meridians and collaterals. In the early 12th century, the rulers of the Northern Song Dynasty ordered physicians and painters to draw pictures by making use of the dead bodies of the executed, and Yang Jie checked and concluded them. It is a relatively early Chinese atlas of the anatomy of the human body, which is no longer extant.

●寸平[cùn píng] 经外穴名。见《针灸孔穴及其疗法便览》。在手背,当腕横纹中央上1寸,向桡侧旁开0.4寸处。〈主治〉心力衰竭,休克等,直刺0.3~0.5寸。

Cunping (EX-UE) An extra point, from *Zhenjiu Kongxue Jiqi Liaofa Bianlan* (*Guide to Acupoints and Acupuncture Therapeutics*). ⟨Location⟩ on the dorsum of the hand, 1 cun above the midpoint of the transverse crease of the wrist, and 0.4 cun lateral to the radial side. ⟨Indications⟩ cardiac failure, shock, etc. ⟨Method⟩ Puncture perpendicularly 0.3～0.5 cun.

●搓法[cuō fǎ] 针刺辅助手法名。十四法之一。用拇食指(加中指)持针作一捻一放的动作。

Twisting An auxiliary method of acupuncture, one of the Fourteen Methods. Hold the needle with the thumb the index finger and the middle finger, twirl the needle and then loosen the grip, and repeat this a few times.

D

●达[dá] 指针刺。见晋代杜预注的《左传》。

Reaching A term, referring to acupuncture, seen in *Zuozhuan* (*Commemtary on the Spring and Autumn Annals*) annotated by Du Yu in the Jin Dynasty.

●打呃[dǎ è] 呃逆的俗称。详见"呃逆"条。

Hiccough The popular name of hiccup. →呃逆(p.92)

●大包[dà bāo] 经穴名。出《灵枢·经脉》。属足太阴脾经,为脾之大络。⟨定位⟩在侧胸部,腋中线上,当第六肋间隙处(图84和图23)。⟨层次解剖⟩皮肤→皮下组织→前锯肌。浅层布有第六肋间神经外侧皮支和胸腹壁静脉的属支。深层有胸长神经的分支和胸背动、静脉的分支或属支。⟨主治⟩胸胁痛、气喘、全身疼痛、四肢无力。斜刺0.5～0.8寸;可灸。

Dabao (SP 21) A meridian point from *Lingshu*: *Jingmai* (*Miraculous Pivot*: *Meridians*), a point on the Spleen Meridian of Foot-Taiyin, and the big collateral of the spleen. ⟨Location⟩ on the lateral side of the chest and on the middle axillary line, in the 6th intercostal space. (Figs. 84 & 23). ⟨Regional anatomy⟩ skin→subcutaneous tissue→anterior serratus muscle. In the superficial layer, there are the lateral cutaneous branches of the 6th intercostal nerve and the tributaries of the thoracoepigastric vein. In the deep layer, there are the branches of the long theracic nerve and the branches or tributaries of the thoracodorsal artery and vein. ⟨Indications⟩ pain in the chest and hypochondrium, asthma, pantalgia, and myasthenia of limbs. ⟨Method⟩ Puncture obliquely 0.5～0.8 cun. Moxibustion is applicable.

●大便秘结[dà biàn bì jié] 即便秘。详见该条。

Dry Stool →便秘(p.24)

●大便不通[dà biàn bù tōng] 即便秘。详见该条。

Difficult Bowel Movement →便秘(p.24)

●大便难[dà biàn nán] 出《素问·至真要大论》。即便秘。详见该条。

Dyschesia Another term for constipation, from *Suwen*: *Zhi Zhenyao Dalun* (*Plain Questions*: *Great Treatise on Extremely True Gists*). →便秘(p.24)

●大脖子[dà bó zī] 即瘿气。详见该条。

Big Neck →瘿气(p.568)

●大补大泻[dà bǔ dà xiè] 针刺手法分类名。出《针灸大成》卷四。与小补小泻相对。指手法较重,刺激量较大的补泻手法。如烧山火、透天凉等法,均属此类。参见"平补平泻"条。

Vigorous Reinforcing and Reducing Method
A needling technique, from Vol. 4 of *Zhenjiu Dacheng* (*A Great Compendium of Acupuncture and Moxibustion*), the opposite of the mild reinforcing and reducing method. It refers to vigorous and strong stimulative techniques of reinforcing and reducing, such as methods of "setting the mountain on fire" and "penetrating heaven coolness" etc.. →平补平泻(p.297)

●大仓[dà cāng] 经穴别名。出《铜人腧穴针灸图

经》即太仓,指中脘穴。详见该条。

Dacang　　Another name for Taicang, a meridin point from *Tongren Shuxue Zhenjiu Tujing* (*Illustrated Manual of Points for Acupuncture and Moxibustion on a Bronze Statue with Acupoints*), referring to the point Zhongwan(RN 12).→中脘(p.614)

●大肠[dà cháng]　　耳穴名。位于耳轮脚上方的内三分之一。用于治疗腹泻、便秘、咳嗽、痤疮。

Large Intestine(MA)　　An auricular point. 〈Location〉on the medial 1/3 of the superior aspect of the helix crus. 〈Indications〉diarrhea, constipation, cough, and acne.

●大肠经[dà cháng jīng]　　手阳明大肠经之简称。详见该条。

Large Intestine Meridian　　Shortened name for the Large Intestine Meridian of Hand-Yangming.→手阳明大肠经(p.401)

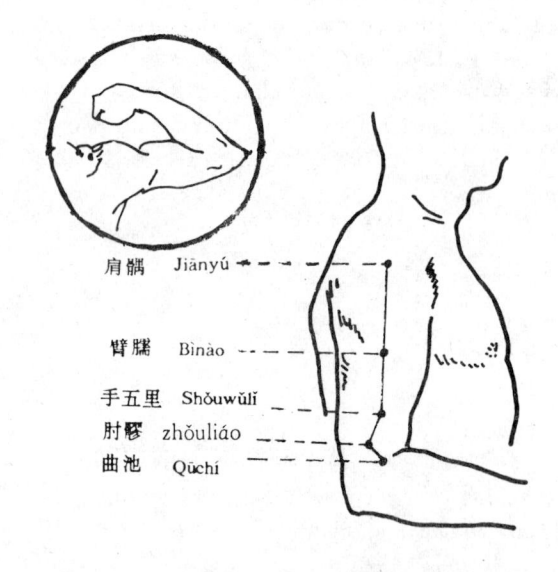

图 6.2　大肠经穴(臂部)

Fig 6.2　Points of Large Intestine Meridian(Arm)

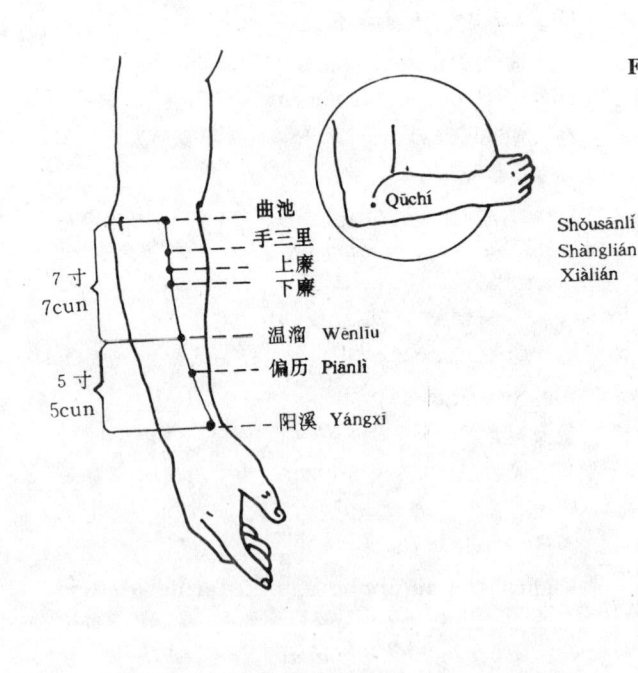

图 6.1　大肠经穴(前臂部)

Fig 6.1　Points of Large Intestine Meridian(Forearm)

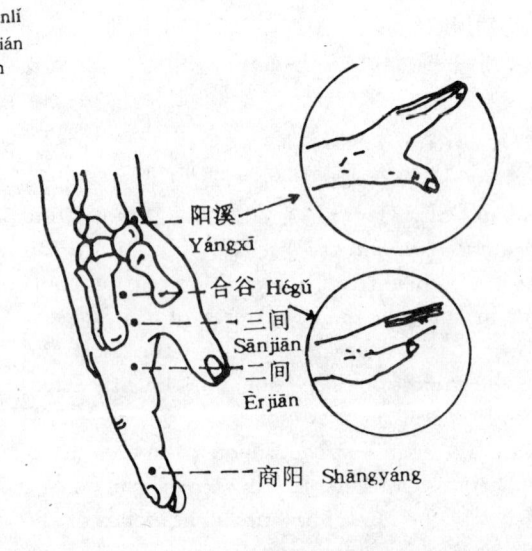

图 6.3　大肠经穴(手部)

Fig 6.3　Points of Large Intestine Meridian(Hand)

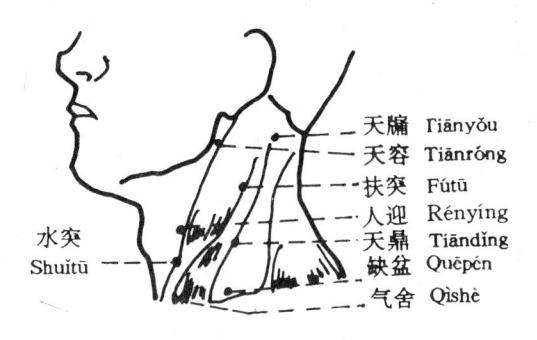

水突 Shuǐtū
天牖 Tiānyǒu
天容 Tiānróng
扶突 Fútū
人迎 Rényíng
天鼎 Tiāndǐng
缺盆 Quēpén
气舍 Qìshè

图 6.4　大肠经和胃经穴（颈部）

Fig 6.4　Points of Large Intestine Meridian & Stomach Meridian (Neck)

●**大肠手阳明之脉**[dà cháng shǒu yáng míng zhī mài]　手阳明大肠经的原名。详见该条。

Large Intestine Hand-Yangming Meridian

The original name for the Large Intestine Meridian of Hand-Yangming. →手阳明大肠经 (p. 401)

●**大肠俞**[dà cháng shū]　经穴名。出《针灸甲乙经》。属足太阳膀胱经，为大肠的背俞穴。〈定位〉在腰部，当第四腰椎棘突下，旁开1.5寸（图7）。〈层次解剖〉皮肤→皮下组织→背阔肌腱膜和胸腰筋膜浅层→竖脊肌。浅层布有第四、五腰神经后支的皮支和伴行的动、静脉。深层有第四、五腰神经后支的肌支和有关动、静脉的分支或属支。〈主治〉腹胀、腹痛、肠鸣、泄泻、便秘、痢疾、腰背疼痛。直刺0.8～1.0寸；可灸。

Dachangshu(BL 25)　A meridian point, originally from *Zhenjiu Jia-Yi Jing*(*A-B Classic of Acupuncture and Moxibustion*), a point on the Bladder Meridian of Foot-Taiyang, the back-shu point of the large intestine. 〈Location〉on the low back, below the spinous process of the 4th lumbar vertebra, 1.5 cun lateral to the posterior midline (Fig. 7). 〈Regional anatomy〉 skin → subcutaneous tissue → aponeurosis of latissimus muscle of back and superficial layer of thoracolumbar fascia → erector spinal muscle. In the superficial layer, there are the cutaneous branches of the posterior branches of the 4th and 5th lumbar nerves and the accompanying arteries and veins. In the deep layer, there are the muscular branches of the posterior branches of the 4th and 5th lumbar nerves and the branches or tributaries of the related lumbar arteries and veins. 〈Indications〉 abdominal distention, abdominalgia, borborygmus, diarrhea, constipation, dysentery, pain in the back and loin. 〈Method〉 Puncture perpendicularly 0.8～1 cun. Moxibustion is applicable.

●**大冲**[dà chōng]　经穴名。出《千金要方》。即太冲。详见该条。

Dachong　Another name for Taichong (LR 3), a meridian point originally from *Qianjin Yaofang* (*Essential Prescriptions Worth a Thousand Gold*). →太冲 (p. 419)

●**大顀**[dà chuí]　经穴别名。出《铜人腧穴针灸图经》。《东医宝鉴》作大椎的别名。详见该条。

Dachui　Another name for Dazhui (DU 14), a meridian point, originally from *Tongren Shuxue Zhenjiu Tujing* (*Illustrated Manual of Points for Acupuncturt and Moxibustion on a Bronze Statue with Acupoints*), as seen in *Dongyi Baojian* (*A Treasured Mirror of Oriental Medicine*). →大椎 (p. 69)

●**大都**[dà dū]　①经穴名。出《灵枢·本输》。属太阴脾经，为本经荥穴。〈定位〉在足内侧缘，当足大趾本节（第一跖趾关节）前下方赤白肉际凹陷处（图39.1和图81）。〈层次解剖〉皮肤→皮下组织→第一趾骨基底部。布有足底内侧神经的趾足底固有神经，浅静脉网，足底内侧动、静脉的分支或属支。〈主治〉腹胀、胃疼、食不化、呃逆、泄泻、便秘、热病无汗、体重肢肿、厥心痛、心烦、不得卧。直刺0.3～0.5寸；可灸。②经外穴名。八邪之一。见《奇效良方》。在手大指、次指虎口赤白肉际处，握拳取之。参见"八邪"条。

1. Dadu(SP 2)　A meridian point, originally from *Lingshu: Benshu* (*Miraculous Pivot: Meridian Points*), the Ying (Spring) point of the Spleen Meridian of Foot-Taiyin. 〈Location〉on the medial border of the foot, in the depression of the junction of the red and white skin, anterior and inferior to the lst metatarsophalangeal joint (Figs. 39.1&81). 〈Regional anatomy〉 skin→subcutaneous tissue→base of

lst phalanx. There are the proper digital plantar nerve of the medial plantar nerve, the superficial venous network and the branches or tributaries of the medial plantar artery and vein. ⟨Indications⟩ abdominal distention, epigastralgia, indigestion, hiccups, diarrhea, constipation, febrile disease without perspiration, heavy sensation and edema in the limbs, precordial pain caused by coldevil, vexation, inability to lie flat. ⟨Method⟩ Puncture perpendicularly 0.3~0.5 cun. Moxibustion is applicable.

2. **Dadu** An extra point, one of the Baxie (EX-UE 9) points, originally from *Qixiao Liangfang*(*Prescriptions of Wonderful Efficacy*). To locate the point, make a fist, the point is at the junction of the red and white skin between the thumb and index fingers. →八邪(p.8)

●大敦[dà dūn] 经穴名。出《灵枢·本输》。属足厥阴肝经，为本经井穴。又名水泉。⟨定位⟩在足踇趾末节外侧，距趾甲角0.1寸(指寸)(图80)。⟨层次解剖⟩皮肤→皮下组织→甲根。布有腓深神经的背外侧神经和趾背动、静脉等结构。⟨主治⟩疝气、缩阴、阴中痛、月经不调、血崩、尿血、癃闭、遗尿、淋证、癫狂、痫证、少腹痛。斜刺0.1~0.2寸，或点刺出血；可灸。

Dadun(LR 1) A meridian point, originally from *Lingshu: Benshu* (*Miraculous Pivot: Meridian Points*), the Jing(Well) point of the Liver Meridian of Foot-Jueyin, also called Shuiquan. ⟨Location⟩ on the lateral side of the distal segment of the great toe, 0.1 cun from the corner of the toenail (Fig. 80). ⟨Regional anatomy⟩ skin→subcutaneous tissue→root of nail. There are the lateral dorsal nerve of the great toe from the deep peroneal nerve and the dorsal digital artery and vein in this area. ⟨Indications⟩ hernia, shrinking of the external genitals, pain in penis, irregular menstruation, metrorrhagia, hematuria, uroschesis, enuresis, stranguria, depressive manic psychosis, epilepsy, pain in the lower abdomen. ⟨Method⟩ Puncture obliquely 0.1~0.2 cun or prick to cause bleeding. Moxibustion is applicable.

●大谷[dà gǔ] 部位名。指肌肉间呈现的大凹陷处。

Big Valley A part of the body, referring to the large depression of muscles.

●大骨[dà gǔ] 经穴名。即京骨。详见该条。

Dagu Another name for the meridian point Jinggu(BL 64). →京骨(p. 207)

●大骨空[dà gǔ kōng] 经外穴名。见《扁鹊神应针灸玉龙经》。在拇指背侧指间关节的中点外(图76)。灸治目痛、目翳、白内障、风眩烂眼、鼻衄、吐泻等。

Dagukong(EX-UE 5) An extra point, originally from *Bian Que Shenying Zhenjiu Yulong Jing* (*Bian Que's Jade Dragon Classic of Acupuncture and Moxibustion*). ⟨Location⟩ on the dorsal side of the thumb, at the centre of the interphalangeal joint (Fig. 76). ⟨Regional anatomy⟩ skin→subcutaneous tissue→tendon of long extensor muscle of thumb. There are the dorsal digital nerve of the radial nerve and the dorsal digital artery and vein in this area. ⟨Indications⟩ pain in the eye, pterygium, cataract, marginal blepharitis, epistaxis, vomiting and diarrhea, etc. ⟨Method⟩ moxibustion.

●大骨孔[dà gǔ kǒng] 即大骨空。详见该条。

Dagukong →大骨空(p. 62)

●大赫[dà hè] 经穴名。出《针灸甲乙经》。属足少阴肾经，为冲脉、足少阴之会。又名阴维、阴关。⟨定位⟩在下腹部，当脐中下4寸，前正中线旁开0.5寸(图40)。⟨层次解剖⟩皮肤→皮下组织→腹直肌鞘前壁→锥状肌上外侧缘→腹直肌。浅层布有腹壁浅动、静脉的分支或属支，第十一、十二胸神经和第一腰神经前支的前皮支及伴行的动、静脉。深层有腹壁下动、静脉的分支或属支，第十一、十二胸神经前支的肌支和相应的肋间动、静脉。⟨主治⟩阴部痛、子宫脱垂、遗精、带下、月经不调、痛经、不孕、泄泻、痢疾。直刺0.8~1.2寸；可灸。

Dahe(KI 12) A meridian point, originally from *Zhenjiu Jia-Yi Jing* (*A-B Classic of Acupuncture and Moxibustion*), a point on the Kidney Meridian of Foot-Shaoyin, the crossing point of the Foot-Shaoyin and Chong Meridians, also named Yinwei and Yinguan. ⟨Location⟩ on the lower abdomen, 4 cun below the centre of the umbilicus and 0.5 cun lateral to the anterior midline. (Fig. 40). ⟨Regional anatomy⟩ skin→subcutaneous tissue→anterior sheath of rectus muscle of abdomen→

superior and lateral border of pyramidal muscle→rectus muscle of abdomen. In the superficial layer, there are the branches or tributaries of the superficial epigastric artery and vein, the anterior cutaneous branches of the anterior branches of the 11th and 12th thoracic and 1st lumbar nerves and the accompanying arteries and veins. In the deep layer, there are the branches or tributaries of the inferior epigastric artery and vein, the muscular branches of the anterior branches of the 11th and 12th thoracic nerves and the related intercostal arteries and veins. 〈Indications〉 pain in the vulva, hysteroptosis, seminal emission, leukorrhea, irregular menstruation, dysmenorrhea, sterility, diarrhea, dysentery. 〈Method〉Puncture perpendicularly 0.8~1.2 cun. Moxibustion is applicable.

●**大横**[dà héng] 经穴名。出《针灸甲乙经》。属足太阴脾经，为足太阴、阴维之会。又名肾气、横文、人横。〈定位〉在腹中部，距脐中4寸（图84和图40）。〈层次解剖〉皮肤→皮下组织→腹外斜肌→腹内斜肌→腹横肌。浅层布有第九、十、十一胸神经前支的外侧皮和胸腹壁静脉属支。深层有第九、十、十一胸神经前支的肌支及伴行的动、静脉。〈主治〉泄泻、痢疾、大便秘结、小腹痛。直刺0.8~1.2寸；可灸。

Daheng (SP 15) A meridian point, from *Zhenjiu Jia-Yi Jing* (*A-B Classic of Acupuncture and Moxibustion*), a point on the Spleen Meridian of Foot-Taiyin, the crossing point of the Foot-Taiyin and Yinwei Meridians, also named Shenqi, Hengwen or Renheng. 〈Location〉 on the middle abdomen, 4 cun to the centre of the umbilicus (Figs. 84&40). 〈Regional anatomy〉 skin→subcutaneous tissue→external oblique muscle of abdomen→internal oblique muscle of abdomen→transverse muscle of abdomen. In the superficial layer, there are the lateral cutaneous branches of the anterior branches of the 9th to 11th thoracic nerves and the tributaries of the thoracoepigastric vein. In the deep layer, there are the muscular branches of the anterior branches of the 9th to 11th thoracic nerves and their accompanying arteries and veins. 〈Indications〉 diarrhea, dysentery, constipation, pain in the lower abdomen. 〈Method〉 Puncture perpendicularly 0.8~1.2 cun. Moxibustion is applicable.

●**大接经法**[dà jiē jīng fǎ] 配穴法之一。见《卫生宝鉴》。是专治中风偏枯的一种特殊配穴法。其从阳引阴，从阴引阳二法，皆取十二经井穴。从阳引阴法，是从足太阳井穴至阴开始，依次取足少阴涌泉、手厥阴中冲、手少阳关冲、足少阳足窍阴、足厥阴大敦、手太阴少商、手阳明商阳、足阳明厉兑、足太阴隐白、手少阴少冲、手太阳少泽，共刺十二穴。从阴引阳法，是从手太阴井穴少商开始，依次取手阳明商阳、足阳明厉兑、足太阴隐白、手少阴少冲、手太阳少泽、足太阳至阴、足少阴涌泉、手厥阴中冲、手少阳关冲、足少阳足窍阴、足厥阴大敦，共刺十二穴。

Method of Connecting Meridians One of the methods for selecting points, originally from *Weisheng Baojian* (*A Treasured Mirror of Health Protection*). A special way of selecting point prescription to treat hemiplegia. Both of its methods, "guiding yin from yang" and "guiding yang from yin" require puncturing the Jing (Well) points of the Twelve Regular Meridians. The former begins at Zhiyin (BL 67), the Jing (Well) point of the Foot-Taiyang Meridian, followed subsequently by Yongquan (KI 1) of Foot-Shaoyin, Zhongchong (PC 9) of the Hand-Jueyin, Guanchong (SJ 1) of the Hand-Shaoyang, Zuqiaoyin (GB 44) of the Foot-Shaoyang, Dadun (LR 1) of the Foot-Jueyin, Shaoshang (LU 11) of the Hand-Taiyin, Shangyang (LI 1) of the Hand-Yangming, Lidui (ST 45) of the Foot-Yangming, Yinbai (SP 1) of the Foot-Taiyin, Shaochong (HT 9) of the Hand-Shaoyin, and Shaoze (SI 1) of the Hand-Taiyang, needling 12 points altogether. The latter begins at Shaoshang (LU 11), the Jing (Well) point of the Hand-Taiyin, followed subsequently by Shangyang (LI 1) of the Hand-Yangming, Lidui (ST 45) of the Foot-Yangming, Yinbai (SP 1) of the Foot-Taiyin, Shaochong (HT 9) of the Hand-Shaoyin, Shaoze (SI 1) of the Hand-Taiyang, Zhiyin (BL 67) of the Foot-Taiyang, Yongquan (KI 1) of the Foot-Shaoyin, Zhongchong (PC 9) of the Hand-Jueyin, Guanchong (SJ 1) of the Hand-Shaoyang, Zuqiaoyin (GB 44) of the Foot-

Shaoyang, and Dadun (LR 1) of the Foot-Jueyin, needling 12 points altogether.

●大巨 [dà jù] 经穴名。出《针灸甲乙经》。属足阳明胃经。又名腋门。〈定位〉在下腹部,当脐中下2寸,距前正中线2寸(图86和图40)。〈层次解剖〉皮肤→皮下组织→腹直肌鞘前壁→腹直肌。浅层布有第十、十一、十二胸神经前支的外侧皮支和前皮支,腹壁浅动脉及腹壁浅静脉。深层有腹壁下动、静脉的分支或属支,第十、十一、十二胸神经前支的肌支。〈主治〉小腹胀满,小便不利,疝气,遗精,早泄,惊悸,不眠,偏枯。直刺0.8～1.2寸;可灸。

Daju (ST 27) A meridian point from *Zhenjiu Jia-Yi Jing* (*A-B Classic of Acupuncture and Moxibustion*), a point on the Stomach Meridian of Foot-Yangming, also called Yemen. 〈Location〉 on the lower abdomen, 2 cun below the centre of the umbilicus and 2 cun lateral to the anterior midline (Figs. 86&40). 〈Regional anatomy〉 skin→subcutaneous tissue→anterior sheath of rectus muscle of abdomen→rectus muscle of abdomen. In the superficial layer, there are the lateral and anterior cutaneous branches of the anterior branches of the 10th to 12th thoracic nerves and the superficial epigastric artery and vein. In the deep layer, there are the branches or tributaries of the inferior epigastric artery and vein and the muscular branches of the anterior branches of the 10th to 12th thoracic nerves. 〈Indications〉 distention of the lower abdomen, oliguria, hernia, seminal emission, premature ejaculation, palpitations due to fright, insomnia, hemiplegia. 〈Method〉 Puncture perpendicularly 0.8～1.2 cun. Moxibustion is applicable.

●大陵 [dà líng] 经穴名。出《灵枢·本输》。属手厥阴心包经,为本经输穴、原穴。又名鬼心、心主、太陵。〈定位〉在腕掌横纹的中点处,当掌长肌腱与桡侧腕屈肌腱之间(图49和图66)。〈层次解剖〉皮肤→皮下组织→掌长肌腱与桡侧腕屈肌腱之间→拇长屈肌腱与指浅屈肌腱、指深屈肌腱之间→桡腕关节前方。浅层布有臂内、外侧皮神经,正中神经掌支,腕掌侧静脉网。深层在掌长肌与桡侧腕屈肌之间的深面可能刺中正中神经。〈主治〉心痛、心悸、胃痛、呕吐、惊悸、癫狂、痫证、胸胁痛、腕关节疼痛、喜笑悲恐。直刺0.3～0.5寸;可灸。

Daling (PC 7) A meridian point from *Lingshu*: *Benshu* (*Miraculous Pivot*: *Meridian Points*), the Shu (Stream) and Yuan (Primary) point of the Pericardium Meridian of Hand-Jueyin, also called Guixin, Xinzhu and Tailing. 〈Location〉 at the midpoint of the crease of the wrist, between the tendons of the long palmar muscle and radial flexor muscle of the wrist (Figs. 49&66). 〈Regional anatomy〉 skin→subcutaneous tissue→between tendons of long palmar muscle and radial flexor muscle of wrist→between tendons of flexor muscle of thumb and superficial flexor muscle of fingers and deep flexor muscle of fingers→distal side of radiocarpal joint. In the superficial layer, there are the medial and lateral cutaneous nerves of the forearm, the palmar branches of the median nerve and the palmar venous network of the wrist. In the deep layer, the median nerve may be injured if the needle is inserted between and beyond the long palmar muscle and the radial flexor muscle of the wrist. 〈Indications〉 cardiac pain, palpitation, stomachache, vomiting, palpitations due to fright, depression, insanity, epilepsy, pain in the chest and hypochondrium, pain in the wrist joint, susceptibility to laughter, sorrow and fear. 〈Method〉 Puncture perpendicularly 0.3～0.5 cun. Moxibustion is applicable.

●大门 [dà mén] 经外穴名。见《千金要方》。在头部,当后发际正中直上3.5寸。〈主治〉半身不遂。沿皮刺0.3～0.5寸;可灸。

Damen (EX-HN) An extra point, originally from *Qianjin Yaofang* (*Essential Prescriptions Worth a Thousand Gold*). 〈Location〉 on the head, 3.5 cun above the midpoint of the posterior hairline. 〈Indication〉 hemiplegia. 〈Method〉 Puncture subcutaneously 0.3～0.5 cun. Moxibustion is applicable.

●大拇指头 [dà mǔ zhǐ tóu] 经外穴名。见《针灸孔穴及其疗法便览》。在手拇指尖端,距爪甲一分处,左右共计二穴。〈主治〉水肿、肾炎。直刺0.1～0.2寸;可灸。

Damuzhitou (EX-UE) An extra point, originally from *Zhenjiu Kongxue Jiqi Liaofa*

Bianlan (*Guide to Acupoints and Acupuncture Therapeutics*). ⟨Location⟩ at the tips of the thumbs of both hands, 0.1 cun from each thumb nail. ⟨Indications⟩ edema and nephritis. ⟨Method⟩ Puncture perpendicularly 0.1~0.2 cun. Moxibustion is applicable.

●**大泉**[dà quán] ①经穴别名。见《千金要方》。即太渊。详见该条。②经外穴名。见《针灸孔穴及其疗法便览》。位于腋前皱襞尽头处。〈主治〉肩臂痛、胸胁痛、痧症等。直刺0.5~1寸。不可向内斜刺过深，免伤肺脏。

1. **Daquan**   Another name of Taiyuan (LU 9), a meridian point, from *Qianjin Yaofang* (*Essential Prescriptions Worth a Thousand Gold*). →太渊 (p. 423)

2. **Daquan**(EX)   An extra point, from *Zhenjiu Kongxue Jiqi Liaofa Bianlan* (*Guide to Acupoints and Acupuncture Therapeutics*). ⟨Location⟩ at the extreme end of the anterior axillary fold. ⟨Indications⟩ pain in the shoulder and back, pain in the chest and hypochondrium and measles, etc. ⟨Method⟩ Puncture perpendicularly 0.5~1.0 cun. Don't obliquely punture too deep toward the medial side in case the lung is injured.

●**大容**[dà róng]   经穴别名。出《西方子明堂灸经》。即天容。详见该条。

Darong   Another name for Tianrong (SI 17), a meridian point from *Xifangzi Mingtang Jiujing* (*Xifangzi's Classic of Moxibustion*). →天容 (p. 433)

●**大腧**[dà shù]   经穴别名。出《灵枢·背腧》。即大杼。详见该条。

Dashu   Another name for Dazhu (BL 11), a meridian point from *Lingshu: Beishu* (*Miraculous Pivot: Back-Shu Points*). →大杼 (p. 68)

●**大溪**[dà xī]   经穴别名。出《千金要方》。即太溪。详见该条。

Daxi   Another name for Taixi (KI 3), a meridian point from *Qianjin Yaofang* (*Essential Prescriptions Worth a Thousand Gold*). →太溪 (p. 420)

●**大泻**[dà xiè]   针刺手法分类名。指用手法较重，刺激量较大的泻法。如透天凉等。

Vigorous Reduction   Name for vigorous reducing manipulations in acupuncture, referring to reducing techniques with strong stimulations, e.g., "cool-producing needling", or "penetrating heaven coolness".

●**大写刺**[dà xiè cì]   《内经》刺法名。出《灵枢·官针》。是九刺之一。指切开引流，排脓放血，泻水的刺法。写通泻，排除泄出的意思，故称大写刺。现属外科范围。

Drainage Needling   A needling technique from *Lingshu: Guanzhen* (*Miraculous Pivot: Official Needles*), one of the nine needlings, referring to the method of removing pus, blood, and water by incision and drainage with needling. Drainage means removing, purging, or getting rid of. Today, this technique is used in surgical therapy.

●**大阴络**[dà yīn luò]   经穴别名。出《铜人腧穴针灸图经》。即漏谷。详见该条。

Dayinluo   Another name for Lougu (SP 7), a meridian point from *Tongren Shuxue Zhenjiu Tujing* (*Illustrated Manual of Points for Acupuncture and Moxibustion on a Bronze Statue with Acupoints*). →漏谷 (p. 256)

●**大迎**[dà yíng]   经穴名。出《灵枢·寒热病》。属足阳明胃经。又名髓孔。〈定位〉在下颌角前方，咬肌附着部的前缘，当面动脉搏动处（图28和图24）。〈层次解剖〉皮肤→皮下组织→降口角肌与颈阔肌→咬肌前缘。浅层布于三叉神经第三支下颌神经的颊神经、面神经的下颌缘支。深层有面动、静脉。〈主治〉牙关紧闭、口㖞、颊肿、齿痛、面肿、牙关脱臼、唇吻瞤动、瘰疬、颈痛。直刺0.2~0.3寸；可灸。

Daying(ST 5)   A meridian point, originally from *Lingshu: Han Re Bing* (*Miraculous Pivot: Cold and Heat Diseases*), a point on the Stomach Meridian of Foot-Yangming, also called Suikong. ⟨Location⟩ Anterior to the mandibular angle, on the anterior border of the masseter muscle, where the pulsation of the facial artery is palpable (Figs. 28 & 24). ⟨Regional anatomy⟩ skin→subcutaneous tissue→depressor muscle of angle of mouth and platysma muscle→anterior border of masseter muscle. In the superficial layer, there are the buccal nerve of the mandibular branch of the trigeminal nerve and the marginal mandibular

branch of the facial nerve. In the deep layer, there are the facial artery and vein. 〈Indications〉 lockjaw, wry mouth, cheek swelling, toothache, facial swelling, mandibular dislocation, lip temor, scrofula, pain in the neck. 〈Method〉Puncture perpendicularly 0.2～0.5 cun. Moxibustion is applicable.

●大羽[dà yǔ]　经穴别名。出《千金要方》。即强间。详见该条。

Dayu　Another name for Qiangjian(DU 18), a meridian point from *Qianjin Yaofang（Essential Prescriptions Worth a Thousand Gold）*. →强间(p. 318)

●大指(趾)次指(趾)[dà zhǐ(zhǐ)cì zhǐ(zhǐ)]　部位名。出《灵枢·经脉》。指食指或足第二趾。

The Second Digit from the Thumb(Big Toe)

　　A part of the body, originally from *Lingshu: Jingmai（Miraculous Pivot: Meridians）*, referring to the index finger or the second toe.

●大指节横纹[dà zhǐ jié héng wén]　经穴名。见《千金要方》又名大指节理。在手拇指掌侧指横纹中点，左右计二穴。灸目卒生翳。

Dazhijiehengwen(EX-UE)　An extra point, seen in *Qianjin Yaofang（Essential Prescriptions Worth a Thousand Gold）*, also named Dazhijieli. 〈Location〉on the palmar side of each thumb, at the midpoint of the transverse crease of the thumb. Moxibustion is used on this point to treat sudden nebula of the eyes.

●大指节理[dà zhǐ jié lǐ]　经外穴别名。见《千金翼方》。即大指节横纹。详见该条。

Dazhijieli　Another name for Dazhijiehengwen(EX-UE), an extra point originally from *Qianjin Yifang（Supplement to the Essential Prescriptions Worth a Thousand Gold）*. →大指节横纹(p. 66)

●大趾聚毛[dà zhǐ jù máo]　经外穴名。见《肘后备急方》。位于踇趾背侧，当趾骨关节部之趾毛中。〈主治〉中风不省人事、头痛、眩晕、疝气、睾丸炎等。直刺0.1～0.2寸；可灸。

Dazhijumao(EX-LE)　An extra point, originally from *Zhouhou Beiji Fang（A Handbook of Prescriptions for Emergencies）*. 〈Location〉on the instep of the 1st toe, in the hair at the phalangeal joint. 〈Indications〉apoplectic coma, headache, vertigo, hernia, testitis, etc. 〈Method〉Puncture perpendicularly 0.1～0.2 cun. Moxibustion is applicable.

●大针[dà zhēn]　针具名。出《灵枢·九针十二原》。古代九针之一。针长四寸，针身粗圆，用于泻水，治关节积液等。后人将此针于火上烧红后刺病，称火针。

Big Needle　Name of a needle, from *Lingshu: Jiu Zhen Shier Yuan（Miraculous Pivot: Nine Needles and Twelve Yuan（Primary）Points）*, one of the nine needles of ancient times, this needle was 4 cun in length, with a thick and round body. It was used to remove water and treat hydrarthrosis. Later, people used to heat the needle to red-hot needle on fire to treat diseases and called it fire needling or red-hot needling.

●大钟[dà zhōng]　经穴名。出《灵枢·经脉》。属足少阴肾经，为本经络穴。又名太钟。〈定位〉在足内侧，内踝后下方，当跟腱附着部的内侧前方凹陷处（图46.1和图81）。〈层次解剖〉皮肤→皮下组织→跖肌腱和跟腱的前方→跟骨。浅层布有隐神经的小腿内侧支皮、大隐静脉的属支。深层有胫后动脉的内踝支和跟支构成的动脉网。〈主治〉咳血、气喘、腰脊强痛、痴呆、嗜卧、足跟痛、二便不利、月经不调。直刺0.3～0.5寸；可灸。

Dazhong(KI 4)　A meridian point from *Lingshu: Jingmai（Miraculous Pivot: Meridians）*, the Luo (Connecting) point of the Kidney Meridian of Foot-Shaoyin, also called Taizhong. 〈Location〉on the medial side of the foot, posterior and inferior to the medial malleolus, in the depression of the medial side of and anterior to the attachment of the Achilles tendon (Figs. 46.1&81). 〈Regional anatomy〉 skin→subcutaneous tissue→anterior side of tendon of plantar muscle and Archilles tendon→calcaneus. In the superficial layer, there are the medial cutaneous branches of the saphenous nerve to the leg and the tributaries of the great saphenous vein. In the deep layer, there is the arterial network formed by the medial malleolus branches and the calcaneal branches of the posterior tibial artery. 〈Indications〉hemoptysis, pain in heel, difficulty in urination and defecation, irregular

menstruation.〈Method〉Puncture perpendicularly 0.3～0.5 cun. Moxibustion is applicable.

●**大中极**[dà zhōng jí] 经穴别名。出《针灸资生经》。即关元。详见该条。

Dazhongji Another name for Guanyuan (RN 4), a meridian point from *Zhenjiu Zisheng Jing* (*Acupuncture-Moxibustion Classic for Saving Life*). →关元(p.148)

●**大肘尖**[dà zhǒu jiān] 部位名。指尺骨鹰嘴部。参见"肘尖"条。

Dazhoujian A part of the body, referring to the area of the olecranon. →肘尖(p.619)

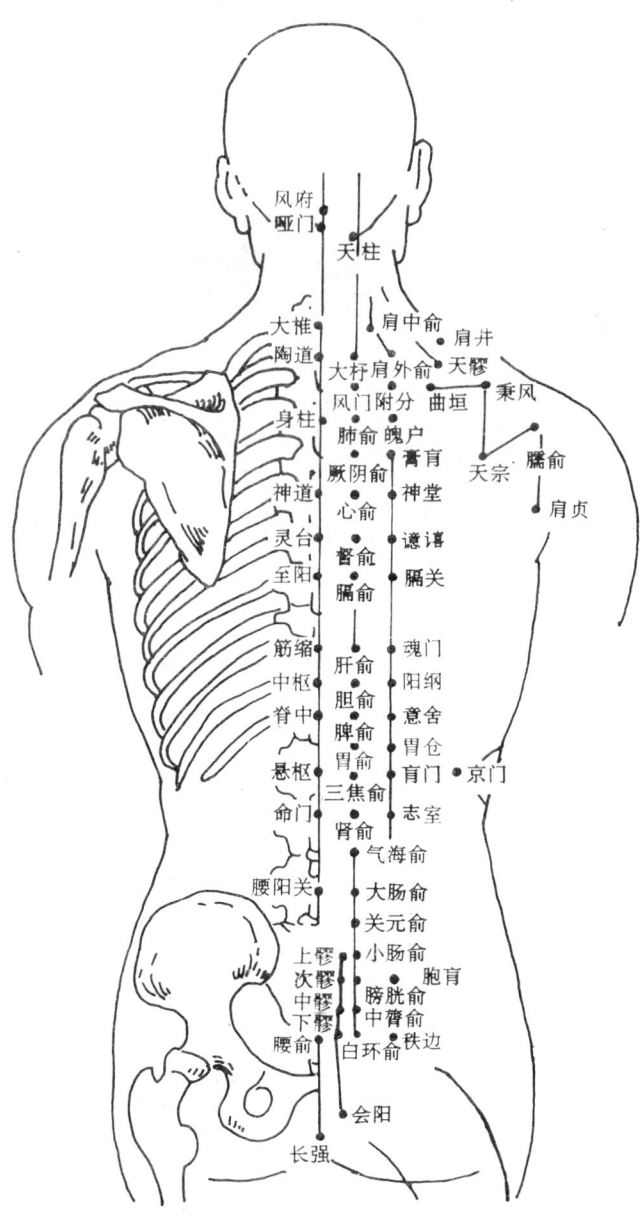

图7 大杼和其他背部穴

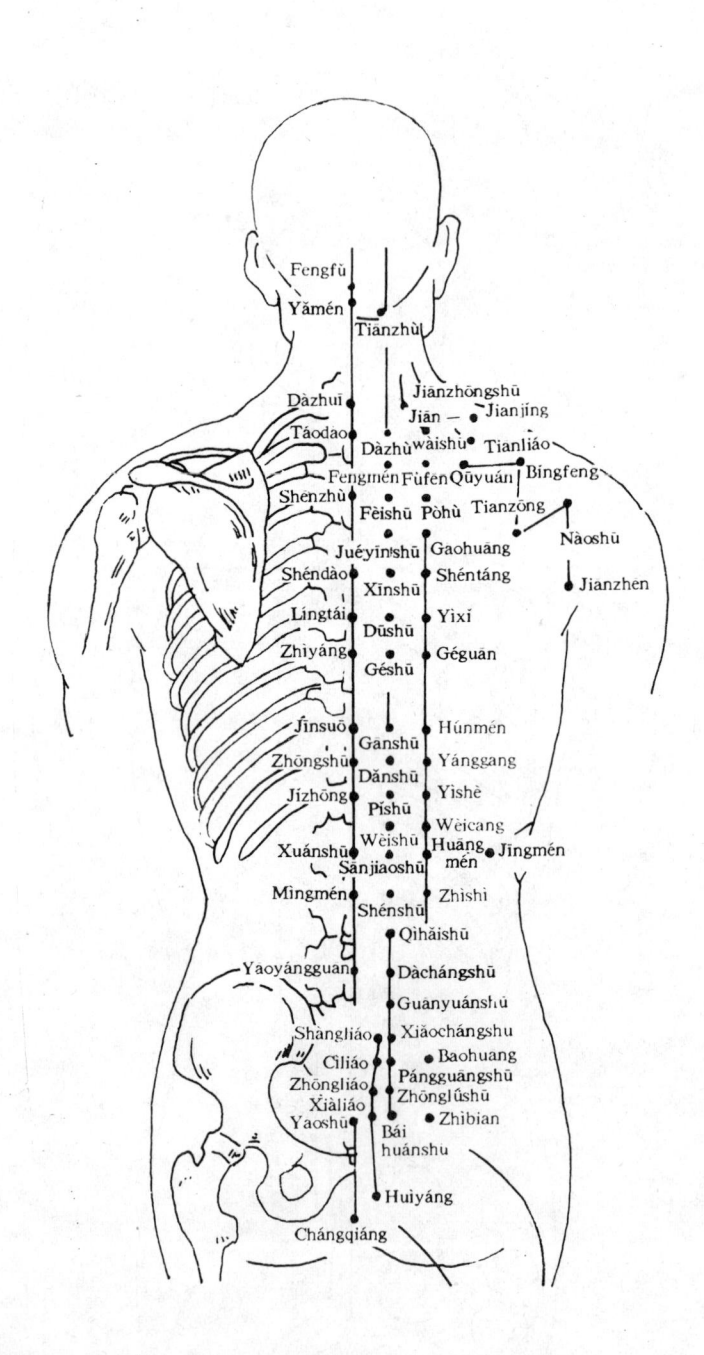

Fig 7 Dazhu and other points of back

●**大杼**[dà zhù] 经穴名。出《灵枢·刺节真邪》。属足太阳膀胱经,为手足太阳之会,督脉别络。又名大腧。八交会穴之骨会。〈定位〉在背部,当第一胸椎棘突下旁开1.5寸。〈层次解剖〉皮肤→皮下组织→斜方肌→菱形肌→上后锯肌→颈夹肌→竖脊肌。浅层布有第一、二胸神经后支的内侧皮支和伴行的肋间后动、静

脉背侧支的内侧皮支。深层有第一、二胸神经后支的肌支和相应的肋间后动、静脉背侧支的分支等结构。〈主治〉咳嗽、发热、鼻塞、头痛、喉痹、肩背痛、颈项强急。斜刺0.5寸～0.8寸;可灸。

Dazhu (BL 11)　A meridian point, from *Lingshu*: *Cijie Zhenxie* (*Miraculous Pivot*: *Acupuncture Principles and Diseases*), a point on the Bladder Meridian of Foot-Taiyang, a crossing point of the Hand- and Foot-Taiyang Meridians, the collateral of the Du Meridian. Also named Dashu, one of the eight influential points for bone. 〈Location〉on the back , below the spinous process of the lst thoracic vertebra, 1.5 cun latral to the posterior midline. 〈Regional anatomy〉skin → subcutaneous tissue → trapezius muscle → rhomboid muscle → superior posterior serratus muscle → splenius muscle of neck → erector spinal muscle. In the superficial layer, there are the medial cutaneous branches of the posterior branches of the lst and 2nd thoracic nerves and the medial cutaneous branches of the accompanying posterior intercostal arteries and veins. In the deep layer, there are the muscular branches of the posterior branches of the lst and 2nd thoracic nerves and the branches of the dorsal branches of the related posterior intercostal arteries and veins. 〈Indications〉cough, fever, stuffy nose, headache, sore throat, pain in the shoulder and back, neck rigidity. 〈Method〉Puncture obliquely 0.5～0.8 cun. Moxibustion is applicable.

●**大炷灸**[dà zhù jiǔ]　灸法术语。又称大壮灸。指用较大的艾炷施灸,艾炷直径不小于三分。古代多用于直接灸,形成灸疮,而为化脓灸。近代则多用于间接灸。

Moxibustion with Big Moxa Cone　A moxibustion term, also called big-cone moxibustion, referring to moxibustion with a big moxa cone, the diameter of which is no less than 0.3 cun. In ancient times, the method was primarily used for direct moxibustion in order to cause blisters, which was known as festering moxibustion. Nowdays, it is mostly used for indirect moxibustion.

●**大壮灸**[dà zhuàng jiǔ]　灸法术语。即大炷灸。详见该条。

Big-Cone Moxibustion　A moxibustion term, synonymous with moxibustion with big moxa cone. →大炷灸(p.69)

●**大椎**[dà zhuī]　经穴名。出《素问·气府论》。为手足三阳、督脉之会。又名百劳、大顀、上杼。〈定位〉在后正中线上,第七颈椎棘突下凹陷中(图12和图7)。〈层次解剖〉针刺经过的层次结构同脊中穴。浅层主要布有第八颈神经后支的内侧支和棘突间皮下静脉丛。深层有棘突间的椎外(后)静脉丛和第八颈神经后支的分支。〈主治〉热病、疟疾、咳嗽、喘逆、骨蒸潮热、项强、肩背痛、腰脊强、角弓反张、小儿惊风、癫狂、痫证、五劳虚损、七伤乏力、中暑、霍乱、呕吐、黄疸、风疹。斜刺0.5～1.0寸;可灸。

Dazhui (DU 14)　A meridian point, originally from *Suwen*: *Qifu Lun* (*Plain Questions*: *On Houses of Qi*), the crossing point of the three yang Meridians of Hand and Foot and the Du meridian, also named Bailao, Dazhui or Shangzhu. 〈Location〉on the posterior midline, in the depression below the 7th cervical vertebra (Figs. 12.1&7). 〈Regional anatomy〉The layer structures of the needle insertion are the same as those in Jizhong (DU 6). In the superficial layer, there are the medial branches of the posterior branches of the 8th cervical nerve and the subcutaneous venous plexus between the adjacent spinous processes. In the deep layer, there are the external (posterior) vertebral venous plexus between the adjacent spinous processes and the branches of the posterior branches of the 7th cervical nerve. 〈Indications〉febrile disease, malaria, cough, dyspnea, hectic fever due to yin-deficiency, stiffness of the nape of the neck and spinal column, pain in the shoulder and back, poisthotonus, infantile convulsions, manic-depressive psychosis, epilepsy, five kinds of impairments caused by overstrain, inertia caused by seven kinds of impairments, sunstroke, cholera morbus, vomiting, jaundice and urticaria. 〈Method〉Puncture obliquely 0.5-1.0 cun. Moxibustion is applicable.

●**代灸膏**[dài jiǔ gāo]　敷贴用方药之一。见《瑞竹堂经验方》。即经药物敷贴穴位,代替艾灸。其方:大附子一个(炮)、吴茱萸、桂皮、木香、蛇床子各9克、马蔺

花18克(焙),研为细末。取药末半匙,面粉半匙,用生姜汁调和为膏状,摊于纸上,临卧贴于脐部或腰眼,次晨去之,每夜如此,如施灸法。可治疗老人衰弱、元气虚冷、脏腑虚滑、腰部冷痛沉重、饮食减少、手足逆冷等症。

Moxibustion Substitute Plaster　One of the prescriptions for application, seen in *Rui Zhu Tang Jingyan Fang* (*Ru Zhu Tang Experienced Prescriptions*), referring to the application of herbs to acupoints instead of moxibution. Prescription: *Fu Zi* (*Radix Aconiti Praeparata*) one large root (processed), *Wu Zhu Yu* (*Fructus Euodiae*) 9g, *Gui Pi* (*Ramulus Cinnamomi*) 9g, *Mu Xiang* (*Radix Aucklandiae*) 9g, *She Chuang Zi* (*Fructus Cnidii*) 9g, *Ma Lin Hua* (*Flos Iridis Chinengis*) 18g (baked). Grind the herbs into a fine powder, use half a spoonful of the powder and half a spoonful of flour to make a paste with ginger juice. Place the paste on a piece of paper, apply it to the navel or Yaoyan (EX-B 7) before sleep. Remove it in the next morning. Apply every night as if moxibustion were being applied. ⟨Indications⟩ senile weakness, coldness due to the deficiency of yuan (primary) qi, asthenia of zang-fu organs, coldness, pain and heavy sensations in the waist, poor appetite, cold limbs, etc.

●代灸涂脐膏[dài jiǔ tú qí gāo]　敷贴用方药之一。见《卫生宝鉴·补遗》。指一种敷贴穴位的膏药,经代替艾灸。其方:附子、马蔺子、蛇床子、肉桂、吴茱萸各等分,研为细末。取药末一匙,面粉一匙,用生姜汁调和为膏状,摊于纸上,贴于关元、气海或脐。自晓至晚,其火力可代艾灸。

Moxibustion Substitute Plaster on Navel
One of the prescriptions for application, seen in *Weisheng Baojian: Buyi* (*A Treasured Mirror of Health Protection: The Supplement*), referring to a soft paste applied to acupoints instead of moxibustion. ⟨Prescription⟩ *Fu Zi* (*Radix Aconiti praeparata*), *Ma Lin Zi* (*Semen Iridis Chinensis*), *She Chuang Zi* (*Fructus Cnidii*), *Rou Gui* (*Cortex Cinnamomi*), *Wu Zhu Yu* (*Fructus Euodiae*). Use equal portions of each herb. Grind them into a fine powder, use a spoonful of the powder and a spoonful of flour, mixed with fresh ginger juice to make a soft paste. Place it on paper, apply it to Guanyuan (RN 4), Qihai (RN 6) or the navel from morning to night. The warmth produced may replace that of moxibustion.

●带脉[dài mài]　①奇经八脉之一。出《灵枢·经别》。其循行,起于季肋下,围绕腰腹一周,前平脐,后平十四椎。②经穴名。出《灵枢·癫狂》。属足少阳胆经,为足少阳、带脉之会。⟨定位⟩在侧腹部,章门下1.8寸,当第十一肋内游离端下方垂线与脐水平线的交点上(图40和图23)。在腹内、外斜肌及腹横肌;有第十二肋间动、静脉;布有第十二肋间神经。⟨主治⟩月经不调、赤白带下、疝气、腰肋痛。直刺0.5~0.8寸;可灸。

1. **Dai Meridian**　One of the eight extra meridians, originally from *Lingshu: Jingbie* (*Miraculous Pivot: Divergent Meridians*). ⟨Course⟩ Originating at the hypochondrium, and running transversely around the waist and abdomen at the level of the navel in the front and of the 14th vertebra in the back.

2. **Daimai** (GB 26)　A meridian point, originally from *Lingshu: Diankuang* (*Miraculous Pivot: Manic-Depressive Psychosis*). A point on the gallbladder meridian of Food-Shaoyang and the crossing point of the Foot-Shaoyang and the Dai Meridians. ⟨Location⟩ on the lateral side of the abdomen, 1.8 cun below Zhangmen (LR 13), at the crossing point of a vertical line through the free end of the 11th rib and a horizontal line through the umbilicus (Figs. 40&23). ⟨Regional anatomy⟩ skin → subcutaneous tissue → external oblique muscle of abdomen → internal oblique muscle of abdomen → transverse muscle of abdomen. In the superficial layer, there are the lateral cutaneous branches of the anterior branches of the 9th to 11th thoracic nerves and the accompanying arteries and veins. In the deep layer, there are the muscular branches of the anterior branches of the 9th to 11th thoracic nerves and the related arteries and veins. ⟨Indications⟩ irregular menstuation, leukorrhea with reddish discharge, hernia, pain in the lumbar and hypochondriac region. ⟨Method⟩ Puncture 0.5~0.8 cun perpendicularly. Moxibustion is applicable.

●带脉病[dài mài bìng]　奇经八脉病候之一。出《难经·二十九难》。见腰腹胀满、带下赤白、脐腹及腰脊痛，下肢萎软不利等。

Diseases of the Dai Meridian　One of the syndromes of the eight extra meridians, originally from *Nan Jing: Ershijiu Nan* (*The Classic of Questions: Qusetion 29*). Manifested as distention and fullness in the lumbar region and abdomen, leukorrhea with reddish discharge, pain in the navel, lumbar and spinal regions, flaccidity and hypoactivity of the lower limbs, etc.

●带五色俱下[dài wǔ sè jù xià]　五色带下的别名。详见该条。

Leukorrhea with Multicolored Discharge　Another name for multicolored vaginal mucoid discharge. →五色带下(p.477)

●带下[dài xià]　①病证名。出《素问·骨空论》。泛指妇科的经、带、胎、产疾病而言。这些疾病均发生在束带以下的部位。②是指妇女阴道内流出的一种粘稠液体，如涕如脓。因与带脉有关，故称带下。据其颜色不同，可分为白带、黄带、赤带、青带、黑带。详见各条。

1. **Below Belt**　Name of a disease, originally from *Suwen: Gu Kong Lun* (*Plain Questions: On apertures of Bones*). Generally referring to gynecological diseases such as those of menstruation, leukorrhea, pregnancy and delivery because all these diseases occur below the belt.

2. **Daixia**　Referring to mucus-like discharge and pus from the vagina. So named because it is related to the Dai (Belt) Meridian. Divided into whitish leukorrhea, leukorrhea with yellowish discharge, leukorrhea with bloody discharge, leukorrhea with greenish discharge and leukorrhea with Darkish discharge. →黄带(p.173)赤带(p.47)、青带(p.320)、黑带(p.163)

●带下病[dài xià bìng]　病证名。见《妇人良方大全》。即带下。根据病因不同，分为脾虚带下、肾虚带下、湿毒带下。详见各条。亦可参见"带下"条。

Leukorrhea Disease　A disease, seen in *Furen Liangfang Daquan* (*A Complete Work of Effective Prescriptions for Women*), i.e. pathogenic leukorrhea. According to the cause, it is divided into: leukorrhea due to deficiency of the spleen, leukorrhea due to deficiency of the kidney, leukorrhea due to damp-heat pathogen, and also called Below Belt. →脾虚带下(p.295)、肾虚带下(p.366)、湿毒带下(p.370).

●带下赤候[dài xià chì hòu]　赤带的别名。详见该条。

Bloody Leukorrhea　Another name for leukorrhea with bloody discharge. →赤带(p.47)

●带下黑候[dài xià hēi hòu]　黑带的别称。详见该条。

Darkish Leukorrhea　Another name for leukorrhea with darkish discharge. →黑带(p.163)

●带下黄候[dà xià huáng hòu]　黄带的别名。详见该条。

Yellowish Leukorrhea　Another name for leukorrhea with yellowish discharge. →黄带(p.173)

●带下青候[dài xià qīng hòu]　青带的别称。详见该条。

Greenish Leukorrhea　Another name for leukorrhea with greenish discharge. →青带(p.320)

●带下五色[dài xià wǔ sè]　五色带下的别名。详见该条。

Vaginal Mucoid Discharge of Five Colors　Another name for multicolored vaginal mucoid discharge. →五色带下(p.477)

●丹熛[dān biāo]　即丹毒。见该条。

Red Fire　→丹毒(p.71)

●丹毒[dān dú]　病证名。出《素问·至真要大论》。又名丹熛、火丹、天火。因患部皮肤红如涂丹，热如火灼，故名。发无定处者，名赤游丹；发于头部者，名抱头火丹；发于小腿者，名流火；发于上者，多为风热化火；发于下者，多为湿热化火。初起证见全不适，恶寒发热，继则皮肤出现红斑，焮热肿胀，色如涂丹，压之褪色，放手后即复原状，常迅速向周围蔓延，有的出现水疱，局部灼痛，痒痛间作，边缘清楚，稍有凸起，与正常皮肤有明显分界，在红斑向四周扩散同时，中央部可逐渐痊愈，而褪为暗红或棕黄色，发生脱屑，周围部分也随之复原。其毒热炽盛者，可出现毒

邪内攻之高热烦躁,神昏谵语,恶心呕吐等。本病多由血分有热,外感风湿邪,内外合邪为病,亦有皮肤破损,感染邪毒而诱发者。临床又可分为风湿丹毒和湿热丹毒。详见各条。

Erysipelas A disease, originally from *Suwen: Zhi Zheng Yao Da Lun (Plain Questions: Great Treatise of Extremely True Gist)*, also named red fire, fire erysipelas, heavenly fire. It is so named because the skin is characterised by bright red coloration and scorching heat. Cases which wander are called migrating erysipelas, cases which manifest on the head are named erysipelas overhead and cases which occur on the leg are named flowing fire. Those occurring on the upper part of the body are mainly caused by fire transformed from wind-heat pathogen. Those occurring on the lower part of the body are mainly caused by fire transformed from dampheat pathogen. In the beginning, the syndrome is manifested by malaise of the body and fever with aversion to cold. Then red maculae appear on the skin with local swelling, scorching heat and bright red coloration. The color fades when the skin is pressed and returns to its original state with the release of pressure. It often spreads quickly. Some cases are accompanied by vesicopustule, local pain and scorching heat, onset of itch and pain at intervals, with a clear margin and slight evagination of the skin. The boundary between the affected skin and normal skin is obvious. When the red maculae spreads, its central part may gradually heal and fade into dim or brown-yellow coloration, then desquamation occurs and the marginal part also recovers. Cases due to excess noxious heat can be marked by high fever, irritability, unconsciousness, delirium, nausea and vomiting caused by attack on the interior of the body by noxious evils. The disease is mostly caused by the presence of noxious heat in the blood system, and affected by external wind, and damp heat, leading to the combination of the exterior and interior pathogens attacking the body. Some cases may be caused by injured skin infected by noxious pathogens. Clinically it can be divived into Erysipelas due to Wind-Heat Pathogens and Eryspelas due to Damp-Heat Pathogens→风热丹毒(p.113)、湿热丹毒(p.371)

●**丹田**[dān tián] ①经穴别名。出《针灸甲乙经》。即石门。见该条。②经穴别名。见《针灸资生经》。即关元。见该条。③经穴别名。见《普济本事方》。即气海。见该条。④部位名。脐下正中之处。

1. **Dantian** Another name for Shimen(RN 5), a meridian point, originally from *Zhenjiu Jia-Yi Jing (A-B Classic of Acupuncture and Moxibustion)*. →石门(p.385)

2. **Dantian** Another name for Guanyuan(RN 4), a meridian point, seen in *Zhenjiu Zisheng Jing (Acupuncture-Moxibustion Classic for Saving Life)*. →关元(p.148)

3. **Dantian** Another name for Qihai(RN 6), a meridian point, seen in *Puji Bengshi Fang (Effective Prescriptions for Universal Relief)*. →气海(p.305)

4. **Dantian**(Red Field) A part of the body, referring to the central area below the navel.

●**单腹胀**[dān fù zhàng] 病证名。见《景岳全书·杂证谟》。即鼓胀。又名蜘蛛鼓。其病以腹部胀大而四肢不肿(或肿亦不甚)为特征。详见"鼓胀"条。

Single Abdominal Distention A disease, seen in *Jingyue Quanshu: Zazheng Mo (Complete Works of Jing Yue: Strategies on Miscellaneous Diseases)*, i.e. tympanites, also named spider-like tympanites. Characterised by an enlarged abdomen without swelling or with mild swelling of the four limbs. →鼓胀(p.146)

●**单鼓**[dān gǔ] 病症名。见《丹溪心法》。即鼓胀。详见该条。

Single Meteorism A disease, seen in *Dan Xi Xinfa (Dan Xi's Experiences)*, i.e. tympanites. →鼓胀(p.146)

●**担截**[dān jié] ①针刺术语。出马丹阳《天星十二穴治杂病歌》。担,指取两穴;截,指独取一穴。②针刺手法名。见《针灸大成》。担,指提法、泻法;截,指按法、补法。

1. **Dan Jie**(Double-Single Acupoint Selection) An acupuncture term, originally from Ma Danyang's *Tianxing Shier Xue Zhi Zabing Ge (Verse on the Treatment of Miscellaneous Diseases with 12 Heavenly-Star*

Points). Dan refers to selecting 2 points and Jie refers to selecting a single point.

2. Lifting-Reducing and Pressing-Reinforcing

A needling technique, seen in *Zhenjiu Dacheng* (*A Great Compendium of Acupuncture and Moxibustion*). Dan refers to the methods of lifting and reducing; jie refers to those of pressing and reinforcing.

● 胆道蛔虫病 [dǎn dào huí chóng bìng] 病名。肠道蛔虫引起的并发症之一。由于胆道蛔虫上窜钻入胆道而致。每因腹泻，便秘，发热妊娠以及不合理的使用驱蛔药物和寒冷刺激等因素引起。古人称为"蚘（蛔）厥"或"虫心痛"。蛔虫钻入胆道后，引起胆道强烈收缩，而突以上腹部（剑突下）绞痛，其则翻滚号叫，全身出汗，其痛有钻顶、撕裂样感觉，常伴有恶心、呕吐。若蛔虫退出胆道，则疼痛会突然缓解，但可再度发作，若蛔虫全部进入胆囊，则疼痛转为持续性胀痛。若蛔虫阻塞胆道，影响胆汁排出或带入细菌，引起炎症则会出现阻塞性黄疸或胆囊炎等并发症，可见寒战，发热等症状。舌苔多白腻，脉弦紧或伏，合并感染时脉弦滑数。治宜疏泄胆气，宽中和胃。取日月、支沟、阳陵泉、迎香透四白。

Ascariasis of Biliary Tract A disease, one of the complications caused by the upward movement of the intestinal ascarids into the biliary tract. The disease is induced by diarrhea, constipation, fever, pregnancy, incorrect application of ascaridole, stimulation due to cold, etc. In ancient times, it was named colic caused by ascarids or epigastric pain due to enterositisis. After the ascarids enter the biliary tract, it can lead to intense contraction of the biliary tract, resulting in the sudden onset of colic in the upper abdomen (below the xiphoid process), in crying with trembling, sweating over the entire body, tearing pain with the sensation of drilling in the head. It is often accompanied by nausea and vomiting. When the ascarids withdraw from the biliary tract, the pain is suddenly relieved but can occur again. If the ascarids enter the gallbladder, persistent pain with distention will occur. If the ascarids obstruct the biliary tract, affecting bile excretion or bringing in bacteria, it will result in inflammation complicated by obstructive jaundice or cholecystitis, generally marked by shiv-

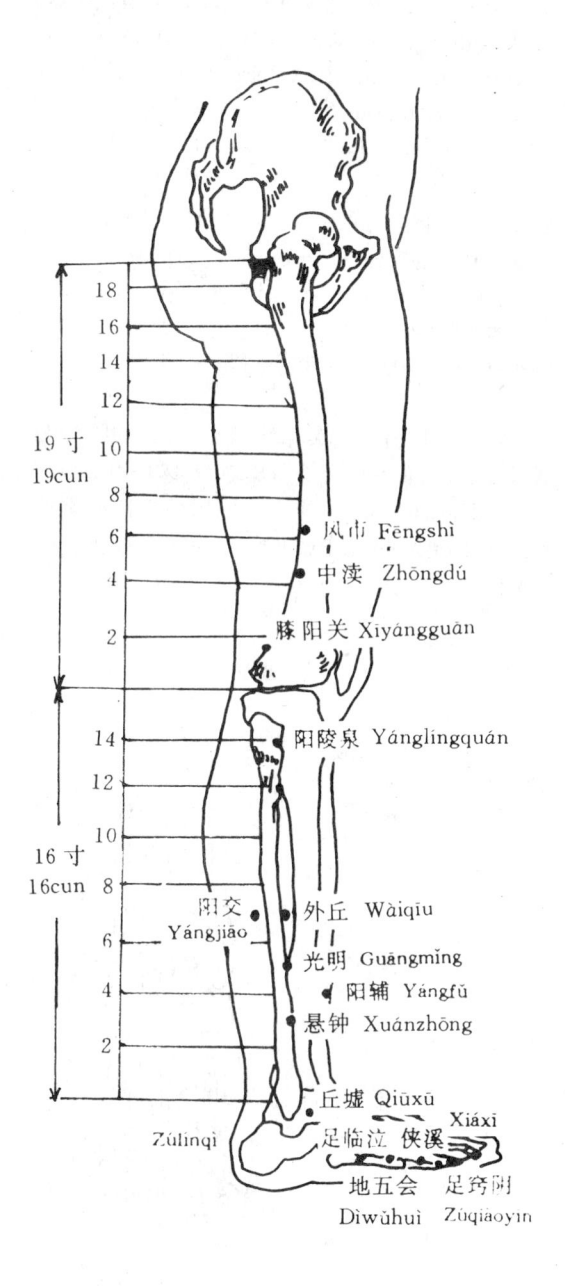

图8.1 胆经穴（下肢部）

Fig 8.1 Points of Gallbladder Meridian (Lower Limb)

ers, fever, a whitegreasy tongue coating, wirytense or deep pulse, or a wiry, slippery and

rapid pulse when complicated with infection. ⟨Treatment principle⟩ Disperse the depressed gallbladder qi, relieve epigastric distention and regulate the stomach. ⟨Point selection⟩ Riyue (GB 24), Zhigou (SJ 6), Yanglingquan (GB 34), Yingxiang (LI 20) through to Sibai (ST 2).

●胆经[dǎn jīng]　足少阳胆经之简称。详见该条。
The Gallbladder Meridian　Shortened form of Gallbladder Meridian of Foot-Shaoyang. → 足少阳胆经(p.633)

●胆囊[dǎn náng]　经外穴名。出《中华外科杂志》。⟨定位⟩在小腿外侧上部,当腓骨小头前下方凹陷处(阳陵泉)直下2寸。⟨层次解剖⟩皮肤→皮下组织→腓骨长肌。浅层布有腓肠外侧皮神经。深层有腓浅神经、腓深神经和胫前支、静脉。⟨主治⟩急慢性胆囊炎、胆石症、胆道蛔虫症、下肢麻痹或瘫痪等。直刺1.0～1.5寸。

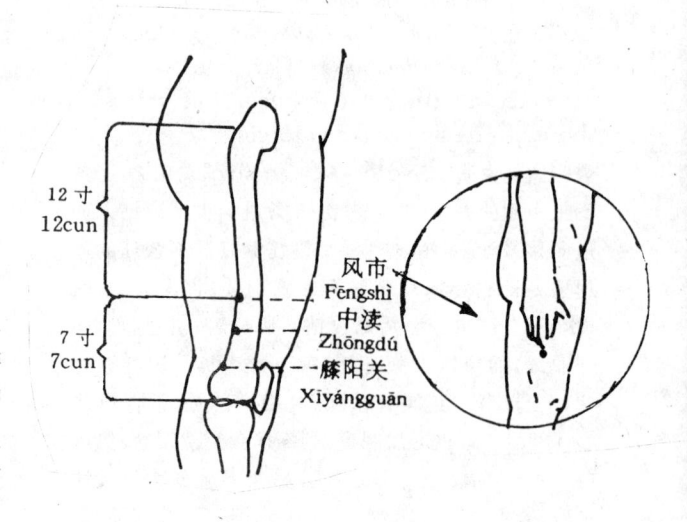

图8.3　胆经穴(大腿部)
Fig 8.3　Points of Gallbladder Meridian(Thigh)

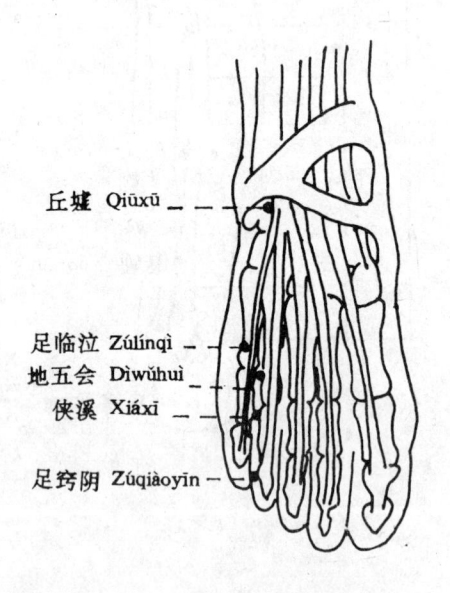

图8.2　胆经穴(足部)
Fig 8.2　Points of Gallbladder Meridian(Foot)

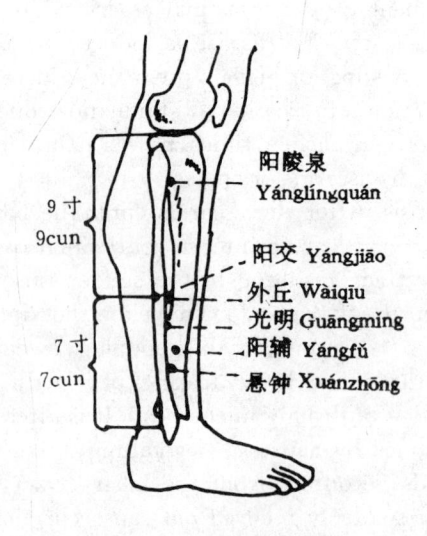

图8.4　胆经穴(小腿部)
Fig 8.4　Points of Gallbladder Meridian(Leg)

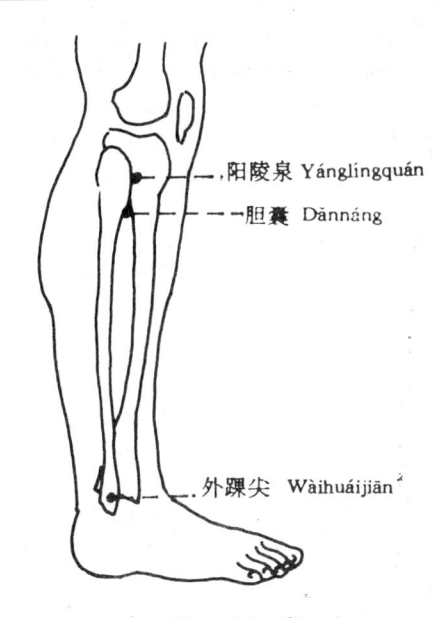

图9 胆囊穴
Fig 9 Dannang point

Dannang (EX-LE 6) An extra point, originally from *Zhonghua Waike Zazhi* (*Chinese Journal of Surgery*). ⟨Location⟩ on the upper part of the lateral surface of the 2 cun directly below the depression anterior and inferior to the head of the fibula [Yanglingquan (GB 34)]. ⟨Regional anatomy⟩ skin→subcutaneous tissue→long peroneal muscle. In the superficial layer, there is the lateral sural cutaneous nerve. In the deep layer, there are the superficial peroneal nerve, the deep peroneal nerve and the anterior tibial artery and vein. ⟨Indications⟩ acute and chronic choleystitis, cholelinthiasis, biliary ascariasis, numbness or paralysis of the lower extremities. ⟨Method⟩ Puncture perpendicularly 1.0～1.5 cun.

●胆俞[dǎn shū] 经穴名。出《针灸甲乙经》。属足太阳膀胱经,为胆的背俞穴。〈定位〉背部,当第十胸椎棘突下,旁开1.5寸(图7)。〈层次解剖〉皮肤→皮下组织→斜方肌→背阔肌→下后锯肌→竖脊肌。浅层布有第十、十一胸神经后支的皮支和伴行的动、静脉。深层有第十、十一胸神经后支的肌支和相应的肋间后动、静脉。深层有第十、十一胸神经后支的肌支和相应的肋间后动、静脉的分支或属支。〈主治〉黄疸、口苦、口干、咽痛、呕吐、胁痛、饮食不下、肺痨、潮热、腋下肿。斜刺0.5～0.8寸;可灸。

Danshu (BL 19) A meridian point, originally form *Zhenjiu Jia-Yi Jing* (*A-B Classic of Acupuncture and Moxibustion*), a point on the Bladder Meridian of Foot-Taiyang, the Back-Shu point of the gallbladder. ⟨Location⟩ on the back, below the spinous process of the 10th thoracic vertebra, 1.5 cun lateral to the posterior midline (Fig. 7). ⟨Regional Anatomy⟩ skin→subcutaneous tissue→trapezius muscle→latissimus muscle of back→inferior posterior serratus muscle→erector spinal muscle. In the superficial layer, there are the cutaneous branches of the posterior branches of the 10th and 11th thoracic nerves and the accompanying arteries and veins. In the deep layer, there are muscular branches of the posterior branches of the 10th and 11th thoracic nerves and the branches or tributaries of the related posterior intercostal arteries and veins. ⟨Indications⟩ jaundice, bitter taste in the mouth, dry mouth, sore throat, vomiting, pain in the hypochondriac region, poor appetite, impairment of the lung, tidal fever and swelling under the arm pit. ⟨Method⟩ Puncture obliquely 0.5～0.8 cun. Moxibustion is applicable.

●胆足少阳之脉[dǎn zú shào yáng zhī mài] 足少阳胆经的原名。详见该条。

The Gallbladder Vessel of Foot-Shaoyang
The original name of the Gallbladder Meridian of Foot-Shaoyang. →足少阳胆经(p.633)

●亶中[dàn zhōng] 经穴别名。见《千金要方》。即膻中。见该条。

Danzhong Another name for Danzhong (RN 17), a meridian point seen in *Qianjin Yaofang* (*Essential Prescriptions Worth a Thousand Gold*). →膻中(p.75)

●膻中[dàn zhōng] ①经穴名。出《灵枢·根结》。属任脉,为心包之募穴,八会穴之气会。又名元儿、元见、上气海、亶中、胸堂。〈定位〉在胸部,当前正中线上,平第四肋间,两乳连线的中点(图43和图40)。〈层次解剖〉皮肤→皮下组织→胸骨体。主要分布有第四肋间神经前皮的胸廓内动、静脉的穿支。〈主治〉咳嗽、气喘、咳唾脓血、胸痹心痛、心悸、心烦、产妇少乳、噎隔、臌胀。平刺0.3-0.5寸;可灸。②部位名。为两乳之间。

1. **Danzhong** (RN 17) A meridian point, o-

riginally from *Lingshu: Gen Jie* (*Miraculous Pivot: Root and Branch*), a point on the Ren Meridian, the Front-Mu point of the Pericardium, the qi influential point of the eight influential points, also named Yuaner, Yuanjian, Shangqihai, Danzhong and Xiongtang. ⟨Location⟩ on the chest at the anterior midline, on the lever of the 4th intercostal space, at the midpoint of the line connecting both nipple (Figs. 43. 1&40). ⟨Regional anatomy⟩ skin → subcutaneous tissue → sternal body. There are the anterior cutaneous branches of the 4th intercostal nerve and the perforating branches of 4th internal thoracic artery and vein in this area. ⟨Indications⟩ cough, dyspnea, cough with bloody sputum, obstruction of the qi in the chest, heart pain, palpitation, irritability, insufficient lactation of parturient, dysphagia, tympanites. ⟨Method⟩ Puncture subcutaneously 0.3~0.5 cun. Moxibustion is applicable.

2. Dan Zhong A part of the body, the region between the breasts.

●当容[dāng róng] 经外穴名。见《千金要方》。在目外眦外方当颧骨突外缘凹陷处。主治目赤肿痛等。针刺0.3~0.5寸；可灸。

Dangrong(EX-HN) An extra point, seen in *Qianjin Yaofang* (*Essential Prescriptions Worth a Thousand Gold*). ⟨Location⟩ lateral to the outer canthus, in the depression on the lateral border of the eye, etc. ⟨Method⟩ Puncture subcutaneously 0.3~0.5 cun. Moxibustion is applicable.

●当阳[dāng yáng] ①经外穴名。见《千金要方》。⟨定位⟩在头前部，当瞳孔直上，前发际上1寸。⟨层次解剖⟩皮肤→皮下组织→枕额肌腹或帽状健膜→疏膜下疏松结缔组织。布有眶上神经和眶上动、静脉的分支或属支。⟨主治⟩头痛、眩晕、感冒、鼻塞、目赤肿痛等。平刺0.3~0.5寸；可灸。②经外穴别名。即太阳。见该条。

1. Dangyang(EX-HN 2) An extra point, seen in *Qianjin Yaofang* (*Essential Prescriptions Worth a Thousand Gold*). ⟨Location⟩ at the frontal part of the head, directly above the pupil, 1 cun above the anterior hairline. ⟨Regional anatomy⟩ skin → subcutaneous tissue → bell of occipitofrontal muscle or epicranial aponeurosis → subaponeurotic loose connective tissue. There are the supraorbital nerve and the branches of tributaries of the supraorbital artery and vein in this area. ⟨Indications⟩ headache, dizziness, common cold, stuffy nose, redness, swelling and pain of eye.

2. Dangyang Another name for the extra point Taiyang (EX-HN 5). → 太阳 (p. 420)

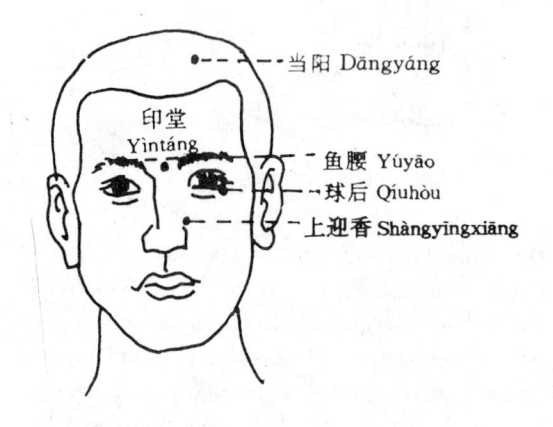

图10 当阳穴
Fig 10 Dangyang point

●导气[dǎo qì] 针刺手法名。出《灵枢·五乱》。①指缓慢进针，再缓慢出针的方法。适用于既不是有余之实证，也不是不足的虚证，只是气机逆乱，而尚未乱及脏腑者。应用此法可以疏导调整经气归于正常，使邪气得祛而不深入，正气恢复，达到治疗疾病的目的。②指促使针刺感应沿着经脉循行路线传导扩散的行气手法，称导气法。参见"行气法"条。

Inducing Qi An acupuncture method, originally from *Lingshu: Wu Luan* (*Miraculous Pivot: Five Disorders of Qi*). Referring to ① the method of slow insertion of the needle and slow withdrawal of the needle, applied to neither excess syndromes nor deficiency syndromes, but to the reverse of qi which has not yet affected zang-fu organs. Apply the method to dredge and regulate the meridian qi to normal, relieve the pathogenic qi in case it gets

deeper and restore the vital-qi, so as to cure thedisease. ② the method of making the needling sensation move along the course of meridian, also called. "qi-guiding method" → "行气法"(p.512)

●捣法[dǎo fǎ] 针刺辅助手法之一。针刺达一定深度后,右手捏持针柄,作较大幅度的连续提插动作。捣时应掌握针刺的方向、深浅距离相同,指力亦应相等。如作小幅度、较快速的提插,其状如颤动者,又称震颤法。其目的是为了加强针感。

Continuous Lifting-Thrusting Technique
One of the auxiliary techniques of acupuncture. Insert the needle to a certain depth, hold the handle of the needle with the right hand and continuously lift and thrust the needle with a large amplitude. During manipulation, be careful to maintain direction and use the same depth and finger force on the needle. Lifting and thrusting the needle with a small amplitude and high frequency, which resembles vibrating the needle, it is also called vibration needling. It's purpose is to strengthen the needling sensation.

●得气[dé qì] 刺法术语。见《内经》,现又称针感。是指进针后,通过一定的手法操作,医生持针的手有沉紧、滞涩的感觉;同时病人的针刺部位产生酸、麻、重、胀的感觉,针刺必须在得气的基础上施行适当的补泻手法,才能获得满意的治疗效果,即"气至而有效"。

Arrival of Qi   A term in acupuncture, seen in *Neijing* (*The Inner Canon of Huangdi*), also called needling sensation or needling reaction. This refers to the tense and heavy feeling felt by the doctor's fingers holding the needle, after the needle is inserted and manipulated; meanwhile, the patient has a sensation of soreness, numbness, heaviness and distention at the needled site. Satisfactory therapeutic effects can be obtained only by applying suitable reinforcing-reducing methods on the basis of the arrival of qi, in other words, only after the arrival of qi does the effect appear.

●灯草灸[dēng cǎo jiǔ] 灸法的一种。出《世医得效方·沙证》。为灯火灸之别称。见该条。

Rush Moxibustion   A moxibustion method, originally from *Shiyi De Xiaofang; Shazheng* (*Effective Prescriptions Handed Down for Generations; Sha-syndrome*), another name for rush-fire cauterization. →灯火灸(p.77)

●灯火灸[dēng huǒ jiǔ] 灸法的一种。见《本草纲目》。又称灯草灸、灯心草灸。用灯心草蘸植物油点火后灸灼穴位。一般宜横对或斜对穴位迅速施灸,蘸油应适量,以防热油下滴引起烫伤。当灯火灼及穴位皮肤时可出现轻微"啪"声,灯火即灭,称为一燋。每穴一般只灸一燋,局部稍起红晕,应保持清洁不使感染。可用于肋腺炎、呃逆、呕吐、阴瘀腹痛、小儿消化不良、功能性子宫出血、手足厥冷等症。

Rush-Fire Cauterization   A moxibustion method, seen in *Bencao Gangmu* (*Compendium of Materia Medica*), also named moxibustion with burning rush, rush moxibustion, or burning-rush cauterization. Dip the rush into vegetable oil, ignite the oiled rush and put it on the acupoints. Moxibustion is usually applied quickly with the rush horizontal or oblique to the points. Not too much oil should be dipped in case the hot oil drips would cause scalding. When the burning rush touches the skin of the acupoints, a "pa" sound should be heard and the fire extinquished. This process is called one "burn", usually one burn is used for each point, turning the local skin reddish; keep the local area clean to avoid infection. 〈Indications〉parotitis, hiccup, vomiting, eruptive disease and abdominal pain, infantile indigestion, dysfunctional uterine bleeding cold extremities, etc.

●灯心草灸[dēng xīn cǎo jiǔ] 灸法的一种。为灯火灸之别称。见该条。

Burning Rush Moxibustion   A moxibustion method, another name for rushfire cauterization. →灯火灸(p.77)

●镝针[dí zhēn] 针具名。出《灵枢·九针十二原》。又称推针。古代九针之一。其长三寸半,针头如黍粟形,圆而微尖。用于按压经脉,治邪居经脉的病症。但不能深入肌肉。

Spoon Needle   An acupuncture needle, originally from *Lingshu: Jiu Zhen Shier Yuan* (*Miraculous Pivot: Nine Needles and Twelve Yuan* (*Primary Points*), also named pushing needles or blunt needle, one of the ancient nine

kinds of needles for acupuncture. The needle, whosehead is shaped like a grain of millet, round but a little tapered, is 3.5 cun long. The needle is used for pressing along meridians to treat diseases caused by evils in the meridians. The needle must not be inserted deeply into muscles.

●骶端[dǐ duān] 骨骼部位名。指骶骨下端,即尾骨。

Sacrum End A part of the skeleton, referring to the bone inferior to the sacrum, i.e., coccyx.

●地仓[dì cāng] 经穴名。出《针灸甲乙经》。属足阳明胃经,为手、足阳明和阳跷之会。又名会维、胃维。〈定位〉在面部,口角外侧,上直瞳孔(图28和图5)。〈层次解剖〉皮肤→皮下组织→口轮匝肌→降口角肌。布有三叉神经的颊支和眶下支、面动、静脉的分支或属支。〈主治〉唇缓不收、眼睑瞤动、口角㖞斜、齿痛颊肿、流涎。直刺0.2寸,或向颊车方向平刺0.5-1寸;可灸。

Dicang(ST 4) A meridian point, originally from *Zhenjiu Jia-Yi Jing* (*A-B Classic of Acupuncture and Moxibustion*), a point on the Stomach Meridian of Foot-Yangming, the crossing point of the Yangming Meridians of Hand and Foot and the Yangqiao Meridian, also named Huiwei or Weihui. 〈Location〉on the face, directly below the pupil, beside the mouth angle (Figs. 28&5). 〈Regional anatomy〉Skin → subcutaneous tissue → orbicular muscle of mouth → depressor muscle of angle of mouth. There are the buccal and infrobital branches of the trigeminal nerve and the branches or tributaries of the gacial artery and vein in this area. 〈Indications〉flabby lip, twitching eyelids, deviation of the mouth, toothache, swelling in the cheek, salivation. 〈Method〉Puncture perpendicularly 0.2 cun, or puncture subcutaneously 0.5～1.0 cun with the tip of the needle directed towards Jiache(ST 6). Moxibustion is applicable.

●地冲[dì chōng] 经穴别名。出《针灸甲乙经》。即涌泉。见该条。

Dichong Another name for Yongquan (KI 1), a meridian point, originally from *Zhenju Jia-Yi Jing* (*A-B Classic of Acupuncture and Moxibustion*). → 涌泉 (p.568)

●地肤子蒸气灸[dì fū zǐ zhēng qì jiǔ] 灸法的一种。取地肤子、蛇床子各30克,苦参、白鲜皮各15克,花椒9克,白矾3克。上药水煎后倒入盆中,对准患部用蒸气熏灸。适于湿疹等症。

Di Fu Zi(*Fructus Kochiae*) **Steaming Moxibustion** A type of moxibustion. Use *Di Fu Zi*(*Fructus Kochiae*)30g, *She Chuang Zi*(*Frutus Cnidii*)30g, *Ku Shen*(*Radicis*)15g, *Bai Xian Pi*(*Cortex Dictamni Radicis*)15g, *Hua Jiao*(*Pericarpium Zanchexyli*)9g and *Bai Fan*(*Alumen*)3g. Decoct them in water, then pour the decoction in a basin and steam the affected area directly. 〈Indications〉eczema, etc.

●地合[dì hé] 经外穴名。出《刺疗捷法》。在承浆穴下方,下颌骨正中向前突起之高点处。〈主治〉头面疔疮、牙痛等。斜刺0.3～0.5寸。

Dihe(EX-HN) An extra point, from *Ciding Jiefa* (*Simple Acupuncture Method for Boils*). 〈Location〉below Chengjiang(RN 24), at the high point of the process at the midpoint of the lower jaw bone. 〈Indications〉furuncle on the face and head, toothache. 〈Method〉Puncture obliquely 0.3～0.5 cun.

●地机[dì jī] 经穴名。出《针灸甲乙经》。属足太阴脾经,为本经郄穴。又名脾舍、地箕。〈定位〉在小腿内侧,当内踝尖与阴陵泉的连线上,阴陵泉下3寸(图39.1和图81)。〈层次解剖〉皮肤→皮下组织→腓肠肌→比目鱼肌。浅层布有隐神经的小腿内侧支和大隐静脉。深层有胫神经和胫后动、静脉。〈主治〉腹胀、腹痛、食欲不振、泄泻、痢疾、月经不调、痛经、女子癥瘕、遗精、腰痛不可俯仰、小便不利、水肿。直刺0.5～1寸;可灸。

Diji(SP 8) A meridian point from *Zhenjiu Jia-Yi Jing* (*A-B Classic of Acupuncture and Moxibustion*), point on the Spleen Meridian of Foot-Taiying, and its Xi(Cleft) point. It is also named Pishe and Diji(地箕). 〈Location〉on the medial side of the leg at the line connecting the medial malleolus and Yinlingquan(SP 9), 3 cun below Yinlingquan (SP 9) (Figs. 39.1&81). 〈Regional anatomy〉skin → subcutaneous tissue → gastrocnemius muscle → soleus muscle. In the superficial layer, there are the medial cutaneous branches of the leg from the

saphenous nerves and the great saphenous vein. In the deep layer, there are the tibial nerve and the posterior tibial artery and vein. 〈Indications〉abdominal distention and pain, poor appetite, diarrhea, dysentery, irregular menstruation, dysmenorrhea, mass in the abdomen of women, nocturnal emission, inability to bend the lumbar area due to lumbago, difficulty in urination, edema. 〈Method〉Puncture perpendicularly 0.5～1.0 cun. Moxibustion is applicable.

●地箕[dì jī]　经穴别名。出《医学入门》。即地机。见该条。

Diji　Another name for Diji(SP 8), a meridian point from *Yixue Rumen*(*An Introduction to Medicine*).→地机(p. 78)

●地神[dì shén]　经外穴名。见《千金要方》。在拇指掌侧掌指关节横纹中点和足大趾跖侧跖趾关节横纹中点处,共四穴。灸自缢死。

Dishen(EX-UE)　Set of extra points seen in *Qianjin Yaofang* (*Essential Prescriptions Worth a Thousand Gold*). 〈Location〉on the palmar side of each thumb, at the midpoint of the crease of the metacarpophalangeal point. Four points in all. 〈Indication〉strangulation. 〈Method〉moxibustion.

●地卫[dì wèi]　经穴别名。出《太平圣惠方》。即涌泉。见该条。

Diwei(KI 1)　Another name for Yongquan (KI 1), a meridian point from *Taiping Shenghui Fang* (*Imperial Benevolent Prescriptions*)→涌泉(p. 568)

●地五[dì wǔ]　经穴别名。出《医学入门》。即地五会。见该条。

Diwu　Another name for Diwuhui(GB 42), a meridian point from *Yixue Rumen*(*An Introduction to Medicine*).→地五会(p. 79)

●地五会[dì wǔ huì]　经穴名。出《针灸甲乙经》。属足少阳胆经。又名地五。〈定位〉在足背外侧,当足四趾本节(第四跖趾关节)的后方,第四、五跖骨之间,小趾伸肌的内侧缘(图81)。〈层次解剖〉皮肤→皮下组织→趾长伸肌腱→趾短伸肌腱外侧→第四骨间背侧肌→第三骨间足底肌。浅层布有足背中间皮神经、足背静脉和跖背动、静脉。深层有趾足底总神经和趾底总动、静脉。〈主治〉头痛、目赤痛、耳鸣、耳聋、胸满、肋痛、腋肿、乳痈、胼痛、跗肿。直刺或斜刺0.5～0.8寸;可灸。

Diwuhui(GB 42)　A meridian point from *Zhenjiu Jia-Yi Jing*(*A-B Classic of Acupuncture and Moxibustion*), a point on the Gallbladder Meridian of Foot-Shaoyang, also named Diwu. 〈Location〉on the lateral side of the instep of the foot, posterior to the 4th metacarophalangeal joint, between the 4th and 5th metatarsal bones, medial to the tendon of the extensor muscle of the little toe(Fig. 81). 〈Regional anatomy〉skin→subcutaneous tissue →tendon of long extensor muscle of toes→lateral side of tendon of short extensor muscle of toes→4th dorsal interosseous muscle 3rd plantar interosseous muscle. In the superficial layer, there are the intermediate dorsal cutaneous nerve of the foot, the venous network of the dorsum of the foot and the dorsal metatarsal artery and vein. In the deep layer, there are the common digital plantar nerve and the common digital plantar artery and vein. 〈Indications〉headache, redness and pain of the eye, tinnitus, deafness, fullness of the chest, pain in the hypochondriac region, swelling of the axilla, acute mastitis, pain of the leg, swelling of the foot. 〈Method〉Puncture obliquely or perpendicularly 0.5～0.8 cun. Moxibustion is applicable.

●颠[diān]　部位名。指头顶部。通作"巅"。

Top　A body part, referring to the top of the head, interchangeable with peak.

●巅上[diān shàng]　经穴别名。出《素问·骨空论》。《针灸聚英》作百会别名。见"百会"条。

Dianshang　Another name for Baihui(DU 20), a meridian point from *Suwen: Gukong Lun*(*Plain Questions On Apertures of Bones*) referred to as Baihui(DU 20)in *Zhenjiu Juying*(*Essentials of Acupuncture and Moxibustion*).→百会(p. 11)

●癫狂[diān kuáng]　病证名。见《丹溪心法·癫狂》。以精神错乱,言行失常为主。癫属阴,多偏于虚,患者多静默;狂属阳,多偏于实,患者多躁动。但癫病经久,痰郁化火,可出现狂症;狂病延久,正气不足,亦可出现癫证。故常癫狂并称。临床可分为癫证、狂症两型。详见各条。

Manic-Depressive Psychosis   A disease, seen in *Danxi Xinfa*: *Diankuang* (*Danxi's Experience*: *Manic-Depressive Psychosis*). Mainly manifested as psychosis and abnormal speech and action. The depressive state is attributed to the disorder or yin mostly due to deficiency, and marked by quiescence of the patient, while the manic state is attributed to the disorder of yang mostly due to excess, manifested by irritability. But the manic syndrome may occur in the lingering depressive cases with fire pathogen from phlegm stagnancy, and the depressive synsrome may occur in the lingering manic case with deficiency of vital-qi, hence the depressive state are generally named together with their symptoms divided into 2 clinical types: Depressive Syndrome and **Manic Syndrome**. →癫症(p. 80)、狂症(p. 235)

●癫痫[diān xián]　病症名。见《千金要方》，卷十四。①为癫症与痫症的合称。癫，指精神错乱一类疾病；痫，指发作性的神志异常疾病。详见"癫症"、"痫症"条。②即痫症。又名风眩。古代癫、痫二字通用。详见"痫症"条。

Epilepsy   1. A disease from Vol. 14 of *Qianjin Yaofang* (*Essential Prescriptions Worth a Thousand Gold*). The combination of depressive psychosis and epilepsy. Depressive psychosis refers to a pathological state of mental confusion, while epilepsy refers to paroxysmal mental disorder. →癫症(p. 80)、痫症(p. 491) 2. Synonymous with epilepsy, which is also named dizziness due to wind pathogen. The words dian and xian were used interchangeably in ancient China. →痫症(p. 491)

●癫证[diān zhèng]　①癫狂症型之一。多由痰气郁结所致。证见精神抑郁，表情淡漠，沉默，多疑、妄想，语无伦次，悲泣无常，甚则妄见妄闻，动作离奇，不知秽洁，苔腻，脉滑。久则气亏耗，惊悸失眠，迷惘呆钝，饮食减少，面色少华，舌质淡，脉细弦。治宜调气化痰，清心安神。取神门、大陵、印堂、膻中、丰隆、三阴交。②即痫症。见该条。

Depressive Psychosis   ①A type of manic-depressive psychosis, mostly due to the stagnation of phlegm and qi. Manifested by emotional depression, apathy, quiescence, doubting, mania, fantasy paraphasis, and tendency towards sadness and weeping. Sometimes accompanied by auditory and visual hallucinations, strange action, or inability to distinguish between dirt and cleanliness. The tongue has greasy fur and the pulse is slippery. Cases of long duration will result in deficiency of qi and blood, marked by insomnia with terror, trance and dullness, poor appetite, dim complexion, pale tongue, thready and taut pulse. ⟨Treatment principles⟩Resolve phlegm by regulating the flow of qi and tranquillize by clearing away heartfire. ⟨Point selection⟩Shenmen(HT 7), Daling (PC 7), Yintang (EX-HN 3), Shanzhong(Ren 17), Fenglong(ST 40)and , Sanyinjiao(SP 6). ②→痫症 (p. 491)

●点刺[diǎn cì]　刺法名。指将针快速刺入后即行退出，针刺较浅，时间短暂，多用于井穴或刺络法中。

Pricking Method   A needling method, referring to swift and superficial insertion followed by the immediate withdrawal of the needle, frequently used for puncturing Jing (Well) points or in blood-letting puncture.

●电热灸[diàn rè jiǔ]　灸法的一种。近代利用电能发热以代替艾炷施灸。先将特制的电灸器接通电流，达到一定温度后，即可在选定部位上进行点灸或来回熨灸。用于风湿痹痛等病。

Electric-Heating Moxibustion   A type of modern moxibustion. Heat is produced by electrical energy instead of moxa cones. First, set up the electric circuit of the specially made electric moxibustion equipment. When it reaches a certain temperature, apply spot or ironing moxibustion to the affected area. ⟨Indication⟩ numbness and pain due to wind-dampness.

●电针法[diàn zhēn fǎ]　针刺手法。出《针灸杂志》1934年第一期。针刺结合电流刺激以治病的方法。系在针刺留针过程中，于有关穴组（两穴为一组）上接通由电针机输出的脉冲电流。有双向脉冲电流（间歇振荡电流）、正弦波、方波等种。其组合方式有连续波、疏密波、断续波、起伏波、锯齿波等。所用频率多为1～1000次/秒，少数达1000次/秒以上。刺激强度以穴位部肌肉刚出现抽动，病人自觉舒适为宜。临床如需对针刺适应症作较长时间刺激时，可选用本法。胸背、上肢穴位使用电针时，不宜将同一对输出的两个电极分别跨于身体两侧。有严重心脏病者，或靠近

延脑、背髓部的穴位应慎用。

Electrotherapy A type of needling therapy from *Zhenjiu Zazhi* (*Journal of Acupunture and Moxibustion*), No. 1, 1934, which combines needling with electric stimulation, i.e., connecting needles of the point group concerned (2 points make up a group) with pulse current from the electric stimulator. There is a dual-directional pulse current (intermittent oscillatory current), sin wave, aquare wave, etc., with characteristics such as continuous wave, sparse-dense wave, intermittent wave, undulatary wave, sawtooth wave, etc. The frequency most commonly used is 1-1000 times/sec. over 1000 times/sec. is used less. Proper intensity of stimulation is marked by a muscular twitch around the point and a comfortable sensation. The therapy can be clinically used for cases requiring long needling stimulations. It's not advisable to connect electrodes from the same output to a point pair on opposite sides of the body when applying the therapy to points on the chest and upper extremities. It should be used with great care for patients with severe heart disease, or points near the medulla oblongata and the spinal cord.

●电针机 [diàn zhēn jī] 针具。应用电脉冲以加强对穴位刺激作用的电子治疗仪器。种类很多，有蜂鸣式电针机，电子管电针机，半导体电针机等数种。蜂鸣式电针机，系利用电铃振荡原理使直流电变成脉冲直流电，再经过感应线圈而产生感应电流的电针器械。所发出的电流波形很窄，如针状，适宜于做电针；但因输出电量不够稳定，频率调制困难，耗电量大和噪音高等缺点，目前很少用。电子管电针机，为电子管产生多种振荡的电针器械。其优点是振荡波形和种类多，频率范围广，工作性能较稳定。缺点是要用交流电源，安全性差，体积较大，防震能力差。目前已少用。半导体电针机，系用半导体元件制作的电针器械。因其不受电源种类限制，具有安全、省电、体小、量轻、耐震等优点，目前临床上最常用。

Electric Stimulator An acupuncture apparatus, a type of electro-therapeutic equipment for strengthening stimulation to the points by applying pulse current. There are many kinds of electric stimulators: buzzer-type, electronic tube or semiconductor electric stimulators. The buzzertype electric stimulator is an electrotherapy instrument made to convert direct current into impulse direct current with the application of the principle of the electric bell oscillation, through the induction coil to produce current. Specific property: narrow needle-shaped wave, available for electric needle. It is now seldom used because of the unsteady current output, the difficult alternation of frequency, a large power consumption and noise. The device with an electronic tube can produce many kinds of oscillation. Advantages: many kinds of oscillating waves, wide range of frequency, stable function. Disadvantages: AC power supply, poor safety, big size, poor resistance to shock. It is seldom used at present. The device with a semiconductor is composed of the components of the semiconductor. Advantages: unlimited in power supply, safe, current-saving, small size, light weight, resistent to shock. It is commonly used in clinic at present.

●电针麻醉 [diàn zhēn má zuì] 针刺法。指用电针刺激达到镇痛效果以进行手术的方法。临床上所用的体针、耳针、鼻针等各种针麻取穴，均可使用本法。参见"针刺麻醉"条。

Electrical Acupuncture Anesthesia An acupuncture method of alleviating pain during surgery with stimulation produced by an electric needle stimulator. It can be applied clinically to points on the body, the ears and the nose for acupuncture anthesia. →针刺麻醉 (p. 588)

●电子温针灸 [diàn zǐ wēn zhēn jiǔ] 灸法的一种。是通过电热作用，使用传统毫针来代替艾卷、艾炷作温针而治疗疾病的一种方法。如最近研制生产的DWJ-Ⅱ型电子温针治疗机和DWR-Ⅲ型电子温针热灸治疗机等。临床上对颈椎病、骨刺、非化脓性肋软骨炎、关节炎、肩周炎、冠心病、偏瘫、坐骨神经痛、支气管哮喘、盆腔炎、不孕症等都有一定疗效。

Moxibustion with Electric Warming Needles
A type of moxibustion therapy with a sheaf of traditional filiform needles warmed with electricity instead of a moxa stick and moxa cone. The DWJ-Ⅱ Electric Needle Warmer and DWR-Ⅲ Electric Hot Moxibustion er

with warm needles are new inventions for this purpose. 〈Indications〉cervical spondylopathy, bone-spur, non-suppurative castochondritis, arthritis, scapulohumeral periarthritis, coronary heart disease, hemiplegia, sciatica, bronchial asthma, pelvic inflammation, sterility, etc.

●雕目[diāo mù] 眼睑下垂的别名。详见该条。

Ptosis of the Eyelid Another name for blepharaptosis. →眼睑下垂(p.535)

●丁德用[dīng dé yòng] 宋代针灸家。著《难经补注》五卷，对经文深奥者均加以绘图说明，对针灸学的阐释有一定贡献。

Ding Deyong An acupuncture and moxibustion expert in the Song Dynasty, compiler of *Nanjing Buzhu* (*Supplementary Notes to the Classic of Difficulties*) in 5 volumes. He illustrated the original texts, and made contributions to the elaboration on acupuncture and moxibustion.

●丁毅[dīng yì] 明代针灸学家。字德刚，精医术，尤擅针灸。著有《医方集》、《宜玉函集》、《兰阁秘方》等。

Ding Yi An acupuncture and moxibustion expert in the Ming Dynasty, who styled himself Degang. Proficient in medical skills, he was especially good at acupuncture and moxibustion, and compiled such books as *Yifang Ji* (*A Collection of Prescriptions*), *Yiyu Hanji* (*Works Which Should be Kept in a Jade Case*), *Lange Mifang* (*Secret Prescriptions of the Chamber of Orchids*), etc.

●疔疮[dīng chuāng] 病证名。见《济生方》。又名疵疮。因其形小，根深，坚硬如钉状，故名。又因发病部位和形状各异，而有人中疔、蛇头疔、红丝疔、虎口疔、下唇疔、鼻疔等名称。多因恣食膏粱厚味及酗酒等，以致脏腑蕴热，火毒结聚；或由肌肤不洁，邪恶外侵，流窜经络，气血郁滞而成。本病初起如粟状，其色或黄或紫，或起水泡、脓疱，根结坚硬如疔，自觉麻痒微痛，继之红肿灼热，肿势蔓延，疼痛增剧，多有寒热。如见壮热烦躁，眩晕，呕吐，神识昏愦者，为疔毒内攻之象，称为疔疮走黄。治宜清热解毒。取身柱、灵台、合谷、委中。生于面部手阳经者加商阳、曲池；生于食指端者，加曲池、迎香；生于面部足少阳经者，加阳陵泉、足窍阴；生于足小趾次趾者，加阳陵泉、听会；如系红丝疔从终点依次点刺至起点，以泄其恶血。疔疮初起，患处切勿挤压、针挑；红肿发硬时忌手术，以免使病情扩散；如已成脓，应予外科处理。

Furuncle A disease seen in *Ji Sheng Fang* (*Recipes for Saving Lives*), also named splinter furuncle since it is small in size, deep-rooted and hard as a nail. It has various names according to the affected parts and the shapes, such as boil on philtrum, snake's head-like furuncle, red-streaked infection, nail-like furuncle in tiger's mouth, furuncle on the lower lip, furuncle of nose, etc. It is mainly due to overeating, a rich fatty diet and excessive drinking, all of which lead to the accumulation of heat in the viscera and stagnation of the firetoxin. Or dirty skin, exterior attack of the toxic pathogen which affects the meridians and collaterals leading to the stagnation of both qi and blood. 〈Manifestations〉yellow or purple millet shaped furuncle with blister, or pustule and a hard root. Symptoms include numbness, itching and slight pain in the initial stages, then redness, swelling and a scorching sensation develop. In most cases, swelling continues and sharp pains with chills and fever develop. Cases with dysphoria due to high fever, dizziness, vomiting and unconsciousness are caused by interior affection of furunculesis. This is called carbuncle complicated by septicemia. 〈Treatment principle〉 Clear heat and toxic material. 〈Point selection〉 Shenzhu (DU 12), Lingtai (DU 10), Hegu (LI 4) and Weizhong (BL 40). Add Shangyang (LI 1) and Quchi (LI 11) when manifested on the Meridian of Hand-Yangming on the face; Quchi (LI 11) and Yingxiang (LI 20) when manifested on the tips of the index fingers; Yanglingquan (SP 9) and Zuqiaoyin (GB 44) when manifested on the Meridian of Foot-Shaoyang on the face; Yanglingquan (SP 9) and Tinghui (GB 2), when manifested on the fourth and fifth toes. Prick a red-streaked infection from end to start to remove the extravasated blood. Avoid squeezing or pricking the affected part in the initial stage. Operations are not indicated for those in the stage of redness and swelling so as to avoid the spread of the furuncle. A surgical

operation is necessary for a pustular furuncle.

●**疔疮走黄**[dīng chāng zǒu huáng] 病证名。见《疮疡经验全书》。又名癀走。多因正气内虚,热毒炽盛;或因失于调治,疔毒走散,入于血分,内攻脏腑而致。证见疮顶黑陷,无脓,肿势散漫,伴有壮热烦躁、眩晕、呕吐、神识昏愦,舌绛苔黄,脉洪数或弦滑。治宜清热解毒凉血。取穴可参见"疔疮"条,并取水沟、大椎、百会、内关、劳宫、血海、膈俞。

Furuncle Complicated by Septicemia A disease seen in *Chuangyang Jingyan Quanshu* (*A Complete Manual of Experiences in the Treatment of Sores*), also called spread of furuncle, mostly due to deficiency of the vital-qi, excess toxic-heat, or mistaken or delayed treatment leading to the spread of furunculosis into the blood system, which internally attacks the viscera. 〈Manifestations〉dark and hollow tip of the furuncle without pus, slow spreading of the swelling, accompanied by irritability due to high fever, dizziness, vomiting, unconciousness, a deep-red tongue with a yellowish coating, full and rapid or taut and slippery pulse. 〈Treatment principle〉Clear heat and toxic material to cool the blood. 〈Point selection〉 (cf. **疔疮 Furuncle**). Add Shuigou (DU 26), Dazhui (DU 14), Baihui (DU 20), Neiguan (PC 6), Laogong (PC 8), Xuehai (SP 10) and Geshu (BL 17).

●**疔毒**[dīng dú] 病名。见《证治准绳》。为疔疮之重者,易发走黄。详见"疔疮"、"疔疮走黄"条。

Furunculosis A disease seen in *Zheng Zhi Zhunsheng* (*Standards for Diagnosis and Treatment*), referring to the serious state of furuncle, which spreads easily. →疔疮(p. 82)、疔疮走黄(p. 83)

●**顶门**[dǐng mén] 经穴名。见《玉龙歌》注。即囟

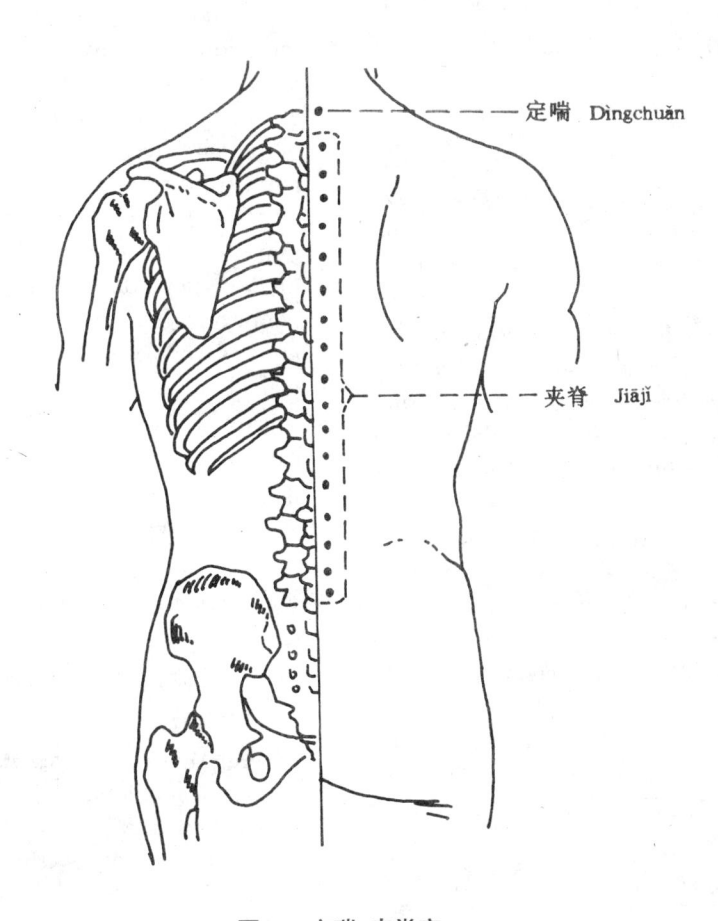

图11 定喘、夹脊穴

Fig 11 Dingchuan and Jiaji points

会。见该条。

Dingmen　Another name for Xinhui (DU 22), a meridian point seen in *Yulong Ge* (*Jade Dragon Verses*).→囟会(p.510)

●顶上回毛[dǐng shàng huí máo]　经外穴名。或释作百会穴。位于头顶回发中点。〈主治〉小儿惊痫、癫痫、脱肛、痔疮出血等。当温灸。

Dingshanghuimao (EX-HN)　An extra point, which can be taken as Baihui (DU 20). 〈Location〉at the midpoint of Huifa of the vertex.〈Indications〉infantile convulsions, epilepsy, prolapse of the rectum and bleeding due to hemorrhoids.〈Method〉mild moxibustion.

●定喘[dìng chuǎn]　经外穴名。出《北京中医》。又名治喘、喘息穴。〈定位〉在背部,当第七颈椎棘突下,旁开0.5寸。〈层次解剖〉皮肤→皮下组织→斜方肌→菱形肌→上后锯肌→颈夹肌→竖脊肌。浅层主要布有第八颈神经后支的内侧皮支。深层有颈深动、静脉和颈横动、静脉的分支或属支及第八颈神经、第一胸神经后支的肌支。〈主治〉哮喘、咳嗽、落枕、荨麻疹等。直刺0.5-1寸;可灸。

Dingchuan (EX-B 1)　Name of an extra point from *Beijing Zhongyi* (*Beijing Traditional Chinese Medicine*), also named Zhichuan and Chuanxi.〈Location〉on the back, below the spinous process of the 7th cevical vertebra, 0.5 cun lateral to the posterior midline.〈Regional anatomy〉skin→subcutaneous tissue→trapezius muscle→rhomboid muscle→superior posterior serratus muscle→splenius muscle of neck→erector spinal muscle. In the superficial layer, there are the medial cutaneous branches of the posterior branch of the 8th cervical never. In the deep layer, there are the branches or tributaries of the deep cervical artery and vein and the transverse cervical artery and vein and the muscular branches of the posterior branches of the 8th cervical and 1st thoracic nerve.〈Indications〉asthma, cough, torticollis, urticaria, etc.〈Method〉Puncture perpendicularly 0.5~1 cun. Moxibustion is applicable.

●定息寸数[dìng xī cùn shù]　出《金针赋》。又称生成息数。见接气通经条。

Location of the Flow of Meridian-Qi　From *Jin Zhen Fu* (*Ode to Gold Needle*), also named location of the course of meridian-qi.→接气通径(p.201)

●东医宝鉴[dōng yī bǎo jiàn]　书名。全书23卷,朝鲜许浚等撰于1610年(明万历三十八年)。作者选摘我国明以前医籍予以分类编纂而成。全书分为内景、外形、杂病、汤液、针灸篇五类,各类均详分细目,记叙了多种病证的证候、病因、治法等内容。书中针灸篇,对针法、灸法、经穴、奇穴、别穴等,均有载述。其它篇中,也有随病记载针灸法。引文均注明出处,便于参考。

Dongyi Baojian (*A Treasured Mirror of Oriental Medicine*)　A book in 23 volumes written by Sui Jin, a Korean and others in 1610 (the 38th year on the reign of Wanli of the Ming Dynasty). The author compiled the book by taking extractions from the medical books of China prior to the Ming Dynasty and classifying them. The book includes five chapters: interior view, exterior body, miscellaneous diseases, decoction, and acupuncture and moxibustion, each of which is catalogued in detail. The syndromes, causes and treatment principles of various diseases are narrated. The chapter on acupuncture and moxibustion records acupuncture and moxibustion methods, meridian points, extra points, other points, etc. The other chapters also record the methods of acupuncture and moxibustion attached to each disease. The author gives sources for all quotations, making reference simple.

●动而伸之[dòng ěr shēn zhī]　刺法用语。见《难经·七十八难》。为针刺法操作的要领。与"推而纳之"相对。系由《灵枢·官能》中泻法"切而转之"、"伸而迎之"的基础上发展而来。意指取得感应后,将针转动并向上抽提,称为泻。其理与《难经·七十八难》中"当泻之时,从荣置气"一致。后世所称的"紧提慢按"的泻法操作,即以此为理论依据。

Lifting While Twirling the Needle　A term for an acupuncture technique seen in *Nan Jing: Qishiba Nan* (*The Classic of Questions: Question 78*). It is the essential technique when performing the reducing method in acupuncture, as opposed to "thrusting while pushing the needle". It was developed on the

basis of the reducing methods of "twirling the needle while the meridian-qi is arriving" and "lifting the needle while the meridian-qi is arriving", which are from *Lingshu*:*Guan Neng*(*Miraculous Pivot*:*Functions and Abilities*). Those techniques refer to the reducing method of lifting while twirling the needle after obtaining the needling response, corresponding to the theory of "directing qi from ying system while performing the reducing method", which is from *Nan Jing*:*Qishiba Nan*(*The Classic of Questions*:*Question 78*). Later generations' manipulation of the reducing method of "swift lifting and slow thrusting" is theoretically based on it.

●动法[dòng fǎ] 针刺手法名。出《难经·七十八难》。①在《针经指南》中列为十四法之一,意指提插。②《针灸问对》中以摇动来解释。

Moving An acupuncture technique from *Nan Jing*:*Qishiba Nan*(*The Classic of Questions*:*Question 78*). ①One of the 14 methods from *Zhenjing Zhinan* (*A Guidebook of Acupuncture Classic*), referring to lifting and thrusting the needle. ②Explained as shaking in *Zhenjiu Wendui*(*Questions and Answers on Acupuncture and Moxibustion*).

●斗肘[dǒu zhǒu] 经外穴名。见《经外奇穴治疗诀》。又称小肘尖。在曲池穴外方,当肱骨外上髁之高点处。灸治臂肘神经痛、偏瘫、神经衰弱等。

Douzhou(EX-UE) An extra point seen in *Jingwai Qixue Zhiliao Jue* (*Pithy Formulas for Treatment with Extra Points*), also named Xiaozhoujian. 〈Location〉At the lateral aspect of Quchi(LI 11), on the tip of the external humeral epicondyle. 〈Indications〉neuralgia of the arm and elbow, hemiplegia and neurosism. 〈Method〉moxibustion.

●豆豉灸[dòu chǐ jiǔ] 为隔豉饼灸之别称。见该条。

Douchi(*Semen Sojae Praeparatum*)**Moxibustion** Another name for *Douchi*(*Semen Sojae Praeparatum*)-cake-separated moxibustion →隔豉饼灸(p.134).

●窦材[dòu cái] 人名。金代医家,真定(今河北正定)人。善针灸,撰《扁鹊心书》三卷,刊于1146年。他倡导多壮灸法及服用热药。

Dou Cai A physician in the Jin Dynasty, a native of Zhending (now Zhengding, Hebei Province). He was trained in acupuncture and moxibustion, and compiled *Bian Que Xinshu* (*Bian Que's Medical Experiences*) in 3 volumes, which was published in 1146. He advocated the use of moxibustion therapy with many cones and taking Chinese drugs of a hot nature.

●窦桂芳[dòu guì fāng] 人名。元代针灸家,字静斋,建安(今属福建)人。1311年校刊《针灸四书》。

Dou Guifang An acupuncture and moxibustion expert in the Yuan Dynasty, a native of Jian An (of today's Fujian Province), who styled himself Jingzhai. He edited *Zhenjiu Si Shu*(*Four Books on Acupuncture and Moxibustion*), which was published in 1311.

●窦汉卿[dòu hàn qīng] 人名。金元时期著名针灸学家,初名杰,字汉卿,后改名默,字子声,广平肥乡(今属河北肥乡)人。以针灸闻名。撰《针经指南》、《流注指要赋》、《标幽赋》等针灸学专著。见《元史》。

Dou Hanqing A famous acupuncture and moxibustion expert in the Jin and Yuan Dynasties, a native of Feixiang, Guanpging (today's Feixiang, Hebei) with Jie as his original name (changed to Mo later), who styled himself Hanqing (changed to Zisheng later). He was famous for his acupuncture techinques, and compiled several monographs on acupuncture and moxibustion including *Zhenjing Zhinan*(*A Guide to the Classic of Acupuncture*), *Liuzhu Zhiyao Fu*(*Ode to the Essentials of Flow*), *Biaoyou Fu*(*Lyrics of Recondite Principles*), Cf. *Yuan Shi* (*History of the Yuan Dynasty*).

●窦氏八穴[dòu shì bā xué] 八脉交会穴的别名。见该条。

Dou's Eight Points Another name for the eight confluence points. →八脉交会穴(p.7)

●督脊[dū jǐ] 经外穴名。见《千金要方》。在背部,当第七颈椎棘突下与尾骨端边线的中点处。灸治癫痫。

Duji(EX-B) An extra point, seen in *Qianjin Yaofang* (*Essential Prescriptions Worth a Thousand Gold*). 〈Location〉on the back, at the midpoint of the line connecting the lower border of the spinous process of the 7th cervi-

cal vertebra and the end of coccyx. ⟨Indication⟩epilepsy. ⟨Method⟩moxibustion.

●督脉[dū mài] ①奇经八脉之一。出《素问·骨空论》。其循行：起于小腹内，下出于会阴部，向后行于脊柱里面，上行达项后风府穴，进入脑部，上至巅顶，沿额下行鼻柱至上齿龈。②奇穴名。出《千金要方》。指神庭穴部位。

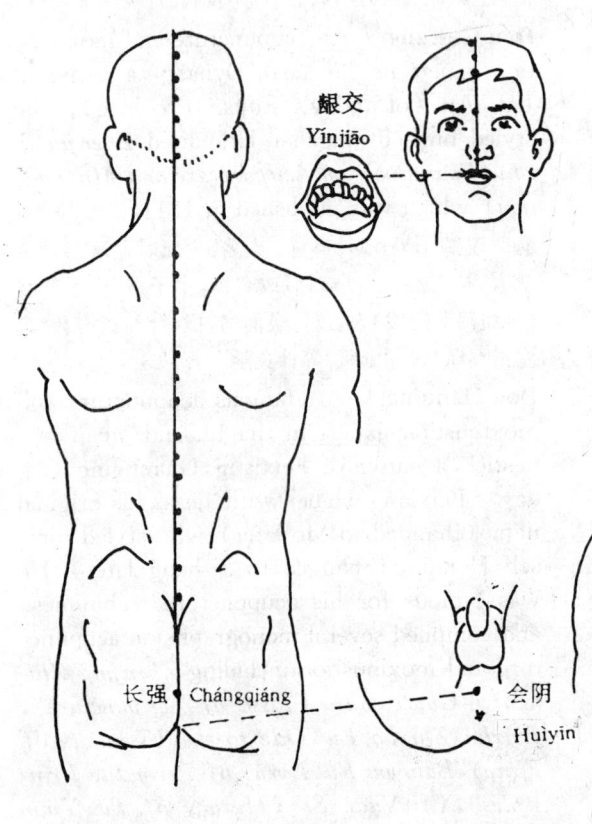

1. Du Meridian One of the eight extra meridians, originally from *Su Wen: Gukong Lun* (*Plain Questions On the Apertures of Bones*). ⟨Course⟩ from the inside of the lower abdomen, descending to the perineum, traveling posteriorly along the interior of the spinal column to Fengfu(DU 16) at the nape of the neck, entering the brain, extending up to the very top of the head and then along the forehead and nose to the superior gums.

2. Dumai(EX-HN) An extra point, originally from *Qianjin Yaofang* (*Essential Prescriptions Worth a Thousand Gold*), referring to the location of Shenting(DU 24).

●督脉病[dū mài bìng] 奇经八脉病候之一。出《素问·骨空论》。因督脉行于脊里及头脑，故病证可见角弓反张以及颈强、癫狂、惊痫、眩晕等。

Diseases of the Du Meridian One of the syndromes of the eight extra meridians, originally from *Suwen: Gukong Lun* (*Plain Questions: On the Apertures of Bones*). Because of the circulation of the Du Meridian inside the spinal column and the brain, the syndrome may be manifested as opisthotonos, stiffness of the neck, manic-depressive disorder, epilepsy induced by terror, dizziness, etc.

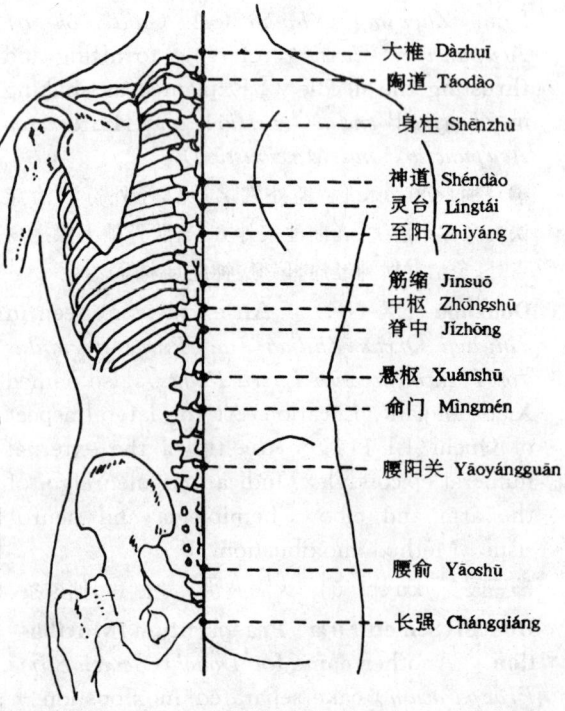

图12.1 督脉
Fig 12.1 The Du Meridian

图12.2 督脉穴（背部）
Fig 12.2 Points of Du Meridian（Back）

Figure labels (图12.3 督脉穴 / Fig 12.3 Points of Du Meridian):

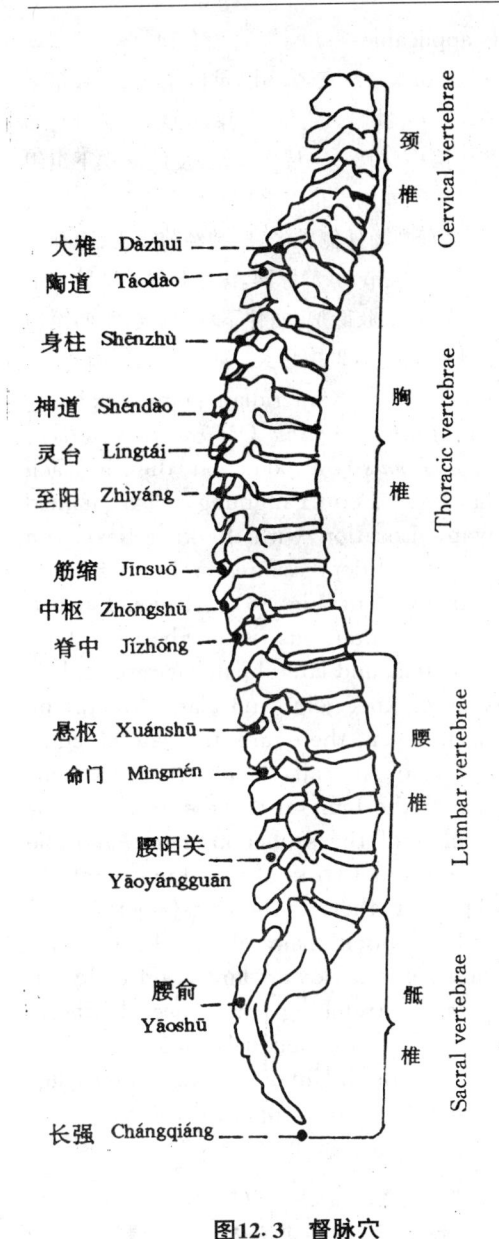

- 大椎 Dàzhuī
- 陶道 Táodào
- 身柱 Shēnzhù
- 神道 Shéndào
- 灵台 Língtái
- 至阳 Zhìyáng
- 筋缩 Jīnsuō
- 中枢 Zhōngshū
- 脊中 Jǐzhōng
- 悬枢 Xuánshū
- 命门 Mìngmén
- 腰阳关 Yāoyángguān
- 腰俞 Yāoshū
- 长强 Chángqiáng

Cervical vertebrae 颈椎
Thoracic vertebrae 胸椎
Lumbar vertebrae 腰椎
Sacral vertebrae 骶椎

the coccyx, it goes up to the nape of the neck along both sides of the spinal column and scatters over the head; the collaterals running downwards reach the regions of the scapulae, go left and right to the Bladder Meridian of Foot-Taiyang, and then enter the muscles on both sides of the spinal column.

●督脉络脉[dū mài luò mài]　即督脉络。详见该条。

Collateral of the Du Meridian　i.e the Du Collateral. →督脉络(p.87)

●督脉络脉病[dū mài luò mài bìng]　十五络脉病候之一。出《灵枢·经脉》。实证见脊强反折，虚证见头垂。取其络穴治疗。

Diseases of Du Collateral　One of the Fifteen Collateral syndromes, originally from *Lingshu: Jingmai* (*Miraculous Pivot: Meridians*). 〈Manifestations〉stiffness of the spinal column and opisthotonos in syndrome of the excess type, and heaviness of the head in syndrome of the deficiency type. 〈Point selection〉the Luo(Connecting) points.

●督脉之别[dū mài zhī bié]　督脉络的别名。见该条。

Branch of the Du Meridian　Another name for the Du collateral. →督脉络(p.87)

●督俞[dū shù]　经穴名。出《太平圣惠方》。属太阳膀胱经。又名高盖。〈定位〉在背部，当第六胸椎棘突下，旁开1.5寸(图7)。〈层次解剖〉皮肤→皮下组织→斜方肌→竖脊肌。浅层布有第六、七胸神经后支的内侧皮支及伴行的动、静脉。深层有第六、七胸神经后支的肌支和相当的肋间后动、静脉侧支的分支或属支。〈主治〉心痛、腹痛、腹胀、肠鸣、呃逆。斜刺0.5～0.8寸；可灸。

Dushu(BL 16)　A meridian point, originally from *Taiping Shenghui Fang* (*Imperial Benevolent Prescriptions*), a point on the Bladder Meridian of Foot-Taiyang, also named Gaogai. 〈Location〉on the back, below the spinous process of the 6th thoracic vertebra, 1.5 cun lateral to the posterior midline (Fig. 7). 〈Regional anatomy〉skin → subcutaneous tissue→trapezius muscle→erector spinal muscle. In the superficial layer, there are the medial cutaneous branches of the posterior branchings of the 6th and 7th thoracic nerves and the

●督脉络[dū mài luò]　十五络脉之一。出《灵枢·经脉》，原称督脉之别。脉从尾闾骨端的长强穴分出，挟着脊柱两侧上至顶部，散布在头上；下行的络脉，下行到肩胛部，左右走向足太阳膀胱经，进入脊柱两旁的肌肉。

Du Collateral　One of the fifteen main collaterals, originally from *Lingshu: Jingmai* (*Miraculous Pivot: Meridians*), originally called the Branch of the Du Meridian. Branching from Changqiang(DU 1), below the tip of

accompanying arteries and veins. In the deep layer, there are the muscular branches of the posterior branches of the 6th and 7th thoracic nerves and the branches or tributaries of the dorsal branches of the related posterior intercostal arteries and veins. 〈Indications〉cardiac pain, abdominal pain and distension, borborygmus, hiccups. 〈Method〉 Puncture obliquely 0.5~0.8 cun. Moxibustion is applicable.

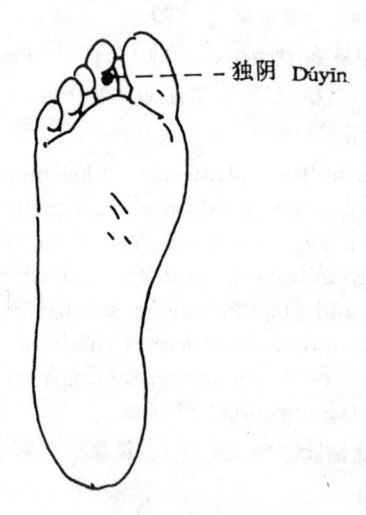

图13 独阴穴
Fig 13 Duyin Point

●**独阴**[dú yīn] 经外穴名。见《奇效良方》。〈定位〉在足第二趾的跖侧远侧趾间关节的中点。〈层次解剖〉皮肤→皮下组织→趾短、长屈肌腱。布有趾足底固有神经,趾底固有动、静脉的分支或属支。〈主治〉女子呕哕、吐血、难产、死胎、胎衣不下、小肠疝气、经血不调等。直刺0.1~0.2寸;可灸。

Duyin(EX-LE 11) An extra point, seen in *Qixiao Liangfang* (*Prescriptions of Wonderful Efficacy*). 〈Location〉on the plantar side of the 2nd toe, at the centre of the distal interphalangeal joint. 〈Regional anatomy〉skin → subcutaneous tissue → tendons of short and long flexor muscles of toes. There are the proper digital plantar nerve and the branches or tributaries of the properdigital artery and vein in this area. 〈Indications〉women's hiccup and vomiting, hemotysis, difficult childbirth, dead fetus, retention of placenta, hernia, irregular menstruation, etc. 〈Method〉 Puncture perpendicularly 0.1~0.2 cun. Moxibustion is applicable.

●**犊鼻**[dú bí] 经穴名。出《灵枢·本输》。属足阳明胃经。又名外膝眼。〈定位〉屈膝,在膝部,髌骨与韧带外侧凹陷中(图86)。〈层次解剖〉皮肤→皮下组织→髌韧带与髌外侧支持带之间→膝关节囊、翼状皱襞。浅层布有腓肠外侧神经,股神经前皮支、隐神经的髌下支和膝关节动、静脉网。深层是膝关节腔。〈主治〉膝关节痛、下肢麻痹、屈伸不利、脚气。稍向髌韧带内方斜刺0.5~1.2寸;可灸。

Dubi(ST 35) A meridian point, originally from *Lingshu*: *Benshu* (*Miraculous Pivot*: *Meridian Points*), a point on the Stomach Meridian of Foot-Yangming, also named Waixiyan. 〈Location〉with the knee flexed, on the knee, in the depression lateral to the patella and its ligament (Fig. 86). 〈Regional anatomy〉skin→subcutaneous tissue→between ligament of patella and lateral patellar retinaculum →capsule of knee joint and alar folds. In the superficial layer, there are the lateral cutaneous nerve of the calf, the anterior cutaneous branches of the femoral nerve, the infrapatellar branches of the saphenous nerve and the arteriovenous network of the knee joint. In the deep layer, there is the cavity of the knee joint. 〈Indications〉pain of the knee joint, numbness of the lower limbs, difficulty in flexing and stretching the knee, heriberi. 〈Method〉Puncture obliquely 0.5~1.2 cun slightly towards the interior of the patellar ligament. Moxibustion is applicable.

●**妒乳**[dù rǔ] 即乳痈。详见该条。

Galactostasis→乳痈(p. 339)

●**短刺**[duǎn cì] 内经刺法名。十二节刺之一。指进针后稍许摇动针柄,逐渐深入至骨所,然后短促提插,以治疗骨痹。

Short-Thrust Needling An acupuncture technique in *Neijing* (*The Canon of Internal Medicine*). One of the Twelve Methods of needling, referring to shaking the handle slightly after inserting the needle, gradually inserting it to the bone, then lifting and thrusting it shortly and quickly for treating osseous rheumatism.

●**断绪**[duàn xù] 不孕的别名。详见该条。

No Posterity Another name for sterility. → 不孕(p.29)

●断针[duàn zhēn] 针刺术语。又称折针。针刺时针身误断在体内。多因针身有损伤,针刺时用力过重,或患者体位突然变动而造成。

Snapping of the Inserted Needle A acupuncture term, also called breaking of the inserted needle, referring to the breaking of the needle body during acupuncture treatment, mostly due to a cracked needle body, over-forced acupuncture manipulation, or a sudden change in the patient's posture.

●对侧取穴[duì cè qǔ xué] 即交叉取穴法。见该条。

Selection of Contralateral Points i. e. method of selecting points across the body. → 交叉取穴(p.193)

●对耳轮[duì ěr lún] 耳廓解剖名称。耳廓边缘内侧与耳轮相对的平行隆起处。

Antihelix An anatomic site on the auricle, parallel projection of the medial side of the auricle edge opposite to the helix.

●对耳轮后沟[duì ěr lún hòu gōu] 耳廓解剖名称。与对耳轮相对应的背凹沟。

Posterior Groove of Antihelix An anatomic site on the auricle, posterior concave sulcus opposite to the antihelix.

●对耳轮上脚[duì ěr lún shàng jiǎo] 耳廓解剖名称。对耳轮上端分叉之上支。

Superior Crus of Antihelix An anatomic site on the auricle, the superior branch of the antihelix.

●对耳轮下脚[duì ěr lún xià jiǎo] 耳廓解剖名称。对耳轮上端分叉之下支。

Inferior Crus of Antihelix An anatomic site on the auricle, the inferior branch of the antihelix.

●对耳屏[duì ěr píng] 耳廓解剖名称。耳垂上部,与耳屏相对的隆起。

Antitragus An anatomic site on the auricle, the upper part of the ear lobe, the projection opposite to the tragus.

●对耳屏后沟[duì ěr píng hòu gōu] 耳廓解剖名称。对耳屏背面的正沟。

Posterior Groove of Antitragus An anatomic site on the auricle, the sulcus at the back side of the antitragus.

●对屏尖[duì píng jiān] 耳穴名。又称平喘、腮腺。位于对耳屏的尖端。具有利肺定喘、清热解毒、驱风邪作用。〈主治〉哮喘、气管炎、腮腺炎、皮肤瘙痒症、副睾炎。

Antitragic Apex(MA) An ear point, also named relieving asthma, or parotid gland. 〈Location〉on the tip of antitragus. 〈Functions〉ventilating the lung and relieving asthma, clearing away heat and detoxifying, and dispersing pathogenic wind. 〈Indications〉asthma, trachitis, parotitis, cutaneous pruritus and epididymitis.

●对应取穴[duì yìng qǔ xué] 取穴法之一。指在与病痛部相对应的远侧部位取穴,包括前后对应、上下对应、左右对应等,为荆虹整体联系的灵活运用。如鼻塞取风池、项强取承浆、头顶痛取涌泉、膝痛取尺泽等。

Corresponding Point Selection One of the methods of point selection, referring to point selection in remote area corresponding to the diseased region, a flexible application of the connection between the meridians and collaterals, including such correspondences as the anterior versus the posterior, superior versus inferior and left versus right, etc. For example, select Fengchi(GB 20)for nasal stuffiness, Chengjiang(RN 24)for stiffness of the neck, Yongquan(KI 1)for parietal headache and Chize(LU 5)for knee pain, etc.

●对症取穴[duì zhèng qǔ xué] 即随症取穴。见该条。

Point Selection in Accordance with the Symptoms → 随症取穴(p.417)

●兑冲[duì chōng] 经穴别名。出《针灸甲乙经》。即神门。见该条。

Duichong Another name for Shenmen(HT 7), a meridian point originally from *Zhenjiu Jia-Yi Jing* (*A-B Classic of Acupuncture and Moxibustion*). → 神门(p.362)

●兑端[duì duān] 经穴名。出《针灸甲乙经》。属督脉。〈定位〉在面部,当上唇的端,人中沟下端的皮肤与唇的移行部(图28和图5)。〈层次解剖〉同水沟穴。

〈主治〉昏迷、晕厥、癫狂、癔病、口㖞唇动、消渴嗜饮、口疮臭秽、齿痛、口噤、鼻塞。斜刺0.2～0.3寸；禁灸。

Duiduan(DU 27) A meridian point originally from *Zhenjiu Jia-Yi Jing* (*A-B Classic of Acupuncture and Moxibustion*), a point on the Du Meridian. 〈Location〉on the face, on the labial tubercle of the upper lip, on the vermilion border between the philtrum and upper lip (Figs. 28&5). 〈Regional anatomy〉the same as the regional anatomy of Shuigou(DU 26)(p. 409). 〈Indications〉coma, syncope, manic-depressive disorder, hysteria, deviation of the mouth and lip, tremor diabetes with polydipsia, ulcer in the mouth with fetid smell, lockjaw, nasal stuffiness. 〈Method〉Puncture obliquely 0.2～0.3 cun. Moxibustion is forbidden.

● 兑骨[duì gǔ] ①经穴别名。出《针灸甲乙经》。即颧髎。见该条。②经穴别名。见《难经·六十六难》。即神门。见该条。③部位名。掌后兑骨，指豆骨。

1. **Duigu** Another name for Quanliao(SI 18), a meridian point originally from *Zhenjiu Jia-Yi Ying* (*A-B Classic of Acupuncture and Moxibustion*). →颧髎(p. 327)

2. **Duigu** Another name for Shenmen(HT 7), a meridian point seen in *Nanjing: Liushiliu Nan* (*The Classic of Questions: Question* 66)→神门(p. 362)

3. A part of the body, at the posterior and of the palm, referring to the pisiform bone.

● 顿灸[dùn jiǔ] 灸法用语。见《千金要方》。指一次灸规定的壮数，与报灸对称。

Draught of Moxibustion A moxibustion method, seen in *Qianjin Yaofang* (*Essential Prescriptions Worth a Thousand Gold*), referring to moxibustion given with a determined number of moxa-cones at one time, as opposed to moxibustion given with a varying number of moxa-cones.

● 顿咳[dùn ké] 病证名。见《医学正传》。又称百日咳、时行顿咳、天哮、疫咳、迫咳，俗称天哮呛、鸡咳。是一种流行于冬春季节的传染病，以五岁以下婴幼儿为多见。多由时行疫毒犯肺，肺气不宣，气郁化热，酿液成痰，阻于气道，气机上逆所致。本病以阵发性发作，连续性咳嗽，咳后伴有吸气性吼声为特征。临床分三期。初咳期：病初与感冒类似，咳嗽、打喷嚏、流鼻涕，吐泡沫样的稀痰，苔薄白，脉浮，指纹淡红。治宜宣肺解表，祛邪止咳。取风门、列缺、合谷。痉咳期：咳嗽逐渐加重，呈阵发性发作，咳则连声不断，咳后有回吼声，至咳出粘痰，或吐出乳食，阵咳始暂时停息。如此反复发作，入夜尤甚，或兼见身热，口干舌燥，便秘溲赤，或痰中带血，鼻中衄血，舌苔黄，脉滑数，指纹紫红。治宜清热泻肺，化痰止咳。取大椎、身柱、尺泽、丰隆。恢复期：咳嗽次数和持续时间逐渐减短，回吼声亦逐渐消失，或咳而无力，痰稀而少，气短声怯，自汗无力，唇色淡白，舌淡苔少，指纹青淡。治宜健脾补肺。取肺俞、脾俞、太渊、足三里。

Paroxysmal Cough A disease, seen in *Yixue Zhengzhuan* (*True Lineage of Medicine*), also named whooping cough, epidemic paroxysmal cough, epidemic cough with asthma, epidemic severe cough, uncontrolled cough, colloquially, also named epidemic cough with dyspnea and chicken cough. An infection disease occurring in winter and spring, mostly seen among children at the age below 5. It is usually due to the epidemic toxin attacking the lung, which leads to the failure to ventilate lung-qi, pathogenic heat induced by the stagnation of qi, and then condensation of the body fluids into phlegm, thus obstructing the respiratory tract, and finally resulting in the reversed flow of qi. It is characterized by paroxysmal continuous cough with an inspiratory roaring. It is divided clinically into 3 stages. At the initial stage it is similar to the common cold, with coughing, sneezing, running nose, thin and frothy sputum, thin and whitish tongue coating, floating pulse and light-red fingerprint. 〈Treatment principle〉Ventilating the lung and relieving exterior syndrome, arresting cough by eliminating the pathogenic factor. 〈Point selection〉Fengmen (BL 12), Lieque (LU 7), and Hegu (LI 4). At the second stage, the stage of spasmodic cough, it is seen as paroxysmal cough gradually aggravated, later developing into continuous cough with an inspiratory roaring; paroxysmal cough will not stop temporarilly until the patient coughs out sticky sputum, or vomits the eaten food or milk. The attacks occur repeatedly, and the syndrome gets worse at night, either accopmanied by fever, dryness of the mouth and

tongue, constipation and deep colored urine, or by bloody sputum, epistaxis, yellowish tongue coating, slippery and rapid pulse, purplish red fingerprint. 〈Treatment principle〉Clear heat from the lung, stop cough by resolving phlegm. 〈Point selection〉Dazhui (DU 14), Shenzhu(DU 12), Chize(LU 5)and Fenglong (ST 40). At the stage of recovery, the cough lessens and its duration gradually shortens, the inspiratory roaring also lightens gradually, vomiting decreases, sputum is thin and reduced. There is a shortness of breath with faint voice, spontaneous perspiration and weakness, pale lip, pale tongue with little coating, light-blue fingerprint. 〈Treatment principle〉Strengthen the spleen and reinforce the lung. 〈Point selection〉Feishu(BL 13), Pishu (BL 20), Taiyuan (LU 9) and Zusanli (ST 36).

●多罐[duō guàn] 拔罐的一种。又称排罐法。指根据病情、病位，适量吸拨数个乃至十数个罐子。用于病变范围比较广泛的疾病。如背部之背俞，常以排罐法拔罐。

Multiple Cupping One method of cupping, also named multiple cupping in alignment, referring to the therapy of proper cupping with several or more cups in accordance with the patient's condition and the site of disease. It is applied to many general diseases, for instance, back-shu points are usually treated with this method.

●多所闻[duō suǒ wén] 经穴别名。出《素问·气穴论》。即听宫。见该条。《针灸聚英》误作听会穴别名。

Duosuowen Another name for Tinggong(SI 19)a meridian point originally from *Suwen*: *Qixue Lun*(*Plain Questions*: *On Loci of Qi*)→听宫(p.439). Misunderstood as another name of Tinghui (GB 2)in *Zhenjiu Juying* (*Essentials of Acupuncture and Moxibustion*).

●夺命[duó mìng] 经外穴名。见《针灸聚英》。又名虾蟆、惺惺。在肩髃与尺泽连线中点，当肱二头肌中。主治昏厥、上臂痛、丹毒等。直刺0.5～1寸。

Duoming(EX-UE) An extra point, seen in *Zhenjiu Juying* (*Essentials of Acupuncture and Moxibustion*), also named Hama, Xingxing. 〈Location〉In the biceps muscle of arm, at the midpoint of the line connecting Jianyu (LI 15)and Chize(LU 5). 〈Indications〉syncope, pain in the forearm, erysipelas, etc. 〈Method〉Puncture 0.5～1 cun perpendicularly.

E

●蛾根[é gēn] 经外穴名。在颌下部，下颌角前1寸处。主治乳蛾，以及咽喉炎等。直刺0.5-1寸。

Egen(EX-HN) An extra point. 〈Location〉in the inferior area of jaw, 1 cun anterior to the angle of mandible. 〈Indications〉tonsillitis, laryngopharyngitis, etc. 〈Method〉Puncture perpendicularly 0.5～1 cun.

●蛾子[é zǐ] 即乳蛾。见该条。

Tonsil like Moth→乳蛾(p. 338)

●额[é] 耳穴名。在对耳屏外侧的前下方。具有镇静止痛作用。〈主治〉头痛、头晕、失眠、多梦。

Forehead(MA) An auricular point. 〈Location〉at the anterior and inferior corner of the external side of antitragus. 〈Functions〉tranquilize and arrest pain. 〈Indications〉headache, dizziness, insomnia, dreamful sleep.

●额颅[é lú] 部位名。见《灵枢·经脉》。又称作额，也称颡，即发下眉上处，俗称前额。

Elu A part of the body, seen in *Lingshu*: *Jingmai* (*Miraculous Pivot*: *Meridians*), also named e or sang, referring to the part above the eyebrow but below the hairline, colloquially named forehead.

●呃逆[è nì] 病证名。古称"哕",俗称"打呃"。是指胃气冲逆而上,出于喉间,呃呃连声、声短而频,连续或间断发作、令人不能自制的一种病证。又名吃逆。据病因的不同可分为胃寒呃逆、胃热呃逆、阳虚呃逆、阴虚呃逆。详见各条。

Hiccup A disease, also called "yue" in ancient times, and now commonly known as "giving out a sound from the throat", referring to adverse rising of the stomach qi causing a shout but frequent sound when it comes through the throat, it is a continuous or intermittent symptom which can not be controlled by oneself, also named "having hiccups". According to the different causes of the disease, it is divided into hiccup due to stomach cold, hiccup due to stomach heat, hiccup due to yang deficiency and hiccup due to yin deficiency. →胃寒呃逆(p. 463)、胃热呃逆(p. 464)、阳虚呃逆(p. 542)、阴虚呃逆(p. 560)

●恶露不尽[è lù bù jìn] 即恶露不绝的别名。见该条。

Persistent Lochia Another name for lochiorrhea. →恶露不绝(p. 92)

●恶露不绝[è lù bù jué] 病证名。见《妇人良方大全》。又称恶露不止、恶露不尽。一般产后恶露持续二至三周尽绝,如仍然持续不断则称为恶露不绝。临床分三种证型。气虚失摄者,多因体弱正虚,产时失血耗气,或产后操劳过早,劳倦伤脾,气虚下陷,冲任不固,不能摄血所致;症见恶露淋漓不绝、量多、色淡红、质清稀、无臭味、小腹下坠、精神倦怠、面色㿠白、舌质淡、脉濡弱;治宜补气摄血,取关元、足三里、三阴交。血热妄行者,多因素体阴虚,复因产时失血,阴血更虚,虚热内生,或过服温燥之品,或肝郁化热,导致热扰冲任,迫血下行所致;症见恶露量多、色红、质稠、有臭味、面色潮红、口干唇燥、舌质红、脉细数;治宜育阴清热,取气海、中极、血海、中都、阴谷。瘀阻胞脉者,多因产后胞脉空虚,寒邪乘虚而入,血因寒凝,瘀阻于内所致;证见恶露淋漓不畅、量少、色紫黯有块、小腹疼痛拒按、舌紫黯有瘀点、脉弦或沉涩;治宜理气活血,取中极、石门、地机、气海。

Lochiorrhea A disease, seen in *Furen Liangfang Daquan*(*A Complete Work of Effective Prescriptions for Women*), also known as persistent lochia, or continuous lochia. It generally lasts two or three weeks after childbirth. If vaginal discharge exceeds two or three weeks, it is called cochiorrhea. There are three clinical types: ① deficiency of qi with failure to control blood. Mostly due to deficiency of the vital qi resulting from loss of blood and qi during delivery or overwork after childbirth, impairing the spleen and leading to the sinking of qi due to deficiency, debility of the Chong and Ren Meridians and failure to control blood. 〈Manifestations〉profuse discharge of lochia with light red color, clear and watery discharge without any foul smell, straining of the lower abdomen, lassitude, pale complexion, pale tongue with soft and weak pulse. 〈Treatment principle〉Invigorate qi to control the blood. 〈Point selection〉Guanyuan (RN 4), Zusanli(ST 36), Sanyinjiao(SP 6). ② bleeding due to blood heat. Mostly caused by prior deficiency of the body-yin, followed by a loss of blood during delivery leading to a worsening of the yin-blood deficiency and generating a fever of the deficiency type, or by overeating warm and dry drugs or food, or by the stagnation of liver-qi transforming into heat and leading to heat which disturbs the Chong and Ren Meridians and makes the blood flow downward. 〈Manifestations〉profuse discharge of lochia with red color, thickness with foul smell, tidal red face, dry mouth and tongue, red tongue with thready and rapid pulse. 〈Treatment principle〉Nourish yin and clear heat. 〈Point selection〉 Qihai(RN 6), Zhongji(RN 3)Xuehai(SP 10), Zhongdu(LR 6)and Yingu(KI 10). ③blood stasis in the uterine collaterals. Mostly due to deficiency of the uterine collaterals after childbirth resulting in the invasion of pathogenic accumulation in the interior. 〈Manifestations〉difficulty in discharging lochia with reduced amount, dark purplish blood with clots, lower abdominal pain when pressed, dark purplish tongue with petechiae, wiry or deep and choppy pulse. 〈Treatment principle〉Regulate qi and activate blood. 〈Point selection〉Zhongji(RN 3), Shimen(RN 5), Diji(SP 8)and Qihai(RN 6).

●恶露不下[è lù bù xià] 病症名。见《肘后备急方》。产后恶露应自然排出体外,如果停留不下,或下亦很

少,称为恶露不下。临床分气滞、血瘀两种证型。气滞者,多因情志不畅,肝气郁结,气机不利,血行受阻所致,症见恶露不下、或流下甚少、小腹胀满而痛、胸胁作胀、苔薄白、脉弦;治宜理气解郁,调和气血,取太冲、间使、气海、关元。血瘀者,多因感受寒邪,饱食生冷,寒则血凝,瘀阻胞脉所致;证见恶露流下甚少、色紫黯、小腹疼痛拒按、痛处有块、舌质紫、脉涩;治宜活血行瘀,取中极、气冲、地机、关元。

Lochiostasis A disease, seen in *Zhouhou Beiji Fang*(*A Hand book of Prescriptions for Emergencies*). Lochia should be excreted naturally after childbirth. If it is stagnated or discharged in small amounts, it is called lochiostasis. This is divided into two clinical types: qi stagnation and blood stasis. The former is mostly due to emotional depression leading to the stagnation of liver qi, disorderly movement of qi followed by the obstruction of blood circulation. 〈Manifestations〉retention of lochia or lochia in small amounts, distention and pain in the lower abdomen, distending sensation in the chest and hypochondrium, thin and whitish coating with wiry pulse. 〈Treatment principle〉Regulate the flow of qi to dissipate blood stasis, and regulate qi and blood. 〈Point selection〉Taichong(LR 3), Jianshi(PC 5), Qihai(RN 6), Guanyuan(RN 4). The latter is mostly due to cold pathogens and cold food intake leading to the stagnation of blood in the uterine collaterals. 〈Manifestations〉very little lochia discharge with dark purplish color, lower abdominal pain when pressed, palpable mass at the paintul place, purplish tongue with uneven choppy pulse. 〈Treatment principle〉Promote blood circulation and remove blood stasis. 〈Point selection〉Zhongji(RN 3), Qichong(ST 30), Diji(SP 8), and Guanyuan(RN 4).

●**恶露不止**[è lù bù zhǐ] 即恶露不绝的别名。详见该条。

Persistent Lochia Another name for lochiorrhea. →恶露不绝(p.92)

●**恶阻**[è zǔ] 病证名。出《诸病源候论》。又名子病、阻病、病儿、病阻、病隔、选饭、妊娠呕吐等。是指妊娠早期出现恶心、呕吐、择饭或食入即吐、甚则呕吐苦水或血性物者称为恶阻。主要是由胃气不降所致。临床分为胃虚恶阻、胃热恶阻、胃寒恶阻、痰滞恶阻、肝热恶阻等。见各条。

Morning Sickness A disease, originally from *Zhubing Yuanhou Lun*(*General Treatise on the Etiology and Symtomatology*), also named sickness during pregnancy, sickness due to fetus, choosing food during pregnancy and vomiting due to sickness during pregnancy and so on. Nausea, vomiting, being choosy about food or vomiting immediately after food intake, even vomiting with gastric secretion or bloody substance, occurring in the early stage of pregnancy, are called morning sickness. It is mainly caused by the failure of stomach qi to descend. In clinic it is divided into morning sickness due to stomach deficiency, morning sickness due to stomach heat, morning sickness due to stomach cold. morning sickness due to the retention of phlegm and morning sickness due to liver heat. →胃虚恶阻(p.469)、胃热恶阻(p.466)、胃寒恶阻(p.463)、痰滞恶阻(p.425)、肝热恶阻(p.125)

●**饿马摇铃**[è mǎ yáo líng] 针刺手法名。见《针灸大成》。与凤凰展翅对称,指捻针时以大指向前为主,缓缓捻转,如饿马无力,故名。大指向前使针向左转,属补法。

Hungry Horse Ringing a Bell A needling technique, seen in *Zhenjiu Dacheng*(*A Great Compendium of Acupuncture and Moxibustion*), mentioned in the same breath with "phoenix spreading the wings". Referring mainly to the thumb's moving forward when the needle is twisted: so slow is the needle twisted, that it is like a hungry horse without strength, thus its name. The thumb moving forward with the needle turning left belongs to reinforcing method.

●**頞**[è] 部位名。又称山根。两目间,鼻之凹陷处,即鼻根部。

E A part of the body, also named shan gen. 〈Location〉between the two eyes, at the depression of the nose, i.e., radix nasi.

●**儿风**[ér fēng] 子痫的别名。见该条。

Epilepsy in a Pregnant Woman Another name for eclampsia gravidarum. →子痫(p.627)

●**儿痉**[ér jìng] 子痫的别名。见该条。

Epileptiform Spasm in a Pregnant woman Another name for eclampsia gravidarum. →子痫(p. 627)

●儿衣不出[ér yī bù chū] 胞衣不下的别名。见该条。

Petardative Delivery of Afterbirth Another name for retention of placenta. →胞衣不下(p. 14)

●儿晕[ér yùn] 子痫的别名。见该条。

Epileptiform Dizziness in a Pregnant Woman Another name for eclampsia gravidarum. →子痫(p. 627)

●儿枕痛[ér zhěn tòng] 产后腹痛的别名。见该条。

Abdominal Pain After Delivery Another name for postpartum abdominal pain. →产后腹痛(p. 33)

●耳[ěr] 外耳之别称。见该条。

Ear Another name for external ear. →外耳(p. 452)

●耳背沟[ěr bèi gōng] 耳穴名。又称降压沟。位于对耳轮上、下脚及对耳轮的耳廓背面呈"Y"形的凹沟。用于治疗高血压、皮肤瘙痒证。

Groove on the Back of Auricle(MA) Name of an ear point, also called groove for lowering blood pressure. 〈Location〉through the backside of the superior antihelix crus and inferior antihelix, in the depression as a "Y" form. 〈Indications〉hypertension and cutaneous puritus.

●耳闭[ěr bì] 即耳聋。见该条。

Bi Syndrome of the Ear →耳聋(p. 95)

●耳垂[ěr chuí] ①经外穴名。出《刺疗捷法》。在耳垂前面中点。〈主治〉锁口疗。直刺0.1寸，或点刺出血。②耳廓解剖名称。耳廓下端无软骨的皮垂。

1. Erchui(EX-HN) An extra point, originally from *Ciding Jiefa* (*Simple Acupuncture Method for Boils*). 〈Location〉at the midpoint of the anterior aspect of the ear lobe. 〈Indication〉mouth-blocking boil. 〈Method〉Puncture perpendicularly 0.1 cun, or prick to cause bleeding.

2. Ear Lobe Anatomical term of the auricle, referring to the inferior part of the auricle which does not contain cartilage.

●耳垂背面[ěr chuí bèi miàn] 耳廓解剖名称。耳垂的背面。

Back Side of the Ear Lobe An anatomical term of the auricle, referring to the posterior aspect of the ear lobe.

●耳疳[ěr gān] 即聤耳。见该条。

Chronic Suppurative Otitis Media →聤耳(p. 439)

●耳骨[ěr gǔ] 经穴别名。见《铜人腧穴针灸图经》。即曲骨。见该条。

Ergu Another name for Qugu (RN 2), a meridian point seen in *Tongren Shuxue Zhenjiu Tujing* (*Illustrated Manual of Points for Acupuncture and Moxibustion on a Bronze Statue with Acupoints*). →曲骨(p. 324)

●耳和髎[ěr hé liáo] 经穴名。出《针灸甲乙经》。原名和髎。属手少阳三焦经，为手足少阳、手太阳之会。〈定位〉在头侧部，当发后缘，平耳廓根之前方，颞浅动脉的后缘(图28)。〈层次解剖〉皮肤→皮下组织→耳前肌→颞筋膜浅层及颞肌。浅层布有耳颞神经，面神经颞支，颞浅动、静脉的分支或属支。深层有颞深前、后神经，均是三叉神经下颌神经的分支。〈主治〉头痛、耳鸣、牙关紧闭、口㖞。斜刺0.3～0.5寸;可灸。

Erheliao(SJ 22) A meridian point, originally from *Zhenjiu Jia-Yi Jing* (*A-B Classic of Acupuncture and Moxibustion*), originally called Heliao. A point on the Sanjiao Meridian of Hand-Shaoyang, the crossing point of the Shaoyang Meridians of Hand and Foot, and hand Taiyang. 〈Location〉on the lateral side of the head, on the posterior margin of the temples, anterior to the anterior border of the root of the ear auricle and posterior to the superficial temporal artery (Fig. 28). 〈Regional anatomy〉skin→subcutaneous tissue→anterior auricular muscle→superficial temporal fascia and temporal muscle. In the superficial layer there are the auriculotemporal nerve, the temporal branches of the facial nerve, and the branches or tributaties of the superficial temporal artery and vein. In the deep layer, there are the anterior and posterior deep temporal nerves from the mandibular division of the trigeminal nerve. 〈Indications〉headache, tinnitus, lockjaw, wry mouth. 〈Method〉Puncture obliquely 0.3～0.5 cun. Moxibustion is applicable.

●耳后发际[ěr hòu fà jì] 经外穴名。见《千金要方》。在耳后颞骨乳突下缘当发际处。灸治瘿气、瘰疬等。

Erhoufaji(EX-HN) An extra point seen in *Qianjin Yaofang* (*Essencial Prescriptions Worth a Thousand Gold*). ⟨Location⟩ at the edge of the mastoid process of the temporal bone behind the ear, on the hairline. ⟨Indications⟩ goiter and scrofula. ⟨Method⟩ moxibustion.

●耳后上沟[ěr hòu shàng gōu] 耳廓解剖名称。对耳轮下脚之背面，三角窝后隆起，与耳甲艇后隆起之间的凹沟。

Retroauricular Upper Groove An anatomical term of the auricle, referring to the groove at the back of the lower crus of antihelix, in the depressed groove between the posterior eminence of the triangular fossa and the posterior eminence of the cymba auriculae.

●耳甲腔[ěr jiǎ qiāng] 耳廓解剖名称。耳轮脚以下的耳腔部分。

Cavity Concha An anatomical term of the auricle, referring to the part below th crus of the helix.

●耳甲腔后隆起[ěr jiǎ qiāng hòu lóng qǐ] 耳廓解剖名称。耳甲腔背面隆起处。

Posterior Eminence of Inferior Concha An anatomical term of the auricle, referring to the eminence at the back of the cavity of concha.

●耳甲艇[ěr jiǎ tǐng] 耳廓解剖名称。耳轮脚以上的耳甲腔部分。

Cymba Auriculae An anatomical term of the auricle, referring to the part of the cavity of concha above the crus of the helix.

●耳甲艇后隆起[ěr jiǎ tǐng hòu lóng qǐ] 耳廓解剖名称。耳甲艇的背面隆起处。

Posterior Eminence of the Cymba Auriculae An anatomical term of the auricle, referring to the eminence at the back of cymba auriculae.

●耳尖[ěr jiān] ①经外穴名。见《奇效良方》。又名耳涌。⟨定位⟩在耳廓的上方，当折耳向前，耳廓上方的尖端处（图56）。⟨层次解剖⟩皮肤→皮下组织→耳廓软骨。布有颞浅动、静脉的耳前支，耳后动、静脉的耳后支，耳颞神经耳前支、枕小神经耳后支和面神经耳支等。⟨主治⟩目赤肿痛、目翳、偏正头痛、颜面疔疮、高热、急性结膜炎、沙眼等。直刺0.1寸，或点刺出血。②经穴别名。出《银海精微》。即率谷，见该条。

1. **Erjian**(EX-HN 6) An extra point seen in *Qixiao Liangfang* (*Prescriptions of Wonderful Efficiency*), also named Eryong. ⟨Location⟩ above the apex of the ear auricle at the tip of the auricle when the ear is folded forward (Fig. 56). ⟨Regional anatomy⟩ skin → subcutaneous tissue → auricular cartilage. There are the anterior auricular branches of the superficial temporal artery and vein, the posterior auricular branches of the posterior auricular artery and vein, the anterior auricular branches of the auriculotemporal nerve, the posterior auricular branches of the lesser occipital never, and the auricular branches of the facial nerve in this area. ⟨Indications⟩ redness of the eyes with swelling and pain, eye nebula migraine and headache, facial furuncle, high fever, acute conjunctivitis, and trachoma. ⟨Method⟩ Puncture perpendicularly 0.1 cun, or prick to cause bleeding.

2. **Erjian** Another name of Shuaigu (GB 8), a meridian point originally from *Yinhai Jingwei* (*Essentials of Ophthalmology*). → 率谷 (p. 408)

●耳孔中[ěr kǒng zhōng] 经外穴名。见《千金要方》。灸治卒中风口㖞。

Erkongzhong (EX-HN) An extra point, seen in *Qianjin Yaofang* (*Essential Presscriptions Worth a Thousand Gold*). ⟨Indication⟩ wry mouth caused by wind-stroke. ⟨Method⟩ moxibustion.

●耳聋[ěr lóng] 病症名。出《素问·缪刺论》等篇。又名耳闭、聋聩。是指听力减退或听觉丧失。耳聋在病机和治疗方面与耳鸣大致相同。详见耳鸣耳聋虚证和耳鸣耳聋实证各条。

Deafness A disease, originally from *Suwen*: *Miuci Lun* (*Plain Questions*: *On Contralateral Needling*), also known as "loss of listening ability" or "Bi syndrome of the ear", referring to hypoacusis or loss of hearing. The pathogeny, pathogenesis and the treatment of deafness are approximately the same as tinni-

tus. →耳鸣耳聋虚证(p. 97)、耳鸣耳聋实证(p. 97)

●耳轮[ěr lún] 耳廓解剖名称。指耳廓边缘向前卷曲的部分。

Helix An anatomical term of the auricle, referring to the part of the auricle edge bending forward.

●耳轮棘[ěr lún jí] 耳廓解剖名称。耳轮与耳轮脚交界处的棘状突起。

Spine of Helix An anatomical term of the auricle, referring to the spinous eminence at the junction of the helix and the crus of helix.

●耳轮脚[ěr lún jiǎo] 耳廓解剖名称。耳轮伸入耳甲腔的横行堤状隆起。

Crus of Helix An anatomical term of the auricle, referring to the transverse dike-shaped eminence where the helix extends into the cavity of concha.

●耳轮脚后沟[ěr lún jiǎo hòu gōu] 耳廓解剖名称。耳甲腔后隆起与耳甲艇后隆起之间的凹沟,于耳轮脚的背面。

Posterior Sulcus to the Crus of Helix An anatomical term of the auricle, referring to the depressed groove at the back of the crus of helix between the posterior eminence of the cavity of concha and the posterior eminence of the cymba auriclae.

●耳轮脚后沟上支和下支[ěr lún jiǎo hòu gōu shàng zhī hé xià zhī] 耳廓解剖名称。耳轮脚后沟在珠形隆起处被分叉为上下两支:上支称耳轮脚后沟上支,下支称耳轮脚后沟下支。

Upper and Lower Branches of Posterior Sulcus to the Crus of Helix An anatomical term of the auricle. Posterior sulcus to the crus of Helix is divided into two parts at the bead-shaped eminence: upper branch of posterior sulcus to the crus of helix and lower branch of posterior sulcus to the crus of helix.

●耳轮结节[ěr lún jié jié] 耳廓表面解剖名称。耳轮后上方稍肥厚的结节状突起。又称达尔文结。

Helix Tubercle An anatomical term of the auricle surface, referring to the slight fleshy node-shaped eminence on the posterior and superior part of the helix, also known as Darwinian tubercle.

●耳轮尾[ěr lún wěi] 耳廓解剖名称。耳轮下端与耳垂相接的无软骨部分。

Cauda Helicis An anatomical term of the auricle, referring to the noncartilaginous part connecting the lower end of the helix and the ear lobe.

●耳轮尾背面[ěr lún wěi bèi miàn] 耳廓解剖名称。耳舟后隆起与耳垂背面之间的平坦部分。

The Back of Cauda Helicis An anatomical term of the auricle, referring to the flat part between the posterior eminence of scapha and the back of the ear lobe.

●耳脉[ěr mài] 早期经脉名。出《帛书》。与手少阳经类似。

Ear Meridian An early name for a meridian originally from *Boshu* (*Silk Book*), similiar to the Meridian of Hand-Shaoyang.

●耳门[ěr mén] 经穴名。出《针灸甲乙经》。属手少阳三焦经。〈定位〉在面部,当耳屏上切迹的前方,下颌骨髁突后缘凹陷处(图28)。〈层次解剖〉皮肤→皮下组织→腮腺。布有耳颞神经,颞浅动、静脉耳前支,面神经颞支等结构。〈主治〉耳聋、耳鸣、聤耳、齿痛、颈颌痛、唇吻强。直刺0.5～1寸;可灸。

Ermen (SJ 21) A meridian point, originally from *Zhenjiu Jia-Yi Jing* (*A-B Classic of Acupuncture and Moxibustion*), a point on the Sanjiao Meridian of Hand-Shaoyang. 〈Location〉 on the face, anterior to the supratragic notch, in the depression behind the posterior border of the condyloid process of the mandible (Fig. 28). 〈Regional anatomy〉 skin → subcutaneous tissue → parotid gland. There are the auriculotemporal nerve, the anterior auricular branches of the superficial temporal artery and vein, and the temporal branches of the facial nerve in this area. 〈Indications〉 deafness, tinnitus, otitis media suppurativa, toothache, pain in the neck and jaw, and stiffness of the lip. 〈Method〉 Puncture perpendicularly 0.5～1 cun. Moxibustion is applicable.

●耳门前脉[ěr mén qián mài] 经外穴名。见《千金翼方》。在耳门穴上、下各1寸处。灸治脾风占候,言声不出。

Ermenqianmai (EX-HN) Two extra points, seen in *Qianjin Yifang* (*Supplement to the Es-*

sential Prescriptions Worth a Thousand Gold). ⟨Location⟩1 cun above or below the point Ermen(SJ 21). ⟨Indications⟩throat affection due to spleen-wind, leading to aphasia. ⟨Method⟩ Moxibustion.

●耳迷根[ěr mí gēn]　耳穴名。位于耳背与乳突交界的根部,耳轮脚对应处。

Root of Ear Vagus(MA)　An auricular point. ⟨Location⟩on the root at the juncture of the backside of the ear and the mastoid process, corresponding to the place of the helix crus.

●耳鸣[ěr míng]　病证名。出《灵枢·海论》等篇。又名耳作蝉鸣。是指自觉耳中鸣响。耳鸣的病因病机及治疗方法与耳聋大致相同。详见"耳鸣、耳聋实证"和"耳鸣、耳聋虚证"各条。

Tinnitus　A disease originally from *Ling Shu:Hai Lun*(*Miraculous Pivot: On Seas*), also named "chirp of cicada in the ear", referring to a subjective feeling of noise in the ears. The aetiology, pathogenesis and treatment of tinnitus are about the same as for deafness. →耳鸣,耳聋实证(p. 97)、耳鸣,耳聋虚证(p. 97)

●耳鸣、耳聋实证[ěr míng ěr lóng shí zhèng]　耳鸣、耳聋证型之一。因暴怒惊恐,肝胆火旺,以致少阳经气闭阻;或痰热郁结,壅遏清窍所致。症见暴病耳聋,或耳中闷胀、鸣声不断、声响如蝉鸣或海潮声,按之不减。肝胆火旺者,多见面赤、口干、烦躁易怒、脉弦;痰热郁结者,多见胸闷痰多、脉滑数。治宜清肝泻火、豁痰通窍。取翳风、听会、中渚、太冲。肝胆火旺配行间、侠溪,痰热郁结配丰隆、劳宫。

Excess-Type Tinnitus and Deafness　One of the syndromes of tinnitus and deafness, caused by the blockage of the Shaoyang Meridian, resulting from emotional upset(violent rage, terror and fear, etc). and flaming up of liver and gallbladder fire, or stagnation of phlegm-heat in external acoustic meatus. ⟨Manifestations⟩ sudden deafness, or distention and choking sensation in the ear, continuous noise in ears like the chirp of a cicada or a tide sound, which can not be released with pressure. Cases with flaming up of liver and gallbladder fire are mostly accompanied by a flushed face, dry mouth, irritability and a wiry pulse;cases with stagnation of phlegm and heat are mostly accompanied by an oppressive feeling in chest, profuse sputum and a slippery rapid pulse. ⟨Treatment principles⟩Reduce the fire of the liver and eliminate phlegm so as to clear the orifice. ⟨Point selection⟩ Yifeng (SJ 17), Tinghui(GB 2), Zhongzhu(SJ 3), and Taichong(LR 3). For cases with flaming up of liver and gallbladder fire, add Xingjian (LR 2), and Xiaxi(GB 43), for cases with stagnation of phlegm and heat, add Fenglong (ST 40)and Laogong(PC 8).

●耳鸣、耳聋虚证[ěr míng ěr lóng xū zhèng]　耳鸣耳聋证型之一。因肾精亏耗,精气不能上达于耳所致。证见久病耳聋,或耳鸣时作时止、声细调低、操劳则加剧,按之鸣声减弱,多兼有头晕、腰酸、遗精、带下、脉虚细。治宜补益肾精。取翳风、听会、肾俞、关元、太溪。

Deficiency-Type Tinnitus and Deafness
One of the syndromes of tinnitus and deafness, caused by the deficiency of kidney essence, causing a failure of the vital essence and energy to reach the ears for nourishment. ⟨Manifestations⟩ protracted deafness, or discontinuous tinnitus with a low sound which can be alleviated by pressing, and is aggravated by overwork. Often accompanied by dizziness, soreness of the waist, seminal emission, morbid leukorrhea and a deficient, thready pulse. ⟨Treatment principle⟩Tonify the kidney essence. ⟨Point selection⟩ Yifeng (SJ 17), Tinghui(GB 2), Shenshu(BL 23), Guanyuan (RN 4) and Taixi(KI 3).

●耳屏[ěr píng]　耳廓解剖名称。耳廓前面的瓣状突起,又称耳珠。

Tragus　An anatomical term of the auricle, referring to the curved flap in front of the auricle, also called the ear pearl.

●耳上[ěr shàng]　①经外穴名。见《千金要方》。在耳尖直上三横指处。灸治小儿暴痫。②耳上发际的别名。见该条。

1. **Ershang**(EX-HN)　An extra point, seen in *Qianjin Yaofang* (*Essential Prescriptions Worth a Thousand Gold*). ⟨Location⟩three-

finger-breadths directly above the apex of the ear. ⟨Indication⟩ sudden onset epilepsy in children. ⟨Method⟩ moxibustion.

2. **Ershang**→耳上发际(p. 100)

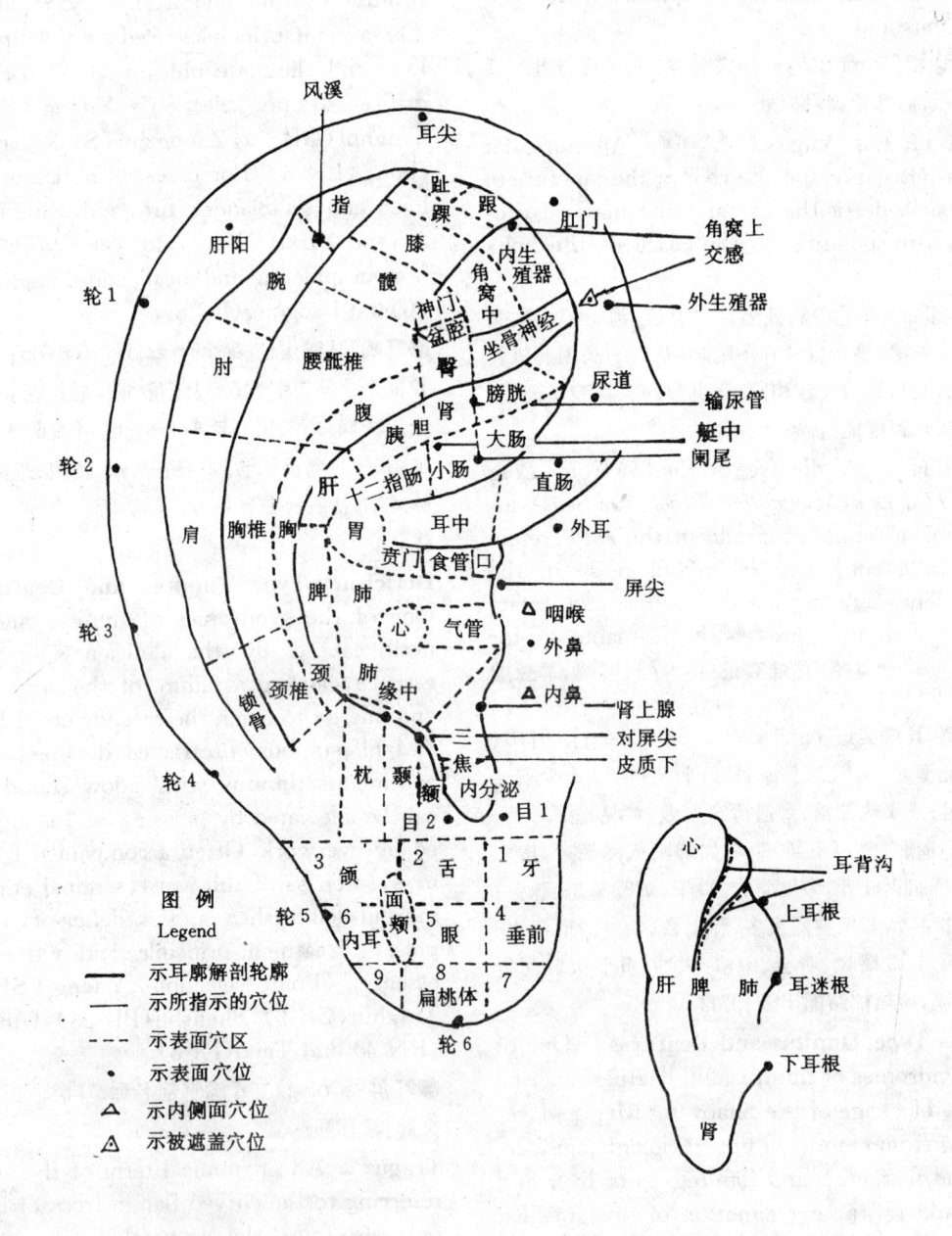

图14 国际标准耳穴分布图

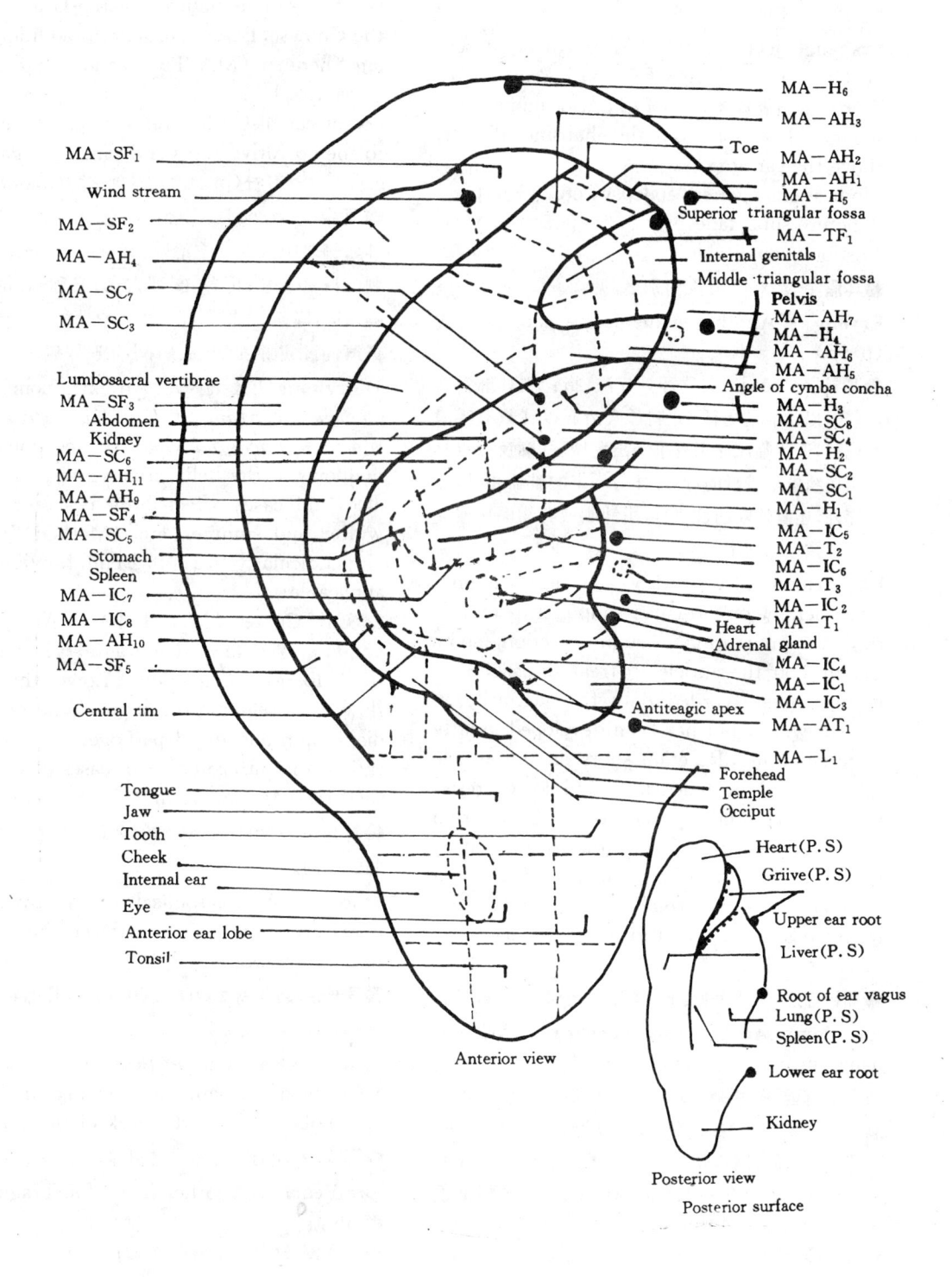

Fig 14 Standard international chart of auricular points

●耳上发际[ěr shàng fà jì] 经外穴名。见《千金要方》。又名耳上。在耳尖直上入发际处。〈主治〉瘿气、癫痫等。沿皮刺0.3～0.5寸；可灸。

Ershangfaji(EX-HN) An extra point seen in *Qianjin Yaofang* (*Essential Prescriptions Worth a Thousand Gold*), also named Ershang. 〈Location〉on the hairline directly above the ear apex. 〈Indications〉goiter, epilepsy, etc. 〈Method〉Puncture subcutaneously 0.3～0.5 cun. Moxibustion is applicable.

●耳涌[ěr yǒng] 耳尖的别名。见该条。

Eryong Another name for Erjian. →耳尖(p. 95)

●耳针[ěr zhēn] 又称耳针疗法。指针刺耳廓反应点(穴)以治病的方法。针刺耳穴治病以往只有零星的记载，近代临床应用有了突出发展。耳廓反应点具有压痛和电阻较低的特点，并与一定的脏器相关，除治疗外，还有诊断的价值。可用针刺或药物贴压或皮内针埋藏方法施术。

Ear Acupuncture Also called ear acupuncture therapy or auricular acupuncture, referring to puncturing certain reaction spots (points) on the auricle to treat disease. This method was recorded only fragmentarily in ancient works, but has been developed greatly in recent times. Reaction spots on the auricle characterized by tenderness and lower resistance are respectively related to the internal organs and so used for diagnoses as well as treatment. Filiform needling, seed-pressing method or intradermal needle embedding techniques may be used for auricular acupuncture.

●耳针疗法[ěr zhēn liáo fǎ] 耳针之别称。见该条。

Ear Points Acupuncture Therapy Another name for ear acupuncture. →耳针(p. 100)

●耳针麻醉[ěr zhēn má zuì] 针麻方法之一。用针刺耳廓特定穴位达到镇痛效果以进行手术的方法。是我国发明的针刺麻醉选穴方法之一。手术时，除取神门和肺穴作为各种手术的基本用穴外，还根据手术部位和有关脏腑器官选取相应穴位。参见"耳针"和"针刺麻醉"条。

Ear Acupuncture Anesthesia One kind of acupuncture anesthesia, referring to puncturing particular ear points to induce analgesia during surgery; one of the ways of selecting points for acupuncture anesthesia invented by the Chinese. Before surgery, in addition to using Shenmen (MA-TF 1) and Lung (MA-JC 1) as the basic points for all operations, the doctor can also select relevant points according to the operative areas and zang-fu organs concerned. →耳针(p. 100)、针刺麻醉(p. 588)

●耳中[ěr zhōng] ①经外穴名。见《千金要方》。在耳轮脚之中点处。〈主治〉马黄黄疸、寒暑疫毒等。直刺0.1～0.2寸；可灸。②耳穴名。又称膈。位于耳轮脚。具有降逆、和胃、利膈、驱风的功能。〈主治〉呃逆、黄疸、消化道病症、皮肤病、小儿遗尿症。

1. **Erzhong**(EX-HN) An extra point seen in *Qianjin Yaofang* (*Essential Prescriptions Worth a Thousand Gold*). 〈Location〉at the midpoint of the helix crus. 〈Indications〉jaundice, and cases affected by pestilent evils in winter and summer, etc. 〈Method〉Puncture perpendicularly 0.1～0.2 cun. Moxibustion is applicable.

2. **Ear Center** (MA-H 1) An auricular point, also named diaphragm. 〈Location〉at the helix crus. 〈Functions〉Lower the adverse flow of qi, regulate the stomach, normalize the diaphragm and expel pathogenic wind. 〈Indications〉hiccup, jaundice, diseases of the digestive tract, dermatosis and infantile enuresis.

●耳舟[ěr zhōu] 耳廓解剖名称。耳轮与对耳轮之间的凹沟。

Scapha An anatomical term of the auricle, referring to the groove between the helix and the outerhelix.

●耳舟后隆起[ěr zhōu hòu lóng qǐ] 耳廓解剖名称。耳舟背面的隆起部分。

Posterior Eminence of Scapha An anatomical term of the auricle, referring to the eminence of scapha on the back of the auricle.

●耳珠[ěr zhū] 为耳屏之别称。见该条。

Ear Pearl Another name for Tragus. →耳屏(p. 97)

●耳作蝉鸣[ěr zuò chán míng] 即耳鸣。见该条。

Chirp of Cicada in the Ear →耳鸣(p. 97)

●二白[èr bái] 经外穴名。见《扁鹊神应针灸玉龙

经》。〈定位〉在前臂掌侧,腕横纹上 4寸,桡侧腕屈肌腱的两侧,一侧各一穴,一臂二穴,左右两臂共四穴(图19)。〈层次解剖〉臂内侧穴:皮肤→皮下组织→掌长肌腱与桡侧腕屈肌腱之间→指浅屈肌→正中神经→拇长屈肌→前臂骨间膜。浅层布有前臂外侧皮神经和前臂正中静脉的属支,深层布有正中神经、正中动脉。臂外侧穴:皮肤→皮下组织→桡侧腕屈肌与肱桡肌腱之间→指浅屈肌→拇长屈肌。浅层布有前臂外侧皮神经和头静脉的属支;深层有桡动、静脉。〈主治〉痔疮、脱肛。直刺0.5~1寸;可灸。

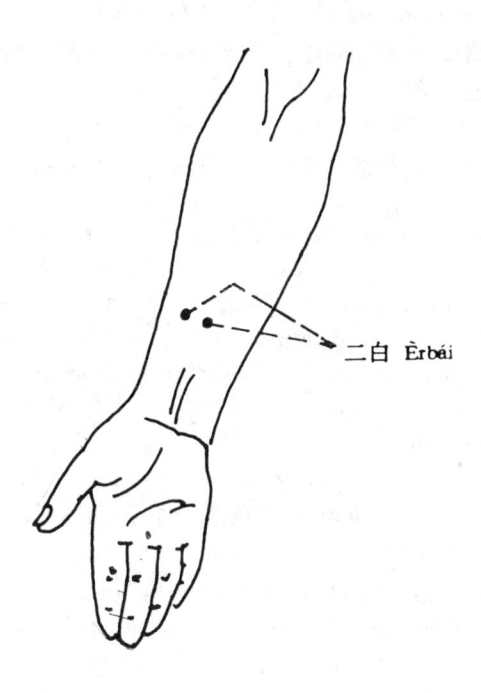

图15 二白穴
Fig 15 Erbai point

Erbai(EX-UE 2)　An extra point, seen in *Bian Que Shenying Zhenjiu Yulong Jing*(*Bian Que's Jade Dragon Classics of Acupuncture and Moxibustion*). 〈Location〉two points on the palmar side of each forearm, 4 cun proximal to the crease of the wrist, on each side of the tendon of the radial flexor muscle of the wrist(Fig. 19). 〈Regional anatomy〉The medial point: skin→subcutaneous tissue→between tendons of long palmar muscle and radial flexor muscle of wrist→superficial digital flexor muscle→median nerve→long flexor muscle of thumb→interosseous membrane of forearm. In the superficial layer, there are the lateral cutaneous nerve of the forearm and the tributaries of the median branhial vein. In the deep layer, there are the median nerve and the median artery. The lateral point: skin→subcutaneous tissue→between radial flexor muscle of wrist and tendon of brachioradial muscle→superficial flexor muscle of fingers→long flexor muscle of thumb. In the superficial layer, there are the lateral cutaneous nerve of the forearm and the tributaries of the cephalic vein. In the deep layer, there are the radial artery and vein. 〈Indications〉hemorrhoids and proctoptosis. 〈Method〉Puncture perpendicularly 0.5~1 cun. Moxibustion is applicable.

●二火[èr huǒ]　出《素问·示从容论》。①指二阳,即阳明。见"二阳"条。②指二阳脏,即心与肺,因其在膈以上之故。见王冰注。

Two Fire　From *Su Wen*: *Shi Congrong Lun* (*Plain Questions*: *Display of Unhurried Manner*) referring to ①the two yang, i.e. Yangming. →二阳(p.102). ②the two yang zang-organs. i.e. the heart and the lung, because the two organs are located above the diaphragm, Cf. Wang Bing's Annotation.

●二间[èr jiān]　经穴名。出《灵枢·本输》。属手阳明大肠经,为本经荥穴。又名间谷、周谷。〈定位〉微握拳,在手食指本节(第2掌指关节)前,桡侧凹陷处(图48和图6)。〈层次解剖〉皮肤→皮下组织→第一蚓状肌腱→示指近节指骨基底部。浅层神经由桡神经的指背神经与正中神经的指掌侧固有神经双重分布。血管有第一掌背动、静脉的分支和示指桡侧动、静脉的分支。深层有正中神经肌支。〈主治〉喉痹、颔肿、䶉衄、目痛、目黄、大便脓血、齿痛口干、口眼歪斜、身热、嗜睡、肩背痛振寒。直刺0.2~0.3寸;可灸。

Erjian(LI 2)　A meridian point originally from *Lingshu*: *Benshu* (*Miraculous Pivot*: *Meridian Points*), the Ying(Spring) point of the Large Intestine Meridian of Hand-Yangming, also named Jiangu, Zhougu. 〈Location〉When a loose fist is made, the point is in the depression on the radial side, distal to the 2nd

metacarpophalangeal joint (Figs. 48&6). ⟨Regional anatomy⟩ skin → subcutaneous tissue → first lumbrical muscle tendon → base of proximal phalanx of index finger. In the superficial layer, there are the dorsal nerve of the radial nerve, the proper palmar digital nerve of the median nerve, the branches of the first dorsal metacarpal artery and vein and the branches of the radial artery and vein of the index finger. In the deep layer, there are the muscular branches of the median nerve. ⟨Indications⟩ inflammation of the throat, submental swelling, rhinallergosis and epistaris, ophthalmalgia, icteric sclera, blood and pus in stool, toothache, dry mouth, deviation of the eye and mouth, fever, sleepiness, pain in the shoulder and back and shivering. ⟨Method⟩ Puncture perpendicularly 0.1～0.2 cun. Moxibustion is applicable.

●二十七气[èr shí qī qǐ]　出《灵枢·九针十二原》。指十二经脉和十五络脉的脉气。

Twenty-Seven Kinds of Qi　Originally from *Lingshu: Jiu Zhen Shier Yuan (Miraculous Pivot: Nine Needles and Twelve Yuan (Primary) Points)*, referring to the twenty-seven kinds of qi flowing in the Twelve Regular Meridians and the Fifteen Collaterals.

●二阳[èr yáng]　经络名。出《素问·阴阳类论》等篇。指阳明，包括足阳明胃经和手阳明大肠经。参见"三阳三阴"条。

The Two Yang　Name of meridians, originally from *Suwen: Yinyang Lei Lun (Plain Questions: On Categories of Yin and Yang)* and other chapters, referring to the Yangming Meridians, including the Stomach Meridian of Foot-Yangming and the Large Intestine Meridian of Hand-Yangming. →三阳三阴(p. 345)

●二阴[èr yīn]　①经络名。出《素问·阴阳类论》等篇。指少阴，包括手少阴心经和足少阴肾经。参见"三阳三阴"条。②指外生殖器（前阴）和肛门（后阴）。出《素问·金匮真言论》。

1. The Two Yin　Name of meridians, originally from *Su Wen: Yinyang Lei Lun (Plain Questions: On Categories of Yin and Yang)* and other chapters, referring to the Shaoyin Meridians including the Heart Meridian of Hand-Shaoyin and the Kidney Meridian of Foot-Shaoyin. →三阴三阳(p. 346)

2. Two Lower Orifices　Referring to the external genital organs and anus, originally from *Suwen: Jingui Zhenyan Lun (Plain Questions: On the Truth of the Golden Chamber)*.

●二趾上[èr zhǐ shàng]　经外穴名。见《类经图翼》。在内庭与陷谷两穴边线之中点处。⟨灸治⟩水肿、牙龈肿痛、鼻衄、足背红肿。

Erzhishang (EX-LE)　An extra point, seen in *Leijing Tuyi (Illustrated Supplements to Classified Canon of Internal Medicine of the Yellow Emperor)*. ⟨Location⟩ at the midpoint of the line connecting Neiting (ST 44) and Xiangu (ST 43). ⟨Indications⟩ edema, swelling and pain of the gum, epistaxis, redness and swelling on the dorsum of the foot. ⟨Method⟩ moxibustion.

●二椎下[èr zhuī xià]　经外穴名，又称无名。位于后正中线，第二胸椎棘突下凹陷处。⟨主治⟩精神病、癫痫、疟疾等。斜刺0.5～1寸，可灸。

Erzhuixia (EX-B)　An extra point, also named Wuming. ⟨Location⟩ on the posterior midline, in the depression of the spinous process of the 2nd thoracic vertebra. ⟨Indications⟩ mental diseases, epilepsy and malarial diseases, etc. ⟨Method⟩ Puncture obiquely 0.5～1 cun. Moxibustion is applicable.

F

●发洪[fā hóng] 灸法术语。出《诸病源候论》卷三十五。指灸疮出血。

Bleeding of Post-Moxibustion Sores A term in moxibustion, originally from Chap. 35 of *Zhubing Yuanhou Lun* (*General Treatise on the Etiology and Symptomatology of Diseases*), referring to the bleeding of sores after festering moxibustion.

●发矇[fā méng] 《内经》刺法名。出《灵枢·刺节真邪》。为刺法五节之一。指对听力、视力减退的耳目病，针刺须在中午的时候，刺听宫穴，使针刺感应达到瞳子，并使其针气的响声传到耳中。其效验有如开发矇聩一样。

Rousing the Blind and Awakening the Deaf An acupuncture technique in *Neijing* (*Canon of Internal Medicine*), originally from *Lingshu: Cijie Zhenxie* (*Miraculous Pivot: Acupuncture Principles and Diseases*), one of the five principles, used for the treatment of ear and eye diseases such as hypoacusis and hapopsia. ⟨Method⟩Puncture Tingong (SI 19) at noon, causing the needling to reach the eyeballs with a sound of the needling sensation reaching the ears at the same time. This method is quite effective, as if rousing the blind and awakening the deaf.

●发泡灸[fā pào jiǔ] ①灸法术语。灸灼穴位皮肤，使之发泡。一般着肤灸时可用小艾炷，灸至皮肤表面稍现黄斑为止；间接灸时可用中等艾炷，灸至局部出现明显红晕为止。灸后渐起小泡，不必挑破，任其自然吸收。②灸法的一种。为天灸之别称。详见该条。

Blistering Moxibustion ①A term in moxibustion, namely, to cauterize the skin around the selected point with an ignited moxa cone to form blisters. In direct moxibustion a small moxa cone is used until a yellowish spot appears on the skin; in indirect moxibustion a moxa cone of medium size is used until obvious redness appears on the skin. After moxibustion, small blisters gradually form on the skin and are absorbed naturally instead of being pricked. ②A kind of moxibustion, another name for medicinal vesiculation. →天灸(p. 432)

●发针[fā zhēn] 针刺手法名。为出针法之别称。详见该条。

Pulling Out the Needle An acupuncture manipulation, another name for withdrawing the needle. →出针法(p. 51)

●发际[fā jì] ①部位名。指头发的边际，在前额的称前发际，在后项的称后发际。②经穴别名。出《普济本事方》。即神庭。见该条。③经外穴名。出《太平圣惠方》。在头部，当前发际正中处。⟨主治⟩小儿风痫、头痛、头晕、目眩等。沿皮刺0.3～0.5寸；可灸。

1. **Hairline** A body part, referring to the hair margin. The hairline on the forehead is the anterior hairline and that at the nape of the neck is the posterior hairline.

2. **Faji** Another name for Shengting (DU 24), a meridian point, originally from *Puji Benshi Fang* (*Effective Prescriptions for Universal Relief*). →神庭(p. 363)

3. **Faji** (EX-HN) An extra point originally from *Taiping Shenghui Fang* (*Imperial Benevolent Prescriptions*). ⟨Location⟩on the head, at the midpoint of the anterior hairline. ⟨Indications⟩ infantile epilepsy, headache, dizziness, etc. ⟨Method⟩Puncture subcutaneously 0.3～0.5 cun. Moxibustion is applicable.

●翻胃[fān wèi] 见宋代朱瑞章《卫生家宝》。即反胃。详见该条。

Upside-Down Stomach The regurgitation of food from the stomach, seen in *Weisheng Jiashi* (*A Book of Health Care for Home Use*), written by Zhu Ruizhang of the Song Dynasty. →反胃(p. 104)

●樊阿[fán ē] 人名。三国时针灸家，彭城（今江苏徐州）人，华佗的学生。他认为胸腹背之间"针不过四

分"的观点可改变,主张深刺。见《后汉书·华佗传》。

Fan E An expert of acupuncture and moxibustion in the period of the Three Kingdoms (A.D. 220-280), a native of Pengcheng (Now Xuzhou, Jiangsu Province) and a pupil of Hua Tuo. He held that the viewpoint that the depth of insertion in the chest, abdomen and back should not exceed 0.4 cun should be changed, allowing for deeper insertion. Cf. *Houhai Shu: Hua Tuo Zhuan* (*The History of the Later Han Dynasty: Biography of Hua Tuo*).

●燔针[fán zhēn] ①刺法术语。见《素问·调经论》。燔,烧的意思。是指针刺入后,用火烧针使暖,为痹证的刺法,以火气祛散寒邪。②针具名。见《针灸大成》。火针之别称。见该条。

1. Heat Needling An acupuncture technique originally from *Sunwen: Tiaojing Lun* (*Plain Questions: On the Regulation of Meridians*), referring to heating the handle of the needle with fire while it remains in the point. This method is used to treat Bi syndromes and to expel pathogenic cold.

2. Heated Needle Another name for the fire needle, an acupuncture instrument, from *Zhenjiu Dacheng* (*A Great Compendium Acupuncture and Moxibustion*). →火针(p.180)

●反胃[fǎn wěi] 病症名。见《景岳全书》。亦称胃反、翻胃。多因脾胃虚冷,命门火衰,不能蒸化水谷所致。症见上腹部疼痛明显,朝食暮吐,暮食朝吐,吐后脘部较为舒畅,神疲乏力,面色少华,舌淡苔白,脉细缓无力。治宜温运脾胃,和胃降逆。取胃俞、脾俞、中脘、章门、梁门、天枢、关元、足三里、肾俞等穴。

Regurgitation of Food from the Stomach A disease, seen in *Jing Yue Quanshu* (*Jing Yue's Complete Works*), also reversing named movement of the stomach, or upside-down stomach. Commonly due to the insufficiency of spleen-yang and the decline of Mingmen (Life-gate) fire, resulting in failure to receive and digest food. 〈Manifestations〉obvious pain in the upper abdomen, vomiting right after eating, comfortable feeling in the stomach after vomiting, exhaustion, dim complexion, pale tongue with white coating, and a thready, leisurely, weak pulse. 〈Treatment principles〉Warm the spleen and stomach, regulate the stomach and check upward adverse flow of the stomach-qi. 〈Point selection〉Weishu (BL 21), Pishu (BL 20), Zhongwan (RN 12), Zhangmen (LR 13), Liangmen (ST 21), Tianshu (ST 25), Guanyuan (RN 4), Zusanli (ST 36) and Shenshu (BL 23).

●返本还原[fǎn běn huán yuán] 子午流注针法用语。指阳经在按时取用五输中所开输穴的同时,须加取与所开井穴同属一经的原穴。其中本是指本日的值日经,原是值日经的原穴。因为原穴是十二经出入的门户,故逢输必开原穴。一般开原穴的时辰,是在开井穴之后的四个时辰,如以胆经为例,在甲戌时开井穴窍阴,到第二天乙日的戊寅时开其原穴丘墟,从戌到寅,正隔四个时辰。所以须知阳经原穴皆在开井穴之后的四个时辰开穴。

Returning Ben and Yuan An acupuncture term related to the midnight-noon ebb-flow theory. It refers to an additional selection of the Yuan (Primary) point on the same Yang meridian that the opened Jing (Well) point belongs to when the Shu (Stream) point on the Yang meridian is selected. Ben refers to the dominant meridian on the day of treatment whereas Yuan refers to the Yuan (Primary) point on the dominant meridian. It is because the Yuan (Primary) point is the door of the twelve regular meridians that the Yuan (Primary) point must be selected once the Shu (Stream) point is open. In general, the Yuan (Primary) point opens 4 two-hour periods after the Jing (Well) point does. For example, on the Gallbladder Meridian, the Jing (Well) point, Zuqiaoyin (GB 44), opens in the period of Jia-Xu (the first of the Ten Heavenly Stems and the eleventh of the Twelve Earthly Branches), and its Yuan (Primary) point, Qiuxu (GB 40), opens at the period of Wu-Yin (the fifth of the Ten Heavenly Stems and the third of the Twelve Earthly Branches) on the following day, (the day of Yi). There is an interval of 4 two-hour periods from Xu (7-9 p.m.) to Yin (3-5 a.m.). Therefore, what should be made clear is that all the Yuan (Primary) points on the Yang meridians open 4 two-hour periods later than the Jing (Well) points on the same meridian.

●范九思[fàn jiǔ sī]　人名。北宋针灸家。精通针术，善治危重病人。曾记载其治喉蛾的验案。见《古今医统》。

Fan Jiusi　An acupuncture and moxibustion expert of the Northern Song Dynasty, who was proficient in acupunture and good at treating patients suffering from imminent and serious diseases. One effective case of his with tonsillitis was recorded in *Gu Jin Yitong* (*The General Medicine of the Past and Present.*)

●范培贤[fàn péi xián]　人名。清末针灸家，字春坡，义乌（今属浙江）人。撰《针灸聚萃》。

Fan Peixian　An acupuncture and moxibustion expert of the Late Qing Dynasty, who styled himself Chunpo, a native of Yiwu (Now in Zhejiang Province), the author of *Zhenjiu Jucui* (*A Colllection of Acupuncture and Moxibustion*).

●范毓䄊[fàn yù yǐ]　人名。清针灸家，字培兰，里籍不详。倡用"太乙针"治病。约雍正时，周雍和据范氏方法编成《太乙神针附方》，此法因而推广。

Fan Yuyi　An acupuncture and moxibustion expert of the Qing Dynasty, who styled himself Peilan. Little is known about his native place. He advocated the application of moxibustion with great monad herbal moxa sticks in treatment. In about the reign of Yong Zheng, Zhou Yonghe compiled *Taiyi Shenzhen Fufang* (*Appended Recipes of Great Monad Herbal Moxa Stick*) on the basis of Fan's method, which therefore spreads extensively.

●放血疗法[fàng xuè liáo fǎ]　即刺血疗法。详见该条。

Blood-Letting Therapy　→刺血疗法(p. 56)

●飞处[fēi chù]　经穴别名。见《神灸经纶》。即支沟。详见该条。

Feichu　Another name for Zhigou (SJ 6), a meridian point, originally from *Shenjiu Jinglun* (*Principles of Magic Moxibustion*). →支沟(p. 600)

●飞法[fēi fǎ]　针刺辅助手法之一。用拇指与食、中指相对捏持针柄，一捻一放。捻时，食、中指内屈，使针顺转（左转）；放时，食、中指外伸，搓动针柄，使针逆转（右转），手指放开时犹如飞鸟展翅，故名。此法可催动经气的到来，使针感增强。

Flying Method　One of the auxiliary manipulations of acupuncture. Hold the handle of the needle with the thumb, the index and middle fingers, twirl the needle and release it. When twirling and releasing the needle, move the index and middle fingers backward, so as to make the needle rotate clockwise (left rotation); extend the index and the middle fingers forward, so as to make the needle rotate counter clockwise (right rotation) while releasing the needle. It is so named because the releasing is done as if a flying bird spreads its wings. It can promote the arrival of meridian qi and strengthen the needling sensation.

●飞虎[fēi hǔ]　经穴别名。见《标幽赋》。即支沟。详见该条。

Feihu　Another name for Zhigou (SJ 6), a meridian point seen in *Biao You Fu* (*Lyrics of Recondite Principles*). →支沟(p. 600)

●飞经走气法[fēi jīng zǒu qì fǎ]　针刺手法名。出《金针赋》。又称龙虎龟凤。指催行经气的一些针刺手法，包括青龙摆尾、白虎摇头、苍龟探穴、赤凤迎源四法。适用于经络气血壅滞之症，或用于在关节附近针刺而不得气者。作为通经接气的催气手法，以促使针刺感应通经过关而达病所。具体操作参见各条。

Methods of Accelerating Qi-Flow over the Meridians　A term in needling techniques, originally from *Jinzhen Fu* (*Ode to Gold Needle*), also named dragon-tiger-tortoise-phoenix. Refers to manipulations which can promote the arrival of the needling sensation and the flow of meridian-qi, includes the following four methods: green dragon wagging its tail, white tiger shaking its head, tortoise exploring a cave and red phoenix greeting the source. 〈Applications〉diseases due to qi-stagnation and blood stasis in the meridian or in cases without a needling response after puncturing near joints. It is a qi-promoting method of connecting qi and dredging the meridians to impel the needling sensation to pass through the joints and reach the affected area of the body. →龙虎龟凤(p. 254)、青龙摆尾(p. 320)、白虎摇头(p. 10)、苍龟探穴(p. 30)、赤凤迎源(p. 47)

●飞腾八法[fēi téng bā fǎ]　按时配穴法的一种。出

《玉龙经》。又称奇经纳甲法。系以八脉八穴配合八卦,按每日各个时辰的天干推算开穴。其法:逢壬、甲时,开公孙(属乾);逢丙时,开内关(属艮);逢戊时,开足临泣(属坎);逢庚时,开外关(属震);逢辛时,开后溪(属巽);逢乙、癸时,开申脉(属坤);逢己时,开列缺(属离);逢丁时,开照海(属兑)。例如甲子日戊辰时,即取足临泣穴;己巳时,即取列缺穴;庚午时,即取外关穴;余皆仿此。参见"灵龟八法"条。

Eight Methods of Soaring A method of point selection according to different times, originally from *Yulong Jing* (*Classic of Jade Dragon*), also called day-prescription of acupoints of extra meridians. It refers to the method of matching the eight points of the eight extra meridians with the eight diagrammatical directions, then selecting the points in accordance with the different days and hours relating to the Heavenly Stems. 〈Method〉at the time of Ren or Jia, puncture Gongsun(SP 4)(relating to Qian); at the time of Bing, puncture Neiguan(PC 6)(relating to Gen); at the time of Wu, puncture Zulinqi(GB 41)(relating to Kan); at the time of Geng, puncture Waiguan(SJ 5)(relating to Zhen); at the time of Xin, puncture Houxi(SI 3)(relating to Xun); at the time of Yi, or Gui, puncture Shenmai(BL 62)(relating to Kun); at the time of Ji, puncture Zhaohai(KI 6)(relating to Dui). e.g. at the time of Wu-Chen on the date of Jia-zi, select Zulinqi(GB 41); at the time of Ji-Si, select Lieque(LU 5); at the time of Geng-Wu, select Waiguan(SJ 5), and so on.
→灵龟八法(p. 248)

●飞扬[fēi yáng] 经穴名。出《灵枢·经脉》。原作飞阳,《针灸甲乙经》作飞扬。属足太阳膀胱经,为本经络穴。又名厥阳。〈定位〉在小腿后面,当外踝后,昆仑穴直上7寸,承山外下方1寸处(图35)。〈层次解剖〉皮肤→皮下组织→小腿三头肌→长屈肌。浅层布有腓肠外侧皮神经,深层有胫神经和胫后动、静脉。〈主治〉头痛、目眩、鼻塞、鼻衄、腰背痛、腿软无力、痔肿痛、癫狂。直刺0.7~1寸;可灸。

Feiyang(BL 58) A meridian point, seen in *Lingshu*: *Jingmai*(*Miraculous Pivot*: *Meridians*), originally referred to as Feiyang(飞阳), as Feiyang(飞扬) in *Zhenjiu Jia-Yi Jing*(*A-B Classic of Acupuncture and Moxibustion*), the Luo (Connecting)point of the Bladder Meridian of Foot-Taiyang, also called Jueyang. 〈Location〉on the posterior side of the leg, 7 cun directly above Kunlun(BL 60) and 1 cun lateral and inferior to Chengshan(BL 57)(Fig. 35). 〈Regional anatomy〉In the superficial layer, there is the lateral cutaneous nerve of calf. In the deep layer, there are the tibial nerve and the posterior tibial artery and vein. 〈Indications〉 headache, dizziness, stuffy nose, epistaxis, pain in the loins and back, myasthenia of legs, hemorrhoids with pain and swelling, manic-depressive psychosis. 〈Method〉Puncture perpendicularly 0.7~1 cun. Moxibustion is applicable.

阳 and 扬 are homonyms in Chinese.

●飞阳[fēi yáng] 经穴别名。出《灵枢·经脉》。即飞扬。详见该条。

Feiyang Another name for Feiyang(BL 58), a meridian point originally from *Ling Shu*: *Jingmai*(*Miraculous Pivot*: *Meridians*).
→飞扬(p. 106)

●飞阳之脉[fēi yáng zhī mài] 经脉名。出《素问·刺腰痛篇》。指足太阳经在小腿部的别络。从外踝上七寸飞扬穴处走向足少阴经复溜之前,上方与阴维郄穴筑宾会合。

Feiyang Meridian A meridian, originally from *Suwen*: *Ci Yaotong Pian* (*Plain Qusetions*: *On Treatment of Lumbago with Acupuncture*), referring to the collateral of the Food-Taiyang Meridian in the leg. It starts at Feiyang(BL 58), 7 cun above the lateral malleous, runs to the area anterior to Fuliu(KI 7) of the Foot-Shaoyin Meridian, and then goes up to meet Zhubin(KI 9), the Xi(Cleft) point of the Yinwei Meridian.

●飞针[fēi zhēn] 针刺方法之一。为砭法之别称。详见该条。

Flying Needling One of the needling techniques, another name for stone needling. →砭法(p. 22)

●非化脓灸[fēi huà nóng jiǔ] 艾炷灸的一种。为无瘢痕灸之别名。详见该条。

Non-Festering Moxibustion One kind of moxibustion with moxa cones, another name for nonscarring moxibustion. →无瘢痕灸(p.

472)

● 铍针 [fēi zhēn]　见《素问·血气形志篇》。为铍针之别称。详见该条。

Pus-Discharging Needle　Seen in *Suwen*: *Xue Qi Xing Zhi Pian* (*Plain Questions*: *On Blood, Qi, Physical and Mental Conditions*), another name for a sword-shaped needle. →铍针 (p. 291)

● 肺 [fēi]　①耳穴名。位于耳背中部内侧。用于治疗哮喘、消化系统病症、发热等。②耳穴名。位于耳甲腔中心凹陷处周围。用于治疗咳喘、声嘶、胸闷、痤疮、皮肤瘙痒症、荨麻疹、扁平疣、便秘、戒烟综合症、单纯性肥胖症。

1. **Lung** (MA)　An auricular point. ⟨Location⟩ on the medial side of the middle region of the back of the ear. ⟨Indications⟩ asthma, diseases of digestive system, fever, etc.
2. **Lung** (MA-IC 1)　An auricular point. ⟨Location⟩ around the central depression of the cavum conche. ⟨Indications⟩ cough and dyspnea, hoarseness, choking ache, cutaneous pruritus, urticaria, flat warts, constipation, stopping smoking, obesity.

● 肺底 [fēi dǐ]　经穴别名。出《循经考穴编》。即灵台。详见该条。

Feidi　Another name for Lingtai (DU 10), a meridian point originally from *Xunjing Kaoxue Bian* (*Studies on Acupoints along Meridians*). →灵台 (p. 249)

● 肺经 [fēi jīng]　手太阴肺经之简称。详见该条。

Lung Meridian　A short name for the Lung Meridian of Hand-Taiyin. →手太阴肺经 (p. 398)

● 肺痨 [fēi láo]　病证名。是一种具有传染性的慢性虚弱性疾病。亦称劳瘵、传尸、传尸痨、尸注、鬼注等。多为机体正气不足，抗病能力不强，感染痨虫所致。初起微有咳嗽，食欲不振，疲乏，体重减轻，或痰中带有少量血丝，舌红苔薄黄，脉浮数。病程长者，咳嗽加剧，两颧及口唇艳红，午后潮热，盗汗，口干多饮，咯血，失眠，胸闷作痛，男子失精，女子经闭，舌红少苔，脉细数。治宜补肺健脾。取太渊、肺俞、膏肓、足三里、三阴交、太溪。盗汗加阴郄，潮热加鱼际，遗精加志室，经闭加血海，肢冷灸关元，咯血加孔最。

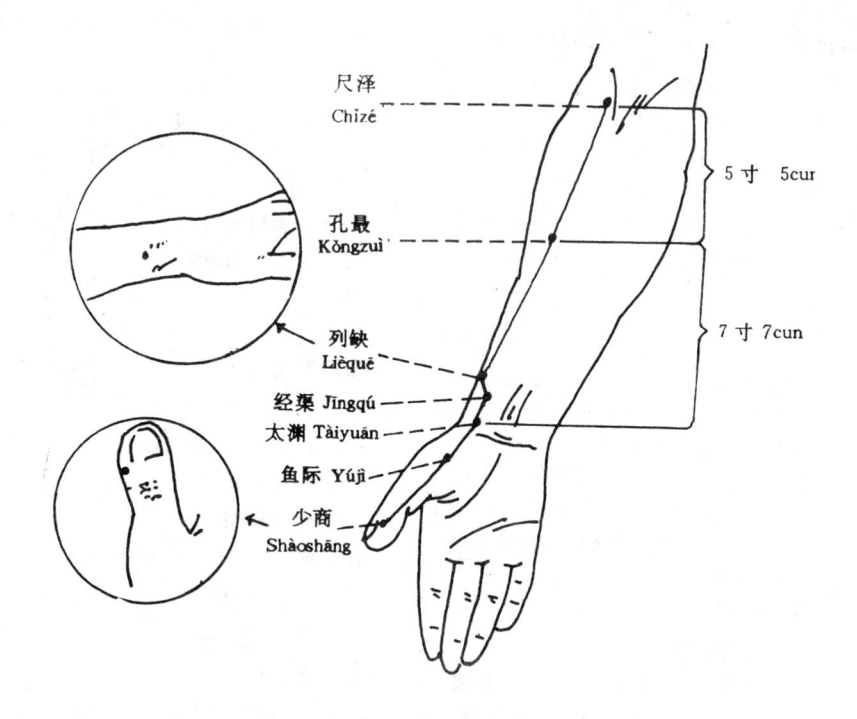

图16　肺经穴
Fig. 16　Points of Lung Meridian

Pulmonary Tuberculosis An infectious and chronic prostrating disease, also called tuberculosis, walking of a corpse, corpse-walking, tuberculosis of a corpse, or tuberculosis of a ghost, etc. Generally due to deficient vital-qi of the body, decline in resistance and the infection of tuberculomyces. 〈Manifestations〉 at the initial stage: slight cough, poor appetite, fatigue, decline in weight, sputum mixed with blood, a red tongue with thin and yellowish coating, and a floating and rapid pulse. Long term cases manifest severe cough, flushing of zygomatic region and lips, afternoon fever, night sweating, dry mouth with a desire to drink a lot, hemoptysis, insomnia, oppressive and painful feeling in the chest, spermatic emission, amenorrhea, a red tongue with little coating, and a thread and rapid pulse. 〈Treatment principle〉 Tonify the lung and strengthen the spleen. 〈Point selection〉 Taiyuan (LU 9), Feishu (BL 13), Gaohuang (BL 43), Zusanli (ST 36), Sanyinjiao (SP 6), Taixi (KI 3). Yinxi (HT 6) is added for night sweating, Yuji (LU 10) for afternoon fever, Zhishi (BL 52) for emission and Xuehai (SP 10) for amenorrhea. Moxibustion is given on Guanyuan (RN 4) for cold limbs, and Kongzui (LU 6) for hemoptysis.

●肺募[fèi mù] ①经外穴名,见《千金要方》。在胸部,当第2肋间隙,约距前正中线1.5寸处。灸治小儿暴痫、胸满、短气等。②脏腑募穴之一。即中府。详见该条。

1. **Feimu** (EX-CA) An extra point, seen in *Qianjin Yaofang* (*Essential Prescriptions Worth a Thousand Gold*). 〈Location〉 on the chest, in the 2nd intercostal space, about 1.5 cun lateral to the anterior midline. 〈Indications〉 sudden onset of infantile epilepsy, fullness in the chest, shortness of breath, etc. 〈Method〉 moxibustion.

2. **Feimu** One of the Front-Mu points of zang-fu organs. →中府(p. 609)

●肺热鼻衄[fèi rè bí nù] 鼻衄症型之一。因肺热上壅所致。症见鼻衄血,兼见鼻燥咽干,发热咳嗽,舌红,脉数。治宜清泻肺热,凉血止血。取天府、孔最、合谷、风府。

Epistaxis due to Lung-Heat A type of epistaxia due to the surging of lung-heat. 〈Manifestations〉 epistaxis accompanied by dry nose and pharynx, fever, cough, red tongue, rapid pulse. 〈Treatment principle〉 Clear heat from the lung to cool blood and stop bleeding. 〈Point selection〉 Tianfu (LU 3), Kongzui (LU 6), Hegu (LI 4), and Fengfu (DU 16).

●肺热津伤痿证[fèi rè jīn shāng wěi zhèng] 痿证证型之一。由肺受热灼,津液耗伤,筋脉失于濡润所致。证见病起发热,或热后突然出现肢体软弱无力,皮肤枯燥,心烦口渴,咳呛少痰,咽干不利,小便黄少,大便干燥,舌质红,苔黄,脉细数。治宜通经活络,清热生津。取肩髃、曲池、合谷、阳溪、髀关、梁丘、足三里、解溪、尺泽、鱼际。

Flaccidity Syndrome due to Lung-Heat Damaging Body Fluid A type of flaccidity syndrome, due to the lung burned by pathogenic heat which leads to the consumption of body fluid, causing a failure to nourish the muscles and vessels. 〈Manifestaions〉 fever, or sudden onset of flaccidity of the limbs after fever, xerosis cutis, irritability, thirst, cough with little sputum, dry pharynx, scanty and deep-coloured urine, dry stool, red tongue with yellowish coating, thready and rapid pulse. 〈Treatment principle〉 Dredge and activate the meridians and collaterals; clear heat to promote the production of the body fluids. 〈Point selection〉 Jianyu (LI 15), Quchi (LI 11), Hegu (LI 4), Yangxi (LI 5), Biguan (ST 31), Liangqiu (ST 34), Zusanli (ST 36), Jiexi (ST 41), Chize (LU 5) and Yuji (LU 10).

●肺手太阴之脉[fèi shǒu tài yīn zhī mài] 手太阴肺经原名。详见该条。

Lung Vessel of Hand-Taiyin The original name for the Lung Meridian of Hand-Taiyin. →手太阴肺经(p. 398)

●肺俞[fèi shū] 经穴名。出《灵枢·背腧》。属足太阳膀胱经,为肺的背俞穴。〈定位〉在背部,当第三胸椎棘突下,旁开1.5寸(图7)。〈层次解剖〉皮肤→皮下组织→斜方肌→菱形肌→上后锯肌→坚脊肌。浅层布有第三、四胸神经后支的内侧皮支的肌支和伴行的肋间后动、静脉侧支的内侧皮支。深层有第三、四胸神经后支的肌支和相应的肋间后动、静脉背侧支的

分支或属支。〈主治〉咳嗽、气喘、胸满、脊背痛、咯血、喉痹、骨蒸、潮热、盗汗、皮肤搔痒。斜刺0.5～0.8寸；可灸。

Feishu(BL 13)　A meridian point, originally from *Lingshu: Beishu* (*Miraculous Pivot: the Back-Shu Points*), the Back-Shu point of the lung on the Bladder Meridian of Foot-Taiyang. 〈Location〉on the back, below the spinous process of the 3rd thoracic vertebra, 1.5 cun lateral to the posterior midline (Fig. 7). 〈Regional anatomy〉skin→subcutaneous tissue→trapezius muscle→rhomboid muscle→suprior serratus muscle→erector spinal muscle. In the superficial layer, there are the medial cutaneous branches of the posterior branches of the 3rd and 4th thoracic nerves and the medial cutaneous branches of the dorsal branches of the accompanying posterior intercostal arteries and veins. In the deep layer, there are the branches or tributaries of the dorsal branches of the related posterior intercostal arteries and veins. 〈Indications〉cough, dyspnea, full sensation in the chest, pain in the spine and back, hemoptysis, sore throat, hectic fever due to yin deficiency, tidal fever, night sweating, cutaneous pruritus. 〈Method〉Puncture obliquely 0.5～0.8 cun. Moxibustion is applicable.

●**肺系**[fèi xì]　出《灵枢·经脉》。①指气管与喉咙。②指肺与喉咙相联系的部位。③肺及其附属器官，如气管、喉、鼻道等。

Pulmonary System　Originally from *Ling Shu: Jing Mai* (*Miraculous Pivot: Meridians*). Referring to ①the larynx and trachea；②the area connecting the lung and the larynx；③the lung and its accessory organs, i.e. larynx, trachea, nasal meatus etc.

●**肺虚哮喘**[fèi xū xiāo chuǎn]　哮喘证型之一。因病久肺气不足，口外不固，气不化津，痰饮蕴肺所致。证见面色㿠白、自汗恶风、息短少气、语言无力、鼻塞喷嚏、疲乏、喉有鼾声、舌质淡红、脉细数无力。治宜补益肺气，化痰平喘。取定喘、膏肓、肺俞、太渊。

Asthma with Wheezing due to Deficiency of the Lung　A type of asthma with wheezing. One to insufficiency of lung-qi resulting from a protracted disease, failure of superficial-qi to protect the body against disease and failure of qi to transport body fluid, leading to stagnation of phlegm in the lung. 〈Manifestations〉pale complexion, spontaneous sweating and aversion to wind, short breath, week speech, stuffy nose, sneezing, fatigue, snore in the larynx, pale tongue, thready, rapid and weak pulse. 〈Treatment principle〉Enrich lung-qi, resolve sputum and relieve asthma. 〈Point selection〉Dingchuan (EX-B 1), Gaohuang (BL 43), Feishu (BL 13) and Taiyuan (LU 9).

●**分刺**[fēn cì]　《内经》刺法名。出《灵枢·官针》。是九刺之一。是指针刺直达肌肉的一种刺法。治疗肌肉的痹证、痿证或陈伤，均可用此法，以调其经气。

Intermuscular Needling　A needling technique in *Nei Jing* (*Internal Classic*), originally from *Ling Shu: Guan Zhen* (*Miraculous Pivot: Official Puncture*), one of the nine needling methods. Refers to the needling technique of inserting the needle directly into the muscle. The method can be used to treat myalgia syndrome, flaccidity or old wound by regulating meridian-qi.

●**分肉**[fēn ròu]　①古代解剖名。见《灵枢·寿夭刚柔》。指筋肉而言。谓腘坚而有分者，肉坚。近人称为骨骼肌。②经穴别名。见《针灸聚英》。即阳辅。详见该条。

1. **Muscle**　An anatomical part in ancient times, seen in *Lingshu: Shouyao Gangrou* (*Miraculous Pivot: Life-Span and Body Constitution*), referring to the muscles and tendons. A strong prominence with obvious fibers means strong muscles which is referred to as skeletal muscle by contemporary people.

2. **Fenrou**　Another name for Yangfu (GB 38), a meridian point seen in *Zhenjiu Juying* (*Essentials of Acupuncture and Moxibustion*.) →**阳辅**(p.536)

●**分中**[fēn zhōng]　经穴别名。出《素问·气穴论》。即环跳。详见该条。

Fenzhong　Another name for Huantiao (GB 30), a meridian point, originally from *Suwen: Qi Xue Lun* (*Plain Questions: On Acupoints*). →**环跳**(p.170)

●**丰隆**[fēng lóng]　经穴名。出《灵枢·经脉》。属足阳明胃经，为本经络穴。〈定位〉在小腿前外侧，当外踝

尖上8寸,条口外,距胫骨前缘二横指(中指)(图60)。〈层次解剖〉皮肤→皮下组织→趾长伸肌→腓骨短肌→小腿骨间膜→胫骨后肌。浅层布有腓肠外侧皮神经。深层有胫前动、静脉的分支或属支和腓深神经的分支。〈主治〉痰多、哮喘、咳嗽、胸疼、头痛、头晕、咽喉肿痛、便秘、癫狂、痫证、下肢痿痹、肿痛。直刺0.5～1.2寸;可灸。

Fenglong(ST 40) A meridian point originally from *Lingshu: Jingmai* (*Miraculous Pivot: Meridians*), a Luo(Connecting) Point of the Stomach Meridian of Foot-Yangming. 〈Location〉on the anteriolateral side of the leg, 8 cun above the tip of the external malleolus, lateral to Tiaokou(ST 38), and two finger breadths (middle finger) from the anterior crest of the tibia (Fig. 60). 〈Regional anatomy〉skin→subcutaneous tissue→long extensor muscle of toes → short peroneal muscle → interosseous membrane of leg → posterior tibial muscle. In the superficial layer, there is the lateral cutaneous nerve of the calf. In the deep layer, there are the branches or tributaries of the anterior tibial artery and vein and branches of the deep peroneal nerve. 〈Indications〉profuse sputum, asthma, cough, pain in the chest, headache, dizziness, sore throat, constipation, manic-depressive psychosis, epilepsy, pain and paralysis, flaccidity, swelling and pain of the lower limbs. 〈Method〉Puncture perpendicularly 0.5～1.2 cun. Moxibustion is applicable.

●风池[fēng chí] 经穴名。出《灵枢·热病》。属足少阳胆经,为足少阳、阳维之会。〈定位〉在项部,当枕骨之下,与风府相平,胸锁乳突肌与斜方肌上端之间的凹陷处(图28和图31)。〈层次解剖〉皮肤→皮下组织→斜方肌和胸锁乳突肌之间→头夹肌→头半棘肌→头后大直肌与头上斜肌之间。浅层布有枕小神经和枕动、静脉的分支或属支。深层有枕下神经等结构。〈主治〉头痛、眩晕、颈项强痛、目赤痛、目泪出、鼻渊、鼻衄、耳聋、气闭、中风、口眼歪斜、疟疾、热病、感冒、瘿气。向对侧眼睛方向斜刺0.5～0.8寸;可灸。

Fengchi(GB 20) A meridian point originally from *Lingshu: Re Bing* (*Miraculous Pivot: Febrile Diseases*), a point on the Gallbladder Meridian of Foot-Shaoyang, the crossing point of the Gallblandder Foot-Shaoyang and Yangwei. 〈Location〉on the nape, below the occipital bone, on the level of Fengfu (DU 16), in the depression between the upper ends of the sternocleidomastoid and trapezius muscles (Figs. 28&31). 〈Regional anatomy〉skin → subcutaneous tissue→between trapezius muscle and strapezius muscle and sternocleidomastoid muscle → splenius muscle of head → semispinal muscle of head → between large posterior straight muscle of head and superior oblique muscle of head. In the superficial layer, there are the lesser occipital nerve and the branches of tributaries of the occipital artry and vein, In the deep layer there is the suboccipital nerver. 〈Indications〉headache, dizziness, pain and stiffness of the neck and nape, conjunctival congestion with pain, lacrimation, rhinorrhea with turbid discharge, epistaxis, deafness, qi-stagnation, apoplexy, deviation of the mouth and eye, malarial disease, febrile disease, common cold, goiter. 〈Method〉Puncture obliquely 0.5～0.8 cun toward the opposite eye. Moxibustion is applicable.

●风齿痛[fēng chǐ tòng] 经外穴名。见《千金要方》。在腕横纹上2.5寸。灸治风齿疼痛。

Fengchitong(EX-UE) An extra point seen in *Qianyin Yaofang* (*Essential Prescriptions Worth a Thousand Gold*). 〈Location〉2.5 cun above the transverse crease of the wrist. 〈Indication〉toothache due to wind pathogen. 〈Method〉moxibustion.

●风耳[fēng ěr] 即聘耳。详见该条。
Otitis Media Suppurativa due to Wind →聘耳(p.439)

●风痱穴[fēng fèi xué] 经外穴名。见《经外奇穴图谱》。在中脘穴下0.5寸一穴,中脘穴旁开1.5寸各一穴,共三穴。灸治风痱不能语,手足不遂等。

Fengfeixue(EX-CA) A set of points, seen in *Jingwai Qixue Tupu* (*An Atlas of Extra Points*). 〈Location〉One point is 0.5 cun below Zhongwan (RN 12); the other two are 1.5 cun lateral to Zhongwan (RN 12), 3 points in all. 〈Indications〉aphonia and hemiplegia after apoplexy, etc. 〈Method〉moxibustion.

●风府[fēng fǔ] 经穴名。出《灵枢·本输》。属督脉，为督脉、阳维之会。又名舌本、曹溪、惺惺、鬼枕、鬼穴。〈定位〉在项部，当后发际正中直上1寸，枕外隆凸直下，两侧斜方肌之间凹陷中（图31和图7）。〈层次解剖〉皮肤→皮下组织→左、右斜方肌腱之间→项韧带（左、右头半棘肌之间）→左、右头后大、小直肌之间。浅层布有枕大神经和第三枕神经的分支及枕动、静脉的分支或属支。深层有枕下神经的分支。主治癫狂、痫证、瘛疭、中风不语、悲恐惊悸、半身不遂、眩晕、颈项强痛、咽喉肿痛、耳痛、鼻衄。伏案正坐位，使头微前倾，项肌放松，向下颌方向缓慢刺入0.5～1寸；可灸。针尖不可向上，以免刺入枕骨大孔，误伤延髓。

Fengfu(DU 16) A meridian point originally from *Ling Shu: Ben Shu*(*Miraculous Pivot: Meridian Points*), a point on the Du Meridian, the crossing point of the Du Meridian and Yangwei Meridian, also called Sheben, Caoxi, Xingxing, Guizhen or Guixue. 〈Location〉on the nape, 1 cun directly above the midpoint of the posterior hairline, directly below the external occipital protuberance, in the depression between the trapezius muscle of both sides (Figs. 31&7). 〈Regional anatomy〉skin→subcutaneous tissue→between left and right tendons of trapezius muscles→nuchal ligament (between left and right semispinal muscles of head)→between left and right larger and lesser posterior straight muscles of head. In the superficial layer, there are the branches of the greater occipital nerve and the 3rd occipital nerve and the branches or tributaries of the occipital artery and vein. In the deep layer, there are the branches of the suboccipital nerve. 〈Indications〉manic-depressive psychosis, epilepsy, hysteria, apoplexy with aphonia, palpitations due to grief, fear and fright, dizziness, pain and stiffness of the neck and nape, sore throat, pain in the ear, epistaxis. 〈Method〉The patient sitting with the head leaning forward slightly and relaxed, the doctor punctures slowly and perpendicularly 0.5～1 cun toward the mandible. Moxibustion is applicable. Puncturing with the needle tip upward is forbidden, in case the needle tip punctures the great occipital foramen to damage the bulb.

●风关[fēng guān] ①部位名。见《针灸大成》卷十。食指第1、2、3节掌面总称三关。其本节称风关，中节称气关，末节称命关。主要用于诊察和按摩。②经外穴名。见《针法穴道记》。风关穴在食指根横纹中，针之见血。主治小儿惊风。

1. **Wind Gate** A body part, seen in Vol. 10 of *Zhenjiu Dacheng*(*A Great Compendium of Acupuncture and Moxibustion*). The 1st, 2nd and 3rd knuckles of the index finger on the palmar side are generally called three gates, of which the 1st knuckle is called Wind Gate, the 2nd Qi Gate and the 3rd Life Gate. They are mainly used for examination, diagnosis and massage.

2. **Fengguan**(EX-UE) An extra point, seen in *Zhen Fa Xue Dao Ji*(*The Acupuncture Manipulations and Acupoints Records*). 〈Location〉at the midpoint of the proximal transverse crease of the index finger. 〈Indication〉infantile convulsion. 〈Method〉Puncture to cause bleeding.

●风寒感冒[fēng hán gǎn mào] 感冒证型之一。由风寒之邪束表，卫阳被阻，肺气壅滞，失于宣肃所致。证见恶寒重、发热轻，无汗，鼻塞流涕，喷嚏，咳嗽，周身酸楚，头痛，舌苔薄白，脉浮紧。治宜疏风散寒，解表宣肺。取风门、风池、列缺、攒竹。

Common Cold due to Wind-Cold Pathogen
A type of common cold, due to wind-cold pathogen tighening the exterior of the body, blocking the superficial yang and clogging lung-qi leading to obstruction of the lung-qi and impairment of the purifying, descending function of the lung. 〈Manifestations〉severe chills, mild fever, anhidrosis, stuffy nose, watery nasal discharge, sneezing, cough, aching feeling of the body, headache, thin and whitish tongue coating, floating and tense pulse. 〈Treatment principle〉Expel wind and cold pathogens, relieve superficial evils to promote the dispersing function of the lung. 〈Point selection〉Fengmen(BL 12), Fengchi(GB 20), Lieque(LU 7) and Zanzhu(BL 2).

●风寒化热鼻渊[fēng hán huà rè bí yuān] 鼻渊证型之一。因风寒袭肺，蕴而化热，肺气失宣，浊液壅于鼻窍所致。证见恶寒发热，头痛鼻塞，多涕色黄，咳嗽

痰多，舌质红，苔薄白，脉浮数。治宜祛风散寒，宣肺开窍。取列缺、合谷、迎香、印堂。

Rhinorrhea due to Heat-Transformation by Wind-Cold Pathogen　A type of rhinorrhea due to the invasion of wind-cold pathogen into the lung, which accumulates and then transforms into heat leading to the obstruction of the lung-qi, and to turbid fluid in nasal cavity. 〈Manifestations〉chills, fever, headache, stuffy nose, abundant yellow nasal discharge, cough with profuse sputum, red tongue with thin, whitish coating, superficial and rapid pulse. 〈Treatment principle〉 Expel wind and cold pathogens and ventilate the lung to dredge nasal orifice 〈Point selection〉 Lieque(LU 7), Hegu(LI 4), Yingxiang(LI 20) and Yintang (EX-HN 3).

●风寒咳嗽[fēng hán ké sòu]　咳嗽证型之一。因风寒犯肺，肺气不宣所致。证见咳嗽痰稀色白，伴鼻塞流涕，恶寒，无汗，头痛，舌苔薄白，脉浮紧。治宜疏风散寒，宣通肺气。取列缺、合谷、风门、外关。

Cough due to Wind-Cold Pathogen　A type of cough, due to the invasion of wind-cold pathogen into the lung leading to the obstruction of the lung-qi. 〈Manifestations〉 cough with watery and white sputum, accompanied by stuffy nose and watery nasal discharge, chill, anhidrosis, headache, thin and whitish tongue coating, superficial and rapid pulse. 〈Treatment principle〉 Expel wind and cold pathogens; facilitate the flow of lung-qi. 〈Point selection〉 Lieque (LU 7), Hegu (LI 4), Pengmen(BL 12) and Waiguan(SJ 5).

●风寒头痛[fēng hán tóu tòng]　头痛证型之一。见《罗氏会约医镜》卷六。由风寒之邪外袭，循太阳经上犯巅顶，清阳之气被遏所致。证见头痛时作，痛连项背，恶风畏寒，遇风加剧，口不渴，舌苔薄白，脉浮紧。治宜疏风散寒。取风池、太阳、风府、列缺、外关。

Headache due to Wind-Cold Pathogen　A type of headache, seen in Vol 6 of *Luoshi Huiyue Yijing*(*Luo's Medical Mirror of Concise Collections*), due to wind-cold pathogen invading the body and attacking the head along the Taiyang meridians, leading to the blockage of lucid yang. 〈Manifestations〉 frequent headache extending to the nape and back, aversion to wind, intolerance of cold, worsening in wind. Lack of thirst, thin, whitish tongue coating and superficial and tense pulse. 〈Treatment principle〉Expel wind and cold pathogens 〈Point selection〉 Fengchi(GB 20), Taiyang(EX-HN 5), Fengfu(DU 16), Lieque(LU 7)and Waiguan(SJ 5).

●风火蛇丹[fēng huǒ shé dān]　蛇丹证型之一。多因风火之邪所致。其证除见蛇丹的一般症状外，疱疹多发于腰部，兼见口苦，头痛、眩晕、烦热易怒，或目赤面红，小溲短赤，苔黄或干腻，脉弦数。治宜清泄风火。取期门、曲泉、足窍阴、中渚，或局部刺络拨罐。参见"蛇丹"条。

Snake-like Herpes Zoster due to Wind-Fire Pathogen　A type of herpes zoster, mostly due to wind-fire pathogen. 〈Manifestations〉In addition to the common symptoms of snake-like herpes zoster, herpes zoster mostly occurs at the waist, accompanied by a bitter taste, headache, dizziness, irritability, susceptibility to anger, flush and red eyes, oligaria with reddish urine, yellow or dry and thick tongue coating, wiry and rapid pulse. 〈Treatment principle〉Dispel wind and remove fire. 〈Point selection〉 Qimen(LR 14), Ququan(LR 8), Zuqiaoyin(GB 44) and Zhongzhu(SJ 3); or cupping with bleeding on the affected area. → 蛇丹(p. 359)

●风火牙痛[fēng huǒ yá tòng]　牙痛证型之一。由风邪外袭经络，郁于阳明而化火，火郁循经上炎所致。证见牙痛甚而龈肿，兼形寒身热。舌苔薄白，脉浮数。治宜疏风清热止痛。取合谷、下关、颊车、外关、风池。

Toothache due to Wind-Fire Pathogen　A type of toothache due to pathogenic wind attacking the meridians, stagnating in Yangming and then transforming into fire, leading to the flame-up of the accumulated fire along meridians. 〈Manifestations〉 toothache with gingival swelling, accompanied by chills and fever, thin and whitish tongue coating, superficial and rapid pulse. 〈Treatment principle〉 Dispel wind and remove heat to alleviate pain. 〈Point selection〉 Hegu (LI 4), Xiaguan (ST 7), Jiache (ST 6), Waiguan (SJ 5) and Fengchi(GB 20).

●风火眼[fēng huǒ yǎn] 即目赤肿痛。详见该条。

Wind-Fire Eyes →目赤肿痛(p. 271)

●风痉[fēng jìng] 即子痫。详见该条。

Convulsions due to Wind Pathogen Another name for eclampsia gravidarum. →子痫(p. 627)

●风门[fēng mén] 经穴名。出《针灸甲乙经》。属足太阳膀胱经，为督脉、足太阳之会。又名风门热府、热府。〈定位〉在背部，当第二胸椎棘突下，旁开1.5寸(图7)。〈层次解剖〉皮肤→皮下组织→斜方肌→菱形肌→上后锯肌→颈夹肌→竖脊肌。浅层布有第二、三胸神经的内侧皮支和伴行的肋间后动、静脉背侧支的内侧皮支。深层有第二、三胸神经后支的肌支和相应的肋间后动、静脉背侧支的分支等。〈主治〉伤风咳嗽、发热、头痛、目眩、多涕、鼻塞、项强、胸背痛、发背痈疽、胸中热。斜刺0.5～0.8寸；可灸。

Fengmen (BL 12) A meridian point, originally from *Zhenjiu Jia-Yi Jing* (*A-B Classic of Acupuncture and Moxibustion*), a point on the Bladder Meridian of Foot-Taiyang, the crossing point of the Du Meridian and Foot-Taiyang Meridian, also called Fengmenrefu or Refu. 〈Location〉on the back, below he spinous process of the 2nd thoracic vertebra, 1.5 cun lateral to the posterior midline (Fig. 7). 〈Regional anatomy〉skin → subcutaneous tissue→trapezius muscle→rhomboid muscle→ superior posterior serratus muscle → splenius muscle of neck→erector spinal muscle. In the superficial layer, there are the medial cutaneous branches of the posterior branches of the 2nd and 3rd thoracic nerves and the medial cutaneous of the dorsal branches of the accompanying intercostal arteries and veins. In the deep layer, there are the muscular branches of the posterior branches of the 2nd 3rd thoracic nerves and the branches of the dorsal branches of the related posterior intercostal arteries and veins. 〈Indications〉cough due to pathogenic wind, fever, headache, vertigo, profuse nasal discharge, stuffy nose, neck rigidity, pain in the chest and back, lumbodorsal carbuncle and cellulitis, hot sensation in the chest. 〈Method〉Puncture obliquely 0.5～0.8 cun. Moxibustion is applicable.

●风门热府[fēng mén rè fǔ]经穴别名。出《针灸甲乙经》。即风门。详见该条。

Fengmenrefu Another name for Fengmen (BL 12), a meridian point originally from *Zhenjiu Jia-Yi Jing* (*A-B Classic of Acupuncture and Moxibustion*). →风门(p. 113)

●风牵偏视[fēng qiān piān shì] 即斜视。详见该条。

Strabismus due to Wind Pathogen Another name for strabismus. →斜视(p. 506)

●风热丹毒[fēng rè dān dú] 丹毒证型之一。多因表气失于卫固，邪毒乘隙而入所致。其证除见丹毒的一般症状外，多发于面，并见发热恶寒，头痛，骨节酸楚，胃纳不香，便秘溲赤，舌红苔薄白或薄黄，脉洪数。治宜疏风、散热、解毒。取曲池、解溪、委中、风门、阿是穴。

Erysipelas due to the Wind-Heat Pathogen One type of erysipelas. Mostly due to the failure of superficial-qi to protect the body against diseases, leading to the invasion of wind-head evils. 〈Manifestations〉Besides the general symptoms and signs of erysipelas, it is commonly seen on the face, accompanied by fever and chills, headache, aching in joints, poor appetite, constipation and deep-coloured urine, red tongue with thin yellow or thin white coating, surging and rapid pulse. 〈Treatment principle〉Dispel wind and clear heat and toxic material. 〈Point selection〉 Quchi(LI 11), Jiexi(ST 41), Weizhong(BL 40), Fengmen(BL 12) and Ashi point.

●风热感冒[fēng rè gǎn mào] 感冒证型之一。由风热之邪侵袭肺卫，肺失清肃，热郁肌肤所致。证见恶寒轻，发热重，有汗不解，鼻塞而干，咽喉肿痛，口渴，咳嗽，咯痰黄稠，舌苔薄黄，脉浮数。治宜疏风清热，清利肺气。取大椎、尺泽、少商、外关。

Common Cold due to Wind-Heat Pathogen One type of common cold, due to the attack of wind-heat evils upon the lung, leading to the failure of the lung-qi to purify and descend, and the stagnation of wind and heat evils in the skin and superficial muscles. 〈Manifestations〉slight chills but severe fever, sweating, stuffy and dry nose, sore throat, thirst, cough with yellow thick sputum, thin yellow tongue coating, superficial and rapid pulse. 〈Treatment principle〉 Expel wind,

clear heat and normalize the function of lung-qi. 〈Point selection〉Dazhui (DU 14), Chize (LU 5), Shaoshang (LU 11), Waiguan (SJ 5).

● 风热咳嗽[fēng rè ké sòu] 咳嗽证型之一。因风热犯肺,肺失清肃所致。证见咳嗽,痰稠或黄,伴口渴,咽痛,鼻流黄涕,或见身热,恶风,有汗,头痛,舌苔薄黄,脉浮数。治宜疏风清热,宣通肺气。取尺泽、合谷、攒竹、大椎。

Cough due to Wind-Heat Pathogen A type of cough due to wind-heat evils attacking the lung, and impairment of the purifying and descending function of the lung. 〈Manifestations〉cough with thick or yellow sputum, accompanied by thirst, sore throat, yellow nasal discharge, fever, aversion to wind, sweating, headache, thin yellow tongue coating, superficial rapid pulse. 〈Treatment principle〉Expel wind, clear heat and relieve functional disturbance of the lung-qi. 〈Point selection〉Chize (LU 5), Hegu (LI 4), Cuanzhu (BL 2), Dazhui (DU 14).

● 风热瘰疬[fēng rè luǒ lì] 瘰疬证型之一。多因感受风热火毒所致。其证除见瘰疬的一般症状外,兼见发热,头痛,骨节酸痛,苔薄黄,脉浮数。治宜疏风清热。取曲池、支沟、肘尖、章门。参见"肝郁瘰疬"条。

Scrofula due to Wind-Heat Pathogen A type of scrofula, mostly due to the invasion of pathogenic wind, heat and fire. 〈Manifestations〉general symptoms and signs of scrofula, accompanied by fever, headache, aching pain in joints, thin yellow tongue coating, superficial and rapid pulse. 〈Treatment principle〉Expel wind and clear heat. 〈Point selection〉Quchi (LI 11), Zhigou (SJ 6), Zhoujian (EX-UE 1) Zhangmen (LR 13). →肝郁瘰疬 (p. 128)

● 风热头痛[fēng rè tóu tòng] 头痛证型之一。见《外台秘要》卷十五。由风热上扰清窍所致。证见头痛而胀,甚则头痛如裂,发热或恶风,面红目赤,口渴欲饮,便秘溲黄。舌红苔黄,脉浮数。治宜疏风清热。取风池、太阳、合谷、陷谷、尺泽、大椎。

Headache due to Wind-Heat Pathogen A type of headache, seen in Vol. 15 of *Waitai Miyao* (*Clandestine Essentials from the Imperial Library*). Due to pathogenic wind-heat moving up to disturb the brain orifices. 〈Manifestations〉distending headache, even splitting headache, fever, aversion to wind, flushed face and conjunctival congestion, thirst relieved by drinking, constipation and deep-colored urine, red tongue with yellow coating, superficial rapid pulse. 〈Treatment principle〉Expel wind and clear heat. 〈Point selection〉Fengchi (GB 20), Taiyang (EX-HN 5), Hegu (LI 4), Xiangu (ST 43), Chize (LU 5) and Dazhui (DU 14).

● 风热咽喉肿痛[fēng rè yān hóu zhǒng tòng] 咽喉肿痛证型之一。因风热犯肺,热邪熏灼肺系所致。证见咽喉红肿疼痛,恶寒发热,咳嗽声嘶,痰多粘稠,喉间如有物梗阻,吞咽不利,苔薄,脉浮数。治宜疏风清热利咽。取少商、尺泽、合谷、曲池。

Sore Throat due to Wind-Heat Pathogen A type of sore throat due to pathogenic wind-heat attacking the lung, and heat evil cauterizing the lung system. 〈Manifestations〉pain and swelling of the throat, chills, fever, hoarseness due to cough, profuse and viscous sputum, obstructed feeling in throat, dysphagia, thin tongue coating, superficial and rapid pulse. 〈Treatment principle〉Expel wind and clear away heat to relieve sore throat. 〈Point selection〉Shaoshang (LU 11), Chize (LU 5), Hegu (LI 4) and Quchi (LI 11).

● 风热眼[fēng rè yǎn] 即目赤肿痛的别名。详见该条。

Eye Disease due to Wind-Heat Pathogen Another name for redness, pain and swelling of the eye. →目赤肿痛 (p. 271)

● 风湿化热型牛皮癣[fēng shī huà rè xíng niú pí xuǎn] 牛皮癣症型之一。多由于风湿热三邪蕴阻肌肤荆忽所致。病程较短,其证除见牛皮癣的一般症状外,患部皮疹伴有潮红,糜烂,湿润和血痂,苔脉黄或黄腻,脉濡数。治宜疏风清热利湿。取阴陵泉、太白、太渊、风池、阿是穴。参见"牛皮癣"条。

Neurodermatitis due to Heat-Transformation of Wind-Damp Pathogen One type of neurodermatitis, mostly caused by the stagnation of wind, damp and heat pathogens in the superficial muscle skin and meridians. 〈Manifestations〉short course of disease, besides the

general symptoms of neurodermatitis, erythra accompanied by flare, anabrosis, wet and blood crusted rashes, thin and yellow or yellow greasy tongue coating, soft and rapid pulse. 〈Treatment principle〉Dispel wind, clear heat and promote diuresis. 〈Point selection〉Yinlingquan (SP 9), Taibai (SP 3), Taiyuan (LU 9), Fengchi (GB 20), Ashi point. →牛皮癣(p. 285)

●风湿头痛[fēng shī tóu tòng] 头痛证型之一。见《赤水玄珠》卷三。由风邪外袭，湿浊上蒙所致。证见头痛如裹，肢体困重，胸闷纳呆，小便不利，大便溏泄，舌苔白腻，脉濡。治宜祛风化湿。取风池、通天、耳和髎、合谷、三阳络、阴陵泉。

Headache due to Wind-Damp Pathogen A type of headache originally seen in Vol. 3 of *Chishui Xuanzhu* (*Black Pearl of the Red River*). Due to the invasion of wind evil, and turbid dampness rising in the head. 〈Manifestations〉headache with a bound feeling all over the head, heavy sensation in the body and limbs, oppressive feeling in the chest, anorexia, diguria, loose stool, white and greasy tongue coating, soft pulse. 〈Treatment principle〉Expel wind and eliminate dampness. 〈Point selection〉Fengchi (GB 20), Tongtian (BL 7), Erheliao (SJ 22), Hegu (LI 4), Sanyangluo (SJ 8), Yinlingquan (SP 9).

●风市[fēng shì] 经穴名。原为经外穴。出《肘后备急方》。《针灸大成》归于少阳胆经。又名垂手。〈定位〉在大腿外侧部的中线上，当腘横纹上7寸。或直立垂手时，中指尖处(图8)。〈层次解剖〉皮肤→皮下组织→髂胫束→股外侧肌→股中间肌。浅层布有股外侧皮神经。深层有旋股外侧动脉降支和股神经的肌支。主治中风半身不遂、下肢痿痹、麻木、遍身搔痒、脚气。直刺1～1.5寸；可灸。

Fengshi (GB 31) A meridian point, originally an extra point, from *Zhouhou Beiji Fang* (*A Handbook of Prescriptions for Emergencies*), classified on the Gallbladder Meridian of Foot-Shaoyang in *Zhenjiu Dazheng* (*A Great Compendium of Acupuncture and Moxibustion*), also called Chuishou. 〈Location〉on the lateral midline of the thigh, 7 cun above the popliteal crease, or at the place touching the tip of the middle finger when the patient stands erect with the arms hanging down freely (Fig. 8). 〈Regional anatomy〉skin→subcutaneous tissue→iliotibial tract→lateral muscle of thigh→intermediate vastus muscle of thigh. In the superficial layer, there is the lateral cutaneous nerve of the thigh. In the deep layer, there are the muscular branches of the descending branches of the lateral circumflex femoral artery and the muscular branches of the femoral nerve. 〈Indications〉hemiplegia due to apoplexy, muscular atrophy of the lower limbs with pain and numbness, general pruritus, beriberi. 〈Method〉Puncture perpendicularly 1～1.5 cun. Moxibustion is applicable.

●风溪[fēng xī] 耳穴名。又称过敏区、荨麻疹点。位于指与腕两穴之间。具有祛风止痒作用。用于治疗荨麻疹、皮肤搔痒症、哮喘、过敏性鼻炎。

Fengxi (MA) An otopoint, also called Allergic Area or Urticaria Point. 〈Location〉at the midpoint between Finger (MA-SF 1) and Wrist (MA-SF 2). 〈Indications〉urticaria, cutaneous praritus, asthma, allergic rhinitis.

●风眩[fēng xuàn] ①癫痫的别称。见《千金要方》。详见"癫痫"条。②指因风邪引起的晕眩。

Feng Xuan ① Another name for epilepsy, seen in *Qianjin Yaofang* (*Essential Prescriptions Worth a Thousand Gold*). →癫痫(p. 80) ② Referring to dizziness due to wind pathogen.

●风岩[fēng yán] 经外穴名。出《山东医刊》。在后发际中点与耳垂下缘连线中点前方0.5寸处。主治癫狂、脏躁、头痛，以及神经衰弱、癔病等。直刺1～1.5寸。

Fengyan (EX-HN) An extra point, originally from *Shandong Yikan* (*Shandong Journal of Medicine*). 〈Location〉at the part 0.5 cun anterior to the midpoint of the line connecting the midpoint of the posterior hairline and the lower border of the earlobe. 〈Indications〉manic-depressive psycnosis, hysteria, headache, neurosis, mythoplasty, etc. 〈Method〉Puncture perpendicularly 1～1.5 cun.

●风眼[fēng yǎn] 经外穴名。见《经外奇穴治疗诀》。在拇指桡侧缘，当指关节横纹头赤白肉际处。〈主治〉心腹烦满、呕吐、呃逆、五指尽痛、屈伸不利、雀目、翳障等。直刺0.1～0.2寸；可灸。

Fengyan (EX-UE)　An extra point, seen in *Jingwai Qixue Zhiliao Jue* (*Pithy Formulas for Treatment with Extra Points*). 〈Location〉 on the radial border of the thumb, at the junction of the red and white skin and at the end of the crease of the phalangeal joint of hand. 〈Indications〉 irritability, fullness of the abdomen, vomiting, hiccup, pain in all fingers, difficulty in bending and extending fingers, night blindness, nebula, etc. 〈Method〉 Puncture perpendicularly 0.1～0.2 cun. Moxibustion is applicable.

●风疹[fēng zhěn]　病名。是一种常见的皮肤病，又有荨麻疹、瘾疹、风疹块等名称。其特征是皮肤上出现鲜红色的瘙痒性风疹团，此起彼伏，疏密不一，发病迅速，但消退也快。本病多因腠理不固，风邪侵袭，遏于肌肤；或体质差异，不耐鱼虾荤腥等食物；或患肠道寄生虫病，导致胃肠积热，外郁肌表所致。临床分为外感风疹和胃热风疹两种。参见各条。

Rubella　A common dermatosis, also called urticaria, hidden rash and wheal, characterized by bright red itching wheals on the skin, which appear here and there with uneven density, quick onset and disappearance. Mostly due to the invasion and obstruction of wind pathogen in the superficial muscles and skin resulting from the failure of the skin straie to resist exterior pathogens; or to constitutional allergies to seafood such as fish, shrimp and meat, oily food, etc.; or to heat accumulation in the stomach and intestines leading to head stagnation in the superficial muscles and skin resulting from intestinal aseariasis. It is clinically divided into two types: rubella due to exterior pathogens and rubella due to stomach heat. →外感风疹(p. 453)、胃热风疹(p. 466)

●风疹块[fēng zhěn kuài]　即风疹。详见该条。

Wheal　→风疹(p. 116)

●锋针[fēng zhēn]　针具名。出《灵枢·九针十二原》。古代九针之一。长一寸六分，针身圆柱状，针尖锋利，呈三棱形。后人称三棱针。用于点刺泻血、排脓。治疗痈肿、热病等。

Lance Needle　An acupuncture needle, originally from *Lingshu: Jiu Zhen Shier Yuan* [*Miraculous Pivot: Nine Needles and Twelve Yuan (Primary) Points*]. The needle is cylindrical, 1.6 cun long. Its sharp tip has a three-edged shape. It is later called the three-edged needle. It is used for bloodletting by pricking and discharging pus. 〈Indications〉 carbuncle, swelling, acute febrile disease, etc.

●冯衢[féng qú]　人名。清代女医家，又名樽宜，江苏丹徒(今镇江)人。擅长挑针，以治痈疽、发背。

Feng Qu　A woman physician of the Qing Dynasty, also named Zun Yi, a native of Dantu (now Zhengjiang, Jiangsu Provines). She was good at applying the pricking therapy to treat lumbodorsal carbuncles and cellulitis.

●冯卓怀[féng zhuó huái]　人名。清代针灸家，于同治年间(1862～1874年)订正《太乙神针方》。

Feng Zhuohuai　An expert of acupuncture and moxibustion in the Qing Dynasty, who amended *Taiyi Shenzhen Fang* (*Recipes of Great Monad Herbal Moxa Stick*) in the reign of Tong Zhi(1862-1874).

●凤凰展翅[fèng huáng zhǎn chì]　针刺手法名。为赤凤迎源之别称。详见该条。

Pheonix Spreading the Wings　An acupuncture technique, another name for red pheonix encountering the sourse. →赤凤迎源(p. 47)

●跗[fū]　部位名。指足背，又称跌或足跌。

Instep　A part of the body, referring to the dorsum of foot, also called dorsum padis or back of foot.

●跗阳[fū yáng]　经穴名。出《针灸甲乙经》。属足太阳膀胱经，为阳跷之郄。〈定位〉在小腿后面，外踝后，昆仑穴直上3寸(图35)。〈层次解剖〉皮肤→皮下组织→腓骨短肌→长屈肌。浅层布有腓肠神经和小隐静脉。深层有胫神经的分支和胫后动、静脉的肌支。主治头重、头痛、腰腿痛、下肢瘫痪、外踝红肿。直刺0.5～1寸；可灸。

Fuyang (BL 59)　A meridian point originally from *Zhenjiu Jiayi Jing* (*A-B Classic of Acupuncture and Moxibustion*), a point on the Bladder Meridian of Foot-Taiyang, the Xi (Cleft) point of the Yangqiao Meridian. 〈Location〉 on the posterior side of the leg, posterior to the lateral malleolus, 3 cun directly above Kunlun (BL 60) (Fig. 35). 〈Regional anatomy〉 skin → subcutaneous tissue → short peroneal muscle → long flexor muscle of great

toe. In the superficial layer, there are the sural nerve and small saphenous vein. In the deep layer, there are the branches of the tibial nerve and the muscular branches of the posterior tibial artery and vein. ⟨Indications⟩heavy sensation in the head, headache, pain in the waist and legs, paralysis of the lower limbs, redness and swelling of the external malleolus. ⟨Method⟩Puncture perpendicularly 0.5~1 cun. Moxibustion is applicable.

●伏白[fú bái] 经穴别名。出《针灸甲乙经》，即复溜。详见该条。

Fubai Another name for Fuliu (KI 7), a meridian point originally from *Zhenjiu Jia-Yi Jing* (*A-B Classic of Acupuncture and Moxibustion*). →复溜(p. 121)

●伏冲之脉[fú chōng zhī mài] 经络名。出《灵枢·岁露》。又名伏膂之脉。指冲脉之伏行于脊内者。因其最深，故名。

Deep-Sited Chong Meridian Name of a meridian, originally from *Lingshu: Sui Lu* (*Miraculous Pivot: On Exopathic Wind and Rain*), also named deep-sited meridian in the spine, referring to the branch of the Chong Meridian with a deep course through the spine. It is so named because of its deep course.

●伏溜[fú liū] 经穴别名。出《千金要方》。即复溜。详见该条。

Fuliu Another name for Fuliu (KI 7), a meridian point originally from *Qianjin Yaofang* (*Essential Prescriptions Worth a Thousand Gold*). →复溜(p. 121)

●伏膂之脉[fú lǚ zhī mài] 经络名。又名伏冲之脉。详见该条。

Deep-Sited Meridian in the Spine Name of a meridian, also named the deep-sited Chong Meridian. →伏冲之脉(p. 117)

●伏兔[fú tù] ①经穴名。出《灵枢·经脉》。属足阳明胃经。又名外勾。⟨定位⟩在大腿前面，当髂前上棘与髌底外侧端的连线上，髌底上6寸(图60)。⟨层次解剖⟩皮肤→皮下组织→股直肌→股中间肌。浅层布有股外侧静脉，股神经前皮支及股外侧皮神经。深层有旋股外侧动、静脉的降支，股神经的肌支。⟨主治⟩腰髋疼痛、腰膝寒冷、麻痹、脚气、疝气、腹胀。直刺0.6~1.2寸；可灸。②人体部位名。出《灵枢·经脉》。指大腿前方肌肉。相当股直肌隆起部。因其形如伏兔，故名。

1. **Futu**(ST 32) A meridian point originally from *Ling Shu: Jingmai* (*Miraculous Pivot: Meridians*), also called waigou, a point on the Stomach Meridian of Foot-Yangming. ⟨Location⟩ on the anterior side of the thigh and on the line connecting the anteriosuperior iliac spine and the superiolateral corner of the patella, 6 cun above this corner (Fig. 60). ⟨Regional anatomy⟩ Skin→subcutaneous tissue→rectus muscle of thigh→intermediate vastus muscle of thigh. In the superficial layer, there are the lateral femoral vein, the anterior cutaneous branches of the femoral nerve and the lateral cutaneous nerve of the thigh. In the deep layer, there are the descending branches of the lateral cirumflex artery and vein and the muscular branches of the femoral nerve. ⟨Indications⟩lumbo-iliac pain, cold lumbar and knee, numbness, beriberi, hernia, abdominal distension. ⟨Method⟩puncture perpendicularly 0.6-1.2 cun. Moxibustion is applicable.

2. **Futu** A part of the body, originally from *Lingshu: Jingmai* (*Miraculous Pivot: Meridians*), referring to the anterior muscles of the thigh, almost equivalent to the prominent portion of the musculus rectus femoris. It is so named in Chinese for its shape resembling a prostrate hare.

●伏羲[fú xī] 人名。传说中中华民族的祖先，教民渔猎、畜牧和医药，据说是九针的创制者。

Fu Xi The legendary ancestor of the Chinese, who taught people how to fish, hunt, raise livestock and use medicine. He is said to have been the inventor of the Nine Needles.

●伏针、伏灸[fú zhēn、fú jiǔ] 针灸术语。指在盛夏三伏天进行针灸。因三伏天气候炎热，阳气升发，一些慢性疾病和秋冬季容易发作的咳嗽、哮喘等症，在此治疗能起到良好的防治作用。

Acupuncture and Moxibustion in the Dog-Days A term for acupuncture and moxibustion, referring to acupuncture and moxibustion in hot, summer days. The method has good preventive and curative effects on some chron-

●扶承[fú chéng] 经穴别名。出《针灸甲乙经》。即承扶。详见该条。

Fucheng Another name for Chengfu (BL 36), a meridian point originally from *Zhenjiu Jia-Yi Jing* (*A-B Classic of Acupuncture and Moxibustion*). →承扶(p.42)

●扶突[fú tū] 经穴名。出《灵枢·本输》。属手阳明大肠经。又名水穴。〈定位〉在颈外侧部，结喉旁，当胸锁乳突肌的前、后缘之间（图6和图28）。〈层次解剖〉皮肤→皮下组织→胸锁乳突肌的胸骨头与锁骨头之间→颈血管鞘的后缘。浅层内有颈横神经，颈阔肌等结构。深层有颈血管鞘。〈主治〉咳嗽、气喘、咽喉肿痛、暴喑、瘿气、瘰疬。直刺0.5~0.8寸；可灸。

Futu (LI 18) A meridian point originally from *Ling Shu: Benshu* (*Miraculous Pivot: Meridian Points*), also named Shuixue, a point on the Large Intestine Meridian of Hand-Yangming. 〈Location〉on the lateral side of the neck, beside the laryngeal protuberance, between the anterior and posterior borders of the sternocleidomastoid muscle (Figs. 6&28). 〈Regional anatomy〉skin→subcutaneous tissue →between sternal head and clavicular head of sternocleidomastoid muscle→posterior border of carotid sheath. In the superficial layer, there are the transverse nerve of the neck and the platysma muscle. In the deep layer, there is the carotid sheath. 〈Indications〉cough, dyspnea, sore throat, sudden loss of voice, goiter, scrofula. 〈Method〉Puncture perpendicularly 0.5~0.8 cun. Moxibustion is applicable.

●浮白[fú bái] 经穴名。出《素问·气穴论》。属足少阳胆经，为足太阳、少阳之会。〈定位〉在头部，当耳后乳突的后上方，天冲与完骨的弧形连线中的1/3与上1/3交点处（图28和图31）。〈层次解剖〉皮肤→皮下组织→帽状腱膜。布有枕小神经和枕大神经的吻合支以及耳后动、静脉。〈主治〉头痛、颈项强痛、耳鸣、耳聋、齿痛、瘰疬、瘿气、臂痛不举、足痿不行。平刺0.5~0.8寸；可灸。

Fubai (GB 10) A meridian point, originally from *Suwen: Qixue Lun* (*Plain Questions: On Loci of Qi*), a point on the Gallbladder Meridan of Foot-Shaoyang, the crossing point of the Meridians of Foot-Taiyang and Foot-Shaoyang. 〈Location〉on the head, posterior and superior to the mastoid process, at the junction of the middle third and upper third of the curved line connecting Tianchong (GB 9) and Wangu (GB 12) (Figs. 28&31). 〈Regional anatomy〉skin→subcutaneous tissue→epicranial aponeurosis. There are the anastomotic branches of the lesser and greater occipital nerves and the posterior auricular artery and vein in this area. 〈Indications〉headache, pain and stiffness of the neck and nape, tinnitus, deafness, toothache, scrofula, goiter, pain when raising the arm, paralytic foot. 〈Method〉Puncture subcutaneously 0.5~0.8 cun. Moxibustion is applicable.

●浮刺[fú cì] 刺法名。见《灵枢·官针》。是十二针刺之一。此法是从旁斜向刺入，而且要浮浅，以治疗肌肉因寒而拘急的病症。因其针刺浮浅，故名。近代应用的皮内针，即由此演变而来。

Superficial Puncture A needling technique, seen in *Ling Shu: Guanzhen* (*Miraculous Pivot: Official Needles*), one of the twelve needlings techniques. 〈Method〉Puncture obliquely and shallowly from the side of the affected area. 〈Indications〉diseases of muscular spasm due to cold. It is so named for its shallow puncture. The modern intradermal needle therapy developed from it.

●浮络[fú luò] 络脉名。出《素问·皮部论》。指位于浅表部的络脉。临床可根据其部位和色泽的变化诊断疾病，也可以进行放血治疗。

Superficial Collaterals Name of one kind of collateral, originally from *Su Wen: Pi Bu Lun* (*Plain Questions: On Cutaneous Regions*), referring to the collaterals in the superficial area. In the clinic, diseases can be diagnosed through changes in their location, color and lustre. The collaterals can also be punctured to cause bleeding.

●浮郄[fú xì] 经穴名。出《针灸甲乙经》。属足太阳膀胱经。〈定位〉在腘横纹外侧端，委阳上一寸，股二头肌腱的内侧（图35）。〈层次解剖〉皮肤→皮下组织→股二头肌腱内侧→腓肠肌外侧头。浅层布有股后

皮神经。深层有腓总神经，腓肠外侧皮神经和膝上外侧动、静脉等。〈主治〉臀股麻木、腘筋挛急。直刺0.5～1寸；可灸。

Fuxi（BL 38） A meridian point originally from *Zhenjiu Jiayi Jing*（*A-B Classic of Acupuncture and Moxibustion*），a point on the Bladder Meridian of Foot-Taiyang.〈Location〉at the lateral end of the popliteal crease, 1 cun above Weiyang（BL 39），medial to the tendon of the biceps muscle of the thigh（Fig. 35）.〈Reginal anatomy〉skin→subcutaneous tissue→medial border of tendon of biceps muscle of thigh→lateral head of gastrocnemius muscle. In the superficial layer, there is the posterior femoral cutaneous nerve. In the deep layer, there are the common peroneal nerve, the tateral cutaneous nerve of the calf and the lateral superior genicular artery and vein.〈Indications〉numbness of gluteal and femoral regions, cramp of tendons in the popliteal fossa.〈Method〉Puncture perpendicularly 0.5～1 cun. Moxibustion is applicable.

●浮肿者治其经[fú zhǒng zhě zhì qí jīng]《内经》取穴法则之一。指对面部浮肿等症，可取用有关经脉五输中的经穴。

Treating Edema by Selecting the Jing（River）Point One of the principles of point selection in *Neijin*（*The Inner Canon of Huangdi*），referring to selecting the Jing（River）point of the Five-Shu Points of relevant meridians to treat fivial edema, etc.

●涪翁[fú wēng] 人名。东汉针灸学家。其针灸造诣很深，著有《针经》、《诊脉法》。均失传。其弟子程高、再传弟子郭玉，均为当时著名针灸家。

Fu Weng An acupuncture-moxibustion expert in the Eastern Han Dynasty. Having a profound knowledge of acupuncture and moxibustion, he compiled *Zhenjing*（*Canon of Acupuncture*）and *Zhenmai Fa*（*Methods of Feeling the Pulse*），both of which are no longer extant. His apprentice Cheng Gao and Cheng Gao's apprentice Guo Yu were both famous acupuncture-moxibustion experts of the time.

●府舍[fǔ shè] 经穴名。出《针灸甲乙经》。属足太阴脾经，为足太阴、厥阴、阴维之会。〈定位〉在下腹部，当脐下4寸，冲门上方0.7寸，距前正中线4寸（图39和图40）。〈层次解剖〉皮肤→皮下组织→腹外斜肌腱膜→腹内斜肌→腹横肌。浅层布有旋髂浅动、静脉的分支或属支，第十一、十二胸神经前支和第一腰神经前支的外侧皮支。深层有第十一、十二胸神经和第一腰神经前支的肌支及伴行的动、静脉。〈主治〉腹痛、疝气、腹满积聚、霍乱、吐泻。直刺0.5～1寸；可灸。

Fushe（SP 13） A meidian point, originally from *Zhenjiu Jiayi Jing*（*A-B Classic of Acupuncture and Moxibustion*），a point on the Spleen Meridian of Foot-Taiyin, the crossing point of the Meridians of Foot-Taiyin and Foot-Jueyin and Yinwei.〈Location〉on the lower abdomen, 4 cun below the centre of the umbilicus, 0.7 cun above Chongmen（SP 12），and 4 cun lateral to the anterior midline（Figs. 39&40）.〈Regional anatomy〉skin→subcutaneous tissue→aponeurosis of external oblique muscle of abdomen→internal oblique muscle of abdomen→transverse muscle of abdomen. In the superficial layer, there are the branches or tributaries of the superficial circumflex iliac artery and vein, the lateral cutaneous branches of the anterior branches of the 11th and 12th thoracic nerves and the 1st lumbar nerve. In the deep layer, there are the anterior branches of the 11th and 12th thoracic nerves and the 1st lumbar nerve and their accompanying arteries and veins.〈Indications〉abdominal pain, hernia, abdominal mass and fullness, cholera morbus, vomiting and diarrhea.〈Method〉Puncture perpendicularly 0.5～1 cun. Moxibustion is applicable.

●府中俞[fǔ zhōng shū] 经穴别名。出《针灸大全》。即中府。详见该条。

Fuzhong Another name for Zhongfu（LU 1），a meridian point, originally from *Zhenjiu Daquan*（*A Complete Work of Acupuncture and Moxibustion*）.→中府（p.609）

●俯伏坐位[fǔ fú zuò wèi] 针灸体位名。患者身体正坐，两臂屈伏于案上，头往前倾或伏于臂上，面部朝下的体位。适用于取后头、项、背部的腧穴。

Sitting in Flexion A posture adopted in acupuncture and moxibustion treatment. The patient sits at the table with his arms pronated

on it, his head bent forward or lying on the arms with the face downward, suitable for selecting points on the back of the head, the nape and the back.

●俯卧位[fǔ wò wèi] 针灸体位名。患者身体俯卧于床,头面、胸腹朝下的体位。适用于取头、项、脊背、腰尻部及下肢背侧和上肢的部分腧穴。

Prone Position A posture adopted in acupuncture and moxibustion treament, referring to a posture the patient takes on the bed with the face, chest and abdomen down. This position is suitable for selecting points on the head, back, lumbar and buttock regions the posterior part of the lower limbs and Shu points in the upper limbs.

●辅骨[fǔ gǔ] 部位名。指膝两侧之骨,其内名内辅,其外名外辅。外辅骨还指腓骨。

Fu Gu A body part, referring to the bones at the two sides of the knee, the inside one is called the medial side-bone of the knee while the outside is called lateral side-bone of the knee, which also refers to the fibule.

●辅助手法[fǔ zhù shǒu fǎ] 针刺术语。与基本手法相对而言。系指针刺操作过程所应用的一些配合手法,用于确定穴位,帮助进出针,调节针刺感应。包括循法、弹法、刮法、摇法、飞法、搗法等。详见各条。

Auxiliary Manipulations A term for acupuncture and moxibustion to the subordinate manipulations applied in the needling process to determine points, help insert and withdraw the needle, and regulate the needling sensation. They include Massage Along Meridian Manipulation, Scraping Manipulation, Shaking Manipulation, Flying Manipulation, Flicking Manipulation, and Lifting-Thrusting Manipulation, etc. →循法(p. 531)、弹法(p. 423)、刮法(p. 146)、摇法(p. 547)、飞法(p. 105)、搗法(p. 77)

●附分[fǔ fēn] 经穴名。出《针灸甲乙经》。属足太阳膀胱经。为手、足太阳之会。〈定位〉在背部,当第二胸椎棘突下,旁开3寸(图7)。〈层次解剖〉皮肤→皮下组织→斜方肌→菱形肌→上后锯肌→竖脊肌。浅层布有第二、三胸神经后支的皮支和伴行的动、静脉。深层有肩胛背神经、肩胛背动、静脉,第二、三在胸神经后支的肌支和相应的肋间动、静脉背侧支的分支或属支。〈主治〉肩背拘急、颈项强痛、肘臂麻木不仁。斜刺0.5～0.8寸;可灸。

Fufen(BL 41) A meridian point, originally from *Zhenjiu Jia-Yi Jing* (*A-B Classic of Acupuncture and Moxibustion*), a point on the Bladder Meridian of Foot-Taiyang and the crossing point of the Taiyang Meridians of Hand and Foot. 〈Location〉on the back, below the spinous process of the 2nd thoracic vertebra, 3 cun lateral to the posterior midline (Fig. 7). 〈Reglonal anatomy〉skin→subcutaneous tissue → trapezius muscle → rhomboid muscle→superior posterior serratus muscle→erector spinal muscle. In the superficial layer, there are the cutaneous branches of the posterior branches of the 2nd and 3rd thoracic nerves and the accompaning arteries and veins. In the deep layer, there are the dorsal scapular nerve, the dorsal scapular artery and vein, the muscular branches of the posterior branches of the 2nd and 3rd thoracic nerves and the branches or tributaries of the dorsal branches of the related posterior intercostal arteries and veins. 〈Indications〉contracting feeling in the shoulder and back, stiffness and pain of the nape and neck and numbness of the elbow and arms. 〈Method〉 Puncture obliquely 0.5～0.8 cun. Moxibustion is applicable.

●附子饼[fù zǐ bǐng] 灸用药饼的一种。见《外科理例·论附子饼》。用附子研为细末,以温水调和作成饼状,厚2～3分,中间可穿刺数孔,以利施灸。

Monkshood Cake A kind of medicinal cake for moxibustion, originally from *Waike Lili*: *Lun Fuzi Bing*(*Theory and Case Reports*: *On External Disease*). To prepare: Grind monkshood into powder and mix it with warm water to make small cakes of about 0.2～0.3 cun thick, then make several holes in the centre for moxibustion.

●附子灸[fù zǐ jiǔ] 间接灸的一种。为隔附子灸之别称。详见该条。

Fu Zi(**Monkshood**) **Moxibustion** Another name for Fu Zi(Monkshood)-separated moxibustion, a form of indirect moxibustion. →隔附子灸(p. 135)

●复留[fù liú] 经穴别名。出《灵枢·本输》。即复

溜。详见该条。

Fuliu　Another name for Fuliu (KI 7), a meridian point, originally from *Lingshu: Benshu* (*Miraculous Pivot: Meridian Points*). → 复溜(p.121)

●复溜[fù liū]　经穴名。见《灵枢·本输》。属足少阴肾经，为本经经穴。又名复留、伏留、昌阳、伏白。〈定位〉在小腿内侧，太溪直上2寸，跟腱的前方(图49和图82)。〈层次解剖〉皮肤→皮下组织→跖肌腱和跟腱前方→拇长屈肌。浅层布有隐神经的小腿内侧皮支，大隐静脉的属支。深层有胫神经和胫后动、静脉。〈主治〉泄泻、肠鸣、水肿、腹胀、腿肿、足痿、盗汗、脉微细时无、身热无汗、腰脊强痛。直刺0.8~1寸；可灸。

Fuliu (KI 7)　A meridian point, originally from *Ling Shu: Ben Shu* (*Miraculous Pivot: Meridian Points*), the Jing (River) point of the Kidney Meridian of Foot-Shaoyin, also named Changyang and Fubai. 〈Location〉on the medial side of the leg, 2 cun directly above Taixi (KI 3), anterior to the achilles tendon (Figs. 49&82). 〈Regional anatomy〉skin→subcutaneous tissue→anterior side of tendon of plantar muscle and Archilles tendon→long flexor of great toe. In the superficial layer, there are the medial cutaneous branches of the saphenous nerve to the leg and the tributaries of the great saphenous vein. In the deep layer, there are the tibial nerve and the posterior tibial artery and vein. 〈Indications〉diarrhea, borborygmus, edema, abdominal distention, swelling in the legs muscular atrophy of the foot, night sweating, feeble thready pulse with frequent intermission, feverish body without sweating, pain and stiffness along the spinal column. 〈Method〉Puncture perpendicularly 0.8~1 cun. Moxibustion is applicable.

●腹[fù]　①耳穴名。位于腰骶椎内侧近耳腔缘。〈主治〉腹痛、腹胀、腹泻、急性腰扭伤。②部位名。胸以下，脐之上下左右都称腹，俗名肚子。又脐以上称上腹；脐以下称少腹或小腹。又说脐下称小腹，脐下两旁为少腹。又说脐以下称小腹。

1. Abdomen (MA)　An auricular point. 〈Location〉on the medial side of the lumbrosacral vertebrae (MA), proximal to the border of the cavum conchae. 〈Indication〉abdominal pain, and distention, diarrhea and acute lumbar muscle sprain.

2. Abdomen　A body part, referring to the region below the chest and around the umbilicus, commonly called the belly. Another interpretation is that the region above the umbilicus is called the upper abdomen and the region below the umbilicus is called the small or lower abdomen; a third interpretation is that the region below the umbilicus is called the small abdomen and the regions beside it are called the lower abdomen; yet another interpretation is that the region below the umbilicus is called the small abdomen.

●腹哀[fù āi]　经穴名。出《针灸甲乙经》。属足太阴脾经，为足太阴、阴维之会。〈定位〉在上腹部，当脐中上3寸，距前正中线4寸(图39和图40)。〈层次解剖〉皮肤→皮下组织→腹外斜肌→腹内斜肌→腹横肌。浅层布有第七、八、九胸神经前支的外侧皮支和胸腹壁静脉的属支。深层有第七、八、九胸神经前支的肌支及伴行的动、静脉。〈主治〉腹痛、肠鸣、消化不良、便秘、痢疾。直刺0.5~1寸；可灸。

Fuai (SP 16)　A meridian point, originally from *Zhenjiu Jia-Yi Jing* (*A-B Classic of Acupuncture and Moxibustion*). A point on the Spleen Meridian of Foot-Taiyin and the crossing point of the Meridians of Foot-Taiyin and Yinwei. 〈Location〉on the upper abdomen, 3 cun above the centre of the umbilicus, and 4 cun lateal to the anterior midline (Figs. 39&40). 〈Regional anatomy〉skin→subcutaneous tissue→external oblique muscle of abdomen→internal oblique muscle of abdomen→transverse muscle of abdomen. In the superficial layer, there are the lateral cutaneous branches of the anterior branches of the 7th of 9th thoracic nerves and the tributaries of the thoracoepigastric vein. In the deep layer, there are the muscular branches of the anterior branches of the 7th to 9th thoracic nerves and their accompanying arteries and veins. 〈Indications〉abdominal pain, borborygmus, indigestion, constipation and dysentery. 〈Method〉Puncture perpendicularly 0.5~1 cun. Moxibustion is applicable.

●腹结[fù jié]　经穴名。出《针灸甲乙经》。属足太阴

脾经。又名腹屈、肠结、肠窟。〈定位〉在下腹部,大横下1.3寸,距前正中线4寸(图39和图40)。〈层次解剖〉皮肤→皮下组织→腹外斜肌→腹内斜肌→腹横肌。浅层有第十、十一、十二胸神经前支的外侧皮支,胸腹壁静脉的属支。深层有第十、十一、十二胸神经前支的肌支及伴行的动、静脉。主治绕脐腹痛、疝气、泄泻。直刺0.8～1.2寸;可灸。

Fujie(SP 14) A meridian point, originally from *Zhenjiu Jia-Yi Jing* (*A-B Classic of Acupuncture and Moxibustion*), a point of the Spleen Meridian of Foot-Taiyin, also named Fuqu, Changjie and Changku. 〈Location〉on the lower abdomen, 1.3 cun below Daheng (SP 15), and 4 cun lateral to the anterior midline(Figs. 39&40). 〈Regional anatomy〉skin→subcutaneous tissue→external oblique muscle of abdomen→internal oblique muscle of abdomen→transverse muscle of abdomen. In the superficial layer, there are the lateral cutaneous branches of the anterior branches of the 10th to 12th thoracic nerves and the tributaries of the thoracoepigastric vein. In the deep layer, there are the muscular branches of the anterior branches of the 10th to 12th thoracic nerves and their accompanying arteries and veins. 〈Indications〉 abdominal pain around the umbilicus, hernia and diarrhea. 〈Method〉Puncture perpendicularly 0.8～1.2 cun. Moxibustion is applicable.

●腹屈[fù qū] 经穴别名。出《针灸甲乙经》。即腹结。详见该条。

Fuqu Another name for Fujie(SP 14), a meridian point originally from *Zhenjiu Jia-Yi Jing*(*A-B Classic of Acupunture and Moxibustion*)→腹结(p.121)

●腹通谷[fù tōng gǔ] 经穴名。出《针灸甲乙经》。原名通谷。属足少阴肾经,为冲脉、足少阴之会。〈定位〉在上腹部,当脐中上5寸,前正中线旁开0.5寸(图40)。〈层次解剖〉皮肤→皮下组织→腹直肌鞘前壁→腹直肌。浅层布有腹壁浅静脉和第六、七、八胸神经前支的前皮支及伴行的动、静脉。深层有腹壁上动、静脉的分支或属支,第六、七、八胸神经前支的肌支和相应的肋间动、静脉。〈主治〉腹痛、腹胀、呕吐、心痛、心悸、胸痛、暴暗。直刺或斜刺0.5～0.8寸;可灸。

Futonggu(KI 20) A meridian point, originally from *Zhenjiu Jia-Yi Jing* (*A-B Classic of Acupuncture and Moxibustion*), originally named Tonggu, a point on the kidney Meridian of Foot-Shaoyin and the crossing point of the Chong Meridian and the Meridian of Foot-Shaoyin. 〈Location〉on the upper abdomen, 5 cun above the centre of the umbilicus and 0.5 cun lateral to the anterior midline (Fig. 40). 〈Regional anatomy〉skin→subcutaneous tissue → anterior sheath of rectus straight muscle of abdomen→rectus muscle of abdomen. In the superficial layer, there are the superficial epigastric vein, the anterior cutaneous branches of the anterior branches of th 6th to 8th thoracic nerves and the accompanying arteries and veins. In the deep layer, there are the branches or tributaries of the superior epigastric artery and vein, the muscular branches of the anterior branches of the 6th to 8th thoracic nerves and the related intercostal arteries and veins. 〈Indications〉abdominal pain and distention, vomiting, precordial pain, palpitations, pain in the chest and sudden loss of voice. 〈Method〉Puncture perpendicularly or obliquely 0.5～0.8 cun. Moxibustion is applicable.

●腹痛[fù tòng] 病证名。出《素问·举痛论》等。泛指腹部疼痛而言。可因寒邪内积,饮食停滞,肝郁气滞,脏腑阳虚所引起。临床分为寒邪腹痛、食滞腹痛、肝郁腹痛、阳虚腹痛四种。详见各条。

Abdominal Pain A disease, originally from *Su Wen*: *Jutong Lun* (*Plain Questions*: *On Acute Pains*) and other resources, generally referring to pain in the abdomen, usually caused by internal accumulation of pathogenic cold, retention of food, stagnation of liver-qi due to qi-stagnancy and yang deficiency of the zang-fu organs. In clinic, it is divided into: abdominal pain due to pathogenic cold, abdominal pain due to retention of food, abdominal pain due to stagnation of liver-qi and abdominal pain due to yang deficiency. →寒邪腹痛(p.157), 食滞腹痛(p.387), 肝郁腹痛(p.127), 阳虚腹痛(p.542)

G

● 干脚气 [gān jiǎo qì]　脚气证型之一。见《太平圣惠方》卷四十五。指脚气病足胫不肿者。因素体阴虚内热,湿热、风毒之邪从热化,伤营血,筋脉失养所致。证见两足无力,腿膝麻木疼痛,时感筋肉挛急,活动欠利,足胫肌肉逐渐萎缩,甚至顽麻萎废,便秘溲黄,舌质淡红,苔薄白或少苔,脉细数。治宜养血滋阴。取解溪、阴市、血海、复溜、照海、悬钟。

Dry Beriberi　One type of beriberi, originally from Vol. 45 of *Taiping Shenghui Fang* (*Imperial Benevolent Prescriptions*), referring to beriberi without swelling of the foot and shank, usually due to costitutional yin-deficiency and internal heat, resulting in the transforming of heat an pathogenic wind into pathogenic dam heat and damaging the ying and blood, leading to the malnutrition of tendons and muscles. ⟨Manifestations⟩ Weakness of both feet, numbness and pain of the lower limbs, frequent feeling of muscular spasm, stiffness when walking, gradual muscular atrophy in the foot and shank, numbness, atrophy and disuse, constipation and yellow urine, pink tongue with a thin white coating or lack of coating and a thready rapid pulse. ⟨Treatment principle⟩ Replenish the blood and nourish the yin. ⟨Point selection⟩ Jiexi (ST 41), Yinshi (ST 33), Xuehai (SP 10), Fuliu (KI 7), Zhaohai (KI 6), and Xuanzhong (GB 39).

● 干呕 [gān ǒu]　症状名。出《金匮要略·呕吐哕下利病脉证并治》。《内经》名哕。又称啘。指患者作呕吐之态,只有声而无物吐出,或仅有涎沫而无食物吐出。

Retching　Name of a symptom, originally from *Jingui Yaolue*: *Outu Yuexia Li Bingmaizheng Bingzhi* (*Synopsis of the Golden Chamber*: *Pulse Conditions, Symptoms and Treatments of Vomiting, Hiccup and Diarrhea*), named hiccough in *Neijing* (*The Inner Canon of Huangdi*), referring to a strong involuntary vomiting of a little saliva and spittle but no food, with a noise which can be heard.

● 干针 [gān zhēn]　针刺术语。指单纯的毫针针刺。在针麻方法中与电针、水针等相对而言。如称"干针得气留针麻醉"。

Acupuncture with Filiform Needle　A term in acupuncture, referring to needling with a filiform needle alone, as opposed to electrical acupuncture, solution-injected acupuncture and other forms of acupuncture used in acupuncture anesthesia. This is what we call "using the filiform needle for inducing the arrival of qi and retaining the needle for anesthesia."

● 甘遂灸 [gān suí jiǔ]　天灸的一种。取甘遂适量研为细末,敷于穴位上。胶布固定;也可用甘遂末加入面粉适量,用温开水调成糊膏状,贴于穴位上,外以油纸覆盖,胶布固定。如敷大椎穴,可治疗疟疾;敷肺俞穴,可治疗哮喘;敷中极,可治疗尿潴留等。

Gansui (Radix Euphorbiae Kansui) Moxibustion　A term of crude herb moxibustion. ⟨Method⟩ Grind the proper amount of dried tuberous root of *Gansui* (*Euphoribae Kansui*) into powder, and apply it on the selected point and then fix it with adhesive plaster, or add the proper amount of flour to the powder of kansui root, and mix them into a paste with warm boiled water, apply the paste to the selected point, cover the paste with oil paper and fix it with adhesive plaster. Apply it to Dazhui (DU 14), for treating malaria, to Feishu (BL 13) for asthma and to Zhongji (RN 3) for uroschesis, etc.

● 肝 [gān]　①耳穴名。位于耳甲艇的外下方。用于治疗胁痛、眩晕、经前期紧张症、月经不调、更年期综合症、高血压、假性近视、单纯性青光眼。②耳穴名。位于耳背中部外侧。用于治疗胸胁胀满,腰背酸痛。

1. **Liver**(MA-SC 5) An auricular point. ⟨Location⟩on the lateral inferior border of the eymba conchae. ⟨Indications⟩ hypochondriac pain, dizziness premenstrual tension, irregular menstruation, menopausal syndrome, hypertension.

2. **Liver**(MA) An auricular point. ⟨Location⟩on the lateral border of the central back auricle. ⟨Indications⟩ fullness in the chest and hypochondrium, soreness in the back and loins.

●肝胆火旺鼻渊[gān dǎn huǒ wàng bí yuān] 鼻渊证型之一。因肝胆火盛，上犯清窍所致。证见鼻塞流涕，涕多黄稠，腥臭难闻，头痛目眩，口苦咽干，舌质红，苔黄，脉弦数。治宜清肝热，泻胆火，通鼻窍。取太冲、风池、印堂、上星、迎香。

Rhinorrhea with Turbid Discharge due to Hyperactivity of Fire in the Liver and Gallbladder A type or rhinorrhea with turbid discharge, caused by hyperactivity of fire in the liver and gallbladder attacking the upper orifices. ⟨Manifestations⟩stuffy nose, yellowish, thick and foul nasal discharge, headache, dizziness, bitter taste, dry throat, red tongue with yellow coating and string-taut rapid pulse. ⟨Treatment principle⟩ Remove heat from the liver, purge the gallbladder of pathogenic fire, clear the nasal passage and relieving stuffy nose. ⟨Point selection⟩Taichong (LR 3), Fengchi(GB 20), Yintang(EX-HN 3), Shangxing (DU 23), and Yingxiang (LI 20).

●肝火鼻衄[gān huǒ bí nǜ] 鼻衄证型之一。因肝火上炎所致。证见鼻衄血，兼见头痛，眩晕，目赤，口苦，烦躁易怒，舌红苔黄，脉弦数。治宜清泄肝热，泻火止血。取兑端、谚谨、攒竹、曲泉、委中、行间。

Epistaxis due to Liver Fire A type of epistaxis due to the flare-up of liver fire. ⟨Manifestations⟩ nasal bleeding, accompanied by headache, dizziness, conjunctival congestion, bitter taste, irritability, red tongue with yellow coating and string-taut rapid pulse. ⟨Treatment principle⟩ Remove heat from the liver and purge the pathogenic fire to stop bleeding. ⟨Point selection⟩Duiduan (DU 27), Yixi(BL 45), Cuanzhu (BL 2), Ququan (LR 8), Weizhong(BL 40), and Xingjian(LR 2).

●肝火犯肺咳血[gān huǒ fàn fèi ké xuè] 咳血证型之一。因肝火犯肺，肺络损伤所致。证见咳嗽，痰中带血，或大口咯血，血色鲜红或紫黯，或胸胁掣痛，烦躁易怒，小便短赤，口苦，苔薄黄，脉弦数。治宜泄肝清肺，和络止血。取肺俞、鱼际、劳宫、行间。

Hemoptysis due to Attack of Liver Fire on the Lung A type of hemoptysis due to attack of liver fire on the lung, resulting in damage to the pulmonary vessels. ⟨Manifestations⟩cough with blood stained sputum, or expectorating blood with a bright red or dark purple color, chest pain radiating to the hypochondrium, irritability, scanty dark urine, bitter taste, thin and yellow tongue coating, string-taut and rapid pulse. ⟨Treatment principle⟩Clear fire from the liver and remove heat from the lung; regulate collaterals and stop bleeding. ⟨Point selection⟩Feishu(BL 13), Yuji (LU 10), Laogong (PC 8) and Xingjian(LR 2).

●肝火咳嗽[gān huǒ ké sòu] 咳嗽证型之一。因肝郁化火，气火上逆犯肺，肺失清肃所致。证见气逆咳嗽，面红，咽喉干燥，咳引胁痛，痰稠难咯，舌苔薄黄少津，脉弦数。治宜平肝降火，清肺化痰。取经渠、尺泽、太冲、液门。

Cough due to Liver Fire A type of cough due to the transformation of depressed liver-qi into fire, resulting in an upward invasion of fire and qi, leading to attack on the lung and impairment of the purifying and descending function of the lung. ⟨Manifestations⟩cough with reversed flow of qi, flushed face, dry throat, cough with hypochondriac pulling pain, thick sputum, difficulty in coughing, thin, yellow tongue coating with little saliva, string-taut and rapid pulse. ⟨Treatment principle⟩Calm the liver and relieve the fire; remove the heat from the lung and dissolve phlegm. ⟨Point selection⟩Jingqu(LU 8), Chize (LU 5), Taichong(LR 3) and Yemen(SJ 2).

●肝火上扰不寐[gān huǒ shàng rǎo bù mèi] 不寐证型之一。因抑郁恼怒，肝火上扰，心神不宁所致。证见头晕而痛，不能入眠，多烦易怒，或伴有胁痛，口苦，舌苔薄黄，脉弦数。治宜平降肝火。取行间、足窍阴、风池、神门。

Insomnia due to Upward Disturbance of Liver Fire　A type of insomnia, resulting from emotional upset, causing upward disturbance of liver-fire, which leads to an unsteadiness of the mind. 〈Manifestations〉 dizziness and headache, sleeplessness, irritability, sometimes accompanied by hypochondriac pain, bitter taste, thin and yellow tongue coating. string-taut and rapid pulse. 〈Treatment principle〉 Calm and suppress liver fire. 〈Point selection〉 Xingjian (LR 2), Zuqiaoyin (GB 44), and Shenmen (HT 7).

●肝火吐血[gān huǒ tù xuè]　吐血证型之一。因肝火炽盛，损伤胃腑所致。证见吐血鲜红或紫黯，口苦胁痛，烦躁易怒，舌质红绛，脉弦数。治宜清肝和胃，泻火止血。取不容、劳宫、梁丘、曲泉、行间、地五会。

Hematermesis due to Liver Fire　A type of hematermesis due to damage of the stomach, resulting from excess liver fire. 〈Manifestations〉 spitting of bright red or dark purple blood, bitter taste, hypochondriac pain, irritability, red or dark red tongue and string-taut rapid pulse. 〈Treatment principle〉 Remove heat from the liver and regulate the stomach; purge fire and stop bleeding. 〈Point selection〉 Burong (ST 19), Laogong (PC 8), Liangqiu (ST 34), Ququan (LR 8), Xingjian (LR 2) and Diwuhui (GB 42).

●肝经[gān jīng]　足厥阴肝经之简称。详见该条。

The Liver Meridian　Short for the Liver Meridian of Foot-Jueyin. →足厥阴肝经 (p. 629)

●肝气呕吐[gān qì ǒu tù]　呕吐证型之一。因肝气不舒，横逆犯胃，胃失和降所致。证见呕吐吞酸，嗳气频繁，胸胁闷痛，舌边红，苔薄腻，脉弦。治宜舒肝和胃。取上脘、阳陵泉、太冲、梁丘、神门。

Vomiting due to Liver Qi　A type of vomiting due to the disorder of liver qi, resulting in transverse attack on the stomach. 〈Manifestations〉 vomiting, acid regurgitiation, frequent eructations, distending pain in the chest and hypochondrium, red border of the tongue, thin and greasy tongue coating and string-taut pulse. 〈Treatment principle〉 Relieve the depressed liver and regulate the stomach. 〈Point selection〉 Shangwan (RN 13), Yanglingquan (GB 34), Taichong (LR 3), Liangqiu (ST 34) and Shenmen (HT 7).

●肝热恶阻[gān rè è zǔ]　恶阻证型之一。多因肝经郁热，邪气犯胃所致。证见妊娠初期，呕吐苦水或酸

图 17.2　肝经穴 (足部)
Fig 17.2　Points of Liver Meridian (Foot)

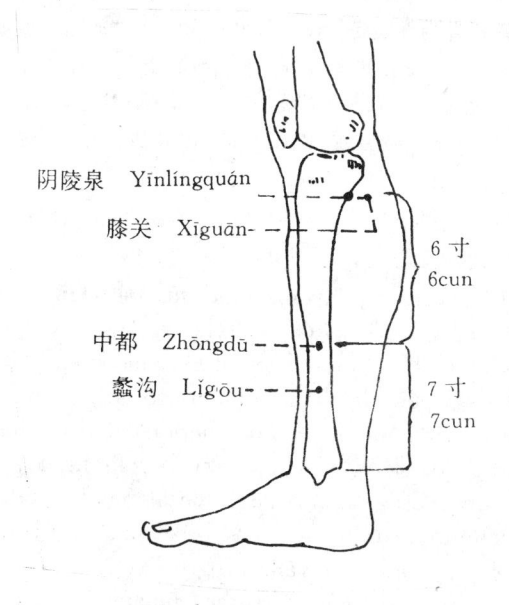

图 17.1　肝经穴 (小腿部)
Fig 17.1　Points of Liver Meridian (Leg)

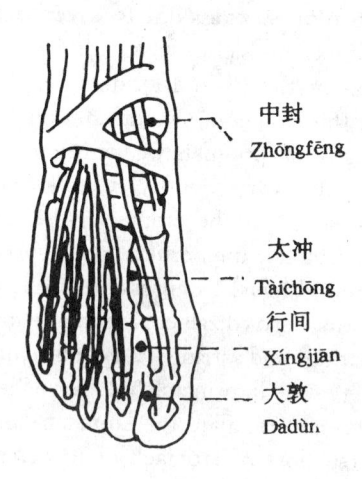

水,口干,口苦,胃脘满闷,胁肋胀痛,嗳气叹息,精神抑郁,头胀头晕,苔微黄,脉弦滑。治宜清肝和胃,降逆止呕。取内关、太冲、中脘、足三里。

Morning Sickness due to Liver Heat A type of morning sickness, mostly due to stagnated heat in the Liver Meridian, leading to attack on the stomach. 〈Manifestations〉in the early stages of pregnancy, vomiting of bilious or acid fluid, dry mouth, bitter taste, fullness and distention in the stomach, distending pain in hypochondrium, eructations, susceptibility to sighing, mental depression, feeling of fullness in the head, dizziness, slight yellowish tongue coating and string-taut and slippery pulse. 〈Treatment principle〉Remove heat from the liver and regulate the stomach; reduce the adverse flow of stomach-qi to arrest vomiting. 〈Point selection〉Neiguan (PC 6), Taichong (LR 3), Zhongwan (RN 12) and Zusanli (ST 36).

●**肝肾不足经闭**[gān shèn bù zú jīng bì] 经闭证型之一。多因素体虚弱,或早婚、分娩过多,损伤肝肾,冲任失养所致。证见超龄月经未至,或先见经期错后,经量逐渐减少,终至闭止,兼见头晕耳鸣,腰膝酸软,口干咽燥,五心烦热,潮热汗出,舌质红,脉弦细。治宜滋补肝肾。取肝俞、肾俞、膏肓俞、然谷、命门、腰眼、阴谷。

Amenorrhea due to Deficiency of the Liver and Kidney A type of amenorrhea due to impairment of the liver and kidney and failure to tonify the Chong and Ren Meridians, caused by a delicate constitution, premature marriage or multiple childbirths. 〈Manifestations〉delayed menarche, or delayed menstrual cycle and gradually diminished discharge of menstruation ending in amenorrhea, accompanied by dizziness, tinnitus, soreness and weakness of the loins and knees, dry mouth and throat, dysphoria with feverish sensation in chest, palms and soles, tidal fever and sweating, red tongue and string-taut and thready pulse. 〈Treatment principle〉Nourish the liver and kidney. 〈Point selection〉Ganshu (BL 18), Shenshu (BL 23), Gaohuangshu (BL 43), Rangu (KI 2), Mingmen (DU 4), Yaoyan (EX-B 7) and Yingu (KI 10).

●**肝肾亏损痛经**[gān shèn kuī sǔn tòng jīng] 痛经证型之一。多因素体虚弱,早婚,分娩过多。损伤肝肾,精亏血少,行经之后血海空虚,冲任胞脉失养所致。证见经期或经后小腹绵绵作痛,按之痛减,经色淡,质清稀,腰背酸痛,头晕耳鸣,面色苍白,精神倦怠,舌质淡,脉沉细。治宜补益肝肾,调补冲任。取肝俞、肾俞、关元、足三里、照海。

Dysmenorrhea due to Impaired Liver-Kidney Essence A type of dysmenorrhea, mostly due to a delicate constitution, premature marriage or multiple childbirths resulting in impairment of the liver and kidney, deficiency of vital essence and lack of blood, emptiness of the Chong Meridian after menstruation, leading to failure to nourish the Chong Meridian, the Ren Meridian and uterine collaterals. 〈Manifestations〉dull pain relieved by pressing in the lower abdomen during or after the menstrual period, thin, pink and scanty menses, soreness and pain in loin and back, dizziness, tinnitus, pale complexion, lassitude, pale tongue and deep thready pulse. 〈Treatment principle〉Tonify the liver and kidney; regulate and invigorate the Chong and Ren meridians. 〈Point selection〉Ganshu (BL 18), Shenshu (BL 23), Guanyuan (RN 4), Zusanli (ST 36), and Zhaohai (KI 6).

●**肝肾阴虚痿证**[gān shèn yīn xū wěi zhèng] 痿证证型之一。由肝肾亏虚,精血不能濡养筋骨经脉所致。证见起病缓慢,下肢痿软无力,腰脊酸软,不能久立,或伴目眩发落,咽干耳鸣,遗精或遗尿,月经不调,甚至步履全废,腿胫大肉渐脱,舌红少苔,脉细数。治宜通经活络,补益肝肾。取肩髃、曲池、合谷、阳溪、髀关、梁丘、足三里、解溪、肝俞、肾俞。

Flaccidity Syndrome due to Deficiency of Liver-Kidney Yin A type of flaccidity syndrome due to deficiency of liver blood and kidney essence, leading to failure to nourish muscles, tendons, bones and meridians. 〈Manifestations〉 slow onset, weakness of the lower limbs, soreness and lassitude along the spinal column, inability to stand long, and even complete inability to walk, progressive muscular atrophy of the legs, often accompanied by dizziness, baldness, dry throat, tinnitus, emission, enuresis, irregular menstruation, red tongue

with little coating and thready and rapid pulse. 〈Treatment principle〉Clear and activate the meridians and collaterals; tonify the liver and kidney. 〈Point selection〉Jianyu(LI 15), Quchi(LI 11), Hegu(LI 4), Yangxi(LI 5), Biguan(ST 31), Liangqiu(ST 34), Zusanli(ST 36), Jiexi(ST 41), Ganshu(BL 18), and Shenshu(BL 23).

●肝俞[gān shū] 经穴名。出《灵枢·背输》。属足太阳膀胱经,为肝的背俞穴。〈定位〉在背部,当第九胸椎棘突下,旁1.5寸(图7)。〈层次解剖〉皮肤→皮下组织→斜方肌→背阔肌→下后锯肌→竖脊肌。浅层布有第九、十胸神经的后支的皮支及伴行的动、静脉。深层有第九、十胸神经后支的肌支和相应的肋间后动、静脉的分支或属支。〈主治〉黄疸、胁痛、吐血、衄血、目赤、目视不明、眩晕、夜盲、癫狂、痫证、脊背痛。斜刺0.5-0.8寸;可灸。

Ganshu(BL 18) A meridian point, originally from *Ling Shu: Beishu* (*Miraculous Pivot: Back Shu Points*), a point on the Bladder Meridian of Foot-Taiyang and the Back-Shu point of the liver. 〈Location〉on the back, below the spinous process of the 9th thoracic vertebra, 1.5 cun lateral to the posterior midline(Fig. 7). 〈Regional anatomy〉skin→subcutaneous tissue→trapezius muscle→latissimus muscle of back→inferior posterior serratus muscle→erector spinal muscle. In the superficial layer, there are the cutaneous branches of the posterior branches of the 9th and 10th thoracic nerves and the accompanying arteries and veins. In the deep layer, there are the muscular branches of the posterior branches of the 9th and 10th thoracic nerves and the branches or tributaries of the related posterior arteries and veins. 〈Indications〉jaundice, hypochondriac pain, epistaxis, conjunctival congestion, blurred vision, dizziness, night blindness, manic-depressive disorder, epilepsy and backache. 〈Method〉Puncture obliquely 0.5~0.8 cun. Moxibustion is applicable.

●肝阳[gān yáng] ①耳穴名。又称肝阳1、肝阳2。位于耳轮结节处。用于治疗头晕、头痛、高血压。②指肝脏的功能活动。

1. **Liver-Yang**(MA) An auricular point, also named Ganyang 1 or Ganyang 2. 〈Location〉at the auricular tubercle. 〈Indications〉dizziness, headache and hypertension.

2. **Liver Yang** Referring to functional activities of the liver.

●肝阳头痛[gān yáng tóu tòng] 头痛证型之一。因肝阳上扰所致。证见头角抽痛(多偏于一侧)、眩晕,面部烘热,多烦善怒,目赤口苦,舌质红,脉弦。常因精神紧张而发病。治宜平肝潜阳。取悬颅、颔厌、合谷、液门、太冲、太溪。

Liver Yang Headache A type of headache due to upward disturbance of hyperactive liver yang. 〈Manifestions〉cramping pain in the temple(mostly inclining to one side), dizziness, paroxysmal fever on the face, irritability, conjunctival congestion, bitter taste, red tongue and string-taut pulse, usually induced by emotional stress. 〈Treatment principle〉Calm the liver and suppress hyperactivity of the liver yang. 〈Point selection〉Xuanlu(GB 5), Hanyan(GB 4), Hegu(LI 4), Yemen(SJ 2), Taichong(LR 3) and Taixi(KI 3).

●肝郁腹痛[gān yù fù tòng] 腹痛证型之一。由肝郁气滞,气机升降不利所致。证见腹痛连两胁,痛无定处,嗳气频频,常在情志不畅时发病,多烦善怒,口苦,苔薄白,脉弦。治宜疏肝理气。取膻中、太冲、内关、阳陵泉。

Abdominal Pain due to Stagnation of Liver-Qi A type of abdominal pain due to qi-stagnation in the liver, resulting in abnormal descent or ascent of qi. 〈Manifestations〉abdominal pain involving the hypochondrim without a fixed region, usually induced by emotional upset, frequent eructations, irritability, bitter taste, white coating and string-taut pulse. 〈Treatment principle〉Relieve the depressed liver and regulate the circulation of qi. 〈Point selection〉Danzhong(RN 17), Taichong(LR 3), Neiguan(PC 6), and Yanglingquan(GB 34).

●肝郁经行先后无定期[gān yù jīng xíng xiān hòu wú dìng qī] 是经行先后无定期的证型之一。多因郁怒伤肝,肝郁气乱,气乱则血亦乱,冲任胞宫蓄溢失常所致。证见经期先后不定,经量或多或少,经色紫黯,经行不畅,胸胁、乳房胀痛,嗳气不舒,喜叹息,舌苔薄白,脉弦。治宜疏肝解郁。取关元、三阴交、太冲、肝

俞、期门、章门。

Irregular Menstruation due to Stagnation of Liver-Qi　A type of irregular menstrual cycle, mostly caused by dysfunction of the liver due to emotional depression and the disorder of qi leading to the disorder of blood circulation and irregularity of the Chong and Ren Meridians and uterus in storing blood. 〈Manifestations〉early or delayed menses without a regular menstrual cycle, profuse or scanty menstrual flow, purplish and dark in color, no free discharge of menses, distending pain in the breast, chest and hypochondrium, eructations, thin and white coating and string-taut pulse. 〈Treatment principle〉Soothe the liver and regulate the cirulation of qi. 〈Point selection〉Guanyuan (RN 4), Sanyinjiao (SP 6), Taichong (LR 3), Ganshu (BL 18), Qimen (LR 14) and Zhangmen (LR 13).

●肝郁经行先期［gān yù jīng xíng xiān qī］　经行先期证型之一。多因情志抑郁，恚怒伤肝，肝郁化热迫血妄行，冲任失守所致。证见经期提前，经量时多时少，色红或紫，或粘稠有块，乳房及小腹胀痛不舒，烦躁易怒等。治宜疏肝解郁清热。取关元、血海、肝俞、期门、三阴交、太冲、曲池、通里。

Preceded Menstrual Cycle due to Stagnation of Liver-Qi　A type of the early menstrual flow, mostly due to dysfunction of the liver caused by emotional depression and irritation, resulting in the depression of liver-qi transforming into pathogenic heat, forcing the blood to go astray and a dysfunction of the Chong and Ren Meridians in storing blood. 〈Manifestations〉early menstrual flow, menstrual blood sometimes profuse and sometimes scant, scarlet or purplish color menstrual blood of a viscous nature or with blood clots, distending pain in the breast and the lower abdomen and irritability. 〈Treatment principle〉Soothe the liver and regulate the circulation of qi and clear heat. 〈Point selection〉Guanyuan (RN 4), Xuehai (SP 10), Ganshu (BL 18), Qimen (LR 14), Sanyinjiao (SP 6), Taichong (LR 3), Quchi (LI 11) and Tongli (HT 5).

●肝郁瘰疬［gān yù luǒ lì］　瘰疬证型之一。多因肝郁气滞所致。证见瘰疬初起，一粒或数粒不等，小如枣核，大如梅子，皮色不变，按之坚硬，推之能移，不热不痛。久则瘰疬逐渐增大，与表皮粘连，有的数个成串，微觉疼痛，将溃时皮肤渐转暗红，疼痛加剧。溃破之后脓水清稀，夹有败絮样物质。兼精神抑郁，胸胁胀痛，脘痞纳呆，苔薄，脉弦。治宜疏肝解郁。取章门、天井、足临泣。

Scrofula due to Stagnation of Liver-Qi　A type of scrofula due to depression of liver-qi. 〈Manifestations〉in the initial stage, manifested as occurrence of one to several swollen lymph nodes with normal skin color, which are hard when pressed, and movable when pushed, some are as big as plums, some are as small as a datestone and they are neither painful nor hot; later, the lymph nodes become more enlarged, some adhere to the skin, others adhere to each other in clusters. The skin over the lymph nodes is dark-red. Before diabrosis there is intense pain. After diabrosis, a thin purulent fluid is discharged. The syndrome is accompanied by mental depression, distending pain in the chest and hypochondrium, fullness in the stomach, anorexia, thin tongue coating and string-taut pulse. 〈Treatment principle〉Soothe the liver and regulate the circulation of qi. 〈Point selection〉Zhangmen (LR 13), Tianjing (SJ 10), and Zulinqi (GB 41).

●肝郁气滞乳少（［gān yù qì zhì rǔ shǎo］　乳少证型之一。多因产后情志不调，肝失条达，气血运行不畅，乳汁壅滞不行所致。证见产后乳汁不行，乳房胀痛，或见精神抑郁，胸闷胀满，食欲减退，苔薄，脉弦。治宜疏肝解郁，佐以通络。取膻中、乳根、少泽、内关、太冲。

Hypogalactia due to Stagnation of Liver-Qi　A type of hypogalactia due to emotional disorder after delivery, resulting in dysfunction of the liver in maintaining the free flow of qi and the disturbance of the qi and blood circulation, leading to the obstruction of milk secretion. 〈Manifestations〉lack of lactation after delivery, distending pain in breasts, mental depression, oppressive feeling in the chest, anorexia, thin tongue coating and string-taut pulse. 〈Treatment principle〉Soothe the liver and regulate the circulation of qi, supported by activating the mammary collaterals. 〈Point se-

lection⟩Danzhong (RN 17), Rugen(ST 18), Shaoze(SI 1), Neiguan (PC 6) and Taichong (LR 3).

●**肝郁乳癖**[gān yù rǔ pǐ] 乳癖证型之一。多因肝郁气滞,血气凝涩,乳络受阻所致。证见乳房有肿块,不红不痛,推之不移。并兼见头晕胸闷,嗳噫不舒,少腹胀痛,行经不畅,苔薄,脉弦。治宜疏肝理气。取屋翳、行间、内关、膻中。

Nodules of Breast due to Stagnation of Liver-Qi A type of nodules in the breast due to depression of liver-qi, resulting in the stagnation of qi and blood, leading to the obstruction of the mammary collaterals. ⟨Manifestations⟩ nodular masses in the breast, which are painless, do not change the skin color, and are unmovable, accompanied by eructations, distending pain in the lower abdomen, no free discharge of menstruation, thin tongue coating and string-taut pulse. ⟨Treatment principle⟩ Soothe the liver and regulate the circulation of qi. ⟨Point Selection⟩ Wuyi (ST 15), Xingjian (LR 2), Neiguan (PC 6), and Danzhong (RN 17).

●**肝郁乳痈**[gān yù rǔ yōng] 乳痈证型之一。多因肝气郁结,阻塞脉络所致。证见初起乳房结块,肿胀疼痛,排乳不畅,同时全身不适,寒热往来。兼见胸闷胁痛,呕逆,纳呆,苔薄,脉弦。若乳部肿胀加剧,掀红疼痛,时时跳痛,此为酿脓征象。治宜疏肝解毒。取期门、行间、外关、天池、肩井。

Acute Mastitis due to Stagnation of Liver-Qi

A type of acute mastitis, mostly due to obstruction of the mammary collaterals, resulting from depression of liver-qi. ⟨Manifestations⟩at onset, nodular masses in the breast with swelling and distending pain, galactostasis, general malaise and alternate chills and fever, accompanied by an oppressive feeling in the chest, hypochondriac pain, vomiting, anorexia, thin tongue coating and string-taut pulse. If the patient's condition aggravates further, there will be severe swelling with enythema, intense pain and constant throbbing pain, which show signs of pyogenesis. ⟨Treatment principles⟩ Soothe the liver and regulate the circulation of qi. ⟨Point selection⟩ Qimen (LR 14), Xingjian (LR 2), Waiguan (SJ 5), Tianchi (PC 1) and Jianjing (GB 21).

●**肝郁胁痛**[gān yù xié tòng] 胁痛证型之一。见《金匮翼·胁痛总论》。多由悲哀恼怒,肝气郁结,失于条达所致。证见痛无定处,胁肋作痛或左或右,常因情志波动时发作,伴有胸闷,嗳噫泛酸,善怒少寐,舌苔薄白,脉弦劲。治宜疏肝解郁。取中庭、肝俞、期门、中渎、侠溪。

Hypochondriac Pain due to Stagnation of Liver Qi A type of hypochondriac pain, seen in *Jingui Yi: Xietong Zonglun* (*Supplement to the Synopsis of the Golden Chamber: Treatise on Hypochondriac Pain*), mostly due to sorrow and anger, leading to the stagnation of liver qi which fails to regulate the functional activities of the liver qi. ⟨Manifestations⟩ unfixed pain in the left or right hypochondriac region, usually caused by emotional upset, accompanied by oppressive feeling in the chest, eructations and acid regurgitation, susceptibility to anger, sleeplessness, thin white tongue coating, wiry and excessive pulse. ⟨Treatment principle⟩Soothe the liver and regulate the cirulation of qi. ⟨Point selection⟩Zhongting (RN 16), Ganshu (BL 18), Qimen (LR 14), Zhongzhu(SJ 3) and Xiaxi(GB 43).

●**肝郁泻**[gān yù xiè] 泄泻证型之一。因肝失条达,横逆乘脾,气机不和,脾失健运所致。证见泄泻每因抑恼怒或情绪紧张而发,肠鸣腹痛,泻后痛减,胸胁胀闷,嗳气食少,舌淡红,苔薄白,脉弦缓。治宜平肝调中,抑木扶土。取中脘、天枢、足三里、内关、期门、太冲、阳陵泉、行间。

Diarrhea due to Stagnation of Liver Qi A type of diarrhea due to stagnation of liver qi, leading to transverse attack on the spleen which causes the disorder of qi and dysfunction of the spleen in circulation. ⟨Manifestations⟩diarrhea, emotional depression and anger or mental stress, borborygmus, abdominal pain relieved after diarrhea, distention and fullness in the chest and hypochondrium, eructations and poor appetite, pink tongue and thin white coating, wiry and leisurely pulse. ⟨Treatment principle⟩Calm the liver and regulate the functions of the spleen, check hyperfunction of the liver and strengthen the spleen. ⟨Point selection⟩ Zhongwan (RN 12), Tianshu (ST 25),

Zusanli(ST 36), Neiguan(PC 6), Qimen(LR 14), Taichong(LR 3), Yanglingquan(GB 34) and Xingjian(LR 2).

●肝足厥阴之脉[gān zú jué yīn zhī mài] 足厥阴肝经的原称。见该条。

Foot-Jueyin Vessel of the Liver The original name of the Liver Meridian of Foot-Jueyin. →足厥阴肝经(p. 629)

●疳[gān] 疳疾的简称。详见该条。

Infantile Malnutrition A short name for infantile malnutrition sickness. →疳疾(p. 130)

●疳病[gān bìng] 即疳疾的别名。详见该条。

Infantile Malnutrition Disease Another name for infantile malnutrition sickness. →疳疾(p. 130)

●疳疾[gān jí] 病证名。出《颅囟经》。又称疳症、疳病,简称疳。是一种由脾胃运化失常所引起的慢性营养障碍性病证。多见于5岁以内的儿童。以面黄肌瘦,毛发焦枯,饮食反常,腹部膨胀,精神萎靡为特征。临床分以下两种证型。①脾胃虚弱型。多因小儿饮食无度,或恣食肥甘生冷,壅滞中焦,损伤脾胃,纳运无权,乳食精微无从运化,以致脏腑肢体缺乏濡养,气阴亏损,而形成疳疾。证见形体干枯羸瘦,精神疲惫,面色萎黄,头发稀疏。肌肤甲错。兼见大便溏泄,完谷不化,腹部凹陷如舟,四肢不温,睡卧不宁,露睛,甚则伴有发育障碍,唇舌色淡,脉细无力。治宜调理脾胃,培中化滞。取中脘、章门、脾俞、胃俞、足三里、公孙、四缝。②感染虫疾型。多因饮食不洁,感染虫疾,耗夺血气,不能濡养脏腑筋肉,日久而形成疳疾。证见形体干枯羸瘦,精神疲惫,面色萎黄,头发稀疏,肌肤甲错。兼见食欲异常,或嗜食无度,不知饥饱,或嗜食异物,脘腹胀大,青筋暴露,经常腹痛,睡中咬牙,舌质淡,脉细弦。治宜消积驱虫。取巨阙、中脘、天枢、百虫窝、足三里。

Infantile Malnutrition Sickness A disease originally from *Lu Xin Jing*(*Classic on Paediatric Diseases*), also named infantile malnutrition syndrome, infantile malnutrition disease, or infantile malnutrition. A chronic dystrophic disease caused by dysfunction of the spleen and stomach in digestion and circulation, mostly occurring in children under the age of five. Characterized by emaciation with sallow complexion, dried and matted hair, heterorexia, abdominal distention and listlessness. Clinically it is divided into: ① Weakness of the spleen and stomach. Mostly due to improper diet, or unrestrained intake of sweet, greasy, raw and cold food. This diet leads to the retention of food in the middle Jiao and impairment of the spleen and stomach, resulting in dysfunction of the spleen and stomach in absorption, digestion and transportation of the nutrient to zang-fu organs and other body parts which then lack nutrients, and are deficient in both qi and yin. 〈Manifestations〉 emaciation with wizened body, listlessness, sallow-complexion, oligotrichia, squamous and dry skin, accompanied by loose stool containing undigested food, boat-shaped abdomen, cold limbs, insomnia with restlessness, sleeping with eyes half closed, maldevelopment, pale lips and tongue, thready and weak pulse. 〈Treatment principle〉Regulate the spleen and stomach, remove food retention by reinforcing the spleen and stomach. 〈Point selection〉 Zhongwan (RN 12), Zhangmen (LR 13), Pishu(BL 20), Weishu(BL 21), Zusanli(ST 36), Gongsun(SP 4), Sifeng(EX-UE 10). ② Infection by parasites. Mostly due to an unclean diet, which contains parasites. The parastes cause the consumption of blood and qi, leading to a failure to mourish zang-fu organs, muscles and tendons. 〈Manifestations〉 emaciation with wizened body, listlessness, sallow complexion, oligotrichia, squamous and dry skin, accompanied by abnormal of appetite, eg. overeating without feeling hungry or full, or addiction to eating strange food, abdominal distention with visible superficial veins, frequent abdominal pain, odontoprisis in spleep, pale tongue, thready and wiry pulse. 〈Treatment principles〉Remove food stagnancy and expel intestinal worms. 〈Point selection〉 Juque (RN 14), Zhongwan (RN 12), Tianshu (ST 25), Baichongwo (EX-LE 3), and Zusanli(ST 36), etc.

●疳证[gān zhèng] 即疳疾。详见该条。

Infantile Malnutrition Syndrome Another name for infantile malnutrition sickness. →疳疾(p. 130)

●感觉区[gǎn jué qū] 头针刺激区之一。在运动区向后移1.5厘米的平行线即是本区。感觉区可分为上、中、下三部。①上部：是感觉区的上1/5，为下肢、头、躯干感觉区。②中部：是感觉区的中2/5，为上肢感觉区。③下部：是感觉区的下2/5，为面感觉区。〈主治〉①上部：对侧腰腿痛、麻木、感觉异常，后头、颈项部疼痛，头晕，耳鸣。②中部：对侧上肢疼痛、麻木、感觉异常。③下部：对侧面部麻木，偏头痛，颞颌关节炎等。

The Sensory Area A stimulation area in scalp acupuncture. 〈Location〉The parallel line, 1.5 cun behind the motor area, is the sensory area, which is divided into three parts. ①The upper 1/5 of this area is the lower limb, head and trunk sensory area; ②the middle 2/5 of this area, the upper limb sensory area; and ③the lower 2/5, the face sensory area. 〈Indications〉①the upper area: contra-lateral lumbar pain, pain of the leg, numbness and patesthesia, occipital headache, pain in the nape region, dizziness and tinnitus. ②the middle area: contra-lateral upper limb pain, numbness and paresthesia. ③the lower area contra-lateral facial numbness, migranie, temporo-mandibular arthritis, etc.

●感冒[gǎn mào] 病证名。见《仁斋直指方·诸风》由风邪侵袭人体所致的外感表证。以鼻塞、流涕、咳嗽、头痛、恶寒、发热为主证。由于体质强弱和受邪的性质不同，又可分为风寒、风热、暑湿感冒三大类。详见各条。

Common Cold A disease seen in *Ren Zhai Zhizhi Fang: Zhu Feng (Renzhai's Straightforward Prescriptions: Diversified Winds)*. An exterior syndrome caused by the attack of pathogenic wind on the human body. 〈Manifestations〉stuffy nose, running nose, cough, headache, chills and fever. Due to differences in constitution and the property of the pathogenic factors, it can be divided into: common cold due to wind-cold pathogen, common cold due to wind-heat pathogen, and common cold due to summer heat-damp pathogen. →风寒感冒(p.111)、风热感冒(p.113)、暑湿感冒(p.407)

●肛门[gāng mén] 耳穴名。又称痔核点。位于与耳轮上脚下缘同水平的耳轮处。用于治疗内外痔。

Anus(MA-H 5) An auricular point, also called Hemorrhoidal Nucleus Point. 〈Location〉on the helix, on the level of the lower border of the superior antihelix crus. 〈Indications〉internal and external hemorrhoids.

●高盖[gāo gài] 经穴别名。出《太平圣惠方》。即督俞。见该条。

Gaogai Another name for Dushu(BL 16), a meridian point originally from *Taiping Shenghui Fang(Imperial Benevolent Prescriptions)*. →督俞(p.87)

●高骨[gāo gǔ] ①经外穴名。见《针灸大成》。在桡骨茎突之高点处。主治手腕痛。平刺0.5～1寸；可灸。②部位名。凡高起之骨统称高骨。一指大指侧臂骨下端，亦有将兑骨与高骨称为手踝骨。

1. Gaogu(EX-UE) An extra point seen in *Zhenjiu Dacheng (A Great Compendium of Acupuncture and Moxibustion)*. 〈Location〉on the high point of the styloid process of the radius. 〈Indications〉pain of the wrist. 〈Method〉Puncture subcutaneously 0.5～1 cun. Moxibustion is applicable.

2. Protuberant Bones Body parts, a general designation for the protuberant bones of the body. One interpretation refers to the styloid process of the radius; another refers to the ulna and other protuberant bones like the carpal and malleolus bones.

●高曲[gāo qū] 经穴别名。出《千金要方》。即商曲。详见该条。

Gaoqu Another name for Shangqu(KI 17), a meridian point originally from *Qianjin Yaofang(Prescriptions Worth a Thousand Gold)*. →商曲(p.350)

●高热[gāo rè] 症状名。为各科急性发热性疾病的主要症状之一。本症多由六淫侵袭肌体所致。包括广义的伤寒、温病等。症见突然发烧，来势凶猛，体温甚至达到四十度以上，可伴有原发病的其它症状。多见于各种细菌或病毒感染的急性炎症或各种传染病，也见于甲亢、中暑、肺结核等。治宜清热祛邪。取大椎、合谷、曲池。如效果不显，可取十宣、曲泽、委中、耳三针，点刺放血；另可酌取风府、厉兑、内陷谷、冲阳、解溪、大陵、足三里、期门、上巨虚、下巨虚。

High Fever Name of a symptom, one of the

cardinal symptoms of acute febrile diseases in all clinical branches including exogenous febrile diseases and epidemic febrile diseases in a broad sense. Mostly due to the six pathogenic factors attacking the body. 〈Manifestations〉sudden fever with tremendous force and a body temperature of up to 40℃. Accompanied by other symptoms of the primary disease commonly seen in various inflammatory or infectious diseases caused by bacteria or viruses. Also seen in hyperthyroidism, heatstroke and pulmonary tuberculosis, etc. 〈Treatment principle〉reduce fever and expel pathogenic factors. 〈Point selection〉Dazhui (DU 14), Hegu(LI 4), Quchi(LI 11). In cases without effect, prick Shixuan(EX-UE 11), Quze (PC 3), Weizhong (BL 40), and three ear points to cause bleeding. In addition, the following points are also applicable: Fengfu (DU 16), Lidui (ST 45), Neixiangu (EX-LE), Chongyang(ST 42), Jiexi(ST 4), Daling (PC 7), Zusanli (ST 36), Qimen (LR 14), Shangjuxu(ST 37) and Xiajuxu(ST 39).

●高热伤阴痉证[gāo rè shāng yīn jìng zhèng] 痉证证型之一。由于高热消烁津液，肝木失于濡养，肝风内动所致。证见高热不解，口噤龂齿，项背强直，甚至角弓反张，手足挛急，口渴引饮，舌苔黄，脉弦数。治宜泄热救阴，平肝熄风。取风府、大椎、曲池、涌泉、太冲、十二井穴。

Convulsive Syndrome due to Impairment of Yin Caused by High Fever A type of convulsive disease, due to excess consumption of body fluid caused by high fever. Results in failure to nourish the liver wood, and stir up of the liver. 〈Manifestations〉persistent high fever, lockjaw and teeth grinding, stiffness of the nape and back, opisthotonus, contracture of hands and feet; thirst relieved by drinking, yellow tongue coating, wiry and rapid pulse. 〈Treatment principle〉Purge heat to rescue the yin, calm the liver to stop wind. 〈Point selection〉Fengfu(DU 16), Dazhui(DU 14), Quchi (LI 11), Yongquan(KI 1), Taichong(LR 3), the Jing(Well) points of the Twelve Regular Meridians.

●高武[gāo wǔ] 人名。明针灸学家，字梅孤，鄞县（今属浙江）人。通天文、乐理、兵法，晚年钻研医学，尤精于针灸。撰《针灸素难要旨》和《针灸聚英》，并自制三具铜人（男、女、童各一具）。

Gao Wu An expert of acupuncture and moxibustion in the Ming Dynasty, who styled himself Mei Gu, a native of Jinxian county (Now in Zhejiang Province), well versed in astronomy, music theory and the art of war. In his later years he began to practice medicine, especially proficient in acupuncture and moxibustion, he wrote *Zhenjiu Su Nan Yaozhi*(*The Essentials of Acupuncture and Moxibustion in "Plain Questions and The Classic of Questions"*) and *Zhenjiu Juying*(*Essentials of Acupuncture and Moxibustion*), and made three bronze statues by himself(a man, a woman and a child.)

●膏肓[gāo huāng] ①经穴名。见《医学入门》。属足太阳膀胱经。又名膏肓俞。〈定位〉在背部，当第四胸椎棘突下，旁开3寸（图7）。〈层次解剖〉皮肤→皮下组织→斜方肌→菱形肌→竖脊肌。浅层布有第四、五胸神经后支的皮支和伴行的动、静脉。深层为肩胛背神经，肩胛背动、静脉，第四、五胸神经后支的肌支和相应的肋间后动、静脉背侧支的分支或属支。主治肺痨、咳嗽、气喘、吐血、盗汗、健忘、遗精、完谷不化、肩胛背痛。斜刺0.5-0.8寸；可灸。②部位名。出《左传·成公十年》。我国古代医学称心脏与隔膜之间的部位为肓，称心尖脂肪为膏。"膏肓"属人体内部深层的部位。

1. Gaohuang(BL 43) A meridian point, seen in *Yixue Rumen* (*An Introduction to Medicine*), a point on the Bladder Meridian of Foot-Taiyang, also named Gaohuangshu. 〈Location〉on the back, below the spinous process of the 4th thoracic vertebra, 3 cun lateral to the posterior midline (Fig. 7). 〈Regional anatomy〉skin→subcutaneous tissue→trapezius muscle→rhomboid muscle→erector spinal muscle. In the superficial layer, there are the cutaneous branches of the posterior branches of the 4th and 5th thoracic nerves and the accompanying arteries and veins. In the deep layer, there are the dorsal scapular nerve, the dorsal scapular artery and vein, the muscular branches of the posterior branches of the 4th and 5th thoracic nerves and the branches or tributaries of the dorsal branches of the relat-

ed posterior intercostal arteries and veins. 〈Indications〉pulmonary tuberculosis, cough, dyspnea, hematemesis, night sweat, amnesia, emission, loose stool containing undigested food, pain in the scapular region and back. 〈Method〉Puncture obliquely 0.5～0.8 cun. Moxibustion is applicable.

2. **Gao Huang**   A body part, originally from *Zuo Zhuan. Cheng Gong Shi Nian*(*Commentary on the Spring and Autumn Annals: The 10th Year of the Reign of Cheng Gong*), In ancient Chinese medicine, the part between the heart and the diaphragm was called huang, and the fat on the cardiac apex called gao. Gao Huang generally refers to the deep part inside the body.

●膏肓俞[gāo huāng shū]　经穴别名。即膏肓。详见该条1。

Gaohuangshu   Another name for a meridian point Gaohuang(BL 43). →膏肓1(p.132)

●膏肓俞穴灸法[gāo huāng shù xué jiǔ fǎ]　书名。又称《灸膏肓俞穴法》,《膏肓灸法》。宋代庄绰撰,一卷,刊于1128年。书中介绍膏肓穴的部位、主治及不同流派的取穴法等,并附有插图。为《针灸四书》之一。

Gaohuangshu Xue Jiufa (**Moxibustion on Gaohuangshu Point**)　A book written by Zhuang Chuo in the Song Dynasty, published in 1128, also named *Jiu Gaohuangshu Xue Fa* (*ditto.*) or *Gaohuang Jufa* (*Moxibustion on Gaohuang*). The book introduces the location, indication and various ways of manipulating Gaohuangshu, and is illustrated. It is one of the *Zhenjiu Si Shu*(*Four Books on Acupuncture and Moxibustion*).

●膏淋[gāo lìn]　病证名,淋证证型之一。出《诸病源候论·淋病诸候》。又名内淋。多由脾肾两虚,清浊不分所致。证见小便混浊如米泔,上有浮油,沉淀有絮状物,或夹凝块,或混有血色、血丝、血块,排尿不畅,口干,苔白微腻,脉濡数。治宜健脾利湿,益肾固涩。取肾俞、脾俞、膀胱俞、气海俞、百会、足三里、关元。

Dysuria with Milky Urine   A type of dysuria, originally from *Zhubing Yuanhou Lun: Lin Bing*(*General Treatise on the Etiology and Symtomatology of Diseases: Causes and Symtoms of Stranguria*), also named inner dysuria. Mostly due to inability to separate the refined essence and turbid urine resulting from a dysfunction of both the spleen and the kidney. 〈Manifestations〉cloudy rice-water-like urine with floating oil and sediment, coagula or bloody color, blood filaments, bloodclots, difficult urination, dry mouth, slight greasy and white tongue coating, soft and rapid pulse. 〈Treatment principle〉Invigorate the spleen and remove dampness by diuresis;tonify the kidney and induce astringency. 〈Point selection〉Shenshu(BL 23), Pishu(BL 20), Pangguangshu(BL 28), Qihaishu(BL 24), Baihui (DU 20), Zusanli (ST 36) and Guanyuan(RN 4).

●割治法[gē zhì fǎ]　治疗方法之一。指切开一定部位的皮肤,摘除少量皮下脂肪,对局部进行适当刺激以治病的方法。有鱼际部割治,膻中部割治等,可用于慢性支气管炎、哮喘、小儿消化不良、疳积、溃疡病、神经官能症等。施治时应严格消毒,防止误伤,并注意创口护理。

Cutting Therapy   A therapeutic technique of cutting through the skin in a particular area and removing a little subcutaneous fat. This induces a stimulation in the local area, e. g. the cutting in the thenar eminence, cutting around Danzhong (RN 17), etc. 〈Indications〉chronic bronchitis, asthma, infantile dyspepsia, infantile malnutrition, peptic ulcer and neurosis, etc. 〈Cautions〉strict sterilization, prevention of accidental injury and careful nursing of the wound.

●阁门[gé mén]　经外穴名。出《扁鹊神应针灸玉龙经》。在耻骨下缘中点,阴茎根旁开3寸处。主治疝气、气上攻心。直刺1-1.5寸;可灸。

Gemen(EX-CA)　An extra point, originally from *Bian Que Shenying Zhenjiu Yulong Jing* (*Bian Que's Jade Dragon Classic of Acupuncture and Moxibustion*). 〈Location〉3 cun lateral to the root of penis, at the midpoint of the lower border of the pubis. 〈Indications〉hernia, reverse-*qi* attacking the heart. 〈Method〉Puncture perpendicularly 1～1.5 cun. Moxibustion is applicable.

●隔巴豆灸[gé bā dòu jiǔ]　即巴豆饼灸。详见该条。

Ba Dou(**Semen Crotonis**)**-Separated Moxi-**

bustion→巴豆饼灸(p.8)

●隔白附子灸[gé bái fù zǐ jiǔ] 间接灸的一种。出《扬起简便方》。将白附子作间隔物而施灸的一种方法。将白附子研为极细末,瓶贮备用。灸治时取白附子末适量,用温水调和如糊膏状。制成圆饼,厚约0.5厘米,敷于神阙穴,上置枣核大艾炷灸之。每次施灸5～10壮,施灸过程中如病人感觉局部灼痛,应立即更换艾炷,谨防烫伤。临床用于治疗疝气。

Bai Fu Zi（Rhizoma Typhonii）-Separated Moxibustion A type of indirect moxibustion with the cake of *Bai Fu Zi Rhizoma Typhonii* placed between the ignited moxa cone and the skin for moxibustion, originally from *Yang Qi Jianbian Fang*（*Yang Qi's Simple and Convenient Prescriptions*）.〈Method〉Grind dried tuber of *Bai Fu Zi*（*Typhonium giganteum*）into powder and put it into a bottle, ready for use. Take a proper amount of the powder, mix it with warm water into paste to make a round cake of 0.5 cun thick, put it, with a moxa cone（big as a date stone）on it, on Shengue（RN 8）for moxibustion, 5—10 cones for each treatment. During moxibustion, if the patient feels a local burning pain, the ignited moxa cone should be replaced immediately by another to prevent burning.〈Indication〉hernia.

●隔苍术灸[gé cāng zhú jiǔ] 间接灸的一种。即苍术灸。详见该条。

Cang Zhu（Rhizoma Athactyloidis）-Separated Moxibustion A form of indirect moxibustion.→苍术灸(p.30)

●隔蟾灸[gé chán jiǔ] 间接灸的一种。见《类经图翼》卷十一。是用蟾蜍作间隔物而施灸的一种灸法。取活蟾蜍一只,破腹去肠(或剥去皮),施患处上置艾炷施灸。适用于瘰疬、疔肿等证。

Toad-separated Moxibustion A form of indirect moxibustion, in which a toad is used as the seperation, originally from *Leijing Tuyi*（*Illustrated Supplementry to the Classified Canon*）.〈Method〉Take a live toad and cut open its belly to remove intestines（or peel its skin）, then place it on the affected part and put a moxa cone on the toad.〈Indications〉scrofula, furuncle with swelling, etc.

●隔豉饼灸[gé chǐ bǐng jiǔ] 间接灸的一种。出《范汪方》。又称豆豉灸。是用豆豉作间隔物而施灸的一种灸法。用豆豉适量捣烂制饼(可用水或黄酒调和),如疮口大,厚约0.6厘米,用细针穿刺数孔,置疮面上放艾炷点燃施灸。临床上适于治疗痈疽发背、顽疮、恶疮肿硬不溃或溃后久不收口、疮面黑暗等证。

Dou Chi（Semen Sojae Praeparatum）-Cake-Separated Moxibustion A form of indirect moxibustion, in which *Dou Chi*（*Semen Sojae Praeparatum*）is used as the separation, originally from *Fan Wang Fang*（*Prescriptions Made by Fan Wang*）, also called *Dou Chi*（*Semen Sojae Prescriptions*）moxibustion.〈Method〉Take a proper amount of *Dou Chi*（*Semen Sojae Praeparatum*）and pound it to make cakes of about 0.6 cm thick each, just the size of the opening of the sore. Mix it with water or yellow wine, punch several holes in the cake with a small needle, then place it on the surface of a sore. Put the ignited moxa cone on the cake for moxibustion.〈Indications〉carbuncle, cellulitis, lumbodorsal carbuncle, obstinate pyogenic sore of skin, hard and non-festering malignant boil with swelling or dark color, etc.

●隔葱灸[gé cōng jiǔ] 间接灸的一种。见《玉机微义》。是用葱作间隔物而施灸的一种方法。即把葱白切成厚0.3～0.5厘米数片,或把葱白捣如泥状,敷于脐中(神阙)及四周,或敷于患处,上置艾炷施灸。一般灸治5～10壮。适用于虚脱、腹痛、尿闭、疝气及乳腺炎等。

Onion-Separated Moxibustion A form of indirect moxibustion in which an onion is used as the separation, originally from *Yuji Weiyi*（*Inscriptions on Jade with Subtle Implications*）.〈Method〉Cut several slices of Chiness green onion, each slice about 0.3～0.5 cm thick, pound it into a jelly, apply the slices or the jelly into and around the umbilicus Shenque（RN 8）, or to the affected area, then place a moxa cone upon it for moxibustion, 5-10 cones for each treatment.〈Indications〉prostration syndrome, abdominal pain, anuresis, hernia and mastitis, etc.

●隔川椒灸[gé chuān jiāo jiǔ] 间接灸的一种。见《古今医鉴》卷十。是用川椒作间隔物而施灸的一种方法。取川椒适量,研为细末,用陈醋调如糊膏状,制

成药饼,厚约0.3厘米,敷于患处,上置艾炷灸之。在灸治过程中,如病人觉施灸处灼痛,可随即更换艾炷再灸。适用于治疗一切肿毒疼痛,跌仆扭伤所致的伤筋积血,腹胀痞满等证。

Chuan Jiao (Pericarpium Zanthexyli)-Separated Moxibustion A form of indirect moxibustion in which pericarpium is used as the separation, originally from *Gujin Yijian* (*A Medical Reference of the Past and Present*), Vol. 1. 〈Method〉Take a proper amount of *Chuan Jiao* (*Pericarpium Zanthoxyli*) and grind it into powder, then mix the powder with mature vinegar into a paste to make cakes of about 0.3 cm thick each, place a cake on the affected area and put a moxa cone on the cake. During moxibustion, if the patient feels a little burning pain, the ignited moxa cone should be replaced by another to continue the treatment. 〈Indications〉all pyogenic infections and pains, injury of muscles and tendons and blood stasis due to tranmatic injury, distention and stuffiness in the abdomen, etc.

●隔矾灸[gé fán jiǔ] 间接灸的一种。见《神灸经纶》卷四。是用皂矾等作间隔物而施灸的一种方法。取皂矾500克(煅)、穿山甲3克(煅存性)、木鳖子8克(煅存性)、乳香、没药各5克,上药共研为细末,瓶贮备用。施灸时取上药末适量,用凉水调和制成饼状,贴于患处,上置艾炷灸之。本法用于治疗外痔和瘘管。

Alumen-Separated Moxibustion A form of indirect moxibustion in which aherbal cake containing black alum and other drugs is used as the separation, originally from Vol. 4 of *Shenjiu Jinglun* (*Principles of Magic Moxibustion*). 〈Method〉Take black alum(calcined) 500g, *Chuan Shan Jia* (*Squama Manitis*) 3g (calcined to keep its property), *Mu Bie Zi* (*Semen Momordicae*)8g(calcined to keep its property), *Ru Xiang* (*Resina Olibani*) 5g, *Mo Yao* (*Resina Commiphroae Myrrhea*) 5g. Grind the herbs into powder and put them in a bottle, well prepared for use. For moxibustion, take out a proper amount of the powder and mix it with cold water to make cakes, then apply one cake to the affected part and place a moxa cone upon the cake for moxibustion. 〈Indications〉extended hemorrhoids and fistula.

●隔附子灸[gé fù zǐ jiǔ] 间接灸的一种。临床上常用的有隔附子片灸和隔附子饼灸两种。①隔附子片灸。取熟附子用水浸透后,切片厚0.3-0.5厘米,中间用细针穿刺数孔,放于穴位或患处,上置艾炷点燃灸之。②隔附子饼灸。将附子切细研末,以黄酒调和作饼如五分硬币大,厚约0.4厘米,中间扎孔,放于穴位上置艾炷灸之。此法适用于治疗各种阳虚病证,如阳痿、早泄、遗精以及疮疡久溃不敛。

Fu Zi (Aconium Carmichaeli)-Separated Moxibustion A form of indirect moxibustion, which is clinically divided into *Fu Zi*(*Aconium Carmicheli*)-slice-separated moxibustion and *Fu Zi* (*Aconium Carmichaeli*)-cake-separated moxibustion. ① *Fu Zi* (*Aconium Carmichaeli*)-slice-separated moxibustion: Infuse processed *Fu Zi*(*Aconium Carmichaeli*) in water and cut it into slices of about 0.3-0.5 cm thick each. Punch several holes in the center with a small needle, then place it on an acupoint or the affected area and put a moxa cone upon the slice for moxibustion. ② *Fu Zi* (*Aconium Carmichaeli*)-cake-separated moxibustion: cut *Fu Zi* (*Aconium Carmichaeli*)into small pieces and grind it into powder, then mix it with yellow wine to make cakes of about 0.4 cm thick each, just the size of a 5-fen coin, punch holes in the center, place one cake on an acupoint and put a moxa cone on the cake for moxibustion. 〈Indications〉various diseases due to insufficiency of yang, e.g. impotence, premature ejaculation, seminal emission and persistent non-astringing sores.

●隔胡椒饼灸[gé hú jiāo bǐng jiǔ] 间接灸的一种。又称胡椒饼灸。用胡椒作间隔物而施灸的一种方法。取白胡椒研末,加适量白面粉,用水调和制成币状圆饼,厚约0.3厘米,中央按成凹陷,内置药末适量(丁香、肉桂、麝香等),将凹陷填平,上置艾炷灸之。临床适用于风寒湿痹痛及局部麻木不仁等病。

Pepper Cake-Separated Moxibustion A form of indirect moxibustion in which pepper is used as the separation, also called pepper-cake moxibustion. 〈Method〉Grind white pepper into powder and mix the powder with a proper amount of flour and water to make coin-like cakes of about 0.3 cm thick, with a depression in the centre. Fill the depression

with a proper amount of drug powder made from *Ding Xiang* (*Flos Syzygii aromatici*), *Rou Gui* (*Cortex Cinnamomi*), *She Xiang* (*Moschus*), etc. Place the dry cake on the affected area with a moxa cone upon it for moxibustion. 〈Indications〉arthralgia due to wind, cold and damp pathogen, local numbness, etc.

●隔姜灸[gé jiāng jiǔ] 间接灸的一种。用姜片作间隔物而施灸的一种方法。取新鲜生姜一块,切成厚约0.3厘米的姜片(大小可根据施灸部位及所选用艾炷大小而定),用细针于中间穿刺数孔,放在施灸的穴位上,上置艾炷点燃施灸。如病人在施灸过程中觉局部有热痛感,可将姜片连同艾炷向上略略提起,稍停放下再灸,亦可随即更换艾炷再灸。灸至局部皮肤潮红湿润为度。一般每次施灸5~10壮,可根据病情反复施灸。适用于一切虚寒病证、呕吐、腹痛、泄泻、遗精、阳萎、早泄、不孕、痛经、面瘫及风寒湿痹等。

Ginger-Separated Moxibustion A form of indirect moxibustion, in which ginger is used as the separation. 〈Method〉Take a piece of fresh ginger, cut a thin slice of it, about 0.3 cm thick (The size of the slice depends on the size of the selected region and the moxa cone). Punch several holes in the center with a small needle, then place it on the selected point with a moxa cone upon it for moxibustion. 〈Cautions〉During moxibustion, if the patient feels a local burning pain, the practitioner may lift the ginger slice, together with the burning moxa cone, for a while, then lay it on the original place again, or may replace the moxa cone with another to continue moxibustion until the local skin becomes flushed and wet. Each treatment generally needs 5-10 cones. This form of moxibustion may be repeated many times according to the patient's condition. 〈Indications〉 all diseases due to cold of insufficiency type, vomiting, abdominal pain, diarrhea, seminal emission, impotence, premature ejaculation, sterility, dysmenorrhea, facial paralysis, and arthralgia due to wind, cold and damp pathogen, etc.

●隔酱灸[gé jiàng jiǔ] 间接灸的一种。出《疮疡经验全书》卷七。用酱作间隔物而施灸的一种方法。操作时病人取坐位,医者将其百会穴上的头发从根部剪去一块,约如中指甲大。然后取干面酱约5克,敷于百会穴处,上置艾炷灸之。可用于治疗脱肛。

Flour Sauce-Separated Moxibustion A form of indirect moxibution, in which flour sauce is used as the separation, originally from Vol. 7 of *Chuang Yang Jingyan Quanshu* (*A Complete Manual of Experience in the Treatment of Sores*). 〈Method〉with the patient sitting, cut off the hair at the root on Baihui (Du 20) so that a piece of the scalp the size of the middle fingernail appears. Then take about 5g. of dried flour sauce and apply it to Baihui (DU 20) with a moxa cone upon it for mixibustion. 〈Indication〉proctoptosis.

●隔韭灸[gé jiǔ jiǔ] 间接灸的一种。见《疡医大全》。用韭菜作间隔物而施灸的一种方法。取韭菜(连根)适量洗净,捣烂如泥状,制成币状圆饼,敷于疮面,上置艾炷点燃灸之。适用于疮疡等证。

Chinese-Chives-Separated Moxibustion A form of indirect moxibustion, in which Chinese chives are used as separation, originally from *Yangyi Daquan* (*A Complete Work of External Diseases*). 〈Method〉wash a proper number of chives (with roots), clean and pound them into jelly to make coin-like cakes, then apply a cake to the surface of sore with a moxa cone upon it, and ignite the moxa cone for moxibustion. 〈Indications〉skin and external diseases, etc.

●隔苦瓠灸[gé kǔ hù jiǔ] 为苦瓠灸之别称。见该条。

Ku Hu (Lagenaria Siceraria)-Separated Moxibustion. →苦瓠灸(p. 234)

●隔面饼灸[gé miàn bǐng jiǔ] 间接灸的一种。见《千金要方》。用面粉饼作间隔物而施灸的一种方法。取面粉适量和水制成面饼,厚约0.5厘米,用细针穿刺数孔,放于患处,上置艾炷灸之。适用于治疗恶疮等。

Flour-Cake-Separated Moxibustion A form of indirect moxibustion, in which the cake is used as separation, originally from *Qianjin Yaofang* (*Essential Prescriptions Worth a Thousand Gold*). 〈Method〉Mix a proper amount of flour and water to make cakes of about 0.5 cm thick each. Pounch several holes in the cake with a small needle. Place the cake

on the affected area with a moxa cone upon for moxibustion.〈Indications〉malignant boil, etc.

●隔木香饼灸[gé mù xiāng bǐng jiǔ] 间接灸的一种。出《外科证治全书》。用木香等作间隔物而施灸的一种方法。取木香末15克,生地30克捣如膏,制成饼状,厚约0.6厘米,将药饼放于患处,上置艾炷灸之。用于治疗扑损闪挫、气滞血瘀等证。

Mu Xiang（Radix Aucklandiae）-Cake-Separated Moxibustion A form of indirect moxibustion, in which a medicinal cake made from radix acuklandiae and other herbs is used as the separation, originally from *Waike Zhengzhi Quanshu*(*A Complete Book on Diagnosis and Treatment of External Diseases*). Take *Mu Xiang*(*Radix Aucklandiae*)15g and *Sheng Di*（*Radix Rehmanniae*）30g, and pound them into paste to make cakes, about 0.6 cm thick each. Place a cake on the affected area with a moxa cone on it for moxibustion.〈Indications〉injury of soft tissue due to external trauma and diseases due to qi stagnancy and blood stasis.

●隔蛴螬灸[gé qí cáo jiǔ] 间接灸的一种。见《外科精义》。用蛴螬作间隔物而施灸的一种方法。取蛴螬一个,剪去两头,贴于疮口,上置艾炷灸之。每个蛴螬灸7壮,7个蛴螬为1疗程。适用于破伤风、疮疡诸证。

Grub-Separated Moxibustion A form of indirect moxibustion, in which a grub is used as the separation, originally from *Waike Jingyi*（*Essence of External Diseases*）.〈Method〉Take a grub, cut off the head and tail, apply it to the opening of the sore, then place a moxa cone on the grub for moxibustion. On each grub, 7 moxa cones can be ignited. A course of treatment is over after seven grubs are used.〈Indications〉tetanus, skin and external diseases, etc.

●隔商陆灸[gé shāng lù jiǔ] 为商陆灸之别称。详见该条。

Shang Lu（Radix Phytolaccae）-Separated Moxibustion Another name for Shang Lu (Radix Phytolaccae)Moxibustion. → 商陆饼灸 (p.350)

●隔蒜灸[gé suàn jiǔ] 间接灸的一种。出《肘后备急方》。用蒜作间物而施灸的一种灸法。常用有两种:①隔蒜片灸。取新鲜独头大蒜,切成厚约0.1-0.3厘米的蒜片,用细针于中间穿刺数孔,放于穴位或患处,上置艾炷点燃施灸,每灸3～4壮后或换去蒜片,继续施灸。②隔蒜泥灸。取新鲜大蒜适量,捣如泥膏状,放于穴位或患处,上置艾炷点燃灸之。均可用于治疗痈、疽、疮、疖、蛇蝎毒虫所伤、腹中积块及肺痨等。

Garlic-Separated Moxibustion A form of indirect moxibustion, originally from *Zhouhou Beiji Fang*（*A Handbook of Prescriptions for Emergencies*）, referring to the method of using garlic as the separation to perform moxibustion. Two kinds of the moxibstion are usually used：① garlic-slice-separated moxibustion.〈Method〉Select fresh, single-clove garlic, cut it into slices of about 0.1～0.3 cm in thickness, prick holes in the center of one slice with a thin needle before placing it on the selected acupoint or the affected region, then put a moxa-cone and burn it on the garlic slice for moxibustion, Substitute a new slice for the used one cones are burned.②mashed-garlic-separated moxibustion.〈Method〉Take a proper amount of fresh garlic, pound it into mashed garlic, place it on the selected acupoint or the affected region, put a moxa cone on it and burn it for moxibustion. Indications of the two methods above：carbuncle, cellulitis, sore, boils, snake, scorpion and insect bite, mass in the abdomen and pulmonary tuberculosis, etc.

●隔葶苈饼灸[gé tíng lì bǐng jiǔ] 间接灸的一种。见《千金要方》。用葶苈子作间隔物而施灸的一种方法。取葶苈子、豆豉适量,捣碎制饼如钱币大,厚约0.6厘米,用针扎数孔,置疮上,再放艾炷灸之。每灸3壮换1个葶苈饼,灸3个饼9壮为1疗程,3日灸1次。适用于瘰疬、痔疮等。

Ting Li Zi(Lepidium Seed)-Cake—Separated Moxibustion A form of indirect moxibustion, originally from *Qianjin Yaofang*(*Essntial Prescriptions Worth a Thousand Gold*), referring to the method of using lepidium seed as the separation to perform moxibustion.〈Method〉Take a proper amount of *Ting Li Zi*(*Lepudium seed*) and *Dou Chi*(*Semen Sojae Praeparatum*), pound them and make them cakes with the size of a coin, and about 0.6

cm in thickness. Prick holes in the cake with a needle before placing it over the sore, then put a moxa cone and burn in on the cake. Use 3 moxa cones for each cake and 9 moxa cones with 3 cakes as one course of treatment, once every three days. 〈Indications〉scrofula, and hemorrhoids, etc.

●隔碗灸[gé wǎn jiǔ] 为碗灸之别称。详见该条。
Bowl-Separated Moxibustion　Another name for bowl moxibustion. →碗灸(p.457)

●隔物灸[gé wù jiǔ] 灸法的一种,为间接灸之别称。详见该条。
Separation Moxibustion　A form of moxibustion, another form for indirect moxibustion. →间接灸(p.192)

●隔香附饼灸[gé xiāng fù bǐng jiǔ] 间接灸的一种。见《外科证治全书》卷五。用香附作间隔物而施灸的一种方法。取生香附研末,加入生姜汁调和,制成圆饼,厚约0.5厘米,放于患处,上置艾炷灸之。适用于痰核、瘰疬、痹证等。
Xiang Fu (Cyperustuber)-Cake-Separated Moxibustion　A form of indirect moxibustion, originally from Vol. 5 of *Waike Zhengzhi Quanshu* (*A Complete Book of Diagnosis and Treatment of External Diseases*), referring to the method of using *Xiang Fu (Cyperustuber)* as the separation to perform moxibustion. 〈Method〉Select fresh *Xiang Fu (Cyperustuber)* and grind it into powder; mix it with fresh ginger juice and make round cakes with it, each being 0.5 cm in thickness. Place a cake on the affected region, and put a buring moxa cone on the cake for moxibustion. 〈Indications〉subcuteneous nodule, scrofula and arthralgia-syndrome, etc.

●隔薤灸[gé xiè jiǔ] 间接灸的一种。出《千金要方》卷二十二。用薤叶作间隔物而施灸的一种方法。取薤叶适量,捣如膏状,敷于患处,上置艾炷灸之。可用于治疗恶露疮。
Xie Ye(Bulbus Allii Macrostemi)-Separated Moxibustion　A form of indirect moxibustion, originally from Vol. 22 of *Qianjin Yaofang* (*Essential Prescriptions Worth a Thousand Gold*), referring to the method of using *Xie Ye(Bulbus Allii Macrostemi)* as the separation to perform moxibustion. 〈Method〉 Take some leaves of *bulbus allii macrostemi*, pound them into a paste and apply it to the affected region with moxa cone on it for moxibustion. 〈Indication〉lochia and sore.

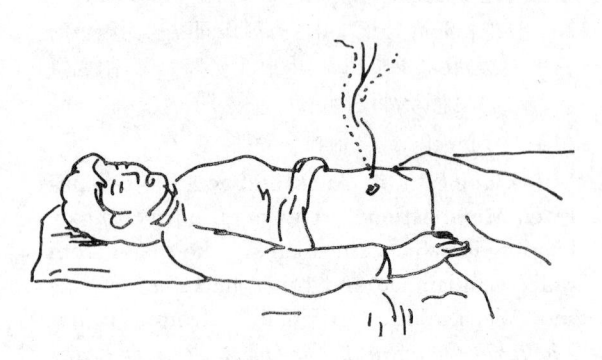

图18　隔盐灸
Fig 18　Salt-separated moxibustion

●隔盐灸[gé yán jiǔ] 间接灸的一种。见《肘后备急方》。用食盐作间隔物而施灸的一种方法。取纯净干燥的食盐适量研细或炒热,纳入脐中,使与脐平,上置艾炷施灸。如患者稍感灼痛,即更换艾炷。也有于盐上放置姜片而再施灸的,以避免食盐受火爆而致烫伤。临床上一般施灸3-9壮,对于急性病症可根据病情多灸,不拘壮数。此法有回阳、救逆、固脱之功效。临床上常用于急性腹泻、呕吐、痢疾、淋病、脱症等。
Salt-Separated Moxibustion　A form of indirect moxibustion, originally from *Zhouhou Beiji Fang* (*A Handbook of Prescriptions for Emergencies*), referring to the method of using salt as the separation to perform moxibustion. 〈Method〉Take a proper amount of pure, dry salt, grind it into powder or fry it, then fill the umbilicus with it to the level of the skin, place a moxa cone on the salt and ignite the moxacone for moxibustion. Change the moxa cone if the patient feels a little scorching pain. Ginger slices are applicable over the salt in this form of moxibustion treatment to avoid scald resulting from the fried salt. In clinical treatment, generally 3-9 moxa cones are used for one treatment. Moxa cones may be applied in moxibustion for acute diseases according to the conditions of the disease. 〈Actions〉recuperating depleted yang, rescuing the patient

●**隔纸灸**[gé zhǐ jiǔ] 间接灸的一种。出《普济方》卷四百二十二。用白纸作间接隔物而施灸的一种方法。将白纸折叠数层,放在冷水中浸湿,将艾炷放于湿纸上,用火点燃,置于患者舌头正中,医生用铜匙放于患者口内上腭以隔住艾烟,患者呼吸如常。此法适用于治疗痰喘、咳嗽、咯脓血等。

Paper-Separated Moxibustion A form of indirect moxibustion, originally from Vol. 422 of *Puji Fang* (*Prescription for Universal Relief*), referring to the method of using white paper as the separation to perform moxibustion. 〈Method〉Fold a piece of paper into several layers, soak it in cold water, then ignite a moxa cone on the wet paper, and place it on the centre of the tongue of the patient. Place a brass spoon at the palate of the patient's mouth in order to prevent the moxa smoke from being sucked so that the patient's breathing can be normal. 〈Indications〉dyspnea with plegm, cough and hemptysis with pus, etc.

●**膈**[gé] 为耳穴耳中之别称。详见该条。

Ge Another term for the ear point, Middle Ear(MA-H)→耳中(p.100)

●**膈关**[gé guān] 经穴名。出《针灸甲乙经》。属足太阳膀胱经。〈定位〉在背部,当第七胸椎棘突下,旁开3寸(图7)。〈层次解剖〉皮肤→皮下组织→斜方肌→菱形肌→竖脊肌。浅层布有第七、八胸神经后支的皮支和伴行的动、静脉。深层有肩胛背神经,肩胛背动、静脉,第七、八胸神经后支的肌支和相应的肋间后动、静脉背侧支的分支和属支。〈主治〉饮食不下、呕吐、嗳气、胸中噎闷、脊背强痛。斜刺0.5～0.8寸;可灸。

Geguan(BL 46) Name of a meridian point, originally from *Zhenjiu Jia-Yi Jing* (*A-B Classic of Acupuncture and Moxibusion*), a point on the Bladder Meridian of Foot-Taiyang. 〈Location〉on the back, below the spinous process of the 7th thoracic vertebra, 3 cun lateral to the posterior midline(Fig. 7). 〈Regional anatomy〉skin→subcutaneous tissue→trapezius muscle→rhomboid muscle→erector spinal muscle. In the superficial layer, there are the cutaneous branches of the posterior branches of the 7th and 8th thoracic nerves and the accompanying arteries and veins. In the deep layer, there are the dorsal scapular nerve, the dorsal scapular artery and vein, the muscular branches of the posterior branches of the 7th and 8th thoracic nerves and the branches or tributaries of the dorsal branches of the related posterior intercostal arteries and veins. 〈Indications〉dysphagia, vomiting, eructations, tight and oppressive feeling in the chest, stiffness and pain along column. 〈Method〉Puncture obliquely 0.5～0.8 cun. Moxibustion is applicable.

●**膈俞**[gé shù] 经穴名。出《灵枢·背腧》。属足太阳膀胱经,八会穴的血会。〈定位〉在背部,当第七胸椎棘突下,旁开1.5寸(图7)。〈层次解剖〉皮肤→皮下组织→斜方肌→背阔肌→竖脊肌。浅层布有第七、八胸神经后支的内侧皮支和伴行的动、静脉。深层有第七、八胸神经后支的肌支和相应肋间后动、静脉背侧支的分支或属支。〈主治〉胃脘胀痛、呕吐、呃逆、饮食不下、气喘、咳嗽、吐血、潮热、盗汗、背痛、脊强。斜刺0.5-0.8寸;可灸。

Geshu(BL 17) A meridian point, originally from *Lingshu*: *Beishu* (*Miraculous Pivot*: *Back-Shu Points*), a point on the Bladder Meridian of Foot Taiyang, the influential point of blood of the Eight Influential Points. 〈Location〉on the back, below the spinous process of the 7th thoracic vertebra, 1.5 cun lateral to the posterior midline(Fig. 7). 〈Regional anatomy〉skin → subcutaneous tissue → trapezius muscle → broadest muscle of back→erector Spinal muscle. In the superficial layer, there are the medial cutaneous branches of the posterior branches of the 7th and 8th thoracic nerves and the accompanying arteries and veins. In the deep layer, there are the muscular branches of the posterior branches of the 7th and 8th thoracic nerves and the branches or tributaries of the dorsal branches of the related posterior intercosal arteries and veins. 〈Indications〉epigastric distension and pain, vomiting, hiccup, difficulty in swallowing, asthma, cough, hemoptysis, afternoon fever, night sweating, pain in the back, stiffness of the spinal column.

〈Method〉Puncture perpendicularly 0.5～0.8 cun. Moxibustion is applicable.

●膈噎[gé yē]　病证名。见《济生方》卷二。即噎膈。详见该条。

Difficutlt Deglutition　Dysphagia a disease originally from Vol. 2 of *Jisheng Fang* (*Recipes for Saving Lives*). →噎膈(p.548)

●葛洪[gě hóng]　人名。东晋著名医药学家、道家，字稚川，号抱朴子，丹阳句容(今属江苏)人。对医学及道家理论有较深研究。著《肘后备急方》，又称《肘后卒救方》，收录的灸治方法不仅范围广，而且大多数是针对急性病证。此外，还著有《神仙传》和《抱朴子内、外篇》。

Ge Hong　A famous physician, pharmacist and Taoist in the Eastern Jin Dynasty, who styled himself Zhichuan, assumed the name of Bao Puzi, a native of Jurong in Danyang(now in Jiangsu province). He did research on the theory of medicine and Taoism, and compiled *Zhouhou Beiji Fang* (*A Handbok of Prescriptions for Emergencies*) which is also named *Zhouhou Cujiu Fang* (*A Handbook of Prescriptions for the Rescue*). The methods of moxibustion treatments recorded in this book are quite extensive and most of them are aimed at acute cases. In addition, he also wrote *Shenxian Zhuan*(*Biographies of Immortals*), and *Bao Puzi Nei/Wai Pian*(*Bao Puzi's Inner Treaties and Outer Treatise*).

●葛可久[gě kě jiǔ]　人名。元代医学家，名乾孙，长洲(今属江苏)人。世医出身，亦长于针灸。著《经络十二论》或[《十二经络(论)》]，已佚。另著《十药神书》、《医学启蒙》等。

Ge Kejiu　A physician in the Yuan Dynasty, also named Qiansun, a native of Changzhou(in Jiangsu Province today)with a family background of doctors for generations, skillful in acupuncture and moxibustion. He compiled *Jingluo Shier Lun*(*On the Twelve Meridians and Collaterals*), also named *Shier Jingluo Lun*[(*On*)*the Twelve Meridians and Collaterals*], which is no longer extant. In addition, he wrote *Shiyao Shenshu*(*A Miraculous Book of Ten Prescriptions*) and *Yixue Qimeng* (*The Enlightenment of Medicine*), etc.

●根结[gēn jié]　出《灵枢·根结》。根，即根本。结，即结聚。经脉以四肢末端(井穴)为根，头面、胸、腹为结。根和结强调经脉以四肢为出发点，突出各经从

表5　　　　　　　　　　　　　　根　　结
Table 5　　　　　　　　**Root and branch**

六　经 Six Meridians	根 Root	结 Branch
太　阳 Taiyang	至　阴 Zhiyin(BL 67)	命门　　　　(目) Mingmen(Jingming,BL 1)(eye)
阳　明 Yangming	厉　兑 Lidui(ST 45)	颡大　　　　(面) Sangda(Touwei,ST 8)(face)
少　阳 Shaoyang	窍　阴 Qiaoyin(GB 44)	窗笼　　　　(耳) Chuanglong(Tinggong,SI 19)(ear)
太　阴 Taiyin	隐　白 Yinbai(SP 1)	太仓　　　　(腹) Taicang(Zhongwan,RN 12)(abdomen)
少　阴 Shaoyin	涌　泉 Yongquan(KI 1)	廉泉　　　　(喉) Lianquan(Lianquan,RN 23)(throat)
厥　阴 Jueyin	大　敦 Dadun(LR 1)	玉英　　　　(胸) Yuying(Yutang,RN 18)(chest)

四肢上达头胸和腹的联系特点。根结的具体部位见表5。

Root and Branch Originally from *Lingshu*: *Gen Jie* (*Miraculous Pivot*: *Root and Branch*). Root is synonymous with source and branch with convergence. The termination of the four extremities, Jing (well) points are taken as the roots of the meridians, and the head, face, chest, and abdomen as the branches. Root and branch lay emphasis on the termination of the four extremities being the source of the meridians, and stress the connecting characteristics of each meridian ascending to the head, the chest and the abdomen from the termination of the four extermities. For the details, see Table 5.

●根溜注入 [gēn liū zhù rù] 出《灵枢·根结》。手足阳经中脉气流行出入的部位。根指四肢末端的井穴，与根结之根相同；溜是流通的意思，指原穴；注是灌注的意思，指经穴；入是由浅入深，指各经的颈部穴及四肢部络穴。详见表6。

Source, Flow, Pour and Entry Originally from *Lingshu*: *Gen Jie* (*Miraculous Pivot*: *Root and Branch*), referring to the regions where the meridian-qi of the yang meridians of the hand and foot begins, flows, pours and enters. Source refers to the Jing (well) points at the termination of the four extremities, (it is the same as the root described in root and branch); flow means circulation, referring to the Yuan (Primary) points; pour means irrigation, referring to Jing (River) points; entry means entrance from the surface to the deep, referring to the acupoints on the neck of each meridian and the Luo (Connecting) points of the four extremities. See Table 6 for details.

●跟 [gēn] 耳穴名。位于对耳轮上脚的内上角。用于治疗足跟痛。

Heel (MA-Ah 1) An ear point. 〈Location〉 at the medial and superior angle of the superi-

表6　　　　　　　　　　根溜注入
Table 6　　　　　　　Source, flow, pour and entry

经名 Meridian	穴位　　Acupoint				
	Source 根	Flow 溜	Pour 注	Entry 入	
				上 Superior	下 Inferior
足太阳 Foot Taiyang	至阴 Zhiyin (BL 67)	京骨 Jinggu (BL 64)	昆仑 Kunlun (BL 60)	天柱 Tianzhu (BL 10)	飞阳 Feiyang (BL 58)
足少阳 Foot Shaoyang	足窍阴 Zuqiaoyin (GB 44)	丘墟 Qiuxu (GB 40)	阳辅 Yangfu (GB 38)	天容 Tianrong (SI 17)	光明 Guangming (GB 37)
足阳明 Foot Yangming	厉兑 Lidui (ST 45)	冲阳 Chongyang (ST 42)	下陵(足三里) Xialing Zusanli (ST 36)	人迎 Renying (ST 9)	丰隆 Fenglong (ST 40)
手太阳 Hand Taiyang	少泽 Shaoze (SI 1)	阳谷 Yanggu (SI 5)	小海 Xiaohai (SI 8)	天窗 Tianchuang (SI 16)	支正 Zhizheng (SI 7)
手少阳 Hand Shaoyang	关冲 Guanchong (SJ 1)	阳池 Yangchi (SJ 4)	支沟 Zhigou (SJ 6)	天牖 Tianyou (SJ 16)	外关 Waiguan (SJ 5)
手阳明 Hand Yangming	商阳 Shangyang (LI 1)	合谷 Hegu (LI 4)	阳溪 Yangxi (LI 5)	扶突 Futu (LI 18)	偏历 Pianli (LI 6)

or crus of the antihelix.〈Indication〉pain in the heel.

●公孙[gōng sūn] 经穴名。出《灵枢·经脉》。属足太阴脾经，为本经络穴。八脉交会穴之一，通于冲脉。〈定位〉在足内侧缘，当第一跖骨基底的前下方(图8和图39)。〈层次解剖〉皮肤→皮下组织→展肌→短屈肌→长屈肌腱。浅层布有隐神经的足内缘支，足背静脉弓的属支。深层有足底内侧动、静脉的分支或属支，足底内侧神经的分支。〈主治〉胃疼、呕吐、饮食不化、肠鸣腹胀、腹痛、痢疾、泄泻、多饮、霍乱、水肿、烦心、失眠、发狂妄言、嗜卧、肠风下血、脚气。直刺0.5～0.8寸；可灸。

Gongsun(SP 4) A meridian point, originally from *Ling Shu: Jingmai (Miraculous Pivot: Meridians)*, the Luo(connecting)point of the Spleen Meridian of Foot Taiyin, one of the Eight confluent Points, connecting with the Chong Meidian.〈Location〉on the inedial border of the foot, anterior and inferior to the proximal end of the lst metatarsal bone(Figs. 8&39).〈Regional anatomy〉skin → subcutaneous tissue → abductor muscle → short flexor → long flexor tendon. In the superficial layer, there are the medial branches of the foot from saphenous nerve and the tributaries of the dorsal venous arch of the foot. In the deep layer, there are the branches or tributaries of the medial platar artery and the branches of the medial plantar artery and vein and the branches of the medial plantar nerve.〈Indications〉gastric pain, vomiting, indigestion of food, borborygmus, abdominal distension and pain, dysentery, diarrhea, excessive drink, cholera morbus, edema, irritability, insomnia, manicpsychosis with ravings, drowsiness, enterorrhagia, beriberi.〈Method〉Puncture perpendicularly 0.5～0.8 cun. Moxibustion is applicable.

●宫冷不孕[gōng lěng bù yùn] 即胞寒不孕的别名。详见该条。

No Fertility with Cold Uterus Another name for Sterility due to Retention of Cold in Uterus.→胞寒不孕(p.13)

●孤府[gū fǔ] 三焦的别称。详见该条。

Solitary Fu Another term for sanjiao.→三焦(p.342)

●谷门[gǔ mén] 经穴别名。出《针灸甲乙经》。即天枢。详见该条。

Gumen Another name for Tianshu(ST 25), a meridian point originally from *Zhenjiu Jia-Yi Jing (A-B Classic of Acupuncture and Moxibustion)*.→天枢(p.434)

●骨度[gǔ dù] 腧穴定位方法之一。骨度折量定位法的简称。详见该条。

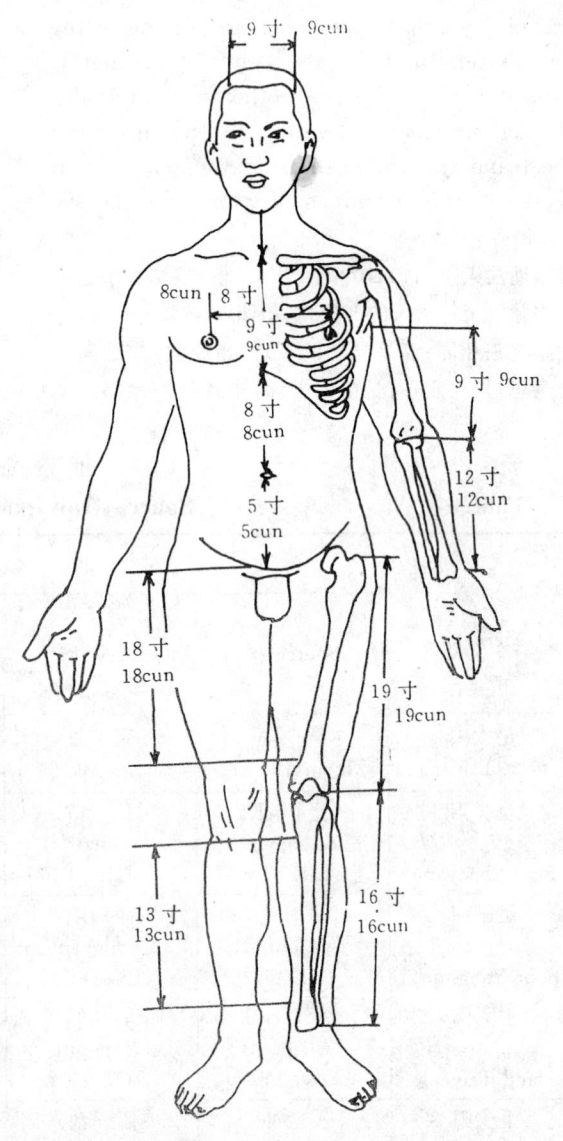

图19.1 骨度分寸(正面)

Fig 19.1 Bone proportional cun(B-cun) (Anterior view)

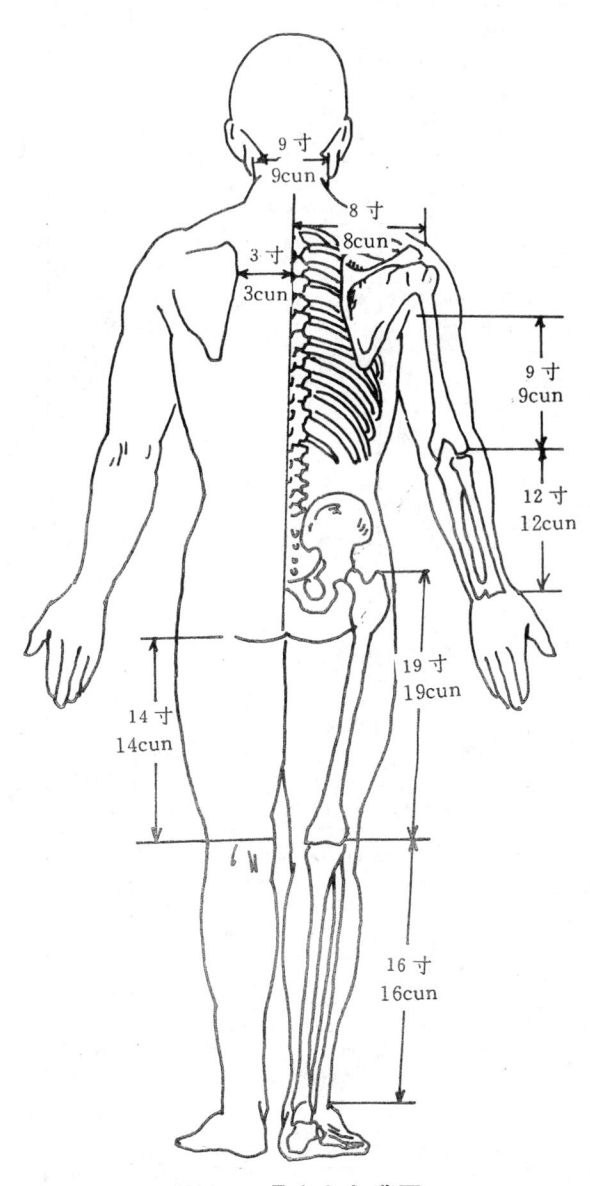

图19.2 骨度分寸(背面)

Fig 19.2 Bone proportional cun (B-cun) (Posterior view)

Bone Measurement One of the methods of locating acupoints, a short form for bone proportional measurement. →骨度折量定位法(p. 143)

●骨度法[gǔ dù fǎ] 腧穴定位方法之一。骨度折量定位法的简称。详见该条。

Bone-Length Measurement One of the methods of locating acupoints, short form for bone proportional measurement. →骨度折量定位法(p. 143)

●骨度折量定位法[gǔ dù zhé liáng dìng wèi fǎ] 腧穴定位方法之一。出《灵枢·骨度》。又称骨度、骨度法。指以体表骨节为主要标志折量全身各部的长度和宽度,定出尺寸,用于经穴定位的方法。即以《灵枢·骨度》规定的人体各部的分寸为基础,并结合历代学者创用的折量分寸(将设定的两骨节点之间的长度折量为一定的等分,每一等分为1寸,十等分为1尺),作为定穴的依据。全身主要"骨度"折量寸见表7(据国家技术监督局1990-06-07发布)。

Bone proportional Measurement One of the methods of locating acupoints, originally from *Lingshu: Gu Du (Miraculous Pivot: Bone Measurement)*, also called bone measmement or bone-length measurement. A method of locating acupoints, in which the proportional cun of width and length of any parts of the body are measured in accordance with the main superficial marks of the bones. In other words, the proportional measurements depend on the measurements of various portions of the human body as are provided in *Lingshu: Gu Du (Miraculous Pivot: Bone Measurement)*, in combination with the proportional measurements created and used by the scholars of the past. The length between the two superficial marks of bones is taken as a definite equal unit, each equal unit is taken as 1 cun, ten equal units as 1 chi. These measurements are the basis of locating acupints. The main bone proportional measurements of the body are shown in Table 7 (issued by the National Technology Supervision Bureau 1990-06-07).

●骨空[gǔ kōng] 腧穴之别名。指骨间空隙,多为腧穴所在。详见该条。

Bone Holes Another name for acupoints, referring to the space between bones, where the acupoints are generally located. →腧穴(p. 407)

表7 全身主要骨度折量寸
Table 7　Main bone proportional measurement of the body

部位 Body Part	起止点 starting and ending points	折量寸 Proportional Measurement	度量法 Method	说明 Explanation
头面部 Head	前发际正中→后发际正中 From the midpoint of the anterior hairline to the midpoint of the posterior hairline	12 寸 12 cun	直 寸 Longitudinal measurement	用于确定头部经穴的纵向距离。 Used for determining the longitudinal distance of the acupoints on the head.
	眉间(印堂)→前发际正中 From the midpoint between the two eyebrows (Yintang EX-HN 3) to the midpoint of the anterior hairline	3 寸 3 cun	直 寸 Longitudinal measurment	用于确定前或后发际及其头部经穴的纵向距离 Used for determining the longitudinal distance between the anterior or posterior hairline and the acupoints on the head.
	第七颈椎棘突下(大椎)→后发际正中 From the depression below the spinous process of the 7th cervical vertebra (Dazhui, DU 14) to the midpoint of the posterior hairline	3 寸 3 cun	直 寸 Longitudinal measurement	
	眉间(印堂)→后发际正中→第七颈椎棘突(大椎) From the midpoint betwoon the two eyebrows (Yintang EX-HN 3) to the midpoint of the posterior hairline to the midpoint of the posterior hairline to the depression below the spinous process of the 7th cervical vertebra (Dazhui DU 14)	18 寸 18 cun	直 寸 Longitiudinal measurement	
	前两额发角(头维)之间 Between the frontal hair corners of the two foreheads(Touwei ST 8)	9 寸 9 cun	横 寸 Transverse measurement	用于确定头前部经穴的横向距离。 Used for determining the transverse distance of the acupoints on the anterior of the head.
	耳后两乳突(完骨)之间 Between the two mastoid processes (Wangu GB 12)	9 寸 9 cun	横 寸 Transvėrse measurement	用于确定头部经穴的下横向距离。 Used for determining the transverse distance of the acupoints on the posterior of the head.
胸、腹胁部 Chest, Abdomen and Rib	胸骨上窝(天突)→胸剑联合中点(歧骨) From the suprasternal fossa of the sternum (Tiantu, RN 22) to the midpoint of the xiphosternal synchondrosis (the 7th costo sternal juncture)	9 寸 9 cun	直 寸 Longitudinal measurement	用于确定胸部任脉穴的纵向距离。 Used for determining the longitudinal distance of the acupoints on the Ren meridian in the chest.
	胸剑联合中点(歧骨)→脐中 from the midpoint of the xiphosternal synchondrosis (the 7th costo sternal juncture) to the centre of the umbilicus	8 寸 8 cun	直 寸 Longitudinal measurement	用于确定上腹部经穴的纵向距离。 Used for determining the longitudial distance of the acupoints in the upper abdomen.
	脐中→耻骨联合上缘(曲骨) From the centre of the umbilicus to the upper border of symphysis pubis (Qugu RN 2)	5 寸 5 cun	直 寸 Longitudinal Measurement	用于确定下腹部经穴的纵向距离 Used for determining the transverse distance of the acupoints in the lower abdomen.
	两乳头之间 Between the two nipples	8 寸 8 cun	横 寸 Transverse measurement	用于确定胸腹部经穴的横向距离。 Used for determining the transverse distance of the acupoints in the chest and abdomen.
	腋窝顶点→第十一肋游离端(章门) From the top of the auxiliary fossa to the free end of the 11th rib(Zhangmen, LR 13)	12 寸 12 cun	直 寸 Longitudinal measurement	用于确定胁部经穴的纵向距离 Used for determining the longitudinal distance of the acupoints in the hypochondriac region.

部 位 Body Part	起止点 starting and ending points	折量寸 Proportional Measurement	度量法 Method	说 明 Explanation
背腰部 Back and Waist	肩胛骨内缘→后正中线 From the medial border of the scapula to the posterior midline	3 寸 3 cun	横 寸 Transverse measurement	用于确定背腰部经穴的横向距离 Used for determining the transverse distance of the acupoints on the back and waist.
	肩峰缘→后正中线 From the acromion border to the posterior midline	8 寸 8 cun	横 寸 Transverse measurement	用于确定肩背部经穴的横向距离。 Used for determining the transverse distance of the acupoints on the shoulder and back.
上肢部 Upper Extremities	腋前、后纹头→肘横纹 From the anterior and posterior ends of the axillary fold to the transverse cubital crease	9 寸 9 cun	直 寸 Longitudinal measurement	用于确定臂部经穴的纵向距离。 Used for determining the longitudinal distance of the acupoints on the arm.
	肘横纹→腕掌侧横纹 From the transverse cubital crease to the transverse wrist crease	12 寸 12 cun	直 寸 Longitudinal Measurement	用于确定前臂部经穴的纵向距离。 Used for determining the longitudinal distance of the acupoints on the forearm.
下肢部 Lower Extremities	耻骨联合上缘→股骨内上髁上缘 From the upper border of symphysis pubis to the upper border to the medial epicondyle of femur	18 寸 18 cun	直 寸 Longitudinal measurement	用于确定下肢内侧足三阴经穴的纵向距离。 Used for determining the longitudinal distance of the acupoints on the three Yin meridians on the medial side of foot.
	胫骨内侧髁下方→内踝尖 From the lower border of the medial condyle of tibia to the tip of medial malleolus	13 寸 13 cun	直 寸 Longitudinal measurement	
	股骨大转子→腘横纹 From the great trochanter of femur to the popliteal transverse crease	19 寸 19 cun	直 寸 Longitudinal measurement	用于确定下肢外后侧足三阳经穴的纵向距离。(臀沟→腘横纹,相当14寸) Used for determining the longitudinal distance of the acupoints on the three Yang meridians on the lateral and posterior side of foot. (gluteal groove → popliteal transverse crease 14 cun)
	横纹→外踝尖 From the popliteal transverse crease to the tip of lateral malleolus	16 寸 16 cun	直 寸 Longitudinal measurement	用于确定下肢外后侧足三阳经穴的纵向距离 Used for determining the longitudinal distance of the acupoints on the three Yang meridints on the lateral-posterior side of foot.

●**骨繇者取之少阳** [gǔ yáo zhě qǔ zhī shào yáng] 《内经》治则之一。繇,音义同摇。指对骨节纵摇动病症的治疗,可从少阳经选穴。
Selection of Shaoyang Points for Bone Convulsion and Shake　One of the treatment principles in *Neijing* (*The Inner Canon of Huangdi*). "繇" means "Shake". The term refers to the treatment for diseases of bone convulsion and shake, in which points on the Shaoyang Meridian can be selected.

●**骨针** [gǔ zhēn] 古针具名。以兽骨制成。1933年在北京周口店山顶洞发现骨针,据考证,距今约十万年左右,说明该时已能制造骨针,并可能用以治病。
Bone Needle　A form of needle used in ancient times, made of animal bones. It was found in 1933 in Shandingdong, Zhoukoudian of Beijing and according to textual research, it must have been made about 100,000 years ago. It has been proved that the bone needle might have been made at that time, and used in the treatemrnt of diseases.

●**骨蒸病灸方** [gǔ zhēng bìng jiǔ fāng] 图书名。唐代崔知悌撰。又名《灸骨蒸方图》、《灸二十二种骨蒸方》、《崔丞相灸劳法》。是较早的一本灸法图册,内容后世针灸书中多有转引。

Guzheng Bing Jiufang(Moxibustion Methods for Consumptive Diseases) A book written by Cui Zhidi in the Tang Dynasty, also named *Jiu Guzheng Fang Tu*(Prescriptions and Diagrams of Moxibustion for Hectic Fever), *Jiu Ershier Zhong Guzheng Fang*(Prescriptions of Moxibustion for 22 Kinds of Hectic Fever), *Cui Chengxiang Jiu Laofa*(Prime Minister Cui's Moxibustion Methods for Consumptive Diseases), an earlier illustrated book on moxibustion. The contents of the book are often quoted in books on acupuncture and moxibustion of later ages.

●鼓胀[gǔ zhàng] 病证名。出《灵枢·水胀》等。一作臌胀。指腹部肿胀膨隆之类的病证。又称单腹胀、单鼓、蜘蛛蛊、胀。临床上根据症候表现的不同，一般分为气鼓、血鼓、水鼓等。详见各条。

Tympanites A disease, originally from *Lingshu: Shuizhang* (*Miraculous Pivot: Edema*), synonymous with bulge. Referring to diseases involving swelling, distension and expansion of the abdomen. Also called distension of side abdomen, tympanites of side abdomen, spider-like tympanites, spider-like distension. It is generally classified as tympanites due to the stagnation of qi, tympanites due to blood stasis and tympanites due to fluid retention depending on the different clinical manifestations. → 气鼓(p. 305)、血鼓(p. 524)、水鼓(p. 409)

●臌胀[gǔ zhàng] 病证名。即鼓胀。详见该条。

Bulge A disease, synonymous with tympanites. → 鼓胀(p. 146)

●固定标志[gù dìng biāo zhì] 体表解剖标志的一种。指各部由骨节和肌肉形成的突起和凹陷，五官轮廓，发际，指（趾）甲，乳头，脐窝等。利用这些标志，可以确定部分腧穴的位置。

Fixed Marks Anatomical marks on the body surface, referring to the prominences, depressions, five sense organs, hairline, nails, nipples, umbilicus, etc, formed by bones and muscles of various portions of the body, with which the locations of some acupoints can be determined.

●刮法[guā fǎ] 针刺辅助手法之一。指针刺达一定深度后，用指甲刮动针柄的操作方法。目的是为加强针感，或使针感传导扩散。①用右手拇指抵压针柄顶端，同时用食指或中指指甲从针柄下端向上刮动，叫单手刮升法。②用左手拇指或食指抵压针柄顶端，右手拇指或食指指甲或从上向下，或从下向上刮动针柄，叫双手刮针法。③以左手拇、食指挟扶针体下端，右手拇指或食指指甲作螺旋形，从下向上刮动针柄，又叫旋刮术。

Scraping An auxiliary acupuncture manipulation. Referring to manipulation by scraping the needle handle with the finger nail after the needle is inserted to a certain depth. 〈Aims〉 Strengthen the needling sensation or conduct and spread the needling sensation. 〈Method〉 ①Place the thumb of the right hand on the top end of the handle, then scrape it upwards with the nail of the index or middle finger of the right hand from its lower end. This is called single-hand upward scraping. ② Place the thumb or the index finger of the left hand on the top end of the handle, then scrape it with the nail of the thumb or the index finger of the right hand from top to bottom, or vice versa. This is called double-hand scraping. ③ Grip the lower part of the needle with the thumb and the index finger of the left hand, then spirally scrape the needle with the nail of the thumb or the index finger of the right hand from bottom to top. This is called spiral scraping.

●关冲[guān chōng] 经穴名。出《灵枢·本输》，属手少阳三焦经，为本经井穴。〈定位〉在手环指末节尺侧，距指甲角0.1寸（指寸）（图44）。〈层次解剖〉皮肤→皮下组织→指甲根。皮下组织内有尺神经指掌侧固有神经的指背支的分支，指掌侧固有动、静脉指背支的动、静脉网。〈主治〉头痛、目赤、耳聋、耳鸣、喉痹、舌强、热病、心烦。浅刺0.1寸，或点刺出血；可灸。

Guanchong(SJ 1) A meridian point originally from *Lingshu: Benshu* (*Miraculous Pivot Meridian Points*), the Jing(Well) point of the Sanjiao Meridian of Hand Shaoyang. 〈Location〉on the ulnar side of the distal segment of the 4th finger, 0.1 cun from the corner of the nail(Fig. 44). 〈Regional anatomy〉 skin→subcutaneous tissue→root of the nail. In the subcutaneous tissue, there are the branches of the dorsal digital branches of the proper palmar digital nerve from the ulnar, and the arteriove-

nous network of the dorsal branches of the proper palmar digital arteries and veins. 〈Indications〉headache, conjunctival congestion, deafness, tinitus, inflammation of the throat, stiffness of the tongue, febrile diseases and irritability. 〈Method〉Puncture subcutaneously 0.1 cun, or prick to cause bleeding. Moxibustion is applicable.

●关刺[guān cì]　《内经》刺法名。出《灵枢·官针》。五刺之一。这种刺法多在关节附近的肌腱上进行针刺,因为筋会于节,四肢筋肉的尽端都在关节附近,故名关刺。可治筋痹证。因针刺较深,必须注意不要伤脉出血。由于肝主筋,所以与肝脏相应。

Joint Puncture　A needling technique in *Neijing*(*The Canon of Internal Medicine*), originally from *Lingshu*:*Guanzhen*(*Miraculous Pivot*:*Official Needles*). One of the five needling techniques, performed by inserting needles on the tendons around the joints. Because tendons gather in the joints, and the terminations of the tendons and muscles of the four extremities are distributed around the joints, the method is named joint puncture. 〈Indications〉muscular rheumatism and pain in the muscles and tendons. Because the needle insertion is deep, attention should be paid to avoiding impairing the meridians and causing bleeding. Since the liver dominates tendons, the method corresponds to the liver organ.

●关阖枢[guān hé shū]　出《灵枢·根结》。《素问·阴阳离合论》等。古时用此来解释经络学说中三阴三阳气机变化的特点。("关"原文作"开",据《黄帝内经太素》卷十及《素问·阴阳离合论》新校正引《九墟》文,改为"关"。方与《灵枢·根结》之"折关败枢"文合。)原意关 是门栓,其变动为开;阖是门扇,其变动为闭;枢是户枢,其变动为转。六经中的太阳居阳分之表,为关;阳明居阳分之里,为阖;少阳居阳分之中,为枢。太阴居阴分之表,为关;厥阴居阴分之里,为阖;少阴居阴分之中,为枢。六经皮部也结合关阖枢命名。

Bolt-Door-Pivot　Originally from *Lingshu*:*Gen Jie*(*Miraculous Pivot*:*Root and Branch*) and *Suwen*:*Yin-Yang Li He Lun*(*Plain Questions*:*On the Parting and Meeting of Yin and Yang*). Used for explaining the characteristics of the qi change of three yin's and three yang's in the theory of meridians and collaterals. ("Bolt" originally was taken as "opening", according to Vol. 10 of *Huang Di Neijing Taisu* (*Comprehensive Notes to the Yellow Emperor's Canon of Internal Medicine*) and *Jiu Xu* (*Nine Earthy Mountains*) quoted in *New Rectification of Suwen*:*Yin-Yang Li He Lun*(*Plain Questions*: *On the Parting and Meeting of Yin and Yang*), "Opening" was corrected as "bolt", which corresponds to the sentence of "broken" bolt and damaged "pivot" in *Lingshu*: *Gen Jie* (*Miraculous Pivot*: *Root and Branch*). Bolt originally meant door bolt, its change meant opening; door meant door plank, its change meant closing; pivot meant door pivot, its change meant transmitting. Of the six meridians the Taiyang Meridians are in the exterior of yangfen, as bolt; yang-ming in the interior of yangfen, as door; shaoyang in the middle of yangfen, as pivot; Taiyin in the exterior of yinfen, as bolt; Jueyin in the interior of yinfen, as door; Shaoyin in the middle of yinfen, as pivot. Cutaneous regions of the six meridians are named in the light of bolt-door-pivot.

●关梁[guān liáng]　经穴别名。出《针灸甲乙经》。即金门。详见该条。

Guanliang　Another name for Jinmen (BL 63), a meridian point originally from *Zhenjiu Jia-Yi Jing* (*A-B Classic of Acupuncture and Moxibustion*). →金门 (p. 203)

●关陵[guān líng]　经穴别名。见《千金要方》。即膝阳关。详见该条。

Guanling　Another name for Xiyangguan (GB 33), a meridian point, originally from *Qianjin Yaofang* (*Essential Prescriptions Worth a Thousand Gold*→膝阳关 (p. 484)

●关门[guān mén]　经穴名。出《针灸甲乙经》。属足阳明胃经。〈定位〉在上腹部,当脐中上3寸,距前正中线2寸(图60和图40)。〈层次解剖〉皮肤→皮下组织→腹直肌鞘前壁→腹直肌。浅层布有第七、八、九胸神经前支的外侧皮支和前皮支,腹壁浅静脉。深层有腹壁上动、静脉的分支或属支,第七、八、九胸神经前支的肌支。〈主治〉腹痛、腹胀、肠鸣泄泻、食欲不振、水肿、遗尿。直刺0.8-1.2寸;可灸。

Guanmen (ST 22) A meridian point originally from *Zhenjiu Jia-Yi Jing* (*A-B Classic of Acupuncture and Moxibustion*). ⟨Location⟩ on the upper abdomen, 3 cun above the centre of the umbilicus and 2 cun lateral to the anterior midline (Figs. 60&40). ⟨Regional anatomy⟩ skin→subcutaneous tissue→anterior wall of vagina musculi recti abdominis. In the superficial layer, there are the lateral and anterior cutaneous branches of the anterior branches of the 7th to 9th thoracic nerves and the superficial epigastric vein. In the deep layer, there are the branches or tributaries of the superior epigastric artery and vein and the muscular branches of the anterior branches of the 7th to 9th thoracic nerves. ⟨Indications⟩ abdominal pain and distension, borborygmus, diarrhea, anorexia, edema, enuresis. ⟨Method⟩ Puncture perpendicularly 0.8-1.2 cun. Moxibustion is applicable.

●关明[guān míng] 即关门。出《千金翼方》。

Guanming Synonymous with Guanmen (ST 22), originally from *Qianjin Yifang* (*A Supplement to the Essential Prescriptions Worth a Thousand Gold*).

●关枢[guān shū] 六经皮部之一，太阳皮部名。出《素问·皮部论》。"关"是关键、门栓的意思，"枢"有枢转的含义。阳经中以太阳为关，故称"关枢"。

Bolt-Pivot One of the cutaneous regions of the six-pair meridians. Name of the cutaneous region of Taiyang, originally from *Su Wen: Pibu Lun* (*Plain Questions: On Cutaneous Regions*). "Bolt" means the crux, and door bolt; "pivot" means transmitting. Taiyang is taken as bolt in the yang meridians, hence the name "pivot".

●关阳[guān yáng] 经穴别名。出《千金要方》。即膝阳关。详见该条。

Guanyang Another name for Xiyangguan (GB 33), a meridian point originally from *Qianjin Yaofang* (*Essential Prescriptions Worth a Thousand Gold*). →膝阳关 (p. 484)

●关仪[guān yí] 经外穴名。见《千金要方》。即膝外侧缘，当腘窝横纹上1寸处。⟨主治⟩小腹绞痛。直刺0.5-1寸；可灸。

Guanyi (EX-LE) An extra point, originally from *Qianjin Yaofang* (*Essential Prescriptions Worth a Thousand Gold*) ⟨Location⟩ on the lateral border of the knee, 1 cun above the popliteal transverse crease. ⟨Indication⟩ colic in the lower abdomen. ⟨Method⟩ Puncture perpendicularly 0.5～1 cun. Moxibustion is applicable.

●关元[guān yuán] 经穴名。出《灵枢·寒热病》。属任脉，为小肠之募穴，足三阴、任脉之会，冲脉所起处。又名次门、三结交、下纪、大中极。⟨定位⟩在下腹部，前正中线上，当脐下3寸（图40）。⟨层次解剖⟩皮肤→皮下组织→腹白线→腹横筋膜→腹膜外脂肪→壁腹膜。浅层主要有第十二胸神经前支的前皮支和腹壁浅动、静脉的分支或属支。深层主要有第十二胸神经前支的分支。⟨主治⟩中风脱证、虚劳冷惫、羸瘦无力、少腹疼痛、霍乱吐泻、痢疾、脱肛、疝气、便血、溺血、小便不利、尿频、尿闭、遗精、白浊、阳萎、早泄、月经不调、经闭、经痛、赤白带下、阴挺、崩漏、阴门搔痒、恶露不止、胞衣不下、消渴、眩晕。直刺0.5-1寸；可灸。

Guanyuan (RN 4) A meridian point, originally from *Lingshu: Han Re Bing* (*Miraculous Pivot: Cold and Heat Diseases*). A point on the Ren Meridian, the Front-Mu point of the small intestine, the crossing point of the three Yin Meridians of the Foot and Ren Merdidian, the place where the Chong meridian starts, also called Cimen, Sanjiejiao, xiaji or Dazhongji. ⟨Location⟩ on the lower abdomen and on the anterior midline, 3 cun below the centre of the umbilicus. (Fig. 40). ⟨Regional anatomy⟩ skin → subcutaneous tissue → linea alba→transverse fascia→extraperitoneal fat→ parietal peritoneum. In the superficial layer, there are the anterior cutaneous branches of the anterior branch of the 12th thoracic nerve and the branches or tributaries of the superficial epigastric artery and vein. In the deep layer, there are the branches of the anterior branch of the 12th thoracic nerve. ⟨Indications⟩ prostration syndrome due to apoplexy, consumptive disease with cold and fatigue feeling, thinness and weakness, pain in the lower area of the abdomen, vomiting and diarrhea due to cholera, dysentery, prolapse of rectum, hernia, hemafecia, hematuria, dysuria, frequent micturation, retention of urine, semi-

nal emission, cloudy urine, impotence, premature ejaculation, irregular menstruation, amenorrhea, dysmenorrhea, leukorrhea with reddish discharge, prolapse of uterus, metrorrhagia and metrostaxis, itching sensation in vagina, persistend lochia, retention of placenta, diabetes, dizziness. 〈Method〉Puncture perpendicularly 0.5～1 cun. Moxibustion is applicable.

●关元俞[guān yuán shù] 经穴名。出《太平圣惠方》。属足太阳膀胱经。〈定位〉在腰部,当第五腰椎棘突下,旁开1.5寸(图7)。〈层次解剖〉皮肤→皮下组织→胸腰筋膜浅层→竖脊肌。浅层布有第五腰神经和第一骶神经后支的皮支及伴行的动、静脉。深层有第五腰神经后支的肌支等结构。〈主治〉腹胀、泄泻、小便不利、遗尿、消渴、腰痛。直刺0.8-1寸;可灸。

Guanyuanshu(BL 26) A meridian point, originally from *Taiping Shenghui Fang*(*Imperial Benevolent Prescriptions*), a point on the Bladder Meridian of Foot Taiyang. 〈Location〉on the low back, below the spinous process of the 5th lumbar vertebra, 1.5 cun lateral to the posterior midline(Fig. 7). 〈Regional anatomy〉 skin→subcutaneous tissue→superficial layer of thoracolummbar fascia→erector spinal muscle. In the superficial layer, there are the cutaneous branches of the posterior branches of the 5th lumbar and 1st sacral nerves and the accompanying arteries and veins. In the deep layer, there are the muscular branches of the posterior branches of the 5th lumbar nerves. 〈Indications〉 abdominal distension, diarrhea, dysuria, enuresis, diabetes, lumbago. 〈Method〉Puncture perpendicularly 0.8～1 cun. Moxibustion is applicable.

●关蛰[guān zhé] 六经皮部之一,太阴皮部名。出《素问·皮部论》,"关"是关键的意思,"蛰"有阴气蛰藏的含义,阴经以太阴为关,故称关蛰。

Bolt-Dormancy One of the cutaneous regions of the six-pair meridians. Name of the cutaneous regions of Taiyin, originally from *Su Wen*: *Pibu Lun*(*Plain Questions*: *On Cutaneous Regions*) "Bolt" means the crux; "dormancy" implies hiding of yin-qi. Taiyin is taken as bolt in the yin meridians, therefore, the name bolt-dormancy.

●镬[guàn] 镬即罐。拔罐用具。一般由泥所烧制成的瓦器。呈圆筒形。

Pot synonymous with cup, an apparatus for cupping. Referring to the cylinder-like pot, made usually of baked clay.

●光明[guāng míng] ①经穴名。出《灵枢·经脉》。属足少阳胆经,为本经络穴。〈定位〉在小腿外侧,当外踝尖上5寸,腓骨前缘(图8)。〈层次解剖〉皮肤→皮下组织→腓骨短肌→前肌间隔→趾长伸肌→拇长伸肌→小腿骨间膜→胫骨后肌。浅层布有腓浅神经和腓肠外侧皮神经。深层有腓深神经和胫前动、静脉。〈主治〉目痛、夜盲、乳胀痛、膝痛、下肢痿痹、颊肿。直刺0.5-0.8寸;可灸。②经穴别名。出《铜人腧穴针灸图经》。即攒竹。详见该条。

1. Guangming(GB 37) A meridian point, originally from *Ling Shu*: *Jing Mai*(*Miraculous Pivot*: *Meridians*), the Luo(connecting) point of the gallbladder meridian of Foot Shaoyang. 〈Location〉on the lateral side of the leg, 5 cun above the tip of the external malleolus, on the anterior border of the fibula(Fig. 8). 〈Regional anatomy〉 skin→subcutaneous tissue→short peroneal muscle→anterior intermuscular septum→long extensor muscle of toes→long extensor muscle of great toe→interosseous membrane of leg→posterior tibial muscle. In the superficial layer, there are the superficial peroneal nerve and the lateral sural cutaneous nerve. In the deep layer, there are deep peroneal nerve and the anterior tibial artery and vein. 〈Indications〉 pain in the eyes, night blindness, distending pain of the breast, pain in the knee, motor impairment and pain of the lower extremities, swelling of the cheek. 〈Method〉Puncture perpendicularly 0.5-0.8 cun. Moxibustion is applicable.

2. Guangming Another name for Cuanzhu (BL 2), a meridian point, originally from *Tongren Shuxue Zhenjiu Tujing*(*Illustrated Manual of Points for Acupuncture and Moxibustion on a Bronze Statue with Acupoints*). →攒竹(p. 58)

●光针[guāng zhēn] 为激光穴位照射法之别称。详见该条。

Light Needling Another term for gentle, lasre irradiation of acupoints. →激光穴位照射法(p. 182)

●归来[guī lái]　经穴名。出《针灸甲乙经》。属足阳明胃经，又名溪穴。〈定位〉在下腹部，当脐中下4寸，距前正中线2寸（图60和图40）。〈层次解剖〉皮肤→皮下组织→腹直肌鞘前壁外侧缘→腹直肌外侧缘。浅层布有第十一、十二胸神经前支和第一腰神经前支的外侧皮支及前皮支，腹壁浅动、静脉的分支或属支。深层有腹壁下动、静脉的分支或属支和第十一、第十二胸神经前支的肌支。〈主治〉少腹疼痛、经闭、阴挺、白带、疝气、茎中痛。直刺0.8-1.2寸；可灸。

Guilai(ST 29)　A meridian point, originally from *Zhenjiu Jia-Yi Jing* (*A-B Classic of Acupuncture and Moxibustion*) a point on the Stomach Meridian of Foot Yangming, also named Xixue. 〈Location〉on the lower abdomen, 4 cun below the centre of the umbilicus and 2 cun lateral to the anterior midline (Figs. 60&40). 〈Regional anatomy〉skin → subcutanneous tissue → lateral border of anteror sheath of rectus muscle of abdomen → lateral border of rectus muscle of abdomen. In the superficial layer, there are the lateral and anterior cutaneous branches of the anterior branches of the 11th and 12th thoracic nerves and the lst lumbar nerve, and the branches or tributaries of the superficial epigastric artery and vein. In the deep layer, there are the branches or tributaries of the inferior epigastric artery and vein, and the muscular branches of the anterior. 〈Indications〉lower-side abdominal pain, amenorrhea, prolapse of uterus, leukorrhea, hernia and pain in penis. 〈Method〉Puncture perpendicularly 0.8~1.2 cun. Moxibustion is applicable.

●鬼藏[guǐ cáng]　十三鬼穴之一。见《千金要方》。男为会阴穴，女为玉门头穴。参见"十三鬼穴"条。

Guicang　One of the 13 ghost points, originally from *Qianjin Yaofang* (*Essential Prescriptions Worth a Thousand Gold*). Huiyin (RN 1) point for male; Yumentou (EX-CA) point for female. →十三鬼穴(p. 379)

●鬼臣[guǐ chén]　经穴别名。十三鬼穴之一。见《千金要方》。又名鬼腿。即曲池穴。

Guichen　Another name for the meridian point Quchi (LI 11), one of the 13 Ghost Points seen in *Qianjin Yaofang* (*Essential Prescriptions Worth a Thousand Gold*), also named Guitui.

●鬼城[guǐ chéng]　经外穴别名。出《千金要方》。即十宣。详见该条。

Guicheng　Another name for Shixuan (EX-UE 11), an extra point originally from *Qianjin Yaofang* (*Essential Prescriptions Worth a Thousand Gold*). →十宣(p. 383)

●鬼床[guǐ chuáng]　十三鬼穴之一。见《千金要方》。即颊车穴。详见该条。参见"十三鬼穴"条。

Guichuang　One of the 13 Ghost Points, seen in *Qianjin Yaofang* (*Essential Prescriptions Worth a Thousand Gold*), i. e. Jiache (ST 6)→颊车(p. 187)、十三鬼穴(p. 379)

●鬼当[guǐ dāng]　经外穴名。见《针灸集成》。在手部当拇指尺侧，指关节横纹头赤白肉际。〈主治〉小儿肠胃病、结膜炎、角膜白翳。直刺0.1-0.2寸；可灸。

Guidang(EX-UE)　An extra point, seen in *Zhenjiu Jicheng* (*A Collection of Acupuncture and Moxibustion*). 〈Location〉on the ulnar side of the thumb of each hand, at the junction of the white and red skin proximal to the end of the transverse crease of the phalangeal joint of hand. 〈Indications〉infantile gastrointestinal disease, coniunctivtis, corneal macula. 〈Method〉Puncture perpendicularly 0.1-0.2 cun. Moxibustion is applicable.

●鬼封[guǐ fēng]　十三鬼穴之一。见《千金要方》。即海泉穴。详见该条。参见"十三鬼穴"条。

Guifeng　One of the 13 Ghost Points, seen in *Qianjin Yaofang* (*Essential Prescriptions Worth a Thousand Gold*), i. e. Haiquan (EX-HN 11). →海泉(p. 154)、十三鬼穴(p. 379)

●鬼宫[guǐ gōng]　十三鬼穴之一。出《千金要方》。即水沟穴。详见该条。参见"十三鬼穴"条。

Guigong　One of the 13 Ghost Points, originally from *Qianjin Yaofang* (*Essential Prescriptions Worth a Thousand Gold*) i. e. Shuigou (DU 26). →水沟(p. 409)、十三鬼穴(p. 379)

●鬼客厅[guǐ kè tīng]　经穴别名。见《千金要方》。即水沟穴。详见该条。

Guiketing　Another mane for Shuigou (DU 26), a meridian point, seen in *Qianjin Yaofang* (*Essential Prescriptions Worth a Thousand Gold*). →水沟(p. 409)

●鬼哭[guǐ kū]　经外穴别名。即鬼眼。详见该条。

Guiku Another name for the extra point, Guiyan(EX-). →鬼眼(p. 152)

●鬼窟[guǐ kū] 十三鬼穴之一。出《针灸大成》。即劳宫。详见该条。参见"十三鬼穴"条。

Guiku One of the 13 Ghost Points, originally from *Zhenjiu Dacheng* (*A Great Compendium of Acupuncture and Moxibustion*). i. e. Laogong(PC 8). →劳宫(p. 237)、十三鬼穴(p. 379)

●鬼垒[guǐ lěi] 十三鬼穴之一。见《千金要方》。即隐白穴。详见该条。参见"十三鬼穴"条。

Guilei One of the 13 Ghost Points, originally from *Qianjin Yaofang* (*Essential Prescriptions Worth a Thousand Gold for Emergencies*). i. e. Yinbai(SP 1). →隐白(p. 565)、十三鬼穴(p. 379)

●鬼路[guǐ lù] ①十三鬼穴之一。见《千金要方》。一指劳宫穴。一指申脉穴。②经穴别名。出《千金要方》。即间使。详见该条。

Guilu① One of the 13 Ghost Points, originally from *Qianjin Yaofang* (*Essential Prescriptions Worth a Thousand Gold*), referring to either Laogong(PC 8)or Shenmai(BL 62). ②. Another name for Jianshi(PC 5), a meridian point, originally from *Qianjin Yaofang* (*Essential Prescriptions Worth a Thousand Gold*)→间使(p. 188)

●鬼禄[guǐ lù] 经外穴别名。出《千金要方》。即悬命。详见该条。

Guilu Another name for Xuanming(EX-HN), an extra point originally from *Qianjin Yaofang* (*Essential Prescriptions Worth a Thousand Gold*). →悬命(p. 519)

●鬼市[guǐ shì] ①十三鬼穴之一。出《千金要方》。即承浆穴。详见该条。参见"十三鬼穴"条。②经穴别名。出《千金翼方》。即水沟。详见该条。

Guishi ①One of the 13 Ghost Points, originally from *Qianjin Yaofang* (*Essential Prescriptions Worth a Thousand Gold*), i. e. Chengjiang(RN 24). →承浆(p. 43)、十三鬼穴(p. 379) ②Another name for Shuigou(DU 26), a meridian point, originally from *Qianjin Yifang* (*Supplement to Essential Prescriptions Worth a Thousand Gold*). →水沟(p. 409)

●鬼舐头[guǐ shì tóu] 即油风。详见该条。

Haircut by Ghost →油风(p. 569)

●鬼受[guǐ shòu] 经穴别名。出《千金要方》。即尺泽。详见该条。参见"十三鬼穴"条。

Guishou Another Name for Chize(LU 5), a meridian point originally from *Qianjin Yaofang* (*Essential Presriptions Worth a Thousand Gold*)→尺泽(p. 46)、十三鬼穴(p. 379)

●鬼堂[guǐ táng] ①十三鬼穴之一。见《千金要方》。即上星穴。详见该条。参见"十三鬼穴"条。②经穴别名。出《千金翼方》。即尺泽。详见该条。

Guitang I One of the 13 Ghost Points, seen in *Qianjin Yaofang* (*Essential Prescriptions Worth a Thousand Gold*), i. e. Shangxing(DU 23). →上星(p. 354)、十三鬼穴(p. 379) ②Another name for Chize(LU 5), a meridian point originally from *Qianjin Yifang* (*Supplement to Essential Prescriptions Worth a Thousand Gold*) →尺泽(p. 46)

●鬼腿[guǐ tuǐ] 出《针灸大成》。鬼臣的别名。详见该条。参见"十三鬼穴"条。

Guitui Another name for Guichen, originally from *Zhenjiu Dacheng* (*A Great Compendium of Acupuncture and Moxibustion*). →鬼臣(p. 150)、十三鬼穴(p. 379)

●鬼邪[guǐ xié] ①经穴别名。出《千金要方》。即足三里。详见该条。②经穴别名。即手三里。详见该条。

Guixie ① Another name for Zusanli(ST 36), a meridian point originally from *Qianjin Yaofang* (*Essential Presciptions Worth a Thousand Gold*). →足三里(p. 632) ②Another name for the meridian point Shousanli(LI 10). →手三里(p. 390)

●鬼心[guǐ xīn] 十三鬼穴之一。出《千金要方》。原注为太渊,《针灸大全》作大陵穴。参见"十三鬼穴"条。

Guixin One of the 13 Ghost Points, originally from *Qianjin Yaofang* (*Essential Prescriptions Worth a Thousand Gold*), initially annotated as Taiyuan(LU 9), which was taken as Daling (PC 7) *in Zhenjiu Daquan* (*A Complete Work of Acupuncture and Moxibustion*). →十三鬼穴(p. 379)

●鬼信[guǐ xìn] ①经外穴名。见《千金要方》。位于手拇指尖端,距指甲0.3寸。主治五尸、水肿。灸七壮。

151

②十三鬼穴之一。见《千金要方》。即少商。参见"十三鬼穴"条。

1. Guixin(EX—UE)　An extra point, seen in *Qianjin Yaofang* (*Essential Prescriptions Worth a Thousand Gold*).〈Location〉at the tip of the thumb, 0.3 cun from the nail.〈Indications〉five corpses and edema.〈Method〉7 moxa cones for moxibustion treatment.

2. Guixin　One of the 13 ghost points, originally from *Qianjin Yaofang* (*Essential Prescriptions Worth a Thousand Gold*), i.e. Shaoshang(LU 11). →十三鬼穴(p. 379)

●鬼穴[guǐ xué]　①指针治癫狂的各穴，有十三鬼穴之称。见"十三鬼穴"条。②经穴别名。出《千金要方》。即风府。详见该条。

Guixue　①Referring to the acupoints selected for treating manic depressive psychosis, the term for the thirteen ghost points. →十三鬼穴(p. 379)
② Another name for Fengfu (DU 16), a meridian point originally from *Qianjin Yaofang* (*Essential Prescriptions Worth a Thousand Gold*). →风府(p. 111)

●鬼眼[guǐ yǎn]　①经外穴名。见《千金要方》。又名手足大指爪甲。手、足大指(趾)桡(胫)侧爪甲根角处，两指(趾)相并取穴。灸治癫痫、精神病、晕厥等。②经外穴别名。指腰眼、鬼哭各穴。参见各条及"十三鬼穴"条。

1. Guiyan(EX—UE&LE)　An extra point, seen in *Qianjin Yaofang* (*Essential Prescions Worth a Thousand Gold*), also named Shouzudazhizhaojia,〈Location〉on the radial (tibial) side of each thumb (big toe), at the corner of the nail root. Puncture the two points when the two thumbs (toes) are side by side.〈Indications〉epilepsy, mental disorder and syncope, etc.〈Method〉moxibustion.

2. Guiyan　Another name for some extra points, referring to Yaoyan(EX-B 7), Guiyan(EX-UE) or Guiku→腰眼(p. 546)、鬼哭(p. 150)、十三鬼穴(p. 379)

●鬼营[guǐ yíng]　出《针灸聚英》。鬼路的别名。详见该条。参见"十三鬼穴"条。

Guiying　Another name for Guilu, originally from *Zhenjiu Juying* (*Essentials of Acupuncture and Moxibustion*). →鬼路(p. 151)、十三鬼穴(p. 379)

●鬼枕[guǐ zhěn]　十三鬼穴之一。出《千金要方》。即风府。详见该条。

Guizhen　One of the 13 Ghost Points, originally from *Qianjin Yaofang* (*Essential Prescriptions Worth a Thousand Gold*). i.e. Fengfu(DU 16)→风府(p. 111)

●鬼注[guǐ zhù]　古病名。见《肘后方》。即肺痨。详见该条。

Ghost Tuberculosis　An archaic name for pulmonary tuberculosis, a disease seen in *Zhou Hou Fang* (*A Handbook of Prescriptions*). →肺痨(p. 107)

●滚刺筒[gǔn cì tǒng]　皮肤针的一种。分柄与滚筒两部，筒壁密布短针，用时手握筒柄，将滚筒在需要刺激的部位来回滚动。适用于须作较大面积浅刺者。参见"皮肤针"条。

Roller Needle　A kind of skin needle, composed of a handle and a roller with rows of short distributed needles.〈Method〉Hold the handle to roll the roller needle back and forth on the areas where stimulation is required, used for shallow puncture on larger surface areas. →皮肤针(p. 292)

●郭玉[guō yù]　人名。东汉针灸学家，字通直，广汉(今属四川)人。早年从程高学针，是涪翁的再传弟子，后任汉和帝的太医丞。用针灸治病，疗效很高。参见《后汉书·郭玉传》。

Guo Yu　An expert of acupuncture and moxibustion in the Eastern Han Dynasty, who styled himself Tongzhi, a native of Guanghan (now in Sichuan Province). He learned acupuncture when he was young from Cheng Gao, and was the regenerative disciple of Fu Wong. Later, he was appointed imperial physician of He Di (of the Han Dynasty). He gave treatment with acupuncture and moxibustion with good therapeutic effects. Cf. *Houhan Shu*: *Guo Yu Zhuan* (*History of the Later Han Dynasty*: *Biography of Guo Yu*)

●郭忠[guō zhōng]　人名。宋针灸学家，字恕甫，兴化(今属江苏扬洲)人。曾为宋广仁宗治愈目疾，得"金针先生"之称。

Guo Zhong　An expert of acupuncture and

moxibustion in the Song Dynasty, who styled himself Shufu, a native of Xinghua (now in Yangzhou, Jiangsu Province), who cured Guangrenzong (Emperor of the Song Dynasty) of his eye disease, and won the title of "Mr. Gold Needle".

●腘[guó] 部位名。指膝关节的后方,俗称腿恋、腿凹或曲瞅。

Popliteal Fossa A part of the body, referring to the posterior of the knee joints, commonly called leg-flexion, leghollow or flexional fossa.

●过梁针[guò liáng zhēn] 经外穴名。见《中医杂志》。指治疗癫狂等精神疾患的十四个经外奇穴。①天灵:在腋窝前缘直上1寸,向内旁开1.5寸,垂膊取之。针5—6寸,微向外斜刺。②腋灵:在腋窝前缘直上0.5寸,肌腱下缘处,针5—6寸。③屈委阳:在屈肘横纹端之稍外方,针1.5—3寸。④尺桡:在前臂伸侧腕横纹至肘横纹的中央,即腕上6.25寸处,针1.5—3寸。⑤中桡:在上肢伸侧,腕横纹上4寸处,针1—2.5寸。⑥寸桡:在上肢伸侧,腕横纹上2寸处,针1—2.5寸。⑦脑根:在外踝与跟腱之间凹陷处。针1—2.5寸。⑧中平:在膝下5寸,胫骨和腓骨之间,针2—6寸。⑨阴委一:在股外侧,腘窝横纹上1寸,股二头肌腱与股外侧肌之间凹陷处,针3-5寸。⑩阴委二:在阴委一上1寸,针3-5寸。⑪阴委三:在阴委二上1寸,针3-5寸。⑫四连:在阴委三上1寸,针3-5寸。⑬五灵:在阴委三上2寸,针3-5寸。⑭灵宝:位于阴委三上3寸,针3-5寸。按以上各穴针刺深度,临床应用时,应根据病人肥瘦、虚实灵活掌握,不宜过深。

Guoliangzhen(EX) Name of a group of extra points, seen in *Zhongyi Zazhi* (*Journal of Traditional Chinese Medicine*), referring to the 14 extra points used to treat manic-depressive psychosis and other mental disorders. ①Tianling(EX-CA). 〈Location〉1.5 cun medial to the point which is 1 cun directly above the anterior end of the axiliary fold, located when the arm is down. Puncture with a lateral oblique insertion of 5-6 cun. ② Yeling (EX-UE). 〈Location〉0.5 cun directly above the anterior end of the auxiliary fold, on the lower border of the tendon. Puncture 5-6 cun. ③Quweiyang (EX-UE). 〈Location〉slightly lateral to the end of the transverse cubital crease. Puncture 1.5-3 cun. ④ Chinao (EX-UE). 〈Location〉on the extension aspect of the forearm, at the middle of the line connecting the midpoint of the transverse crease of the wrist and the transverse cubital crease, i.e. 6.25 cun above the wrist. Puncture 1.5-3 cun. ⑤Zhongnao(EX-UE). 〈Location〉on the extension aspect of the arm, 4 cun above the transverse crease of the wrist. Puncture 1-2.5 cun. ⑥Cunnao (EX-UE). 〈Location〉on the extension aspect of the arm, 2 cun above the transverse crease of the wrist. Puncture 1-2.5 cun. ⑦Naogen(EX-LE). 〈Location〉in the depression between the external malleolus and tendon calcaneus. Puncture 1-1.2 cun. ⑧ Zhongping(EX-LE). 〈Location〉:5 cun below the knee, between the fibula and the tibia. Puncture 2-6 cun. ⑨ Yinwe1 (EX-LE). 〈Locaion〉on the lateral aspect of the thigh, 1 cun above the transverse crease of the popliteal fossa, on the depression between the tendon of the biceps muscle of thigh and musculus vastus lateralis. Puncture 3-5 cun. ⑩ Yinwei2 (EX-LE). 〈Location〉1 cun above Yinweil (EX-LE). Puncture 3-5 cun. ⑪Yinwei3(EX-LE). 〈Location〉1 cun above Yinwei2 (EX-LE) Puncture 3-5 cun. ⑫ Silian (EX-LE). 〈Location〉1 cun above Yinwei3 (EX-LE). Puncture 3-5 cun. ⑬Wuling(EX-LE). 〈Location〉2 cun above Yinwei3(EX-LE). Puncture 3-5 cun. ⑭ Lingbao (EX-LE). 〈Location〉3 cun above Yinwei3 (EX-LE). Puncture 3-5 cun. In clinical application, the insertion depth of these points should be applied flexibly, according to the fat or thin physical condition, and deficiency or excess conditions of the patient. The insertion should not be too deep.

●过门[guò mén] 经穴别名。见《针灸大成》。即三阳络。详见该条。

Guomen Another name for Sanyangluo(SJ 8), a meridian point seen in *Zhenjiu Dacheng* (*A Great Compendium of Acupuncture and Moxibustion*). →三阳络(p.345)

●过敏区[guò mǐn qū] 风溪之别称。详见该条。

Allergic Area(MA) Another name for Fengxi(MA). →风溪(p.115)

● 过期经行 [guò qī jīng xíng] 经行后期的别名。详见该条。

Delayed Menstrual Period Another name for delayed menstruation. →经行后期(p. 214)

H

● 虾蟆 [há má] ①经外穴别名。即夺命。见该条。②间接灸的一种。即隔蟾灸。见该条。

1. Hama Another name for Duoming, (EX-UE)an extra point. →夺命(p. 91)

2. Toad A form of indirect moxibustion, i.e. toad-separated moxibustion. →隔蟾灸(p. 134)

● 蛤蟆瘟 [há má wēn] 即痄腮的别名。详见该条。

Pyogenic Inflammation of Cheeks →痄腮 (p. 583)

● 骸关 [hái guān] 部位名。指膝关节。

Pass of Tibia A part of the body, referring to the knee joint.

● 海底 [hǎi dǐ] 经穴别名。出《医方六集·神照集》。即会阴。见该条。

Haidi Another name for Huiyin (RN 1), a meridian point originally from *Yifang Liu Ji: Shenzhao Ji* (*Six Collections of Prescriptions, Collection Under God's Brightness*). →会阴(p. 178)

● 海泉 [hǎi quán] 经外穴名。见《针灸大全》。〈定位〉在口腔内,当舌下系带中点处(图20)。〈层次解剖〉粘膜→粘膜下组织→舌肌。布有下颌神经的舌神经、舌下神经和面神经鼓索的神经纤维及舌动脉的分支舌深动脉和舌静脉的属支舌深静脉。〈主治〉呕吐、呃逆、重舌肿胀、舌缓不收、喉闭、腹泻、消渴等。点刺出血。

Haiquan (EX-HN 11) An extra point, seen in *Zhen Jiu Da Quan* (*A Complete Work of Acupuncture and Moxibustion*). 〈Location〉 in the mouth, at the midpoint of the frenulum of the tongue (Fig. 20). 〈Regional anatomy〉 mucosa → submucous tissue → lingual muscle. There are the lingual nerve from the mandibular nerve, the hypoglossal nerve, the nervous bines of the tympanic cord from the facial nerve, the deep lingual artery from the lingual artery, and the deep lingual veins to the lingual vein in this area. 〈Indications〉 vomiting, hiccup, double tongue due to tumefaction, abscess of sublingual gland, flaccid tongue, inflammation of the throat, diarrhea, diabetes, etc. 〈Method〉 Prick the point to cause bleeding.

● 害蜚 [hài fēi] 六经皮部之一,阳明皮部名。出《素问·皮部论》。"害"古与盍、阖通用,应读"阖";"蜚"是阳气正动之意。阳经以阳明为阖,故称"害蜚"。

Haifei One of the cutaneous regions of the six meridians. Name of the cutaneous region of *Yangming*, originally from *Su Wen: Pibu Lun* (*Plain Questions: Cutaneous Regions*). In ancient times, "*Hai*(害)" Was interchangeable with "*He*(盍阖)", and it should be pronounced as "*He*" (closing); "*Fei*" meant the moving of yang-qi. Among Yang Meridians, yangming is for "*He*" (closing). Its cutaneous region was therefore called "Haifei".

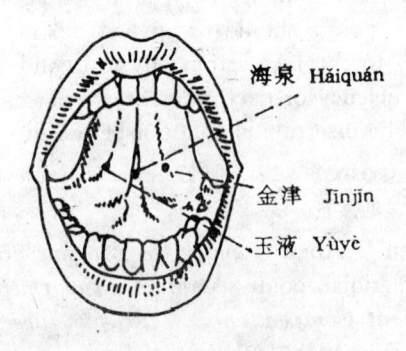

图 20 海泉、金津和玉液穴
Fig 20 Haiquan, Jinjin and Yuye points

●含腮疮[hán sāi chuāng]　即痄腮的别名。见该条。
Sore inside Cheek　Another name for mumps.→痄腮(p.583)

●寒府[hán fǔ]　经穴别名。出《素问·骨空论》王冰注。《中国针灸学》列为膝阳关的别名。见"膝阳关"条。

Hanfu　Another name for a meridian point, originally from Wang Bing's annotation on *Suwen*: *Gukong Lun* (*Plain Questions*: *On the Aperters of Bones*). Taken as another name for the point Xiyangguan (GB 33) in *Zhongguo Zhenjiuxue* (*Chinese Acupuncture and Moxibustion*).→膝阳关(p.484)

●寒霍乱[hán huò luàn]　病证名。霍乱证型之一。见《霍乱论》。又称寒气霍乱。多因阳气素虚，内伤生冷，外感寒湿所致。证见或吐或泻，或吐泻不止，脘腹绞痛，四肢厥冷，甚则唇青，两腿转筋，舌淡苔白，脉沉迟细。治宜和中温胃散寒。取中脘、天枢、关元、神阙、足三里。

Cholera Morbus due to Cold　Name of a disease, a type of acute vomiting and diarrhea, seen in *Huoluan Lun* (*Treatise on Cholera Morbus*), also named Cholera Morbus due to cold-qi. Mostly caused by constitutional Yang deficiency, internal damage by cold and raw food, and invasion of exogenous cold dampness.〈Manifestations〉vomiting, diarrhea, or vomiting and diarrhea without break, colic pain in abdomen, cold limbs, purplish lips and spasm of legs in severe case, pale tongue with white coating, deep, slow and thready pulse.〈Treatment principle〉Regulate the middle-jiao, warm the stomach and dispel cold.〈Point selection〉Zhongwan (RN 12), Tianshu (ST 25), Guanyuan (RN 4), Shenque (RN 8) and Zusanli (ST 36).

●寒积胃痛[hán jī wèi tòng]　胃痛证型之一。多因胃阳不足，冷饮内伤，阴寒凝结所致。证见胃痛暴作，恶寒喜暖，脘腹得温则痛减，遇寒则痛增，口和不渴，或喜热饮，舌苔薄白，脉弦紧。治宜温胃散寒止痛。针中脘、足三里、内关、公孙、梁丘。

Stomachache due to Accumulation of Cold　A type of stomachache, mostly caused by the deficiency of stomach-yang, internal damage by cold drink, or the accumulation of yin-cold.〈Manifestations〉sudden pain of the stomach, aversion to cold and preference for warmth. The pain in the epigastrium is relieved when warm and aggravated when cold. Lack of thirst with a normal sense in the mouth, preference for warm drink, thin and white tongue coating, wiry and tense pulse.〈Treatment principle〉Warm the stomach, dispel cold and alleviate pain.〈Point selection〉Zhongwan (RN 12), Zusanli (ST 36), Neiguan (PC 6), Gongsun (SP 4) and Liangqiu (ST 34).

●寒结[hán jié]　即冷秘。见该条。
Cold-Accumulation　Constipation of cold type.→冷秘(p.241)

●寒厥[hán jué]　厥证证型之一。出《素问·厥论》等篇。指因阳虚阴盛而引起的厥证。一名冷厥。证见面青身冷，蜷卧，口不干不渴，下利清谷，四肢厥逆，意识蒙胧，苔薄白，脉沉细。治宜回阳救逆。针百会、气海，灸神阙。

Cold Limbs　One of the Jue-syndromes, originally from *Suwen*: *Jue Lun* (*Plain Questions*: *On Jue-Syndromes*). Referring to the Jue-syndrome due to preponderance of yin resulting from yang deficiency, also named cold Jue-syndrome.〈Manifestations〉purple face, chills, huddling up, absence of thirst, diarrhea with undigested food in stool, cold limbs, haziness, thin and white tongue coating, deep, thready and slow pulse.〈Treatment principle〉Recuperate depleted yang and rescue the patient from collapse.〈Point selection〉Baihui (DU 20) and Qihai (RN 6); moxibustion on Shenque (RN 8).

●寒凝血滞经闭[hán níng xuè zhì jīng bì]　是经闭的证型之一。多因饮冷受寒，邪气客于胞宫，血脉凝滞所致。证见经闭不行，形寒肢冷，小腹冷痛，喜得温暖，苔白，脉沉迟。治宜温经散寒行血。取中极、地机、关元、气海。

Amenorrhea due to Blood Stasis Caused by Accumulation of Pathogenic Cold　One of the syndromes of menoschesis. Mostly caused by cold drink or external pathogenic cold, which invades the uterus and causes blood stagnation.〈Manifestations〉menoschesis, aversion to cold, cold limbs, pain and cold sen-

sation in the lower abdomen, preference for warmth, white tongue coating, deep and slow pulse. ⟨Treatment principle⟩ Expel pathogenic cold by warming the meridians and promote blood circulation. ⟨Point selection⟩ Zhongji (RN 3), Diji(SP 8), Guanyuan(RN 4) and Qihai(RN 6).

●寒疟[hán nüè]　疟疾证型之一。出《素问·疟论》。多因寒气内伏,秋凉再感疟邪所致。证见热少寒多,口不渴,胸脘痞闷,神疲体倦,苔白腻,脉弦。治宜和解表里,温阳达邪。取陶道、曲池、间使、中渚、丘墟。

Algid Malaria　One of the syndromes of malaria, originally from *Suwen: Nüe Lun (Plain Questions: On Malaria Diseases)*. Mostly caused by latent pathogenic cold in the interior, and the invasion of malarial evils in cold autumn. ⟨Manifestations⟩ light fever and great chills, absence of thirst, stuffiness in the chest and epigastrium, lassitude and fatigue, white and greasy tongue coating, wiry pulse. ⟨Treatment principle⟩ Harmonize and regulate the exterior and interior; warm yang to dispel pathogenic factors. ⟨Point selection⟩ Taodao (DU 13), Quchi (LI 11), Jianshi (PC 5), Zhongzhu(SJ 3) and Qiuxu(GB 40).

●寒气霍乱[hán qì huò luàn]　见《症因脉治》。即寒霍乱。见该条。

Cholera Morbus due to Cold-Qi　Seen in *Zheng Yin Mai Zhi (Syndromes, Causes, Pulse Conditions and Treatments)*, i. e. cholera morbus due to cold. →寒霍乱(p.155)

●寒疝[hán shàn]　疝气证型之一。出《金匮要略》。由寒湿之邪侵犯任脉、肝经,凝滞于少腹、睾丸、阴囊等部,血气痹阻所致。证见少腹睾丸牵掣绞痛,甚则上攻胸胁,痛甚欲绝,茎缩囊冷,形寒,手足欠温,面色苍白,舌淡苔白,脉弦紧或沉伏。治宜温化寒湿,疏通经脉。取期门、大敦、足三里、气海。

Periumbilical Colic and Testalgia due to Invasion of Cold　One of the syndromes of hernia, originally from *Jin Gui Yao Lue (Synopsis of the Golden Chamber)*. Due to the stagnation of qi and blood resulting from cold-dampness attacking the Ren and the Liver Meridians, and the pathogenic factors accumulating in the lower abdomen, testicle and scrotum, etc. ⟨Manifestations⟩ colic pain of testicle and lower abdomen, even radiating to the chest and hypochondrium, shock due to severe pain, contraction of penis, cold scrotum, chills, cold limbs, pale complexion, pale tongue with white coating, wiry and tense pulse or deep and floating pulse. ⟨Treatment principle⟩ Expel pathogenic cold and dampness and dredge the meridians. ⟨Point selection⟩ Qimen (LR 14), Dadun(LR 1), Zusanli (ST 36) and Qihai (RN 6).

●寒湿痢[hán shī lì]　痢疾证型之一。因寒湿留滞肠中,气机阻滞,传导失常所致。证见痢下白多赤少,或为纯白粘冻,常有稀水糟粕,形寒,发热不甚,口中粘腻,不渴,苔白腻,脉濡缓。治宜温化寒湿,疏调肠胃。取合谷、天枢、上巨虚、中脘、气海、阴陵泉。

Dysentery Due to Cold-Dampness　One of the syndromes of dysentery. Due to the stagnation of qi and disordered transportation, which are caused by the retention of cold and dampness in the intestines. ⟨Manifestations⟩ white mucus in stool with a little blood, or pure white mucus, or watery stool, cold limbs, slight fever, viscid feeling and taste lesseness in the mouth, absence of thirst, white and greasy tongue coating, soft and leisurely pulse. ⟨Treatment principle⟩ Expel pathogenic cold and dampness with warmth; regulate the intestines and stomach. ⟨Point selection⟩ Hegu (LI 4), Tianshu (ST 25), Shangjuxu (ST 37), Zhongwan (RN 12), Qihai (RN 6) and Yinlingquan(SP 9).

●寒湿凝滞痛经[hán shī níng zhì tòng jīng]　痛经证型之一。多在经期受寒饮冷,坐卧湿地,寒湿伤于下焦,客于胞宫,经血为寒湿所凝,经血下行受阻所致。证见经前或经行期间小腹冷痛,按之痛甚,重则连及腰脊,得热痛减,经水量少,色黯,常伴有血块,苔薄白,脉沉紧。治宜温寒利湿,通经止痛。取中极、水道、地机。

Dysmenorrhea due to Cold-Dampness　One of the syndromes of dysmenorrhea. Mostly due to the attack of external pathogenic cold or intake of cold drinks, sitting and sleeping in damp places during menstrual period, invasion of cold and dampness into the lower jiao and the uterus, and the failure of menstrual blood to flow because of the stagnation of blood.

⟨Manifestations⟩cold sensation and pain in the lower abdomen before menses or during the menstrual period, which is aggravated by pressure, pain radiating to the lower back and spine, and relieved by warmth, hypomenorrhea, dark menses with clots, thin and white tongue coating, deep and tense pulse. ⟨Treatment principle⟩ Expel pathogenic cold and dampness, dredge the meridians to relieve menalgia. ⟨Point selection⟩Zhongji(RN 3), Shuidao(ST 28)and Diji(SP 8).

●寒湿泻[hán shī xiè] 泄泻证型之一。多因感受寒湿或风寒之邪，侵袭肠胃，传化失常所致。证见泻下清稀，甚至如水样，腹痛肠鸣，脘闷纳少，或兼有寒热头痛，肢体酸痛，舌苔薄白或白腻，脉濡缓。治宜和中化湿，疏风散寒。取中脘、天枢、足三里、合谷、阴陵泉。

Cold-Damp Diarrhea One of the syndromes of diarrhea. Mostly due to the invasion of cold-dampness and wind-cold pathogens into the intestine and stomach, which lead to a disorder of digestion and transportation. ⟨Manifestations⟩loose or watery stool, abdominal pain, borborygmus, fullness in the stomach, lack of hunger, headache accompanying chills and fever, and aching pain of limbs, thin and white, or white and greasy tongue coating, soft and slow pulse. ⟨Treatment principle⟩Regulate the functions of the middle-jiao, promote digestion, expel wind, cold and dampness pathogens. ⟨Point selection⟩ Zhongwan(RN 12), Tianshu(ST 25), Zusanli(ST 36), Hegu(LI 4) and Yinlingquan (SP 9).

●寒湿腰痛[hán shī yāo tòng] 腰痛证型之一。多因寒湿之邪客于经络，气血阻滞所致。证见腰部重痛，痠麻，或拘急强直不可俯仰，或痛连骶、臀、股、腘。疼痛时轻时重，患部恶冷，天气寒冷、阴雨则发作，舌苔白腻，脉沉。治宜祛寒利湿，温经通络。取肾俞、委中、腰阳关、秩边、阴陵泉。

Lumbar Pain due to Cold and Dampness One of the syndromes of lower back pain due to the stagnation of qi and blood, which is caused by the invasion of cold and dampness into the meridians and collaterals. ⟨Manifestations⟩ weighty pain of loins, soreness and numbness of the waist, stiffness or spasm of the waist, pain radiating to the sacrum, buttock, thigh and popliteal fossa, changing pain with aversion to cold in the affected region, attcks occurring during cold and rainy days, white and greasy tongue coating, deep pulse. ⟨Treatment principle⟩Dispel cold and damp, promote the flow of qi by warming the meridians and dredging the collaterals. ⟨Point selection⟩ Shenshu (BL 23), Weizhong (BL 40), Yaoyangguan (DU3), Zhibian (BL 54) and Yinlingquan(SP 9).

●寒吐[hán tù] 小儿呕吐证型之一。见《幼科全书》。即小儿因胃中虚冷而致的呕吐。证见呕吐，吐出物为清涎夹奶，或不消化食物，四肢不温，舌淡苔白，脉细无力。治宜温中止呕。取建里、中脘、足三里。

Vomiting due to Cold One of the syndromes of infantile vomiting, seen in *Youke Quanshu*(*A Complete Work of Pediatrics*). Due to cold of the deficient type in the stomach. ⟨Manifestations⟩vomiting with milk and undigested food or sialemesis, cold limbs, pale tongue with white coating, thready and weak pulse. ⟨Treatment principle⟩Warm the middle-Jiao to stop vomiting. ⟨Point selection⟩ Jianli(RN 11), Zhongwan(RN 12)and Zusanli(ST 36).

●寒邪腹痛[hán xié fù tòng] 腹痛症型之一。多因寒邪内侵，阳气不运，气血被阻所致。证见腹痛急暴，腹部喜温怕冷，便溏或泄泻，腹中雷鸣，小便清白，口不渴，四肢欠温，苔白腻，脉沉紧。治宜散寒理气。取中脘、足三里、大横、公孙。

Abdominal Pain due to Pathogenic Cold One of the syndromes of abdominal pain. Due to the invasion of pathogenic cold which hinders the functions of Yang-qi and causes the stagnation of qi and blood. ⟨Manifestations⟩acute abdominal pain with aversion to cold and preference for warmth, loose stools or diarrhea, strong borborygmus, clear urine, absence of thirst, cold limbs, white and greasy tongue coating, deep and tense pulse. ⟨Treatment principle⟩Dispel cold and regulate qi. ⟨Point selection⟩ Zhongwan (RN 12), Zusanli (ST 36), Daheng(SP 15) and Gongsun(SP 4).

●寒饮哮喘[hán yǐn xiāo chuān] 哮喘证型之一。由于风寒与痰饮互结,阻遏气道所致。证见呼吸困难,喉中有痰鸣音,咳逆痰少,质稀色白,或带泡沫,形寒无汗,或兼头痛身痛,多在冬季或受寒发作,舌苔白滑,脉紧或浮紧。治宜散寒宣肺平喘。取列缺、尺泽、风门、肺俞。

Asthma due to Retention of Cold Fluid
One of the syndromes of asthma due to the mingling of phlegm and pathogenic wind-cold blocking the respiratory tract. 〈Manifestations〉dyspneic respiration, rale in the throat, cough with little, whitish, clear and thin sputum, or with frothy sputum, aversion to cold, anhidrosis, headache, pantalgia, mostly occurring in winter or when attacked by pathogenic cold, white tongue coating with fluid, tense or superficial and tense pulse. 〈Treatment principle〉Dispel cold and facilitate the flow of the lung-qi to relieve asthma. 〈Point selection〉Lieque(LU 7), Chize(LU 5), Fengmen(BL 12) and Feishu(BL 13).

●寒则留之[hán zé liú zhī] 针灸治疗原则之一。出《灵枢·经脉》。与"热则疾之"相对,指寒证可通过留针达到温散寒邪的作用。参见"热则疾之"、"留针"条。

Long Retention of the Needle for Cold Syndromes One of the principles of acupuncture treatment, originally from *Lingshu: Jingmai (Miraculous Pivot: Meridians)*, opposite to the principle of "quick removal of the needle for heat syndromes". Referring to dispelling the pathogenic cold which can be relieved by retaining the needle in the treatment of cold-syndrome. →热则疾之(p. 332)、留针(p. 251)

●扞皮开腠理[hàn pí kāi còu lǐ] 进针方法之一。见《灵枢·邪客》。指顺着筋肉的缝隙,以左手撑开皮肤,右手轻轻地进针而缓缓刺入,使病人没有惊恐的感觉,而又有好的针感。

Stretch Skin to Open the Striae One of the methods of needle insertion, seen in *Lingshu: Xieke (Miraculous Pivot: Pathogenic Factors)*. Stretch the skin with the left hand along the suture of tendons and muscles, and insert the needle gently and slowly with the right hand. As a result, a good needling sensation appears without frightening the patient.

●旱莲草灸[hàn lián cǎo jiǔ] 天灸的一种。用新鲜旱莲草捣烂如泥膏状,敷于穴位,然后用胶布固定即可。敷灸时间约为1~4小时,以局部充血潮红或起泡为度。适用于治疗疟疾等证。

Han Lian Cao(Herb Eclipta) Moxibustion
A form of medicinal vesiculation. Pound fresh *Han Lian Cao(Herb Eclipta)* into paste, apply it to the selected acupoint, and fix it with adhesive plaster for about 1~4 hours or until the appearance of hyperemia and a flush on the local skin, or the formation of a blister. It is used to treat malaria, etc.

●颔[hàn] 部位名。颏下结喉上,两侧肉之空软处,下颌底与甲状软骨之间。

Submental Region A part of the body, referring to the fleshy part between the chin and the Adam's apple, i. e. the part between the base of the mandible and thyroid cartilage.

●颔厌[hàn yàn] 经穴名。出《针灸甲乙经》。属足少阳胆经,为手足少阳、足阳明之会。〈定位〉在头部鬓发上,当头维与曲鬓弧形连线的上1/4与下3/4交点处(图28)。〈层次解剖〉皮肤→皮下组织→耳上肌→颞筋膜→颞肌。浅层布有耳颞神经,颞浅动、静脉顶支。深层有颞深前、后神经的分支。〈主治〉头痛、眩晕、目外眦痛、齿痛、耳鸣、惊痫、瘛疭。向后平刺0.3~0.4寸;可灸。

Hanyan(GB 4) A meridian point, originally from *Zhenjiu Jia-Yi Jing (A-B Classic of Acupuncture and Moxibustion)*, a point on the Gall-bladder Meridian of Foot-Shaoyang, the crossing point of Hand-Shaoyang, Foot-Shaoyang and Foot-Yangming Meridians. 〈Location〉on the head, in the hair above the temples, at the junction of the upper fourth and lower three fourths of the curved line connecting Touwei(ST 8) and Qubin(GB 7) (Fig. 28). 〈Regional anatomy〉skin→subcutaneous tissue→superior auricular muscle→temporal fascia→temporal muscle. In the superficial layer, there are the auriculotemporal nerve and the parietal branches of the superficial temporal artery and vein. In the deep layer, there are the branches of the anterior and posterior deep temporal nerves. 〈Indications〉headache, dizziness, pain of outer canthus, toothache, tinnitus, epilepsy induced by ter-

ror, clonic convulsions. 〈Method〉 Puncture subcutaneously and backward 0.3～0.4 cun. Moxibustion is applicable.

● **毫针**[háo zhēn] 针具名。见《灵枢·九针十二原》。古代九针之一。其长一寸六分或三寸六分,针身细小如毫毛,针尖纤细如蚊喙。具有通经络,益精气的作用。治寒热、痹痛。为现代最常用的一种针具,临床上所用毫针多采用不锈钢制造,也有用金、银或其他合金制造者。其结构分为五部分：①针柄。手持针之处,用紫铜丝或铝丝绕成,其外形有盘龙柄、佛手柄、平柄和管柄等；②针尾。指针柄上端；③针尖。指针体前端的锋利部分,又称针芒。其形如松针,圆而不钝,尖而不锐；④针体。指介于针尖与针柄之间针的本体部分；⑤针根。指针身与针柄连接部分。毫针有大小不同的规格,参见"毫针规格"条。

Filiform Needle An acupuncture instrument, seen in *Lingshu: Jiu Zhen Shier Yuan* [*Miraculous Pivot: Nine Needles and Twelve Yuan(Primary)Points*]. One of the Nine Needles in ancient times, which is 1.6～3.6 cun long, its body is like a fine hair, and its tip is like the rostrum of a mosquito. It has the function of clearing the meridians and replenishing vital essence and qi, and is used to treat chills and fever, and arthralgia-syndrome. It is currently the most commonly used needling instrument. Most of the filiform needles used in clinic are made of stainless steel, although some are made of gold, silver or other alloys. The needle is composed of five parts: ①Handle: the part that the hand catches hold of, coiled with red copper or aluminium wire. According to their shapes, there are coiled dragon handles, Buddha's-hand handles, smooth handles and tube handles. ②Tail: referring to the upper end of the handle. ③Tip: referring to the sharp point of the needle body, also named

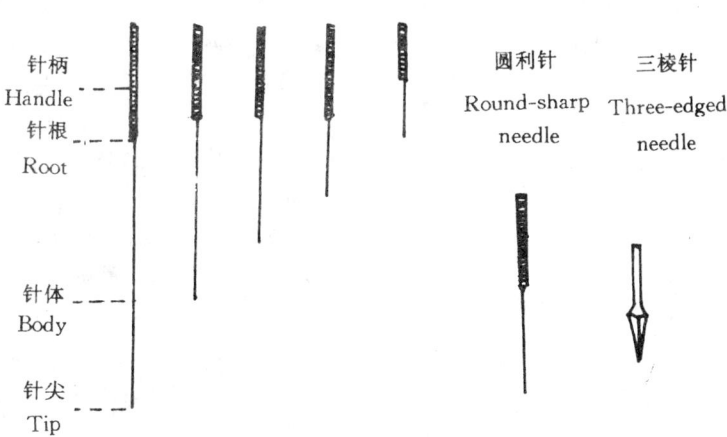

图21 毫针、圆利针和三棱针

Fig 21 Filiform needles, round-sharp needle, and three-edged needle

表8 毫针规格

Table 8   Specifications of filiform needles

新规格(毫米) New Standard (mm) \ 旧规格(寸) Old Standard (cun)		0.5	1	1.5	2	2.5	3	4	4.5	5	6
针身长 Length of the Body		15	25	40	50	65	75	100	115	125	150
针柄长 Length of the handle	长 long	25	35	40	40	40	40	55	55	55	56
	中 medium			30	35	35					
	短 short	20	25	25	30	30	30	40	40	40	40
GAUGE											
号数 Size No.		26	27	28	29	30	31	32	33	34	35
直径(毫米) Diameter (mm)		0.45	0.42	0.38	0.34	0.32	0.30	0.28	0.26	0.23	0.32

Zhenmang (awn of the needle) like a pine-needle in shape, it is round but not blunt, and it is pointed but not too sharp. ④Body: referring to the part between the hand and the tip. ⑤Root: referring to the connecting part between the body of needle and the handle of needle. The specifications of filiform needles vary. → 毫针规格(p.160)

● 毫针刺[háo zhēn cì]　刺法术语。为毫针针刺之简称。

Filiform Needle Acupuncture　A term in acupuncture, short for techniques of filiform needle acupuncture.

● 毫针刺法[háo zhēn cì fǎ]　针刺术语。毫针在针灸治疗中最为常用。毫针刺法是针刺治疗必须掌握的技能。其中包括进针法、基本手法、辅助手法以及补泻手法等。详见各条。

Techniques of Filiform Needle Acupuncture

A term in acupuncture. Filiform needles are most commonly used in acupuncture therapy, the techniques of the needle which must be mastered include, Insertion of the Needle, Fundamental Manipulation Techniques, Auxiliary Manipulation Techniques, Reinforcing and Reducing Methods in Acupuncture, etc. → 进针法(p.206)、基本手法(p.182)、辅助手法(p.120)、补泻手法(p.27)

● 毫针规格[háo zhēn guī gé]　刺法用语。毫针规格包括毫针针身的长短和粗细(详见表8)。临床上以25～75毫米长和28～30号最常应用。

Specifications of Filiform Needles　A term in acupuncture, including the length and the gauge of filiform needles. (See Table 8). Clinically, needles of 25～75 mm in length and those numbered from 28～30 are most commonly used.

● 禾髎[hé liáo]　经穴别名。出《针灸甲乙经》。即口禾髎。见该条。

Heliao　Another name for Kouheliao (LI 19), a meridian point originally from *Zhenjiu Jia-Yi Jing* (*A-B Classic of Acupuncture and Moxibustion*). → 口禾髎(p.292)

● 合谷[hé gǔ]　经穴名。出《灵枢·本输》。属手阳明大肠经，为本经原穴。又名虎口、合骨。〈定位〉在手背，第1、2掌骨间，当第二掌骨桡侧的中点处(图48和图6)。〈层次解剖〉皮肤→皮下组织→第一骨间背侧肌→拇收肌。浅层布有桡神经浅支、手背静脉网的桡侧部和第一掌背动、静脉的分支或属支。深层有尺神经深支的分支等结构。〈主治〉头痛、眩晕、目赤肿痛、鼻衄、鼻渊、齿痛、耳聋、面肿、疔疮、咽喉肿痛、失喑、牙关紧闭、口眼㖞斜、痄腮、指挛、臂痛、半身不遂、发热恶寒、无汗、多汗、咳嗽、经闭、滞产、胃痛、腹痛、便秘、痢疾、小儿惊风、瘾疹、疥疮、疟疾。直刺0.5～0.8寸;可灸。

Hegu (LI 4)　A meridian point, originally from *Lingshu: Benshu* (*Miraculous Pivot: Meridian Points*), the Yuan (Primary) point of the Large Intestine Meridian of Hand-Yangming, also named Hukou and Hegu (合骨).

⟨Location⟩ on the dorsum of the hand, between the 1st and 2nd metacarpal bones, and on the radial side of the midpoint of the 2nd metacarpal bones, and on the radial side of the midpoint of the 2nd metacarpal bone (Figs. 48&6). ⟨Regional anatomy⟩ skin → subcutaneous tissue → first dorsal interosseous muscle → adductor muscle of thumb. In the superficial layer, there are the superficial branches of the radial nerve, the radial part of the dorsal venous network of the hand and the branches of tributaries of the first dorsal metacarpal artery and vein. In the deep layer, there are the deep branches of the ulnar nerve. ⟨Indications⟩ headache, dizziness, redness, swelling and pain of the eye, epistaxis, nasal sinusitis, rhinorrhea, toothache, deafness, swelling of the face, furuncle, sore throat, aphasia, trismus, deviation of the mouth and the eye, mumps, finger contracture, pain of the arm, hemiplegia, fever with chills, anhidrosis, hidrosis, cough, amenorrhea, delayed labour, gastric pain, abdominal pain, constipation, dysentery, infantile convulsion, urticaria, scabies, malarial disease. ⟨Method⟩ Puncture perpendicularly 0.5~0.8 cun. Moxibustion is applicable.

●合谷刺[hé gǔ cì] 《内经》刺法名。出《灵枢·官针》。五刺之一。这种刺法是刺在肌肉比较丰厚处,当进针后,退至浅层又依次再向两旁斜刺,形如鸡爪的的分叉。本法刺于分肉之间,脾主肌肉,故能应合脾气。临床上用于治疗痹证。

Hegu Puncture A needling technique in *Neijing* (*The Inner Canon of Huangdi*) originally from *Lingshu: Guanzhen* (*Miraculous Pivot: Official Needles*), one of the five needling techinques applied to the points lying on thick muscles. ⟨Manipulation⟩ Lift the needle to the shallow area after insertion, and then insert the needle obliquely to both sides, the insertion is shaped like the claw of a chicken. This technique develops in response to the diseases associated with the spleen, by virtue of the fact that the spleen is in control of muscles. Clinically, it is used to treat arthralgia syndromes.

●合谷疔[hé gǔ dīng] 即虎口疔。详见该条。

Nail-like Boil at Hegu Area → 虎口疔(p. 168)

●合谷疽[hé gǔ jū] 即虎口疽。详见该条。

Deeply-Rooted Carbuncle at Hegu Area → 虎口疽(p. 168)

●合骨[hé gǔ] 经穴别名。即合谷。见该条。

Hegu Another name for the meridian point Hegu(LI 4). → 合谷(p. 160)

●合颅[hé lú] 经穴别名。见《外台秘要》。即脑户。见该条。

Helu Another name for Naohu(DU 17), a meridian point seen in *Waitai Miyao* (*Clandestine Essentials from the Imperial Library*). → 脑户(p. 276)

●合穴[hé xué] 五腧穴之一。合穴位于肘膝关节附近,喻脉气汇集,如水流汇入江河,用于气逆泄泻。

He (Sea) Point One of the Five Shu points, located near the elbow or knee. "Sea" here is a metaphor for the gathering of meridian-qi like the flow of water into the river and sea. The point is used to treat the reversed flow of qi and diarrhea.

●合阳[hé yáng] 经穴名。出《针灸甲乙经》。属足太阳膀胱经。⟨定位⟩在小腿后面,当委中与承山的连线上,委中下2寸(图35)。⟨层次解剖⟩皮肤→皮下组织→腓肠肌→跖肌。浅层布有小隐静脉,股后皮神经和腓肠内侧皮神经。深层有动、静脉和胫神经。⟨主治⟩腰脊痛引腹、下肢酸痛、麻痹、崩漏、疝痛。直刺0.5~1寸;可灸。

Heyang(BL 55) A meridian point, originally from *Zhenjiu Jia-Yi Jing* (*A-B Classic of Acupuncture and Moxibustion*), a point on the Bladder Meridian of Foot-Taiyang. ⟨Location⟩ on the posterior side of the leg, on the line connecting Weizhong (BL 40) and Chengshan (BL 57), 2 cun below Weizhong (BL 40) (Fig. 35). ⟨Regional anatomy⟩ skin → subcutaneous tissue → gastrocnemius muscle → plantar muscle. In the superficial layer, there are the small saphenous vein, the posterior cutaneous nerve of the thigh and the medial cutaneous nerve of the calf. In the deep layer, there are the popliteal artery and vein and the tibial nerve. ⟨Indications⟩ lumbar and spinal pain exending to the abdomen, aching pain of the lower extremities, paralysis and arthralgia

●合治内腑[hé zhì nèi fǔ] 《内经》取穴原则之一。出《灵枢·邪气脏腑病形》。指足三阳经上的六腑下合穴,主治六腑病。因手足六阳经脉的经气是从六腑下合穴处别入于内属于六腑。六腑下合穴:足三里,治胃病;上巨虚,治大肠病;下巨虚,治小肠病;委阳,治三焦病;委中,治膀胱病;阳陵泉,治胆病。(参见"治腑者治其合"条)。

Employing He(Sea)Points to Treat Disorders of Fu Organs   A point-selecting principle from *Neijing*(*The Inner Canon of Huangdi*),originally from *Lingshu: Xieqi Zang-Fu Bingxing* (*Miraculous Pivot: Pathogenic Evils, Zangfu Organs and Manifestations*), referring to the fact that the lower He(Sea) points on the three yang meridians of the foot are mainly used for the treatment of diseases of the six fu organs. Because the meridian-qi of the six yang meridians of the hand and foot flows from the lower He(sea) points of the six fu organs the qi belongs to the six fu organs. Of these six points, Zusanli(ST 36)is used for the treatment of stomach diseases; Shangjuxu(ST 37) for large intestine diseases; Xiajuxu (ST 39) for small intestine diseases; Weiyang(BL 39) for sanjiao diseases; Weizhong(BL 40)for bladder diseases; and Yanglingquan (GB 34) for gallbladder diseases. →治腑者治其合(p. 606)

●何若愚[hé ruò yú]   人名。金代针灸家,精于针灸,倡导子午流注针法,著《流注指微论》。为便于记诵,改写为《流注指微针赋》,阎明广作注释,收载于《子午流注针经》中,刊于1153年。

He Ruoyu   An acupuncturist in the Jin dynasty, who specialised in acupuncture and moxibustion, initiated the acupuncture technique of midnight-noon ebb-flow, wrote *Liu Zhu Zhi Wei Lun* (*Treatise on the Subtleties of Flow*). For easy reading and reciting, the book was revised and reentitled *Liu Zhu Zhi Wei Zhen Fu*(*Acupuncture Ode to the Subtleties of Flow*), which was annotated by Yan Mingguang and included in the book *Zi Wu Liu Zhu Zhen Jing*(*Acupuncture Classic on Midnight-noon Ebb-flow*), which was published in 1153.

●和髎[hé liáo]   经穴别名。出《针灸甲乙经》。即耳和髎。见该条。

Heliao   Another name for Erheliao(SJ 22), a meridian point originally from *Zhenjiu Jia-Yi Jing* (*A-B Classic of Acupuncture and Moxibustion*).→耳和髎(p. 94)

●核骨[hé gǔ]   骨骼部位名。指大趾本节后内侧隆起的圆骨,即第一蹠骨小头部。

Walnut-Like Bone   Name of a bone. The nodular process on the medial aspect of the lst metatarsophalangeal joint, i. e. the head of the lst metatarsal bone.

●核桃灸[hé táo jiǔ]   间隔灸的一种。以核桃壳为垫隔物,上置艾柱施灸。治肩背、腰胁、手臂、腿膝、环跳贴骨处疼痛。

Walnut Moxibustion   A form of indirect moxibustion, with walnut shells as the separation, on which the moxa cone is placed and moxibustion is applied.〈Indications〉pain of the shoulder, back, loin, hypochondrium, hand, arm, leg, knee, or hip.

●颌(hé)   耳穴名。位于3区,参见牙条。用于治疗牙痛、下颌关节功能紊乱。

Jaw(MA)   An auricular point.〈Location〉on the 3rd area of the ear lobe. →牙(p. 533)〈Indications〉toothache, functional disorder of mandibular articulation.

●髑骬[hé gàn]   ①经穴别名。出《针灸甲乙经》。即鸠尾。见该条。②骨骼名。指胸骨剑突部分。

1. **Hegan**   Another name for Jiuwei (RN 15), a meridian point originally from *Zhenjiu Jia-Yi Jing*(*A-B Classic of Acupuncture and Moxibustion*).→鸠尾(p. 219)
2. Dovetail part of the skeleton, referring to the xiphoid process of the sternum.

●鹤顶[hé dǐng]   ①经外穴名。出《针灸集成》。又名膝顶。〈定位〉在膝上部,髌底的中点上方凹陷处(图二十九)。〈层次解剖〉皮肤→皮下组织→股四头肌腱。浅层布有股神经前皮支和大隐静脉的属支。深层有膝关节的动、静脉网。〈主治〉膝痛、足胫无力、下肢瘫痪、脚气等。针0.5～1寸;可灸。②经外穴名。出

《陈修园医书七十二种·考正穴法》。在头顶部,自鼻尖直上入发际3.5寸,与督脉前顶同位。

1. Heding(EX-LE 2)   An extra point originally from *Zhenjiu Jicheng* (*A Collection of Acupuncture and Moxibustion*), also named Xiding. 〈Location〉above the knee, in the depression at the midpoint of the upper border of the patella (Fig. 29). 〈Regional anatomy〉skin→subcutaneous tissue→tendon of quadriceps muscle of thigh. In the superficial layer, there are the anterior cutaneous branches of the femoral nerve and the tributaries of the great saphenous vein. In the deep layer, there is the arteriovenous network of the knee joint. 〈Indications〉knee pain, weakness of foot and leg, paralysis of lower extremities, beriberi, etc. 〈Method〉Puncture 0.5～1 cun. Moxibustion is applicable.

2. Heding(EX-HN)   An extra point originally from *Chen Xiuyuan Yishu Qishier Zhong: Kaozheng Xuefa* (*Seventy-Two Medical Works of Chen Xiuyuan: Textual Studies on Acupoints*). 〈Location〉on the head, 3.5 cun directly above the midpoint of the anterior hairline, same as Qianding(DU 21).

●**黑带**[hēi dài]   病证名。见《傅青主女科》。又称带下黑候。指妇女从阴道经常流出黑豆水色粘稠或稀或腥臭的液体,也有在赤白带下中杂有黑色,连绵不断。多因热盛熏蒸,伤及任、带二脉,肾水亏虚所致。治宜泻火清热。取带脉、中极、阴陵泉、下髎、行间、间使。

Blakish Discharge   A disease seen in *Fu Qingzhu Nuke* (*Fu Qingzhu's Obsterrics and Gynecology*), also named leukorrhea with blackish discharge. Refers to black soybean water-like liquid discharging from the vagina of a woman, which is ropy, dilute and often stinks, or to continuous black bloody vaginal discharge or leukorrhea. Mostly caused by the domination of heat which leads to injuries of Ren and Du Meridians and deficiency of kidney-Yin. 〈Treatment principle〉Clear heat and reduce fire. 〈Point selection〉Daimai(GB 26), Zhongji(RN 3), Yinlingquan(SP 9), Xialiao(BL 34), Xingjian(LR 2), and Jianshi(PC 5).

●**横刺**[héng cì]   沿皮刺之别称。见该条。

Transverse Insertion   Another name for subcutaneous or horizontal insertion. →沿皮刺(p.535)

●**横骨**(héng gǔ)   ①经穴名。出《针灸甲乙经》。属足少阴肾经,为冲脉、足少阴之会。又名下极、下横。〈定位〉在下腹部,当脐中下5寸,前正中线旁开0.5寸(图40)。〈层次解剖〉皮肤→皮下组织→腹直肌鞘前壁→锥状肌→腹直肌。浅层布有髂腹下神经前皮支,腹壁浅静脉的属支。深层有腹壁下动、静脉的分支或属支和第十一、十二胸神经前支的分支。〈主治〉阴部痛、少腹痛、遗精、阳痿、遗尿、小便不通、疝气。直刺0.8～1.2寸;可灸。②骨骼部位名。一指耻骨联合部;一指舌骨。③经外穴别名。即屈骨端。见该条。

1. Henggu(KI 11)   Originally from *Zhenjiu Jia-Yi Jing* (*A-B Classic of Acupuncture and Moxibustion*), a point on the kidney meridian of Foot-Shaoyin, the crossing point of the Chong and Foot-Shaoyin meridians also named Xiaji or Xiaheng. 〈Location〉on the lower abdomen, 5 cun below the center of the ubilicus and 0.5 cun lateral to the anterior midline(Fig. 40). 〈Regional anatomy〉skin→subcutaneous tissue→anterior sheath of rectus muscle of abdomen→pyramidal muscle→rectus muscle of abdomen. In the superficial layer, there are the anterior cutaneous branches of the iliohypogastric nerve and the tributaries of the superficial epigastric vein. In the deep layer, there are the branches or tributaries of the inferior epigastric artery and vein and the branches of the anterior branches of the llth and 12th thoracic nerves. 〈Indications〉pain of the pudendum, pain of the lower abdomen, nocturnal emission, impotence, enuresis, retention of urine, hernia. 〈Method〉Puncture perpendicularly 0.8-1.2 cun. Moxibustion is applicable.

2. Transverse Bone   Name of a bone, referring to pubic symphysis or the hyoid bone.

3. Henggu   Another name for the extra point Quguduan(EX-CA). →屈骨端(p.326)

●**横户**[héng hù]   经穴别名。出《针灸甲乙经》。即阴交。见该条。

Henghu   Another name for Yinjiao(RN 7), a meridian point originally from *Zhenjiu Jia-*

● 横三间寸 [héng sān jiān cùn]　灸法术语。见《千金要方·灸例》。指以三分宽度的艾炷三个并列，加上中间的间隙，两端的距离共一寸。临床多用于化脓灸法。

One-Cun Distance with Three Cones Side by Side　A kind of moxibustion, seen in *Qianjin Yaofang: Jiuli (Essential Treasured Prescriptions: Conventions of Moxibustion)*. Place three moxa cones side by side in a line, each standing on end and covering a width of 0.3 cun the total distance they cover, together with the little gaps between them is one cun. Clinically, this method is mostly used in festering moxibustion.

● 横舌 [héng shé]　经穴别名。出《外台秘要》。即哑门。见该条。

Hengshe　Another name for *Yamen* (DU 15), a meridian point originally from *Waitai Miyao (Clandestine Essentials from the Imperial Library)*. →哑门 (p.533)

● 横文 [héng wén]　①指大横穴。见《千金要方》、《千金翼方》。参见"大横"条。②即横纹。见该条1。

1. Hengwen　Referring to the point Daheng (SP 15), originally from *Qianjin Yaofang (Essential Prescriptions Worth a Thousand Gold)* and *Qianjin Yifang (Supplement to the Essential Treasured Prescriptions Worth a Thousand Gold)*. →大横 (p.63)

2. Transverse Crease　→横纹 1. (p.164)

● 横纹 [hén wén]　①又作横文，也称约纹。指皮肤皱纹，作为定穴的依据，如腕横纹等。②经外穴名。见《千金翼方》。在脐侠相去7寸。灸治多汗、四肢不举少力。

1. Transverse Crease　It can be written as 横文 in Chinese. Also named blinding crease, referring to wrinkles of the skin, used for locating acupoints, e.g. the transverse crease of the wrist, etc.

2. Hengwen (EX-CA)　An extra point, seen in *Qianjin Yifang (Supplement to the Essential Prescriptions Worth a Thousand Gold)*. ⟨Location⟩ 7 cun lateral to the umbilicus. ⟨Indications⟩ hidrosis, weakness and limited movement of limbs. ⟨Method⟩ moxibustion.

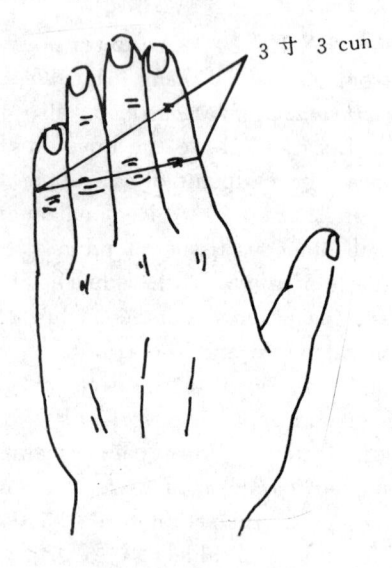

图22　横指同身寸
Fig 22　Finger-Breadth Cun

● 横指同身寸 [héng zhǐ tóng shēn cùn]　同身寸的一种。又名一夫法。即患者尺侧手四指并拢，以其中指中节横纹为准，其四指的宽度作为三寸。

Finger-Breadth Cun　A kind of finger measurement, also named Yi Fu Method (Four-Finger cun). The width the four fingers (index, middle, ring and little) cover when brought close together side by side, at the level of the dorsal skin crease of the proximal interphalangeal joint of the middle finger, is taken as 3 cun.

● 衡络之脉 [héng luò zhī mài]　经脉名。出《素问·刺腰痛篇》。指足太阳经在大腿后外侧的支脉。此支脉横过环跳部，下经浮郄、委阳，会合于委中。

Transverse Meridian　Name of a meridian from *Suwen: Ci Yaotong Pian (Plain Questions: On Treatment of Lumbago with Acupuncture)*. Refers to the branch of the Meridian of Foot-Taiyang in the posterior lateral side of the thigh. It traverses Huantiao (GB 30), goes down through Fuxi (BL 38) and Weiyang (BL 39), and joins the meridian at Weizhong (BL 40)

● 红丝疔 [hóng sī dīng]　疔疮的一种。见《证治准绳》。又名红线疔、血丝疔。因火毒凝聚，或破伤感染

所致。多起于手脚,初起局部红肿疼痛,继而红线由上臂前侧或小腿内侧向上走窜,重者可伴寒热、头痛、乏力。相当于急性淋巴管炎。治宜清热解毒。取穴见"疔疮"条。

Red-Streaked Infection　A kind of nail-like infection seen in *Zheng Zhi Zhun Sheng*(*Standards for Diagnosis and Treatment*). Also called red-thread infection or blood-streaked infection, due to accmulation of fire-evil or infection from external injuries. It usually appears on the hands and the feet with local redness, swelling, and pain, and then a red line extends upward along the anterior side of the upper arm or the medial side of the leg. It may be accompanied by chills, fever, headache and sluggishness in severe cases. It corresponds to acute lymphangitis. 〈Treatment principle〉Clear heat and toxic material. For point selection, see **Furuncle**(疔疮)(p. 82).

●红外线灸[hóng wài xiàn jiǔ]　为红外线照射法之别称。见该条。

Infrared Moxibustion　Another name for infrared radiation. →红外线照射法(p. 165)

●红外线穴位照射法[hóng wài xiàn xué wèi zhào shè fǎ]　为红外线照射法之别称。见该条。

Infrared Radiation on Points　Another name for infrared radiation. →红外线照射法(p. 165)

●红外线照射法[hóng wài xiàn zhào shè fǎ]　现代针灸疗法之一。又称红外线穴位照射法,或称红外线灸。是用红外线照射穴位以治疗疾病。其法以白布遮去其它部位,露出穴位部,用红外线发生器进行照射,以病人有舒服的温热感和皮肤出现淡红色为度。可用于哮喘、慢性支气管炎、风湿性关节炎、腱鞘炎、产后缺乳等症。对高热、心血管机能不全、有出血倾向或局部温觉障碍者,不可使用。

Infrared Radiation　A modern acupuncture and moxibustion therapy, also called infrared radiation on points or infrared moxibustion. A method of treating diseases by radiating the points with infrared rays. 〈Manipulation〉Cover the patient with white cloth leaving the point exposed, radiate the point with infrared rays until a warm sensation is felt by the patient and the local skin becomes light red. 〈Indications〉asthma, chronic bronchitis, rheumatic arthritis, tenosynovitis, puerperal agalactosis, etc. 〈Contraindications〉high fever, cardiac insufficiency, hemorrhagic tendency, and thermohypoesthesia.

●红线疔[hóng xiàn dīng]　即红丝疔。见该条。

Red-Thread Infection→红丝疔(p. 165)

●红眼[hóng yǎn]　即目赤肿痛。详见该条。

Red Eye　Another name for the disease with redness, swelling and pain of the eye. →目赤肿痛(p. 271)

●喉闭[hóu bì]　见《三因方》。即喉痹。详见该条。

Sore Throat　Seen in *Sanyin Fang*(*Prescriptions Based on Three Categories of Pathogenic Factors*). →喉痹(p. 165)

●喉痹[hóu bì]　病证名。出《素问·阴阳别论》等篇。一作喉闭,参见咽喉肿痛条。

Inflammation of the Throat　A disease, from *Suwen: Yinyang Bielun*(*Plain Questions: Supplementary Exposition of Yin and Yang*), etc., also named sore throat. →咽喉肿痛(p. 534)

●喉蛾[hóu é]　即乳蛾。详见该条。

Moth-Like Throat→乳蛾(p. 338)

●后顶[hòu dǐng]　经穴名。出《针灸甲乙经》。属督脉。又名交冲。〈定位〉在头部,当后发际正中直上5.5寸(脑户上3寸)(图28和图31)。〈层次解剖〉皮肤→皮下组织→帽状腱膜→腱膜下疏松组织。布有枕大神经以及枕动、静脉和颞浅动、静脉的吻合网。〈主治〉头痛、眩晕、项强、癫狂、痫证、烦心、失眠。平刺0.5~0.8寸;可灸。

Houding(DU 19)　A meridian point, on the Du Meridian, originally from *Zhenjiu Jia-Yi Jing*(*A-B Classic of Acupuncture and Moxibustion*), also named Jiaochong. 〈Location〉on the head, 5.5 cun directly above the midpoint of the posterior hairline and 3 cun above Naohu(DU 17)(Figs. 28&31). 〈Regional anatomy〉 skin → subcutaneous tissue → epicranial aponeurosis → subaponeurotic loose tissue. There are the great occipital nerve and the anastomotic network of the occipital arteries and veins with the superficial temporal arteries and veins in this area. 〈Indications〉headache, dizziness, neck rigidity, manic-depressive dis-

●后关[hòu guān] 经穴别名。出《针灸大全》。即听会。见该条。

Houguan Another name for Tinghui (GB 2), a meridian point originally from *Zhenjiu Daquan* (*A Complete Work of Acupuncture and Moxibustion*). →听会(p. 439)

●后曲[hòu qǔ] 经穴别名。见《外台秘要》。即瞳子髎。见该条。

Houqu Another name for Tongziliao (GB 1), a meridian point seen in *Waitai Miyao* (*Clandestine Essentials from the Imperial Library*). →瞳子髎(p. 443)

●后神聪[hòu shén cōng] 经外穴名。出《类经图翼》。在头部中线上,当前、后发际连线的中点处。〈主治〉中风、头痛、眩晕、癫痫等。沿皮刺0.3～0.5寸;可灸。

Houshencong (EX-HN) An extra point originally from *Leijing Tuyi* (*Illustrated Supplements to Classified Canon of Internal Medicine of the Yellow Emperor*). 〈Location〉 on the midline of the head, at the midpoint of the line connecting the anterior and posterior hairline. 〈Indications〉 apoplexy, headache, dizziness, epilepsy, etc. 〈Method〉 Puncture subcutaneously 0.3～0.5 cun. Moxibustion is applicable.

●后溪[hòu xī] 经穴名。出《灵枢·本输》属手太阳小肠经,为本经输穴;八脉交会穴之一,通于督脉。〈定位〉在手掌尺侧,微握拳,当小指本节(第五掌指关节)后的远侧掌横纹头赤白肉际(图48和图65)。〈层次解剖〉皮肤→皮下组织→小指展肌→小指短屈肌。浅层布有尺神经手背支、尺神经掌支和皮下浅静脉等。深层有小指尺掌侧固有动、静脉和指掌侧固有神经。〈主治〉头项强痛、耳聋、目赤目翳;肘臂及手指挛急、热病、疟疾、癫狂、痫证;盗汗、目眩、目眦烂、疥疮。直刺0.5～0.8寸;可灸。

Houxi (SI 3) A meridian point, on the small Intestine Meridian of Hand-Taiyang, originally from *Lingshu: Benshu* (*Miraculous Pivot: Meridian Points*), the Shu (Stream) Point of the meridian, one of the Eight Confluent Points communicating with the Du Meridian. 〈Location〉 at the junction of the red and white skin along the ulnar border of the hand, at the ulnar end of the distal palmar crease, proximal to the 5th metacarpophalangeal joint when a hollow fist is made (Figs. 48&65). 〈Regional anatomy〉 skin→subcutaneous tissue→abductor muscle of 5th finger→short flexor muscle of 5th figer. In the superficial layer, there are the dorsal branches of the ulnar nerve, the palmar branches of the ulnar nerve and the subcutaneous superficial vein. In the deep layer, there are the proper ulnar palmar artery and vein and the proper palmar digital nerve of the 5th finger. 〈Indications〉 pain and rigidity of the head and neck, deafness, redness of the eye, blurred vision; contracture of the elbow, arm and finger, febrile disease, malaria, depressive psychosis, mania, epilepsy; night sweating, dizziness and vertigo, blepharitis angularis and scabies. 〈Method〉 Punctrue perpendicularly 0.5～0.8 cun. Moxibustion is applicable.

●后腋[hòu yè] 经外穴别名,即后腋下穴。见该条。

Houye Another name for the extra point Houyexiaxue (EX-B). →后腋下穴(p. 166)

●后腋下穴[hòu yè xià xué] 经外穴名。见《类经图翼》。又名后腋。在腋后纹头处。〈主治〉颈项瘰疬、肩背挛急不举、喉风喉痹等。直刺0.5～1寸;可灸。

Houyexiaxue (EX-B) An extra point, seen in *Leijing Tuyi* (*Illustrated Supplements to Classified Canon of Internal Medicine of the Yellow Emperor*), also called Houye. 〈Location〉 at the end of the crease, posterior to the axilla. 〈Indications〉 neck lymphnoditis, shoulder and back region contracting, being unable to raise arms, acute throat trouble, and inflammation of the throat, etc. 〈Method〉 Puncture perpendicularly 0.5～1 cun. Moxibustion is applicable.

●候气[hòu qì] ①针刺术语。见《针灸大成》。指针刺时于适当深度候取感应,又称待气。其法主要是停针以待气至,如仍不得气,则可改变针刺深度和方向,并适当用提插等法。又可分为浅部候气和深部候气。②指针刺须候四时八正之气。见《素问·八正神明论》。参见"八正"条。③指诊脉候气。见《素问·离合真邪论》。

Waiting for Qi ① An acupuncture term seen in *Zhenjiu Dacheng*(*Great Compendium of Acupuncture and Moxibustion*), also named waiting for the arrival of qi, or waiting for the appearance of needling sensation. Refers to waiting for the response at a suitable depth after inserting the needle. 〈Method〉Stop puncturing to wait for qi; change the depth or direction of the insertion if the sensation is not achieved and properly apply the lifting and thrusting method, etc. It is divided into two forms: waiting for qi in the superficial area, and waiting for qi in the deep area. ②Referring to waiting for the qi of the four seasons and the qi of the eight solar terms, seen in *Suwen*: *Bazheng Shenming Lun* (*Plain Questions*: *On Eight Natural Qi and Divinity*). →八正(p.8)③Referring to waiting for qi while feeling the pulse, seen in *Suwen*: *Lihe Zhenxie Lun* (*Plain Questions*: *On the Expelling and Parting of Evil-Qi From Vital-Qi*).

●候时[hòu shí]　针刺术语。见《灵枢·卫气》。指针刺须等待合适的时间。此说为以后子午流注针法所本。

Waiting for the Proper Time An acupuncture term, seen in *Lingshu*: *Weiqi*(*Miraculous Pivot*: *Defensive Qi*), refers to waiting for a suitable time for acupuncture treatment, the foundation of the acupuncture technique of midnight-noon ebb-flow in later ages.

●呼吸补泻[hū xī bǔ xiè]　针刺手法名。见《素问·离合真邪论》。是以进、出针时配合病人呼吸来分别补泻的方法。即呼气时进针，吸气时出针，针气相顺为补；吸气时进针，呼气时出针，针气相逆为泻。

Reinforcing or Reducing by Means of Respiration A needling technique, seen in *Suwen*: *Lihe Zhenxie Lun*(*On the Expelling and Parting of Evil-Qi from Vital-Qi*). A method of inserting and removing the needle in coordination with the breathing of the patient in order to reduce or reinforce. To reinforce, insert the needle on inspiration, remove the needle on exhalation. To reduce, insert the needle on exhalation and remove the needle on inspiration.

●狐疝[hú shàn]　疝气证型之一。出《灵枢·五色》。又名小肠气、阴狐疝。多由劳累过度，强力负重，络脉损伤，气虚下陷所致。证见少腹部与阴囊牵连坠胀疼痛，甚者睾丸立则下坠，卧则入腹，重疝以手推托才能使坠物回收入腹。常因反复发作，久延失治，出现食少、短气、疲乏等兼证。治宜补气升陷，止痛。取归来、带脉、维道、关元。

Inguinal Hernia One of the syndromes of hernia, originally from *Lingshu*: *Wu Se* (*Miraculous Pivot*: *Five Colors*), also called qi of the small intestine, or yin-type hernia. Mostly caused by sinking of *qi* due to deficiency, and injury of the collaterals resulting from overwork or carrying too much weight. 〈Manifestations〉tugging and down-bearing sensation and distending pain of the lower abdomen and scrotum. Occasionally, the testis comes out when the patient is in the standing position; and enters into the abdomen when the patient is in the lying position. For serious hernia, the prolapsed substance can only be put back into the abdomen with the help of the hand. There may be a lack of appetite, shortness of breath, fatigue, etc., because of repeated attacks or a protracted course of disease. 〈Treatment principle〉Tonify and elevate the spleen-qi, and alleviate pain. 〈Point selection〉Guilai(ST 29), Daimai(GB 26), Weidao (GB 28)and Guanyuan(RN 4).

●胡椒饼灸[hú jiāo bǐng jiǔ]　即隔胡椒饼灸。详见该条。

Peper Cake Moxibustion →隔胡椒饼灸(p.135)

●虎口[hǔ kǒu]　①经穴别名。出《针灸甲乙经》。即合谷。见该条。②经外穴名。见《备急千金要方》。位于合谷穴前方赤白肉际处。〈主治〉头痛、烦热、眩晕、失眠、盗汗、心痛、牙痛、小儿唇紧，以及扁桃体炎等。斜刺0.3～0.5寸；可灸。③指两手拇指与食指之间的部位。

1. Hukou Another name for Hegu(LI 4), a meridian point from *Zhenjiu Jia-Yi Jing*(*A-B Classic of Acupuncture and Moxibustion*). →合谷 Hegu(LI 4)(p.160)

2. Hukou(EX-UE) An extra point, seen in *Beiji Qianjin Yaofang*(*Essential Prescriptions for Emergencies Worth a Thousand Gold*).

⟨Location⟩ at the junction of the red and white skin anterior to Hegu (LI 4). ⟨Indications⟩ headache, dysphoria with smothering sensation, dizziness, insomnia, night sweating, precordial pain, toothache, lockjaw in children, and tonsillitis, etc. ⟨Mehthod⟩ Puncture obliquely 0.3~0.5 cun. Moxibustion is applicable.

3. **Tiger's Mouth** Part of the hand, referring to the area between the thumb and index finger.

●虎口百丫[hǔ kǒu bǎi yā] 即虎口疔。见该条。

Pustule in Tiger's Mouth Nail-like furuncle in tiger's mouth →虎口疔(p.168)

●虎口疔[hǔ kǒu dīng] 病证名。出《证治准绳·疡医》。又名合谷疔、虎口白丫、丫叉毒、手叉发、病蟹叉、虎口疽、合谷疽、手丫刺、丫刺毒、虎丫毒、擘蟹毒、拍蟹毒、丫指等。生于手大指,次指歧骨间合谷穴处。由阳明经湿热凝结而成。初起黄色小泡,或结豆粒硬块,焮赤肿痛,根深坚韧,或漫肿色青,木痛坚硬,重者可继发红丝疔。参见"疔疮"条。

Nail-Like Furuncle in Tiger's Mouth Name of a disease, from *Zheng Zhi Zhunsheng: Yang Yi* (*Standard of Diagnosis and Treatment: Skin External Diseases*), also named nail-like boil at Hegu area, pustule in tiger's mouth, poison at fork area, carbuncle of hand, forelegs of a diseased crab, deep-rooted carbuncle in tiger's mouth, deep-rooted carbuncle at Hegu area, thorn at the hand, poisonous thorn at fork area, pyogenic infection at the area of tiger's mouth, thumb-crab poison, clappingcrab poison, fork-finger, etc. It appears at Hegu (LI 4) area, between the thumb and index finger. It is caused by the accumulation of damp-heat in the Yangming Meridian. At the begining, a small yellowish blister or lenticular gelosis, with redness, pain and swellings appear. It can be deep-rooted, tough and tensile, or swelling with blue color, painful and hard. A serious one may lead to red-streaked infection. →疔疮(p.82)

●虎口毒[hǔ kǒu dú] 即虎口疔。见该条。

Poison at the Area of Tiger's Mouth →虎口疔(p.168)

●虎口疽[hǔ kǒu jū] 即虎口疔。见该条。

Deep-Rooted Carbuncle in Tiger's Mouth →虎口疔(p.168)

●虎丫毒[hǔ yā dú] 即虎口疔。见该条。

Pyogenic Infection at the Area of Tiger's Mouth →虎口疔(p.168)

●花翳白陷[huā yì bái xiàn] 即目翳的别名。详见该条。

Nebula Another name for blurred vision, or kerato malacia. →目翳(p.273)

●华盖[huá gài] 经穴名。出《针灸甲乙经》。属任脉。⟨定位⟩在胸部,当前正中线上,平第一肋间(图40)。⟨层次解剖⟩皮肤→皮下组织→胸大肌起始腱→胸骨柄与胸骨体之间(胸骨角)。主要布有第一肋间神经前皮支和胸廓内动、静脉的穿支。⟨主治⟩咳嗽、气喘、胸痛、胁肋痛、喉痹、咽肿。平刺0.3~0.5寸;可灸。

Huagai(RN 20) A meridian point, originally from *Zhenjiu Jia-Yi Jing* (*A-B Classic of Acupuncture and Moxibustion*), a point on the Ren Meridian. ⟨Location⟩ on the chest and on the anterior midline, on the level of the lst intercostal space (Fig. 40). ⟨Regional anatomy⟩ skin→subcutaneous tissue→origm of greater pectoral muscle→between manubrium of sternum and sternal body (sternal angle). There are the anterior cutaneous branches of the lst intercostal nerve and the perforating branches of the internal thoracic artery and vein in this area. ⟨Indications⟩ cough, asthma, chest pain, pain in hypochondriac region, inflammation of the throat, and tonsilitis. ⟨Method⟩ Puncture subcutaneously 0.3~0.5 cun. Moxibustion is applicable.

●滑精[huá jīng] 病证名。见《景岳全书·杂证谟》。又名精滑。多因思欲不遂,房事过度,肾元亏损,精关不固所致。少数则因下焦湿热而起。证见无梦而遗,甚则见色流精,滑泄频仍,腰部酸冷,面色㿠白,神疲乏力,或兼阳萎、自汗、短气,舌淡苔白,脉细或细数。治宜补益肾气,固涩精关。取气海、三阴交、志室、肾俞。

Spermatorrhoea A disease, seen in *Jingyue Quanshu: Zazheng Mo* (*Jingyue's Complete Works: Strategies on Miscellaneous Diseases*), also named involuntary seminal emission, mostly caused by unsatisfied sexual intemper-

ance in sexual life, deficiency of the kidney, and uncontrolled gate of essence. Sometimes caused by lower-jiao damp-heat. 〈Manifestations〉emission without dream, or even worse emission at the sight of a female, frequent emission, aching and cold in lumbar region, pale complexion, lassitude with impotence, spontaneous perspiration, or shortness of breath, pale tongue and white coating, thready and rapid pulse. 〈Treatment principle〉Tonify the kidney qi so as to control the gate of essence. 〈Point selection〉Qihai (RN 6), Sanyinjiao (SP 6), Zhishi(BL 52) and Shenshu(BL 23).

●滑肉门[huá ròu mén] 经穴名。出《针灸甲乙经》。属足阳明胃经。〈定位〉在上腹部,当脐中上1寸,距前正中线2寸(图60和图40)。〈层次解剖〉在腹直肌及其鞘处;有第9肋间动、静脉分支及腹壁下动、静脉;布有第9肋间神经分支。〈主治〉癫狂、呕吐、胃疼。直刺0.8~1.2寸;可灸。

Huaroumen (ST 24) A meridian point, from *Zhenjiu Jia-Yi Jing* (*A-B Classic of Acupuncture and Moxibustion*), a point on the Stomach Meridian of Foot-Yangming. 〈Location〉 on the upper abdomen, 1 cun above the centre of the umbilicus and 2 cun lateral to the anterior midline (Figs. 60&40). 〈Regional anatomy〉 skin→subcutaneous tissue→anterior sheath of rectus muscle of abdomen→rectus muscle of abdomen. In the superficial layer, there are the lateral and anterior cutaneous branches of the anterior branches of the 8th to 10th thoracic nerves and the periumbilical venous network. In the deep layer, there are the branches of tributaries of the superior epigastric artery and vein and the muscular branches of the anterior branches of the 8th to 10th thoracic nerves. 〈Indications〉 manic-depressive psychosis, vomiting, and stomachache. 〈Method〉 Puncture perpendicularly 0.8~1.2 cun. Moxibustion is applicable.

●滑寿[huá shòu] 人名。元代著名医学家,字伯仁,晚号樱宁生,祖籍襄城(今河南襄城),迁居仪真(今江苏仪征),后定居余姚(今属浙江)。精读《内经》等古医书,对针灸亦很有研究,他认为督、任二脉应与十二经相提并论,对经络腧穴理论提出新见解,著《十四经发挥》。该书刊于1341年。

Hua Shou A famous physician in the yuan Dynasty, who styled himself Boren, and assumed the name of Ying Ningsheng, a native of Xiangcheng County (now Xiangcheng in Henan Province). His family moved to Yizhen (today's Yizheng in Jiangsu Province) and later settled down in Yuyao(now in Zhejiang Province). He read *Neijing*(*The Canon of Internal Medicine*) and other ancient medical books intensively, and was proficient in acupuncture and moxibustion as well. He believed that the Du and Ren Meridians should be mentioned and discussed together with the Twelve Regular Meridians and put forward new ideas on the theory of meridians and collaterals and points. He wrote *Shisi Jing Fahui* (*An Elaboration of the Fourteen Meridians*), which was published in 1341.

●化脓灸[huà nóng jiǔ] 艾炷灸的一种,又称瘢痕灸。系以艾炷直接灸灼穴位皮肤,渐致化脓,最后留有瘢痕。一般每穴灸5~9壮之后,再用灸疮膏药(淡膏药)封贴,每日更换膏药一次,约经4~7天,灸处化脓起疱,形成灸疮。多用于哮喘、慢性肠胃病等顽固性、疼痛性病证的治疗。

Festering Moxibustion A method of moxibustion with moxa cones, also called scarring moxibustion. A moxa cone is burnt directly on the skin at the acupuncture point, so that the skin festers and a scar is left. After using five to nine moxa cones on a point, put an adhesive plaster for post-moxibustion on it. Renew the plasters every day. After four to seven days, suppuration and blisters should occur at the point. Then post-moxibustion sores form. It is mostly used for the treatment of asthma, chronic enterogastric diseases and other obstinate.

●华佗[huà tuó] 人名。东汉末杰出的医学家,又名旉,字元化,沛国谯(今安徽亳县)人。在医学上有很高的成就,通晓内、外、妇、儿等科,尤精于外科与针灸,他首创外科手术治疗,用酒服"麻沸散"进行全身麻醉,施行腹腔手术,收到较好效果;同时,在针灸方面,他创"华佗夹脊穴",直沿用至今。另还创造了"五禽戏",以模仿虎、熊、鹿、猿、鸟的动作和姿态活动肢体,来达到防病健身的目的。史料记载华佗著有《枕中灸刺经》等多种医书。均佚。在《肘后备急方》、《千

金要方》、《医心方》中保留有他关于针灸的部分佚文。《中藏经》是后人托华佗之名的作品。

Hua Tuo An outstanding physician in the late years of the Eastern Han Dynasty. His other name is Hua Fu, he styled himself Yuanhua. He was from Qiaoxian County of Pei State (now Boxian county, Anhui Province). He made remarkable achievements in medicine and was proficient in internal medicine, surgery, gynecology and pediatrics, particularly in surgery and acupuncture and moxibustion. He initiated surgical operations, performed general anesthesia by getting the patient drink Ma Fei in alcohol for operations on the abdominal cavity and gained results. Meanwhile, in the field of acupuncture and moxibustion, the "Huatuojiaji Points" (Hua Tuo's paravertebral points) which he invented are still in use today. He also created five-animal boxing, a method of exercising the extremities by imitating the motions and postures of tigers, deer, bears, monkeys and birds to prevent diseases and strengthen the body. It is recorded in historical data that he compiled *Zhenzhong Jiuci Jing* (*Canon of Moxibustion and Acupuncture Preserved in Pillow*), and many other medical works, all of which have been lost. Preserved in *Zhouhou Beiji Fang* (*A Handbook of Prescriptions for Emergencies*), *Qianjin Yaofang* (*Essential Prescriptions Worth a Thousand Gold*) and *Yixin Fang* (*The Heart of Medical Prescriptions*) are some extant parts of what he wrote on acupuncture and moxibustion. *Zhong Zang Jing* (*Canon of the Stored Treasures*) is a work produced by later generations under Hua Tuo's name.

● 华佗夹脊 [huà tuó jiā jí] 夹脊的别名。见该条。

Huatuojiaji Another name for Jiaji (EX-B 2)→夹脊 (p.186)

● 华佗穴 [huá tuó xué] 经外穴别名。见《针灸学简编》。即夹脊穴。见该条。

Hua Tuo Points Another name for Jiaji (EX-B2), a set of extra points seen in *Zhen jiuxue Jianbian* (*Concise Book of Acupuncture and Moxibustion*). →夹脊 (p.186)

● 踝 [huái] ①耳穴名。位于跟与膝两穴之中部。用于治疗踝部疾患、踝关节扭挫伤。②部位名。足上胫下隆起之骨，内侧为内踝，为胫骨之下端，外侧为外踝，是胫骨下端。

1. **Ankle** (MA-AH 2) An auricular point. 〈Location〉at the middle point between Heel (MA-AH 1) and Knee (MA-AH 3). 〈Indications〉ankle diseases, sprain of ankle.

2. **Ankle** A part of the body, the projected bone below the tibia and above the foot, i.e. the inferior end of tibia; the medial one is the medial mallacolus and the lateral one is the lateral malleolus.

● 踝骨 [huái gǔ] 骨骼部位名。指胫、腓骨下端的内踝和外踝，又指尺骨茎突和桡骨茎突的高点。

Malleolus Name of a skeletal locality, referring to the medial malleolus and the lateral malleolus at the lower end of the tibia and fibula, also referring to the high point of the styloid progress of the ulna and of radius.

● 踝尖 [huái jiān] 经外穴别名。见《类经图翼》。即内踝尖。见该条。

Huaijian Another name for Neihuaijian (EX-LE), an extra point from *Leijing Tuyi* (*Illustrated Supplements to Classified Canon of Internal Medicine of the Yellow Emperor*). →内踝尖 (p.279)

● 环铫 [huán diào] 经穴别名。出《千金翼方》。即环跳。见该条。

Huandiao Another name for Huantiao (GB 30), a meridian point from *Qianjin Yifang* (*Supplement to Essential Prescriptions Worth a Thousand Gold*). →环跳 (p.170)

● 环岗 [huán gǎng] 经外穴别名。即团岗。见该条。

Huangang Another name for the extra point Tuangang (EX-B). →团岗 (p.449)

● 环谷 [huán gǔ] 经外穴别名。出《灵枢·四时气》。即神阙。见该条。

Huangu Another name for Shenque (RN 8), a meridian point, from *Lingshu: Sishi Qi* (*Miraculous Pivot: Qi of Four Seasons*). →神阙 (p.363)

● 环跳 [huán tiào] 经穴名。出《针灸甲乙经》。属足少阳胆经，为足少阳、太阳经之会。又名髋骨、分中、髀厌、髋骨、环铫。〈定位〉在股外侧部，侧卧屈股，当股骨大转子最凸点与骶管裂孔连线的外1/3（图8和图23）。〈层次解剖〉皮肤→皮下组织→臀大肌→坐骨

huán 环 huán

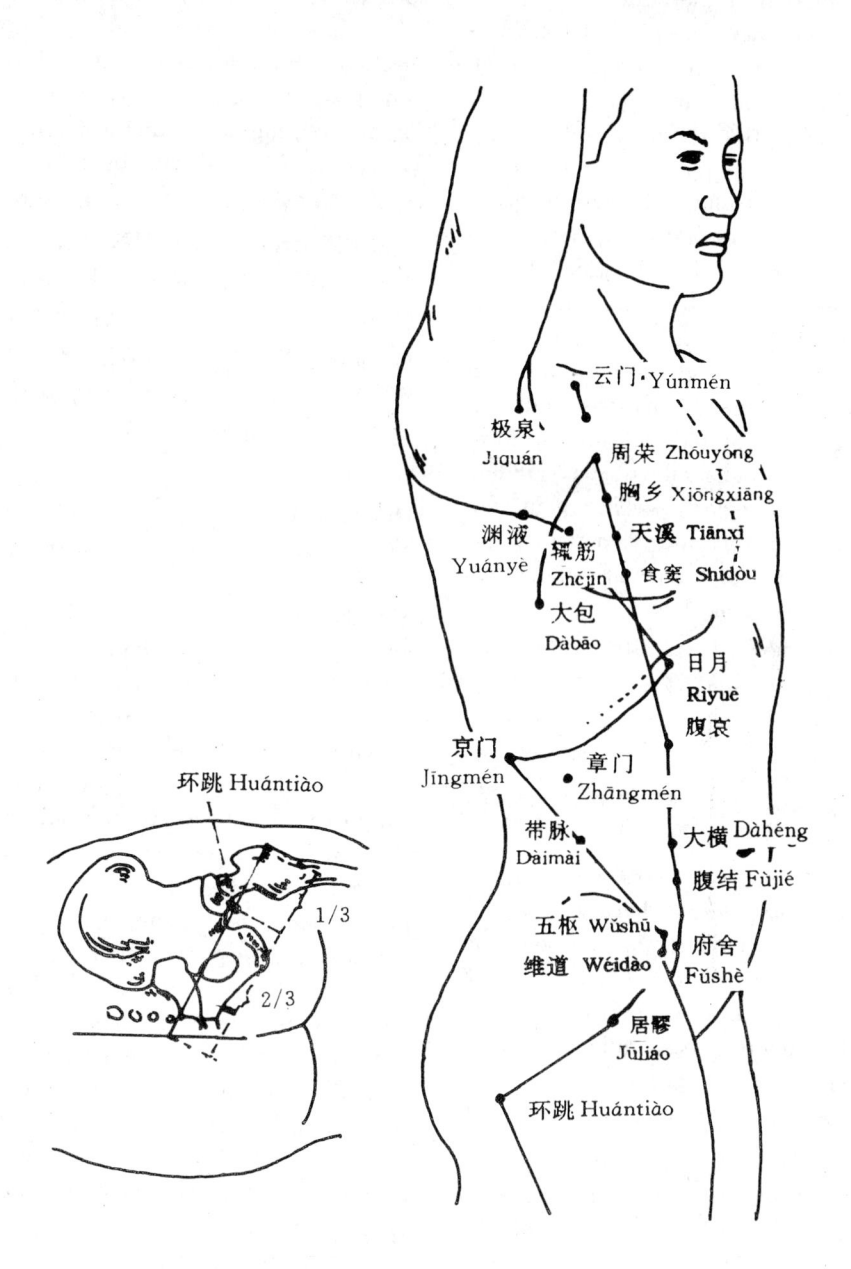

图23 环跳和其他胸腹部穴

Fig 23 Huantiao and other points of chest and abdomen

神经→股方肌。浅层布有臀上皮神经。深层有坐骨神经,臀下神经,股后皮神经和臀下动、静脉等。〈主治〉腰胯疼痛、半身不遂、下肢痿痹、遍身风疹、闪挫腰疼、膝踝肿痛不能转侧。直刺2～2.5寸;可灸。

Huantiao(GB 30) A meridian point, from *Zhenjiu Jia-Yi Jing* (*A-B classic of Acupuncture and Moxibustion*), a point on the Gallbladder Meridian of Foot-Shaoyang, the crossing point of the Foot-Shaoyin and Foot-Taiyang Meridians. Other names for it are Bingu, Fenzhong, Biyan, Kuangu, or Huandiao. 〈Location〉 on the lateral side of the

171

thigh, at the junction of the middle third and lateral third of the line connecting the prominence of the great trochanter and the sacral hiatus when the patient is in a lateral recumbent position with the thigh flexed (Figs. 8 & 23). 〈Regional anatomy〉 skin→subcutaneous tissue→greatest gluteal muscle→sciatic nerve→quadrate muscle of thigh. In the superficial layer, there is the superior clunial nerve. In the deep layer, there are the sciatic nerve, the inferior gluteal nerve, the posterior cutaneous nerve of the thigh, and the inferior gluteal artery and vein. 〈Indications〉 lumbar and hip pain, hemiplegia, flaccidity and numbness of lower limbs, general rubella, sudden sprain in the lumbar region, swelling, pain and limited movement of the ankle and the knee. 〈Method〉 Puncture perpendicularly 2～2.5 cun. Moxibustion is applicable.

● 环跳针 [huán tiào zhēn] 长针之别称。见该条。

Huantiao Needle Another name for a long needle. →长针(p. 40)

● 环中 [huán zhōng] 经外穴名。见《中国针灸学》。在环跳穴与腰俞穴连线之中点。〈主治〉坐骨神经痛。直刺1～1.5寸；可灸。

Huanzhong (EX) An extra point, from *Zhongguo Zhenjiuxue* (*Chinese Acupuncture and Moxibustion*). 〈Location〉 at the midpoint of the line connecting Huantiao (GB 30) and Yaoshu (DU 2). 〈Indication〉 sciatica neuralgia. 〈Method〉 Puncture perpendicularly 1～1.5 cun. Moxibustion is applicable.

● 缓风 [huǎn fēng] 病证名。脚气的古称。见《类证治裁·脚气》。详见"脚气"条。

Slow Wind A disease, the archaic name of beriberi, from *Leizheng Zhicai: Jiaoqi* (*Differential Diagnosis and Treatment of Diseases: Beriberi*). →脚气(p. 200)

● 患门 [huàn mén] 经外穴名。见《外台秘要》。在背部，当第5胸椎突两旁各开1.5寸处。灸治五劳七伤、骨蒸潮热、面黄肌瘦、饮食无味、咳嗽、遗精、盗汗、心痛、胸背引痛等。

Huanmen (EX-B) An extra point, from *Waitai Miyao* (*Clandestine Essentials from the Imperial Library*). 〈Location〉 on the back, 1.5 cun lateral to the spinous process of the 5th thoracic vertebra. 〈Indications〉 five kinds of strains and seven kinds of impairments, hectic fever, emaciation with sallow complexion, poor appetite, cough, seminal emission, night sweating, precordial pain, chest and back pain, etc. 〈Method〉 moxibustion.

● 肓门 [huāng mén] 经穴名。出《针灸甲乙经》。属足太阳膀胱经。〈定位〉在腰部，当第一腰椎棘突下，旁开3寸(图7)。〈层次解剖〉皮肤→皮下组织→背阔肌腱膜→竖脊肌→腰方肌。浅层布有第一、二腰神经后支的外侧皮支和伴行的动、静脉。深层有第一、二腰神经后支的肌支和第一腰动、静脉背侧支的分支或属支。〈主治〉上腹痛、痞块、便秘、妇人乳疾。直刺0.8～1寸；可灸。

Huangmen (BL 51) A meridian point, from *Zhenjiu Jia-Yi Jing* (*A-B Classic of Acupuncture and Moxibustion*), a point of the Bladder Meridian of Foot-*Taiyang*. 〈Location〉 on the low back, below the spinous process of the 1st lumbar vertebra, 3 cun lateral to the posterior midline (Fig. 7). 〈Regional anatomy〉 skin→subcutaneous tissue→aponeurosis of latissimus muscle of back→erector spinal muscle→lumbar quadrate muscle. In the superfical layer, there are the lateral cutaneous branches of the posterior branches of the 1st and 2nd lumbar nerves and the accompanying arteries and veins. In the deep layer, there are the muscular branches of the posterior branches of the 1st and 2nd lumbar nerves and the branches or tributaries of the dorsal branches of the 1st lumbar artery and vein. 〈Indications〉 epigastric pain, abdominal masses, constipation, female mastosis. 〈Method〉 Puncture perpendicularly 0.8～1 cun. Moxibustion is applicable.

● 肓募 [huāng mù] 经外穴名。见《千金要方》。从乳头斜度至脐，中屈去半，从乳头下行，度头是穴。灸治腹中积块疼痛、黄疸、病后虚弱等。

Huangmu (EX-CA) An extra point, seen in *Qianjin Yaofang* (*Essential Prescriptions Worth a Thousand Gold*). 〈Location〉 The point is directly below the nipple (Ruzhong, ST17), the distance from the nipple to the point is half of the distance from the nipple to the navel. 〈Indications〉 abdominal masses with pain, jaundice, and asthenia after disease,

etc. 〈Method〉moxibustion.

●**肓俞**[huāng shù] 经穴名。出《针灸甲乙经》。属足少阴肾经，为冲脉、足少阴经之会。〈定位〉在中腹部，当脐中旁开0.5寸（图40）。〈层次解剖〉皮肤→皮下组织→腹直肌鞘前壁→腹直肌。浅层布有脐周皮下静脉网，第九、十、十一胸神经前支的前皮支及伴行的动、静脉。深层有腹壁上、下动、静脉吻合形成的动、静脉网，第九、十、十一胸神经前支的肌支及相应的肋间动、静脉。〈主治〉腹痛、呕吐、腹胀、痢疾、泄泻、便秘、疝气、月经不调、腰脊痛。直刺0.8～1.2寸；可灸。

Huangshu(KI 16) A meridian point, from *Zhenjiu Jia-Yi Jing (A-B Classic of Acupuncture and Moxibustion)*, a point on the Kidney Meridian of Foot-Shaoyin, the crossing point of the Chong and Foot-Shaoyin Meridians. 〈Location〉on the middle abdomen, 0.5 cun lateral to the centre of the umbilicus (Fig. 40). 〈Regional anatomy〉skin→subcutaneous tissue→anterior sheath of rectus muscle of abdomen→rectus muscle of abdomen. In the superficial layer, there are the periumbilical subcutaneous venous network, the anterior cutaneous branches of the anterior branches of the 9th to 11th thoracic nerves and the accompanying arteries and veins. In the deep layer, there are the arteriovenous network formed by the anastomosis of the superior epigastric arteries and veins with the inferior epigastric arteries and veins, the muscular branches of the anterior branches of the 9th to 11th thoracic nerves and the related intercostal arteries and veins. 〈Indications〉abdominal pain, vomiting, abdominal distention, dysentery, diarrhea, constipation, hernia, irregular menstruation, and pain along the spinal column. 〈Method〉Puncture perpendicularly 0.8～1.2 cun. Moxibuation is applicable.

●**皇甫谧**[huáng fǔ mì] 人名。魏晋间医学家、文学家，字士安，幼名静，自号玄晏先生，安定朝那（今甘肃灵台）人。中年患风痹后专心攻医学，尤精于针灸。他在《素问》、《针经》、《明堂孔穴针灸治要》的基础上，著成《针灸甲乙经》。总结了晋以前的针灸学成就，是我国现存最早的针灸学专著。

Huangfu Mi A physician and writer in the Wei and Jin Dynasties, who was named Jing as a child and styled himself Shian. His assumed name was Mr. Xuanyan. He was from Chaona, Anding County (now Lingtai, Gansu Province), After contracting migrating athralgia in middle age, he went out for and specialized in medicine, particularly in acupuncture and moxibustion. On the basis of *Suwen (Plain Questions)*, *Zhenjing (Canon of Acupuncture)*, and *Ming Tang Kongxue Zhenjiu Zhiyao (An outline of Points for Acupuncture and Moxibustion)*, he compiled *Zhenjiu Jia-Yi Jing (A-B Classic of Acupuncture and Moxibustion)*, which summarized the achivements in acupuncture and moxibustion prior to the Jin Dynasty and was the earliest treatise on acupuncture and moxibustion in China.

●**黄带**[huáng dài] 病证名。见《傅青主女科》。又称带下黄候。指阴道内流出淡黄色稠粘的液体，甚则色浓如茶汁，或有臭秽气味。多因体内湿邪过盛，湿郁化热，伤及任、带二脉所致。治宜清热利湿解毒。取足三里、三阴交、阴陵泉、带脉、下髎、行间。

Leukorrhea with Yellowish Discharge A disease, from *Fu Qingzhu Nüke (Fu Qingzhu's Obstetrics and Gynecology)*, also named yellowish leukorrhea. Referring to the thick, yellowish liquid flowing out of vagina. In serious cases, the liquid is like tea, or has a foul smell. It is often caused by excessive dampness, the change from damp stagnancy to heat, and injury to the Ren and Du Meridians. 〈Treatment principle〉Reduce fever, remove dampness by diuresis, and detoxify. 〈Point selection〉Zusanli(ST 36), Sanyinjiao(SP 6), Yinlingquan(SP 9), Daimai(GB 26), Xialiao(BL 34) and Xingjian(LR 2).

●**黄疸**[huáng dǎn] 病证名。出《素问·平人气象论》等篇。又称黄瘅。以目黄，尿黄，皮肤黄为主要特征。多由感受时邪，湿浊外入，或饮食不节，湿浊内生致使脾不健运，肝失疏泄，胆汁外溢而发黄。临床上分为阳黄和阴黄。详见各条。

Jaundice A disease, from *Suwen: Pingren Qixiang Lun (Plain Questions: On Normal People's Physiology)*, and other writings, also named Huang Dan. Characterized by yellowish sclera skin, and yellowish urine. 〈Pathology〉

dampness (seasonal factors) from the outside or produced in the interior due to improper diet, leading to dysfunction of the spleen in transportation and transformation, and the stagnation of liver-qi followed by the abnormal outflow of bile which turns into jaundice. Clinically, it is divided into yang jaundice and yin jaundece. →阳黄(p. 538)、阴黄(p. 555)

●黄瘅[huáng dàn] 病症名。出《素问·玉机真藏论》等篇。即黄疸。详该条。

Huang Dan A disease, from *Suwen*: *Yu ji Zhen Zang Lun* (*Plain Questions*: *On Miraculous Pulse Phenomena and Essential Zang-Organs*) and other writings, i.e. jaundice. →黄疸 (p. 173)

●黄帝[huáng dì] 人名。传说中中华民族的祖先,为有熊国君少典之子,姓公孙,名轩辕。相传黄帝为我国文化之创始者,凡兵器、舟车、弓箭、衣服等皆为黄帝所作,其中也包括医药。据载黄帝与其臣子岐伯等医家讨论医药,而创造了医药。故许多医书均假托黄帝之名。

Huang Di (**The Yellow Emperor**) The lengendary ancestor of the Chinese, the son of Shaodian, the king of You Xiong State. His surname was Gongsun and personal name Xuanyuan. His name is also translated into the Yellow Emperor. It is said that Huangdi was the founder of the Chinese culture that he developed weapons, boats and vehicles, bows and arrows garments, etc. and also medicine. It was recorded that he discussed medicine with his official Qi Bo and other physicians, and created medicines. That is why many medical books were written under his name.

●黄帝九虚内经[huáng dì jiǔ xū nèi jīng] 书名。见《宋史·艺文志》。似即指《灵枢》。

Huang Di Jiu Xu Neijing (**The Yellow Emperor's Inner Canon in Nine Parts**) A book, from *Song Shi*: *Yi Wen Zhi* (*History of the Song Dynasty*: *Records of Art and Culture*), referring seemingly to *Lingshu* (*Miraculous Pivot*).

●黄帝明堂灸经[huáng dì míng táng jiǔ jīng] 书名。原书出唐代或唐以前,撰人不详。北宋末年(1127年)刊有单行本。书中分别载成人及小儿常用要穴的灸法及经验,并附腧穴图40余幅。元代(1311年)窦桂芳辑入《针灸四书》中。

Huangdi Mingtang Jiujing (**The Yellow Emperor's Classic of Mingtang Chart and Moxibustion**) A book, written in or before the Tang Dynasty, author unknown. A separate edition was published in the late years of the Northern Song Dynasty (1127), in which, moxibustoin methods and experiences of the commonly used important points for adults and children were stated with more than forty illustrated drawings of acupoints. It was edited into *Zhenjiu Si Shu* (*Four Books on Acupuncture and Moxibustion*) by Dou Guifang in the Yuan Dynasty (1311).

●黄帝明堂偃侧人图[huáng dì míng táng yǎn cè rén tú] 书名。撰人不详。见《隋书·经籍志》。又有《曹氏黄帝十二经明堂偃侧人图》十二卷。为三国、晋初时曹翕撰。书佚。见《新唐书·艺文志》。

Huangdi Mingtang Yan Ce Retu (**The Yellow Emperor's Mingtang Chart of Anterior and Lateral Views**) Title of a book, whose author is unknown, seen in *Sui Shu*: *Jing ji Zhi* (*Book of the Sui Dynasty*: *Records of Classics and Books*). Another book is *Caoshi Huangdi Shier Jing Mingtang Yan Ce Rentu* (*Cao's Charts of Anterior and Lateral Views for Illustrating the Points of the Yellow Emperor's Twelve Meridians*) in twelve volumes, written by Cao Xi in the late years of the Three Kingdoms and early years of the Jin Dynasty, no longer extant. Cf. *Xin Tang Shu*: *Yi Wen Zhi* (*New Book of the Tang Dynasty*: *Records of Art and Literature*).

●黄帝内经[huáng dì nèi jīng] 书名。简称《内经》。包括《灵枢》(九卷)和《素问》(九卷)两部分,共十八卷。约成书于战国至秦、汉时期,假托黄帝之名。是我国现存最早的一部医学理论著作。书中有关针灸经络、腧穴、刺灸、治疗的论述,为后世针灸学的发展奠定了基础。

Huangdi Neijing (**The Yellow Emperor's Canon of Internal Medicine**) Title of a book, called *Neijing* (*The Inner Canon of Huangdi*) for short, including *Lingshu* (*Miraculous Pivot*) (in nine volumes) and *Suwen* (*Plain Questions*) (in nine volumes), eighteen volumes in all, completed during the

period between the Warring States and the Qin and Han Dynasties under Yellow Emperor's name. It is the earliest work on medical theories extant in China. Its expositions on meridians and collaterals, acupoints, acupuncture and moxibustion, and treatments laid a good foundation for the development of the theory of acupuncture and moxibustion in later ages.

●黄帝内经明堂［huáng dì nèi jīng míng táng］ 书名。见"黄帝内经明堂类成"条。

Huangdi Neijing Mingtang（The Yellow Emperor's Inner Classic Acupoints） Title of a book, also entitled *Huangdi Neijing Mingtang Leicheng（Classification of Acupoints of the Yellow Emperor's Inner Classic）*. →黄帝内经明堂类成(p.175)

●黄帝内经明堂类成［huáng dì nèi jīng míngtáng lèi chéng］ 书名。又称《黄帝内经明堂》，十三卷，是《黄帝明堂经》的一种注本。由杨上善撰注。前十二卷论十二经脉腧穴，末一卷论奇经八脉。唐曾规定其为学针灸的主要课本。现仅存卷一。见《旧唐书·经籍志》。

Huangdi Neijing Mingtang Leicheng（Classification of Acupoints of the Yellow Emperor's Inner Classic）. Title of a book, also entitled *Huangdi Neijing Mingtang（The Yellow Emperor's Inner Classic of Acupoints）* in 13 volumes, an annotated version of *Huangdi Ming Tang Jing（The Yellow Emperor's Classic of Acupoints）* with notes by Yang Shangshan. The first 12 volumes discuss the twelve regular meridians and acupoints, and the last volume deals with the eight extra meridians. It was made the principal textbook for the study of acupncture and moxibustion in the Tang Dynasty. Of all the 13 volumes, only Vol. 1 is extant. Cf. *Jiu Tangshu: Jing Ji Zhi（Old Book of the Tang Dynasty: Records of Classics and Books）*.

●黄帝内经太素［huáng dì nèi jīng tài sù］ 书名。简称《太素》，隋唐间杨上善编注。原为三十卷，现已残缺，仅存二十三卷。是注释《内经》的早期传本，本书不仅保存了《内经》的一部分旧貌，且在校释文字、引证文献上，都有一定参考价值。

Huangdi Neijing Taisu（Comprehensive Notes to the Yellow Emperor's Inner Canon Title of a book, called *Taisu（Comprehensive Notes）* for short. It was compiled and annotated by Yang Shangshan in the Sui and Tang Dynasties. Of all the original 30 volumes, only 23 now exist. It is an earlier annotated version of *Neijing（The Inner Canon of Huangdi）*, which not only reserves some original appearances of *Neijing（Canon of Internal Medicine）*, but also has some reference value in the check and interpretation of wording and citation of documents.

●黄帝岐伯论针灸要诀［huáng dì qí bó lùn zhēn jiǔ yào jué］ 书名。又作《岐伯论针灸要诀》，撰人不详。书佚。见宋《崇文总目》。

Huangdi Qibo Lun Zhenjiu Yaojue（Essentials of Acupuncture and Moxibustion Expounded in Verse by the Yellow Emperor and Qi Bo） Title of a book, also entitled *Qi Bo Lun Zhenjiu Yaojue（Essentials of Acupuncture and Moxibustion Expounded in Verse by Qi Bo）*, author unknown; lost, Cf. *Chongwen Zongmu（Chong Wen Complete Catalogue）* of the Song Dynasty.

●黄帝十二经脉明堂五藏人图［huáng dì shí èr jīng mài míng táng wǔ zàng rén tú］ 书名。又名《黄帝十二经脉明堂五藏图》，撰人不详。书佚。见《隋书·经籍志》。

Huangdi Shier Jingmai Mingtang Wu Zang Rentu（The Yellow Emperor's Chart of Twelve Meridians, Acupoints and Five Zang-Organs as Shown on Human Figure） Title of a book, also entitled *Huangdi Shier Jingmai Mingtang Wu Zang Tu（The Yellow Emperor's Chart of Twelve Meridians, Acupoints and Five Zang-Organs）*, author unknown, lost. Seen in *Sui Shu: Jing Ji Zhi（Book of the Sui Dynasty: Records of Classics and Books）*.

●黄帝针灸虾蟆忌［huáng dì zhēn jiǔ há má jì］ 书名。又名《黄帝虾蟆经》、《明堂虾蟆图》。一卷，汉时作品，撰人不详，为现存较早的针灸文献。全书以插图为主，主要讨论按月的盈亏定刺灸禁忌的部位。见《隋书·经籍志》。

Huangdi Zhenjiu Hama Ji（Frog Contraindications of the Yellow Emperor's Acupuncture and Moxibustion） Title of a book, also entitled *Huangdi Hama Jing（The Yellow*

Emperor's Frog Classic) and *Mingtang Hama Tu* (*Charts of Frog with Acupoints*), a single-volume work of the Han Dynasty, author unknown. It is an earlier existing version of the acupuncture and moxibustion literature. The book, most of which is illustrations, mainly discusses the improper acupoints in acupuncture and moxibustion according to the phases of the moon. Seen in *Sui Shu: Jing Ji Zhi* (*Book of the Sui Dynasty: Records of Classics and Books*).

●黄蜡灸 [huáng là jiǔ] 灸法的一种。出《肘后备急方》卷七。其方法是先以面粉调和，用湿面团沿着疮疡肿根围成一圈，高出皮肤3厘米左右，圈外围布数层，防止烘肤，圈内放入上等蜡片约1厘米厚，随后以铜勺（或铁勺）盛灰火在蜡上烘烤，使黄蜡熔化，皮肤有热痛感即可。若疮疡毒较深，可随灸随添黄蜡，以添到周围满为度。若灸时蜡液沸动，病人施灸处先有痒感，随后痛不可忍，立即停止治疗。灸完洒冷水少许于蜡上，冷却后揭去围布，面团及黄蜡。此法与近代蜡疗相似。适用于风寒湿痹、无名肿毒、痈疖、臁疮等。

Yellow Wax Moxibustion A moxibustion technique, from Vol. 7 of *Zhouhou Beiji Fang* (*A Handbook of Prescriptions for Emergencies*), (also termed scalding with melted wax). ⟨Method⟩ Mix wheat flour and water, enclose the skin and external diseases and pyogenic infections with the dough about 3 cm high, then put several layers of cloth around the wet flour to prevent the skin from being burnt. Put first-class wax flakes of about 1 cm thick within the circle. Lay a copper or iron spoon of charcoal fire on the wax until the wax melts and a local scorching pain is felt. If the sore is severe, more yellow wax can be added until the enclosure is full. If the wax boils and the patient feels itching on the skin where the moxibustion is applied, and then has an unbearable pain, stop the treatment immediately. After treatment, pour cold water on the wax to cool it, then remove the cloth, the dough and the yellow wax. This method is similar to the kerotherapy used in modern times. ⟨Indications⟩ arthralgia-syndrome due to wind-cold-dampness, innominate inflammatory swelling, carbuncle and furuncle, and ecthyma, etc.

●黄石屏 [huáng shí píng] 人名。清末针灸家，名灿，清江（今属江西）人。精于针术。

Huang Shiping An acupuncture-moxibustion expert in the late Qing Dynasty, also named Huang Can, from Qingjiang (Now of Jiangxi Province), proficient in acupuncture.

●黄土饼灸 [huáng tǔ bǐng jiǔ] 隔饼灸的一种。见《千金要方》。指以净土水和为泥，捻作饼子，以粗艾大作炷灸泥土，一炷易一饼子。《东医宝鉴》称之为黄土饼灸。

Loess-Cake-Separated Moxibustion A kind of cake-separated moxibustion, from *Qianjin Yaofang* (*Prescriptions Worth a Thousand Gold*), referring to moxibustion which uses coarse moxa-cones and mud-cakes made of clean earth and water, one cake for each moxa-cone. It was named loess-cake-separated moxibustion in *Dongyi Baojian* (*Treasured Mirror of Oriental Medicine*).

●黄士真 [huáng shì zhēn] 人名。元代针灸家，号峨眉山人。撰《琼瑶真人八法神针》。参见该条。

Huang Shizhen An acupuncture-moxibustion expert in the Yuan Dynasty, who assumed the name Man in the Emei Mountains. He wrote *Qiongyaozhenren Ba Fa Shenzhen* (*Eight Methods of Miraculous Needling of the Pretty Jade Taoist*). →琼瑶真人八法神针 (p. 322)

●黄液上冲 [huáng yè shàng chōng] 目翳的别名。详见该条。

Hypopyon Another name for blurred vision →目翳(p. 273)

●黄中子 [huáng zhōng zǐ] 人名。元代艾师。见《铁崖先生古乐府》卷六。

Huang Zhongzi A moxibustion physician in the Yuan Dynasty. Seen in Vol. 6 of *Tieya Xiansheng Guyuefu* (*Mr. Tieya's Ancient Musical Poems*).

●癀走 [huáng zǒu] 即疔疮走黄。详见该条。

Spread of Furuncle →疔疮走黄(p. 83)

●恢刺 [huī cì] 刺法名。见《灵枢·官针》。是十二刺之一。恢，是宽廓、扩大的意思。对筋肉拘急等病证，

刺其附近,采用或前或后斜刺和提举针体等方法,以疏通经气。这是一针多用的刺法,类似近代临床上应用的多向透刺法。

Lateral Puncture　An acupuncture method, from *Lingshu: Guanzhen* (*Miraculous Pivot: Official Needles*), one of the Twelve Needlings. Using oblique insertions and lifting the needle in order to dredge the meridians and activate the circulation of qi for the treatment of muscle spasm. It is similar to the penetration needling in many directions used in contemporaty times.

●回发五处[huí fā wǔ chù]　经外穴名。见《千金要方》。在头顶旋毛正中及其前、后、左、右共五处。先用绳量患者两口角间长度,再量两鼻孔外缘间长度,以其全长的中点置于头顶旋毛正中,前后与头正中线合,两端是穴;再以此绳与正中线成十字交叉,左右两端也是穴。灸治头风眩晕。

Huifawuchu(EX-HN)　A set of five extra points, from *Qianjin Yaofang* (*Prescriptions Worth a Thousand Gold*). 〈Location〉 of the five points, one is in the centre of the eddy of hair, and the other four respectively on its front, back, left and right sides. First, measure the distances between the angles of the mouth and the lateral borders of the two nostrils with a rope. With the midpoint of the total length of the two distances overlap midpoint eddy of hair, and the same length of rope overlapping the median cephalic line, the two ends of the rope will be on the points; put the rope across the median cephalic line vertically and the two ends will be on another two points. 〈Indications〉 severe headache and dizziness. 〈Method〉moxibustion.

●回骨[huí gǔ]　经穴别名。见《铜人腧穴针灸图经》。即曲骨。见该条1。

Huigu　Another name for Qugu(RN 2), a meridian point from *Tongren Shuxue Zhenjiu Tujing* (*Illustrated Manual of Points for Acupuncture and Moxibustion on a Bronze Statue with Acupoints*). →曲骨1. (p.326)

●回气[huí qì]　经外穴名。出《千金要方》。又名*迴气。在骶骨尖端。灸治痔疮、便血、大便不禁等。

Huiqi(回气)(EX-B)　An extra point, from *Qianjin Yaofang* (*Essential Prescriptions Worth a Thousand Gold*), also named Huiqi (迴气). 〈Location〉 on the sacral apex. 〈Indications〉 hemorrhoid, hemafecia, and fecal incontinence, etc. 〈Method〉moxibustion.

●回旋灸[huí xuán jiǔ]　艾条灸的一种。将燃着的艾条空悬于穴位部,作往复回旋的移动,给以较大范围的温热刺激。

Revolving Moxibustion　A kind of moxa-stick moxibustion done by swinging the lighted end of a moxa stick while hanging it over the selected acupoint in order to give a warm-heat stimulation to a wider area.

●迴气[huí qì]　经外穴别名。出《千金翼方》。即回气。见该条。

Huiqi　Another name for Huiqi(回气)(EX-B), an extra point from *Qianjin Yifang* (*A Supplement to the Essential Prescriptions Worth a Thousand Gold*)→回气(p.177)

●蚘厥[huí jué]　古病名。出《伤寒论·辨厥阴病脉证并治》。指因蛔虫而引起的发作性腹痛,烦躁,手足厥冷等病证。详见"胆道蛔虫病"条。

Colic Caused by Ascariasis　Ancient name of a disease, from *Shanghan Lun: Bian Jueyin Bing Mai Zheng Bing Zhi* (*Treatise on Cold-Induced Diseases: Pulse Conditions, Differentiation of Syndromes, and Treatments of Jueyin Diseases*). Referring to paroxysmal abdominal pain, fidgetiness, and cold limbs, etc , caused by ascarides. →胆道蛔虫病(p.73)

●会[huì]　腧穴别名。见该条。

Gathering Sites　An earlier name for acupoints. →腧穴 **Acupoints**(p.406)

●会额[huì é]　经穴别名。出《针灸甲乙经》。即脑户。见该条。

Huie　An other name for Naohu(DU 17), a meridian point from *Zhenjiu Jia-Yi Jing* (*A-B Classic of Acupuncture and Moxibustion*). →脑户(p.276)

●会维[huì wéi]　经穴别名。出《针灸甲乙经》。即地仓。见该条。

Huiwei　Another name for Dicang(ST 4), a meridian point from *Zhenjiu Jia-Yi Jing* (*A-B Classic of Acupuncture and Moxibustion*). →地仓(p.78)

●会阳[huì yáng]　经穴名。出《针灸甲乙经》。属足太阳膀胱经。又名利机。〈定位〉在骶部,尾骨端旁开0.5寸(图7)。〈层次解剖〉皮肤→皮下组织→臀大肌→提肛肌腱。浅层布有臀中皮神经。深层有臀下动、静脉的分支或属支和臀下神经。〈主治〉带下、阳萎、痢疾、泄泻、便血、痔疾。直刺0.8～1寸;可灸。

Huiyang (BL 35)　A meridian point, from *Zhenjiu Jia-Yi Jing* (*A-B Classic of Acupuncture and Moxibustion*), a point on the Bladder Meridian of Foot-Taiyang, also called Liji. 〈Location〉 on the sacrum, 0.5 cun lateral to the tip of the coccyx (Fig. 7). 〈Regional anatomy〉 skin→subcutaneous tissue→greatest gluteal muscle→tendon of levator ani muscle. In the superficial layer, there is the middle clunial nerve. In the deep layer, there are the branches or tributaries of the inferior gluteal artery and vein and the inferior gluteal nerve. 〈Indications〉 leukorrhea, impotence, dysentery, hemafecia, and hemorrhoid. 〈Method〉 Puncture perpendicularly 0.8～1 cun. Moxibustion is applicable.

●会阴[huì yīn]　①经穴名。出《针灸甲乙经》。属任脉,为任、督、冲三脉之会。又名屏翳、平翳、下极、下极之俞、海底、鬼藏。〈定位〉在会阴部,男性当阴囊根部与肛门连线的中点。女性当大阴唇后联合与肛门连线的中点(图4)。〈层次解剖〉皮肤→皮下组织→会阴中心腱。浅层布有股后皮神经会阴支,阴部神经的会阴神经分支。深层有阴部神经的分支和阴部内动、静脉的分支或属支。〈主治〉溺水窒息、昏迷、癫狂、惊痫、小便难、遗尿、阴痛、阴痒、阴部汗湿、脱肛、阴挺、疝气、痔疾、遗精、月经不调。直刺0.5～1寸,孕妇慎用;可灸。②部位名。

〈1〉**Huiyin** (RN 1)　A meridian point, from *Zhenjiu Jia-Yi Jing* (*A-B Classic of Acupuncture and Moxibustion*), a point on the Ren Meridian, the crossing point of the Ren, Du and Chong Meridians, also called Pingyi (屏翳), Pingyi (平翳), Xiaji, Xiajizhishu, Haidi and Guizang. 〈Location〉 on the perineum, at the midpoint between the posterior border of the scrotum and anus in men and between the posterior commissure of the large labia and anus in women (Fig. 4). 〈Regional anatomy〉 skin→subcutaneous tissue→central tendon of perineum. In the superficial layer, there are perineal branches of the posterior femoral cutaneous nerve and the perineal nervous branches of the pudendal nerve. In the deep layer, there are the branches of the pudendal nerve and the branches or tributaries of the internal pudendal artery and vein. 〈Indications〉 drowning asphyxia, coma, manic-depressive psychosis, epilepsy induced by terror, dyuria, enuresis, perineal pain, pruritus genitalium, wet in pudendal region, proctoptosis, prolapse of uterus, hernia, hemorrhoid, seminal emission, and irregular menstruation. 〈Method〉 Puncture perpendicularly 0.5～1 cun, careful application in pregnant women. Moxibustion is applicable.

〈2〉**Perineum**　A part of the body.

●会阴之脉[huì yīn zhī mài]　经脉名。出《素问·刺腰痛篇》。指足太阳经从腰中通过骶部的一支。

Perineum Meridian　A meridian, from *Suwen: Ci Yaotong Pian* (*Plain Questions: On Treatment of Lumbago with Acupuncture*). Referring to a branch of the Foot-Taiyang Meridian which passes through the loin and sacral region.

●会原[huì yuán]　经穴别名。出《针灸甲乙经》。即冲阳。见该条。

Huiyuan　Another name for Chongyang (ST 42), a meridian point from *Zhenjiu Jia-Yi Jing* (*A-B Classic of Acupuncture and Moxibustion*). →冲阳 (p.49)

●会宗[huì zōng]　经穴名。出《针灸甲乙经》。属手少阳三焦经,为本经郄穴。〈定位〉在前臂背侧,当腕背横纹上3寸,支沟尺侧,尺骨的桡侧缘(图48和图44)。〈层次解剖〉皮肤→皮下组织→尺侧腕伸肌→示指伸肌→前臂骨间膜。浅层有前臂后皮神经,贵要静脉的属支等结构。深层有前臂骨间后动、静脉的分支或属支,前臂骨间后神经的分支。〈主治〉耳聋、痫证、上肢肌肤痛。直刺0.5～1寸;可灸。

Huizong (SJ 7)　A meridian point, from *Zhenjiu Jia-Yi Jing* (*A-B Classic of Acupuncture and Moxibustion*), the Xi (Cleft) point of the Sanjiao Meridian of Hand-Shaoyang. 〈Location〉 on the dorsal side of the forearm, 3 cun proximal to the dorsal crease of

the wrist, on the ulnar side of Zhigou(SJ 6) and on the radial border of the ulna (Figs. 48&44). ⟨Regional anatomy⟩ skin→subcutaneous tissue→ulnar extensor muscle of wrist → extensor of index finger → interosseous membrane of forearm. In the superficial layer, there are the posterior cutaneous nerve of the forearm and the tributaries of the basilic vein. In the deep layer, there are the branches or the tributaries of the posterior interosseous artery and vein of the forearm and the branches of the posterior interossous nerve of the forearm. ⟨Indications⟩ deafness, epilepsy, and pain of the upper extremities. ⟨Method⟩ Puncture perpendicularly 0.5～1 cun. Moxibustion is applicable.

●绘图经络图说[huì tú jīng luò tú shuō] 图书名。明代张明绘著,全本一折册,刊于1630年。内有彩色经络图十四幅,脏腑图一幅。每图对经络、俞穴均有说明,后附骨度法和脏腑总论。

Huitu Jingluo Tushuo(Illustrated Manual of Meridians and Collaterals) Title of an illustrated book, drawn and written by Zhang Ming in the Ming Dynasty, a folding edition, published in 1630. There are 14 color drawings of meridians and collaterals, and 1 drawing of the zang-fu organs. There are captions about meridians, collaterals, acupoints for each drawing; a bone-length measurement, and a general introduction to the zang-fu organs is appendixed to the book.

●魂户[hún hù] 经穴别名。见《太平圣惠方》。即魄户。见该条。

Hunhu Another name for Pohu(BL 42), a meridian point, from *Taiping Shenghui Fang (Imperial Benevolent Prescriptions)*. →魄户(p.298)

●魂门[hún mén] 经穴名。出《针灸甲乙经》。属足太阳膀胱经。⟨定位⟩在背部,当第九胸椎棘突下,旁开3寸(图7)。⟨层次解剖⟩皮肤→皮下组织→背阔肌→下后锯肌→竖脊肌。浅层布有第九、十胸神经后支的外侧皮支和伴行的动、静脉。深层有第九、十胸神经后支的肌支和相应肋间后动、静脉背侧支的分支和属支。⟨主治⟩胸胁胀满、背痛、饮食不下、呕吐、肠鸣泄泻。斜刺0.5～0.8寸;可灸。

Hunmen(BL 47) A meridian point, from *Zhenjiu Jia-Yi Jing(A-B Classic of Acupuncture and Moxibustion)*, a point on the Bladder Meridian of Foot-Taiyang. ⟨Location⟩ on the back, below the spinous process of the 9th thoracic vertebra, 3 cun lateral to the posterior midline (Fig. 7). ⟨Regional anatomy⟩ skin→ subcutaneous tissue → latissimus muscle of back → in ferior posterior serratus muscle → erector spinal muscle. In the superficial layer, there are the lateral cutaneous branches of the posterior branches of the 9th and 10th thoracic nerves and the accompanying arteries and veins. In the deep layer, there are the muscular branches of the posterior branches of the 9th and 10th thoracic nerves and the branches or tributaries of the dorsal branches of the related posterior intercostal arteries and veins. ⟨Indications⟩ fullness in the chest and hypochondrium, backache, anorexia, vomiting, borborygmus and diarrhea. ⟨Method⟩ Puncture obliquely 0.5～0.8 cun. Moxibustion is applicable.

●魂舍[hún shè] 经外穴名。出《千金要方》。在腹部,当脐中旁开1寸处。主治泄痢脓血、肠炎、消化不良、习惯性便秘等。直刺0.5～1寸;可灸。

Hunshe (EX-CA) An extra point, from *Qianjin Yaofang (Essential Prescriptions Worth a Thousand Gold)*. ⟨Location⟩ on the abdomen, 1 cun lateral to the centre of the umbilicus. ⟨Indications⟩ dysentery with blood and pus in the stool, enteritis, dyspepsia, and habitual constipation, etc. ⟨Method⟩ Puncture perpendicularly 0.5～1 cun. Moxibustion is applicable.

●混合痔[hùn hé zhì] 即内外痔。见该条。
Mixed Hemorrhoid→内外痔(p.280)

●混睛障[hùn jīng zhàng] 目翳的别名。见该条。
Interstitial keratitis Another name for blurred vision. →目翳(p.273)

●活动标志[huó dòng biāo zhì] 体表解剖标志的一种。指各部的关节、肌肉、肌腱,皮肤随着活动而出现的空隙、凹陷、皱纹、尖端等。利用这些标志,可以确定部分腧穴的位置。

Moving Landmarks One of the anatomic

marks of body surface, referring to lacunas, pittings, wrinkles and prominences, etc, appearing at the joints, muscles, tendons and skin. With these landmarks, the location of some acupoints can be determined.

●活人妙法针经[huó rén miào fǎ zhēn jīng] 书名。明代徐廷璋撰，二卷。已佚。参见"徐廷璋"条。

Huoren Miaofa Zhenjing (Acupuncture Canon of Magical Methods for Saving Life)   A book, written by Xu Tingzhang in the Ming Dynasty, 2 volumes, no longer extant. →徐廷璋(p.517)

●火柴头灸[huǒ chái tóu jiǔ] 灸法的一种。是将火柴擦燃后，快速按在穴位上进行焠烫的一种灸法。适用于治疗流行性腮腺炎等。

Match-Head Moxibustion   A moxibustion technique of cauterizing the selected point rapidly with a burning match. Used to treat mumps, etc.

●火带疮[huǒ dài chuāng] 即缠腰火丹。见该条。

Burning Sores Along Belt →缠腰火丹(p.31)

●火丹[huǒ dān] 即丹毒。见该条。

Fire-Erysiplelas   →丹毒(p.71)

●火罐法[huǒ guàn fǎ] 拔罐法的一种。又称火罐气。利用点火燃烧法排除罐内空气，形成负压，将罐吸附在体表上。常用的有投火法和闪火法两种。前者用木纸片点燃后投入罐内，随即覆盖吸附处；后者用镊子夹住沾有95%酒精的棉球，点燃后伸入罐内瞬即退出，速将罐口覆罩在选定部位上。参见"拔罐法"条。

Fire Cupping   One of the cupping methods, also called cupping with heated air. That is, to burn fire in the cup, driving away the air to create a negative pressure inside, thus producing suction of the cup to the skin. There are two types of fire cupping in common use: the fire-throwing cupping and the fire-twinkling cupping. The first method is carried out by putting a burning piece of wood or paper into the cup and applying it to the proper area at once; the latter one is done by clamping a cotton ball soaked in 95% alcohol with forceps, igniting the cotton ball, putting it into the cup and quickly turning it around inside the cup. Then immediately take the cotton out and place the cup on the selected positions. →拔罐法(p.9)

●火罐气[huǒ guàn qì] 拔罐法的一种。为火罐法之别称。见该条。

Cups with Heated Air   One of the cupping methods, another name for fire cupping. →火罐法(p.180)

●火逆[huǒ nì] 灸法术语。出《伤寒论》。指误用灸法治疗而引起的变证。

Deterioration due to Fire   Moxibustion term from *Shanghan Lun* (*Treatise on Febrile Diseases*), referring to the deterioration of a case due to misuse of moxibustion.

●火眼[huǒ yǎn] 即目赤肿痛。详见该条。

Fiery Eye   Another name for the disease with redness, swelling and pains of the eye. →目赤肿痛(p.271)

●火针[huǒ zhēn] 针具名。又称燔针、烧针。一般用较粗的不锈钢针，如圆利针或24号粗、2寸长的不锈钢针。也有特别的火针，如弹簧式火针、三头火针以及用钨合金所制的火针等。弹簧式火针，进针迅速并易于掌握针刺深度。三头火针，常用于对体表痣、疣的治疗。

Fire Needle   A needling instrument, also called red-hot needle or heated needle. Usually a thicker needle made of stainless steel, e.g. round-sharp needle or a stainless-steel needle No. 24 in thickness and 2 cun in length is used. There are also special fire needles such as spring fire needles, three-head fire needles and fire needles made of tungsten alloy. A spring fire needle can make the needle insertion quick and the depth of puncture easy to control. A three-head fire needle is often used to treat nevus and verruca on body surface.

●火针疗法[huǒ zhēn liáo fǎ] 针刺方法名。是指用火烧红的针尖迅速刺入穴内，以治疗疾病的一种方法。具有温经散寒，通经活络的作用。主要用于治疗痈肿脓疡未溃、瘰疬、疣、痣、息肉等病症。

Fire Needling   An acupuncture method, also called red-hot needling, pyro-puncture, or heated needling. That is, to puncture a point quickly with a red-hot needle to treat diseases. It has the functions of warming the meridians and dispelling cold, clearing

and activating meridians and collaterals. 〈Indicatons〉carbuncle and furuncle with pus-pocket which doesn't ulcerate, scrofula, nevus verruca, polyp, etc.

●火珠疔[huǒ zhū dīng] 即鼻疔中红者。见该条。

Fire Bead-like Furuncle Red colored furuncle inside the nose. →鼻疔(p. 18)

●或中[huò zhōng] 经穴别名。见《千金要方》。即彧中。见该条。

Huozhong Another name for Yuzhong (KI 26), a meridian point from *Qianjin Yaofang* (*Essential Prescriptions Worth a Thousand Gold*). →彧中(p. 575)

●霍乱[huò luàn] 病证名。出《素问·王乱》等篇。是以起病急骤，卒然发作，上吐下泻，腹痛或不痛为特征的疾病。因饮食生冷不洁，或感受寒邪，暑湿，疫疠之气所致。临床有寒霍乱和热霍乱之辨。详见各条。

Cholera Morbus A disease, from *Suwen*: *Wangluan* (*Plain Questions*), and other chapters. Refers to a group of diseases characterized by sudden and drastic vomiting and diarrhea and abdominal pain in some cases, caused by uncooked, cold and dirty food, affection of cold, summer-heat, dampness and extremely infectious noxious epidemic factors. It is clinically divided into two types: cold and heat. →寒霍乱(p. 155)、热霍乱(p. 330)

J

●机关[jī guān] 经穴别名。见《针灸聚英》。即颊车。见该条1。

Jiguan Another name for Jiache (ST 6), a meridian point, from *Zhenjiu Juying* (*Essentials of Acupuncture and Moxibustion*). →颊车1(p. 187)

●鸡冠疮[jī guān chuāng] 阴挺的别名。见该条，参见子宫脱垂条。

Cockscomb Sore Another name for prolapse of uterus and vagina. →阴挺(p. 559)、子宫脱垂(p. 625)

●鸡咳[jī ké] 即顿咳。详见该条。

Chicken Cough →顿咳(p. 90)

●鸡子灸[jī zǐ jiǔ] 间接灸法的一种。见《寿世保元》卷十。是用鸡子作间隔物而施灸的一种方法。即将鸡子一个，煮熟，对半切开，取半个(去蛋黄)盖于患处，于蛋壳上置炷灸之。以病人感觉局部热痒为度。适于发背、痈疽初起诸症。

Egg Moxibustion A type of indirect moxibustions, from Vol. 10 of *Shoushi Baoyuan* (*Longevity and Life Preservation*), referring to using an egg as the separation for moxibustion. Cut a boiled egg in half, cover the affected area with one half (without the yolk) of the egg, and apply moxibustion with a moxa cone on the eggshell until the patient gets the sensation of heat and itching. 〈Indications〉lumbodorsal cellulitis, carbuncle and cellulitis at early stage, etc.

●鸡足针法[jī zú zhēn fǎ] 刺法名。①《灵枢·卫气失常》谓"鸡足取之"。指上取人迎、天突、喉中，下取三里、气冲，中取章门。上中下三取之，若鸡足之分三岐。②《灵枢·官针》谓"左右鸡足"。指针斜刺进针后，退回浅部又分别向两旁斜刺，如鸡爪分叉的一种刺法。参见"合谷刺"条。

Chicken Claw Acupuncture A technique used in acupuncture. ① *Lingshu*: *Weiqi Shichang* (*Miraculous Pivot*: *Abnormalities of Defensive Qi*) says: Select points like the branching of a chicken claw. In other words, puncture Renying (ST 9), Tiantu (KI 27) and Houzhong (EX-HN) for the upper portion of the body, Zusanli (ST 36), Qichong (ST 30) for the lower portion, Zhangmen (LR 13) for the middle portion. The points of these three portions are just like the three branches of a chicken claw. ② *Lingshu*: *Guanzhen* (*Miracu-

181

lous Pivot:Official Needles)records: Left and right insertions are like chicken claw, that is after an oblique insertion, lift the needle to the shallow part, and insert the needle to both sides obliquely, like the claws of a chicken. → 合谷刺(p. 161)

●积聚痞块穴[jī jù pǐ kuài xué] 经外穴名。见《类经图翼》。在腰部,当第2腰椎棘突下旁开4寸处。〈主治〉积聚痞块、胃痛、肠鸣、消化不良、经闭、遗精等。直刺0.5～1寸;可灸。

Jijupikuaixue（EX-B） An extra point, from Leijng Tuyi (Supplements to Illustrated Classified Canon of Internal Medicine of the Yellow Emperor).〈Location〉on the lower back, below the spinous process of the 1st lumbar vertebra, 4 cun lateral to the posterior midline. 〈Indications〉 abdominal masses, etc.〈Method〉Puncture perpendicularly 0.5～1 cun. Moxibustion is applicable.

●积吐[jī tǔ] 病证名。见《证治准绳·幼科》。是指食积不消而引起的呕吐。症见小儿呕吐不消化食物,或吐黄酸水,面微黄,脉沉滑。治宜消积导滞,调理脾胃。取中脘、脾俞、胃俞、足三里、建里、四缝。

Vomiting due to Retained Food A disease, from Zhengzhi Zhunsheng:Youke (Standards for Diagnosis and Treatment: Pediatrics). Refers to vomiting caused by retention of food in the stomach, characterized by infantile vomiting with undigested food or yellow and sour water, sallow complexion, deep and slippery pulse. 〈Treatment principle〉Promote digestion and remove stagnancy, and regulate the function of the spleen and stomach.〈Point selection〉 Zhongwan (RN 12), Pishu (BL 20), Weishu (BL 21), Zusanli (ST 36), Jianli (RN 11) Sifeng(EX-UE 10).

●基本手法[jī běn shǒu fǎ] 针刺手法分类名。与辅助手法、综合手法相对而言,系指针刺手法中一些主要的、单一的方法,包括提插法、捻转法。详见各条。

The Fundamental Manipulation A term used to describe the basic needling techniques, which are more basic and simple than the auxiliary and comprehensive manipulations of acupuncture. The fundamental manipulation techniques include lifting-thrusting technique and twirling technique. →辅助手法(p. 120)、综合手法(p. 628)、提插法(p. 428)、捻转法(p. 283)

●箕门[jī mén] 经穴名。出《针灸甲乙经》。属足太阴脾经。〈定位〉在大腿内侧,当血海与冲门连线上,血海上6寸(图81)。〈层次解剖〉皮肤→皮下组织→股内侧肌。浅层布有股神经前皮支,大隐静脉的属支。深层有股动、静脉,隐神经和股神经股支。〈主治〉小便不利、遗尿、鼠蹊肿痛、阴囊湿疹。避开动脉,直刺0.5～1寸;可灸。

Jimen(SP 11) A meridian point from Zhenjiu Jia-Yi Jing (A-B Classic of Acupuncture and Moxibustion), a point on the Spleen Meridian of Foot-Taiyang. 〈Location〉 on the medial side of the thigh and on the line connecting Xuehai (SP 10) and Chongmen (SP 12), 6 cun above Xuehai (SP 10) (Fig. 81). (Lower Limbs). 〈Regional anatomy〉skin→subcutaneous tissue→medial vastus muscle of thigh. In the subcutaneous layer, there are the anterior cutaneous branches of the femoral nerve and the tributaries of the great saphenous vein. In the deep layer, there are the femoral artery and vein, the saphenous nerve and the muscular branches of the femoral nerve.〈Indications〉 dysuria, enuresis, swelling and pain in the groin, eczema of scrotum. 〈Method〉 Avoid the artery. Puncture perpendicularly 0.5～1 cun. Moxibustion is applicable.

●箕坐位[jī zuò wèi] 针灸体位名。适用于针灸下肢内、外侧的穴位。

Sitting Position Like a Winnowing Pan Posture for acupuncture and moxibustion, used when the points on the medial or lateral side of the lower limbs are chosen for acupuncture and moxibustion.

●激光穴位照射法[jī guāng xué wèi zhào shè fǎ] 又称激光针、光针。为利用激光器所发生的受激辐射光照射穴位以治病的方法。激光的特点是:发散角小,方向性强,能量密度高,强度大,能穿透皮肤而作用于深部。小剂量激光能产生光、热、机械、电磁等效应。常用的激光有氦—氖激光、氢离子激光、氦—镉激光等。

Laser Irradiation of Acupoints Also named laser acupuncture, or light-beam acupuncture.

A therapy carried out by illuminating the acupoints with stimulated radiation from a laser, characterized by a small diverging angle, definite direction, high energy density, high intensity, ability to pass through the skin so as to act on deep areas. A small amount of laser can produce light, heat, mechanic and electromagnetic effects. Helium-neon laser, hydrogenion laser, helium-acadmium laser, etc., are frequently used.

●激光针[jī guāng zhēn] 激光穴位照射法之别称。见该条。

Laser Acupuncture Another name for laser Irradiation of Acupoints. →激光穴位照射法(p. 182)

●极泉[jí quán] 经穴名。出《针灸甲乙经》。属手少阴心经。〈定位〉在腋窝顶点,腋动脉搏动处(图23)。〈层次解剖〉皮肤→皮下组织→臂丛、腋动脉、腋静脉→背阔肌腱→大圆肌。浅层有肋间臂神经分布。深层有桡神经、尺神经、正中神经、前臂内侧皮神经、臂内侧皮神经、腋动脉、腋静脉等结构。〈主治〉心痛、胸闷、心悸、气短、心悲不舒、干呕、胁肋疼痛、咽干烦渴、目黄、瘰疬、肘臂冷痛、四肢不举。避开动脉,直刺0.2～0.5寸;可灸。

Jiquan (HT 1) A meridian point, from *Zhenjiu Jia-Yi Jing* (*A-B Classic of Acupuncture and Moxibustion*), a point on the Heart Meridian of Hand-Shaoyin. 〈Location〉 at the apex of the axillary fossa, where the pulsation of the axillary artery is palpable. (Fig. 23). 〈Regional anatomy〉 skin → subcutaneous tissue → brachial plexus and axillary artery and vein → tendon of latissimus muscle of back → teres major muscle. In the superficial layer, there is the intercostobrachial nerve. In the deep layer, there are the radial nerve, the ulnar nerve, the median nerve, the medial cutaneous nerve of forearm, the medial cutaneous nerve of the arm and the axillary artery and vein. 〈Indications〉 cardialgia, oppressive feeling in chest, palpitations, shortness of breath, depression and grief, retching, pain in costal and hypochondriac regions, dry throat, excessive thirst, icteric sclera, scrofula, cold-pain in elbow, inability to raise the limbs. 〈Method〉 Avoid artery. Puncture perpendicularly 0.2～0.5 cun. Moxibustion is applicable.

●急惊风[jí jīng fēng] 病证名。见《小儿药证直诀》。以发病迅速,症情急暴为特点。根据病因临床分三种类型。①外感时邪型。多因小儿肌肤薄弱,腠理不密,极易感受时邪,化火生风,内陷厥阴所致。②痰火积滞型。多因乳食不节,积滞胃肠,痰浊内生,气机壅阻,郁而化热,热极生风所致。③暴受惊恐型。多因小儿神气怯弱,元气未充,如乍见异物,乍闻怪声,或不慎跌仆等,暴受惊恐,恐则气下,惊则气乱,神无所依所致。本病在发作前常有壮热面赤,烦躁不宁,摇头弄舌,咬牙龁齿,睡中易惊,或昏沉嗜睡等先兆。但为时短暂,很快即出现急惊风的症状。神志昏迷,两目上视,牙关紧闭,颈项强直,角弓反张,四肢抽搐,关纹青紫等。外感惊风者,兼见发热、头痛、咳嗽、咽红,或恶心呕吐,或口渴烦躁。治宜清热祛邪,开窍熄风。取大椎、合谷、太冲、阳陵泉、十二井穴。痰火积滞者,兼见发热、腹胀腹痛、呕吐、喉间痰鸣、便秘或大便腥臭,挟有脓血。治宜清热豁痰,开窍熄风。取水沟、颊息、中脘、丰隆、神门、太冲。暴受惊恐者,兼见身不热,四肢欠温,夜卧不宁,或昏睡不醒,醒后哭啼易惊。治宜镇惊安神。取前顶、印堂、神门、涌泉。

Acute Infantile Convulsion A disease, from *Xiaoer Yaozheng Zhijue* (*Key to Therapeutics of Children's Diseases*), characterized by sudden occurance and drastic changes. Clinically, it is divided into three types according to different causes: 1. Acute infantile convulsion due to affection by seasonal expathogenic factors, infants with thin and weak muscles and skin, loose striae of skin will be easily affected by seasonal expathogenic factors. As a result, these evils will transform to fire and produce internal wind, which means that the Jueyin Meridian has been affected. 2. Acute infantile convulsion due to stagnation and accumulation of phlegm-fire, as a result of improper feeding of the infant, retention of food in the stomach and intestines, occurrences of phlegm in the interior, qi stagnation, which will transform to heat, and when the heat becomes extremely strong, the internal wind will be stirred. 3. Acute infantile convulsion due to sudden terror and fear. Being timid and short of primordiae qi, infants may be frightened. For instance, when they see a strange object, or hear a

strange noise, or suddenly fall to the ground, fear and fright will appear in their minds. Fear makes qi descend, while fright will lead to the disorder of qi movement. In this way, the mind can not be settled in the heart. Before the onset of the disease, there are usually some premonitory symptoms as high fever, flushed face, dysphoria and restlessness, shaking the head and playing with the tongue, gnashing, easily frightened during sleep, drowness, etc.. Not long after these pre-monitory symptoms, the symptoms of convulsions will appear: unconsionsness, upward staring of eyes, trismus, stiffness, opisthotonus, tic of limbs, purple and blue color to the veins on the radial side of the index finger, etc.. If the convulsion is due to external factors, accompanying symptoms or signs will be fever, headache, cough, congestion in throat, or nausea, vomiting, thirst, dyphoria. This type of patient should be treated by clearing heat and eliminating evils, causing resuscitation and calming the endopathic wind. 〈Points used〉Dazhui (DU 14), Hegu (LI 4), Taichong (LR 3), Yanglingquan (GB 34), and the twelve Jing (well) points. Patients with phlegm-fire accompanied by fever, abdominal distention and pain, vomiting, rale in the throat, constipation or smelly stools with pus and blood should be treated by removing heat-phlegm causing resuscitation and calming the endopathic wind. 〈Points used〉Shuigou (DU 26), Luxi (SJ 19), Zhongwan (RN 12), Fenglong (ST 40), Shenmen (HT 7), and Taichong (LR 3). Patients with sudden fear and fright accompanied by other symptoms like cool body and limbs, restlessness at night, or stupor, crying and being easily frightened after waking up should be treated by relieving muscular spasm and tranquilizing the mind. 〈Points used〉Qianding (DU 21), Yintang (EX-HN 3), Shenmen (HT 7) and Yongquan (KI 1).

●急脉[jí mài] 经穴名。出《素问·气府论》。属足厥阴肝经。〈定位〉在耻骨结节的外侧,当气冲下方腹股沟股动脉搏动处,前正中线旁2.5寸(图40)。〈层次解剖〉皮肤→皮下组织→耻骨肌→闭孔外肌。浅层布有股神经前支,大隐静脉和腹股沟浅淋巴结。深层有阴部外动、静脉的分支或属支,闭孔神经前支等结构。〈主治〉疝气、阴挺、阴茎痛、少腹痛、股内侧痛。直刺0.5~1寸;可灸。

Jimai (LR 12) A meridian point from *Suwen: Qifu Lun (Plain Questions: On Houses of Qi)*, a point on the Liver Meridian of Foot-Jueyin. 〈Location〉lateral to the pubic tubercle, lateral and inferior to Qichong (ST 30), in the inguinal groove where the pulsation of the femoral artery is palpable, 2.5 cun lateral to the anterior midline (Fig. 40). 〈Regional anatomy〉 skin → subcutaneous tissue → pectineal muscle → lateral obturator muscle. In the superficial layer, there are the anterior cutaneous branches of the femoral nerve, the great saphenous vein and the superficial inguinal lymph nodes. In the deep layer, there are the external pudendal artery and vein, the branches or tributaries of the medial femoral circumflex artery and vein, and the anterior branches of the obturator nerve. 〈Indications〉hernia, prolapse of uterus, pain in penis, lower abdominal pain and pain in the medial side of thigh. 〈Method〉Puncture perpendicularly 0.5 ~1 cun. Moxibustion is applicable.

●疾而徐则虚[jí ěr xú zé xū] 针刺泻法要领。与补法"徐而疾则实"对举。语出《灵枢·九针十二原》。指迅速地进针,缓慢地出针,能使邪气虚,即为泻。后世泻法一进三退,或一进二退,即出于此。参见"徐疾补泻"条。又指泻法要迅速地出针,缓慢按住针孔。参见"开阖补泻"条。

Rapid-Yet-Slow Needling Weakens Evil-Qi An essential needling tenchnique for reducing. The opposite of "Slow-Yet-Rapid Needling Makes Body-qi Strong." From *Lingshu: Jiu Zhen Shier Yuan [Miraculous Pivot: Nine Needles and Twelve Yuan (Primary) Points]* i.e., to insert the needle rapidly and withdraw it slowly; a reducing technique for eliminating pathogenic factors, so the evils inside the body become weak. The reducing methods of acupuncture used in later times such as thrusting once and lifting three times and withdrawing after inserting are evolved from this technique. →徐疾补泻(p. 517). Referring to the reducing technique of the rapid withdrawl of the needle and slow pressing of

the needle hole. →开阖补泻(p. 230)

●集合刺[jí hé cì]　齐刺之别称。见该条。

Gathering Puncture　Another name for assembling puncture. →齐刺(p. 300)

●脊背五穴[jǐ bèi wǔ xué]　经外穴名。见《千金要方》。第2胸椎棘突高点一穴，骶骨尖端一穴，两穴连线中点处有一穴，再以此穴为顶点，以上两穴连线1/6为一边，作一等边三角形，底边呈水平，下两角顶点二穴，共五穴。〈主治〉癫疾、惊痫等。用灸法。

Jibeiwuxue（EX-B）　A set of five extra points on the back, from *Qianjin Yaofang* (*Essential Prescriptions Worth a Thousand Gold*). 〈Location〉 the first point, at the spinous process of the 2nd thoracic vertebra, the second point, at the sacral apex (lower end of sacrum), the third point, at the midpoint between the two points mentioned above, then take 1/6 of the distance from the first point to the third point as the side of an equalateral triangle, and put the top of the triangle on the third point and keep the base horizontal. There are another two points at the tops of the two bases angles. There are five points in all. 〈Indications〉 disorder of head, epilepsy induced by terror, infantile convulsion, etc.. 〈Method〉 Apply moxibustion to the five points.

●脊骨解中[jǐ gǔ jiě zhōng]　奇穴名。见《千金要方》。位于后正中线，与乳头平高之脊骨上。〈主治〉咳嗽。可灸。

Jigujiezhong（EX-B）　An extra point, seen in *Qianjin Yaofang* (*Essential Prescriptions Worth a Thousand Gold*). 〈Location〉 on the posterior midline, at the vertebra which is on the same level as nipples. 〈Indication〉 cough. 〈Method〉 Moxi-bustion is applicable.

●脊内俞[jǐ nèi shù]　经穴别名。出《太平圣惠方》。即中膂俞。见该条。

Jineishu　Another name for Zhonglushu (BL 29), a meridian point from *Taiping Shenghui Fang* (*Imperial Benevolent Prescriptions*). →中膂俞(p. 612)

●脊三穴[jǐ sān xué]　脊上三个穴的合称。见《针灸经外奇穴治疗诀》。后正中线哑门穴下1寸处一穴，陶道穴一穴，第5腰椎棘突下一穴。〈主治〉脑脊髓膜炎、腰背神经痛等。各直刺0.5～1寸；可灸。

Jisanxue（EX-B）　A general name for the three points on the spinal column, seen in *Zhenjiu Jingwai Qixue Zhiliao Jue* (*Pithy and Rhythmic Formulas of Extraordinary Points*). 〈Location〉 At the posterior midline 1 cun below Yamen (Du 15), the second is Taodao (Du 13), and the third is below the spinous process of the 5th lumbar vertebra. 〈Indications〉 Erebrospinal meningitis, lumbodorsal neuralgia, etc. 〈Method〉 Puncture perpendicularly 0.5～1 cun. Moxibustion is applicable.

●脊俞[jǐ shù]　经穴别名。出《太平圣惠方》。《针灸大全》作脊中别名。见"脊中"条

Ji shu　Another name for Jizhong (Du 6), a meridian point from *Taiping Shenghui Fang* (*Imperial Benevolent Prescriptions*) and *Zhenjiu Daquan* (*A Complete Work of Acupuncture and Moxibustion*). →脊中(p. 185)

●脊髓1[jǐ suí yī]　耳穴别名。即上耳根，见该条。

Spinal Cord 1（MA）　Another name for the ear point. Upper Root of Auricle. →上耳根(p. 351)

●脊中[jǐ zhōng]　经穴名。出《针灸甲乙经》。属督脉。又名神宗、脊俞。〈定位〉在背部，当后正中线上，第十一胸椎棘突下凹陷中(图12和图7)。〈层次解剖〉皮肤→皮下组织→棘上韧带→棘间韧带。浅层主要布有第十一胸神经后支的内侧皮支和伴行的动、静脉。深层有棘突间的椎外(后)静脉丛，第十一胸神经后支的分支和第十一肋间后动、静脉背侧支的分支或属支。〈主治〉腰脊强痛、黄疸、腹泻、痢疾、小儿疳积、痔疾、便血、癫痫。斜刺0.5～1寸。

Jizhong（DU 6）　A meridian point from *Zhenjiu Jia-Yi Jing* (*A-B Classic of Acupuncture and Moxibustion*), a point on the Du Meridian, also named Shenzong or Jishu. 〈Location〉 on the back and on the posterior midline, in the depression below the spinous process of the 11th thoracic vertebra (Figs. 12&7). 〈Regional anatomy〉 skin → subcutaneous tissue → supraspinal ligament → interspinal ligament. In the superficial layer, there are the medial cutaneous branches of the posterior branches of the 11th thoracic nerve and the accompanying artery and vein. In the deep

layer, there are the external (posterior) vertebral venous plexus between the adjacent spinous processes, the branches of the posterior branches of the 11th thoracic nerve and the branches or tributaries of the dorsal branches of the 11th. posterior intercostal artery and vein. 〈Indications〉stiffness and pain along the spinal column, jaundice, diarrhea, dysentery, malnutrition of children, hemorrhoid, hemafecia, epilepsy. 〈Method〉Puncture obliquely 0.5～1 cun.

●忌穴[jì xué] 见《千金翼方》。指某一日时不能施行针灸的穴位。古代有针灸择日、择时之说。认为某日时宜针灸，或不宜针灸，或某部忌针灸。据此提出忌穴。

Inapplicable Points Seen in *Qianjin Yifang* (*A Supplement to the Prescriptions Worth a Thousand Gold*), referring to points, to which acupuncture and moxibustion can not be applied at certain times. It was said that acupuncture and moxibustion should be applied on selected dates and at certain times, and some points should not be punctured on some days or at some time-periods. These points are accordingly termed inapplicable points.

●季胁[jì xié] ①经穴别名。出《针灸大全》。即章门。见该条。②部位名。指胁之下缘，胁下软肋的部分。

〈1〉**Jixie** Another name for Zhangmen (LR 13), a meridian point, from *Zhenjiu Daquan* (*The Complete Works on Acupuncture and Moxibustion*). →章门(p. 585)

〈2〉**Hypochondrium** The area where the floating ribs are.

●夹白[jiā bái] 经穴别名。即侠白。见该条。

Jiabai Another name for the meridian point Xiabai (LU 4). →侠白(p. 485)

●夹持进针[jiā chí jìn zhēn] 进针法之一。其法：手指消毒后，左手拇、食指夹住针身下段，露出针尖；对准穴位，右手捏持针柄，两手同时配合用力，将针快速刺到穴位。适用于长针直刺。

Pinching Needle Method A method for the insertion of needles. 〈Manipulations〉After disinfecting the fingers, hold the lower part of the needle with the thumb and index finger of the left hand, fix the needle tip correctly over the point, and hold the needle handle with the right hand, with the concerted force of the two hands, the needle is inserted quickly into the point. This technique is suitable for perpendicular insertion of long needles.

●夹持押手[jiā chí yā shǒu] 押手方式之一。指在肌肉浅薄部位进针时，左手的拇、食二指将皮肤捏起，以利进针。

Pinching Technique A technique of inserting the needle with the help of the pressing hand. That is, to hold up the skin with the left thumb and index finger to maintain the insertion of the needle at points with thin muscle.

●夹脊[jiā jǐ] 经外穴名。见《针灸集成》。又作华佗穴、华佗夹脊。〈定位〉在背腰部，当第一胸椎至第五腰椎棘突下两侧，后正中线旁0.5寸，一侧17穴，左右共34穴(图11)。〈层次解剖〉因各穴位位置不同，所涉及肌肉、血管、神经也不尽相同。一般的层次结构是：皮肤→皮下组织→浅层肌(斜方肌、背阔肌、菱形肌、上后锯肌、下后锯肌)→深层肌(竖脊肌、横突棘肌)。浅层内分别布有第一胸神经至第五腰神经后支的内侧皮支和伴行的动、静脉。深层布有第一胸神经至第五腰神经后支的肌支，肋间后动、静脉或腰动、静脉背侧支的分支或属支。〈主治〉上肢疾患，胸1至胸8夹脊穴。胸部疾患，胸6至腰5夹脊穴。腹部疾患，腰1至腰5夹脊穴。下肢疾患，亦可参照相应背俞穴应用。毫针斜刺0.3～0.5寸，或用梅花针叩刺；可灸。

Jiaji (EX-B 2) A set of extra points, seen in *Zhenjiu Jicheng* (*A Collection of Acupuncture and Moxibustion*), also named Huatuo points or *Huatuo jiaji*. 〈Location〉on the back and low back, 17 points on each side, below the spinous processes from the lst thoracic to the 5th lumbar vertebrae, 0.5 cun lateral to the posterior midline (Fig. 11). 〈Regional anatomy〉The related muscles, blood vessels and nerves are not totally alike because the location of each point is different. The layer structures are usually: skin→subcutaneous tissue→superficial muscles (trapezius muscle, latissimus muscle)→deep muscles (erector spinal muscle, transversospinal muscle). In the

superficial layer, there are the medial cutaneous branches of the posterior branches of the lst thoracic nerve to the 5th lumbar nerve and the accompanying arteries and vein. In the deep layer, there are the muscular branches of the posterior branches of the lst thoracic nerve to the 5th lumbar nerve, the branches or tributaries of the dorsal branches of the posterior intercostal arteries and veins or lumbar arteries and veins respectively. ⟨Indications⟩ the points from the first to the third thoracic vertebra: diseases related to the upper limbs; points from the 1st to the 8th thoracic vertebra: diseases related to the thoracic area; points from the 6th thoracic vertebra to the 5th lumbar vertabra: diseases related to the abdomen; points from the lst to the 5th lumbar vertebra: diseases related to the lower limbs. Or these points can be used with reference to the lower limbs. Or, these points can be used with reference to the back-shu points of the same level. ⟨Method⟩ Puncture obliquely 0.3～0.5 cun or tap with a plumb-blossom needle. Moxibustion is applicable.

●夹惊吐[jiā jīng tù] 惊吐的别名。详见该条。
Vomiting in Infancy due to Fright Another name for vomiting in infancy induced by fright. →惊吐(p. 217)

●颊[jiá] ①耳穴名。位于5、6区交界周围,参见牙条。用于治疗周围性面瘫、痤疮、三叉神经痛、扁平疣。②部位名。面两旁称颊。

1. **Cheek**(MA) An auricular point. ⟨Location⟩ round the border line of the fifth and sixth sections of the ear. →牙(p. 533) ⟨Indications⟩ peripheral facial paralysis, ache, trigeminal neuralgia, flat wart.

2. **Cheek** A body part, namely, the lateral sides of the face.

●颊车[jiá chē] ①经穴名。出《素问·气府论》、《灵枢·经脉》。属足阳明胃经。又名曲牙、齿牙、机关、鬼床。⟨定位⟩在面颊部,下颌角前上方约一横指(中指),当咀嚼时咬肌隆起,按之凹陷处(图28)。⟨层次解剖⟩皮肤→皮下组织→咬肌。布有耳大神经的分支,面神经下缘颌支的分支。⟨主治⟩口眼歪斜、颊肿、齿痛、牙关紧闭、失音、颈项强痛。直刺0.3～0.4寸,或向地仓方向斜刺0.7～0.9寸;可灸。②部位名。指下颌骨的下颌支,或指其全骨。

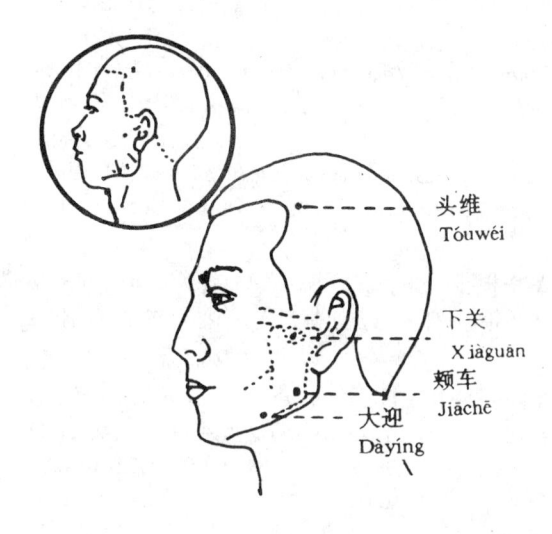

图24 颊车、下关和头维穴
Fig. 24 Jiache, Xiaguan and Touwei Points

1. **Jiache**(ST 6) A meridian point from *Suwen: Qifu Lun*(*Plain Questions: On Houses of Qi*) and *Lingshu: Jingmai*(*Miraculous Pivot: Meridians*), a point on the Stomach Meridian of Foot-Yangming, also called Quya, Chiya, Jiguan or Guichuang. ⟨Location⟩ on the cheek, one finger breadth (middle finger) anterior and superior to the mandibular angle, in the depression where the masseter muscle is prominent (Fig. 28). ⟨Regional anatomy⟩ skin → subcutaneous tissue → masseter muscle. There are the branches of the great auricular nerve and the marginal mandibular branches of the facial nerve in this area. ⟨Indications⟩ facial paralysis, swelling of cheek, toothache, trismus, aphonia, stiffness and pain of neck. ⟨Method⟩ Puncture perpendicularly 0.3～0.4 cun, or obliquely in the direction of Dicang (ST 4) 0.7～0.9 cun. Moxibustion is applicable.

2. Mandible A body part, referring to the mandible, or the alveolus of the mandible.

● 颊里[jiá lǐ] 经外穴名。出《千金要方》。在口腔内，颊粘膜上，当口解平开1寸处。〈主治〉黄疸、瘟疫、口疮、齿龈溃烂等。斜刺0.1～0.2寸。或点刺出血。

Jiali(EX-HN) An extra point, from *Qianjin Yaofang* (*Essential Prescriptions Worth a Thousand Gold*). 〈Location〉in the mouth, on the buccal mucosa, 1 cun alteral to the mouth angle. 〈Indications〉jaundice, pestilence, aphthae in children, ulceration of gums. 〈Method〉Puncture obliquely 0.1～0.2 cun, or prick to cause bleeding.

● 甲根[jiǎ gēn] 经外穴名。见《针灸集成》。在足蹰指爪甲内、外根角处两侧四穴。〈主治〉疝气。直刺0.1寸。

Jiagen(EX-LE) A set of four extra points, seen in *Zhenjiu Jicheng* (*A Collection of Acupuncture and Moxibustion*). 〈Location〉four points on the medial and lateral corners of each big toe. 〈Indication〉hernia. 〈Method〉Puncture perpendicularly 0.1 cun.

● 胛缝[jiǎ fèng] 经外穴名。见《医学纲目》。在背部，当肩胛骨内缘上下尽处，左右共四穴。〈主治〉肩胛神经痛、肩胛风湿痛。向外沿皮刺1寸；可灸。

Jiafeng(EX-B) A set of four extra points, seen in *Yixue Gangmu* (*An Outline of Medicine*). 〈Location〉on the back, at the superior and inferior ends of the medial border of the scapula, 4 points, altogether, 2 on each side. 〈Indications〉scapularneuralgia and rheumatilgia. 〈Method〉Puncture obliquely toward the lateral side 1 cun. Moxibustion is applicable.

● 间谷[jiān gǔ] 经穴别名。出《针灸甲乙经》。即二间。见该条。

Jiangu Another name for Erjian(LI 2), a meridian point from *Zhenjiu Jia-Yi Jing* (*A-B Classic of Acupuncture and Moxibustion*). → 二间(p.101)

● 间使[jiān shǐ] 经穴名。出《灵枢·本输》。属手厥阴心包经，为本经经穴。又名鬼路、鬼营。〈定位〉在前臂掌侧，当曲泽与大陵的连线上，腕横纹上3寸。掌长肌腱与桡侧腕屈肌腱之间(图49和图66)。〈层次解剖〉皮肤→皮下组织→桡侧腕屈肌腱与掌长肌腱之间→指浅屈肌→指深屈肌→旋前方肌→前臂骨间膜。浅层有前臂内、外侧皮神经分支和前臂正中静脉。深层布有正中神经。正中神经伴行动、静脉，骨间前动脉、神经等结构。〈主治〉心痛、心悸、胃痛、呕吐、热病、烦躁、疟疾、癫狂、痫证、腋肿、肘挛、臂痛。直刺0.5～1寸；可灸。

Jianshi(PC 5) A meridian point from *Lingshu: Benshu* (*Miraculous Pivot: Meridian Points*), the Jing(river) point of the Pericardium Meridian of Hand-Jueyin, also named Guilu or Guiying. 〈Location〉the palmar side of the forearm at the line connecting Quze(PC 3) and Daling(PC 7), 3 cun above the crease of the wrist, between the tendons of the long palmar muscle and radial flexor muscle of the wrist(Figs. 49&66). 〈Regional anatomy〉skin → subcutaneous tissue → between tendons of radial flexor muscle of wrist and long palmar muscle → superficial flexor muscle of fingers → deep flexor muscle of fingers → quadrate pronate muscle → interosseous membrane of forearm. In the superficial layer, there are the branches of the lateral and medial cutaneous nerves and the median vein of the forearm. In the deep layer, there are the median nerve and the accompanying artery and vein and the anterior interosseous artery and nerve. 〈Indications〉cardialgia, palpitations, stomachache, vomiting, febrile disease, dysphoria, malarial disease, manic-depressive psychosis, epilepsy, swelling in armpit, spasm of elbow, brachialgia. 〈Method〉Puncture perpendicularly 0.5～1 cun. Moxibustion is applicable.

● 肩[jiān] ①部位名。指颈项之下，左右两侧都称肩，是上肢和躯干的连属处。②耳穴名。将耳舟部分为六等分，自上而下，第四、五等分为肩。用于治疗肩部疼痛、肩关节周围炎、胆石症。

1. Shoulder A part of the body. Both the right and left sides below the neck and the nape, the juncture of the trunk and arms.

2. Shoulder(MA-SF 4) An auricular point. 〈Location〉Divide the scapha into 6 equal parts and the 4th and 5th parts are the shoulder (MA-SF 4). 〈Indications〉shoulder pain, scapulohumeral periarthritis, gallstones, etc..

● 肩胛[jiān jiǎ] 部位名。肩下成片之骨。现称肩胛

骨。

Scapula A blade-shaped bone inferior to shoulder, also named bladebone or shoulderblade.

●**肩尖**[jiān jiān] ①经穴别名。见《外科枢要》。即肩髃。见该条。②经外穴别名。见《经外奇穴图谱》。即肩头。见该条。

Jianjian Another name for ① Jianyu (LI 15), a meridian point seen in *Waike Shuyao* (*Essentials of External Diseases*). →肩髃(p. 191) ② Jiantou(EX-UE), an extra point seen in *Jingwai Qixue Tupu* (*An Atlas of Extra Points*). →肩头(p. 190)

●**肩解**[jiān jiě] 部位名。①出《灵枢·经脉》。肩端之骨节解处，即肩关节。②《素问·气穴论》等。指肩井、秉风等穴处，即肩胛冈上部。

Dividing Area of Shoulder ① A part of the body from *Lingshu: Jingmai* (*Miraculous Pivot: Meridians*), referring to the part between the arm and the trunk, i.e. shoulder joint. ② From *Suwen: Qixue Lun* (*Plain Questions: On Loci of Qi*), referring to the area where Jianjing (GB 21), Bingfeng (SI 12), etc. are located, i.e. the part above the spine of scapula.

●**肩井**[jiān jǐng] ①经穴名。出《针灸甲乙经》。属足少阳胆经，为手少阳、阳维之会。又名膊井。〈定位〉在肩上，前直乳中，当大椎与肩峰端连线的中点上（图7）。〈层次解剖〉皮肤→皮下组织→斜方肌→肩胛提肌。浅层布有锁骨上神经及颈浅动、静脉的分支或属支。深层有颈横动、静脉的分支或属支和肩胛背神经的分支。〈主治〉肩背痹痛、手臂不举、颈项强痛、乳痛、中风、瘰疬、难产、诸虚百损。直刺0.5～0.8寸，深部正当尖，慎不可深刺；可灸。②经穴别名。出《外科大成》。即肩髃。见该条。

1. **Jianjing** (GB 21) A meridian point from *Zhenjiu Jia-Yi Jing* (*A-B Classic of Acupuncture and Moxibustion*), a point on the Gall Bladder Meridian of Foot-Shaoyang and the crossing point of Hand-Shaoyang and Yangwei Meridians, also named Bojing. 〈Location〉on the shoulder, directly above the nipple, at the midpoint of the line connecting Dazhui (DU 14) and the acromion (Fig. 7). 〈Regional anatomy〉skin → subcutaneous tissue → trapezius muscle → levator muscle of scapula. In the superficial layer, there are the supraclavicular nerve and the branches or tributaries of the superficial cervical artery and vein. In the deep layer, there are the branches or tributaries of the transverse cervical artery and vein and the branches of the dorsal scapular nerve. 〈Indications〉numbness and pain of the shoulder and back, inability to raise hands and arms, stiffness and pain of the neck, mammary abscess, apoplexy, scrofula, dystocia, various conditions of deficiency and impairment. 〈Method〉Puncture perpendicularly 0.5～0.8 cun. Since the apex of lung is right beneath the point, deep needling should be avoided. Moxioustion applicable.

2. **Jianjing** Another name for Jianyu (LI 15), a meridian point from *Waike Dacheng* (*A Great Compendium of External Diseases*). →肩髃(p. 191)

●**肩聊**[jiān liáo] 经穴别名。见《太平圣惠方》。即肩髎。见该条。

Jianliao Another name for Jianliao (SJ 14), a meridian point, seen in *Taiping Shenghui Fang* (*Imperial Benevolent Prescriptions*). →肩髎(p. 189)

●**肩髎**[jiān liáo] 经穴名。出《针灸甲乙经》。属手少阳三焦经。又名肩聊。〈定位〉在肩部，肩髃后方，当臂外展时，于肩峰后下方呈现凹陷处（图48和图44）。〈层次解剖〉皮肤→皮下组织→三头肌→小圆肌→大圆肌→背阔肌腱。浅层布有锁骨上外侧神经。深层有腋神经和旋肱后动、静脉。〈主治〉臂痛、肩重不能举。直刺0.5～1寸；可灸。

Jianliao (SJ 14) A meridian point, from *Zhenjiu Jia-Yi Jing* (*A-B Classic of Acupuncture and Moxibustion*), a point on the Sanjiao Meridian of Hand-Shaoyang, also named Jianliao (SJ 14). 〈Location〉on the shoulder, posterior to Jianyu (HI 15), in the depression inferior and posterior to the acromion when the arm is abducted (Figs. 48&44). 〈Regional anatomy〉skin → subcutaneuos tissue → deltoid muscle → teres minor muscle → teres major muscle → tendon of latissimus muscle of back. In the superficial layer, there is the lateral supracla vicular nerve. In the deep layer, there are the axillary nerve and

the posterior circumflex humeral artery and vein. ⟨Indications⟩brachialgia, heavy sensation of shoulder and inability to raise arms. ⟨Method⟩Puncture perpendicularly 0.5~1.0 cun. Moxibustion is applicable.

●肩脉[jiān mài] 早期经脉名。出《帛书》。与手太阳经类似。

Shoulder Meridian An early name of a meridian, from *Bo Shu* (*Silk Book*), similar to the Meridian of Hand-Taiyang.

●肩内俞[jiān nèi shū] 经外穴名。见《腧穴学概论》。位于肩髃穴与云门穴连线之中点直下1寸处。⟨主治⟩肩臂痛不举。直刺0.5~1寸。可灸。

Jianneishu(EX-UE) An extra point, seen in *Shuxuexue Gailun*(*An Outline of Acupoints*). ⟨Location⟩1 cun straight below the midpoint of the line connecting Jianyu (LI 15) and Yunmen (LU 2). ⟨Indication⟩inablility to raise arms due to pain in the shoulder and arm. ⟨Method⟩Puncture perpendicuary 0.5~1.0 cun. Moxibustion is applicable.

●肩内髃[jiān nèi yú] 经外穴名。见《经外奇穴汇编》。在胸壁外上方，中府穴外侧0.5寸处。⟨主治⟩肩臂疼痛。直刺0.5~1寸；可灸。

Jianneiyu(EX-CA) An extra point, seen in *Jingwai Qixue Huibian*(*Expository Manual of Extra Points*). ⟨Location⟩in the superior lateral part of the thoracic wall, 0.5 cun lateral to Zhongfu(LU 1). ⟨Indication⟩pain in the shoulder and arm. ⟨Method⟩Puncture perpendicularly 0.5~1 cun. Moxibustion is applicable.

●肩凝症[jiān níng zhèng] 即漏肩风。详见该条。

Frozen Shoulder. →漏肩风(p. 257)

●肩俞[jiān shū] 经外穴名。见《腧穴学概论》。在肩部，当肩髃与云门穴连线之中点。⟨主治⟩肩疼痛不举等。直刺0.5~1寸；可灸。

Jianshu(EX) An extra point, seen in *Shu xuexue Gailun*(*An Outline of Acupoints*). ⟨Location⟩ on the shoulder, on the midpoint of the line conneceng Jianyu(LI 15) and Yumen(LU 2). ⟨Indication⟩ inablility to raise arm due to pain in the shoulder and arm, etc. ⟨Method⟩Puncture perpendicularly 0.5~1.0 cun. Moxibustion is applicable.

●肩头[jiān tó] 经外穴名。见《备急千金要方》。又名肩尖。位于肩锁关节的凹陷中，即肩髃的内上方处。⟨主治⟩瘰疬、牙痛、肩臂酸痛，以及肩关节及其周围软组织炎等。直刺0.5~1寸。艾炷灸3—7壮；或温灸5~15分钟。

Jiantou(EX-UE) An extra point seen in *Beiji Qianjin Yaofang*(*Essential Prescriptions for Emergencies Worth a Thousand Gold*), also named Jianjian. ⟨Location⟩in the process of the acromioclavicular joint, i. e. medial and superior to Jianyu(LI 15). ⟨Indications⟩tinea, toothache, aching pain in the shoulder omarthritis and periarthritis of shoulder. ⟨Method⟩ Puncture perpendicularly 0.5~1 cun. Give moxa-cone moxibustion for 3~7 cones, or mild-warm moxibustion with moxa stick for 5~15 minutes.

●肩外俞[jiān wài shū] 经穴名。出《针灸甲乙经》。属手太阳小肠经。⟨定位⟩在背部，当第一胸椎棘突下，旁开3寸(图7)。⟨层次解剖⟩皮肤→皮下组织→斜方肌→菱形肌。浅层有第一、二胸神经后支的皮支和伴行的动、静脉。深层分布有颈横动、静脉。深层分布有颈横动、静脉的分支或属支和肩胛背神经的肌支。⟨主治⟩肩背酸痛、颈项强急、上肢冷痛。斜刺0.3~0.6寸；可灸。慎勿深刺，免伤肺脏。

Jianwaishu(SI 14) A meridian point from *Zhenjiu Jia-Yi Jing* (*A-B Classic of Acupuncture and Moxibustion*), a point on the small Intestine Meridian of Hand-Taiyang. ⟨Location⟩ on the back, below the spinous process of the lst thoracic vertebra, 3 cun lateral to the posterior midline(Fig. 7). ⟨Regional anatomy⟩ skin → subcutaneous tissue → trapezius muscle → rhomboid muscle. In the superficial layer, there are the cutaneous branches of the posterior branches of the lst and 2nd thoracic nerves and their accompanying arteries and veins. In the deep layer, there are the branches or tributaries of the transverse cervical artery and vein and muscular branches of the dorsal scapular nerve. ⟨Indications⟩ pain and soreness in the shoulder and back, stiff neck, cold-pain in arm. ⟨Method⟩ Puncture obliquely 0.3~0.6 cun. ⟨Moxibustion⟩ is applicable. Avoid deep needling for fear of injuring the lung.

● 肩髃[jiān yú] ①经穴名。出《针灸甲乙经》。属手阳明大肠经,为手阳明、阳蹻交会穴。又名中间井、肩骨、偏骨、尚骨、偏肩、肩头、肩井。〈定位〉在肩部,三角肌上,臂外展,或向前平伸时,当肩峰前下方凹陷处(图48和图6)。〈层次解剖〉皮肤→皮下组织→三角肌→三角肌下囊→冈上肌腱。浅层有锁骨上外侧神经、臂外侧上皮神经分布。深层有旋肱后动、静脉和腋神经的分支。〈主治〉肩臂疼痛、手臂挛急、肩中热、半身不遂、风热瘾疹、瘰疬诸瘿。直刺0.5～0.8寸;可灸。②人体部位名。指肩关节上方。

1. **Jianyu**(LI 15) A meridian point, from *Zhenjiu Jia-Yi Jing*(*A-B Classic of Acupuncture and Moxibustion*), a point on the Large Intestine Meridian of Hand-Yangming, and the crossing point of the Hand-Yangming and Yangqiao Meridians, also named Zhongjianjing, Jiangu Piangu, Shanggu, Pianjian, Jiantou, or Jianjing. 〈Location〉on the shoulder, superior to the deltoid muscle, in the depression anterior and inferior to the acromion when the arm is abducted or raised to the level of the shoulder(Figs. 48&.6). 〈Regional anatomy〉skin→subcutaneous tissue→deltoid muscle → subdeltoid bursa → supraspinous muscle tendon. In the superficial layer, there are the lateral supraclavicular nerve and the superior lateral cutaneous nerve of the arm. In the deep layer, there are the posterior humeral circumflex artery and vein and the branches of the axillary nerve. 〈Indications〉pain in the shoulder and arm, contracture of hand and arm, heat sensation in shoulder, hemiplegia, urticaria due to pathogenic wind-heat, scrofula and various goiter. 〈Method〉Puncture perpendicularly 0.5～0.8 cun. Moxibustion is applicable.

2. **Top of Shoulder** A body part, referring to the upper part of the shoulder joint.

● 肩贞[jiān zhēn] 经穴名。出《灵枢·气穴论》。属手太阳小肠经。〈定位〉在肩关节后下方,臂内收时,腋后纹头上1寸(指寸)(图48和图65)。〈层次解剖〉皮肤→皮下组织→三角肌后份→肱三头肌长头→大圆肌→背阔肌腱。浅层有第二肋间神经的外侧皮支和臂外侧上皮神经分布。深层有桡神经等结构。〈主治〉肩胛痛、手臂痛麻、不能举、缺盆中痛、瘰疬、耳鸣、耳聋。直刺0.4～1寸;可灸。不宜向胸侧深刺,以免损伤肺脏。

Jianzhen(SI 9) A meridian point, from *Lingshu*: *Qixue Lun* (*Miraculous Pivot*: *On Loci of Qi*), a point on the Small Intestine Meridian of Hand-Taiyang. 〈Location〉Posterior and inferior to the shoulder joint, 1 cun above the posterior end of the axillary fold with the arm abducted (Figs. 48&.65). 〈Regional anatomy〉 skin→subcutaneous tissue→posterior part of deltoid muscle→long head of brachial triceps muscle→teres major muscle→tendon of latissimus muscle of back. In the superficial layer, there are the lateral cutaneous branch of the 2nd intercostal nerve and the superior lateral cutaneous nerve of the arm. In the deep layer, there is the radial nerve. 〈Indications〉 scapular pain, painful and numb hands and arms which can not be raised, pain in supraclavicular fossa, scrofula, tinnitus, deafness. 〈Method〉 Puncture perpendicularly 0.4～1.0 cun. Moxibustion is applicable. Do not needle deeply toward the chest for fear of injuring the lung.

● 肩中俞[jiān zhōng shū] 经穴名。出《针灸甲乙经》。属手太阳小肠经。〈定位〉在背部,当第七颈椎棘突下,旁开2寸(图7)。〈层次解剖〉皮肤→皮下组织→斜方肌→菱形肌。浅层有第八神经后支,第一胸神经后支的皮支分布。深层有副神经,肩胛背神经的分支和颈横动、静脉。〈主治〉咳嗽、气喘、肩背疼痛、唾血、寒热、目视不明。斜刺0.3～0.6寸;可灸。慎勿深刺,免伤肺脏。

Jianzhongshu(SI 15) A meridian point, from *Zhenjiu Jia-Yi Jing* (*A-B Classic of Acupuncture and Moxibustion*) on the Small Intestine Meridian of Hand-Taiyang. 〈Location〉 on the back, below the spinous process of the 7th cervical vertebra, 2 cun lateral to the posterior midline (Fig. 7). 〈Regional anatomy〉 skin→subcutaneous tissue→trapezius muscle→rhomboid muscle. In the superficial layer, there are the posterior branches of the 8th cervical nerve and the cutaneous branches of the posterior branches of the lst thoracic nerve. In the deep layer, there are the accessory nerve, the branches of the dorsal scapular nerve and the transverse cervical artery and vein. 〈Indications〉 cough, asthma,

pain of shoulder and back, spitting blood, fever and chills, poor vision. ⟨Method⟩ Puncture obliquely 0.3~0.6 cun. Moxibustion is applicable. Avoid deep needling for fear of injuring the lung.

●肩柱[jiān zhù] 经外穴别名，即肩柱骨。见该条。
Jianzhu Another name for the extra point Jianzhugu(EX-B). →肩柱骨(p.192)

●肩柱骨[jiān zhù gǔ] 经外穴名。出《奇效良方》。又名肩柱。在肩部，当肩胛骨肩峰突起之高点处。⟨主治⟩瘰疬肩臂痛、手不能举动等。用灸法。
Jianzhugu(EX-B) An extra point, from *Qixiao Liangfang* (*Prescriptions of Wonderful Efficacy*), also named Jianzhu. ⟨Location⟩ on the shoulder, on the high point of the process of the scapular acromion. ⟨Indications⟩ scrofula, pain of shoulder and arm, inability to raise and move hand. ⟨Method⟩ moxibustion.

●睑废[jiǎn fèi] 眼睑下垂的别名。详见该条。
Dysfunction of Eyelid →眼睑下垂(p.535)

●间隔灸[jiàn gé jiǔ] 为间接灸之别称。见该条。
Separated Moxibution Another name for indirect moxibustion. →间接灸(p.192)

●间接灸[jiàn jiē jiǔ] 艾炷灸的一种。见《肘后备急方》。又称隔物灸、间隔灸。指在艾炷下穴位上衬隔药物施灸的一种方法。这样可以避免灸伤皮肤，又可以发挥艾与药物的双重作用。根据所隔药物不同，可分称为隔姜灸、隔蒜灸、隔盐灸、隔附子饼灸等多种。详见各条。
Indirect Moxibustion A form of moxa-cone moxibustion, seen in *Zhouhou Beiji Fang* (*A Handbook of Prescriptions for Emergencies*), also named separated moxibustion, or insulated moxibustion. Place certain barriers between the acupoint and moxa cone to prevent the fire from burning the skin and make use of the effects of both moxa and the barrier chosen. According to the materials used for separation, indirect moxibustion is divided into ginger-separated moxibustion, garlic-separated moxibustion, salt-separated moxibustion and *Fu Zi* monkshood-cake-separated moxibustion, etc.. →隔姜灸(p.136)、隔蒜灸(p.137)、隔盐灸(p.138)、隔附子灸(p.135), etc..

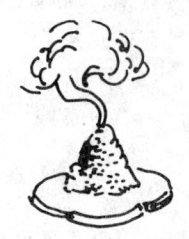

图25 间接灸
Fig. 25 Indirect moxibustion

●建里[jiàn lǐ] 经穴名。出《针灸甲乙经》。属任脉。⟨定位⟩在上腹部，前正中线上，当脐中上3寸(图43和图40)。⟨层次解剖⟩皮肤→皮下组织→腹白线→腹横筋膜→腹膜外脂肪→壁腹膜。浅层主要布有第八胸神经前支的前皮支及腹壁浅静脉的属支。深层主要有第八胸神经前支的分支。⟨主治⟩胃脘疼痛、腹胀、呕吐、食欲不振、肠中切痛、水肿。直刺0.5~1寸；可灸。
Jianli(RN 11) A meridian point, from *Zhenjiu Jia-Yi Jing* (*A-B Classic of Acupuncture and Moxibustion*), a point on the Ren Meridian. ⟨Location⟩ on the upper abdomen and on the anterior midline, 3 cun above the centre of the umbilicus (Figs. 43&40). ⟨Regional anatomy⟩ skin→subcutaneous tissue→linea alba→transverse fascia→extraperitoneal fat tissue→parietal peritoneum. In the superficial layer, there are the anterior cutaneous branches of the anterior branch of the 8th thoracic nerve and the tributaries of the superficial epigastric vein. In the deep layer, there are the branches of the anterior branch of the 8th thoracic nerve. ⟨Indications⟩ epigastralgia, abdominal distention, vomiting, anorexia, pain in intestines, edema. ⟨Method⟩ Puncture perpendicularly 0.5~0.1 cun. Moxibustion is applicable.

●剑巨[jiàn jù] 经外穴名。出《外科大成》。在前臂屈侧，当腕横纹上3.2寸，当掌长肌腱与桡侧腕屈肌腱之间。⟨主治⟩马刀。直刺0.5~1寸；可灸。
Jianju(EX-UE) An extra point from

Waike Dacheng (*A Great Compendium of External Diseases*). 〈Location〉on the flexor side of the forearm, 3.2 cun proximal to the crease of the wrist, between the tendons of the long palmar muscle and the radial flexor muscle of the wrist. 〈Indication〉sabre and beadstring shaped scrofulae. 〈Method〉Puncture perpendicularly 0.5～1.0 cun. Moxibustion is applicable.

●剑针[jiàn zhēn] 即铍针。见该条。

Sword-Shaped Needle Another name for stiletto needle. →铍针(p.291)

●楗[jiàn] 部位名。即股骨。出《素问·骨空论》："辅骨上横骨下为楗。"又名髀骨。

Femur A part of the body, originally from *Suwen: Gukong Lun* (*Plain Questions: On the Apertures of Bones*): "The part above the condyle and below symphysis pubis is called femur (Jian)". It is also called the bone of the thigh.

●箭头针[jiàn tóu zhēn] 即镵针。见该条。

Arrow-Head Needle →镵针(p.31)

●姜椒蒸气灸[jiāng jiāo zhēng qì jiǔ] 药物蒸气灸法之一。取生姜、辣椒各等份，水煎后用蒸气熏灸患部，候水温后再洗患部。适于冻伤。

Steaming with a Decoction of Ginger and Chili A form of medicinal steaming therapy. Decoct equal amounts of fresh ginger and chili, then heat the affected area with the steam of the decoction, wash the area when the decoction becomes warm. 〈Indication〉frostbite.

●畺尾[jiāng wěi] 经穴别名。出《西方子明堂经》。即长强。见该条。

Jiangwei Another name for Changqiang (DU 1), a meridian point from *Xi Fang Zi Mingtang Jing* (*Xi Fang Zi's Classic of Acupoints*). →长强(p.39)

●降压点[jiàng yā diǎn] 角窝上之别称。见该条。

Point for Lowering Blood Pressure (MA) Another name for the superior triangular fossa (MA). →角窝上(p.199)

●交叉取穴[jiāo chā qǔ xué] 取穴法之一。又称对侧取穴。其法有二：①左右交叉，即某一侧的病痛选取其另一侧穴位。《内经》中所载巨刺、缪刺，皆属此类取穴法。参见该条。②左右上下交叉，即左上肢病痛选取右下肢穴位，左下肢病痛选取右上肢的穴位等。

Selection of Contralateral Points A method of selecting points, also called selection of points on the opposite side, including two aspects: ①left and right crossing, i.e. to treat pains on one side of the body by needling points on the other side of the body. Both the opposing needling and the contralateral needling recorded in *Neijing* (*Canon of Internal Medicine*) belong to this kind of acupuncture. →巨刺(p.225)、缪刺(p.270) ②left-right and upper-lower crossing, i.e. to treat pains on the left arm by needling points on the right leg; and pains on the left leg by needling poins on the right arm.

●交冲[jiāo chōng] 经穴别名。出《针灸甲乙经》。即后顶。见该条。

Jiaochong Another name for Houding (DU 19), a meridian point originally from *Zhenjiu Jia-Yi Jing* (*A-B Classic of Acupuncture and Moxibustion*). →后顶(p.165)

●交感[jiāo gǎn] 耳穴名。位于对耳轮下脚的末端。具有解痉镇痛、滋阴潜阳作用。〈主治〉内脏疼痛、心悸、自汗、植物神经功能紊乱、胃肠痉挛、心绞痛、输尿管结石绞痛。并为耳针麻醉之常用穴。

Sympathetic (MA-AH 7) An auricular point. 〈Locations〉at the end of the inferior antihelix crus. 〈Function〉Relieve spasm and pain, nourish yin and suppress hyperactive yang. 〈Indications〉pain of the internal organs, palpitations, spontaneous perspiration, vegetative nerve functional disturbance, gastrointestinal spasm, angina pectoris, colic of ureter stone, one of the common points for auriculoacupuncture anesthesia.

●交会穴[jiāo huì xué] 经穴分类名。见《针灸甲乙经》。指两经或数经相交会合的腧穴。其中，主要的一经即腧穴所归属的一经称为本经，相交的经称为他经。交会穴大多分布在头面躯干部。交会穴不但能治本经的疾病，还能兼治所交会经脉的疾病。

Crossing Point A category of meridian points, seen in *Zhenjiu Jia-Yi Jing* (*A-B Classic of Acupuncture and Moxibustion*), re-

表9 经 脉 交 会 穴 表
Table 9   Crossing Points

经 属 Meridians	穴 名 Name of Points	交会经脉 Crossed Meridians
手太阴 Hand-Taiyin	中 府 Zhōngfǔ(LU 1)	手足太阴之会 Crossing Point of Hand-Taiyin and Foot-Taiyin
手阳明 Hand-Yangming	臂 臑 Bìnào(LI 14)	手阳明络之会 Crossing Point Hand-Yangming collaterals
	肩 髃 Jiānyú(LI 15)	手阳明、阳跷脉之会 Crossing Point of Hand-Yangming and Yangqiao Meridian
	巨 骨 Jùgǔ(LI 16)	
	迎 香 Yíngxiāng(LI 20)	手足阳明之会 Crossing Point of Hand-Yangming and Foot-Yangming
足阳明 Foot-Yangming	承 泣 Chéngqì(ST 1)	阳跷、任脉、足阳明之会 Crossing Point of Yangqiao, Ren Meridian and Foot-Yangming
	巨 髎 Jùliáo(ST 3)	阳跷、足阳明之会 Crossing Point of Yangqiao Meridian and Foot-Yangming
	地 仓 Dìcāng(ST 4)	阳跷、手足、阳明之会 Crossing Point of Yangqiao Meridian, Hand-Yangming and Foot-Yangming
	下 关 Xiàguān(ST 7)	足阳明,足少阳之会 Crossing Point of Foot-Yangming and Foot-Shaoyang
足阳明 Foot-Yangming	头 维 Tóuwéi(ST 8)	足少阳、足阳明之会 Crossing Point of Foot-Shaoyang and Foot-Yangming
	气 冲 Qìchōng(ST 30)	冲脉起于气冲 Chong Meridian originally from Qìchōng(ST 30)
足太阴 Foot-Taiyin	三阴交 Sānyīnjiāo(SP 6)	足太阴,足厥阴,足少阴之会 Crossing Points of Foot-Taiyin, Foot-Jueyin and Foot-Shaoyin
	冲 门 Chōngmén(SP 12)	足厥阴,足太阴之会 Crossing Point of Jueyin and Foot-Taiyin
	府 舍 Fǔshě(SP 13)	足太阴、阴维、足厥阴之会 Crossint Point of Foot-Taiyin, Yinwei and Foot-Jueyin
	大 横 Dàhéng(SP 15)	足太阴、阴维 Crossing Point of Foot-Taiyin and Yinwei
	腹 哀 Fù'āi(SP 16)	
手太阳 Hand-Taiyang	天 容 Tiānróng(SI 17)	手太阳脉气所发 Origin of qi of Hand-Shaoyang Meridian
	臑 俞 Nàoshū(SI 10)	手太阳,阳维,阳跷之会 Crossing Point of Hand-Taiyang, Yangwei and Yangqiao
	秉 风 Bǐngfēng(SI 12)	手阳明,手太阳,手足少阳 Crossing Point of Hand-Yangming, Hand-Taiyang Hand-Shaoyang and Foot-Shaoyang
	颧 髎 Quánliáo(SI 18)	手少阳,手太阳之会 Crossing Point of Hand-Shaoyang and Hand-Taiyang
	听 宫 Tīnggōng(SI 19)	手足少阳,手太阳之会 Crossing Point of Hand-Shaoyang, Foot-Shaoyang, and Hand-Taiyang

经 属 Meridians	穴 名 Name of Points	交会经脉 Crossed Meridians
足太阳 Foot-Taiyang	睛 明 Jīngmíng(BL 1)	手足太阳、足阳明之会 Crossing Point of Hand-Taiyang, Foot-Taiyang and Foot-Yangming
	大 杼 Dàzhū(BL 11)	足太阳、手太阳之会 Crossing Point of Foot-Taiyang and Hand-Taiyang
	风 门 Fēngmén(BL 12)	督脉、足太阳之会 Crossing Point of Du Meridian and Foot-Taiyang
	附 分 Fùfēn(BL 41)	手太阳、足太阳之会 Crossing Point of Hand-Taiyang and Foot-Taiyang
	上 髎 Shàngliáo(BL 31)	足太阳、足少阳之络 Collateral of Foot-Taiyang and Foot-Shaoyang
	跗 阳 Fūyáng(BL 59)	阳跷之郄 Xi(Cleft) Point of Yangqiao Meridian
	申 脉 Shēnmài(BL 62)	阳跷所生 Yangqiao Meridian begins here.
	仆 参 Púcān(BL 61)	足太阳、阳跷所会 Crossing Point of Foot-Taiyang and Yangqiao Meridian
	金 门 Jīnmén(BL 63)	阳维所别属也 Pertaining Point of Yangwei Meridian
足少阴 Foot-Shaoyin	大 赫 Dàhè(KI 12)	冲脉、足少阴之会 Crossing Point of Chong Meridian and Foot-Shaoyin
	气 穴 Qìxué(KI 13)	冲脉、足少阴之会 Crossing Point of Chong Meridian and Foot-Shaoyin
	四 满 Sìmǎn(KI 14)	冲脉、足少阴之会 Crossing Point of Chong Meridian and Foot-Shaoyin
	中 柱 Zhōngzhù(KI 15)	冲脉、足少阴之会 Crossing Point of Chong Meridian and Foot-Shaoyin
	肓 俞 Huāngshū(KI 16)	冲脉、足少阴之会 Crossing Point of Chong Meridian and Foot-Shaoyin
	商 曲 Shāngqū(KI 17)	冲脉、足少阴之会 Crossing Point of Chong Meridian and Foot-Shaoyin
	横 骨 Hénggǔ(KI 11)	冲脉、足少阴之会 Crossing Point of Chong Meridian and Foot-Shaoyin
	石 关 Shíguān(KI 18)	冲脉、足少阴之会 Crossing Point of Chong Meridian and Foot-Shaoyin
	阴 都 Yīndū(KI 19)	冲脉、足少阴之会 Crossing Point of Chong Meridian and Foot-Shaoyin
	腹通谷 Fùtōnggǔ(KI 20)	冲脉、足少阴之会 Crossing Point of Chong Meridian and Foot-Shaoyin
	幽 门 Yōumén(KI 21)	冲脉、足少阴之会 Crossing Point of Chong Meridian and Foot-Shaoyin
	照 海 Zhàohǎi(KI 6)	阴跷脉所生 Yinqiao Meridian begins here.
	交 信 Jiāoxìn(KI 8)	阴跷之郄 Xi(Cleft) Point of Yinqiao Meridian
	筑 宾 Zhùbīn(KI 9)	阴维之郄 Xi(Cleft) Point of Yinwei Meridian

经　属 Meridians	穴　名 Name of Points	交会经脉 Crossed Meridians
手厥阴 Hand-Jueyin	天　池 Tiānchí (PC 1)	手厥阴、足少阳之会 Crossing Point of Hand-Jueyin and Foot-Shaoyang
手少阳 Hand-Shaoyang	臑　会 Nàohuì (SJ 13)	手阳明之络 Collateral of Hand-Yangming
	丝竹空 Sīzhúkōng (SJ 23)	足少阳脉气所发 Origin of the qi of Foot-Shaoyang Meridian
	天　髎 Tiānliáo (SJ 15)	手少阳、阳维之会 Crossing Point of Hand-Shaoyang and Yangwei Meridian
	翳　风 Yìfēng (SJ 17)	手足少阳之会 Crossing Point of Hand-Shaoyang and Foot-Shaoyang
	角　孙 Jiǎosūn (SJ 20)	手足少阳之会 Crossing Point of Hand-Shaoyang and Foot-Shaoyang
	耳和髎 Ěrhéliáo (SJ 22)	手足少阳，手太阳之会 Crossing Point of Hand-Shaoyang, Foot-Shaoyang and Hand-Taiyang
足少阳 Foot-Shaoyang	瞳子髎 Tóngzǐliáo (GB 1)	手太阳，手足少阳之会 Crossing Point of Hand-Taiyang, Hand-Shaoyang and Foot-Shaoyang
	上　关 Shàngguān (GB 3)	手少阳，足阳明 Crossing Point of Hand-Shaoyang and Foot-Yangming
	颔　厌 Hànyàn (GB 4)	手少阳、足阳明之会 Crossing Point of Hand-Shaoyang and Foot-Yangming
	听　会 Tīnghuì (GB 2)	手少阳脉气所发 Origin of the qi of Hand-Shaoyang Meridian
	悬　厘 Xuánlí (GB 6)	手足少阳，阳明之会 Crossing Point of Hand-Shaoyang, Foot-Shaoyang, Hand-Yangming and Foot-Yangming
	曲　鬓 Qūbìn (GB 7)	足太阳、足少阳之会 Crossing Point of Foot-Taiyang and Foot-Shaoyang
	天　冲 Tiānchōng (GB 9)	足太阳、足少阳之会 Crossing Point of Foot-Taiyang and Foot-Shaoyang
	率　谷 Shuàigǔ (GB 8)	足太阳、足少阳之会 Crossing Point of Foot-Taiyang and Foot-Shaoyang
	浮　白 Fúbái (GB 10)	足太阳、足少阳之会 Crossing Point of Foot-Taiyang and Foot-Shaoyang
	头窍阴 Tóuqiàoyīn (GB 11)	足太阳、足少阳之会 Crossing Point of Foot-Taiyang and Foot-Shaoyang
	完　骨 Wángǔ (GB 12)	足太阳、足少阳之会 Crossing Point of Foot-Taiyang and Foot-Shaoyang
	本　神 Běnshén (GB 13)	足少阳、阳维之会 Crossing Point of Foot-Shaoyang and Yangwei
	阳　白 Yángbái (GB 14)	足少阳、阳维之会 Crossing Point of Foot-Shaoyang and Yangwei
	头临泣 Tóulínqì (GB 15)	足太阳、足少阳、阳维之会 Crossing Point of Foot-Taiyang, Foot-Shaoyang and Yangwei
	目　窗 Mùchuāng (GB 16)	足少阳、阳维之会 Crossing Point of Foot-Shaoyang and Yangwei
	正　营 Zhèngyíng (GB 17)	足少阳、阳维之会 Crossing Point of Foot-Shaoyang and Yangwei
	承　灵 Chénglíng (GB 18)	足少阳、阳维之会 Crossing Point of Foot-Shaoyang and Yangwei

经属 Meridians	穴 名 Name of Points	交会经脉 Crossed Meridians
	脑 空 Nǎokōng(GB 19)	足少阳,阳维之会 Crossing Point of Foot-Shaoyang and Yangwei
	风 池 Fēngchí(GB 20)	足少阳,阳维之会 Crossing Point of Foot-Shaoyang and Yangwei
	肩 井 Jiānjǐng(GB 21)	足少阳,阳维之会 Crossing Point of Foot-Shaoyang and Yangwei
	日 月 Rìyuè(GB 24)	足太阳、足少阳之会 Crossing Point of Foot-Taiyang and Foot-Shaoyang
	环 跳 Huántiào(GB 30)	足少阳,足太阳二脉之会 Crossing Point of Foot-Shaoyang and Foot-Taiyang
	带 脉 Dàimài(GB 26)	足少阳,足太阳二脉之会 Crossing Point of Foot-Shaoyang and Dai Meridian
	五 枢 Wǔshū(GB 27)	足少阳,足太阳二脉之会 Crossing Point of Foot-Shaoyang and Dai Meridian
	维 道 Wéidào(GB 28)	足少阳,带脉之会 Crossing Point of Foot-Shaoyang and Dai Meridian
	居 髎 Jūliáo(GB 29)	阳跷、足少阳之会 Crossing Point of Yangqiao and Foot-Shaoyang
	阳 交 Yángjiāo(GB 35)	阳维之郄 Xi(Cleft) Point of Yangwei Meridian
足厥阴 Foot-Jueyin	章 门 Zhāngmén(LR 13)	足厥阴、足少阳之会 Crossing Point of Foot-Jueyin and Foot-Shaoyang
	期 门 Qīmén(LR 14)	足太阴、厥阴、阴维之会 Crossing Point of Foot-Taiyin, Foot-Jueyin and Yinwei
任脉 Ren Meridian	承 浆 Chéngjiāng(RN 24)	足阳明、任脉之会 Crossing Point of Foot-Yangming and Ren Meridian
	廉 泉 Liánquán(RN 23)	阴维、任脉 Crossing Point of Yinwei and Ren Meridian
	天 突 Tiāntū(RN 22)	阴维、任脉 Crossing Point of Yinwei and Ren Meridian
	上 脘 Shàngwǎn(RN 13)	任脉、足阳明、手太阳之会 Crossing Point of Ren Meridian, Foot-Yangming and Hand-Taiyang
	中 脘 Zhōngwǎn(RN 12)	手太阳、少阳、足阳明所生,任脉之会 Hand-Taiyang, Hand-Shaoyang and Foot-Yangming begin here, the Crossing Point of them and Ren Meridian
	下 脘 Xiàwǎn(RN 10)	足太阴、任脉之会 Crossing Point of Foot-Taiyin and Ren Meridian
	阴 交 Yīnjiāo(RN 7)	任脉、冲脉之会 Crossing Point of Ren and Chong Meridians
	关 元 Guānyuán(RN 4)	足三阴、任脉之会 Crossing Point of three Yin Meridians of Foot and Ren Meridian
	中 极 Zhōngjí(RN 3)	足三阴、任脉之会 Crossing Point of three Yin Meridians of Foot and Ren Meridian
	曲 骨 Qūgǔ(RN 2)	任脉、足厥阴之会 Crossing Point of Ren Meridian and Foot-Jueyin
	会 阴 Huìyīn(RN 1)	任脉、别络、夹督脉、冲脉之会 Crossing Point of Ren Meridian, Large Collatereals, Du Meridian and Chong meridian

经属 Meridians	穴名 Name of Points	交会经脉 Crossed Meridians
督脉 Du Meridian	神庭 Shénting (DU 24)	督脉、足太阳、阳明之会 Crossing Point of Du Meridian, Foot-Taiyang and Foot-Yangming
	水沟 Shuǐgōu (DU 26)	督脉、手、足阳明之会 Crossing Point of Du Meridian, Hand-Yangming and Foot-Yanming
	百会 Bǎihuì (DU 20)	督、足太阳之会 Crossing Point of Du and Foot-Taiyang
	脑户 Nǎohù (DU 17)	督、足太阳之会 Crossing Point of Du and Foot-Taiyang
	风府 Fēngfǔ (DU 17)	督脉、阳维之会 Crossing Point of Du Meridian and Yangwei
	哑门 Yǎmén (DU 15)	督脉、阳维之会 Crossing Point of Du Meridian and Yangwei
	大椎 Dàzhuī (DU 14)	手足三阳、督脉之会 Crossing Point of Three Yang Meridians of Hand and Three Yang Meridians of Hand and Du Meridian
	陶道 Táodào (DU 13)	督脉、足太阳之会 Crossing Point of Du Meridian and Foot-Taiyang
	长强 Chángqiáng (DU 1)	督脉、别络、足少阴所结 Du Meridian, Large Collaterals and Foot-Shaoyin gather here.

ferring to the points where two or several meridians intersect and meet. The principal meridian that the point belongs to is called the pertaining meridian, while meridians which intersect with this meridian are called other meridian. Most of the crossing points are distributed on the head, face and trunk. They may be used to treat not only the disorders of their pertaining meridians but also the crossing meridians.

●交经八穴 [jiāo jīng bā xué] 八脉交会八穴的别名,见该条。

Eight Crossing Points Another name of the Eight Confluent Points of the Eight Meridians. →八脉交会八穴 (p. 7)

●交经缪刺 [jiāo jīng miù cì] 刺法之一。见《标幽赋》。指左病取右,右病取左的交叉取穴刺法。本自《内经》刺法,参见"缪刺"、"巨刺"条。

Crossing Needling One of the methods of acupuncture, seen in *Biao You Fu* (*Lyrics of Recondite Principles*), referring to the selection of contralateral points, that is, selecting points contralateral to the affected side, a needling technique, originating from *Nei Jing* (*Canon of Internal Medicine*). →缪刺 (p. 270)、巨刺 (p. 225)

●交信 [jiāo xìn] 经穴名。出《针灸甲乙经》。又名内筋。属足少阴肾经,为阴跷脉的郄穴。〈定位〉在小腿内侧,当太溪直上2寸,复溜前0.5寸,胫骨内侧缘的后方(图81和图46)。〈层次解剖〉皮肤→皮下组织→趾长屈肌→胫骨后肌后方→拇长屈肌。浅层布有隐神经的小腿内侧皮支,大隐静脉的属支。深层有胫神经和胫后动、静脉。〈主治〉月经不调、崩漏、阴挺、泄泻、大便难、睾丸肿痛、五淋、疝气、阴痒、泻痢赤白及膝、股、腨内廉痛。直刺0.8~1寸;可灸。

Jiaoxin (KI 8) A meridian point, originally from *Zhenjiu Jia-Yi Jing* (*A-B Classic of Acupuncture and Moxibustion*), also called neijin, a point on the Kidney Meridian of Foot-Shaoyin, the Xi (Cleft) point of Yinqiao Meridian. 〈Location〉 on the medial side of leg, 2 cun above Taixi (KI 3) and 0.5 cun anterior to Fuliu (KI 7), posterior to the medial border of the tibia (Figs. 81&46). 〈Regional anatomy〉 skin → subcutaneous tissue → long flexor muscle of toes → posterior side of posterior tibial muscle → long flexor muscle of great toe. In the superficial layer, there are the medial cutaneous branches of the saphenous nerve to the leg and the tributaries of the

great saphenous vein. In the deep layer, there are the tibial nerve and the posterior tibial artery and vein. 〈Indications〉 irregular menstruation, metrorrhagia and metrostasis, prolapse of uterus, diarrhea, constipation, painful and swollen testis, five types of stranguria, hernia, pruritus vulvae, dysentery, and pain in medial side of knee, thigh and leg. 〈Method〉 Puncture perpendicularly 0.8~1 cun. Moxibustion is applicable.

●交仪[jiāo yí]　经穴别名。出《千金要方》。即蠡沟。见该条。

Jiaoyi　Another name for Ligou(LR 5), a meridian point from *Qianjin Yaofang*(*Essential Prescriptions Worth a Thousand Gold*).→蠡沟(p.242)

●椒饼灸[jiāo bǐng jiǔ]　为隔胡椒饼灸之别称。见该条。

Pepper-Cake Moxibustion　Another name for pepper-cake separated moxibustion.→隔胡椒饼灸(p.135)

●焦蕴稳[jiāo yùn wěn]　人名。明针灸家,海州(今属江苏)人。其针法有奇效。事见《海州志》。

Jiao Yunwen　An acupuncture-moxibustion expert in the Ming Dynasty, a native of Haizhou (now of Jiangsu Province). It was recorded in *Haizhou Zhi* (*Records of Haizhou*) that his acupuncture therapy was miraculous and highly effective.

●角[jiǎo]　①部位名。额角,指额骨结节;头角,指顶骨结节。②角法的简称。即拔罐法的古代称谓。

1.**Angle**　A part of the body, frontal angle, referring to the frontal tubercle; angle of head, referring to the tubercle of parietal bone, namely the parietal angle.
2.**Horn**　the simpler name for horn cupping, the archaic name for cupping.

●角法[jiǎo fǎ]　拔罐法之古称。见该条。

Horn Cupping　The archaic name for cupping.→拔罐法(p.9)

●角孙[jiǎo sūn]　经穴名。出《灵枢·寒热病》。属手少阳三焦经,为手足少阳、手阳明之会。〈定位〉在头部,折耳廓向前,当耳尖直上入发际处(图44、图65和图28)。〈层次解剖〉皮肤→皮下组织→耳上肌→颞筋膜浅层及颞肌。布有耳颞神经的分布,颞浅动、静脉

耳前支。〈主治〉耳部肿痛、目赤肿痛、目翳、齿痛、唇燥、项强、头痛。平刺0.3~0.5寸;可灸。

Jiaosun(SJ 20)　A meridian point, originally from *Lingshu*: *Han Re Bing* (*Miraculous Pivot*: *Cold and Heat Diseases*), a point on the Sanjiao Meridian of Hand-Shaoyang, the crossing point of the Hand-Shaoyang, Foot-Shaoyang and Hand-Yangming Meridians. 〈Location〉 on the head, above the ear apex within the hairline (Figs. 44, 65&28). 〈Regional anatomy〉 skin→subcutaneous tissue→superior auricular muscle→superficial temporal facia and temporal muscle. There are the branches of the auriculotemporal nerve and the anterior auricular branches of the superficial temporal artery and vein in this area. 〈Indications〉 swelling and pain in the ear, redness, swelling and pain of the eye, blurred vision, toothache, dry lips, rigidity of the neck, headache. 〈Method〉 Puncture subcutaneously 0.3~0.5 cun. Moxibustion is applicable.

●角窝上[jiǎo wō shàng]　耳穴名。又称降压点。位于三角窝内上方。具有平肝熄风作用。〈主治〉高血压。

Superior Triangular Fossa(MA)　An auricular point, also called Lowering Blood Pressure Point. 〈Location〉 on the interior superior border of the triangular fossa. 〈Function〉 Calm the liver to stop wind. 〈Indication〉 Hypertension.

●角窝中[jiǎo wō zhōng]　耳穴名。位于三角窝中三分之一。具有清热平喘作用。〈主治〉喘息。

Middle Triangular Fossa(MA)　An auricular point. 〈Location〉at middle 1/3 of the triangular fossa. 〈Function〉 Clear heat to relieve asthma. 〈Indication〉 asthma.

●角针[jiǎo zhēn]　针具名。以塑料、胶木或金属制成,呈圆锥型,有似小艾炷,其高度与底面直经均为1分。使用时,将针尖按于穴上,底面与皮肤面相平,再以胶布固定。用法与"皮内针"相类似。

Horn Needle　A needle, made of plastics, bakelite or metal, with a shape of a circular cone like a small moxa cone, the height and diameter of the basal surface are about 1 fen. 〈Usage〉 Press the tip of the needle on the point and keep the basal surface level with the

skin, then fix it with adhesive plaster. The needle is used in a way similiar to the cutaneous needle.

●脚气[jiǎo qì] 病名。见《诸病源候论》卷十三。古名缓风，又称脚病弱。以足胫软弱乏力，步履艰难为主要症状。因外感湿邪风毒，或饮食厚味所伤，积湿生热，流注于足胫所致。可分为湿脚气、干脚气、脚气冲心三种。详见各条。

Beriberi A disease, seen in *Zhubing Yuanhou Lun* (*General Treatise on Etiology and Symptomatology of Diseases*), named mild wind in ancient times, also called foot asthenia. 〈Main symptoms〉 myosthenia of lower limbs, difficulty in walking. 〈Etiology and pathology〉 Invasion of wind-wet evil, or impairment due to a rich, fatty diet, leading to an accumulation of dampness and producing heat. The damp-heat flows downward to the lower limbs. It can be divided into three types: dry beriberi, wet beriberi, and cardiac beriberi. →干脚气(p. 123)、湿脚气(p. 370)、脚气冲心(p. 200)

●脚气八处灸[jiǎo qì bā chù jiǔ] 出《千金方》。指灸治脚气的八个经验效穴。指风市、伏兔、犊鼻、膝眼、足三里、上廉、下廉、绝骨八穴。

Moxibustion at Eight Points for Beriberi Originally from *Qianjin Fang* (*Prescriptions Worth a Thousand Gold*), referring to the eight effective points for treating beriberi with moxibustion. The points are Fengshi(GB 20), Futu(ST 32), Dubi(ST 35), Xiyan(EX-LE 5), Zusanli(ST 36), Shanglian(LI 9), Xialian(LI 8), and Juegu[i. e. Xuanzhong(GB 39)].

●脚气冲心[jiǎo qì chōng xīn] 脚气证型之一。见《外台秘要》卷十八。又称脚气攻心、脚气入心。由于湿毒上攻心胸所致。证见足胫肿痛或萎细麻木，步行乏力，突然气急、心悸、恶心呕吐，胸中懊憹。重证则神昏烦躁，语言错乱，唇舌发绀，脉细数无力。治宜降气泻肺，泄毒宁心。取尺泽、膻中、劳宫、神门、足三里、涌泉。

Cardiac Beriberi One kind of beriberi, originally from Vol. 18 of *Waitai Miyao* (*Clandestine Essentials from the Imperial Library*), also called beriberi attacking the heart, or beriberi entering the heart due to wet pathogens attacking the heart. 〈Manifestations〉 Edema and pain in the foot and leg, atrophy and numbness of the foot, weakness of walking, accelerated respiration, palpitations, nausea and vomiting, restlessness, severe cases manifest coma delirium, dysphoria, cyanosis of lip and tongue, rapid thready and weak pulse. 〈Treatment principle〉 Keep qi moving downward, reduce the pathogenic lung fire, clear poisons and ease mental anxiety. 〈Point selection〉 Chize(LU 5), Tanzhong(RN 17), Laogong(PC 8), Shenmen(HT 7), Zusanli(ST 36) and Yongquan(KI 1).

●脚气攻心[jiǎo qì gōng xīn] 见《奇效良方》卷三十九。即脚气冲心。见该条。

Beriberi Attacking the Heart Another name for cardiac beriberi, a disease seen in Vol. 39 of *Qixiao Liangfang* (*Prescriptions of Wonderful Efficacy*). →脚气冲心(p. 200)

●脚气入心[jiǎo qì rù xīn] 出《医宗金鉴》卷三十九。即脚气冲心。见该条。

Berberi Entering the Heart Another name for cardiac beriberi, a disease from Vol. 39 of *Yizong Jinjian* (*Gold Mirror of Orthodox Medical Lineage*). →脚气冲心(p. 200)

●脚弱[jiǎo ruò] 即脚气。见该条。

Foot-Asthenia →脚气(p. 200)

●痎疟[jiē nüè] 病证名。出《素问·疟论》等。即疟疾。见该条。

Malaria A disease originally from *Suwen: Nüe Lun* (*Plain Questions: Malarial Disease*), another name for malarial disease. →疟疾(p. 287)

●接骨[jiē gǔ] 经外穴别名。即接脊。见该条。

Jiegu Another name for the extra point Jieji (EX-B). →接脊(p. 200)

●接脊[jiē jǐ] 经外穴名。出《太平圣惠方》。又名接骨。在背部，后正中线上，当第12胸椎棘突下凹处。〈主治〉小儿痢疾、脱肛、癫痫、消化不良等。斜刺0.5～1寸；可灸。

Jieji(EX-B) An extra point, originally from *Taiping Shenghui Fang* (*Imperial Benevolent Prescriptions*), another name for Jiegu. 〈Location〉 on the back, at the posterior midline, in the depression below the spinous process of

the 12th thoraic vertebra. 〈Indications〉 infantile dysentery, proctoptosis, epilepsy and indigestion, etc. 〈Method〉 Puncture obliquely 0.5~1 cun. Moxibustion is applicable.

●接经取穴[jiē jīng qǔ xué] 取穴法之一。又称同名经取穴。十二经脉中,手足同名经脉上下相连结。根据这种关系,对其一经脉的病变,可取与其相连接的手经或足经上的穴位来进行治疗。

Selection of Points on Connected Meridians A method of selecting acupoints, also called selection of points on meridians of the same name. Among the twelve regular meridians, the meridians of the hand and foot with the same name are connected. (For instance, Hand-Yangming and Foot-Yangming meridians are all Yangming meridians). Based on this relationship, the diseases of one meridian can be treated with the points on the connected hand or foot meridian.

●接气通经[jiē qì tōng jīng] 根据各经脉不同长度,按呼吸次数规定运用针刺手法所需要的时间。出《流注指微针赋》。其法依照《灵枢·脉度》所载的经脉长度,结合《灵枢·五十营》所载的每一呼吸气行长度,提出各经的行针时间须结合呼吸次数,以便经气流通,上下相接。这种方法是据古代文献推算气血运行的理论而创立的。

Dredging the Meridians by Connecting Meridian Qi The time that the application of the needling manipulation takes is determined by the different lengths of meridians and the frequency of respiration. The method is from *Liuzhu Zhiwei Zhen Fu* (*Acupuncture Ode of the Subtleties of Flow*), based on the lengths of meridians as recorded in *Lingshu: Mai Du* (*Miraculous Pivot: Courses and Lengths of Meridians*), and the distance that qi travels per respiration, as in *Lingshu: Wushiying* (*Miraculous Pivot: Fifty Circulatory Cycles*), the method points out that the manipulation time of the needle should correlate with the number of respiration times in order to make the meridian qi flow and connect. This technique was established in accordance with the theories of calculating the circulation of qi and blood in ancient works.

●节[jié] ①部位名。指骨节。见《素问·五脏生成》。

②指穴位,为穴位的通称。见《灵枢·九针十二原》。

Jie ① A body part, referring to joints, seen in *Suwen: Wuzang Shengcheng* (*Plain Questions: On the Five Viscera in the Relation to Their Part in Perfecting Life*). ② Referring to acupoints, a general name for acupoints, seen in *Lingshu: Jiu Zhen Shier Yuan* [*Miraculous Pivot: Nine Needles and Twelve Yuan (Primary) Points*].

●截肠[jié cháng] 即脱肛。见该条。

Blockage of Rectum →脱肛(p. 450)

●截根疗法[jié gēn liáo fǎ] 挑治法之别称。见该条。

Root-Cutting Therapy Another name for pricking therapy. →挑治法(p. 438)

●截疟[jié nüè] 经外穴名。见《千金要方》。在胸部,当乳头直下4寸。〈主治〉疟疾、胸胁串痛等。用灸法。

Jienüe (EX-CA) An extra point, seen in *Qianjin Yaofang* (*Essential Prescriptions Worth a Thousand Gold*). 〈Location〉 on the chest, 4 cun directly below the nipple. 〈Indications〉 malaria, wandering pain in the chest and hypochondrium. 〈Method〉 moxibustion.

●解惑[jiě huò] 《内经》刺法名。出《灵枢·刺节真邪》。为刺法五节之一。指中风偏枯一类病后,血气偏虚(正气),实者有余(邪气),左右轻重不相称,身体不能倾斜反侧或俯伏,甚则神志昏乱、意识模糊之类病证,可泻其有余之邪,补其正气的不足,使之达到阴阳平衡。其用针之效验如突然解除迷惑一样迅捷。

Dispelling of Perplexity An acupuncture method in *Neijing* (*The Inner Canon of Huangdi*), from *Ling shu: Cijie Zhenxie* (*Miraculous Pivot: Acupuncture Principles and Diseases*), one of the Five Acupuncture Methods. When patients have windstroke or hemiplegra, the qi and blood (body resistance qi) are deficient and the pathogenic qi (or evil qi) is in excess, therefore, the left and right sides of the body are not balanced. Patients are unable to turn their bodies or lie prostrate, and sometimes have a loss of consciousness. At this time, the excessive evil qi should be reduced and the body resistance qi strength-

ened, so as to balance yin and yang. The efficiency of acupuncture is as quick as the sudden dispelling of doubts.

●解脉[jiě mài] 出《素问·刺腰痛篇》。①指经脉。《医学读书记》谓解脉系指带脉,乃传写之误。②指部位。在膝筋肉分间郄外廉之横脉,即委中(郄中)、委阳穴处。

Jiemai From *Suwen: Ci Yaotong Pian*(*Plain Questions: On Treatment of Lumbago with Acupuncture*), referring to. ①a meridian. In *Yixue Dushu Ji* (*Reading Records of Medicine*), Jiemai is called Dai Meridian, an error in copying. ②a part of the body, vessels in the popliteal fossa, among the muscles and tendons, at the positions where Weizhong(BL 40) and Weiyang(BL 39) are located.

●解溪[jiě xī] 经穴名。出《灵枢·本输》。属足阳明胃经,为本经经穴。又名草鞋带穴。〈定位〉在足背与小腿交界处的横纹中央凹陷中,当拇长伸肌腱与趾长伸肌腱之间(图60.5和图60.3)。〈层次解剖〉皮肤→皮下组织→拇长伸肌腱与趾长伸肌腱之间→距骨。浅层布有足背内侧皮神经及足背皮静脉。深层有腓深神经和胫前动、静脉。〈主治〉头面浮肿、面赤、目赤、头痛、眩晕、腹胀、便秘、下肢痿痹、癫疾、胃热谵语、眉棱骨痛。直刺0.4～0.8寸;可灸。

Jiexi(ST 41) A meridian point, from *Lingshu: Benshu* (*Miraculous Pivot: Meridian Points*), the Jing(River)point of the Stomach Meridian of Foot-Yangming, also called Caoxiedai point. 〈Location〉 in the central depression of the crease between the instep of the foot and leg, between the tendons of the long extensor muscle of the great toe and the long extensor muscle of the toes(Figs. 60. 5&60. 3). 〈Regional anatomy〉 skin→subcutaneous tissue → between tendons of long extensor muscle of great toe and long extensor muscle of toes→talus. In the superficial layer, there are the medial dorsal cutaneous nerves and the subcutaneous veins. In the deep layer, there are the deep peroneal nerve and the anterior tibial artery and vein. 〈Indications〉 edema in the face and hand, flushed face and eye, headache, dizziness, abdominal distention, constipation, paralysis and pain of legs, epilepsy, delirium due to heat in the stomach and supra-orbital pain. 〈Method〉 Puncture perpendicularly 0.4～0.8 cun. Moxibustion is applicable.

●巾针[jīn zhēn] 古代生活用针具。出《灵枢·九针论》。巾,指头巾。此针短小,用于固定巾帛,故名。九针之一的镵针的形状仿自此针。

Scarf Needle A needle used in daily life in ancient times, originally from *Lingshu: Jiu Zhen Lun* (*Miraculous Pivot: On Nine Needles*). "Scarf" means a long strip of material worn over the head. The needle is short and used for fixing the scarf, hence the name. The shape of the shear needle, one of the nine classical needles, is modelled on this one.

●金疮痉[jīn chuāng jìng] 即破伤风。见该条。

Convulsion due to Wound by a Metalic Tool
→破伤风(p. 298)

●金津[jīn jīn] 经外穴名。见"金津玉液"条。

Jinjin(EX-HN 12) An extra point. →金津玉液(p. 202)

●金津玉液[jīn jīn yù yè] 经外穴名。见《医经小学》。〈定位〉在口腔内,当舌下系带左右两侧的静脉上。左侧为金津,右侧为玉液(图20)。〈层次解剖〉粘膜→粘膜下组织→颏舌肌。布有下颌神经的颌神经,舌下神经和面神经鼓索的神经纤维及舌动脉的分支舌深动脉,舌静脉的属支舌深静脉。〈主治〉舌肿痛、口疮、喉痹、失语、呕吐、腹泻、黄疸、消渴,以及口腔溃疡、舌炎、扁桃体炎、急性胃肠炎等。点刺出血。

Jinjin(EX-HN 12), **Yuye**(EX-HN 13) A pair of extra points, originally from *Yijing Xiaoxue*(*Elementary Collection of Medical Classics*). 〈Location〉 in the mouth, on the vein on the left side (Jinjin), and on the right side (Yuye) of the frenulum of the tongue(Fig. 20). 〈Regional anatomy〉mucosa→submucous tissue → genioglossus muscle. There are the gnathic nerve from the mandibular nerve, the hypoglossal nerve, the nervous fibres of the tympanic cord from the facial nerve, the deep lingual artery of the lingual artery and the deep lingual veins to the lingual vein in this area. 〈 Indications 〉 pain and swelling of tongue, aphtha, inflammation of the throat, aphasia, vomiting, diarrhea, jaundice, diabetes, aphthosis, glossitis, tonsillitis, and acute gastroenteritis. 〈Method〉 Prick to cause

bleeding.

●金孔贤[jīn kǒng xián] 人名。明代医家,义乌(今属浙江)人。著《经络发明》。书佚。见《浙江通志》。

Jin Kongxian A physician in the Ming Dynasty, a native of Yiwu (now in Zhejiang Province), the author of *Jingluo Faming* (*Invention on Meridians*), which has been lost, seen in *Zhejiang Tongzhi* (*Annals of Zhejiang Province*).

●金兰循经[jīn lán xún jīng] 为《金兰循经取穴图解》的简称。详见该条。

Jinlan Xunjing (Gold Orchid Book on Meridians) A short name for *Jinlan Xunjing Quxue Tujie* (*Gold Orchid Book With Illustrations for Selecting Points along Meridians*). → 金兰循经取穴图解(p. 203)

●金兰循经取穴图解[jīn lán xún jīng qǔ xué tú jiě] 书名。又称《金兰循经》。元代忽泰必烈著,其子光济铨次,一卷,刊于1303年。其首为脏腑前后二图,记载三阴三阳走属。后论十四经流注且附注释、插图。原书已佚。据载,《十四经发挥》即以此为蓝本著成。

Jinlan Xunjing Quxue Tujie (Gold Orchid Book with Illustrations for Selecting Points along Meridians) A one-volume book, also named *Jinlan Xunjing* (*Gold Orchid Book on Meridians*), written by Hutai Bilie in the Yuan Dynasty, annotated by his son, Hutai Guangji, published in 1303. At the beginning of the book are two pictures of zang-fu organs from the front and back illustrating the distribution and courses of three Yin and three Yang Meridians, followed by a discussion on the cyclical flow of qi and blood in the fourteen meridians with illustrations. The original book is lost. It was recorded that *Shisi Jing Fahui* (*An Elaboration of the Fourteen Meridians*) was compiled on the basis of this book.

●金门[jīn mén] 经穴名。出《针灸甲乙经》。属足太阳膀胱经。为本经郄穴,又名关梁、梁关。〈定位〉在足外侧,当外踝前缘直下,骰骨下缘处(图35.2)。〈层次解剖〉皮肤→皮下组织→腓骨长肌腱及小趾展肌。布有足背外侧皮神经,足外侧缘静脉(小隐静脉)。〈主治〉癫痫、小儿惊风、腰痛、外踝痛、下肢痿痛。直刺0.3～0.5寸;可灸。

Jinmen (BL 63) A meridian point, originally from *Zhenjiu Jia-Yi Jing* (*A-B Classic of Acupuncture and Moxibustion*), the Xi (Cleft) point of the Bladder Meridian of Foot-Taiyang, also called Guanliang, or Liangguan. 〈Location〉 on the lateral side of the foot, directly below the anterior border of the external malleolus, on the lower border of the cuboid bone (Fig. 35.2). 〈Regional anatomy〉 skin → subcutaneous tissue → tendon of long peroneal muscle and abductor muscle of little toe. There are the lateral dorsal cutaneous nerve of the foot and the lateral vein of the foot (the small saphenous vein) in this area. 〈Indications〉 epilepsy, infantile convulsion, pain in the lower back and lateral malleolus, pain and flaccidity of the lower extremities. 〈Method〉 Puncture perpendicularly 0.3～0.5 cun. Moxibustion is applicable.

●金滕玉匮针经[jīn téng yù guì zhēn jīng] 书名。又称《玉匮针经》。三国时吕博(即吕广)撰,已佚。见宋代《崇文总目》。

Jinteng Yugui Zhenjing (Acupuncture Canon of the Gold Bag and Jade Chamber) A book, also called *Yugui Zhenjing* (*Canon of Acupuncture of the Jade Chamber*), written by Lü Bo (Lü Guang) in the Three Kingdoms period (AD 220-280), no longer extant, seen in *Chongwen Zongmu* (*Chong Wen Complete Catalogue*) of the Song Dynasty.

●金冶田[jīn yě tián] 人名。清针灸学家。对灸法深有研究。雷少逸传其学著成《灸法秘传》。参见《灸法秘传》条。

Jin Yetian An expert of acupuncture and moxibustion in the Qing Dynasty, who had great achievements in moxibustion. According to his theory and experience, Lei Shaoyi wrote *Jiufa Michuan* (*Secretly Bequeathed Methods of Moxibustion*). → 灸法秘传(p. 223)

●金针[jīn zhēn] 针具名。①专指用金质制的医用针具。②泛指金属制的医用针具。

1. Gold Needle A kind of needle, made of gold for medical use.

2. Metal Needle A general term given to needles made of metal for medical use.

●金针赋[jīn zhēn fù] 针灸歌赋名。始载《针灸大

全》,全名为《梓歧风谷飞行走气撮要金针赋》。主要论述取穴治疗方法及补泻手法。其中提出烧山火、透天凉等针法,对后世有一定影响。

Jinzhen Fu(Ode to Gold Needle) A ballad on acupuncture and moxibustion, originally recorded in *Zhenjiu Daquan(A Complete Work of Acupuncture and Moxibustion)*, the full name being *Ziqi Fenggu Feixing Zouqi Cuoyao Jinzhen Fu(Ode to Gold Needle Dealing with Ziqi's Essence of Accelerating Qi Circulation over the Meridians like Strong Wind in a Valley)*. Mainly discussing the principles of point selection, treatment and tonification or purgation in acupuncture and moxibustion. The needling methods of setting the mountain on fire and penetrating-heaven coolness were put forward in this book, which have had a great influence on later generations.

●**筋束**[jīn sù] 经穴别名。出《医学入门》。即筋缩。见该条。

Jinshu Another name for Jinsuo (DU 8), a meridian point originally from *Yixue Rumen (An Introduction to Medicine)*. →筋缩(p. 204)

●**筋缩**[jīn suō] 经穴名。出《针灸甲乙经》。属督脉,又名筋束。〈定位〉在背部当后正中线上,第九胸椎棘突下凹陷中(图12.2和图7)。〈层次解剖〉针刺经过的层次结构同脊中穴。浅层主要布有第九胸神经后支的内侧皮支和伴行的动、静脉。深层有棘突间的椎外(后)静脉丛,第九胸神经后支的分支和第九肋间后动、静脉背侧支的分支或属支。〈主治〉癫狂、惊痫抽搐、脊强、背痛、胃痛、黄疸、四肢不收、筋挛拘急。斜刺0.5～1寸;可灸。

Jinsuo(DU 8) A meridian point originally from *Zhenjiu Jia-Yi Jing (A-B Classic of Acupuncture and Moxibustion)*, a point on the Du Meridian, also called Jinsu. 〈Location〉on the back and on the posterior midline, in the depression below the spinous process of the 9th thoracic vertebra (Figs. 12. 2&7). 〈Regional anatomy〉The layer structures of the needle insertion are the same as those in Jizhong (DU 6). In the superficial layer, there are the medial cutaneous branches of the posterior branches of the 9th thoracic nerve and the accompanying artery and vein. In the deep layer, there are the external (posterior) vertebral venous plexus between the adjacent spinous processes, the branches of the posterior branches of the 9th thoracic nerve and the branches or tributaries of the dorsal branches of the 9th posterior intercostal artery and vein. 〈Indications〉manic-depressive disorders, epilepsy, clonic convulsions, stiffness of the back, pain in the lower back, pain in the stomach, jaundice, flaccidity of the limbs in paralysis, spasm of muscles. 〈Method〉Puncture obliquely 0.5～1 cun. Moxibustion is applicable.

●**筋之府**[jīn zhī fǔ] 部位名。指膝部。因其为大筋所聚,故名。

House of Tendons A body part, referring to the knee. It is so named because it is the region where big tendons gather.

●**紧按慢提**[jǐn àn màn tí] 针刺手法名。出《金针赋》。即急插缓提之意。紧按刺激较重,慢提刺激较轻,故亦称重插轻提。

Swift Insertion and Slow Lifting An acupuncture manipulation term, originally from *Jinzhen Fu(Ode to Gold Needle)*, meaning inserting the needle quickly and lifting it slowly in the course of puncturing. It is also named heavy insertion and gentle lifting because swift insertion can achieve stronger stimulation while slow lifting can achieve lighter stimulation.

●**紧提慢按**[jǐn tí màn àn] 针刺手法名。出《金针赋》。即急提缓插之意。紧提刺激较重,慢按刺激较轻,故亦称重提轻插。

Swift Lifting and Slow Insertion An acupuncture manipulation term, originally from *Jinzhen Fu(Ode to Gold Needle)*, meaning lifting the needle quickly and inserting it slowly. It's also named heavy lifting and gentle insertion because heavy lifting can achieve stronger stimulation while slow insertion can achieve lighter stimulation.

●**进**[jìn] 针刺基本手法之一。先将针刺入肌肉部分,根据浅部、较深部、深部,假设为天、人、地三部。所谓"进",即将针从浅部(天部)刺到较深部(人部)或深部(地部),向下刺入的操作过程。《内经》内谓之"推",近代又称为"插"。目的是为了取得针感。参见

持针姿势
Right way to hold a needle

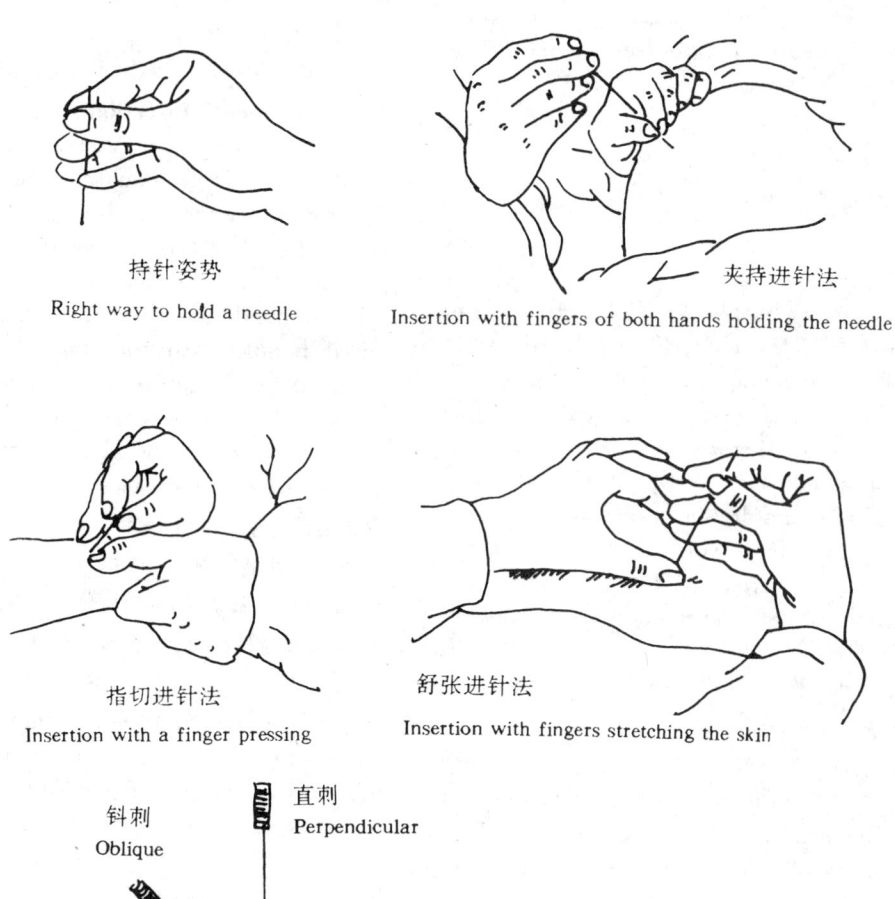

夹持进针法
Insertion with fingers of both hands holding the needle

指切进针法
Insertion with a finger pressing

舒张进针法
Insertion with fingers stretching the skin

斜刺 Oblique
直刺 Perpendicular
横刺 Horizontal
外关 Wàiguān 支沟 Zhīgōu 三阳络 Sānyángluò
针刺的角度
Angle of insertion

图26 进 针 法
Fig. 26 Method of needle insertion

"进法"条。

Insertion One of the basic acupuncture manipulations. First, insert the needle into the muscle; the layers of heaven, human and earth correspond to the shallow, fairly deep and deep parts. Needle insertion is the process of

inserting the needle into the muscle from the superficial part (the heaven layer) into the fairly deep part (the human layer) or the deep part (the earth layer). It was called "pushing" in *Neijing* (*Canon Internal Medicine*) and it is called "sticking in" in modern times. Its purpose is to gain the needling sensation. →进法 (p. 206)

●进法 [jìn fǎ]　针刺手法名。《针经指南》列为十四法之一,谓"进"。《针灸大成》列为十二法之一,谓"进针"。后世之补法三进,泻法一进,均指此而言。参见"进"条。

Method of Insertion　An acupuncture manipulation term. In *Zhenjing Zhinan* (*Guide to the Classics of Acupuncture*), it is listed as one of the fourteen manipulations of acupuncture, called insertion. In *Zhenjiu Dacheng* (*A Great Compendium of Acupuncture and Moxibustion*), it is listed as one of the Twelve Manipulations of acupuncture and called needle insertion. Both the reinforcing method with three thrusting and reducing method with one thrusting of later generations refer to this. →进 (p. 204)

●进针 [jìn zhēn]　针刺手法名。出《针灸大成》,为十二手法之一。参见"进法"。

Inserting the Needle　An acupuncture manipulation term, form *Zhenjiu Dacheng* (*A Great Compendium of Acupuncture and Moxibustion*) one of the twelve needing methods. →进法 (p. 206).

●进针法 [jìn zhēn fǎ]　刺法用语。将针刺入穴位皮下的方法。根据针刺部位的深浅和针身长短的不同,进针方法可灵活掌握。一般要求穿透皮肤时要快,以减轻疼痛感。常用的毫针进针法有:指切进针、提捏进针、舒张进针、夹持进针等。

Method of Needle Insertion　A term in acupuncture, referring to the method of inserting a needle into the skin layer at the acupoint. It can be flexibly mastered according to the depth of the area to be punctured and the length of the needle. Generally it is required that the insertion should be quick enough so as to ease the painful sensation. The common methods of the filiform needle insertion are as follows: finger press insertion, pinch needle insertion, pinch skin needle insertion and tight skin needle insertion.

●进针管 [jìn zhēn guǎn]　针刺辅助用具。系一种用金属或塑料制成的小圆管。管腔可通过毫针,管身应略短于选用的毫针。使用时左手将针管按于穴位上,右手以指弹压管腔露出的针柄,使针迅速刺入皮内,随后去其针管再进行运针。此法可减轻进针的痛感。

Tube for Needle Insertion　An auxiliary tool used in acupuncture. A small tube made of metal or plastic. It should be made so that the filiform needle may go through it and its body should be a bit shorter than the needle. In application, hold the pipe on the acupoint with the left hand, and flick and suppress the exposed handle with the fingers of the right hand so as to get the needle into the skin quickly. After removing the tube, apply the needling manipulation. This method can ease the painful sensation of insertion.

●进针器 [jìn zhēn qì]　针刺辅助工具。一种利用弹簧装置将针迅速刺入皮下以减轻痛感的针刺辅助工具。塑料或金属制成,结构可分置针管、弹簧盒、调节杆和拉条等几部分。将针刺入皮下后,再予手法运针。

Appliance for Needle-Insertion　An auxiliary tool used in acupuncture, which can cause the needle to go quickly into the skin by means of a spring apparatus, thereby easing the painful sensation. It is made of metal or plastic, and composed of a tube, a spring case, a regulating lever and brace. Apply acupuncture manipulations after the needle is inserted into the skin.

●近部取穴 [jìn bù qǔ xué]　即近道取穴。见该条。

Point selection near the Affected Region　→近道取穴 (p. 206)

●近道取穴 [jìn dào qǔ xué]　取穴法之一。又称近部取穴、就近取穴,简称近取。与远道取穴相对。指在病痛的局部或邻近部选穴。

The Combination of Local Points　One of the methods of point selection, also called point selection near the affected region or local point selection, or shortened to local selection. It is the opposite of distant point selection. The method means selecting points in or near

the affected region.

● 近节段取穴 [jìn jié duàn qǔ xué] 现代取穴法的一种。指在临床治疗和针麻时，选用与病痛或手术部位属于同一或邻近的脊髓节段所支配的穴位。局部取穴、邻近取穴均可归属此类。如胸腔病症或手术选取上肢穴，腹腔病症或手术选取下肢穴，也属于此类。在针刺麻醉中，颅脑手术取颧髎，甲状腺手术取扶突，颈部胸部手术取合谷、内关等均是。参见"远节段取穴"条。

Nearby Neural Segment Point Selection
One of the methods of point selection, referring to selecting acupoints located at the same or neighbouring spinal neural segment, as the disease or the area to be operated on pertains to in clinical treatment or acupuncture anesthesia. Local point selection or nearby point selection both belong to this method. Point selection on the upper limbs for diseases or operations of the chest, on the lower limbs for diseases or operations of the abdomen, or for acupuncture anesthesia, the selection of Quanliao (SI 18) for crani ocerebal operations, of Futu (LI 18) for thyroid operations, and of Hegu (LI 4) and Neiguan (PC 6) for operations of the chest or neck are all examples of this method. →远节段取穴 (p. 577)

● 近取 [jìn qǔ] 近道取穴的简称。见该条。

Local Selection The short form for local point selection. →近道取穴 (p. 206)

● 近视 [jìn shì] 即能近怯远症。详见该条。

Short-Sightedness →能近怯远症 (p. 282)

● 噤口痢 [jìn kǒu lì] 痢疾证型之一。见《丹溪心法》。多由疫毒痢、湿热痢演变而来。因湿浊热毒蕴结肠中，邪毒盛实，胃阴复伤，和降失常。或因久病脾胃两伤，中气败损所致。证见下痢，饮食不进，恶心呕吐，甚则消瘦，神疲，舌苔黄腻，脉濡数。治宜祛邪降逆、疏调肠胃。取合谷、天枢、上巨虚、中脘、内关、内庭。

Fasting Dysentery One type of dysentery, seen in *Danxi Xinfa* (*Danxi's Experience*). Generally developing from fulminant dysentery or dysentery due to damp-heat. Caused by the retention of damp-heat in the large intestine, excess pathogens impaired stomach-yin and the failure of the stomach-qi to descend, or to the impairment of both the spleen and stomach resulting from prolonged illness and qi-deficiency in the middle-jiao. 〈Manifestations〉 dysentery, anorexia, nausea and vomiting, in severe cases, emaciation and listlessness yellowish and greasy tongue coating, relaxed and rapid pulse. 〈Treatment principle〉 Remove pathogenic factors and descend the adversed-qi, coordinate the function of the stomach and intestine. 〈Point selection〉 Hegu (LI 4), Tianshu (ST 25), Shangjuxu (ST 37), Zhongwan (RN 12), Neiguan (PC 6) and Neiting (ST 44).

● 京骨 [jīng gǔ] ①经穴名。出《灵枢·本输》。属足太阳膀胱经，为本经原穴，又名大骨。〈定位〉在足外侧，第五跖骨粗隆下方，赤白肉际处（图35.2）。〈层次解剖〉皮肤→皮下组织→小趾展肌。布有足背外侧皮神经，足外侧缘静脉。〈主治〉癫痫、头痛、目翳、项强、腰腿疼、膝痛、脚挛。直刺0.3～0.5寸；可灸。②骨骼部位名。指第五跖骨粗隆。

1. **Jinggu** (BL 64) A meridian point, originally from *Lingshu*: *Benshu* (*Miraculous Pivot*; *Meridian Points*), the Yuan (Primary) Point of Bladder Meridian of Foot-Taiyang, also called Dagu. 〈Location〉 on the lateral side of the foot, below the tuberosity of the 5th metatarsal bone, at the junction of the red and white skin (Fig. 35.2). 〈Regional anatomy〉 skin→subcutaneous tissue→abductor muscle of little toe. There are the lateral dorsal cutaneous nerve of the foot and the lateral vein of the foot (the small saphenous vein) in this area. 〈Indications〉 epilepsy, headache, blurred vision, neck rigidity, pain in the lower back, leg and knee, spasm of feet. 〈Method〉 Puncture perpendicularly 0.3～0.5 cun. Moxibustion is applicable.

2. **Jinggu** A bone, referring to the tuberosity of the 5th metatarsal bone.

● 京门 [jīng mén] 经穴名。出《针灸甲乙经》。属足少阳胆经，为肾之募穴。又名气府、气俞。〈定位〉在侧腰部，章门后1.8寸，当第十二肋骨游离端的下方（图7和图23）。〈层次解剖〉皮肤→皮下组织→腹外斜肌→腹内斜肌→腹横肌。浅层布有第十一、十二胸神经前支的外侧皮支及伴行的动、静脉。深层有第十一、十二胸神经前支的肌支和相应的肋间、肋下动、静

脉。〈主治〉肠鸣、泄泻、腹胀、腰胁痛。斜刺0.5~0.8寸；可灸。

Jingmen (GB 25)　A meridian point, originally from *Zhenjiu Jia-Yi Jing* (*A-B Classic of Acupuncture and Moxibustion*), a point on the Gallbladder Meridian of Foot-Shaoyang, the Front-Mu point of the kidney, also named Qifu, Qishu. 〈Location〉on the lateral side of the waist, 1.8 cun posterior to Zhangmen (LR 13), below the free end of the 12th rib (Figs. 7&23). 〈Regional anatomy〉skin→subcutaneous tissue→external oblique muscle of abdomen→internal oblique muscle of abdomen→transverse muscle of abdomen. In the superficial layer, there are the lateral cutaneous branches of the anterior branches of the 11th and 12th thoracic nerves and the accompanying arteries and veins. In the deep layer, there are the muscular branches of the anterior branches of the 11th and 12th thoracic nerves and the related intercostal and subcostal arteries and veins. 〈Indications〉borborygmus, diarrhea, abdominal distension, pain in the loin and hypochondriac region. 〈Method〉Puncture obliquely 0.5~0.8 cun. Moxibustion is applicable.

●经闭 [jīng bì]　病名。出《妇人良方大全》。又名不月、月闭、不月水、月水不来、月经不通、血闭、月事不来、月事不通、月不通、月使不来、月水不通、月经不行、经水不行、经水不通、经闭不利、经脉不行、经脉不通、经候水行、歇、歇经等。包括女子暗闭，女子暗闭经。指女子年龄超过18岁，仍不见月经来潮，或曾来过月经，但又连续闭止三个月以上，除妊娠、哺乳期等生理性闭经外，均称之为经闭。临床有血亏，肝肾不足，脾胃虚弱，气滞血瘀，寒凝血滞，痰湿阻滞等不同类型。详见各条。

Amenorrhea　A disease, originally *Furen Liangfang Daquan* (*A Complete Work of Effective Prescriptions for Women*), also called no menses, menses stoppage, no menstrual blood, no arrival of menstrual flow, obstruction of menses, blood stoppage, disappearance of menses, obstruction of menstruation, blocked menses, no arrival of menses, obstruction of menstrual flow, obstructed menstruation, obstructed menstrual flow, obstruction of menstrual flow, menstrual stop and retention, no flow of menstrual blood, obstruction of menstrual blood, no flow of menses, pause, or menopause, etc. It includes secret stoppage of women and women's secret stoppage of menses. All those who have never menstruated until they are over 18 years old or those who ever had menstruation and have had no menses for three successive months or more, except in pregnancy or breast feeding, are patients with amenorrhea. Amenorrhea can be clinically divided into the following types—amenorrhea due to blood deficiency, amenorrhea due to deficiency of the liver and kidney, amenorrhea due to weakness of the spleen and stomach, amenorrhea due to stagnation of qi and blood stasis, amenorrhea due to blood stasis caused by accumulation of pathogenic cold and Amenorrhea due to stagnation of phlegm-dampness, etc. →血亏经闭(p. 525)、肝肾不足经闭(p. 126)、脾胃虚弱经闭(p. 295)、气滞血瘀经闭(p. 315)、寒凝血滞经闭(p. 155)、痰湿阻滞经闭(p. 425)

●经闭不利 [jīng bì bù lì]　即经闭。详见该条。

Amenorrhea due to Menstual Disorder　→经闭(p. 208)

●经别 [jīng bié]　十二经别之简称。见该条。

Divergent Meridians　Shortened term for Divergent Meridians of the Twelve Regular Meridians. →十二经别(p. 376)

●经不调 [jīng bù tiáo]　即月经不调。详见该条。

Abnormal Menstruation　→月经不调(p. 578)

●经迟 [jīng chí]　即经行后期。详见该条。

Later Menstruation than Usual　→经行后期(p. 214)

●经断前后诸症 [jīng duàn qián hòu zhū zhèng]　即绝经前后诸证。详见该条。

Menopausal Syndromes　→绝经前后诸证(p. 228)

●经候不调 [jīng hòu bù tiáo]　即月经不调。详见该条。

Irregular Menstrual Flow→月经不调(p. 578)

●经候不行 [jīng hòu bù xíng]　即经闭。详见该条。

No Flow of Menses　→经闭(p. 208)

●经候不匀 [jīng hòu bù yún]　即月经不调。详见该

条。

Disorder of Menstruation →月经不调 (p. 578)

●经后腹痛 [jīng hòu fù tòng] 即痛经。详见该条。

Abdominal Pain After Menstruation. →痛经 (p. 444)

●经筋 [jīng jīn] 十二经筋之简称。见该条。

Tendons The simple name for muscles along the Twelve Regular Meridians. →十二经筋 (p. 377)

●经乱 [jīng luàn] 即经行先后无定期。详见该条。

Menstruation Irregularity →经行先后无定期 (p. 214)

●经络 [jīng luò] 人体运行气血的通道。出《灵枢·经脉》。包括经脉和络脉两部分，其中纵行的干线称为经脉，由经脉分出网络全身各个部位的分支称为络脉。经络的主要内容有：十二经脉、十二经别、奇经八脉、十五络脉、十二经筋、十二皮部等。其中经脉方面以十二经脉为主，络脉方面以十五络脉为主，它们纵横交贯，遍布全身，将人体内外、脏腑、肢节联成了一个有机的整体。详见各条。

Meridians and Collaterals The pathways for the circulation of qi and blood throughout the human body, originally form *Lingshu: Jingmai* (*Miraculous Pivot: Meridians*), composed of two parts—meridians and collaterals. The ones running longitudinally are termed meridians; the ones branching out of the meridians and connecting all portions of the body are termed collaterals. This system of meridians and collaterals includes: Twelve Regular Meridians, Branches of the Twelve Regular Meridians Eight Extra Meridians, Fifteen Collaterals, Muscles along the Twelve Regular Meridians and Twelve Cutaneous Regions, etc. Among them, the Twelve Regular Meridians are the main meridians, while the Fifteen Collaterals are the main collaterals. They run in length and breadth, scattering throughout the whole body and connecting the interior and exterior, zang-fu organs and extremities, thus forming an organic integrity.

●经络感传现象 [jīng luò gǎn chuán xiàn xiàng] 又称经络现象、经络敏感现象或针灸感应现象。指感觉沿经络循行路线传导或循经出现的各种皮肤病症。这种现象在某些人身上可因针刺、艾灸、通电、按压等刺激穴位或在气功练功的过程中产生，其感觉因刺激原和个体之不同而有所差异。如针刺多感酸、胀、重、麻；艾灸则现热气感；低频脉冲电可有电麻感；按压可有胀、麻感等。感传一般呈带状、线状或放射状，其路线与经络主干的分布基本相符，有的还出现表里经之间，手足同名经之间的互传现象。感传速度一般缓慢，能为受试者清楚描述，而且可呈双向性传导，这种传导可被机械压迫或局部注射麻醉剂所阻断，刺激一旦停止，感传也就逐渐减弱乃至消失。经络感传现象的另一种表现，有沿经抽痛，皮疹，脱毛和引起皮肤出现红线、白线、皮丘带、过敏带、麻木带等特异现象。经络感传现象对于研究经络实质，有重要意义。

Meridian Transmission Phenomenon Also named meridian phenomenon, acupuncture reaction phenomenon, referring to the transmission of the sensation induced during needling along the course of the meridians, or all kinds of cutaneous diseases ocurring along the meridians. In some people, the phenomenon may result from needling, moxibustion, electrification, and pressure, stimulating acupoints or in the process of practising qi gong. The sensations may vary due to different stimuli and constitutions. For instance, soreness, distension, heaviness and numbness are mostly caused by needling; scorching heat by moxibustion; siderant numbness by low frequency pulse current; distension and numbness by pressure, etc. The sensations are generally transmitted in the shape of belt, thread and radioactivity; the transmitting routes basically conform with how the meridians and collaterals distribute, some times mutual transmission between the meridian of interior and exterior and between the hand and foot of the same name meridians occurs. The speed of transmission is generally slow and can clearly be depicted by tests. The sensations may also present two way conduction which can be blocked by machinery pressing and local injection of anesthetics. In this case the transmission will, as soon as the stimulation stops, fade until it is gone altogether. Another phenomenon of meridian transmission may be

manifested by twitching pain along the meridians, skin rash, trichomadesis and by some peculiar symptoms such as redline whiteline skin rash zone, allergic zone, numbness zone and so on. Meridian transmission phenomenon is very significant for research of the essence of meridians and collaterals.

● 经络汇编 [jīng luò huì biān] 书名。明清间翟良撰，两卷，刊于1628年。此书以十四经排列顺序，联系脏腑、经络、经穴予以论述，并附脏腑经脉图、手足经起止图、内景图、奇经八脉论、歌诀等。另对经络的许多概念有所阐发。

Jingluo Huibian (A Collection of Meridians and Collaterals) A book in 2 volumes, written by Zhai Liang in the Ming and Qing Dynasties, published in 1628. The book includes the order of the Fourteen Meridians, an exposition on the connections of the zang-fu meridians and meridian points. Attached to the book are illustrations of zang-fu and meridians, an illustration of the start and end of hand and foot meridians, an illustration of the inner situation, a theory on the Eight Extra Meridians, and some verses, etc., In addition, many approaches on meridians are expounded in it.

● 经络笺注 [jīng luò jiān zhù] 书名。明代韦编编撰，男明辅校订，两卷，成书于1636年，未刊行。其以形体为纲，从头至足分为六十六纲，每纲中又分小目，分别归属于相应脏腑、经络。

Jingluo Jianzhu (Notes and Commentary on Meridians and Collaterals) A book in 2 volumes written by Wei Bian in the Ming dynasty and collated by Nan Mingfu, completed in 1636, but not published. In the book, the shape of the human body was taken as the key link, the portions from head to foot were divided into 66 key-links, each of which was in turn subdivided into a certain number of items, which pertain respectively to their corresponding zang-fu organs and meridians.

● 经络经穴玻璃人 [jīng luò jīng xué bō lí rén] 教具名。为直立健康男子，透过有机玻璃外壳能看到骨骼、内脏、十四经循行路线及三百六十一个穴位的位置。其中的脏腑、经络均可发光。1958年由上海医学模型厂与上海中医学院协作制作。

Glass Statue with Meridians and Acupoints A teaching instrument modelled on a standing healthy man with bones, internal organs, courses of the fourteen meridians and the locations of 361 acupoints which can be seen through the outer covering made of plexiglass, and among them, both the zang-fu organs and the acupoints can glow. It was made by Shanghai Medical Model Factory in cooperation with Shanghai College of Traditional Chinese Medicine in 1958.

● 经络考 [jīng luò kǎo] 书名。明代张三锡撰，一卷。为《医学六要》之一。其采用多部著作，对经络穴位进行考订。该书刊于1609年。

Jingluo Kao (Study on Meridians and Collaterals) A book of a single volume written by Zhang Sanxi in the Ming Dynasty, one part of *Yixue Liu Yao (Six Essentials of Medicine)*. A number of works were employed for the checking of the meridians and acupoints. It was published in 1609.

● 经络敏感现象 [jīng luò mǐn gǎn xiàn xiàng] 又称经络感传现象。见该条。

Meridian Sensation Phenomenon →经络感传现象 (p. 209)

● 经络全书 [jīng luò quán shū] 书名。由明代沈子禄《经络分野》与徐师曾的《经络枢要》合编而成。清代尤乘重辑订，共四册，刊于1688年。

Jingluo Quanshu (A Complete Work on Meridians and Collaterals) A book compiled from *Jingluo Fen Ye (Separate Expositions of Meridians and Collaterals)* by Shen Zilu and *Jingluoshu Yao (Essentials of Meridians and Collaterals)* by Xu Shizeng in the Ming Dynasty. It was compiled and checked again by You Cheng in the Qing. Dynasty It was recompiled into four volumes and published in 1688.

● 经络枢要 [jīng luò shū yào] 书名。明代徐师曾撰。全书分原病、阴阳、脏腑、营卫、经络、常经（即十二经）、奇经、人迎、气口、三部、诊脉、清浊、客感、传变十四篇，并引各家之论，加以发挥。参见"经络全书"条。

Jingluo Shuyao (The Pivot of Meridians and Collaterals) A book written by Xu Shizeng in the Ming Dynasty, including 14 chapters—

the Origin of Diseases, Yin-Yang, Zang-Fu, Ying-Wei, Meridians and Collaterals, Regular Meridians (i. e. the 12 Regular Meridians), Extra Meridians, Renying, Qi-Emersion, Three Portions, Pulse-Feeling Clearness and Turbidity, Affection by Exopathogen and Transmission. Viewpoints of different schools were cited and elaborated in the book. →经络全书(p. 210)

●经络现象[jīng luò xiàn xiàng] 又名经络感传现象。见该条。

Meridian Phenomenon Also named meridian transmission. →经络感传现象(p. 209)

●经络穴区带[jīng luò xué qū dài] 指疾病反映于体表的敏感带和区域,其部位与经络穴位相符而较宽广。临床上可在相关的穴区带内查找敏感点(穴)进行针灸等法治疗,故称经络穴区带疗法。

Acupuncture Zone of Meridians Referring to the sensitive zone and area represented on the body surface due to diseases. The location of the zones and areas are in conformity with the positions of the acupoints, but are a little wider. In clinic the methods of acupuncture and moxibustion are adopted for the treatment of diseases by looking for the sensitive points in the related acupoint zone; thus acupoint zone therapy is named.

●经脉[jīng mài] 出《灵枢·经脉》等。是运行气血的主要通道。"经"有路经的意思,是经络系统中大的、纵行的主干道,其部位多循行于深部,包括十二经脉与奇经八脉等。参见"经络"条。

Meridians Originally from *Lingshu*: *Jing Mai*(*Miraculous Pivot*; *Meridians*), the principal pathway for the flow of qi and blood. In the meridian system, "经" means "passage", referring to the major conduits which are distributed longitudinally and circulate in the deep area of the body, includes the twelve meridians and the eight extra meridians, etc. →经络(p. 209)

●经脉不调[jīng mài bù tiáo] 即月经不调。详见该条。

Irregular Menstrual Vessel Another name for irregualr menstruation. →月经不调(p. 578)

●经脉不通[jīng mài bù tōng] 即经闭。详见该条。

Obstruction of Menstrual Blood Another name for amenorrhea. →经闭(p. 208)

●经脉不行[jīng mài bù xíng] 即经闭。详见该条。

No Flow of Menstrual Blood Another name for amenorrhea. →经闭(p. 208)

●经脉分图[jīng mài fēn tú] 书名。清代吴之英撰,罗绍骥绘图,四卷,刊于1900年。为《寿栎庐丛书》之六。其经脉次序按手足三阳三阴排列,与一般按流注顺序不同。后论奇经,并作了经络穴位的考释。

Jingmai Fentu (Illustrated Book on Meridians) A book in 4 volumes, written by Wu Zhiying in the Qing Dynasty with illustrations by Luo Shaoji, published in 1900, the 6th volume of *Shou Yuelu Congshu*(*A Series of Books of Shou Yuelu*). In the book meridians are arranged in order of the three yangs and three yins of hand and foot, which is different from the usual order of circulation. In the latter part of the book, the extra meridians are expounded. The locations of the acupoints were checked and interpreted.

●经脉分野[jīng mài fēn yě] 书名。明代沈子禄撰。书中按部位分述经络的循行分布。其内容为《类经图翼》汲取。参见"经络全书"条。

Jingmai Fenye (Separate Exposition on Meridians) A book, written by Shen Zilu in the Ming Dynasty, in which the courses and distributions of the meridians are discussed according to where the meridians lie. *Leijing Tuyi*(*Illustrated Supplementary to the Classified Canon*) is a derivation of its contents. →经络全书(p. 210)

●经脉图考[jīng mài tú kǎo] 书名。清代陈惠畴撰,四卷,刊于1878。卷一,总论人体内景、周身骨度、经脉循行要穴等;卷二—三,论十二经脉经穴循行主病、图象及歌诀;卷四,论奇经的循行主病及诸部经络循行发明。对各部经脉考证详细,并附插图。

Jingmai Tukao (An Illustrated Book on Meridians) A book in 4 volumes, written by Chen Huichou in the Qing Dynasty, published in 1878. Vol. I includes a general comment on the inner situation of the human body, bone-lengths and the chief points of the meridians. Vols. II and III deal with a study on the syndromes occurring in the circulations

of the twelve regular meridians and pictures of their circulations and verses. Vol. IV is a study of the syndromes occurring in the circulation of the extra meridians and an elucidation of the circulation of meridians and collaterals of each part. A detailed research is made on the meridians of each part with illustrations attached.

●经脉之海[jīng mài zhī hǎi] 又称冲脉。见该条。

Sea of Meridians Also called Chong Meridian. →冲脉(p. 48)

●经门四花[jīng mén sì huā] 组合穴名。见《医学入门》。见"四花"条。

Jing Men Sihua A set of acupoints, seen in *Yixue Rumen(An Introduction to Medicine)*. →四花(p. 414)

●经气[jīng qì] 出《素问·离合真邪论》。指经络中传导输注的气，也称脉气，又称真气。属人体的正气。包括先天之气与后天之气，即人体生命活动的根本肾气(原气)和水谷精微所化生的营气、卫气，以及天阳之气等。针灸治疗对经气十分注重，所谓候气、得气、调气及失气等，均关系到经气。

Meridian Qi Originally from *Suwen: Lihe Zhenxie Lun(Plain Questions: Treatise on the Parting and Meeting of That Which is Beneficial and That Which is Harmful)*. Refers to the qi flowing in the meridians and collaterals, also named vessel qi or genuine qi and acquired qi, or the kidney qi[Yuan(primary) qi] of all vital activities of the human body and ying qi, wei qi, and natural yang qi derived from food essense, etc. Much attention is paid to meridian qi in acupuncture and moxibustion therapy. "Waiting for qi", "arrival of qi", "regulating qi," "loss of qi" and so on are all related to meridian qi.

●经气不调[jīng qì bù tiáo] 即月经不调。详见该条。

Irregular Menstrual Qi Another name for irregular menstruation. →月经不调(p. 578)

●经前便血[jīng qián biàn xuě] 病证名。见《简明中医妇科学》。指每月行经前一、二日，大便下血。多因素嗜辛辣燥热之物，热郁肠中。大肠与胞宫并域而居，当行经之前，胞中气血俱盛，引动肠中郁热，迫血下行所致。症见经前大便下血，色深红，面赤唇干，咽燥口苦，渴喜冷饮，头晕心烦，经行量少，色紫红稠粘等。治宜清热凉血止血。取大肠俞、上巨虚、血海、承山、次髎、二白。

Hemafecia Before Menstruation A disease, seen in *Jianming Zhongyi Fukexue(A Concise Gynecology of Traditional Chinese Medicine)*, referring to bloody stools one or two days before each menstrual period. Mostly caused by the excessive intake of pungent, dry and hot foods, and prolonged stagnation of heat in the intestine. The large intestine and the uterus are neighbours in the same region and before menstruation, the excessive qi and blood in the uterus can induce the stagnation of heat in the intestine, which leads to the extravasation of blood. 〈Manifestations〉 bloody stools before menstruation with dark-red colour, flushed complexion and dryness of the lip, dry throat, bitter taste, thirst relieved by cold drinks, dizziness and irritability, scanty and sticky menstruation with purplish red color, etc. 〈Treatement principle〉 Clear heat, remove heat from blood and arrest bleeding. 〈Point selection〉 Dachangshu(BL 25), Shangjuxu(ST 37), Xuehai(SP 10), Chengshan(BL 57), Ciliao(BL 32) and Erbai(EX-UE 2)

●经前腹痛[jīng qián fù tòng] 即痛经的别名。详见该条。

Lower Abdominal Pain Before Menstruation Another name for dysmenorrhea. →痛经(p. 444)

●经前脐下痛[jīng qián qí xià tòng] 病证名。指经前三、五日，脐下作痛如刀刺，寒热交作，经血下如黑豆汁样。多因寒湿凝滞所致。治宜温经化湿。取关元、气海、足三里、三阴交。

Pain Below the Umbilicus Before Menstruation A disease, referring to a stabbing pain below the umbilicus 3-5 days before menstruation, and alternate attacks of chills and fever. The menses appears as if it were the juice of black soya bean. Mostly due to the coagulation of cold and damp. 〈Treament principle〉Warm the meridians and resolve dampness. 〈Points selection〉 Guanyuan(RN 4), Qihai(RN 6), Zusanli(ST 36) and Sanyinjiao(SP 6).

●经渠[jīng qú]　经穴名。出《灵枢·本输》。属手太阴肺经,为本经经穴。〈定位〉在前臂掌面桡侧,桡骨茎突与桡动脉之间凹陷处,腕横纹上1寸(图48和图16)。〈层次解剖〉皮肤→皮下组织→肱桡肌腱尺侧缘→旋前方肌。浅层布有前臂外侧皮神经和桡神经浅支。深层有桡动、静脉。〈主治〉咳嗽、气喘、喉痹、胸部胀满、掌中热、胸背痛。直刺0.2～0.3寸;禁灸。

Jingqu (LU 8)　A meridian point originally from *Lingshu: Benshu* (*Miraculous Pivot: Meridian Points*), the Jing(River)point of the Lung Meridian of Hand Tai-yin. 〈Location〉on the radial side of the palmar surface of the forearm, 1 cun above the crease of the wrist, in the depression between the styloid process of the radius and radial artery (Figs. 48&16). 〈Regional anatomy〉skin→subcutaneous tissue→ulnar border of tendon of brachioradial muscle→quadrate pronator muscle. In the superficial layer, there are the lateral cutaneous nerve of the forearm and the superficial branches of the radial nerve. In the deep layer, there are the radial artery and vein. 〈Indications〉cough, dyspnea, sore throat, distension and fullness in the chest, feverish sensation in the palm, pain in the chest and back. 〈Method〉Puncture perpendicularly 0.2～0.3 cun. Moxibustion is forbidden.

●经始[jīng shǐ]　经穴别名。出《针灸甲乙经》,即少冲。见该条。

Jingshi　Another name for Shaochong (HT 9), a meridian point originally from *Zhenjiu Jia-Yi Jing* (*A-B Classic of Acupuncture and Moxibustion*). →少冲(p. 356)

●经水[jīng shuǐ]　出《灵枢·经水》。又称十二经水。指当时大地上的清、渭、海、湖、汝、渑、淮、江、河、济、漳等十二条河流,用水流来比喻十二经脉气血运行的情况。

Meridian Waters　Originally from *Lingshu: Jing Shui* (*Miraculous Pivot: Meridian Waters*), also named Twelve Meridian Waters, referring to the twelve rivers on earth at that time, the Qing, Wei, Hai, Hu, Ru, Sheng, Huai, Jiang, He, Ji and Zhang, the flow of which is used to show how the qi and blood of the Twelve Regular Meridians flow.

●经水不定[jīng shuǐ bù dìng]　即月经不调。详见该条。

Unfixed Amount of Menstrual Flow→月经不调(p. 578)

●经水不调[jīng shuǐ bù tiáo]　即月经不调。详见该条。

Irregular Menstrual Flow　→月经不调(p. 578)

●经水不通[jīng shuǐ bù tōng]　即经闭。详见该条。

Obstruction of Menstrual Flow　Another name for amenorrhea. →经闭(p. 208)

●经水不行[jīng shuǐ bù xíng]　即经闭。详见该条。

No Menstrual Flow　Another name for amenorrhea. →经闭(p. 208)

●经水后期[jīng shuǐ hòu qī]　即经行后期。详见该条。

Postponed Menstrual Cycle　Another name for delayed menstrual cycle. →经行后期(p. 214)

●经水否涩[jīng shuǐ pǐ sè]　即月经过少。详见该条。

Hard Menstruation Flow　Another name for scanty menstruation. →月经过少(p. 579)

●经水涩少[jīng shuǐ sè shǎo]　即月经过少。详见该条。

Difficult and Scanty Menstruation　Another name for scanty menstruation. →月经过少(p. 579)

●经水无常[jīng shuǐ wú cháng]　①月经不调的别名。详见该条。②经行先后无定期的别名。详见该条。

Disorder of Menstrual Flow　Another name for ①irregular menstruation. →月经不调(p. 578)②menstruation in an unfixed (either preceded or delayed) period. →经行先后无定期(p. 214)

●经水先后无定期[jīng shuǐ xiān hòu wú dìng qī]　经行先后无定期的别名。详见该条。

Irregular Menstrual Flow　Another name for menstruation in an unfixed (either preceded or delayed) period. →经行先后无定期(p. 214)

●经水先期[jīng shuǐ xiān qī]　即经行先期的别名。详见该条。

Preceded Menstrual Flow　Another name for preceded menstrual cycle. →经行先期(p. 214)

●经隧[jīng suì]　经络名。出《素问·调经论》等。经

隧，指潜布于体表以下，运行气血的经络通道。

Human Tunnels An archaic name for meridians and collaterals, originally from *Suwen: Tiaojing Lun* (*Plain Questions: On the Regulations of Meridians*). "Tunnels" here refers to the meridians and collaterals which distribute beneath the skin for circulating qi and blood.

●经外奇穴[jīng wài qí xué] 经外穴的别名。见该条。

Extraordinary Points →经外穴(p.214)

●经外穴[jīng wài xué] ①腧穴分类名。见"腧穴"条。②系指尚未纳入十四经系统，但其临床有奇效的穴位。又称经外奇穴，简称奇穴，或称奇输。是在"阿是穴"的基础上发展而来的。其有明确位置，并有定名的，称有名奇穴；一些仅有明确位置，但尚未定名的则称为无名奇穴。前者居多，而后者为数较少。这类腧穴的主治性能较单纯，多数对某些病证有特殊的疗效。

Extra Points ①A category of acupoints. →腧穴(p.) ②Referring to the points which are not classified into the Fourteen Meridians, but have magical clinical effect. They are also called extraordinary points, magical points or magical acupoints. These points developed from "Ashi Points". The ones with definite locations and names are called namable extra points, and the ones with definite locations without names are called namelsss extra points. Of all these points, the former have the majority and the latter the minority. The indications of these points are simple, and most of them have special effects for certain diseases.

●经行腹痛[jīng xíng fù tòng] 即痛经。详见该条。

Abdominal Pain During Menstruation Another name for dysmenorrhea. →痛经(p.444)

●经行后期[jīng xíng hòu qī] 病名。又称月经落后、经水后期、经迟、过期经行等。指月经来潮比正常周期推迟一周以上。临床有血虚经行后期，血寒经行后期，肾虚经行后期，气滞经行后期，血瘀经行后期。详见各条。

Delayed Menstruation A disease, also called postdated menstruation, postponed menstrual cycle, later-than-usual menstruation or delayed menstrual period, etc., referring to the occurrence of menstruation over a week later than normal. Clinically, it is divided into delayed menstruation due to blood deficiency, delayed menstruation due to cold in blood, delayed menstruation due to kidney deficiency, delayed menstruation due to qi stagnation, and delayed menstruation due to blood stagnation. →血虚经行后期(p.528)、血寒经行后期(p.525)、肾虚经行后期(p.366)、气滞经行后期(p.314)、血瘀经行后期(p.530)。

●经行或前或后[jīng xíng huò qián huò hòu] 即经行先后无定期。详见该条。

Either Preceded or Delayed Menstruation →经行先后无定期(p.214)

●经行先后无定期[jīng xíng xiān hòu wú dìng qī] 病名。又称经行或前或后、经乱、经水先后无定期、经水无常、经血不定等。指月经来潮或提前，或错后，经期不规律。多因肝郁，肾虚所致。详见"肝郁经行先后无定期"、"肾虚经行先后无定期"条。

Menstruation in an Unfixed (Either Preceded or Delayed) Period A disease, also called either preceded or delayed menstruation, disordered menstruation, menstrual flow in an unfixed (either preceded or delayed) period, uncertain menstruation, or changeable menstruation, etc. The menstrual period occurs irregularly, sometimes earlier or sometimes later than the due date. It is mostly caused by liver-qi stagnation and kidney deficiency. →肝郁经行先后无定期(p.127)、肾虚经行先后无定期(p.366)

●经行先期[jīng xíng xiān qī] 病名。又称月经先期、一月经再行、经水先期、经早等。指月经来潮比正常周期提前一周以上，甚或一月两至者。临床有血热经行先期，虚热经行先期，气虚经行先期，肝郁经行先期等。详见各条。

Preceded Menstrual Cycle A disease, also named antedated menstruation, two menstruations in a month, preceded menstrual cycle, earlier-than-usual menstrual period, etc. Refers to menstruation occurring over a week earlier than normal, or menstruation occurring twice a month. Clinically, it is divided into advanced menstrual period due to heat in blood, and preceded menstrual period due to deficient heat, preceded menstrual period due to qi defi-

ciency, preceded menstrual period due to liver-qi stagnation. →血热经行先期(p. 527)、虚热经行先期(p. 516)、气虚经行先期(p. 310)、肝郁经行先期(p. 128)

●经穴[jīng xué] ①五腧穴之一。经穴多位于腕踝关节以上,喻脉气流注,象水之长流。用于气喘、咳嗽、寒热、咽喉不利等。参见"五腧穴"条。②十四经穴的简称。参见"十四经穴"条。

1. **Jing (River) Points** One of the Five Shu Points, mostly located above the ankle and wrist. They are imaged as the flow of water, representing the circulation of qi in the meridians. Jing (River) points are used to treat asthma, cough, chill and fever, sore throat, etc. → 五腧穴(p. 479)

2. **Meridian Points** A short form for the points on the Fourteen Meridians. →十四经穴(p. 380)

●经穴测定[jīng xué cè dìng] 近代从皮肤的电现象研究,发现穴位部的皮肤电阻一般较低,利用经穴测定仪可测定穴位的导电量,分析各经代表性穴位的导电量高低,可以推断各经气血的盛衰现象。其代表穴位多采用原穴或井穴、郄穴及背俞穴等。测定须在安静的情况下进行,注意避免各种干扰因素,根据测定的结果,分析左右两侧经穴导电量的高低和差数。一般以高出其他穴位1/3者为高数,低出1/3者为低数。高数多表示病情属实,低数表示属虚,左右两侧同名经穴相差数在一倍以上者,表示该经有病变。此法仍应参合四诊八纲进行综合分析,才能得出比较正确的结论。

Acupoint Electrometry It has been found in Recent studies on the skin electricity that the electric resistance of the skin of a point is usually lower than that of the skin areas without points. The electrical conductivity of a point may be determined by an acupoint surveying apparatus. Analysing the conductivity of representative points of each meridian helps the doctor to know whether the condition of qi and blood in each meridian is weak or strong. The representative points are the Yuan (Primary) points, Jing (Well) points, Xi (Cleft) points, or Back-Shu points. Analysis must be carried out in a quiet environment without interference. With the results, compare the electrical conductivities of two sides. Usually, the conductivity of a point 1/3 higher than that of other points is considered high, and 1/3 lower than that of other points low. A high indicates excess, and a low number indicates deficiency. Difference between two points of the same name on two sides of the body is also important, indicating that the meridian has a disease. This method should also be combined with the four diagnostic methods and the eight principles so as to get a comprehensive analysis of the condition, and then a correct conclusion can be drawn.

●经穴发明[jīng xué fā míng] 书名。明代徐春甫撰。其另撰《针灸直指》,同编入《古今医统》第六、七卷,成书于1556年。

Jingxue Faming (Invention on Meridian Points) A book written by Xu Chunfu in the Ming Dynasty, who was also the author of *Zhenjiu Zhizhi (Straightforward Exposition of Acupuncture and Moxibustion)*. The two books mentioned above were put together into Vols. 6 and 7 of *Gu Jin Yi Tong (The General Medicine of the Past and Present)*.

●经穴汇解[jīng xué huì jiě] 书名。日本原昌克撰,八卷,刊于1893年。引用二十八种书籍,分部、经详考穴位,并收集263个奇穴,是一部考证穴位的专书。

Jingxue Huijie (Collective Exposition on Meridian Points) A book of 8 volumes on the points, written by a Japanese Hara Masakatsu, published in 1893. The author quoted from 28 books, gave detailed textual studies on the points and collected 263 extra points. This is a special book on the study of points.

●经穴诊断法[jīng xué zhěn duàn fǎ] 指通过经络、穴位的检查以诊断病症的方法。有体表按诊、皮肤电测定(经穴测定)及知热感度测定等,而以前者为主。其中包括体表的审视,用指切、循摸、抚扣、按压等方法,判断经络穴位温度的变异和气血虚实现象,指导针灸治疗。临床上一般用拇指的指腹,沿经络部位轻轻滑动,或用拇、食指轻轻撮捏,以探索浅层的异常反应;用稍重的按压、揉动的方法,以探索较深层的异常反应。要求用力均匀,并注意左右对比。常以检查背腰部经穴为主,兼及胸腹和四肢部分

经穴,包括俞、募、郄、合等穴的所在。按诊所见的异常反应,如皮下触到结节或索条状物,称为阳性反应物;局部有疼痛或酸胀等敏感反应则称压痛点;还有局部肌肤呈隆起、凹陷、松弛,以及颜色、温度的变异等。根据不同的现象,可分析、推断有关脏器的病症。例如呼吸系统疾病,常在肺俞、中府、孔最等部出现反应,再结合其他穴位的异常反应,可作出患有某一病症的推断。这些有诊断作用的反映点,还可作为针灸治疗的选穴。此外,经穴测定(穴位电测定)和知热感度测定,系此法的近代发展。详见各条。

Diagnosis by Examining the Meridians and Points   A method of diagnosis through examining, detecting and palpating the meridians and acupoints, including superficial palpation, dermometry (acupoint electrometry) and heat sensimetry, with the former as the main method. Superficial palpation includes observation of the skin, finger pressing, touching the skin with hand, palpating and stroking. With these methods, we can determine the variation of the temperature of acupoints and meridians, so as to guide acupuncture treatment. In clinic, the belly of the finger is usually used to palpate and slide along the meridians, or to pinch up the skin with the thumb and index fingers in order to detect abnormal reactions of the shallow part. Stronger pressure and massage are used to determine abnormal changes of the deep part. The force exerted should be even and the comparison of the two sides of the body should be noted. The points on the back and lumbar regions are mainly examined, and some of the meridian points on the chest, abdomen and limbs are also used. These points include the back-Shu points, Front-Mu points, Xi (Cleft) points, He (Sea) points, etc. Abnormal reactions include: positive reactant which means that node or cord-like objects are felt, tender spots or sensitive reactions like pain, soreness and distention. Local projections, pittings, or flaccidity, change of color and temperature, etc, should also be noted. The above mentioned abnormal reactions will help the doctor to analyse and deduce the conditions of the internal organs. For instance, if the patient has a disease of the respiratory system, abnormal reactions will be found at Feishu (BL 13), Zhongfu (LU 1), and Kongzui (LU 6) points, and after consideration of the reactions of other points, a certain disease could be diagnosed. These reactive spots are helpful for diagnosis and can also guide the selection of points in acupuncture treatment. In addition, acupoint electrometry and heat sensimetry are newly developed methods. →经穴测定(p. 215)、知热感度测定(p. 601)

●**经穴纂要**[jīng xué zuǎn yào]   书名。日本小阪元祐(荣升)撰,五卷,刊于1810年。卷(首)前列"骨度";卷一—三为十二经脉及奇经的经穴考,内容详细并附插图;卷四论脏腑;卷五论周身各穴,诸穴异名等。其引用书籍较多。

Jingxue Zuanyao (Essentials of Meridian Points)   A book in five volumes, written by a Japanese, Kosaramotosuke, published in 1810. At the beginning of the book, bone measurements are listed. Volumes 1-3 deal with the study on the points of the twelve regular meridians and extra meridians with detailed explanations and illustrations. Vol, 4 is a discussion on zang-fu organs. Vol, 5 discusses the names of points and the points of different names. This book has quotations from many other books.

●**经血不定**[jīng xuè bù dìng]   即经行先后无定期。详见该条。

Unfixed Menstrual Period   →经行先后无定期(p. 214)

●**经验取穴**[jīng yàn qǔ xué]   取穴法之一。根据临床实践经验而选取有效穴位。多选取奇穴。如小儿疳积刺四缝,目视不明取翳明等。

Empirical Selection of Points   A method of selecting points. To select effective points according to clinical experiences. The points are usually extra points (magical points). For instance, puncturing Sifeng (EX-UE 10) for infantile malnutrition, and selecting Yiming (EX-HN 14) for poor vision, etc.

●**经早**[jīng zǎo]   即经行先期。详见该条。

Earlier-Than-Usual Menstruation   Another name for preceded menstrual cycle. →经行先期(p. 214)

● 经乍来乍多[jīng zhà lái zhà duō] 即月经过多。详见该条。

Profuse Menstruation Another name for menorrhagia. →月经过多(p. 579)

● 经乍来乍少[jīng zhà lái zhà shǎo] 即月经过少。详见该条。

Scanty Menstruation Another name for hypomenorrhea. →月经过少(p. 579)

● 经中[jīng zhōng] 经外穴名。又名阴都。出《针灸集成》。在气海穴旁开3寸。〈主治〉二便不通,五淋,带下,月经不调,腹泻等。直刺1~1.5寸;可灸。

Jingzhong (EX-CA) An extra point, also called Yindu, originally from *Zhenjiu Jicheng* (*A Compendium of Acupuncture and Moxibustion*). 〈Location〉3 cun lateral to Qihai(RN 6). 〈Indication〉retention of urine and stool, five types of straguria, leukorrhea, irregular menstruation. diarrhea, etc. 〈Method〉Puncture perpendicularly 1~1.5 cun. Moxibustion is applicable.

● 惊风[jīng fēng] 病名。见《小儿药证直诀》。又称惊厥。是儿科常见疾病之一。以搐、搦、掣、颤、反、引、窜、视等八个主要证候为其特征。临床分急惊风、慢惊风。详见各条。

Infantile Convulsion A disease, originally seen in *Xiaoer Yaozheng Zhijue* (*Key to Differentiation and Treatment of Children's Diseases*), one of the common diseases seen in children. It is marked by eight manifestations: convulsion of the limbs, intermittent clenching of the hands, shaking of the shoulders, tremors of hands and feet, opisthotonos with stiffness of the neck and arching of the body, spasmatic contractions of the arms, upward rotation of the eyes, squint or eyes staring or widely open. It is clinically divided into acute infantile convulsion and chronic infantile convulsion. →急惊风(p. 183),慢惊风(p. 263)

● 惊膈吐[jīng gé tù] 惊吐的别名。详见该条。

Vomiting due to Fright →惊吐(p. 217)

● 惊悸[jīng jì] 病证名。见《诸病源候论》。指由于惊骇而悸,或心悸易惊,恐惧不安的病证。参见心悸条。

Palpitation due to Fright A disease, originally seen in *Zhubing Yuanhou Lun* (*General Treatise on the Etiology and Symptomatology of Diseases*), referring to palpitations caused by fright, susceptibility to panic with fright, uneasiness due to fright. →心悸(p. 509)

● 惊厥[jīng jué] 惊风的别名。详见该条。

Convulsion due to Fright →惊风(p. 217)

● 惊吐[jīng tù] 小儿呕吐证型之一。见《小儿卫生总微论方》。又称夹惊吐、惊膈吐。多因惊吓,而致食随气逆,导致呕吐。症见呕吐清水稀涎,面色清白,精神倦息,发热不高,睡卧不安,不思乳食,或睡卧不宁,手足轻微抽搐,脉弦细,舌淡,苔白腻等。治宜镇惊安心、安神止吐。取内关、公孙、曲池、合谷、足三里、太冲、水沟。

Vomiting in Children due to Fright One type of vomiting in children, seen in *Xiaoer Weisheng Zongwei Lunfang* (*General Discussion on the Health Care and Prescriptions for Infants*), also called vomiting in children by frightening or vomiting due to fright. It is mostly due to fright causing the adverse flow of qi followed by the regurgitation of food. 〈Manifestations〉watery vomitus, pallor, listlessness, low fever, uneasy sleep leading to anorexia or light intermittent convulsion of the four limbs, taut and thready pulse, pale tongue with whitish and greasy coating. 〈Treatment principle〉Tranquilize the mind and arrest vomiting. 〈Point selection〉Neiguan (PC 6), Gongsun (SP 4), Quchi (LI 11), Hegu (LI 4), Zusanli (ST 36), Taichong (LR 3) and Shuigou (DU 26).

● 睛明[jīng míng] 经穴名。出《针灸甲乙经》。属足太阳膀胱经,为手足太阳、足阳明、阴跷、阳跷之会。又名泪孔、泪空、精明。〈定位〉在面部,目内眦角稍上方凹陷处(图28和图5)。〈层次解剖〉皮肤→皮下组织→眼轮匝肌→上泪小管上方→内直肌与筛骨眶板之间。浅层布有三叉神经眼支的滑车上神经,内眦动、静脉的分支或属支。深层有眼动、静脉的分支或属支,眼神经的分支和动眼神经的分支。〈主治〉目赤肿痛、憎寒头痛、目眩、迎风流泪、内眦痒痛、胬肉攀睛、目翳、目视不明、近视、夜盲、色盲。针刺时嘱病人闭目,左手将眼球推向外侧固定,针沿眼眶边缘缓缓刺入0.3~0.5寸。不宜作大幅度提插、捻转,出针后按压针孔片刻,以防出血;禁灸。

Jingming (BL 1) A meridian point, original-

ly from *Zhenjiu Jia-Yi Jing* (*A-B Classic of Acupuncture and Moxibustion*), a point on the Bladder Meridian of Foot-Taiyang, the crossing point of Hand and Foot-Taiyang, Foot-Yangming, Yinqiao and Yangqiao meridians, also called Leikong(泪孔), Leikong(泪空), Jingming. 〈Location〉 on the face, in the depression slightly above the inner canthus (Figs. 28&5). 〈Regional anatomy〉 skin → subcutaneous tissue → orbicular muscle of eye → upper side of superior lacrimal duct → between internus muscle of the eye and orbital lamina of ethmoid bone. In the superficial layer, there are the supratrochlear nerve of the ophthalmic branches of the trigeminal nerve, and the branches or tributaries of the angular artery and vein. In the deep layer, there are the branches or tributaries of the ophthalmic artery and vein, the branches of the ophthalmic nerve and the branches of the oculomotor nerve. 〈Indications〉 redness, swelling and pain of the eye, aversion to cold, headache, dizziness, lacrimation, itch in the inner canthus, pterygium, nebula, blurred vision, myopia, night blindness, color blindness. 〈Method〉 Have the patient close his eyes before puncture, push the eyeball to the lateral side and hold it with the left hand. Puncture slowly 0.3～0.5 cun along the border of the orbit. It is not advisable to twirl or lift and thrust the needle to a large extent. Press the puncture site for a while after the withdrawal of the needle to avoid bleeding. Moxibustion is forbidden.

●睛中[jīng zhōng]　经外穴名。见《针灸大成》。位于黑眼珠正中。〈主治〉一切内障、年久不能视物。近代金针拨障术，即源于此穴的应用。

Jingzhong(EX-HN)　An extra point, originally seen in *Zhenjiu Dacheng* (*A Great Compendium of Acupuncture and Moxibustion*). 〈Location〉 at the midpoint of the pupil. 〈Indications〉 all kinds of internal oculopathy, a long-time inability to see. Modern cataractopiesis with a gold(metal) needle is derived from the application on this acupoints.

●精宫[jīng gōng]　①经穴别名。见《医学入门》。即志室。见该条。②经穴别名。出《医学原始》。即命门。见该条。③为内生殖器之别称，见该条。

1. **Jinggong**　Another name for Zhishi(BL 52), a meridian point seen in *Yixue Rumen* (*An Introduction to Medicine*). →志室(p. 605)
2. Another name for Mingmen(DU 4), a meridian point originally from *Yixue Yuanshi* (*Origin of Medicine*). →命门(p. 270)
3. **Palace of Essence**　Another name for internal genital organs. →内生殖器(p. 280)

●精滑[jīng huá]　病证名。见《丹溪心法》。即滑精。见该条。

Incontinence of Seminal Fluid　A disease, seen in *Dan Xi Xinfa* (*Danxi's Experience*), synonymous with spermatorrhea. →滑精(p. 168)

●精露[jīng lù]　经穴别名。出《针灸甲乙经》。即石门。见该条。

Jinglu　Another name for Shimen(RN 5), a meridian point, originally from *Zhenjiu Jia-Yi Jing* (*A-B Classic of Acupuncture and Moxibustion*). →石门(p. 385)

●精明[jīng míng]　经穴别名。出《备急千金要方》。即睛明。见该条。

Jingming　Another name for Jingming(BL 1), a meridian point originally from *Beiji Qianjin Yaofang* (*Essential Prescriptions Worth a Thousand Gold for Emergencies*). →睛明(p. 217)

●井穴[jǐng xué]　五腧穴之一。井穴多位于手足之端，喻脉气起始有如泉水初出。用于心下满胀。

Jing (Well) Point　One of the Five Shu points, mostly located on the distal ends of the hands and feet (fingertips and toetips), describing the origin of meridian-qi like water from the well, used to treat fullness below the head (gastric fullness).

●颈[jǐng]　耳穴名。位于颈椎穴内侧近耳胫缘。〈主治〉落枕、斜颈、颈部肿痛。

Neck(MA-AH 10)　An auricular point. 〈Location〉 on the border of cavum conchae, anterior to Cervical Vertebrae(MA-AH 8). 〈Indications〉 stiff neck, torticollis, swelling and pain of neck.

●颈百劳[jǐng bǎi láo]　经外穴名。出《针灸资生经》。〈定位〉在颈部，当大椎直上2寸，后正中线旁开1

寸(图61)。〈层次解剖〉皮肤→皮下组织→斜方肌→上后锯肌→头颈夹肌→头半棘肌→多裂肌。浅层布有第四、第五颈神经后支的皮支。深层有第四、第五颈神经后支的分支。〈主治〉瘰疬、气喘、咳血、百日咳、肺痨、妇人产后浑身病、落枕等。直刺0.3～0.6寸；可灸。

Jingbailao(EX-HN 15) An extra point, originally from *Zhenjiu Zisheng Jing* (*Acupuncture-Moxibustion Classic for Saving Life*). 〈Location〉on the nape, 2 cun directly above Dazhui(DU 14) and 1 cun lateral to the posterior midline (Fig. 61). 〈Regionsal anatomy〉skin→subcutaneous tissue→trapezius muscle→superior posterior seratus muscle→splenius muscles of head and neck→semispinal muscle of head→multifidus muscle. In the superficial layer, there are the cutaneous branches of the posterior branches of the 4th and 5th cervical nerves. In the deep layer, there are the branches of the posterior branches of the 4th and 5th cervical nerve. 〈Indications〉scrofula, asthma, hemoptysis, chin cough, pulmanery tuberculosis, general aching after childbirth, stiff neck, etc. 〈Method〉Puncture perpendicularly 0.3～0.6 cun. Moxibustion is applicable.

●颈臂[jǐng bì] 经外穴名。见《芒针疗法》。在颈部，当锁骨内1/3与外2/3交点向上1寸，胸锁乳突肌锁骨头后缘处。〈主治〉上肢瘫痪、麻木、肩臂风湿痛等。直刺0.5～1寸。禁向下深刺，免伤肺尖。

Jingbi(EX-HN) An extra point, seen in *Mangzhen Liaofa* (*Elongated Needle Therapy*). 〈Location〉on the neck, 1 cun above the point on the junction of the medial 1/3 and lateral 2/3 of clavicle, on the posterior border of the clavicular head of m. sternocleidomastoideus. 〈Indications〉paralysis and numbness of upper limbs, pain in arm and shoulder, etc. 〈Method〉Puncture perpendicularly 0.5～1 cun; deep downward insertion is not allowed for fear of injuring the lungs.

●颈冲[jǐng chōng] 经穴别名。出《千金翼方》。即臂臑。见该条。

Jingchong Another name for Binao (LI 14), a meridian point originally from *Qianjin Yifang* (*Supplement to the Essential Prescriptions Worth a Thousand Gold*). →臂臑(p.21)

●颈中[jǐng zhōng] 经穴别名。出《千金翼方》。即臂臑。见该条。

Jingzhong Another name for Binao (LI 14), a meridian point originally from *Qianjin Yifang* (*Supplement to the Essential Prescriptions Worth a Thousand Gold*). →臂臑(p.21)

●颈椎[jǐng zhuī] 耳穴名。位于轮屏切迹至对耳轮上、下脚分叉处分为五等份，下五分之一为颈椎。具有强脊益髓作用。〈主治〉落枕、颈椎综合症。

Cervical Vertebrae(MA-AH 8) An auricular point. 〈Location〉on the antihelix, a curved line from the helix-tragic notch to the bifurcation of the superior and inferior antihelix crura can be divided into five equal parts. The lower 1/5 of it is cervical vertebrae. 〈Functions〉Strengthen the spine and tonify the marrow. 〈Indications〉stiff neck, cervical spondylotic syndrome.

●痉[jìng] 病名。出《灵枢·经筋》等。又称痓，即痉证。见该条。

Convulsion A disease, originally from *Lingshu: Jingjin* (*Miraculous Pivot: Muscles along Meridians*), also called spasm, synonymous with convulsion syndrome. →痉证(p.219)

●痉证[jìng zhèng] 病名。是以项背强直、口噤、四肢抽搐、角弓反张为主症的一种病证。又称痉。多由津血虚少，筋脉失养所致。临床分为高热伤阴痉证和热入营血痉证。详见各条。

Convulsion Syndrome A disease, whose syndrome is manifested mainly by lockjaw, convulsion of limbs, opisthetonos, also called convulsion. Mainly due to malnutrition of tendons, muscles and meridians resulting from deficiency of blood and body fluid. Clinically, there are convulsions due to severe heat damaging yin, and convulsions due to heat entering the ying and blood. →高热伤阴痉证(p.132)、热入营血痉证(p.331)

●鸠尾[jiū wěi] ①经穴名。出《灵枢·九针十二原》。属任脉，为本经络穴，膏之原。又名尾翳，髑骬。〈定位〉在上腹部，前正中线上，当胸剑结合部下1寸(图43和图40)。〈层次解剖〉皮肤→皮下组织→腹白线→腹横筋膜→腹膜外脂肪→壁腹膜。浅层主要有第七胸神经前支的前皮支。深层主要有第七胸神经前支

的分支。〈主治〉心痛、心悸、心烦、癫痫、惊狂、胸中满痛、咳嗽气喘、呕吐、呃逆、反胃、胃痛。斜向下刺0.5～1寸；可灸。②骨骼名。指胸骨剑突。

1. **Jiuwei**(RN 15)　　A meridian point, originally from *Ling Shu*: *Jiu Zhen Shier Yuan* (*Miraculous Pivot*: *Nine Needles and Twelve Yuan* (*Primary*) *Points*, the Luo (connecting) point of the Ren Meridian, th source of Gao (the region below the heart), also named Weiyi, Heyu. 〈Location〉 on the upper abdomen and on the anterior midline, 1 cun below the xiphistemal synchondrosis (Figs. 43&40). 〈Reginal anatomy〉 skin → subcutaneous tissue → linea alba → transverse fascia → extraperitoneal fat tissue → parietal peritoneum. In the superficial layer, there are the anterior cutaneous branches of the anterior branch of the 7th thoracic nerve. In the deep layer, there are the branches of the anterior branch of the 7th thoracic nerve. 〈Indications〉 cardiac pain, palpitation, dysphoria, epilepsy, mania, fullness and pain in the chest, cough, asthma, vomiting, hiccup, stomachache. 〈Method〉 Puncture obliquely downward 0.5～1 cun. Moxibustion is applicable.

2. **Processus Xiphoideus**　　A part of the skeleton, referring to the process of the sternum.

● 鸠尾骨端[jiū wěi gǔ duān]　　经外穴名。见《千金要方》。在前正中线上，当胸骨剑突尖下缘处。〈主治〉小儿疳瘦、小儿囟陷、小儿消化不良。用灸法。

Jiuweiguduan（EX-CA）　　An extra point, seen in *Qianjin Yaofang* (*Essential Prescriptions Worth a Thousand Gold*). 〈Location〉 on the anterior midline and on the inferior border of the tip of the xiphoid process of the sternum. 〈Indication〉 infantile malnutrition, sunken fontanel and indigestion. 〈Method〉 moxibustion.

● 九部针经[jiǔ bù zhēn jīng]　　书名。作者不详，一卷，已佚。见《隋书·经籍志》。

Jiu Bu Zhenjing (*A Collection of Nine Acupuncture Classics*)　　A book, whose author is not identified, single-volume, no longer extant, originally recorded in *Suishu*: *Jing Ji Zhi* (*The History of the Sui Dynasty*: *Records of Classics and Works*).

● 九刺[jiǔ cì]　　《内经》刺法分类。出《灵枢·官针》。指九类不同性质的病变，应运用九种不同的刺法。包括输刺、远道刺、经刺、络刺、分刺、大泻刺、毛刺、巨刺、焠刺。

The Nine Needlings　　A category of acupuncture techniques in *Neijing* (*The Inner Canon of Huangdi*), originally from *Ling shu*: *Guanzhen* (*Miraculous Pivot*: *Official Needles*), referring to the nine different needling methods employed for treating nine kinds of diseases. They include shu needling, distant needling, meridian needling, collateral needling, intermuscular needling, drainage needling, skin needling, opposite needling and heat needling.

● 九宫尻神[jiǔ gōng kāo shén]　　古代针灸宜忌说之一。出《针经指南》。简称尻神。系以九宫八卦为依据，按病人年龄来推算人神所在部位，从而避忌刺灸。一岁起坤宫，避忌外踝；二岁当震宫，避忌齿、指、腨；三岁当巽宫，避忌头、口、乳；四岁当中宫，避忌肩尻；五岁当乾宫，避忌面、目、背；六岁当兑宫，避忌膊、手；七岁当艮宫，避忌项、腰；八岁当离宫，避忌膝、肋；九岁当坎宫，避忌脐、肘、脚；十岁复起坤宫，依次轮转。此为行年尻神所在部位，不宜刺灸。

Kao Vitality in Nine Palaces　　An ancient theory about the compatibility and incompatibility of acupuncture and moxibustion, simply called kao vitality, originally from *Zhenjing Zhinan* (*A Guide to the Classics of Acupuncture*). The theory used the Nine Palaces and Eight Diagrams to reckon where the human vitality is located according to the age of the patient so as to avoid acupuncture and moxibustion at these points. Beginning in the Kun Palace at the age of 1, the lateral malleolus is forbidden; in the Zhen Palace at 2, the tooth, finger and clif are forbidden; in the Xun Palace at 3, the head, mouth and breast are forbidden; in the Zhong Palace at 4, the shoulder and buttocks are forbidden; in the Qian Palace at 5, the face, eye and back are forbidden; in the Dui Palace at 6, the arm and hand are forbidden; in the Gen Palace at 7, the nape and waist are forbidden; in the Li Palace at 8,

the knee and rib are forbidden; in the Kan Palace at 9, the navel, elbow and foot are forbidden. At beginning again in the Kun Palace and so on. Each of these positions is the place where the kao vitality of human beings lies, and where acupuncture and moxibustion are forbidden.

●九卷[jiǔ juàn]　书名。《灵枢》的古称。见"灵枢"条。

Jiu Juan(Nine Volumes)　The archaic name of *Lingshu*(*Miraculous Pivot*).→灵枢(p. 249)

●九灵[jiǔ líng]　书名。《灵枢经》的古称之一。见该条。

Jiu Ling　A book, one of the archaic titles of *Lingshu Jing*(*The Canon of Miraculous Pivot*).→灵枢经(p. 249)

●九六补泻[jiǔ liù bǔ xiè]　针刺补泻法。出《金针赋》。指结合九六数的补泻法，即以九或六作为基数，一般补法用九阳数，泻法用六阴数。如补法用三九二十七，或七七四十九(少阳)，或九九八十一(老阳)数。泻法用三六一十八，或六六三十六(少阴)，或八八六十四(老阴)数。作为捻轻、提插的次数标准。

Nine-Six Reinforcing-Reducing　A reinforcing-reducing method of acupuncture, originally from *Jinzhen Fu*(*Ode to Gold Needle*), referring to the reinforcing-reducing method combined with the numbers 9 and 6, i. e., with 9 or 6 respectively taken as the basic numbers. Generally, the reinforcing method adopts nine yang numbers, whereas the reducing method adopts six yin numbers. For instance, the reinforcing method adopts numbers such as 27(3 times 9), or 7 times 7 is 49 (shaoyang), or 9 times 9 is 81 (laoyang); the reducing method adopts numbers such as 3 times 6 is 18, or 6 times 6 is 36(shaoyin), or 8 times 8 is 64(laoyin), the numbers serve as a standard of times for twirling lifting and thrusting the needle.

●九六数[jiǔ liù shù]　刺法用语。古代《易经》中以九为阳数，六为阴数。后世刺法的补法操作以九为基数；泻法操作则以六为基数。参见"九六补泻"条。

Nine-Six Number　A term for acupuncture technique. In ancient times 9 is taken as a yang number in *Yi Jing*(*The Book of Change*) and 6 as a yin number. In later ages 9 is taken as a basic number for reinforcing manipulation of acupuncture technique and 6 as a basic number for reducing.→九六补泻(p. 221)

●九曲[jiǔ qū]　九曲中府的简称。见该条。

Jiuqu　The short name for Jiuquzhongfu (EX-CA).→九曲中府(p. 221)

●九曲中府[jiǔ qū zhōng fǔ]　经外穴名。见《千金要方》。位于腋窝正中直下，第7肋间隙下3寸处。〈主治〉恶风邪气遁尸，内有瘀血、胸肋疼痛、腹痛等。斜刺0.3～0.5寸；可灸。

Jiuquzhongfu（EX-CA）　An extra point, seen in *Qianjin Yaofang*(*Essential Prescriptions Worth a Thousand Gold*).〈Location〉on the middle axillary line, 3 cun below the 7th intercostal space.〈Indications〉aversion to wind induced by excessive pathogenic factors, blood stasis in the interior, pain in the chest and rib, and abdominal pain, etc.〈Method〉Puncture obliquely 0.3～0.5 cun. Moxibustion is applicable.

●九虚[jiǔ xū]　书名。即《灵枢》的别称。见"灵枢"条。

Jiu Xu(Nine Mysteries)　A book, another name for *Lingshu*(*Miraculous Pivot*).→灵枢(p. 249)

●九宜[jiǔ yí]　刺法术语。出《灵枢·五禁》。指九针的运用，根据其形状特点各有其适应的范围。

Nine Compatibilities　An acupuncture technique, originally from *Lingshu*: *Wu Jin*(*Miraculous Pivot*: *Five Incompatibilities*). The term refers to the application of nine needles, based on their shapes, to different indications.

●九针[jiǔ zhēn]　古代针具分类名。出《内经》。指镵针、圆针、鍉针、锋针、铍针、圆利针、毫针、长针、大针等九种不同的针具。《灵枢·九针十二原》、《灵枢·九针论》等篇，对其形状和用途有具体论述。详见"九针"各条。

Nine Needles　A category of ancient needles, originally from *Neijing*(*The Canon of Internal Medicine*). Nine different needles are involved, shear needle, round-point needle, spoon needle, lance needle, stiletto needle, round-sharp needle, filiform needle, long needle and big needle. The shape and application

1	2	3	4	5	6	7	8	9
大针	长针	毫针	圆利针	铍针	锋针	鍉针	圆针	镵针

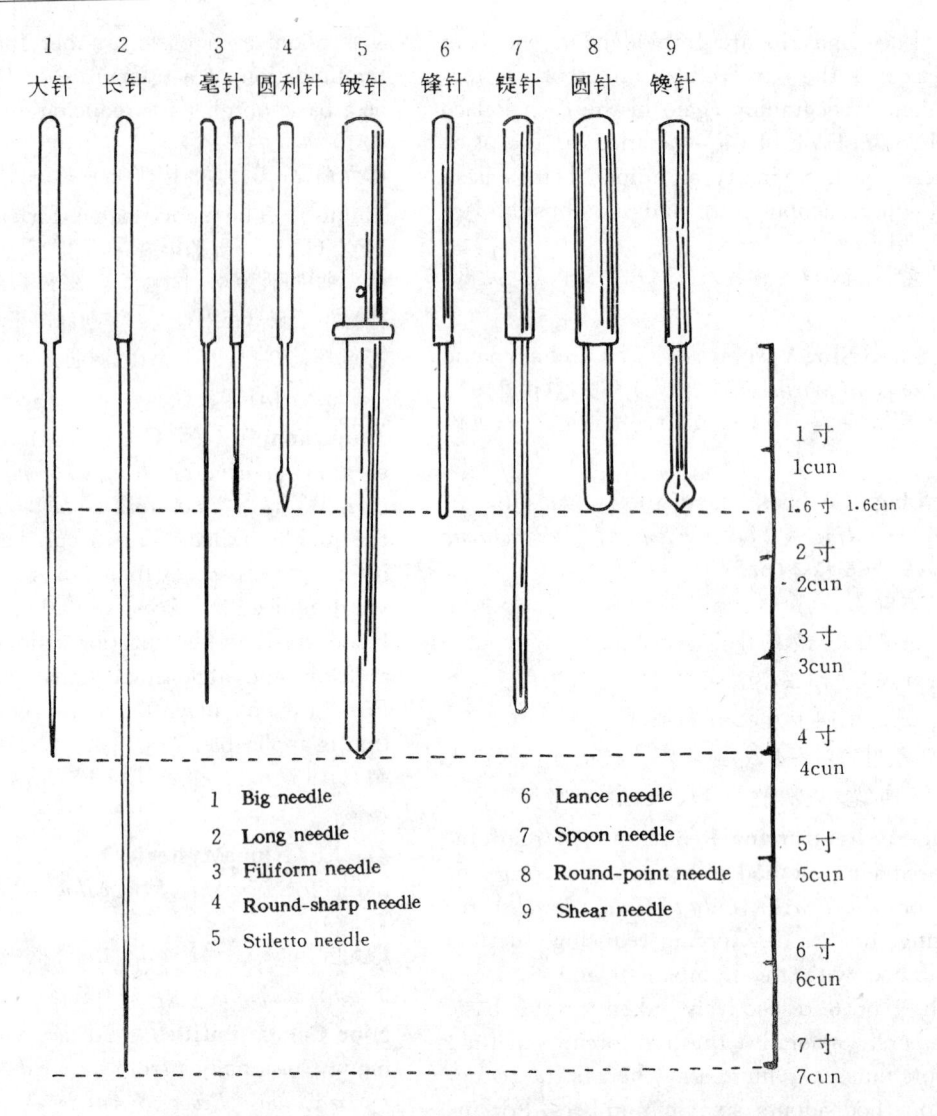

1 Big needle
2 Long needle
3 Filiform needle
4 Round-sharp needle
5 Stiletto needle
6 Lance needle
7 Spoon needle
8 Round-point needle
9 Shear needle

图27 古代九针 Fig. 27 The ancient nine needles

of each needle are discussed in detail in *Lingshu: Jiuzhen Shier Yuan* [*Miraculous Pivot: Nine Needles and Twelve Yuan (Primary) Points*] and *Lingshu: Jiuzhen Lun* (*Miraculous Pivot: On Nine Needles*), etc. →镵针(p. 31)、圆针(p. 576)、鍉针(p. 77)、锋针(p. 116)、铍针(p. 291)、圆利针(p. 576)、毫针(p. 159)、长针(p. 40)、大针(p. 66)

●灸瘢[jiǔ bān] 灸法术语。见《抱朴子·仙药》。因灸治而造成的瘢痕。

Post-Moxibustion Scar A moxibustion term, seen in *Bao Puzi: Xianyao* (*Bao Puzi's Drugs for Becoming Celestials*), referring to the scar induced by moxibustion.

●灸板[jiǔ bǎn] 灸用器具。见《外科图说》。为穿有数孔的长板，上置艾绒，用以施灸。

Plate for Moxibustion A tool for moxibustion, seen in *Waike Tushuo* (*Illustrated Explanation of External Diseases*). It is a plate with a few holes in it, in which moxa wool is put.

●灸疮[jiǔ chuāng] 灸法术语。见《金匮要略》。灸治后局部因灼伤而出现的无菌性化脓状态。一般灸疮经3—5周后结痂愈合。在此期间须保持疮面清洁，勤换膏药，以防继发感染。参见"化脓灸"条。

Post-Moxibustion Sore A moxibustion term, seen in *Jinggui Yaolüe* (*Synopsis of the Golden Chamber*), referring to a bacterial suppuration

due to the burning of the local skin after moxibustion. Generally, the score scabs and heals in 3 to 5 weeks' time, during which, the surface of the sore should be kept clean and the adhesive plaster should be renewed regularly in case secondary infection occurs. →化脓灸 (p. 169)

●灸疮膏药[jiǔ chuāng gāo yào] 见《针灸资生经》。化脓灸法所用膏药,于直接灸后敷贴局部,以促发灸疮和保护疮面。

Adhesive Plaster for Post-Moxibustion Sore Seen in *Zhenjiu Zisheng Jing* (*Acupuncture Moxibustion Classic for Saving Life*), referring to the adhesive plaster for moxibustion with suppuration. After direct moxibustion, the plaster is put on the region in order to induce the formation of the post-moxibustion sore and protect its surface.

●灸刺[jiǔ cì] 针灸术语。指灸法和刺法。古书中多有此称。

Moxibustion-Acupuncture A term in acupuncture and moxibustion, referring to moxibustion and acupuncture technique. It is so termed in many of the ancient books.

●灸癜风[jiǔ diàn fēng] 经外穴名。见《千金要方》。在手中指掌侧,远侧指节横纹中点稍前方处。〈主治〉白癜风。用灸法。

Jiudianfeng (EX-UE) An extra point, seen in *Qianjin Yaofang* (*Essential Prescriptions Worth a Thousand Gold*). 〈Location〉 on the palmar side of the middle finger, slightly distal to the midpoint of the crease of the distal interphalangeal articulation. 〈Indication〉 vitiligo. 〈Method〉 moxibustion.

●灸法[jiǔ fǎ] 治病方法的一种。古称灸焫,又称艾灸。指利用艾绒或其它药物以烧灼、熏熨体表的一定部位,以温热的刺激,来防治疾病的方法。灸法具有悠久的历史,在治疗上有针、药所不及的特点。其作用归纳起来有以下几点。①温通经气,祛散寒邪。②温补益气,扶阳固脱。③行气活血,消瘀散结。④预防疾病,保健强身。多用于一些慢性久病,以及阳气不足的疾病。如久泻、久痢、久疟、痰饮、冷哮、阳痿、痹痛等,其适应证十分广泛。近代,随着灸法的临床应用又有所发展。

Moxibustion A therapy, named cauterization and moxa moxibustion in ancient times, referring to the therapeutic technique with heat stimulation of applying ignited mugwort or other medical herbs to a certain part of the body. The technique, with its long history, has some special treatment characteristics which are somewhat superior to acupuncture and medicines. Its effects can be summed up as follows: ① It expels cold evil by warming the meridians and promoting the flow of qi. ② It warms and invigorates qi, strengthens yang and relieves prostration syndrome. ③ It promotes qi and blood circulation, removes blood stasis and disperses accumulation of pathogens. ④ It prevents diseases, protects heals and strengthens the body. 〈Indications〉 It's widely applied to the treatment of some chronic and yang-deficiency diseases, such as chronic diarrhea, protracted dysentery, chronic malaris, phlegm retention, asthma of cold type, impotence, pain due to stagnation, etc. At present, with the development of the clinical application of moxibuston, it is facing splendid prospects in modern times.

●灸法秘传[jiǔ fǎ mì chuán] 书名。清代金冶田传,雷少逸编,刊于1883年。内容有:正面穴图,背面穴图,指节图,灸盏图,灸药神方,灸法禁忌,应灸七十症等。书中介绍了一种将特制的药艾放入银质的"灸盏"中进行灸疗的方法。书末附刘国光的"太乙神针方"和"雷火针法",其为灸法专书。

Jiufa Michuan (*Secretly Bequeathed Method of Moxibustion*) A monograph on moxibustion, imparted by Jin Yetian and compiled by Lei Shaoyi in the Qing Dynasty, and published in 1883. It includes drawings of front acupoints, drawings of back acupoints, a drawing of the knuckles, a drawing of a moxibustion plate, wonderful prescriptions for moxibustion, the contraindications of moxibustion, etc. The book introduces a moxibustion plate made of silver. *Taiyi Shenzhen Fang* (*Recipes of Great Monad Herbal Moxa Stick*), and *Leihuo Zhenfa* (*Moxibustion with Thunder-Fire Herbal Moxa Stick*) written by Liu Guoguang are appendixed at the end of the book.

●灸感[jiǔ gǎn] 灸法术语。指病人因施用灸法而出

现的温热或麻木、虫行等感觉,有时也可向某一方向传布或扩散。

Moxibustion Sensation A term of moxibustion, refers to feelings such as warmth, heat, and numbness after moxibustion. Such feelings can sometimes diffuse or spread in a certain direction.

●**灸花**[jiǔ huā] 灸法术语。见《针灸集成》。指灸疮的化脓状态。

Post-Moxibustion Pox A term of moxibustion, seen in *Zhenjiu Jicheng* (*A Compendium of Acupuncture and Moxibustion*), referring to the suppuration of post-moxibustion sore.

●**灸火木**[jiǔ huǒ mù] 施灸材料。见《黄帝虾蟆经》。古代灸治注重点火源,认为松、柏、竹、桔、榆、枳、桑、枣的火皆伤血脉骨髓肌肉,不宜作为施灸的热源。参见"八木火"条。

Moxibustion Wood Material for moxibustion, seen in *Huang Di Hama Jing* (*The Yellow Emperor's Frog Classic*), In ancient times, the kindling material for moxibustion was taken seriously, and it was thought that the fire of pine, cypress, bamboo, orange, elm, trifoliate orange, mulberry and jujube would impair the blood vessels, bone marrow and muscles, and could not be the source of heat for moxibustion. →八木火(p.8)

●**灸痨**[jiǔ láo] 经外穴名。见《中国针灸学》。以足中趾尖经足心至腘窝横纹之长为度,自鼻尖向后沿正中线量至脊背尽处标点,此点旁开半口寸处是穴。主治虚劳盗汗、咳嗽、咳吐脓血、面黄消瘦、神疲乏力等。用灸法。

Jiulao(EX-B) An extra point, seen in *Zhong Guo Zhenjiuxue* (*Chinese Acupuncture and Moxibustion*). 〈Location〉 Take the distance between the tip of the 3rd toe and the popliteal line (via the plantar centre) as the measurement. Measure along the posterior midline with the point on it, which is on the level with the nasal apex, as the starting point, half a mouth cun lateral to the ending point of the measurement on the back is Jiulao (EX-B) point. 〈Indcatons〉 night sweat, cough with sticky sputum and blood, emaciation with sallow complexion, mental fatigue and inertia, etc. caused by consumption.

〈Method〉 moxibustion.

●**灸疗器**[jiǔ liáo qì] 为温灸器之别称。见该条。

Moxibustion Apparatus →温灸器(p.470)

●**灸器灸**[jiǔ qì jiǔ] 灸法的一种。用特制的灸器盛放点燃的艾绒在穴位上进行熨灸或熏灸。用灸器施灸,可以较长时间连续地给穴位以温热刺激。一般用于腹部、腰背部。有温中散寒,调和气血等作用。治疗寒性的腹痛、腰痛、腹泻、腹胀等症。

Moxibustion with Apparatus A method of moxibustion on the acupoints with the ignited mugwort in the special moxibustion apparatus. Moxibustion with apparatus can give a continuous warm stimulation to the acupoint for a longer period of time and is commonly applied to the abdomen, the waist and the back. 〈Functions〉 Warm the middle-jiao to dispel cold, regulating qi and blood, etc. 〈Indications〉 abdominal pain, lumbago, diarrhea and abdominal distention caused by cold, etc.

●**灸焫**[jiǔ ruò] 灸法术语。出《素问·异法方宜论》。焫,又作爇,火烧的意思。灸焫为灸法之古称。见该条。

Moxibustion Cauterization A term of moxibustion, originally from *Su Wen*: *Yi Fa Fang Yi Lun* (*Plain Questions*: *On Variation of Methods in Accordance with Geographical Locations*). Cauterization, also named ignition, means burning. Moxibustion cauterization is the archaic name for moxibustion. →灸法(p.223)

●**灸师**[jiǔ shī] 见《昌黎先生集》卷七。指专门施行灸法的医师。

Moxibustionist A doctor specializing in treatment with moxibustion, seen in Vol. 7 of *Changli Xiansheng Ji* (*Changli's Anthology*).

●**灸哮**[jiǔ xiāo] 经外穴名。见《针灸聚英·杂病歌》。位于背部,以绳环颈下垂至胸骨剑突尖,环转向背,绳之中点平喉结,绳端着脊骨中处是穴。主治哮喘、咳嗽,以及支气管炎等。用灸法。

Jiuxiao(EX-B) An extra point, seen in *Zhenjiu Juying*: *Zabing Ge* (*Essentials of Acupuncture and Moxibustion*: *Verses on Miscellaneous Diseases*). 〈Location〉 Put a rope round the nape with the rest dropped to the xiphoid process of the strenum, then turn the

ring backwards with the midpoint of the dropped length overlapping the Adam's apple, and the point on the vertebra touched by the end of the rope is Jiuxiao (EX-B) point. ⟨Indications⟩ asthma, cough and bronchitis, etc. ⟨Method⟩ moxibustion.

●**灸血病**[jiǔ xuè bìng] 经外穴名。见《千金要方》。《中国针灸学》列作奇穴,名灸血病。位于第三骶椎嵴之高点处。灸治吐血、衄血、便血、血崩及其他血症。

Jiuxuebing An extra point, seen in *Qianjin Yaofang (Essential Prescriptions Worth a Thousand Gold)*, taken as an extra point in *Zhongguo Zhenjiuxue (Chinese Acupuncture and Moxibustion)*. ⟨Location⟩ on the tip of the crest of the 3rd sacral vertebra. ⟨Indications⟩ spitting blood, apstaxis, hematochezia, metrorrhagia, etc. ⟨Method⟩ moxibustion.

●**灸盏**[jiǔ zhǎn] 灸具名。见《灸法秘传》。为温灸器的一种,与近代所用的艾斗相类似。参见"艾斗"条。

Moxibustion Plate A moxibustion apparatus, seen in *Jiufa Michuan (Secretly Bequeathed Method of Moxibustion)*, a kind of mild-moxibustionizers similiar to the moxa dipper used in modern times. →艾斗(p. 1)

●**灸罩**[jiǔ zhào] 灸具名。见《外科图说》。为圆锥形罩子,上有一孔,罩于施灸的艾炷上。

Moxibustion Cover A moxibustion apparatus, seen in *Waike Tushuo (Illustrated Explanation of External Diseases)*. A tapered cover with a hole in the top. used to cove the moxa cone of moxibustion.

●**居髎**[jū liáo] 经穴名。出《针灸甲乙经》。属足少阳胆经,为阳跷、足少阳之会。⟨定位⟩在髋部,当髂前上棘与股骨大转子最凸点连线的中点处(图64)。⟨层次解剖⟩皮肤→皮下组织→阔筋膜→臀中肌→臀小肌。浅层布有臀上皮神经和髂腹下神经外侧皮支。深层有臀上动、静脉的分支或属支和臀上神经。⟨主治⟩腰腿痹痛、瘫痪、足痿、疝气。直刺或斜刺1.5～2寸;可灸。

Juliao(GB 29) A meridian point, originally from *Zhenjiu Jia-Yi Jing (A-B Classic of Acupuncture and Moxibustion)*, a point on the Gallbladder Meridian of Foot-Shaoyang, the Crossing point of the Meridian of Foot-Shaoyang and the Yangqiao Meridian. ⟨Location⟩ on the hip at the midpoint of the line connecting the anteriosuperior iliac spine and the prominence of the great trochanter (Fig. 64). ⟨Regional anatomy⟩ skin→subcutaneous tissue→fascia lata→middle gluteal muscle→least gluteal muscle. In the superficial layer, there are the superior clunial nerve and the lateral cutaneous branches of the iliohypogastric nerve. In the deep layer, there are the branches or tributaries of the superior gluteal artery and vein and the superior gluteal nerve. ⟨Indications⟩ pain in the waist and lower extremities due to stagnation, paralysis, foot flaccidity and hernia. ⟨Method⟩ Puncture perpendicularlly or obliquely 1.5～2 cun. Moxibustion is applicable.

●**局部取穴**[jú bù qǔ xué] 取穴法之一。指在病痛所在的部位上选经穴、经外穴、阿是穴等。例如肘痛取曲池,膝痛取膝眼,眼病取睛明,鼻塞取迎香,胃痛取中脘,遗尿取中极等。

Local Point Selection One of the point selection methods, referring to the selection of the meridian points, extra points, or Ashi points, etc. in the affected area, e. g. Quchi(LI 11) selected for the pain in elbow, Xiyan(EX-LE 4 & 5) for knee pain, Jingming(BL 1) for eye diseases, Yingxiang(LI 20) for stuffy nose, Zhongwan(RN 12) for gastralgia, Zhongji(RN 3) for enuresis, etc.

●**巨处**[jù chù] 经穴别名。出《医学入门》。即五处。见该条。

Juchu Another name for Wuchu(BL 5), a meridian point originally from *Yixue Rumen (An Introduction to Medicine)*. →五处(p. 475)

●**巨刺**[jù cì] 《内经》刺法名。出《灵枢·官针》。是九刺之一。指左侧病痛取右侧穴,右侧病痛取左侧穴的交叉刺法。可治疗病在经脉的病症。临床上对中风后遗症、坐骨神经痛等症,常用交叉取穴法。巨刺与缪刺在应用上有所不同,参见"缪刺"条。

Opposite Needling A needling technique in *Neijing (The Canon of Internal Medicine)*, originally from *Lingshu: Guanzhen (Miraculous Pivot: Official Needles)*, one of the Nine Needlings, referring to the crossing needling technique, in which points on the right side are selected for diseases on the left and *vice*

versa. The method can be applied to the treatment of diseases in the meridian. The technique is commonly used for treating sequel of apoplexy and sciatica. There are some differences in application between crossing needling and contralateral needling. →缪刺(p. 270)

●巨骨[jù gǔ] ①经穴名。出《素问·气府论》。属手阳明大肠经。〈定位〉在肩上部,当锁骨肩峰端与肩胛冈之间凹陷处(图48)。〈层次解剖〉皮肤→皮下组织→肩锁韧带→冈上肌。浅层有锁骨上外侧神经等分布。深层布有肩胛上神经的分支和肩胛上动、静脉的分支或属支。〈主治〉肩背、手臂疼痛、不得屈伸、瘰疬、瘿气、惊痫吐血。直刺0.4~0.6寸; 不可深刺,以免刺入胸腔,造成气胸。可灸。②部位名。指肩端横于膺上之大骨,又称缺盆骨,现称锁骨。

1. **Jugu**(LI 16) A meridian point, originally from *Suwen*: *Qifu Lun* (*Plain Questions*: *On Houses of Qi*), a point of the Large Intestine Meridian of Hand-Yangming. 〈Location〉 on the shoulder, in the depression between the acromial extremity of the clavicle and scapular spine (Fig. 48). 〈Regional anatomy〉 skin → subcutaneous tissue → acromioclavicular ligament→supraspinous muscle. In the superficial layer, there is the lateral supraclavicular nerve. In the deep layer, there are the branches of the suprascapular nerve and the branches or tributaries of the suprascapular artery and vein. 〈Indications〉 pain in shoulder, back and upper limbs, difficulty in flexion and extension of the upper limbs, scrofula, goiter, epilepsy due to terror, and spitting blood. 〈Method〉 Puncture perpendicularly 0.4~0.6 cun; too deep puncture is inapplicable, lest it should reach the thoracic cavity and causes a pneumothorax. Moxibustion is applicable.

2. **Huge Bone** A part of the body, referring to the big bone at the shoulder which is horizontally above the breast, also named bone of suraclavicular fossa, now called the clavicle.

●巨搅[jù jiǎo] 经外穴别名。见《中国针灸学》。即巨觉。见该条。

Jujiao Another name for Chenjue(EX-B), an extra point seen in *Zhongguo Zhenjiuxue* (*Chinese Acupuncture and Moxibustion*). →巨觉(p. 226)

●巨窌[jù jiāo] ①经穴别名。即巨髎。见该条。②经穴别名。出《针灸甲乙经》。即丝竹空。见该条。

Jujiao Another name for ① the meridian point Juliao (ST 3). →巨髎(p. 226) ② Sizhukong(SJ 23), a meridian point originally from *Zhenjiu Jia-Yi Jing* (*A-B Classic of Acupuncture and Moxibustion*). →丝竹空(p. 412)

●巨觉[jù jué] 经外穴别名。出《千金要方》。即臣觉。见该条。

Jujue Another name for Chenjue(EX-), an extra point originally from *Qianjin Yaofang* (*Essential Prescriptions Worth a Thousand Gold*). →臣觉(p. 226)

●巨髎[jù liáo] 经穴名。出《针灸甲乙经》。属足阳明胃经,为阳跷、足阳明之会。〈定位〉在面部,瞳孔直下,平鼻翼下缘处,当鼻唇沟外侧(图28和图5)。〈层次解剖〉皮肤→皮下组织→上唇肌,有上唇方肌,深层为犬齿肌;有面动静脉及眶下动,静脉会合支;布有眶下神经支及面神经颊支。〈主治〉口眼歪斜、眼睑瞤动、鼻衄、齿痛、唇颊肿、目翳。直刺0.3~0.6寸;可灸。

Juliao(ST 3) A meridian point, originally from *Zhenjiu Jia-Yi Jing* (*A-B Classic of Acupuncture and Moxibustion*), a point on the Stomach Meridian of Foot-Yangming, the crossing point of the Yangqiao Meridian and the Stomach Meridian of Foot-Yangming. 〈Location〉 on the face, directly below the pupil, on the level of the lower border of the nasal ala, beside the nasolabial groove (Figs. 28&5). 〈Regional anatomy〉 skin → subcutaneous tissue→levator muscle of upper lip→levator muscle of angle of mouth. There are the infraorbital nerve of the maxillary nerve, the buccal branches of the facial nerve, the anastomotic branches formed by the branches or tributaries of the facial artery and vein and the infraorbital artery and vein in this area. 〈Indications〉 deviation of the eye and mouth, twitching of eyelids, epistaxis, toothache, swelling of the lips and cheeks, and nephelium. 〈Method〉 Puncture perpendicularly 0.3~0.6 cun. Moxibustion is applicable.

●巨阙[jù què] 经穴名。出《脉经》。属任脉,为心之募穴。〈定位〉在上腹部,前正中线上,当脐中上6寸

(图43.2和图40)。〈层次解剖〉皮肤→皮下组织→腹白线→腹横筋膜→腹膜外脂肪→壁腹膜。浅层主要布有第七胸神经前支的前皮支和腹壁浅静脉。深层主要有第七胸神经前支的分支。〈主治〉胸痛、心痛、心烦、惊悸、尸厥、癫狂、痫证、健忘、胸满气短、咳逆上气、腹胀暴痛、呕吐、呃逆、噎膈、吞酸、黄疸、泄利。直刺0.5~1寸;可灸。

Juque(RN 14)   A meridian point, originally from *Mai Jing* (*The Pulse Classic*), a point on the Ren Meridian, the Front-Mu Point of the heart. 〈Location〉on the upper abdomen and on the anterior midline, 6 cun above the centre of the umbilicus (Figs. 43. 2&40). 〈Regional anatomy〉 skin → subcutaneous tissue → linea alba → transverse fascia → extraperitoneal fat tissue → parietal peritoneum. In the superficial layer, there are the anterior cutaneous branches of the anterior branch of the 7th thoracic nerve and the superficial epigastric vein. In the deep layer, there are the branches of the anterior branch of the 7th thoracic nerve. 〈Indications〉 chest pain, precordial pain, vexation, palpitation due to fright, corpse-like syncope, manic-depressive psychosis, epilepsy, amnesia, full sensation in chest with short breath, cough with dyspnea, abdominal distention and sudden pain, vomiting, hiccup, dysphagia, acid regurgitation, jaundice, diarrhea and dysentery. 〈Method〉Puncture perpendicularly 0. 5 ~1 cun. Moxibustion is applicable.

●**巨阙俞**[jù què shù]   经外穴名。见《千金翼方》。在背部,当第4、5胸椎棘突之间。主治胸膈中气、咳嗽、喘息;以及支气管炎,神经衰弱等。用灸法。

Jiuqueshu(EX-B)   An extra point seen in *Qianjin Yifang* (*A Supplement to the Prescriptions Worth a Thousand Gold*). 〈Locations〉on the back, between the 4th and 5th thoracic vertebrae spinous processes. 〈Indications〉 qi-stagnation in the chest, cough, dyspnea, bronchitis, neurasthenia, etc. 〈Method〉moxibustion.

●**巨虚**[jù xū]   ①经穴别名。即上巨虚。见该条。②经穴别名。即下巨虚。见该条。

Juxu   Another name for ① the meridian point Shangjuxu(ST 37). →上巨虚(p. 352)② the meridian point Xiajuxu(ST 37). →下巨虚(ST 39)(p. 489).

●**巨虚上廉**[jù xū shàng lián]   经穴别名。出《灵枢·本输》。即上巨虚。见该条。

Juxushanglian   Another name for Shangjuxu(ST 37), a meridian point originally from *Lingshu*: *Benshu* (*Miraculous Pivot*: *Meridian Points*). →上巨虚(p. 352)

●**巨虚下廉**[jù xū xià lián]   经穴别名。出《灵枢·本输》。即下巨虚。见该条。

Juxuxialian   Another name for Xiajuxu(ST 39), a meridian point originaly from *Lingshu*: *Benshu* (*Miraculous Pivot*: *Meridian Points*) →下巨虚(p. 489)

●**巨阳**[jù yáng]   ①太阳经的别名。出《素问·热论》。巨,意为巨大,指足太阳经连于督脉,主持一身阳气,故称巨阳。马王堆汉墓帛书医经又写作"钜阳",意义相同。《素问·五脏生成篇》中手、足太阳,分别称"手巨阳"、"足巨阳"。②经穴别名。指申脉穴。详见该条。

1. **Great Yang**   Another name for the Taiyang Meridian, originally from *Suwen*: *Re Lun* (*Plain Questions*: *On Febrile Diseases*), referring to the Meridian of Foot Taiyang, connected with the Du meridian, governing the yang-qi of the whole body, thus named great yang. Enormous yang(钜阳) was named synonymously with great yang(巨阳) in the silk-copied medical classic, unearthed from a Han tomb in Mawangdui In *Suwen*: *Wu Zang Sheng Cheng Pian* (*Plain Questions*: *Physiology and Pathology of the Five Zang-Organs*), the Hand- and Foot-Taiyang were called respectively Hand Great Yang and Foot Great Yang.

2. **Juyang**   Another name for the meridian point Shenmai(BL 62). →申脉(p. 359)

●**巨针**[jù zhēn]   针具名。原指九针中的大针。近代有以不锈钢制成的巨针,针体直径为0.5~1毫米,长度有3寸、5寸,1尺等数种。用于沿皮下横刺和肌腱部刺,以治疗瘫痪和肌肉挛缩等症。

Giant Needle   A type of acupuncture apparatus, originally referring to the big needle among the nine needles. In modern times, there are giant needles made of stainless steel, the needle body 0. 5-1 mm in diameter, 3 cun or 5

cun or 10 cun in length, etc. The needles are used to puncture subcutaneously and puncture the muscles and tendons to treat the diseases of paralysis, muscular spasm, etc.

●聚毛[jù máo]　部位名。又称丛毛，三毛。指大趾爪甲后方有毛处。

Crowded Hairs　A part of the body, also called clumpy hairs or three hairs, referring to hairs growing in the part proximal to the nail of the big toe.

●聚泉[jù quán]　经外穴名。出《奇效良方》。〈定位〉在口腔内，当舌背正中缝的中心处。〈层次解剖〉舌粘膜→粘膜下疏松结缔组织→舌肌。布有下颌神经的舌神经，舌下神经和鼓索的神经纤维以及舌动、静脉的动、静脉网。〈主治〉哮喘、咳嗽、消渴、舌强，以及舌肌麻痹等。直刺0.1～0.2寸；或点刺出血。

Juquan (EX-HN 10)　An extra point originally from *Qixiao Liangfang* (*Prescriptions of Wonderful Efficacy*). 〈Location〉in the mouth, at the midpoint of the dorsal midline of the tongue. 〈Regional anatomy〉tongue mucosa→submucous loose connective tissue→lingual muscle. There are the lingual nerve from the mandibular nerve, the hypoglossal nerve, the nervous fibers of the tympanic cord, and the arteriovenous network of the lingual artery and vein in this area. 〈Indications〉asthma, cough diabetes, stiffness of the tongue, paralysis and numbness of the tongue muscle, etc. 〈Method〉Puncture perpendicularly 0.1～0.2 cun, or prick to cause bleeding.

●撅[juē]　刺法用语。见《针灸大成》。撅与"撅"通，在刺法用语中有重插轻提（紧提慢按）的意思。

Spading　A term in acupuncture, seen in *Zhenjiu Dacheng* (*A Great Compendium of Acupuncture and Moxibustion*). Spading means digging, referring to thrusting the needle with force and lifting the needle lightly. (Lifting quickly and thrusting slowly).

●绝产[jué chǎn]　即不孕。详见该条。

No Delivery　Another name for sterility.→不孕(p.29)

●绝骨[jué gǔ]　①经穴别名。出《难经·四十五难》。即悬钟。见该条。②经穴别名。出《素问·刺疟篇》王冰注。即阳辅。见该条。③部位名。指外踝上方，当腓骨与腓骨长短肌之间的凹陷处。

1. **Juegu**　Another name for Xuanzhong (GB 39), a meridian point originally from *Nanjing*: *Sishiwu Nan* (*The Classic of Questions*: *Question 45*).→悬钟(p.519)

2. **Juegu**　Another name for Yangfu (GB 38), a meridian point originally from Wang Bing's notes on *Suwen*: *Ci Nüe Pian* (*Plain Questions*: *Acupuncture Methods for Malarial Diseases*).→阳辅(p.536)

3. **Bone End**　A part of the body, referring to the depression between the fibula and in the peroneus longus and the peroneus brevis, above the external malleolus.

●绝经前后诸证[jué jīng qián hòu zhū zhèng]　病证名。见《金匮要略·妇人杂病脉证并治》。妇女在四十九岁左右，月经开始终止，称为绝经。有些妇女在绝经期前后，往往出现一些症状，如经行紊乱，头晕，心悸，烦躁，出汗，情志异常等，名为绝经前后诸证。主要由于妇女绝经前后，天癸将竭，肾气衰弱，冲任虚损，精血不足，以致脏腑经络失于濡养和温煦所致。临床分四类。①肝阳上亢型。多因肾阴不足，肝失所养所致。证见头晕目眩，心烦易怒，烘热汗出，腰膝酸软，经来量多，或淋漓漏下，舌质红，脉弦细而数。治宜平肝潜阳，益水涵木。取太冲、太溪、百会、风池。②心血亏损型。多因劳心过度，营血暗伤，心失濡养所致。证见心悸怔忡，失眠多梦，五心烦热，舌红少苔，脉细数。治宜补益心血，交通心肾。取心俞、脾俞、肾俞、三阴交。③脾胃虚弱型。多因肾阳虚衰，脾胃失于温养所致。证见面色㿠白，神倦肢怠，纳少腹胀，大便溏泄，面浮肢肿，脉沉细无力。治宜补脾养胃。取脾俞、胃俞、中脘、章门、足三里。可加灸。④痰气郁结型。多因脾失健运，痰湿阻滞所致。证见胸闷吐痰，脘腹胀满，嗳气吞酸，呕恶食少，苔腻，脉滑。治宜理气化痰。取膻中、中脘、气海、支沟、丰隆、三阴交。

Climacterium　A disease, seen in *Jingui Yaolüe*: *Furen Zabing Mai Zheng Bing Zhi* (*Synopsis of the Golden Chamber*: *Pulse Conditions, Symptoms and Treatments of Woman's Miscellaneous Diseases*). Women stop menstruation at the age of about 49, which is called menopause. Before or after the period of menopause, some symptoms commonly appear, such as irregular menstruation, dizzi-

ness, palpitation, irritability, sweating, abnormal emotional changes, etc., which is called climacterium. This is because of the near exhaustion of the congenital essence of women, deficiency of the kidney-qi, insufficiency and impairment of the Chong and Ren Meridians, consumption of the essence and blood, which finally fails to nourish and warm the zang-fu organs, meridians and callaterals. It is clinically divided into four types: ①hyperactivity of liver-yang caused by deficiency of kidney-yin, failing to nourish the liver. 〈Manifestation〉 dizziness and blurring of vision, vexation and susceptibility to anger, hectic fever with sweating, lassitude in the loins and knee, profuse menstruation or dribbling meotrostaxis, red tongue, wiry, thready and rapid pulse. 〈Treatment principle〉 Calm the liver and suppress the sthenic yang, nourish the liver by tonifying the kidney. 〈Point selection〉 Taichong(LR 3), Taixi(KI 3), Baihui(DU 20), Fengchi(GB 20). ②General debility of the heartblood. Mostly due to overthinking, gradual impairment of ying-blood failing to nourish the heart. 〈Manifestations〉 severe palpitation, insomnia, frequent dreams, dysphoria due to feverish sensation in the chest, palms and soles, red tongue with little coating, thready and rapid pulse. 〈Treatment principle〉 Invigorate the heart and enrich the blood, restore the normal coordination between the heart and kidney. 〈Point selection〉 Xinshu(BL 15), Pishu(BL 20), Shenshu(BL 23), Sanyinjiao(SP 6). ③Weakness of the spleen and stomach. Mostly due to collapse of kidney-yang, failing to reinforce and warm the spleen and stomach. 〈Manifestations〉 pallor lassitude and inertia, anorexia and abdominal distention, loose stool, edema of the face and limbs, deep, thready and weak pulse. 〈Treatment principle〉 Tonify the spleen and replenish the stomach. 〈Point selection〉 Pishu(BL 20), Weishu(BL 21), Zhongwan(RN 12), Zhangmen(LR 13), Zusanli(ST 36). 〈Method〉 Besides acupuncture, moxibustion is applicable. ④Stagnation of pathogenic phlegm and qi. Mostly due to dysfunction of the spleen in transporting, leading to stagnation of phlegm and dampness. 〈Manifestations〉 oppressive feeling in the chest and expedoration, fullness and distension of the abdomen and epigastrium, belching, acid regurgitation, nausea and vomiting, loss of appetite, greasy tongue coating, slippery pulse. 〈Treatment principle〉 Regulate the flow of qi to resolve phlegm. 〈Point selection〉 Danzhong(RN 17), Zhongwan(RN 12), Qihai(RN 6), Zhigou(SJ 6), Fenglong(ST 40), Sanyinjiao(SP 6).

●绝阳[jué yáng] 经穴别名。出《针灸甲乙经》。即商阳。见该条。

Jueyang Another name for Shangyang(LI 1), an extra point originally from *Zhenjiu Jia-Yi Jing* (*A-B Classic of Acupuncture and Moxibustion*). →商阳(p. 350)

●绝孕穴[jué yùn xué] 经外穴名。见《太平圣惠方》。在腹部,当脐下2.3寸处。主治妇人绝子、小儿深秋冷痢不止。用灸法。

Jueyunxue (EX-CA) An extra point, seen in *Taiping Shenghui Fang* (*Imperial Benevolent Prescriptions*). 〈Location〉 on the abdomen, 2.3 cun below the umbilicus. 〈Indications〉 women's sterility, children's lingering dysentery with cold sensation in late autumn. 〈Method〉 moxibustion.

●绝子[jué zǐ] 不孕的别名。详见该条。

No offspring Another name for sterility. →不孕(p. 29)

●厥[jué] 病证名。详见"厥证"条。

Syncope A disease. →厥证 Syncope Syndrome. (p. 230)

●厥俞[jué shù] 经穴别名。出《针灸大成》。即厥阴俞。见该条。

Jueshu Another name for Jueyinshu(BL 14), a meridian point originally from *Zhenjiu Dacheng* (*A Great Compendium of Acupuncture and Moxibustion*). →厥阴俞(p. 230)

●厥阳[jué yáng] 经穴别名。出《针灸甲乙经》。即飞扬。见该条。

Jueyang Another name for Feiyang(BL 58), a meridian point originally from *Zhenjiu Jia-Yi Jing* (*A-B Classic of Acupuncture and Moxibustion*). →飞扬(p. 106)

●厥阴俞[jué yīn shū] 经穴名。出《千金要方》。属足太阳膀胱经,为心包的背俞穴。又名厥俞、阙俞。〈定位〉在背部,当第四胸椎棘突下,旁开1.5寸(图7)。〈层次解剖〉皮肤→皮下组织→斜方肌→菱形肌→竖脊肌。浅层布有第四、五胸神经后支的内侧皮支和伴行的肋间后动、静脉背侧支。深层有第四、五胸神经后支的肌支和相应的肋间后动、静脉背侧支的分支或属支。〈主治〉心痛、心悸、胸闷、咳嗽、呕吐。斜刺0.5～0.8寸;可灸。

Jueyinshu (BL 14) A meridian point, originally from *Qianjin Yaofang* (*Essential Prescriptions Worth a Thousand Gold*), a point on the Bladder Meridian of Foot-Taiyang, the Back Shu-Point of the pericardium, also named Jueshu or Queshu. 〈Location〉 on the back, below the spinous process of the 4th thoracic vertebra, 1.5 cun lateral to the posterior midline (Fig. 7). 〈Regional anatomy〉 skin → subcutaneous tissue → trapezius muscle → rhomboid muscle → erector spinal muscle. In the superficial layer, there are the medial cutaneous branches of the posterior branches of the 4th and 5th thoracic nerves and the dorsal branches of the accompanying posterior intercostal arteries and veins. In the deep layer, there are the muscular branches of the posterior branches of the 4th and 5th thoracic nerves and the branches or tributaries of the dorsal branches of the related posterior intercostal arteries and veins. 〈Indications〉 precordial pain, palpitation, stuffiness of the chest, cough, vomiting. 〈Method〉 Puncture obliquely 0.5～0.8 cun. Moxibustion is applicable.

●厥证[jué zhèng] 病证名。简称厥。出《素问·厥论》等。是以突然昏倒,不省人事,四肢厥冷为主证的一种病证。一般昏厥时间较短,醒后无后遗症,但也有一厥不复而导致死亡者。由于阴阳失调,气机逆乱所引起。临床分气厥、血厥、寒厥、热厥、痰厥。详见各条。

Syncope Syndrome A disease with the simple name of syncope, originally from *Suwen*: *Jue Lun* (*Plain Questions*: *On Jue-Syndromes*), referring to disease mainly manifested as sudden fainting, unconsciousness and cold limbs. Usually syncope only lasts a short time leaving no sequela after it is gone. But there are some cases in which the patients die. It is caused by the imbalance of yin and yang, and sudden disorder of qi. It is clinically divided into syncope due to qi, syncope due to blood, syncope due to cold, syncope due to heat and syncope due to phlegm. →气厥(p. 308)、血厥(p. 525)、寒厥(p. 155)、热厥(p. 331)、痰厥(p. 424)

●橛骨[jué gǔ] ①经穴别名。见《针灸聚英》。即长强。见该条。②骨骼名。指尾骨。

1. Juegu Another name for Changqiang (DU 1), a meridian point seen in *Zhenjiu Juying* (*Essentials of Acupuncture and Moxibustion*). →长强(p. 39)

2. Stake-Like Bone A part of a skeleton, referring to coccyx.

●䐃肉[jùn ròu] 部位名。指隆起的肌肉。

Bulging Muscles A part of the body, referring to the prominent muscles.

K

●开阖补泻[kāi hé bǔ xiè] 针刺补泻法之一。出《内经》。于起针时开放孔穴或揉闭孔穴,以区分补泻。即行泻法时,出针开其针孔,不加揉按,为开;行补法时,出针后闭其针孔,加以揉按,为阖。

Reinforcing and Reducing Achieved by Keeping the Hole Opened or Closed One of the acupuncture reinforcing-reducing methods, originally from *Neijing* (*The Canon of Internal Medicine*), referring to distinguishing reinforcing or reducing depending on the hole being kept open or closed while withdrawing the needle without giving massage on the point,

keep the hole open, which means opening. While performing the reinforcing method, withdraw the needle and massage the point to make the hole close, which means closing.

●开阖枢[kāi hé shū] 又名关阖枢。见该条。

Opening-Closing-Pivot　Also named bolt-door-pivot. →关阖枢(p. 147)

●看部取穴[kàn bù qǔ xué] 取穴法之一。见《针灸大成》。对头身部病症，按经选取有关的穴位。《医学入门》所载：上部病多取手阳明经，中部足太阴，下部足厥阴，前膺足阳明，后背足太阳，即属此法。

Point Selection According to the Affected Area　One of the methods for point selection, seen in *Zhengjiu Dacheng* (*A Great Compendium of Acupuncture and Moxibustion*), referring to selecting points on related meridians for treating the diseases of the head and body. What is recorded in *Yixue Rumen* (*An Introduction to Medicine*)—in most cases, select the Hand-Yangming Meridian for diseases of the upper part, the Foot-Taiyin for the middle part, the Foot-Jueyin for the lower part, the Foot-Yangming for the prothorax, and the Foot-Taiyang for the back—pertains to this method.

●尻[kāo] 部位名。指骶骨和尾骨。

Buttock　A part of the body, referring to the sacrum and coccyx.

●尻神[kāo shén] 九宫尻神的别名。详见该条。

Human Vitality　→九宫尻神(p. 220)

●考正周身穴法歌[kǎo zhèng zhōu shēn xué fǎ gē] 书名。一卷，清代廖润鸿撰。本书将全身十四经经穴及经外奇穴编成五言歌诀，并加注释，便于初学者习诵，末附铜人图两张。现存清刊本(善成堂刊)。

Kaozheng Zhoushen Xuefa Ge (Verse on Methods of Textual Research on Points of the Whole Body)　A book in one volume, written by Liao Runhong of the Qing Dynasty, in which the Fourteen Meridian points and extra points of the whole body were written into verses of five characters in a line with annotation, convenient for beginners to remember. Two pictures of the acupoints on the bronze figure were attached at the end. The extant book was published in Shan Cheng Tang in the Qing Dynasty.

●颗粒式皮内针[kē lì shì pí nèi zhēn] 针具名。皮内针的一种，又称麦粒型皮内针。按针身长短分五分和一寸两种，粗细如毫针，尾部呈颗粒样。使用时用镊子夹住针体，轻缓沿皮刺入0.3～0.8寸，然后用胶布固定。

Granular Intradermal Needle　A needling apparatus, a kind of intradermal needle, also called a wheat-shaped intradermal needle. This kind of needle is divided into two kinds by length, i. e. 0.5 cun and 1 cun in length, the diameter of the needles is like the filiform needle, the handle of the needle is granular. 〈Method〉 Grip the body of the needle with a pair of tweezers, mildly puncture 0.3～0.8 cun subcutaneously, then fix it with adhesive cloth.

●咳嗽[ké sòu] 病证名。出《素问·五脏生成论》。肺经疾患之主要证候。咳，指肺气上逆作声；嗽，指咯吐痰液。有声有痰为咳嗽。咳嗽的发生，或因外邪犯肺，或因其他脏腑先病累及于肺而致。咳嗽的分类有风寒咳嗽、风热咳嗽、燥热咳嗽、肝火咳嗽、痰湿咳嗽、阴虚咳嗽等。详见各条。

Cough　A disease, originally from *Suwen*: *Wu Zang Sheng Cheng Lun* (*Plain Questions*: *Physiology and Pathology of the Five Zang-Organs*), the main syndrome of the disease of the Lung Meridian. Cough means tussis with gargling. Tussis refers to the abnormal rising of the lung-qi with sound. Gargling refers to spitting with sputum. The tussis with sound and sputum is called cough with gargling. It is due to invasion of the lung by external pathogenic factors, or the affection of the lung by the disease of the other organs. It is clinically divided into cough due to wind-cold pathogen, cough due to wind-heat pathogen, cough due to dry-heat pathogen, cough due to the liver fire, cough due to phlegm-dampness and cough due to yin-deficiency. →风寒咳嗽(p. 112)风热咳嗽(p. 114)燥热咳嗽(p. 583)肝火咳嗽(p. 124)痰湿咳嗽(p. 424)阴虚咳嗽(p. 561)

●咳嗽血[ké sòu xuè] 即咳血，见该条。

Cough with Blood　→咳血(p. 232)

●咳血[ké xuè] 病证名。见《丹溪心法》。指血因咳

嗽而出，或痰中带血，或咯纯血。又称嗽血、咳嗽血。多因肝火犯肺或阴虚火旺所致。临床可分为肝火犯肺咳血和阴虚火旺咳血。详见各条。

Hemoptysis A disease, seen in *Danxi Xinfa* (*Danxi's Experience*), referring to coughing with fresh blood, also called gargling with blood and coughing with blood. It is mostly due to invasion of the lung by liver-fire, or hyperactivity of fire due to yin-deficiency. Clinically, it is divided into hemoptysis due to invasion of lung by liver-fire and hemoptysis due to hyperactivity of fire due to yin-deficiency.
→肝火犯肺咳血(p. 124)阴虚火旺咳血(p. 560)

●客主人[kè zhǔ rén] 经穴别名。出《素问·气府论》。即上关。见该条。

Kezhuren Another name for Shangguan (GB 3), an extra point originally from *Suwen*: *Qifu Lun* (*Plain Questions*: *On House of Qi*). →上关(p. 352)

●孔广培[kǒng guǎng péi] 人名。清代针灸家，字筱亭，萧山（属浙江）人。同治十一年（1872年），刊其所撰《太乙神针集解》。

Kong Guangpei An expert of acupuncture and moxibustion in the Qing Dynasty, who styled himself Xiaoting, a native of Xiaoshan (now in Zhejiang Province). His *Taiyi Shenzhen Jijie* (*Exposition on Methods of Moxibustion with Great Monad Herbal Stick*) was published in the 11th year of the reign of Tong Zhi (1872).

●孔穴[kǒng xué] 腧穴的别名。见该条。

Holes Another name for acupoint. →腧穴 (p. 407)

●孔最[kǒng zuì] 经穴名。出《针灸甲乙经》。属手太阴肺经，为本经郄穴。〈定位〉在前臂掌面桡侧，当尺泽与太渊连线上，腕横纹上7寸（图49）。〈层次解剖〉皮肤→皮下组织→肱桡肌→桡侧腕屈肌→指浅层肌与旋前圆肌之间→拇长屈肌。浅层内布有头静脉和前臂外侧皮神经的分支。深层有桡动、静脉，桡神经浅支等结构。〈主治〉咳嗽、气喘、咯血、咽喉肿痛、失音、热病无汗、头痛、肘臂挛痛、痔疮。直刺0.5～0.8寸；可灸。

Kongzui (LU 6) A meridian point, originally from *Zhenjiu Jia-Yi Jing* (*A-B Classic of Acupuncture and Moxibustion*), the *Xi* (Cleft) Point of the Lung Meridian of Hand-Taiyin. 〈Location〉on the radial side of the palmar surface of the forearm, and on the line connecting Chize (LU 5) and Taiyuan (LU 9), 7 cun above the cubital crease (Fig. 49). 〈Regional anatomy〉 skin→subcutaneous tissue→brachioradial muscle→radial flexor muscle of wrist→between superficial flexor muscle of fingers and round pronator muscle→long flexor muscle of thumb. In the superficial layer, there are the cephalic vein and the branches of the lateral cutaneous nerve of the forearm. In the deep layer, there are the radial artery and vein and the superficial branches of the radial nerve. 〈Indications〉cough, dyspnea, hemoptysis, sore throat, loss of voice, anhidrosis in febrile disease, headache, the contracture and pain of the elbow and arm, and hemorrhoid. 〈Method〉Puncture perpendicularly 0.5～0.8 cun. Moxibustion is applicable.

●控脑砂[kòng nǎo shā] 即重症鼻渊。详见"鼻渊"条。

Serious Sinusitis with Purulent Discharge i. e. serious rhinorrhea with turbid discharge →鼻渊(p. 19)

●口[kǒu] 耳穴名。位于外耳道口后上方。具有清心火、除风邪作用。主治面瘫、口腔炎、胆囊炎、胆石症、戒断综合证。

Mouth (MA-ICS) An otopoint, which has the function of clearing heat fire, and removing pathogenic wind. 〈Location〉on the posterior and superior border of the orifice of the external auditory meatus. 〈Indications〉facial paralysis, stomatitis, cholecystitis cholelithiasis, abstinence syndrome.

●口寸[kǒu cùn] 经外奇穴比量法之一。见《千金要方》，系以患者本人两口角之间的距离作为一寸。

Mouth-Width Measurement One of the methods of locating extra points, from *Qianjin Yaofang* (*Essential Prescriptions Worth a Thousand Gold*). The mouth of the patient measures one cun between its two corners.

●口禾髎[kǒu hé liáo] 经穴名。出《针灸甲乙经》。属手阳明大肠经。又名禾髎、顑、长频、长髎、长颊、长频。〈定位〉在上唇部，鼻孔外缘直下，平水沟穴（图5和图28）。〈层次解剖〉皮肤→皮下组织→口轮匝肌。

浅层有上颌神经的眶下神经分支等结构。深层有上唇动、静脉和面神经颊支等分布。〈主治〉鼻疮息肉、鼻衄、鼻塞、鼻流清涕、口㖞、口噤不开。直刺0.2～0.5寸；禁灸。

Kouheliao(LI 19)　A meridian point, originally from *Zhenjiu Jia-Yi Jing* (*A-B Classic of Acupuncture and Moxibustion*), a point on the Large Intestine Meridian of Hand-Yangming, also named Heliao, Zhuo, Changpin, Changliao, Changjia, and Changhui. 〈Location〉on the upper lip, directly below the lateral border of the nostril, on the level of Shuigou (Du 26) (Figs. 5 & 28). 〈Regional anatomy〉skin→subcutaneous tissue→orbicular muscle of mouth. In the superficial layer, there are the branches of the infraorbital nerve of the maxillary nerve and so on. In the deep layer, there are the artery and vein of the upper lip and the buccal branches of the facial nerve. 〈Indications〉pyogenic infection of nose, nasal polyp, epistaxis, stuffy nose, watery nasal secretion, wry mouth, lockjaw. 〈Method〉Puncture perpendicularly 0.2～0.5 cun. Moxibustion is forbidden.

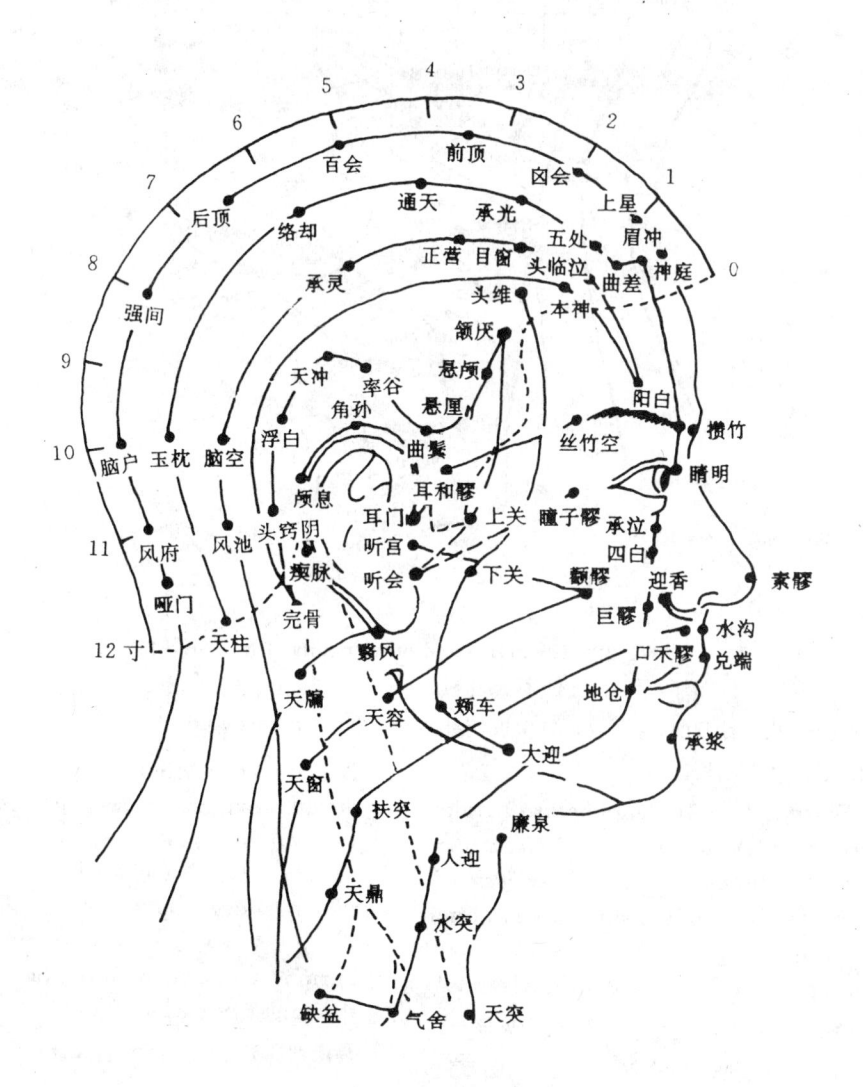

图28　口禾髎和其它头面部穴

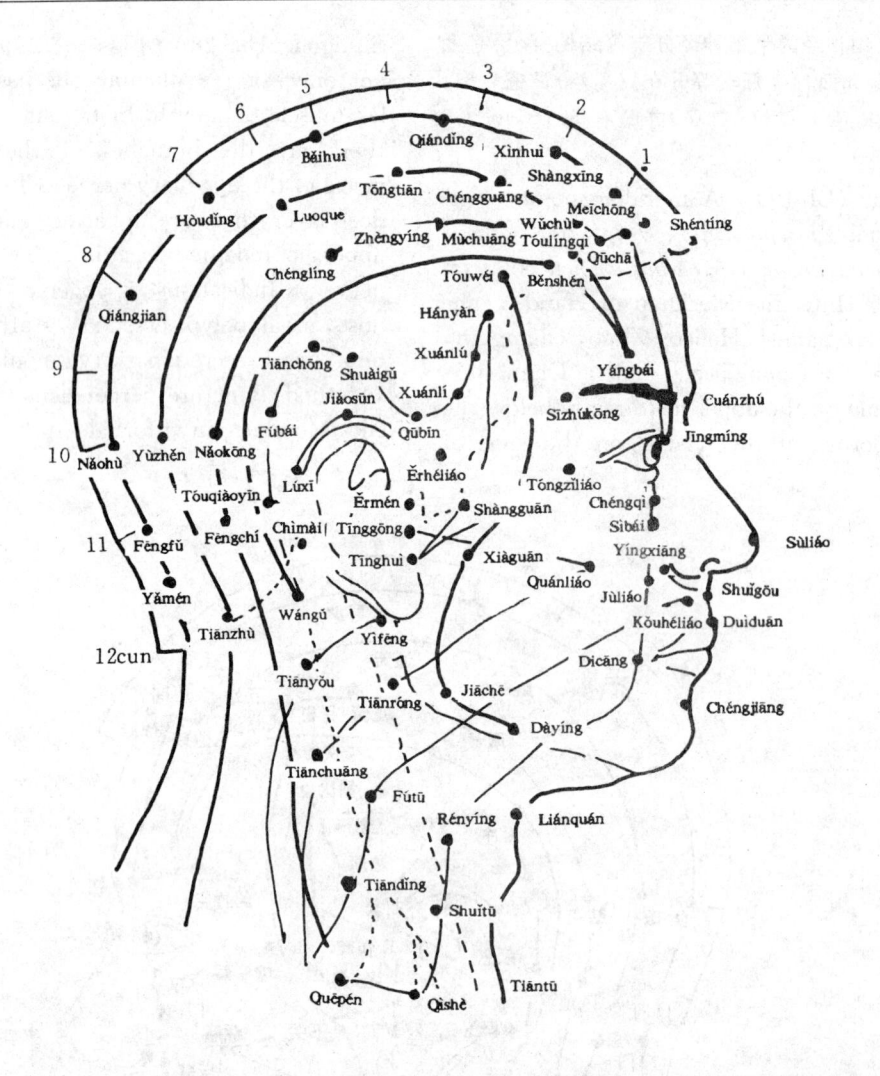

Fig. 28 Kouheliao and other points of head and face

●口温 [kǒu wēn] 针刺手法名。见《针灸大成》。十二字手法之一。指在针刺前,将针放入口中以使针热的一种方法,近代多不用。

Mouth Warming An acupuncture manipulation seen in *Zhenjiu Dacheng* (*A Great Compendium of Acupuncture and Moxibustion*), one of the twelve-word manipulations, referring to warming the needle inside the mouth before insertion, which is seldom used now.

●口眼歪斜 [kǒu yǎn wāi xié] 即面瘫。详见该条。

Deviation of the Eye and Mouth →面瘫(p. 266)

●苦瓠灸 [kǔ hú jiǔ] 间接灸的一种。见《串雅外编》。又称隔苦瓠灸。是用苦瓠作间隔物而施灸的一种灸法。取新鲜苦瓠一个,切片贴于疮上,上置艾炷灸之。可用于治疗痈疽。

Balsam Pear Moxibustion One form of indirect moxibustion, seen in *Chuanya Waibian* (*Treatises on Internal and External Folk Medicine*), also named balsam pear-separated moxibustion. Apply moxibustion by putting a slice of a raw balsam pear on the sore and a burning moxa cone on the balsam pear for the treatment of carbuncle.

●库房 [kù fáng] 经穴名。出《针灸甲乙经》。属足阳明胃经。〈定位〉在胸部,当第一肋间隙,距前正中线4寸(图40)。〈层次解剖〉皮肤→皮下组织→胸大肌→胸小肌。浅层布有锁骨上神经,肋间神经的皮支。深

层有胸肩峰动、静脉的分支或属支,胸内、外侧神经的分支。〈主治〉咳嗽、气逆、咳唾脓血、胸胁胀痛。向内斜刺0.5～0.8寸;可灸。

Kufang(ST 14) A meridian point originally from *Zhenjiu Jia-Yi Jing* (*A-B Classic of Acupuncture and Moxibustion*), a point on the Stomach Meridian of Foot-Yangming. 〈Location〉 on the chest, in the lst intercostal space, 4 cun lateral to the anterior midline(Fig. 40). 〈Regional anatomy〉 skin→subcutaneous tissue→greater pectoral muscle→smaller pectoral muscle. In the superficial layer, there are the supraclavicular nerve and the cutaneous branches of the intercostal nerve. In the deep layer, there are the branches or tributaries of the thoracoacromial artery and vein and the branches of the medial pectoral and lateral pectoral nerves. 〈Indications〉 cough, reversed flow of Qi, spitting pus and blood with cough, distending pain in the chest and hypochondrium. 〈Method〉 Puncture obliquely 0.5～0.8 cun towards the interior. Moxibustion is applicable.

●**快插进针**[kuài chā jìn zhēn] 进针方法之一。为注射式进针之别称。见该条。

Quick Needle Insertion A form of needle insertion in acupuncture, another name for injecting insertion of the needle. →注射式进针(p. 621)

●**髋**[kuān] 耳穴名。位于对耳轮上脚的下三分之一处。可用于治疗髋关节疼痛、坐骨神经痛。

Hip(MA-AH 4) An otopoint. 〈Location〉 at the inferior 1/3 of the superior antihelix crus. 〈Indications〉 pain in the hip joint, sciatica.

●**髋骨**[kuān gǔ] ①骨骼部位名。又称胯骨。左右髋骨与骶骨通过韧带形成一个完整的骨性环,即骨盆,由髂骨、坐骨和耻骨所组成。②经穴别名。见《针方六集·神照集》。即环跳。见该条。③经外穴名。见《类经图翼》。〈定位〉在大腿前面下部,当梁丘两旁各1.5寸,一侧二穴,左右共四穴(图29)。〈层次解剖〉外侧髋骨穴:皮肤→皮下组织→股外侧肌。浅层布有股神经前皮支和股外侧皮神经。深层有旋股外侧动、静脉降支的分支或属支。内侧髋骨穴:皮肤→皮下组织→股内侧肌。浅层布有股神经前皮支。深层有股深动脉的肌支等。〈主治〉两脚红肿疼痛、寒湿走注、腿痛举动不得等。斜刺或直刺0.5～1.0寸;可灸。

1. **Hip Bone** A part of the skeleton, also called Kuangu. Both the left and right hip bones form a complete osseous circle, i.e. the bony pelvis, by connecting the sacral bone through ligament. The hip bone is composed of the iliac bone, the ischium and the pubic bone.

2. **Kuangu** Another name for Huantiao(GB 30), a meridian point seen in *Zhenfang Liu Ji: Shen Zhao Ji*(*Six Collections of Acupuncture Prescriptions: Collection under Illumination of the Deity*). →环跳(p. 170)

3. **Kuangu**(EX-LE 1) An extra point, seen in *Leijing Tuyi*(*Illustrated Supplements to the Classified Canon of Internal Medicine of the Yellow Emperor*). 〈Location〉 two points on each thigh, in the lower part of the anterior surface of the thigh, 1.5 cun lateral and medial to Liangqiu(ST 34)(Fig. 29). 〈Regional anatomy〉 Kuangu(EX-LE 1)on the lateral side: skin→subcutaneous tissue→lateral muscle of thigh. In the superficial layer, there are the anterior cutaneous branches of the femoral nerve and the lateral cutaneous nerve of the thigh. In the deep layer, there are the branches or tributaries of the descending branches of the lateral circumflex femoral artery and vein. Kuangu(EX-LE 1)on the medial side: skin→subcutanecous tissue→medial of thigh. In the superficial layer, there are the anterior cutaneous branches of the femoral nerve. In the deep layer, there are the muscular branches of the deep femoral artery and vein. 〈Indications〉 red swelling and pain of the feet, migratory arthralgia due to cold-dampness, inability to raise the leg due to pain. 〈Method〉 Puncture obliquely or perpendicularly 0.5～1.0 cun. Moxibustion is applicable.

●**狂证**[kuáng zhèng] 癫狂证型之一。出《素问·癫狂》。多因七情郁结,五志化火,痰蒙心窍所致。证见面色垢赤,喧扰不定,打人毁物,多怒,高傲自居,无理争辩。甚则赤身露体,不避亲疏,登高而歌,狂乱不可制约,舌苔黄腻,脉滑数。久则郁火伤阴,烦躁善

惊,少寐,形瘦神倦,舌红少苔,脉细数。治宜平肝泻火,清心豁痰。取劳宫、水沟、丰隆、大钟、内庭、行间。久则伤阴加太溪、三阴交。

Mania A type of manic-depressive psychosis originally from *Suwen*: *Diankuang* (*Plain Questions*: *Manic-Depressive Psychosis*), due to stagnation of seven emotions, pathogenic fire caused by the disorders of five emotions, mental confusion due to phlegm. 〈Manifestations〉 dirty and flushed complexion, restlessness, beating others, destroying things, irritability, arrogance, unjustifiable debate, or, even worse, the patient will be naked without avoiding people around him, whether they are intimate or not and ascend to a height to sing, accompanied by uncontrollable madness. The tongue has a yellowish and greasy coating, the pulse is slippery and rapid. Lingering cases are manifested by impairment of yin due to stagnated fire, dysphoria, susceptibility to fright, insomnia, thirst, spiritlessness, red tongue with thin coating, thready and rapid pulse. 〈Treatment principle〉 Calm the liver and purge intense heat; remove heat from the heart and eliminate phlegm for resuscitation. 〈Point selection〉 Laogong(PC 8), Shuigou(DU 26), Fenglong(ST 40), Dazhong(KI 4), Neiting(ST 44), Xingjian(LR 2), add Taixi(KI 3) and Sanyinjiao(SP 6) for lingering cases whose yin-fluid is injured.

●昆仑[kūn lún] 经穴名。出《灵枢·本输》。属足太阳膀胱经,为本经经穴。又名下昆仑、上昆仑。〈定位〉在足部外踝后方,当外踝尖与跟腱之间的凹陷处(图35.2)。〈层次解剖〉皮肤→皮下组织→跟腱前方的疏松结缔组织中。浅层布有腓肠神经和小隐静脉。深层有腓动、静脉的分支或属支。〈主治〉头痛、项强、目眩、鼻衄、疟疾、肩背拘急、腰痛、足跟痛、小儿痫证、难产。直刺0.5~1寸;可灸。

Kunlun (BL 60) A meridian point from *Lingshu*: *Benshu* (*Miraculous Pivot*: *Meridian Points*), a point on the Bladder Meridian of Foot-Taiyang, also named Xiakunlun and Shangkunlun. 〈Location〉 posterior to the lateral malleolus, in the depression between the tip of the external malleolus and achilles tendon (Fig. 35.2). 〈Regional anatomy〉 skin → subcutaneous tissue → loose connective tissue anterior to achilles tendon. In the superficial layer, there are the sural nerve and small saphenous vein. In the deep layer, there are the branches or tributaries of the peroneal artery and vein. 〈Indications〉 headache, stiff-nape, dizziness, epistaxis, malarial disease, contracture of shoulder and back, lumbago, pain in the heel, epilepsy in children and dystocia. 〈Method〉 Puncture perpendicularly 0.5~1.0 cun. Moxibustion is applicable.

L

●拉罐法[lā guàn fǎ] 为推罐法之别称。见该条。

Pulling Cupping Another name for cupping by pushing the cup. →推罐法(p. 449)

●喇嘛穴[lǎ ma xué] 经外穴名。见《北京中医》。在肩胛部,当天宗与腋后皱襞尽端连线上,距天宗1.5寸处,主治咽喉炎。直刺0.5~1寸。

Lama(EX-B) An extra point, seen in *Beijing Zhongyi*(*Traditional Chinese Medicine In Beijing*). 〈Location〉 on the scapula and on the line connecting Tianzong(SI 11) and the extreme end of the posterior axillary line, 1.5 cun from Tianzong (SI 11). 〈Indication〉 laryngopharyngitis. 〈Method〉 Puncture perpendicularly 0.5~1.0 cun.

●兰门[lán mén] 经外穴名。见《针灸大成》,在曲骨两旁各3寸。主治膀胱七疝、奔豚。直刺0.5~1.0寸;可灸。

Lanmen(EX-CA) Two extra points origi-

nally from *Zhenjiu Dacheng* (*A Great Compendium of Acupuncture and Moxibustion*). ⟨Location⟩ 3 cun lateral to Qugu(RN 2). ⟨Indications⟩ seven forms of hernia of the urinary bladder and sensation of gas rushing. ⟨Method⟩ Puncture perpendicularly 0.5~1.0 cun. Moxibustion is applicable.

●拦江赋[lán jiāng fù]　针灸歌赋名。见《针灸聚英》。拦江,拦截水流,即截用要穴的意思。其讲八脉八穴及合谷、复溜、期门等穴的应用。

Lan Jiang Fu (Intercepting-River Fu) A verse about acupuncture and moxibustion, seen in *Zhenjiu Juying* (*Essentials of Acupuncture and Moxibustion*). "Intercepting river", or "intercepting water flow", refers to interception of important points. It mentions the application of Eight Confluence Points, Hegu(LI 4), Fuliu(KI 7) and Qimen(LR 14), etc.

●阑尾[lán wěi]　①经外穴名。见《新中医药》。⟨定位⟩在小腿前侧上部,当犊鼻下5寸,胫骨前缘旁开一横指。⟨层次解剖⟩皮肤→皮下组织→胫骨前肌→小腿骨间膜→胫骨后肌。浅层布有腓肠外侧皮神经和浅静脉。深层有腓深神经和胫前动、静脉。⟨主治⟩急、慢性阑尾炎,急、慢性肠炎,下肢麻木或瘫痪,足下垂等。直刺1.0~1.5寸。②耳穴名。位于大、小肠两穴之间。用于治疗单纯性阑尾炎,腹泻。

1. **Lanwei**(EX-LE 7) An extra point seen in *Xin Zhong yiyao* (*New Traditional Chinese Medicine and Herb*). ⟨Location⟩ at the upper part of the anterior surface of the leg, 5 cun below Dubi(ST 35), one finger breadth lateral to the anterior crest of the tibia. ⟨Regional anatomy⟩ skin→subcutaneous tissue→anterior tibial muscle→interosseous membrane of leg→posterior tibial muscle. In the superficial layer, there are the lateral sural cutaneous nerve and the superficial veins. In the deep layer, there are the deep peroneal nerve and the anterior tibial artery and vein. ⟨Indications⟩ acute and chronic appendicitis, acute and chronic enteritis, numbness or paralysis of the lower limbs and foot drop, etc. ⟨Method⟩ Puncture perpendicularly 1.0~1.5 cun.

2. **Appendix**(MA) An otopoint. ⟨Location⟩ between Large Intestine(MA-SC 4) and Small Intestine(MA-SC 2). ⟨Indications⟩ simple appendicitis and diarrhea.

●劳宫[láo gōng]　经穴名。出《灵枢·本输》。属手厥阴心包经,为本经荥穴。又名五里、掌中、鬼营、鬼窟。⟨定位⟩在手掌心,当第二、三掌骨之间偏于第三掌骨,握拳屈指时中指尖处(图49和图45)。⟨层次解剖⟩皮肤→皮下组织→掌腱膜→分别在桡侧两根指浅、深屈肌腱之间→第二蚓状肌桡侧→第一骨间掌侧肌和第二骨间背侧肌。浅层布有正中神经的掌支和手掌侧静脉网。深层有指掌侧总动脉,正中神经的指掌侧固有神经。⟨主治⟩中风昏迷、中暑、心痛、癫狂、痫证、口疮、口臭、鹅掌风。直刺0.3~0.5寸;可灸。

Laogong(PC 8) A meridian point, originally from *Lingshu: Benshu* (*Miraculous Pivot: Acupoints*), Ying(Spring) Point of the Pericardium Meridian of Hand-Jueyin, also named Wuli, Zhangzhong, Guiying or Guiku. ⟨Loca-

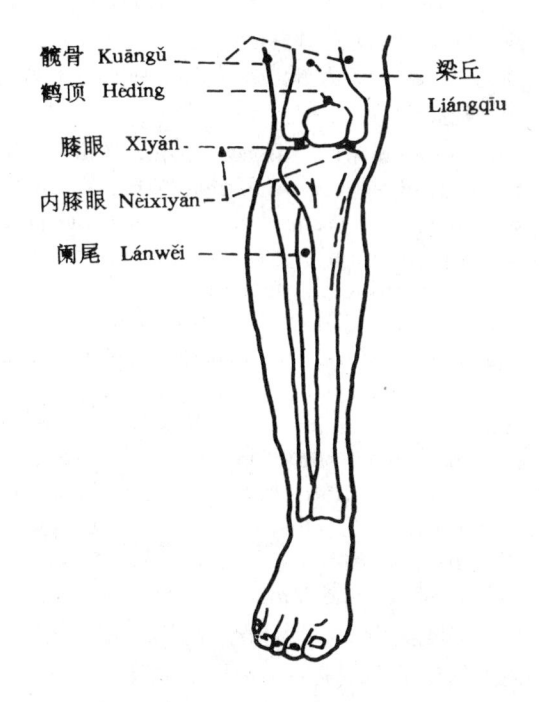

髌骨 Kuāngǔ
鹤顶 Hèdǐng
膝眼 Xīyǎn
内膝眼 Nèixīyǎn
阑尾 Lánwěi
梁丘 Liánqiū

图29　阑　尾　穴
Fig. 29　Lanwei point

tion〉at the centre of the palm, between the 2nd and 3rd metacarpal bones, but closer to the latter, and touching the tip of the middle finger when a fist is made(Figs. 49&45).〈Regional anatomy〉skin→subcutaneous tissue→palmar aponeurosis→between tendons of superficial and deep flexor muscle of fingers on radial side→radial side of second lumbrical muscle→first palmar interosseous muscle and second dorsal interosseous muscle. In the superficial layer, there are the palmar branches of the median nerve and the venous network of the palmar side. In the deep layer, there are the common palmar digital artery and the proper palmar digital nerve of the median nerve.〈Indications〉apoplectic coma, heatstroke, precardial pain, manic-depressive disorder, epilepsy, aphthae, foul breath, tinea unguium.〈Method〉Puncture perpendicularly 0.3~0.5 cun. Moxibustion is applicable.

●劳淋[láo lìn]　淋证证型之一。多由诸淋日久，或久病体虚，或劳伤过度，以致脾肾两虚，湿浊不去而致。证见小便不甚赤涩，但淋沥不已、时作时止，遇劳即发、腰酸膝软、神疲之力、舌质淡、脉虚弱。治宜健脾利湿，益肾固涩。取肾俞、膀胱俞、脾俞、足三里、关元、三阴交。可加灸。

Stranguria Induced by Overstrain　One type of stranguria, mostly due to lingering stranguria, valetudinarianism, or serious internal injury caused by overstrain, which leads to deficiency of both the spleen and the kidney and lingering pathogenic dampness.〈Manifestations〉slightly dark and difficult but dribbling urination which occurs from time to time especially when overstrained, lassitude in loin and knees, both mental and manual fatigue, pale tongue, feeble and weak pulse.〈Treatment principle〉Invigorate the kidney and induce astringency.〈Point selection〉Shenshu (BL 23), Pangguangshu (BL 28), Pishu (BL 20), Zusanli (ST 36), Guangyuan (RN 4), Sanyinjiao (SP 6).〈Method〉Moxibustion is applicable.

●劳疟[láo nüè]　疟疾之一。出《金匮要略》。由正气虚衰，劳损之体，又感疟邪所致。证见倦怠乏力、短气懒言、食少、面色萎黄、形体消瘦，遇劳则疟发、寒热时作、舌质淡、脉细无力。治宜扶正祛邪，益气养血。取陶道、曲池、足三里、外关、脾俞、胃俞、气海俞、关元俞。

Malaria with General Debility　A form of malarial disease originally from *Jingui Yaolüe* (*Synopsis of the Golden Chamber*), due to vital-qi deficiency, internal injury caused by overstrain followed by affection of the pathogenic factor of malarial disease.〈Manifestations〉lassitude, acratia, short breath, disliking speaking, anorexia, sallow complexion, thinness, reoccurrence of malarial disease whenever overstrained, alternate attack of chills and fever, pale tongue, thready and weak pulse.〈Treatment principle〉Strengthen the body resistance and eliminate pathogenic factors, supplement qi and nourish blood. 〈Point selection〉Taodao(DU 13), Quchi(LI 11), Zusanli(ST 36), Waiguan(SJ 5), Pishu (BL 20), Weishu(BL 21), Qihaishu(BL 24), Guanyuanshu(BL 26).

●劳伤月经过多[láo shāng yuè jīng guò duō]　是月经过多的证型之一。多因经期不慎，过度劳伤，冲任受损所致。证见月经过多，并持续时间较长、血色黯、面色萎黄、体倦乏力、腰腹酸坠，治宜固冲止血。取气海、肾俞、足三里、三阴交、隐白。

Menorrhagia with Internal Injury Caused by Overstrain　A type of manorrhagia usually caused by carelessness during menstrual period, serious internal injury caused by overstrain, resulting in the impairment of Chong and Ren Meridians.〈Manifestations〉menorrhagia with dark red menstruation, lingering longer than usual, sallow complexion, lassitude, acratia, sensation of aching and weighing in the loin and abdomen.〈Treatment principle〉Reinforce the Chong meridian and arrest bleeding.〈Point selection〉Qihai (RN 6), Shenshu (BL 23) Zusanli (ST 36), Sanyinjiao (SP 6), and Yinbai (SP 1).

●劳损腰痛[láo sǔn yāo tòng]　腰痛证型之一。多因跌仆闪挫，经气受损，或弯腰劳作过度，气血运行不利，气滞血瘀所致。证见多有陈伤宿疾、劳累时加剧、腰部强直酸痛，其痛固定不移、转侧俯仰不利，胭中常有络脉瘀血、舌脉多无变化。治宜活血化瘀，通络定痛。取膈俞、次髎、三阴交、肾俞、委中。

Lumbar Pain due to Internal Injury Caused by Overstrain A type of lumbar pain mostly due to traumatic injury, sprain and contusion, impairment of the meridian qi, or overwork with the body bent, abnormal flowing of qi and blood stasis. ⟨Manifestations⟩ affection of old trauma and chronic disease of the loin which becomes more serious with overwork, aching pain of the loin when forced to straighten, difficulty in turning about, bending and lying on the back, frequent blood stasis of collaterals in popliteal fossa, usually with normal pulse and tongue. ⟨Treatment principle⟩ Promote blood circulation to remove blood stasis and pain, clear collaterals to relieve pain. ⟨Point selections⟩ Geshu (BL 17), Ciliao (BL 32), Sanyinjiao (SP 6), Shenshu (BL 23) and Weizhong (BL 40).

●劳瘵[láo zhài] 病证名。见《三因极一病证方论·劳瘵叙论》。即肺痨。见该条。

Tuberculosis Another name of a consumptive disease, seen in *Sanyin Jiyi Bingzheng Fanglun*: *Laozhai Xulun* (*Treatise on the Three Categories of Pathogenic Factors of Diseases and the Prescriptions*: *Introduction to Tuberculosis*). →肺痨(p. 107)

●老鼠疮[lǎo shǔ chuāng] 即瘰疬。详见该条。

Mouse Sore →瘰疬(p. 258)

●落枕[lào zhěn] ①病证名。古称失枕。多由睡眠姿势不当，枕头高低不适，致使颈部关节、筋肉长时间过度牵拉而致。证见早晨起床后突然感到一侧颈项强直，不能俯仰转侧，患部酸楚疼痛，或向同侧肩背及上臂放散，或兼有头痛怕冷等症状，局部肌肉紧张、压痛明显，但无红肿发热。治宜调气活血，舒筋散寒。取风池、天柱、落枕穴、后溪、悬钟。②经外穴名，又名项强。在颈部当天容与天柱穴连线之中点。主治落枕、偏头痛、肩背痛、胃痛等，直刺0.5～1.0寸。

1. Stiffneck A disease, of which the archaic term is loss from pillow, frequently due to improper sleeping posture and the height of the pillow, which leads to overdrawing of cervical joints or tendon and muscles. ⟨Manifestations⟩ sudden stiffness on one side of the neck and nape after getting up in the morning, inability to bend, lift or turn the head, aching pain of the affected part, which may spread to the shoulder and the back of the same side or be accompanied by headache, intolerance of cold; local muscular tone and obvious pressing tenderness without reddness, swelling and fever. ⟨Treatment principle⟩ Promote the flow of qi and blood circulation, relax muscles and dispel cold. ⟨Point selection⟩ Fengchi (GB 20), Tianzhu (BL 10), Laozhen (EX-HN), Houxi (SI 3), Xuanzhong (GB 39).

2. Laozhen (EX-HN) An extra point, also named Xiangqiang. ⟨Location⟩ on the cervical part and at the midpoint between Tianrong (SI 17) and Tianzhu (BL 10). ⟨Indications⟩ stiffneck, migraine, pain of shoulder and back, stomachache, etc. ⟨Method⟩ Puncture perpendicularly 0.5～1.0 cun.

●雷丰[léi fēng] 人名。晚清医家，字少逸，衢州（今属浙江）人。著《时病论》、《灸法秘传》。

Lei Feng A physician in the Late Qing Dynasty who styled himself Shao Yi, a native of Quzhou (now in Zhejiang), and compiler of *Shi bing Lun* (*Treatise on Seasonal Diseases*) and *Jiufa Michuan* (*Secretly Bequeathed Method of Moxibustion*).

●雷火神针[léi huǒ shén zhēn] 药艾条之一。见《本草纲目》。所含药物以沉香、木香、乳香、茵陈、羌活、干姜、穿山甲、麝香等为主。适用于风寒湿痹、寒性腹痛、痛经等。其制作和操作方法与太乙神针相同。参见"太乙神针"条。

Thunder-Fire Miraculous Needle A type of medicinal moxa roll, seen in *Bencao Gangmu* (*Compendium of Materia Medica*) composed mainly of *Chen Xiang* (*Aquilaria Agallocha*) *Mu Xiang* (*Aucklandia lappa*), *Ru Xiang* (*Boswellia carterii*), *Yin Chen* (*Artemisia capillaris*), *Qiang Huo* (*Notoptergium forbesii*), fresh ginger (dried), *Chuan Shan Jia* (*Manis pentadactyla*) and *She Xiang* (*Moschus berezovskii*), etc., used for treating maladies such as arthralgia due to wind-cold-dampness, abdominal pain of cold nature, dysmenorrhea, etc. Its construction and manipulation are the same as those of Taiyi moxa-cigar. →太乙神针(p. 421)

●雷火针法[léi huǒ zhēn fǎ] ①为雷火神针之别称，

见该条。②书名,清代刘国光辑,收载于《灸法秘传》。详见"灸法秘传"条。

1. Moxibustion with Thunder-Fire Herbal Moxa Stick →雷火神针(p.239)

2. Leihuo Zhenfa (Moxibustion with Thunder-Fire Herbal Moxa Stick) A book compiled by Liu Guoguang of the Qing Dynasty, which is included in *Jiufa Michuan (Secretly Bequeathed Method of Moxibustion)*. →灸法秘传(p.223)

●肋头[lèi tóu] 经外穴名。见《类经图翼》。在胸骨两侧缘,当第1及第2肋骨头下缘处,左右共四穴。主治瘰疬、咳嗽、哮喘、呃逆,以及肋间神经痛、支气管炎等。斜刺0.3~0.5寸;可灸。

Leitou (EX-CA) A set of extra points originally seen in *Leijing Tuyi (Illustrated Supplements to Classified Canon of Internal Medicine of the Yellow Emperor)*. 〈Location〉 on both lateral borders of the sterna, on the inferior edges of the 1st and 2nd rib-heads; 2 on each side, 4 points in all. 〈Indications〉 abdominal mass, cough, asthma, hiccup, intercostal neuralgia, bronchitis, etc. 〈Method〉 Puncture obliquely 0.3~0.5 cun. Moxibustion is applicable.

●肋䏶[lèi xià] 经外穴名。见《类经图翼》。在胸部,约当第4肋间隙处,乳头向外旁开4寸。主治腹痛、胁肋痛等。可灸。

Leixia (EX-CA) An extra point originally from *Leijing Tuyi (Illustrated Supplements to Classified Canon of Internal Medicine of the Yellow Emperor)*. 〈Location〉 on the chest, approximately in the 4th intercostal space, 4 cun lateral to the nipple. 〈Indications〉 abdominal pain and pain in hypochondriac region. 〈Method〉 Moxibustion is applicable.

●泪空[lèi kōng] 经穴别名。出《针灸聚英》。即睛明。见该条。

Leikong Another name for Jingming (BL 1), a meridian point originally from *Zhenjiu Juying (Essentials of Acupuncture and Moxibustion)*. →睛明(p.217)

●泪孔[lèi kǒng] 经穴别名。出《针灸甲乙经》,即睛明,见该条。

Leikong Another name for Jingming (BL 1), a meridian point originally from *Zhenjiu Jia-Yi Jing (A-B Classic of Acupuncture and Moxibustion)*. →睛明(p.217)

●类经[lèi jīng] 书名。明代张介宾(景岳)撰,三十二卷,刊于1624年。本书为分类研究《内经》的著作,将《内经》分为摄生、阴阳、藏象、脉色、经络、标本、气味、论治、疾病、针刺、运气、会通十二类。并对其原文进行研究和注释,为研究《内经》的重要参考书。

Leijing (Classified Canon) A 32-volume book by Zhang Jiebin (Jingyue) of the Ming Dynasty, published in 1624. It is a classified study of *Neijing (The Inner canon of Huangdi)*. It divides *Neijing (The Inner Canon of Huangdi)* into 12 classifications—health preserving, Yin and Yang, state of viscera, state of pulse, meridians and collaterals, superficiality and origin, the nature and taste of a drug, therapy, diseases, acupuncture and the doctrine on five elements, motion and six kinds of natural factors, and bringing things together and understanding them thoroughly. It is a study and annotation of the original and an important reference book for the study of *Neijing (The Canon of Internal Medicine)*.

●类经附翼[lèi jīng fù yì] 书名。明张介宾撰,刊于1624年,四卷。为《图翼》的附篇,分医易、律原、求正录、针灸歌赋等内容。

Leijing Fuyi (An Addition to Supplements to Illustrated Classified Canon of Internal Medicine of the Yellow Emperor) A 4-volume book written by Zhang Jiebin of the Ming Dynasty and published in 1624. It is a supplement to *Tuyi (Supplements to Illustrated Classified Canon of Internal Medicine of the Yellow Emperor)*. It includes such contents as medicine and changes, Lü Yuan, seeking the correct, and verses on acupuncture and moxibustion, etc.

●类经图翼[lèi jīng tú yì] 书名。明张介宾撰,十一卷,刊于1624年。以图解方式补《类经》注文之不足。主要为运气(卷1-2)和针灸(卷3-11)两部分,针灸部分包括经络腧穴、要穴歌及灸法等,且有附图,有重要参考价值。

Leijing Tuyi (Supplements to Illustrated Classified Canon of Internal Medicine of the Yellow Emperor) An 11-volume book by

Zhang Jiebin of the Ming Dynasty, published in 1624. It made up for the shortness of the annotations to *Leijing* (*Classified Canon of Internal Medicine of the Yellow Emperor*) by presenting illustrations. It mainly involves two parts—doctrine on five-element motion and six kinds of natural factors (Vols. 1 & 2) and acupuncture and moxibustion (Vols. 3-11). The latter includes the theory of meridians, collaterals and acupoints, verses about important acupoints and moxibustion, with attached illustrations. It is of great reference value.

●冷秘[lěng bì] 便秘证型之一,见《济生方》。又名阴结、寒结。因脾肾阳虚,阴寒凝结,温运无力所致,证见大便艰难不易排出、甚则脱肛、腹中冷痛、面色白、小便清白频数、四肢欠温、腰膝酸软、舌淡苔白、脉沉迟。治宜补肾助阳。取气海、照海、石门、肾俞、关元俞。

Constipation of Cold Type A type of constipation seen in *Jisheng Fang* (*Recipes for Saving Lives*), also named yin-accumulation or cold-accumulation, usually caused by yang deficiency of both the spleen and the kidney, accumulation of severe pathogenic cold, and weak transportation due to the deficiency of warmth. ⟨Manifestations⟩ dyschesia, proctoptosis, cold pain in the abdomen, pale complexion, clear, whitish and frequent urine, cold limbs, lassitude in the loin and knees, pale tongue with whitish coating, deep and slow pulse. ⟨Treatment principle⟩ Reinforce the kidney and support yang. ⟨Point selection⟩ Qihai (RN 6), Zhaohai (KI 6), Shimen (RN 5), Shenshu (BL 23), Guanyuanshu (BL 26).

●冷灸[lěng jiǔ] 灸法的一种,又称无热灸。与热灸相对而言,泛指药物敷贴等不用任何热源,以进行灸治的方法。参见"热灸"条。

Cold Moxibustion A form of moxibustion by applying medicine on certain acupoints without any heat resources, also named moxibustion without heat. It is the opposite of heat moxibustion. →热灸(p. 330)

●冷厥[lěng jué] 见《类证活人书·问手足逆冷》即寒厥,见该条。

Chilly Limbs Seen in *Leizheng Huoren Shu: Wen Shouzu Nileng* (*A Book of Differential Diagnosis and Treatment for Saving Lives: Inquiry about Cold Extremities*) →寒厥 (p. 155)

●冷瘴[lěng zhàng] 瘴疟之一,由素体阳虚,复感瘴毒疟邪,以致瘴毒湿浊壅闭,蒙蔽心神所致。证见寒甚热微、或但寒不热、或呕吐腹泻,甚则神昏不语、苔白厚腻,脉弦。治宜解毒除瘴,蠲湿化浊,兼清心开窍之法。取陶道、后溪、间使、液门、公孙、内关、足三里、水沟。

Cold Malignant Malaria A type of malignant malaria due to constitutional yang deficiency and the affection of mountainous evil air and damp-evil, and disturbance of vitality. ⟨Manifestations⟩ cold sensation with little or no warmth, vomiting, diarrhea, or even coma and speechlessness, whitish, thick and greasy tongue coating, taut pulse. ⟨Treatment principle⟩ Detoxicate and remove mountainous evil air, dampness, turbid qi, and heat from the heart to restore to consciousness. ⟨Point selection⟩ Taodao (DU 13), Houxi (SI 3), Jianshi (PC 5), Yemen (SJ 2), Gongsun (SP 4), Neiguan (PC 6), Zusanli (ST 36) and Shuigou (DU 26).

●冷针[lěng zhēn] 针刺用语。①与温针相区别,指单纯的针刺方法。②为白针之别称。见该条。

1. Cold Needling A term of acupuncture, differentiated from warm needling referring to pure needling.

2. Cold Needling Another name for ordinary needle. →白针(p. 11)

●离左酉南[lí zuǒ yǒu nán] 见《标幽赋》。离,八卦之一,方位正南,代表午。离左,指午时之后;酉南,指酉时之前。即当未申二时(3.00~7.00p. m时),意指午后酉前(相当于下半月)。取月相由盈转亏,以喻人之气血由盛而衰,因其午后气血之基础为实,在向虚转变过程中,应顺势用泻法。

Left to Li and South to You Seen in *Biaoyou Fu* (*Lyrics of Recondite Principles*). Li, one of the Ba Gua (the 8 Diagrams) due south, stands for the Wu period (1p. m ~ 3p. m), "left to Li" refers to the time after the Wu period (11a. m ~ 1p. m), whereas "south to You" refers to the time prior to the You period (5p. m ~ 7p. m), in other words the time

covering the Wei and Shen periods (roughly 3.00~7.00p.m), or, the time "after Wu and prior to You" (corresponding to the 2nd half of a month). The moon phase which is from waxing to waning is here compared to the qi and blood of a human being, the process of which is from prosperity to decline. Since excess is the essential of qi and blood after moon time, the reducing method should be used along with the turning from excess to deficiency.

●蠡沟[lí gōu] 经穴名。出《灵枢·经脉》。属足厥阴肝经，为本经络穴。又名交仪。〈定位〉在小腿内侧，当足内踝尖上5寸，胫骨内侧面的中央（图81和图80）。〈层次解剖〉皮肤→皮下组织→胫骨骨面。浅层布有隐神经的小腿内侧皮支和大隐静脉。〈主治〉月经不调、赤白带下、阴挺、阴痒、疝气、小便不利、睾丸肿痛、小腹满、腰背拘急不可仰俯、胫部酸痛。平刺0.5~0.8寸，可灸。

Ligou (LR 5) A meridian point originally from *Lingshu*: *Jingmai* (*Miraculous Pivot*: *Meridians*), the Luo(Connecting) Point of the Liver Meridian of Foot-Jueyin, also named Jiaoyi. 〈Location〉 on the medial side of the leg, 5 cun above the tip of the medial malleous, on the midline of the medial surface of the tibia (Figs. 81&80). 〈Regional anatomy〉 skin → subcutaneous tissue → medial surface of tibia. There are the medial cutaneous branches of the leg from the saphenous nerve and the great saphenous vein in this area. 〈Indications〉 irregular menstruation, leukorrhea with reddish discharge, prolapse of uterus, pruritus vulvae, hernia, difficulty in urination, painful and swollen testis, fullness of the lower abdomen,, contracture in the back and loin leading to the inability to bend forward and backward, aching pain in the tibia. 〈Method〉 Puncture subcutaneously 0.5~0.8 cun. Moxibustion is applicable.

●李浩[lí hào] 人名。金代针灸家，李源之子。其常于山东一带行医，治病有显效。著有《素问钩玄》、《仲景或问》、《伤寒钤法》等书。参见"李源"、"窦汉卿"条。

Li Hao An expert of acupuncture and moxibustion in the Jin Dynasty, son of Li Yuan. He practised medicine in Shandong Province and was always achieving obvious effects. He complied *Suwen Gouxuan* (*Profundities of Plain Questions*), *Zhongjing Huowen* (*A Study on Puzzles from Zhongjing's Book*) and *Shanghan Qianfa* (*Key Methods for Cold-Induced Diseases*), etc. →李源 (p.243)、窦汉卿 (p.85)

●李梦周[lí mèng zhōu] 人名。清代针灸家，鄞县（今属浙江）人。精针术，治病多验。事见《鄞县志》。

Li Mengzhou An expert of acupuncture and moxibustion in the Qing Dynasty, from Jinxian County (now in Zhejiang Province). Proficient in acupuncture techniques, he gained good effects. For details see *Jinxian Zhi* (*Annals of Jinxian County*).

●李守道[lí shǒu dào] 人名。明代针灸家，字存吾，浦城（今属福建）人。据说治中痰痫症有特效。事见《建宁府志》。

Li Shoudao An expert of acupuncture and moxibustion in the Ming Dynasty, who styled himself Cunwu, from Pucheng (of Fujian Province today). He is said to have been especially effective in the treatment of epilepsy due to phlegm. For details see *Jianningfu Zhi* (*Annals of Jianningfu*).

●李守先[lí shǒu xiān] 人名。清针灸家，字善述，长葛（今属河南）人。撰《针灸易学》二卷，为清代较通俗的针灸著作。

Li Shouxian An expert of acupuncture and moxibustion in the Qing Dynasty from Changge (of Henan Province today), who styled himself Shanshu, compiler of *Zhenjiu Yixue* (*Acupuncture and Moxibustion Is Easy to Learn*) in 2 volumes, which was a popular book about acupuncture and moxibustion in the Qing Dynasty.

●李学川[lí xué chuān] 人名。清代针灸家，字三源，别号邓尉山人，吴县（今属江苏）人。历经四十余年，终于于嘉庆二十年（1815年）撰成《针灸逢源》一书，为清代针灸佳作。

Li Xuechuan An acupuncture-moxibustion expert in the Qing Dynasty, from Wuxian County (of Jiangsu Province today), who styled himself Sanyuan and assumed the name

of Dengwei, the Mountainous Man. His *Zhenjiu Fengyuan* (*The Origin of Acupuncture and Moxibustion*), which was completed, after more than 40 years of hard work, in 1815, the 20th year in the reign of Jiaqing, was an excellent work of acupuncture and moxibustion in the Qing Dynasty.

●李玉[lǐ yù] 人名。明代针灸家,字成章,官六安卫(今安微六安)*千户。善骑射,尤精于方药针灸,其治学严谨,疗效显著,号称神针。

Li Yu An acupuncture-moxibustion expert in the Ming Dynasty who styled himself Chengzhang,* Qian Hu in Liuanwei (now Liuan County, Anhui Province). He was good at riding horse especially proficient in recipes, acupuncture and moxibustion, meticulous with studies, and often created notable curative effects. As a result, he won the name of Miraculous Needle.

*(*qian hu*) an army officer in the Yuan Dynasty, in command of 1,120 soldiers.

●李源[lǐ yuán] 人名。金代针灸家,蔡邑(今河南汝南)人。精于针灸术,传其子李浩,为窦默所师承,撰成《流注指微赋》。

Li Yuan An acupuncture-moxibustion expert in the Jin Dynasty from Caiyi (now Runan, Henan Province). Proficient in acupuncture techniques, he passed them on to his son, Li Hao. Teacher of Dou Mo, who compiled *Liuzhu Zhiwei Fu* (*Ode to the Subtleties of Flow*).

●里内庭[lǐ nà tíng] 经外穴名。见《中国针灸学》。在足底部,当第2、3趾骨间,与内庭穴相对处。主治足趾疼痛、小儿惊风、癫痫、胃痛等,直刺0.3～0.5寸;可灸。

Lineiting (EX-LE) An extra point, seen in *Zhongguo Zhenjiuxue* (*Chinese Acupuncture and Moxibustion*). 〈Location〉on the sole, between the 2nd and the 3rd metatarsal bones, opposite to Neiting (ST 44). 〈Indications〉pain of toes, infantile convulsion, epilepsy, stomachache. 〈Method〉Puncture perpendicularly 0.3～0.5 cun. Moxibustion is applicable.

●理瀹骈文[lǐ yuè pián wén] 书名。又名《外治医说》,一册,不分卷,清代吴尚光撰,刊于1870年。本书正文以骈文体写成,是一部以膏药为主的外治专书,提倡内病外治,亦有灸法内容,具有简、便、验、廉的特点。

Liyue Pianwen (**A Rhymed Discourse on External Therapies**) (1870) A single-volume book compiled by Wu Shangguang in the Qing Dynasty, also entitled *Waizhi Yishuo* (*Theories on External Diseases*). Written in the style of *Pianwen* (a rhythmical prose characteristic of parallelism and ornateness), the book is a monograph about external treatment with adhesive plaster, advocating treating internal diseases externally. Also included in the book is some information about moxibustion. It is quite simple, convenient, efficacious and cheap.

●厉兑[lì duì] 经穴名。出《灵枢·本输》。属足阳明胃经,为本经井穴。〈定位〉足第二趾末节外侧,距趾甲角0.1寸(指寸)(图60.3和图60.5)。〈层次解剖〉皮肤→皮下组织→甲根。布有足背内侧皮神经的趾背神和趾背动、静脉网。〈主治〉面肿、口㖞、齿痛、鼻衄、鼻流黄涕、胸腹胀满、足胫寒冷、热病、梦魇、癫狂。直刺0.1寸,或点刺出血;可灸。

Lidui (ST 45) A meridian point, originally from *Lingshu: Benshu* (*Miraculous Pivot: Meridian Points*), the Jing (Well) point of the Stomach Meridian of Foot-Yangming. 〈Location〉on the lateral side of the distal segment of the 2nd toe, 0.1 cun from the corner of the toenail (Figs. 60.3&60.5). 〈Regional anatomy〉skin→subcutaneous tissue→root of nail. There are the dorsal digital nerve of the medial dorsal pedal cutaneous nerve and the dorsal digital arteriovenous network in this area. 〈Indications〉edema of the face, wry mouth, toothache, epistaxis, yellow nasal discharge, distention and full sensation in the chest and abdomen, cold feet and legs, febrile disease, nightmare, manic-depressive disorder. 〈Method〉Puncture perpendicularly 0.1 cun, or prick to cause bleeding. Moxibustion is applicable.

●利机[lì jī] ①经穴别名。出《针灸甲乙经》。即会阳。见该条。②经穴别名。出《针灸甲乙经》。即石门。见该条。

Liji Another name for ①Huiyang(BL 35), a meridian point originally from *Zhenjiu Jia-Yi Jing* (*A-B Classic of Acupuncture and Moxibsution*). →会阳(p. 178) ②Shimen(RN 5), a meridian point originally from *Zhenjiu Jia-Yi Jing* (*A-B Classic of Acupuncture and Moxibustion*). →石门(p. 385)

●疬子颈[lì zǐ jǐng]
Scrofulous Neck →瘰疬(p. 258)

●痢疾[lì jí] 病证名。见《济生方》。又称肠澼、下利、滞下。夏秋季节常见的急性肠道传染病。多因外受湿热疫毒之气，内伤饮食生冷，积滞于肠中所致。以大便次数增多、腹痛、里急后重、下粘液及脓血样便为特征。一般分为湿热痢、寒湿痢、疫毒利、噤口痢、休息痢五种类型，详见各条。

Dysentery A disease, seen in *Jisheng Fang* (*Recipes for Saving Lives*), also named qi from intestine, diarrhea or difficulty in defecation, a common acute intestinal infectious disease in summer and autumn. Usually due to the affection by exopathic damp-heat and internal injury caused by raw and cold food, accumulation of cold in intestine. 〈Manifestations〉 frequent stools, abdominal pain, tenesmus, mucus, pus and bloody stools. It is divided into five types: dysentery due to damp-heat pathogen, cold-damp dysentery, fulminant dysentery, fasting dysentery and chronic dysentery with frequent relapse. →湿热痢(p. 371)、寒湿痢(p. 156)、疫毒痢(p. 552)、噤口痢(p. 207)、休息痢(p. 514)

●廉泉[lián quán] ①经穴名。出《针灸甲乙经》。属任脉，为阴维、任脉之会。又名本池、舌本。〈定位〉在颈部，当前正中线上，结喉上方，舌骨上缘凹陷处(图40和图58)。〈层次解剖〉皮肤→皮下组织→(含颈阔肌)→左、右二腹肌前腹之间→下颌舌骨肌→颏舌骨肌→颏舌肌。浅层布有面神经颈支和颈横神经上支的分支。深层有舌动、静脉的分支或属支，舌下神经的分支和下颌舌骨肌神经等。〈主治〉舌下肿痛、舌根急缩、舌纵涎出、舌强、中风失语、舌干口燥、口舌生疮、暴喑、喉痹、聋哑、咳嗽、哮喘、消渴、食不下。直刺0.5～0.8寸，不留针；可灸。②经外穴名。见《素问·刺疟篇》、《灵枢·卫气》。均以舌下的脉络为廉泉。③指舌下腺，能分秘粘液。见《灵枢·口问》。

1. Lianquan(RN 23) A meridian point of the Ren Meridian, from *Zhenjiu Jia-Yi Jing* (*A-B Classic of Acupuncture and Moxibustion*), the crossing point of Yinwei and Ren Meridians, also named Benchi and Sheben. 〈Location〉 on the neck at the anterior midline, above the laryngeal protuberance, in the depression above the upper border of the hyoid bone (Figs. 40&58). 〈Regional anatomy〉 skin→subcutaneous tissue (including platysma)→between bilateral anterior bellies of digastric muscles→mylohyoid muscle→geniohyoid muscle → genioglossus muscle. In the superficial layer, there are the cervical branches of the facial nerve and the branches of the superficial layer, there are the cervical branches of the facial nerve of the neck. In the deep layer, there are the branches or tributaries of the lingual artery and vein and the branches of the hypoglossal and mylohyoid nerve. 〈Indications〉 swelling and pain of the subglossal region, sudden shortened root of tongue, salivation with flaccid tongue and mouth, soreness of tongue and mouth, sudden loss of voice, inflammation of the throat, deafness, alalia, cough, asthma, diabetes, difficulty in swallowing. 〈Method〉 Puncture perpendicularly 0.5～0.9 cun without retaining the needle. Moxibustion is applicable.

2. Lianquan(EX-HN) An extra point, seen in *Suwen*: *Cinüe Pian* (*Plain Questions*: *Acupuncture Methods for Malarial Diseases*) and *Lingshu*: *Weiqi* (*Miraculous Pivot*: *Defensive Qi*). The blood vessel under the tongue is regarded as Lianquan in both books.

3. Sublingual Gland The body part which can secrete mucus, seen in *Lingshu*: *Kouwen* (*Miraculous Pivot*: *Questions*).

●练针法[liàn zhēn fǎ] 指练习针刺手法的一些方法。因毫针针具比较细软，如不经练习，很难做到对其运用自如。学习时需要训练指力和熟练手法，掌握好技巧后再应用于临床治疗。常用的练针法有：①纸垫练针：将草纸折叠成小方块，用线扎紧，做成纸垫，用毫针捻转刺入，反复进行，以锻炼指力。②棉纱球练针：用纱布将棉花裹紧成小球，在上面反复练习进针、提插和捻转等各种手法，以达到熟练的程度。

Acupuncture Drills Drills on acupuncture manipulation. Fairly thin and pliable needling

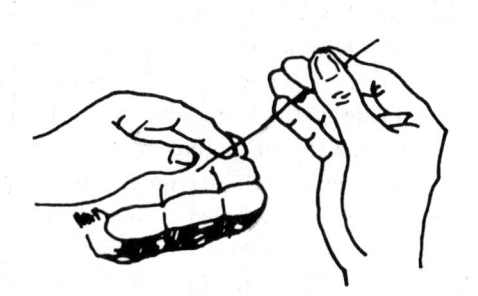

纸垫练针　Drills with a paper pad

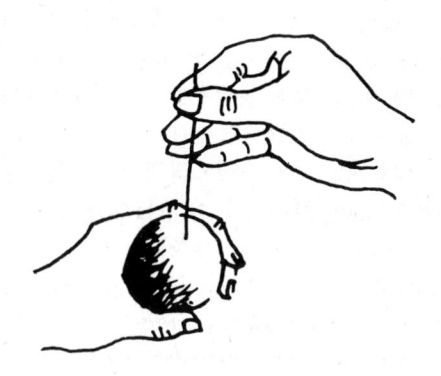

棉纱球练针　Drills with a cotton ball

图30　练针法
Fig. 30　Acupuncture drills

instruments such as filiform needles are very difficult to handle skillfully without drills, one should train the strength of his fingers and master acupuncture manipulation and techniques before applying them in clinic. The commonly used drills are as follows: ① Puncturing drills on a paper pad: Fold a piece of strawboard into a small square, tie it tightly into a pad. Insert the needle into the pad by twirling and do the same repeatedly to train the strength of fingers. ② Puncturing drills with a cotton ball: Wrap cotton tightly with gauze and make it a small ball, on which techniques such as inserting, lifting, thrusting, twirling, etc may be repeatedly drilled until they are skillfully mastered.

●炼脐法[lián qí fǎ]　间接灸的一种。见《医学入门》卷二。即蒸脐治病法。见该条.

Training-Navel Method　A form of indirect moxibustion, seen in Vol. 2 of *Yixue Rumen* (*An Introduction to Medicine*), i. e. steaming-navel method. →蒸脐治病法(p. 599)

●梁关[liáng guān]　经穴别名。出《针灸聚英》。即金门,见该条。

Liangguan　Another name for Jinmen (BL 63), a meridian point from *Zhenjiu Juying* (*Essentials of Acupuncture and Moxibustion*). →金门(p. 203)

●梁门[liáng mén]　经穴名。出《针灸甲乙经》。属足阳明胃经。〈定位〉在上腹部,当脐中上4寸,距前正中线3寸(图60.4和图40)。〈层次解剖〉皮肤→皮下组织→腹直肌鞘前壁→腹直肌。浅层布有第七、八、九胸神经前支的外侧皮支和前皮支及腹壁浅静脉。深层有,腹壁上动、静脉的分支或属支,第七、八、九胸神经前支的肌支。主治胃疼、呕吐、食欲不振、大便溏。直刺0.5～1寸;可灸。

Liangmen (ST 21)　A meridian point, originally from *Zhenjiu Jia-Yi Jing* (*A-B Classic of Acupuncture and Moxibustion*), a point on the Stomach Meridian of Foot-Yangming. 〈Location〉on the upper abdomen, 4 cun above the centre of the umbilicus and 2 cun lateral to the anterior midline (Figs. 60.4 & 40). 〈Regional anatomy〉skin→subcutaneous tissue→anterior sheath of rectus muscle of abdomen→rectus muscle of abdomen. In the superficial layer, there are the lateral and anterior cutaneous branches of the anterior branches of the 7th to 9th thoracic nerves and the superficial epigastric vein. In the deep layer, there are the branches or tributaries of the superior epigastric artery and vein and the muscular branches of the anterior branches of the 7th to 9th thoracic nerves. 〈Indications〉 stomachache, vomiting, anorexia, loose stool. 〈Method〉 Puncture perpendicularly 0.5～1.0 cun. Moxibus-

tion is applicable.

●梁丘[liáng qiū] 经穴名。出《针灸甲乙经》。属足阳明胃经,为本经郄穴。〈定位〉屈膝,在大腿前面,当髂前上棘与髌底外侧端的连线上,髌底上2寸(图60.5)。〈层次解剖〉皮肤→皮下组织→股直股肌腱与股外侧肌之间→股中间肌腱的外侧。浅层布有旋股外侧皮神经的前皮支和股外侧皮神经。深层有旋股外侧动、静脉的降支和股神经的肌支。主治胃痛、膝肿痛、下肢不遂、乳痈,直刺0.5~1寸;可灸。

Liangqiu (ST 34)　A meridian point, originally from *Zhenjiu Jia-Yi Jing* (*A-B Classic of Acupuncture and Moxibustion*), the Xi (Cleft) point of the Stomach Meridian of Foot-Yangming. 〈Location〉 with the knee flexed, on the anterior side of the thigh and on the line connecting the anterior superior iliac spine and the superiolateral corner of the patella, 2 cun above this corner (Fig. 60.5). 〈Regional anatomy〉 skin→subcutaneous tissue →between tendons of rectus muscle of thigh and lateral vastus muscle of thigh→lateral side of the tendon of intermediate vastus muscle of thigh. In the superficial layer, there are the anterior cutaneous branches of the femoral nerve and the lateral cutaneous nerve of the thigh. In the deep layer, there are the descending branches of the lateral circumflex femoral artery and vein and the muscular branches of the femoral nerve. 〈Indications〉 stomachache, swelling and pain of the knee, paralysis of the lower limbs, acute mastitis. 〈Method〉 Puncture perpendicularly 0.5~1.0 cun. Moxibustion is applicable.

●两叉骨[liǎng chà gǔ]　部位名。肩胛与肩峰相连处。即肩锁关节处。

Bifid Bone　A part of the body, referring to the part where the scaplula and acromion link, i.e. where the acromioclavicular joint lies.

●两手研子骨[liǎng shǒu yán zǐ gǔ]　经外穴别名。出《类经图翼》。即研子,见该条。

Liangshouyanzigu　Another name for Yanzi (EX-UE), an extra point from *Leijing Tuyi* (*Supplements to Illustrated Classified Canon of Internal Medicine of the Yellow Emperor*). →研子(p. 535)

●髎髎[liáo liáo]　经外穴名。见《经外奇穴汇编》。在膝关节内侧,当阴陵泉直下3寸处。主治崩中漏下、月经不调、腿内廉风疮痒痛。直刺0.5~1寸;可灸。

Liaoliao (EX-LE)　An extra point seen in *Jingwai Qixue Huibian* (*An Expository Manual of Extra Acupoints*). 〈Location〉 on the medial side of the knee joint, 3 cun inferior to Yinlingquan (SP 9). 〈Indications〉 metrorrhagia and metrostaxis, irregular menstruation, itch and pain in the medial side of the leg due to wind-sore. 〈Method〉 Puncture perpendicularly 0.5~1.0 cun. Moxibustion is applicable.

●列缺[liè quē]　经穴名。出《灵枢·经脉》。属手太阴肺经,为本经络穴,八脉交会穴之一,通任脉。又名童玄、腕劳。〈定位〉在前臂桡侧缘,桡骨茎突上方,腕横纹上1.5寸。当肱桡肌与拇长展肌腱之间(图49和图16)。〈层次解剖〉皮肤→皮下组织→拇长展肌腱→肱桡肌腱→旋前方肌。浅层布有头静脉、前臂外侧皮神经和桡神经浅支。深层有桡动、静脉的分支。〈主治〉咳嗽、气喘、咽喉痛、掌中热、半身不遂、口眼歪斜、偏正头痛、项强、惊痫、溺血、小便热、阴茎痛、牙痛。向肘部斜刺0.2~0.3寸;可灸。

Lieque (LU 7)　A meridian point originally from *Lingshu: Jingmai* (*Miraculous Pivot: Meridians*), the Luo (Connecting) point of the Lung Meridian of Hand-Taiyin, and one of the Eight Confluence Points, connected with the Ren Meridian, also named Tongxuan or Wanlao. 〈Location〉 on the radial side of the forearm, proximal to the styloid process of the redius, 1.5 cun above the crease of the wrist, between the brachioradial muscle and tendon of the long abductor muscle of the thumb (Figs. 49&16). 〈Regional anatomy〉 skin → subcutaneous tissue→long abductor muscle of thumb → tendon of brachioradial muscle → quadrate pronator muscle. In the superficial layer, there are the cephalic vein, the lateral cutaneous nerve of the forearm and the superficial branches of the radial nerve. In the deep layer, there are the branches of the radial artery and vein. 〈Indications〉 cough, asthma, sore throat, feverish sensation in the palm, hemiplegia, deviation of the eye and mouth, migraine, aching all over the head, stiff neck,

epilepsy induced by terror, hematuria, burning sensation during urination, pain in the penis and toothache. 〈Method〉 Puncture obliquely 0.2～0.3 cun towards the elbow. Moxibustion is applicable.

●**邻近取穴**[lín jìn qǔ xué] 取穴法之一。又称四周取穴。指在靠近病变部位的周围选取有关穴位进行治疗,其范围较局部取穴为广。例如:眼病取太阳、腕痛取外关、膝痛取阴市、阳陵泉等。

Nearby Point Selection One of the point selection methods, also named point selection around the affected region, which means the selection of relevant points near the diseased area for acupuncture. The range is larger than that of local point selection, e. g. select Taiyang（EX-HN 5）for ophthalmopathy; Waiguan(SJ 5) for pain in the wrist; Yinshi (ST 33) and Yanglingquan(GB 34)for pain in the knee joint, etc.

●**临泣**[lín qì] 经穴名。有二:一在头,一在足,同属足少阳胆经。为便于区分,《圣济总录》称前者为目临泣,后者足临泣。《针灸资生经》则改"目临泣"为"头临泣"。详见各条。

Linqi A pair of meridian points on the Gallbladder Meridian of Foot-Shaoyang, one on the head, the other on the foot. In order to distinguish them, *Shengji Zonglu* (*Imperial Medical Encyclopaedia*) names the former Mulinqi and the latter Zulinqi(GB 41). And *Zhenjiu Zisheng Jing*(*Acupuncture and Moxibustion for Saving Life*) changes Mulinqi into Toulinqi (GB 15). → 目临泣(p. 272)、足临泣(p. 631)、头临泣(p. 444)

●**淋泉**[lìn quán] 经外穴名。见《针灸集成》,在骶部,当后正中线上,尾骨尖端上1口寸,旁开0.5口寸处。主治淋证。用灸法。

Linquan（EX-B） An extra point seen in *Zhenjiu Jicheng* (*Collection of Acupuncture and Moxibustion*). 〈Locattion〉 1 mouth-cun above the tip of coccyx and 0.5 mouth-cun lateral to it, on the sacral region. 〈Indication〉 stranguria. 〈Method〉 moxibustion.

●**淋证**[lìn zhèng] 病证名。出《素问·六元政纪大论》。指小便频数、短涩淋沥、小腹尿道刺痛胀痛的病证。根据病机和症状的不同,临床上一般分为热淋、石淋、气淋、血淋、膏淋、劳淋六种类型。详见各条。

Stranguria A disease originally from *Suwen*: *Liuyuan Zhengji Dalun* (*Plain Questions*: *on the Laws of the Six Climate Changes*). 〈Manifestations〉 frequency of micturition, dribbling urination, stabbing and distending pain in the lower abdomen and urethra. According to different pathogensis and symptoms, it is clinically divided into 6 types: stranguria due to heat, stranguria caused by the passage of urinary stone, stranguria caused by disorder of qi, stranguria complicated by hematuria, stranguria marked by chyluria, and stranguria induced by overstrain. →热淋(p. 331)、石淋(p. 385)、气淋(p. 308)、血淋(p. 526)、膏淋(p. 133)、劳淋(p. 238)

●**灵道**[líng dào] 经穴名。出《针灸甲乙经》。属手少阴心经,为本经经穴。〈定位〉在前臂掌侧,当尺侧腕屈腱的桡侧缘,腕横纹1.5寸(图49和图67)。〈层次解剖〉皮肤→皮下组织→尺侧腕屈肌与指浅屈肌之间→指深屈肌→旋前方肌。浅层布有前臂内侧皮神经,贵要静脉属支等分布。深层有尺动、静脉和尺神经等。主治心悸怔忡、心痛、悲恐、善笑、暴喑、舌强不语、腕臂挛急、足跗上痛、头昏目眩。直刺0.3～0.4寸;可灸。

Lingdao（HT 4） A meridian point, originally from *Zhenjiu Jia-Yi Jing* (*A-B Classic of Acupuncture and Moxibustion*), the Jing (River) point of the Heart Meridian of Hand-Shaoyin. 〈Location〉 on the palmar side of the forearm and on the radial side of the tendon of the ulnar flexor muscle of the wrist, 1.5 cun proximal to the crease of the wrist (Figs. 49&67). 〈Regional anatomy〉 skin→subcutaneous tissue→between ulnar flexor muscle of wrist and superficial flexor muscle of fingers → deep flexor muscle of fingers → quadrate pronator muscle. In the superficial layer, there are the medial cutaneous nerve of the forearm and the tributaries of the basilic vein. In the deep layer, there are the ulnar artery and vein and the ulnar nerve. 〈Indications〉 palpitations, severe palpitations, cardiodynia, susceptibility to laughter due to sorrow and fear, sudden loss of voice, inability to speak due to stiffness of the tongue, contracture of the

wrist and the arm, pain in the back of the foot, dizziness. ⟨Method⟩ Puncture perpendicularly 0.3～0.4 cun. Moxibustion is applicable.

● 灵光赋[líng guāng fù] 针灸歌赋名。见《针灸大全》、《针灸聚英》。为七言韵语，内容与《席弘赋》相似。

Lingguang Fu (Ode to the Brilliance of Gods) A verse of acupuncture and Moxibustion seen in *Zhenjiu Daquan* (*A Complete Work of Acupunture and Moxibustion*) and *Zhenjiu Juying* (*Essentials of Acupuncture and Moxibustion*), rhythmic with 7 characters to each line. The content is similar to *Xi Hong Fu* (*Ode to Xi Hong*).

● 灵龟八法[líng guī bā fǎ] 又名奇经纳卦法、灵龟飞腾。是一种按时取穴的针刺方法。它是运用古代哲学九宫八卦学说，结合人体奇经八脉气血会合，取其与十二经脉相通的八个经穴，按照日时干支的推演数字变化，采用相加、相除的方法，按时取穴的一种针刺方法。灵龟八法的组成包括：①九宫八卦，八卦是古人取阴阳之象，结合自然界的天、地、水、火、风、雷、山、泽作成的。把八卦的名称和图象结合四方，即成九宫。由于八卦各有方位，配合九宫，根据戴九履一，左三右七，二四为肩，八六为足，五十居中的九宫数字，每宫再配上一条奇经及其配属的穴位，就成为坎一联申脉，照海坤二五，震三属外关，巽四临泣数，乾六是公孙，兑七后溪府，艮八系内关，离九列缺主。②八脉交会。在四肢部位的十二经上有八个经穴与八脉相通：小肠经的后溪通于督脉，肺经的列缺通于任脉，脾经的公孙通于冲脉，胆经的临泣通于带脉，肾经的照海通于阴跷，膀胱经的申脉通于阳跷，心包经的内关通于阴维，三焦经的外关通于阳维。③八法逐日干支代数：甲己辰戌丑未十，乙庚申酉九为期，丁壬寅卯八成数，戊癸巳午七相宜，丙辛亥子亦七数，逐日干支即得知。④八法临时干支代数：甲己子午九宜用，乙庚丑未八无疑，丙辛寅申七作数，丁壬卯酉六须知，戊癸辰戌各有五，已亥单加四共齐，阳日除九阴除六，不及零余下推。运用灵龟八法，是将日、时的干支数字共同加起来，得出四个数字的和数，然后按照阳日用九除，阴日用六除的公式去除干支的和数，再将它的余数，求得八卦所分配的某穴的数字，就是当时应开的腧穴。它的公式是：(日干数＋日支数＋时干数＋时支数)÷9(阳)或6(阴)＝商……(余数)。

Eight Methods of the Intelligent Turtle Also called the method of associating extrameridians with eight diagrams or soaring of the intelligent turtle. A needling method of selecting acupoints according to the time, which is determined, with the application of the theory of Jiu Gong (the Nine Palaces) and Ba Gua (the Eight Diagrams) in ancient philosophy. In association with the theory of the confluence of qi and blood from the 8 Extra Meridians, selecting the eight meridian points connected with the 12 Regular Meridians by means of addition and division of the deduced varying numerals according to the day and the hour in terms of the heavenly stems and earthly branches. The method is composed of ① Jiu Gong (the Nine Palaces) and Ba Gua (the Eight Diagrams). The Eight Diagrams are made up of symbols of Yin and Yang adopted by the ancient people in association with sky, earth, water, fire, wind, thunder, mountain and lake in nature. The names and diagrams of Ba Gua form the Jiu Gong by associating the four sides. Each of the Eight Diagrams has its own direction, and, in combination with Jiu Gong, according to the numerals in it (the principle is like this: the head is 9 and the foot is 1; left 3 and right 7; 2 and 4 stand for the shoulders; 8 and 6 refer to the feet; and 5 and 10 lie in the centre). Associated with each of the 9 palaces is one of the 8 extra meridians and its corresponding acupoint as well, thus forming the follwing verse:

Kan-1 is connected with Shenmai (BL 62);

Zhaohai (KI 6) relates to *Kun*-2 and -5;

Zhen-3 pertains to Waiguan (SJ 5);

Xun-4 refers to Zulinqi (GB 41);

Qian-6 is of Gongsun (SP 4);

Dui-7 is where Houxi (SI 3) lies;

Gen-8 is the location of Neiguan (PC 6); and

Li-9 belongs to Lieque (LU 7).

② the 8 Confluence Points: There are 8 meridian point on the 12 Regular Meridians at the extremities connecting with the extra meridians: Houxi (SI 3) of the Small Intestine

Meridian connects with the Du Meridian; Lieque(LU 7) of the Lung Meridian with the Ren Meridian; Gongsun(SP 4) of the Spleen Meridian with the Chong Meridian; Zulinqi (GB 41) of the Gallbladder Meridian with Dai Meridian; Zhaohai (KI 6) of the Kidney Meridian with the Yinqiao Meridian; Shenmai (BL 62) of the Bladder Meridian with the Yangqiao Meridian; Neiguan (PC 6) of the Pericardium Meridian with the Yinwei Meridian; Waiguan (SJ 5) of the Sanjiao Meridian with the Yangwei Meridian. ③numerals representing the heavenly stems and earthly branches of the eight methods in terms of the successive Jia, Ji, Chen, Xu, Chou and Wei are of 10, Yi, Geng, Shen and You are of 9, Ding, Ren, Yin and Mao are of 8, Wu, Gui, Si, Wu, Bing, Xin, Hai and Zi are of 7. ④temporary numerals representing the heavenly stems and earthly branches of the Eight Methods: Jia, Ji, Zi and Wu are 9; Yi, Geng, Chou and Wei are 8, Bing, Xin, Yin and shen are 7, Ding, Ren, Mao and You are 6, Wu, Gui, Chen and Xu are 5, and Yi and Hai are 4. Divide the sum by 9 on a Yang day or by 6 on a Yin; the remainder is the due numeral standing for the one in Ba Gua indicating the point to be used. The application of the eight methods of intelligent turtle means adding the four numerals representing the heavenly stems and earthly branches of the dates and hours, and then dividing it by 9 if it's a Yang date, or by 6 if it's a Yin date, to get the number of the points distributed to the eight diagorams accrding to the remainder. The point is the one which should be used at the time. The formula is: (numeral of the heavenly stem of the date + number of the earthly branch of the date + number of the heavenly stem of the hour + number of the earthly branch of the hour)÷9 (Yang) or 6(Yin)=the quotient……(the remainder).

●灵龟飞腾[líng guī fēi téng] 灵龟八法之别称。见该条。

Soaring of the Intelligent Turtle →灵龟八法 (p.248)

●灵墙[líng qiáng] 经穴别名。见《备急千金要方》。即灵墟。见该条。

Lingqiang Another name of Lingxu (KI 24), a meridian point seen in *Beiji Qianjin Yaofang* (*Essential Prescriptions for Emergencies Worth a Thousand Gold*). →灵墟 (p.250)

●灵枢[líng shū] 书名。又名《灵枢经》、《九卷》、《针经》、《九灵》、《九墟》与《素问》合称《黄帝内经》。宋代史崧以家藏旧本校刊后,将《灵枢》分二十四卷、八十一篇,论及九针、经络、俞穴、刺法、治疗等,是针灸学的经典著作,为我国现存最早的针灸文献之一。现行本为十二卷。

Ling Shu (Miraculous Pivot) A book, also entitled *Ling Shu Jing* (*Classic of Miraculous Pivot*), *Jiu Juan* (*Nine Volumes*), *Zhenjing* (*Canon of Acupuncture*), *Jiu Ling* (*Nine Divinities*), and *Jiu Xu* (*Nine Earthy Mountains*). It is, together with *Su Wen* (*Plain Questions*), jointly named *Huangdi Neijing* (*The Yellow Emperor's Inner Cannon*). Shi Song of the Song Dynasty, after revising his home-preserved old edition, divided *Lingshu* (*Miraculous Pivot*) into 81 chapters in 24 volumes, dealing with nine needles, meridians and collaterals, acupoints, needling methods and therapies, etc. It is a classic of acupuncture, one of the earliest monographs on acupuncture and moxibustion extant in our country. The present-day version of the book is in 12 volumes.

●灵枢经[líng shū jīng] 书名,即《灵枢》。见该条。

Ling Shu Jing (The Canon of Miraculous Pivot) →灵枢 (p.249)

●灵枢经脉翼[líng shū jīng mài yì] 书名,明代夏英撰,三卷,内容是根据滑寿的《十四经发挥》等来注释《灵枢》的原文,个人见解较少。

Ling Shu Jingmai Yi (Supplement to the Meridians of the Miraculous Pivot) A book in 3 volumes written by Xia Ying in the Ming Dynasty, the content of which is an annotation to the original text of *Lingshu* (*Miraculous Pivot*) on the basis of *Shisi Jing Fahui* (*An Elaboration of the Fourteen Meridians*) by Hua Shou, and which lacks his personal ideas.

●灵台[líng tái] 经穴名。出《素问·气府论》王冰注。属督脉,又名肺底。〈定位〉在背部,当后正中线

上，第六胸椎棘突下凹陷中（图12.1和图7）。〈层次解剖〉针刺穿过的层次结构同脊中穴。浅层主要布有第六胸神经后支的内侧皮支和伴行的动、静脉。深层有棘突间的椎外（后）静脉丛，第六胸神经后支的分支和第六肋间后动、静脉背侧支的分支或属支。〈主治〉咳嗽、气喘、项强、背痛、身热、疔疮。斜刺0.5～1寸；可灸。

Lingtai(DU 10)　A meridian point, originally from *Su Wen*: *Qi Fu Lun*(*Plain Questions*: *On Houses of Qi*) annotated by Wang Bing, a point on to Du Meridian, also named Feidi. 〈Location〉 on the back and on the posterior midline, in the depression below the spinous process of the 6th thoracic vertebra (Figs. 12.1 & 7). 〈Regional anatomy〉 The layer structures of the needle insertion are the same as those in Jizhong(DU 6). In the superficial layer, there are the medial cutaneous branches of the posterior branches of the 6th thoracic nerve and the accompanying artery and vein. In the deep layer, there are the external (posterior) vertebral venous plexus between the adjacent spinous processes, the branches of the posterior branches of the 6th thoracic nerve and the branches or tributaries of the dorsal branches of the 6th posterior intercostal artery and vein. 〈Indications〉 cough, dyspnea, stiffness of the neck, back pain, fever furuncle and sore. 〈Method〉 Puncture obliquely 0.5～1 cun. Moxibustion is applicable.

●灵墟[líng xū]　经穴名。出《针灸甲乙经》。属足少阴肾经，又名灵墙。〈定位〉在胸部，当第三肋间隙，前正中线旁开2寸（图40）。〈层次解剖〉皮肤→皮下组织→胸大肌。浅层布有第三肋间神经的前皮支，胸廓内动、静脉的穿支。深层有胸内、外侧神经的分支。〈主治〉咳嗽、气喘、痰多、胸胁胀痛、呕吐、乳痈。斜刺或平刺0.5～0.8寸；可灸。

Lingxu(KI 24)　A meridian point, orginally from *Zhenjiu Jia-Yi Jing* (*A-B Classic of Acupuncture and Moxibustion*), a point on the Kidney Meridian of Foot-Shaoyin, also named Lingqiang. 〈Location〉 on the chest, in the 3rd intercostal space, 2 cun lateral to the anterior midline (Fig. 40). 〈Regional anatomy〉 skin → subcutaneous tissue → greater pectoral muscle. In the superficial layer, there are the anterior cutaneous branches of the 3rd intercostal nerves and the perforating branches of the internal thoracic artery and vein. In the deep layer, there are the branches of the medial and lateral pectoral nerves. 〈Indications〉 cough dyspnea abundant expectoration, pain and distension in the chest and hypochondriac region, vomiting, mastitis. 〈Method〉 Puncture obliquely or subcutaneously 0.5～0.8 cun. Moxibustion is applicable.

●陵后[líng hòu]　经外穴名。见《针灸孔穴及其疗法便览》。在小腿外侧、当腓骨小头后缘下方凹陷中。〈主治〉腓神经痛、膝关节炎、坐骨神经痛、下肢麻痹或瘫痪。直刺0.5～1寸；可灸。

Linghou(EX-LE)　An extra point, seen in *Zhenjiu Kongxue Jiqi Liaofa Bianlan*(*Guide to Acupoints and Acupuncture Therapeutics*). 〈Location〉 on the lateral side of the leg, in the depression inferior to the posterior border of the small head of the fibula. 〈Indictions〉 peroneal neuralgia, gonitis, sciatica, palsy or paralysis of the lower limbs. 〈Method〉 Puncture perpendicularly 0.5～1.0 cun. Moxibustion is applicable.

●刘党[liú dǎng]　人名。宋代道家、针灸家，号琼瑶真人。参见"琼瑶发明神书"条。

Liu Dang　A Taoist and an acupuncture-moxibustion expert in the Song Dynasty, who styled himself Qiongyao Zhenren. →琼瑶发明神书(p.321)

●刘瑾[liú jǐn]　人名。明代医家，字永怀，号恒庵，南昌（属江西）人。从陈会学针灸术，后应宁献王之命重新校订和补辑陈会的《广爱书》，并改名为《神应经》。

Liu Jin　A medical doctor in the Ming Dynasty, who styled himself Yonghuai, and assumed the name of Heng'an, a native of Nanchang, (in Jiangxi Province). He learned techniques of acupuncture and moxibustion from Chen Hui and later, took orders from the king of Ning Xian, to rectify and supplement *Guang'ai Shu*(*Great Fraternity to Patients*) written by Chen Hui, and changed its title into *Shenying Jing*(*Classic of God Merit*).

●刘完素[liú wán sù]　人名。金代著名医家，"金元四大家"之一。字守真，自号通玄处士，河间（今河北河间）人，故又称刘河间。其著有《素问玄机原病式》、

《素问病机气宜保命集》、《宣明论方》等书,强调火热病机,善用寒凉之品。其不仅发挥了《内经》经旨,亦很注重针灸治疗。

Liu Wansu A famous medical expert of the Jin Dynasty, one of "the four great experts in the Jin and Yuan Dynasties", who styled himself Shouzhen, and assumed the name of Tong Xuan Chu Shi himself, a native of Hejian, (now Hejian, Hebei province), also named Liu Hejian. He wrote *Su Wen Xuanji Yuan Bing Shi* (*Exploration to Mysterious Etiology in Plain Questions*)、*Su Wen Bingji Qiyi Baoming Ji* (*Collection of Pathology, Five Motions, Six Climate Changes and Health Preserving from Plain Questions*) and *Xuanming Lunfang* (*Prescriptions and Expositions*), etc. in which he emphasized the pathogenesis of fire and heat and was favorable to using cold and cool drugs. Not only did he develop the essential of *Neijing* (*The Canon of Internal Medicine*), but he also stressed acupuncture and moxibustion therapy.

●刘元宾[liú yuán bīn] 人名。北宋医家,字子仪,自号通真子,安福(今属江西)人。精通方脉,著有《通真子补注王叔和脉诀》、《通真子续注脉赋》、《脉诀机要》、《脉要新括》、《诊脉须知》、《通真子伤寒诀》、《伤寒括要》、《神巧万全方》等,并著有《洞天针灸经》,已佚。

Liu Yuanbin A physican in the Northern Song Dynasty, styling himself Ziyi and assuming the name of Tong Zhen Zi, a native of Anfu (now in Jiangxi Province). He was skillful in prescription and pulse-taking. He wrote *Tong Zhen Zi Buzhu Wang Shuhe Maijue* (*Supplementary Notes to Wang Shuhe's Verse of Pulse-Taking Given by Tong Zhenzi*), *Tongzhenzi Xuzhu Maifu* (*Continued Notes to Pulse-taking in Verse Given by Tong Zhenzi*), *Maijue Jiyao* (*Essentials of Pulse-Taking in Verse*), *Maiyao Xinkuo* (*New Development on Essentials of Pulse-Taking*), *Zhenmai Xuzhi* (*Notice for Pulse-Taking*), *Tong Zhenzi Shanghan Jue* (*Febrile Diseases in Verse Written by Tong Zhenzi*), *Shanghan Kuoyao* (*Contracted Essentials of Febrile Diseases*), *Shenqiao Wanquan Fang* (*Miraculous Prescriptions for All Kinds of Diseases*), etc. He also wrote *DongTian ZhenJiu Jing* (*Dong Tian Classic on Acupunctre and Moxibustion*), which was already lost.

●流火[liú huǒ] 发于小腿的丹毒,详见"丹毒"条。
Running Fire Erysipelas occuring in the shank. →丹毒(p.71)

●流气法[liú qì fǎ] 即留气法,见该条。
Qi-Flowing Method →留气法(p.251)

●流注八穴[liú zhù bā xué] 八脉交会八穴的别名。见该条。
Eight Ebb-Flow Points →八脉交会穴(p.7)

●流注指微赋[liú zhù zhǐ wēi fù] 针灸歌赋名。金代何若愚作,初载于《子午流注针经》中。是关于子午流注法的早期著作,现辑入《针灸四书》中。
Liuzhu Zhiwei Fu (Lyrics of Flow) A verse of acupuncture and moxibustion, written by He Ruoyu in the Jin Dynasty, recorded first in *Ziwu Liuzhu Zhenjing* (*Acupuncture Classic on Midnight-noon Ebb-flow*), an earlier writing on midnight-noon ebb-flow, which is now included in *ZhenJiu Sishu* (*Four Books on Acupuncture and Moxibustion*).

●留[liú] 针刺基本手法之一,指将针留置于穴内。参见"留针"条。
Retention one of the basic manipulations for needling, referring to the retention of the needle in the acupoint. →留针(p.251)

●留气法[liú qì fǎ] 针刺手法名。又名流气法。见《针灸聚英》。其法须先进针7分深处,行紧按慢提九数;得气后进入1寸深处,略作伸提动作,再退回原处。反复施行,用以破气散结。
Qi-Moving Method A needling technique also called qi-flowing method, seen in *Zhenjiu Juying* (*Essentials of Acupuncture and Moxibustion*). 〈Method〉 First insert the needle 0.7 cun, then perform quick thrust and slow lift of the needle 9 times. Insert the needle 1 cun deep after the needling reaction has been obtained, lift the needle slightly and then insert it to the original place. Perform all this repeatedly so as to relieve the stagnation of qi and resolve masses.

●留针[liú zhēn] 针刺术语,又名置针。针刺穴位后一般需留置适当的时间,其长短依病情和刺法的特点而定。毫针在留针时间内可间歇运针,或使用温针、电针等,留针的目的是为了加强针刺的作用和便

于继续行针施术。

Retention of the Needle   A term of needling technique, also named placing the needle. The needle will be placed in the point for an appropriate period of time after it is inserted. The patient's condition and needling characteristics decide the duration of retaining the needle. Intermittent manipulation can be given when the filiform needle is retained, or acupuncture with the needle warmed by burning moxa and electrotherapy can also be applied. Retaining the needle is on the purpose of strengthening the action of needling and making it easy to manipulate the needle continuously.

●硫磺灸[liú huáng jiǔ]   灸法的一种。见《太平圣惠方》卷六十一。是用硫磺作为施灸材料的一种灸法。〈方法〉硫磺一块，其大小依疮口大小而定，放于疮口上，另取少量硫磺放在火上烧之，用银钗脚挑起放于硫磺块上。反复操作3～5遍。用于治疗疮疡久不愈合，形成瘘管者。

Sulphur Cauterization   A form of cauterization, seen in Vol. 61 of *Taiping Shenghui Fang* (*Imperial Benevolent Prescriptions*), a method of using sulphur, whose size depends on how big the sore is, and place it on the sore. Take another small amount of sulphur, ignite it and put it on the previous sulphur piece with a silver fork. Repeat the manipulation 3～5 times for each treatment. 〈Indication〉 prolonged skin and external diseases with fistula formed on the diseased area.

●硫朱灸[liú zhū jiǔ]   灸法的一种。见《本草纲目拾遗》卷二。又称香砂灸。用麝香3克、劈砂6克、硫磺9克，研为细末，将硫磺用温火化开，加入麝午、劈砂，离火搅拌均匀，在光石上摊作薄片，切如米如栖的小块，贮藏在瓶内备用。施灸时将药片放在患处，点燃施灸。又法加樟脑1.5克，如前法制成硫朱锭备用。近代有以制硫磺18克，朱砂粉15克制成灸锭，安于穴位上，每月一粒。年老体弱及儿童用半粒。用治风寒湿痹、伤痛、脘腹痛寒等证。

Sulphur-Cinnabaris Cauterization   A form of cauterization, seen in Vol. 2 of *Bencao Gangmu Shiyi* (*A Supplement to Compendium of Materia Medica*), also called *Moschus-Cinnabaris Cauteriztaion*. 〈Method〉 Take *Moschus* 3g, *Cinnabaris* 6g, *sulphur* 9g and grind them into fine powder. Melt the *sulphur* on a gentle fire, then remove the fire and mix the *sulphur* with the *Moschus* and *Cinnabaris*, spread the mixture on a smooth stone to make thin slices. Cut the slices into pieces as small as rice grains, then keep them in bottles for use. while performing the cauterization, put the drug-slices on the diseased area and ignite them. 〈Another method〉 Add *Camphora* (1.5g) to the above mentioned drugs, make ingot-shaped *sulphur-Cinnabaris* tablets for use in the same way as is mentioned above. In recent years, an ingot-shaped tablet is made with 18g of *sulphur* and 15g of *Cinnabaris* powder for cauterization, and is placed on the selected acupoint, one piece a month, half a piece for the aged or the weak or children. 〈Indications〉 arthralgia-syndrome due to wind, cold an damp pathogen, pain due to injury, and epigastric pain and cold, etc.

●六缝[liù fèng]   经外穴名。见《腧穴学概论》。在手掌侧，当第2、3、4、5指近端指关节各1穴（即四缝穴），以及拇指掌指关节横纹中点和指节横纹中点各一穴，每手六穴，两手共十二穴。〈主治〉疗疮、小儿疳积等。直刺0.1～0.2寸，或点刺挤出黄白色粘液。

Liufeng (EX-UE)   A set of extra points, seen in *Shuxuexue Gailun* (*An Outline of Acupoints*). 〈Location〉 four points [i. e. Sifeng (EX-UE 10)], on the palmer side, at the centre of the proximal interphalangeal joints of the 2nd to 5th fingers, and the other two points, at the midpoints of the transverse crease of the metacarpophalangeal joint and the interphalangeal joint of the thumb 6 points on each hand, 12 points in all. 〈Indications〉 furuncles, malnutrition and indigestion in children, etc. 〈Method〉 Puncture perpendicularly 0.1～0.2 cun, or prick to squeeze out yellowish and whitish mucus.

●六腑下合穴[liù fǔ xià hé xué]   下合穴的别名，见该条。

Lower Confluent Points of the Six Fu Organs
   Another name for the Lower Confluent Points. →下合穴(p. 487)

●六合[liù hé] ①经别名。出《灵枢·经别》。经别按十二经脉的表里关系分成的六对组合，故名。即以足太阳经别与足少阴经别为一合，足少阳经别与足厥阴经别为二合，足阳明经别与足太阴经别为三合，手太阳经别与手少阴经别为四合，手少阳经别与手厥阴经别为五合，手阳明经别与手太阴经别为六合。②指天地之间，上下、四方为六合。见《素问·生气通天论》

1. Six Pairs of Combinations Name of divergent meridians, originally from *Lingshu：Jing Bie* (*Miraculous Pivot：Divergent Meridians*). It is so named due to the division of the divergent meridians into 6 pairs of combinations in accordance with the exterior-interior relationship of the Twelve Regular Meridians. The divergent meridians of Foot-Taiyang and Foot-Shaoyin are the first pair of combinations; those of Foot-Shaoyang and Foot-Jueyin are the second; those of Foot-Yangming and Foot-Taiyin are the third, those of Hand-Taiyang and Hand-Shaoyin are the fourth, those of Hand-Shaoyang and Hand-Jueyin are the fifth, those of Hand-Yangming and Hand-Taiyin are the sixth.

2. Liuhe Referring to the space between heaven and earth, namely, superior and inferior and the four directions north, south, east and west, originally from *Suwen：Sheng Qi Tongtian Lun* (*Plain Questions：On the Relations between Life Activities and Nature*).

●六华[liù huá] 经外穴名。见《经外奇穴治疗诀》。即八华穴中的上六穴。详见"八华"条。

Liuhua (EX-B) A set of extra points, seen in *Jingwai Qixue Zhiliao Jue* (*Treatment of Extra Points In Rhyme*), referring to the six upper Bahua Points. →八华(p. 5)

●六经[liù jīng] ①出《黄帝内经》。即太阳经、阳明经、少阳经和太阴经、少阴经、厥阴经的合称。六经又可分为手六经和足六经，计十二经脉。②《伤寒论》则以太阳、阳明、少阳、太阴、少阴、厥阴六经，作为外感热病辨证分型的纲领。

Six Meridians ① Originally from *Huang Di Neiing* (*The Yellow Emperor's Inner Canon*), the general term for Meridians of Taiyang, Yangming, Shaoyang, and Taiyin, Shaoyin and Jueyin. The six meridians can be subdivided into the six meridians of hand and the six meridians of foot, 12 meridians in all. ② In *Shanghan Lun* (*Treatise on Febrile Disease*), meridians of Taiyang, Yangming, Shaoyang, Taiyin, Shaoyin and Jueyin are taken as the guiding principle in the differentiation of exopathogen and febrile diseases.

●六经标本[liù jīng biāo běn] 十二经标本的别名。见该条。

Superficialities and Origins of the Six Meridians →十二经标本(p. 375)

●六经皮部[liù jīng pí bù] 部位名。出《素问·皮部论》。十二皮部按手足同名经相合，则称六经皮部。六经皮部各有专名：太阳皮部称关枢，阳明皮部称害蜚，少阳皮部称枢持，太阴皮部称关蛰，少阴皮部称枢儒，厥阴皮部称害肩。参见"皮部"。

Cutaneous Regions of the Six Meridians A part of the body, originally from *Su Wen：Pibu Lun* (*Plain Queations：On Cutaneous Regions*) The twelve cutaneous regions are called cutaneous regions of the six meridians with the hand and foot meridians of the same name going together. Each cutaneous region of the six meridans has a particular name：bolt-pivot for cutaneous region of Taiyang, door-movement for cutaneous region of Yangming, pivot-hold for cutaneous region of Shaoyang, bolt-hiding for cutaneous region of Taiyin, pivot-mildness for cutaneous region of Shaoyin, door-bearing for cutaneous region of Jueyin. →皮部(p. 291)

●龙颔[lóng hàn] ①经穴别名。即中府，见该条。②经外穴名。又名龙头，位于鸠尾穴上1.5寸。〈主治〉心痛冷气、胃寒、胃痛、心窝痛、喘息，平刺0.2-0.3寸；可灸。

1. Longhan Another name for Zhongfu(DU 1). →中府(p. 609)

2. Longhan (EX-CA) An extra point, also named Longtou. 〈Location〉1.5 cun directly above Jiuwei (RN 15).〈Indications〉cardiac pain with chills, cold and pain in the gastric region, epigastric pain, dyspnea.〈Method〉Puncture subcutaneously 0.2～0.3 cun. Moxibustion is applicable.

●龙虎龟凤[lóng hǔ guī fèng] 针刺手法。为飞经走气之别称。见该条。

Dragon-Tiger-Turtle-Phoenix A needling technique, another name of accelerating flow of qi over meridians. →飞经走气法(p.105)

●龙虎交腾[lóng hǔ jiāo téng] 针刺手法名。出《医学入门》。龙虎，指左右捻转；交腾，指经气流通。其法：先一左(顺)一右(逆)捻针三九二十七次；得气后，大指向前转针并下按，再以大指弹动针尾催气，行下按上提动作以行气。用于赤眼、痛肿初起等热症。

Dragon-Tiger Alternate Prance A needling technique, originally from *Yixue Rumen*(*Elementary Medicine*), "dragon-tiger" means twirling the needle left and right; "alternate prance" refers to the flow of the meridian qi. ⟨Method⟩ First, twist the needle to the left (clockwise), and right (counter clockwise) for 27(3×9) times ; after the needling reaction has been obtained, twist and thrust the needle with the thumb moving forward and downward, then vibrate the tail of the needle with the thumb to promote the arrival of qi, thrust and lift the needle to promote the flow of qi. ⟨Indications⟩ heat diseases, such as redness of the eye, onset of the carbuncle.

●龙虎交战[lóng hǔ jiāo zhàn] 针刺手法名。出《金针赋》。龙指左转，虎指右转，反复进行故称交战。〈其法〉先以左转为主，即大指向前较用力地捻九数。再以右转为主，即食指向前较用力地捻六数。反复施行。也可分浅、中、深三部重复进行。用于痛证。

Dragon-Tiger's Alternate Fight A term for a needling technique, originally from *Jinzhen Fu*(*Lyrics of Golden Needle*). "Dragon" refers to twirling the needle left, while "tiger" refers to twirling the needle right, this repeated manipulation is called alternate fight. ⟨Method⟩ First, mainly twirl the needle left, twisting the needle forcefully with the thumb moving forward for 9 times, then mainly twirl the needle right, twisting the needle forcefully with the index finger moving forward for 6 times. It can also be performed repeatedly in three parts: superficial, medium and deep. ⟨Indication⟩pain syndrome.

●龙虎升降[lóng hǔ shēng jiàng] 针刺手法名。又名龙虎升腾。出《针灸大成》卷四。龙虎，指左右捻转；升降，指气行上下。〈其法〉先用右手大指向前捻针；进穴后，再用左手大指向前捻针；得气后又向左向右转针，并用下按上提动作，使气行。气未盛，可反复操作。

Dragon-Tiger Ascending and Descending A needling technique, also named dragon-tiger ascending and prancing, originally from Vol. 4 of *Zhenjiu Dacheng*(*A Great Compendium of Acupuncture and Moxibustion*), "dragon-tiger" refers to twirling the needle left and right, ascending and descending" refers to qi flowing upwards and downwards. ⟨Method⟩ First, twist the needle with the right thumb moving forward; after the needle is inserted, twist the needle with the left thumb moving forward; after needling reaction has been obtained, twirl the needle left and right again and do the thrust and lift simutanously to promote the flow of qi. Manipulate it repeatedly unless an abundant flow of qi appears.

●龙虎升腾[lóng hǔ shēng téng] ①针刺手法名。出《针灸问对》。龙虎，指左右盘旋的动作；升腾，指经气运行。〈其法〉进针以后，先在浅部做左盘动作一圈并下按。再做右盘动作一圈并下按，再用中指按捺针身如拔弩机之状，如此反复九次；然后将针插入深部，做右盘并上提动作一圈，再做左盘并上提动作一圈，再以中指按捺针身作弩法。如此反复六次。还可结合手指按压，使经气运行。属飞经走气之法，可用于气滞血凝各证。②为龙虎升降之别称。见该条。

Dragon-Tiger Ascending and Prancing ① A needling technique, originally from *Zhenjiu Wendui*(*Questions and Answers on Acupuncture and Moxibustion*). "Dragon-tiger" means the movements of spiraling left and right;"ascending and prancing" means the flow of meridian qi. ⟨Method⟩After inserting the needle, make it spiral one circle to left in the shallow part and press it simutaneously, reverse the needle in the same way and then push the needle with the middle finger as if drawing a bow. Repeat 9 times. After that insert the needle to the deep part, make it spiral one circle to the end lift it simutaneously, reverse the needle in the same manner, and also push the needle as if drawing a bow. Repeat 6 times.

Besides, it can be applied in combination with the finger-pressing method so as to promote the flow of qi, which pertains to the method of accelerating the flow of qi over the meridians. 〈Indications〉diseases due to stagnation of qi and blood stasis. ②Another name for dragon-tiger ascending and descending. →龙虎升降 (p. 254)

●龙泉[lóng quán]　经穴别名。出《备急千金要方》。即该条。

Longquan　Another name for Rangu (KI 2), a meridian point originally from *Beiji Qianjin Yaofang* (*Essential Prescriptions for Emergencies Worth a Thousand Gold*). →然谷 (p. 329)

●龙泉疔[lóng quán dīng]　即人中疔。见该条。

Boil on Dragon Stream　→人中疔(p. 333)

●龙衔素[lóng xián sù]　人名。里籍不详。《隋书·经籍志》载有《龙衔素针经》，已佚。在《医心方》中有引文。

Long Xiansu　A medical doctor, whose family background is unknown. The book of *Long Xiansu Zhenjing* (*Long Xiansu's Acupuncture Classic*), which is no longer existant, was included in *Suishu: Jing Ji Zhi* (*Sui History Book: Annals of Classics*), but quotations of his book can be seen in *Yixin Fang* (*The Heart of Medical Prescriptions*).

●龙玄[lóng xuán]　经外穴名。见《针灸大成》。在前臂桡侧腕横纹上2寸，列缺穴上方0.5寸之静脉外。〈主治〉手痛、中风口㖞、下牙痛。用灸法，禁针。

Longxuan　(EX-UE)　An extra point, seen in *Zhenjiu Dacheng* (*A Great Compendium of Acupuncture and Moxibustion*). 〈Location〉2 cun above the transverse crease of the wrist, on the radial side of the forearm, on the part where the vein is, 0.5 cun above Lieque (LU 7). 〈Indications〉pain in the hand, deviation of mouth due to apoplexy, pain of the lower teeth. 〈Method〉moxibustion. Acupuncture is forbidden.

●龙渊[lóng yuān]　经穴别名。出《针灸甲乙经》。即然谷。见该条。

Longyuan　Another name for Rangu (KI 2), a meridian point originally from *Zhenjiu Jia-Yi Jing* (*A-B Classic of Acupuncture and Moxibustion*). →然谷 (p. 329)

●聋聩[lóng kuì]　即耳聋。详见该条。

Obstruction of the Ear→耳聋(p. 95)

●聋哑[lóng yǎ]　病证名。聋和哑是不同的两种症状。因聋而致哑者，称为聋哑。以听力丧失，不会说话为主症。多由先天禀赋不足，或后天感受温邪热毒，误治失治，邪毒壅滞络脉，闭阻清窍，以致幼时两耳失聪，不能学习语言，遂成聋哑。也有因跌仆损伤、巨响震动而致者，治宜通络开窍。一般原则先治聋，后治哑，或聋哑兼治。聋，取耳门、听会、听宫、翳风、中渚、外关；哑，取哑门、廉泉、通里。

Deaf-mutism　A disease. Deafness and mutism are two different symptoms. Mutism resulting from deafness is called deaf-mutism, characterized by loss of aural ability and failure to speak. Mostly due to congenital defect or attacks of warm and heat pathogens, delayed or incorrect treatment leading to the stagnation of pathogens in the collaterals, which blocks the lucid orifices, thus resulting in the deafness of both ears in childhood, inability to learn a language and eventually in deaf-mutism. In addition, some cases are caused by traumatic injury and vibration due to an enormous sound. 〈Treatement principle〉Remove obstruction in the meridians and open orifices. Treat deafness before mutism or treat both simultaneously according to general principle. 〈Point selection〉for the treatment of deafness: Ermen (SJ 21), Tinghui (GB 2), Tinggong (SI 19), Yifeng(SJ 17), Zhongzhu (SJ 3), Waiguan (SJ 5); for the treatment of mutism: Yamen(DU 15), Lianquan (RN 23), Tongli(HT 5).

●癃[lóng]　病证名。指小便不利。见癃闭条。

Retention of Urine　A disease, referring to difficulty in urination. →癃闭(p. 255)

●癃闭[lóng bì]　病证名。出《素问·五常政大论》。又名癃、闭癃。指排尿困难，点滴难下，甚则闭涩不通的病证。本病临床上分虚、实两种。见"癃闭实证"、"癃闭虚证"各条。

Uroschesis　A disease, originally from *Suwen: Wu Changzheng Dalun* (*Plain Questions: On the Routines and Laws of the Five*

Evolutive Phases), also named retention of urine,or blockage of urination,referring to the disease of difficulty in urination,difficult dribbling urination and even blocked urination. Clinically, it is divided into two kinds:excess syndrome of uroschesis and deficiency syndrome of uroschesis. →癃闭实证(p. 256)、癃闭虚证(p. 256)

●癃闭实证[lóng bì shí zhèng] 癃闭证型之一。多因中焦湿热移注膀胱,阻遏膀胱气化所致。证见小便阻塞不通,努责无效,少腹胀急而痛,烦躁口渴,舌质红,苔黄腻,脉数。若因湿毒上犯,可见喘息、心烦、神昏等症。治宜清热利湿,行气活血。取三阴交、阴陵泉、膀胱俞、中极。湿毒上犯喘息者,加尺泽、少商。心烦,加内关。神昏,加水沟、中冲。

Excess Syndrome of Uroschesis A type of uroschesis, mostly due to the blockage of qi transformation of the urinary bladder caused by the transmission of damp-heat from the middle-jiao to the urinary bladder.〈Manifestations〉blockage of urination,lower abdominal distension and pain,irritability and thirst,red tongue with yellowish and greasy coating, rapid pulse. In the cases of damp pathogen,it may manifest as:dyspnea,irritability,and coma, etc .〈Treatment principle〉Clear heat and remove dampness,promote the flow of qi and blood circulation.〈Point selection〉Sanyinjiao(SP 6), Yinlingquan(SP 9), Pangguangshu(BL 28) and Zhongji(RN 3);for asthma due to rising of damp pathogen, add Chize (LU 5) and Shaoshang(LU 11);for irritability, add Neiguan (PC 6); for coma, add Shuigou(DU 26) and Zhongchong(PC 9).

●癃闭虚证[lóng bì xū zhèng] 癃闭证型之一。多因老年肾虚,命门火衰,或中气不足,使膀胱输化不利所致。证见小便淋沥不爽、排出无力、甚则点滴难出,伴有小腹膨隆、面色㿠白,腰酸膝软,神气怯弱,少气乏力,大便不坚、时觉肛坠、舌淡、脉细无力。治宜温补脾肾,益气启闭。取阴谷、肾俞、三焦俞、气海、委阳、脾俞。

Deficiency Syndrome of Uroschesis A type of uroschesis, mostly caused by deficiency of the kindey among aged people, the decline of fire from the gate of life, or by deficiency of qi in the middle-jiao, which leads to disturbance in qi transformation of the urinary bladder. 〈Manifestations〉dribbling urination,weakness in discharging urine,even difficulty in dribbling urination accompanied with fullness and bulge of the lower abdomen,pale complexion,soreness of the waist and lassitude of the knee joint,timidness,shortness of breath and fatigue, loose stools, sometimes with a falling sensation in the anus,pale tongue,and thready and weak pulse. 〈Treatment principle〉Warm and invigorate the spleen and kindey, replenish qi to promote diuresis. 〈Point selection〉Yingu(KI 10),Shenshu(BL 23), Sanjiaoshu (BL 22), Qihai (RN 6), Weiyang(BL 39) and Pishu(BL 20).

●楼英[lóu yīng] 人名。元明间医学家,一名公爽,字全善,浙江萧山人。著《医学纲目》四十卷,内载针灸基本理论和治法,论经络有独到见解。

Lou Ying A physician in the Yuan-Ming Dynasties, assuming the name Gongshuang and styling himself Quanshan,a native of Xiaoshan in Zhejiang Province,compiler of *Yixue Gangmu*(*An Outline of Medicine*)in 40 volumes,in which the basic theory and treatment principles of acupuncture and moxibustion were recorded, and the approaches to the meridians and collaterals were new and original.

●漏谷[lòu gǔ] 经穴名。出《针灸甲乙经》。属足太阴脾经。又名太阴络、足太阴络、大阴络。〈定位〉在小腿内侧,当内踝尖与阴陵泉的连线上,距内踝尖6寸,胫骨内侧缘后方(图39.4和图81)。〈层次解剖〉皮肤→皮下组织→小腿三头肌→趾长屈肌→胫骨后肌。浅层布有隐神经的小腿内侧皮支和大隐静脉。深层有胫神经和胫后动、静脉。〈主治〉腹胀、肠鸣、偏坠、腿膝厥冷、麻痹不仁,足踝肿痛,小便不利。直刺0.5 ~0.8寸;可灸。

Lougu(SP 7) A meridian point, originally from *Zhenjiu Jia-Yi Jing* (*A-B Classic of Acupuncture and Moxibustion*), a point on the Spleen Meridian of Foot-Taiyin, also named Taiyinluo, Zutaiyinluo, Dayinluo.〈Location〉 on the medial side of the leg and on the line connecting the tip of the medial malleolus and Yinlingquan(SP 9),6 cun from the tip of the medial malleolus, posterior to the medial bor-

der of the tibia (Figs. 39. 4&81). 〈Regional anatomy〉skin→subcutaneous tissue→triceps muscle of calf→long flexor muscle of toes→posterior tibial muscle. In the superficial layer, there are the medial cutaneous branches of the leg from the saphenous nerve and the great saphenous vein. In the deep layer, there are the tibial nerve and the posterior tibial artery and vein.〈Indications〉abdominal distension, borborygmus, swelling with bearing down pain of one testis, cold, numbness and paralysis of the knee and leg, swelling and pain of the foot and ankle, dysuria.〈Method〉Puncture perpendicularly 0.5~0.8 cun. Moxibustion is applicable.

●漏肩风[lòu jiān fēng] 病证名。又称肩凝证，多因营卫虚弱，局部感受风寒，或劳累闪挫，气血阻滞所致。初病时单侧或双侧肩部酸痛，并可向颈部和上肢放散，日轻夜重，患肢畏风寒、手指麻胀，肩关节呈不同程度的僵直。手臂上举、外展、后伸等动作均受限，日久可致肌肉萎缩。治宜祛风散寒，化湿通络。取风池、肩髃、肩髎、肩贞、臂臑、曲池、外关、条口透承山等。

Omalgia A disease, also known as frozen shoulder, mostly due to deficiency of ying and wei, local attack by wind and cold, or sprain in labour leading to stagnation of qi and blood. Aching pain in one or two shoulders at onset, radiating to the neck and the upper limbs, better in daytime and worse at night, aversion to wind and cold on the affected side, numbness and distension of the fingers, stiffness of the shoulder joint in a certain degree, difficulty and limit in raising the arm, extending the arm outward and stretching it backward, prolonged illness may result in muscular atrophy.〈Treatment principle〉Expel wind and dispel cold; remove dampness and dredge meridians.〈Point selection〉Fengchi(GB 20), Jianyu(LI 15), Jianliao(SJ 14), Jianzhen(SI 9); Binao (LI 14), Quchi (LI 11), Waiguan (SJ 5), Tiaokou(ST 38)through Chengshan(BL 57).

●漏阴[lòu yīn] 经外穴名。见《千金要方》。在内踝下0.5寸微动脉上。主治崩漏、赤白带下，直刺0.3~0.5寸；可灸。

Louyin (EX-LE) An extra point, seen in *Qianjin Yaofang* (*Essential Prescriptions Worth a Thousand Gold*).〈Location〉0.5 cun below the medial malleolus, where the arteriole is.〈Indications〉metrorrhagia and metrostaxis, leukorrhea with reddish discharge.〈Method〉Puncture perpendicularly 0.3~0.5 cun. Moxibustion is applicable.

●颅息[lú xī] 经穴名。出《针灸甲乙经》。属手少阳三焦经，又名颅囟。〈定位〉在头部，当角孙至翳风之间，沿耳轮连线的上、中1/3的交点处(图28)。〈层次解剖〉皮肤→皮下组织→耳后肌。布有耳大神经，枕小神经，面神经耳后支，耳后动、静脉的耳支分布。〈主治〉头痛、耳鸣、耳痛、小儿惊痫、呕吐涎沫。平刺0.3~0.5寸；可灸。

Luxi(SJ 19) A meridian point, originally from *Zhenjiu Jia-Yi Jing* (*A-B Classic of Acupuncture and Moxbustion*), a point on the Sanjiao Meridian of Hand-Shaoyang, also named Luxin.〈Location〉on the head, at the junction of the upper third and middle third of the line connecting Jiaosun(SJ 20) and Yifeng (SJ 17) along the curve of the ear helix(Fig. 28).〈Regional anatomy〉skin→subcutaneous tissue→posterior auricular muscle. There are the great auricular nerve, the lesser occipital nerve, the posterior auricular branches of the facial nerve, and the auricular branches of the posterior auricular artery and vein in this area.〈Indications〉headache, tinnitus, earache, infantile convulsion, vomiting with salivation.〈Method〉Puncture subcutaneously 0.3~0.5 cun. Moxibustion is applicable.

●颅囟[lú xìn] 经穴别名。见《针灸大全》。即颅息，见该条。

Luxin Another name for *Luxi*(SJ 19), a meridian point seen in *Zhenjiu Daquan* (*A Complete Work of Acupuncture and Moxibustion*).→颅息(p.257)

●鹭鸶咳[lù sī ké]
Egret Cough
cough.→顿咳(p

●吕广[lǚ guǎng]
博，吴赤乌二年(23
《金韬玉鉴经》、《募

Lu Guang A p

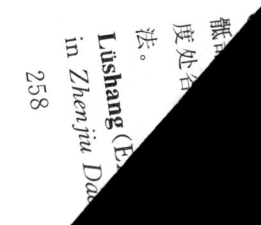

Wu during the period of Three Kingdoms, also named Lu Bo, minister of imperial medical affairs in the second year of Chiwu's reign (A.D. 239). He wrote *Yugui Zhenjing* (*Canon of Acupuncture of the Jade Chamber*), *Jintao Yujian Jing* (*Canon of the Gold Bag and Jade Basin*) and *Mu Shu Jing* (*Classic of Front-Mu and Back-Shu Points*). These works have already been lost. He once annotated *Nanjing* (*Classic of Questions*).

●吕夔[lǚ kuí] 人名。明代医家,本姓承,因依舅改姓吕,字大章,江阴(今属江苏)人。嘉靖时曾在太医院任职。著有《经络详据》、《运气发挥》、《脉理明辨》、《治法捷要》等书,均已佚。

Lü Kui A physician in the Ming Dynasty. His surname was Cheng, but was changed into Lü according to his maternal uncle. He styled himself Dazhang and was a native of Jiangyin (in Jiangsu Province today). He once worked in the Institute of Imperial Physicians during the reign of Jiajing. He wrote *Jingluo Xiangju* (*Detailed Grounds for Meridians and Collaterals*), *Yunqi Fahui* (*Elaboration on the Theory of Five Elements' Motion and Six Climate Variation Factors*), *Maili Mingbian* (*Clear Explanation on the Mechanism of Pulses*) and *Zhifa Jieyao* (*Essentials of Therapy*). These works have been lost already.

●吕细[lǚ xì] ①经穴别名。出《卫生宝鉴·流注(通玄)指要赋》。即太溪。见该条。②经外穴别名。见《针灸集成》。即内踝尖,见该条。

Lüxi Another name for ① Taixi (KI 3), a meridian point originally from *Weisheng Baojian: Liuzhu* (*Tongxuan*) *Zhiyao Fu* (*Main Rules in Medical and Health Service: Lyrics of Outline in Circulation of Qi*). →太溪(p. 420) ② Neihuaijian (EX-LE 8) an extra point, seen in *Zhenjiu Jicheng* (*A Collection of Acupuncture and Moxibustion*). →内踝尖(p. 279)

●闾上[lǘ shàng] 经外穴名。见《针灸大成》。在尾部,当尾骨尖端直上一中指及左右旁开1/2中指长__一穴,共三穴。主治痔疮、肠风下血等。用灸

(X-B) A set of extra points, seen __cheng (*A Great Compendium of Acupuncture and Moxibustion*). ⟨Location⟩ on the caudal, one middle-finger length directly above the tip of the coccyx, and half of the middle-finger length beside the point, 3 points in all. ⟨Indications⟩ hemorrhoid, hematochezia. ⟨Method⟩ moxibusiton.

●膂[lǚ] 部位名,脊旁劲起之肉,脊柱两旁之肌群。

Paravertebral Musculature of Back A part of the body, referring to the flesh bulged muscles beside the spine and muscle group beside the spinal column.

●轮1、轮2、轮3、轮4、轮5、轮6[lún yī lún èr lún sān lún sì lún wǔ lún liù] 耳穴名。位于自耳轮结节下缘至耳垂下缘中点划分五等份共六穴,由上而下依次为轮1、轮2、轮3、轮4、轮5、轮6。具有清热止痛、平肝熄风作用。用于治疗发热、上感、扁桃体炎、高血压。

Helix 1(MA), Helix 2(MA), Helix 3(MA), Helix 4(MA), Helix 5(MA), Helix 6(MA)
Ear points. ⟨Location⟩ one in each of the six areas formed when the part from the lower border of the node of the helix to the midpoint of the lower border of the ear lobe is evenly separated with five lines, 6 points in all. The order from the superior to the inferior is: Helix 1, Helix 2, Helix 3, Helix 4, Helix 5, and Helix 6. ⟨Actions⟩ Clear heat to stop pain and calm the liver to stop wind. ⟨Indications⟩ fever, upper respiratory tract infection, tonsillitis hypertention.

●瘰疬[luǒ lì] 病证名。出《灵枢·寒热》。又名鼠瘘、老鼠疮、疬子颈等。小的为瘰,大的为疬。多因肝火久郁,虚火内灼,炼液为痰,或受风火邪毒,结于颈项、腋、胯之间。临床可分为肝郁瘰疬、阴虚瘰疬、风热瘰疬。详见各条。

Scrofula A disease, originally from *Lingshu: Han Re* (*Miraculous Pivot: Febrile Diseases*), also named mouse fiscula, mouse sore, cervical scrofula, etc. The smaller one as small scrofula, the bigger one as big scrofula. Mostly caused by prolonged stagnation of liver-fire, internal burning of asthenic fire, which decocts the body fluid into phlegm, or attack by wind and fire pathogens, which stagnate in the neck, armpit and between the waist and thigh. It can be divided clinically into scrofula due to the stagnation of liver-qi, scrofula due

to yin-deficiency and scrofula due to wind-heat pathogen. →肝郁瘰疬(p.128)、阴虚瘰疬(p.561)、风热瘰疬(p.114)

●络[luò] ①络脉名。出《灵枢·经脉》泛指各类络脉,如罗网状,无处不到,由大而小。通常分别络、浮络、血络、孙络和丝络等类。它们的作用是加强表里经的联系,并通达经脉未能行经的器官和组织。②专指别络。出《素问·调经论》。③连络。出《灵枢·经脉》。如手太阴之脉,起于中焦,向下连络大肠。

1. **Collaterals** Originally from *Lingshu: Jingmai* (*Miraculous Pivot: Meridians*), generally referring to all kinds of collaterals running everywhere like a network from large to small, usually divided into large collaterals, superficial collaterals, superficial venules minute collaterals, and thready collaterals. 〈Functions〉Strengthen the relationship between the interior meridian and exterior meridian, and run to the organs and tissues which the meridians fail to pass through.

2. **Large Collaterals** Originally from *Suwen: Tiao Jing Lun* (*Plain Questions: Regulating the Meridians*).

3. **Connecting** Originally from *Ling Shu: Jingmai* (*Miraculous Pivot: Meridians*). For instance, the Lung Meridian of the Hand-Taiyin starts from the middle jiao and runs posteriorly to connect the large intestine.

●络刺[luò cì] 刺法名。见《灵枢·官针》,指刺络放血法,与经刺相对。临床上多用于实证、热证。参见"刺络"条。

Collateral-Pricking A needling technique, seen in *Ling Shu: Guanzhen* (*Miraculous Pivot: Official Needles*), referring to the method of blood-letting puncture, the opposite of puncturing the meridians, mostly used for treating excess syndrome and heat-syndrome. →刺络(p.55)

●络脉[luò mài] 经络名。出《灵枢·脉度》。指由经脉分出的网络全身的分支。络脉以十五络为主体,也包括孙络、血络、浮络等,有沟通经脉,运行气血,反应和治疗疾病的作用。详见各条。

Collateral Branch of the Large Merdian Name for meridians and collaterals, originally from *Ling Shu: Mai Du* (*Miraculous Pivot: Measurement of Meridians*), referring to the branches derived from the meridians and netted throughout the human body. The Fifteen Collaterals are the main ones; and the minute collaterals, superficial venules and superficial collaterals are also included. 〈Function〉Connect meridians, transport qi and blood, manifest and treat diseases. →十五络(p.382)、孙络(p.417)、血络(p.526)、浮络(p.118)

●络气[luò qì] 指行于络脉的气,与经气相对而言。参见"脉气"条。

Collateral Qi The qi which flows in the collaterals, as opposed to the meridian qi. →脉气(p.263)

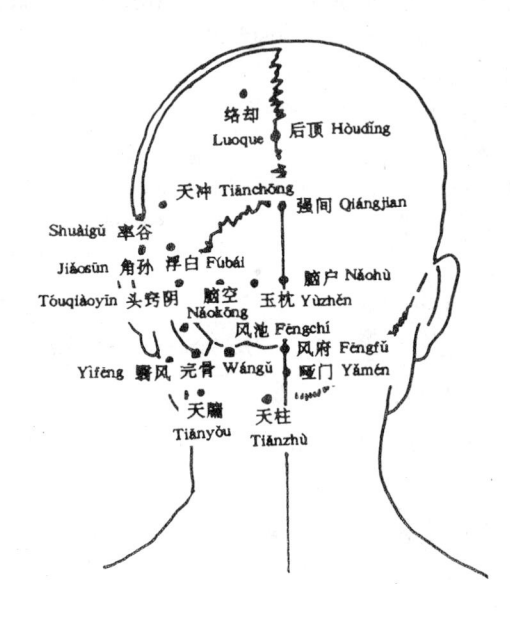

图31 络却和其它后头部穴

Fig. 31 Luoque and other points of occiput

●络却[luò què] 经穴名。出《针灸甲乙经》。属足太阳膀胱经,又名强阳、脑盖、络郄。〈定位〉在头部,当前发际正中直上5.5寸,旁开1.5寸。按语:本穴位置,唐以后诸文献均曰"在通天后一寸半"。今从其说,定位如上(图28)。〈层次解剖〉皮肤→皮下组织→帽状腱膜。浅层布有枕大神经和枕动、静脉。深层为腱膜下疏松组织和颅骨外膜。〈主治〉眩晕、耳鸣、鼻塞、口㖞、癫狂、痫证、目视不明、项肿、瘿瘤。平刺0.3~0.5寸;可灸。

Luoque (BL 8) A meridian point, originally

from *Zhenjiu Jia-Yi Jing* (*A-B Classic of Acupuncture and Moxibustion*), a point on the Bladder Meridian of Foot-Taiyang, also known as Qiangyang, Naogai, Luoxi. ⟨Location⟩ on the head, 5.5 cun directly above the midpoint of the anterior hairline and 1.5 cun lateral to the midline (Fig. 28). ⟨Regional anatomy⟩ skin→subcutaneous tissue→epicranial aponeurosis. In the superficial layer, there are the greater occipital nerve and the occipital artery and vein. In the deep layer, there are the subaponeurotic loose connective tissue and the pericranium. ⟨Indications⟩ dizziness, tinnitus, stuffy nose, deviation of the mouth, manic-depressive psychosis, epilepsy, blurred vision, swelling of the neck, goiter. ⟨Method⟩ Puncture subcutaneously 0.3~0.5cun. Moxibustion is applicable.

●络郄 [luò xì] 经穴别名。见《医学入门》，即络却。见该条。

Luoxi Another name for Luoque (BL 8), a meridian point seen in *Yixue Rumen* (*An Introduction to Medicine*). →络却 (p. 259)

●络穴 [luò xué] 经穴分类名。出《灵枢·经脉》。络脉在由经脉别出的部位各有一个腧穴，称为络穴。它具有联络表里两经的作用。十二经的络穴皆位于肘膝关节以下，加上任脉、督脉及脾之大络穴，共计十五穴。故称为"十五络穴"。见表9。

Luo (Connecting) Points A term for the classification of the acupoints, originally from *Ling Shu: Jingmai* (*Miraculous Pivot: Meridians*). A point at a certain place on the meridians from which each collateral branch is called Luo (Connecting) Point. ⟨Function⟩ Connect the two meridians of the exterior and the interior. The Luo (Connecting) Point of the Twelve Regular Meridians are all located below the joints of the elbow and knee. Add the Luo (Connecting) Points of Ren and Du Meridians and the large Luo (Connecting) Point of the Spleen, and there are 15 points in all, which are named the Fifteen Luo (Connecting) Points. See Table 9.

表9 十五络穴表

Table 9　　Distribution of the Fifteen Luo (Connecting) Points

手三阴经 Three Yin Meridians of Hand	肺经 Lung Meridian	列缺 Lieque (LU 7)	心经 Heart Meridian	通里 Tongli (HT 5)	心包经 Pericardium Meridian	内关 Neiguan (PC 6)
手三阳经 Three Yang Meridians of Hand	大肠经 Large Intestine Meridian	偏历 Pianli (LI 6)	小肠经 Small Intestine Meridian	支正 Zhizheng (SI 7)	三焦经 Sanjiao Meridian	外关 Waiguan (SJ 5)
足三阳经 Three Yang Meridians of Foot	胃经 Stomach Meridian	丰隆 Fenglong (ST 40)	膀胱经 Bladder Meridian	飞扬 Feiyang (BL 58)	胆经 Gallbladder Meridian	光明 Guangming (GB 37)
足三阴经 Three Yin Meridians of Foot	脾经 Spleen Meridian	公孙 Gongsun (SP 4)	肾经 Kidney Meridian	大钟 Dazhong (KI 4)	肝经 Liver Meridian	蠡沟 Ligou (LR 5)
任、督、脾大络 Ren & Du Meridians, Large Luo (Connecting) Point of the Spleen	任脉 Ren Meridian	鸠尾 Jiuwei (RN 15)	督脉 Du Meridian	长强 Chang qiang (DU 1)	脾大络 Large Collateral of the Spleen	大包 Dabao (SP 21)

M

●麻叶灸[má yiè jiǔ] 灸法的一种。见《串雅外编》。将采集新鲜的麻花、麻叶捣烂,做成圆柱状,放于病变部施灸。用于治疗瘰疬。

Cauterization with Folium Cannabis A form of cauterization, seen in *Chuanya Waibian(External Treatise on Folk Medicine)*. Collect the fresh Flos and Folium Cannabis, pound them to make cannabis cones, ignite the cone on the diseased area for cauterization. ⟨Indication⟩scrofula.

●马丹阳[mǎ dān yáng] 金代道家、针灸家(1123~1183年)。初名从义,字宜甫,后改名钰,字元宝,号丹阳顺化真人,故世称马丹阳。著有《天星十二穴治杂病歌》。流传较广。

Ma Dangyang A Taoist and an expert of acupuncture and moxibustion (1123-1183) in the Jin Dynasty. Formerly he was named Congyi and his self-styled name was Yifu; later he changed his name into Yu and his self-styled name into Yuanbao, and assumed the name Danyang Shun Hua Zhen Ren. Therefore, Ma Danyang was known for generations. He wrote *Tianxing Shier Xue Zhi Zabing Ge(A Verse on the Treatment of Miscellaneous Diseases with the Twelve Heaven-Star Points)*, which is widely spread.

●马丹阳十二穴[mǎ dān yáng shí èr xué] 指十二经验效穴。《针灸大全》载《马丹阳天星十二穴并治杂病歌》,特将这十二个穴的定位及主治用歌赋的形式描述。这十二个穴是足三里、内庭、曲池、合谷、委中、承山、太冲、昆仑、环跳、阳陵泉、通里和列缺。《针灸聚英》对此十二穴亦有载述,只是文字略异,又题《薛真人天星十二穴歌》。

Ma Danyang's Twelve Points The twelve effective acupoints. *Ma Dangyang Tianxing Shier Xue Bing Zhi Zabing Ge(A Verse on the Twelve Heaven-Star Point Employed by Ma Danyang to Treat Miscellaneous Diseases)*, which was recorded in *Zhenjiu Daquan (A Complete Work of Acupuncture and Moxibustion)*, depicted the locations and indications of these points in the form of verse. They are: Zusanli(ST 36), Neiting(ST 44), Quchi(LI 11), Hegu(LI 4), Weizhong(BL 40), Chengshan(BL 57), Taichong(LR 3), Kunlun(BL 60), Huantiao(GB 30), Yanglingquan(GB 34), Tongli(HT 5) and Lieque(LU 7). They were also recorded and described in *Zhenjiu Juying(Essentials of Acupunctre and Moxibustion)*, but with a slight difference in the writing style, which was entitled *Xue Zhen Ren Tianxing Shier Xue Ge(Verse on Twelve Heaven-Star Points by Xue Zhen Ren)*.

●马嗣明[mǎ sì míng] 南北朝至隋初医家。《北史》有传。医术精妙,治病多奇效,著作不明。

Ma Siming A physician in the Northern and Southern Dynasties and early Sui Dynasty. His excellent medical skills and miraculous therapeutic effects are recorded in *Beishi (The Northern History)*. His works are unknown.

●马王堆汉墓帛书[mǎ wáng duī hàn mù bó shū] 文献名。1973年,长沙马王堆三号汉墓出土大量帛书,其中有很多医学文献。帛书抄写年大约在秦汉之际。这些文献原无篇名和书名,整理者依据内容分别给以命名,即:《足臂十一脉灸经》、《阴阳十一脉灸经》甲本、《脉法》、《阴阳脉死候》、《五十二病方》,以上五种合一卷帛书;《却谷食气》、《阴阳十一脉灸经》乙本,《导引图》,以上三种合为一卷帛书;《养生方》,《杂疗方》、《胎产书》,以上三种合为一卷帛书。其中称为《十一脉灸经》者为有关经脉的最早文献,或称《帛书经脉》,可与《灵枢·经脉》相互印证。参见"十一脉灸经"条。

Ancient Book Copied on Silk Discovered in the Tomb of Han Dynasty of Mawangdui Historical documents excavated in 1973 from No. 3 Tomb of Han Dynasty of Mawangdui in

Changsha, among which, there are a lot of medical documents. These ancient books were copied on silk during the Qin and Han Dynasties. These documents bear no titles originally, those who put them in order entitled them respectively according to their contents. They are: *Zu Bi Shiyi Mai JiuJing* (*Moxibustion Classic on Eleven Meridian of the Arm and Foot*), *YinYang Shiyi Mai Jiuing* (*A Book of Moxibustion Classic on Eleven Meridians of Yin-Yang*), *Maifa* (*Principles of Pulse*), *Yin-Yang Mai Sihou* (*Death Syndrome of Yin-Yang Pulse*), *Wushier Bingfang* (*Prescriptions for 52 Diseases*), the above five were bound up into 1 volume copied on silk. *Quegu Shiqi* (*Abandoning Food and Living on Qi*), *Yinyang Shiyi Mai Jiujing* (*Book of Moxibusiton Classic on Eleven Meridians of Yinyang*), *Daoyin Tu* (*A Map for Physical and Dreathing Exercises*), these three were bound up into one. *Yangsheng Fang* (*Prescriptions for Health-Care*) *Za Liao Fang* (*Treating Miscellaneous Diseases*), *Taichan Shu* (*A Book for Midwifery*) these three were bound up into one. *Shiyi Mai Jiujing* (*Moxibustion Classic on Eleven Meridians*) is the earliest document on the meridians, It is also called *Boshu Jingmai* (*Ancient Book Copied on Silk on the Meridians*), which can be confirmed with *Ling Shu*: *Jingmai* (*Miraculous Pivot*: *Meridians*). →十一脉灸经(p. 384)

●马衔铁针[mǎ xián tiě zhēn] 针具名。指用马衔铁制成的医用针具,《针灸聚英》卷三"铁针"条载:"《本草》云:马衔铁无毒"。

Tinplate Needle A kind of needle, referring to a form of medical needle made of tinplate. It was recorded in the entry of "iron needle" in Vol. 3 of *Zhenjiu Juying* (*Essentials of Acupuncture and Moxibustion*): "In *Bencao* (*Compendium of Materia Medica*), it was said that tinplate was nontoxic."

●埋线疗法[mái xiàn liáo fǎ] 又名穴位埋线法,将铬制羊肠线埋入穴位皮下或肌肉深层,利用它的持续刺激作用以治病。一般采用特制埋线针,选取腹背及四肢肌肉丰满处的穴位,每次埋线1~2穴,可用于消化性溃疡、慢性胃炎、慢性支气管炎、哮喘、神经官能症、小儿麻痹后遗症等。

Catgut Embedding Also known as catgut embedding at acupoints. 〈Method〉Embed a piece of catgut subcutaneously or in the deeper layer of muscle at a certain point for therapeutic purposes to cause continuous stimulation. Generally, a specially made needle for embedding is used, the acupoints on the abdomen, back and the four limbs where the muscles are well-developed are selected, 1 or 2 points for embedding each time. 〈Indications〉 pepticulcer, chronic gastritis, chronic bronchitis, asthma, psychoneurosis and sequela of infantile paralysis, etc.

●埋针疗法[mái zhēn liáo fǎ] 针灸疗法之一。用镊子夹住皮内针,针尖对准穴位,轻缓刺入皮内0.3~0.8寸,然后用胶布固定。留针时间长短视具体情况而定。

Needle-Embedding One of the acupuncture therapies. 〈Method〉Grip the cutaneous needle with a pair of tweezers, place the tip of the needle directly on the selected acupoint, then insert the needle slowly 0.3-0.8 cun. Fix the needle with adhesive plaster. The duration of retaining needle depends on the specific conditions.

●麦粒灸[mài lì jiǔ] 灸法术语。见《扁鹊心书》。即小炷灸。因用如麦粒大的小艾炷施灸,故名。

Moxibustion with Wheat Grain-Like Moxa-cone A term for moxibustion, seen in *Bianque Xinshu* (*Bian Que's Medical Experiences*), i.e, moxibustion with a small moxa-cone which is about the size of a wheat grain.

●麦粒肿[mài lì zhǒng] 针眼的别名。详见该条。

Wheat Grain-Like Swelling Another name for hordeolum. →针眼(p. 597)

●脉[mài] ①经络名。出《素问·脉要精微论》等,指脉管,为气血运行的通道。②指脉搏、脉象。出《灵枢·邪气脏腑病形》。③五不女之一。出《广嗣纪要·择配篇》,指女子无月经或因月经不调致原发性不孕症。

1. **Meridians** Originally from *Suwen*: *Maiyao Jingwei Lun* (*Plain Questions*: *Treatise on the Importance of the Pulse and the Subtle Skill of Its Examination*), referring to the vessels which are the passages through which qi and blood circulate.

2. Pulse Condition From *Lingshu: Xieqi Zangfu Bingxing* (*Miraculous Pivot: Pathogenic Evils, Zang-Fu Organs and Manifestations*).

3. Primary Infertility One of the five types of female sterility, from *Guangsi Jiyao: Zepei Pian* (*Summary of Flourishing Offsprings: On Selection of Spouse*), referring to the congenital infertility due to amenorrhea or irregular menstruation.

●脉度[mài dù] 指经脉的长度。见《灵枢·脉度》,手三阳经从手至头,各长5尺;手三阴经从手至胸中,各长3尺5寸;足三阳经从足上至头,各长8尺;足三阴经从足至胸中,各长6尺5寸,阴阳跷脉,从足至目,各长7尺5寸。督脉、任脉,各长4尺5寸。经脉长度是以身长7尺5寸来计算,即以内度为基础,所以说"先度其骨节之大小、广狭、长短,而脉度定矣"。

Measurement of Meridians Referring to the length of the meridians, seen in *Ling Shu: Maidu* (*Miraculous Pivot: Measurement of Meridians*), each of the three yang meridians of hand from the hand to the head is measured 5 chi; each of the three yin meridians from the hand to the chest is measured 3.5 chi; each of the three yang meridians of foot from the foot to the head is measured 8 chi, each of the three yin meridians of foot from the foot to the chest is measured 6.5 chi. Meridians of yinqiao and yangqiao from the foot to the eye are measured 7.5 chi; Du and Ren Meridians are measured 4.5 chi each. The length of the meridian is measured by taking the height of 7.5 chi as the standard stature. In other words, it is based on bone-length. Therefore, "first measure the size, width and length of the bones, then the measurement of meridians is decided".

●脉气[mài qì] 指经络之气。分称经气、络气,详见各条。

Vessel-Qi The qi of meridians and collaterals, respectively called meridian qi and collateral qi. →经气(p.212)、络气(p.259)

●慢惊风[màn jīng fēng] 病证名。见《证治准绳·幼科》。又称天吊风,以发病缓慢、无热,抽搐时发时止,缓而无力为其特点。多因大吐大泻之后,或脾胃素弱,化源不足;或热病伤阴,肾阴不足,肝血亏损,木失濡养,虚风内动所致,证见面黄肌瘦、形神疲惫、四肢倦怠或厥冷,呼吸微弱,囟门低陷,昏睡露睛、时有抽搐。脾阳虚弱者还可大便稀薄,色青带绿,足跗和面部浮肿,脉缓无力。肝肾阴亏者还可见神倦虚烦、面色潮红、舌光少苔、脉沉细而数,治宜培土益肾、熄火定惊。取脾俞、胃俞、肝俞、气海、足三里、太冲、百会、印堂、筋缩。

Chronic Infantile Convulsion A disease, seen in *Zhengzhi Zhunsheng: Youke* (*Standard for Diagnosis and Treatment: Pediatrics*), also known as convulsion due to natural pathogenic wind. Characterized by gradual onset, without fever, intermittent spasm of the limbs relaxed and weak limbs, mostly caused by insufficiency of the mutrient due to weakness by stirring-up of endopathic wind of deficiency due to deficiency of the liver-blood, which fails to nourish wood. 〈Manifestations〉 sallow complexion and emaciation, listlessness, lauguishness and cold of the four limbs, weak breath, depression of the limbs. Cases of deficiency of the spleen-yang are manifested by watery stools with cyanotic colour, edema of foot and face, moderate pulse. Cases of insufficiency of liver-yin and kidney-yin are marked with fatigue, restlessness, pink complexion, smooth tongue with little coating, deep, thready and rapid pulse. 〈Treatment principle〉Invigorate the spleen and kidney, remove fire to arrest convulsion. 〈Point selection〉Pishu (BL 20), Weishu (BL 21), Ganshu (BL 18), Shenshu (BL 23) Qihai (RN 6), Taichong (LR 3) Baihui (DU 20), Yintang (EX-HN 3) and Jinsuo (DU 8).

●芒针[máng zhēn] 针具名,是在古代九针中的长针基础上发展而来的。近代用不锈钢丝制造,针身细长有如麦芒,故名,长度分5寸、7寸、10寸、15寸等数种,用于深刺和沿皮下横刺法。

Elongated Needle A needling instrument, developed from the long needle in ancient times. In recent years, it is made of the screw of stainless steel. It is so named because of its long and thin appearance like awn of wheat. The needles vary in length-5 cun, 7 cun, 10 cun and 15 cun and so on, suitable for deep puncture and subcutaneous transverse

needling.

● 芒针疗法 [máng zhēn liáo fǎ] 针刺治疗方法之一,指用芒针深刺穴位的治疗方法,使用时,以右手持针柄捻转,左手扶持针体下压协同缓慢进针,一般腹部用直刺,腰、臀、肘、膝关节部用斜刺,头面、胸背部用沿皮刺,适用于精神病,风湿痹痛,月经不调等。

Therapy with Elongated Needle One of the acupuncture therapies, referring to the deep puncture at an acupoint with an elongated needle for therapeutic purposes. 〈Method〉To start with, hold and twirl the handle of the needle with the right hand, hold and thrust the body of the needle with the left hand to help insert the needle slowly. Generally, puncture the points on the abdomen perpendicularly; puncture the points on the lower back, buttock, elbow and knee joints obliquely; puncture the points on the head, face, chest and back subcutaneously. 〈Indications〉mental disorder, althralgia-syndrome due to wind-dampness and irregular menstruation.

● 盲肠穴 [máng cháng xué] 经外穴名。见《腧穴学概论》。在腹右侧,当髂前上棘与脐连线的中点处,〈主治〉肠痈、腹泻等,直刺1～1.5寸;可灸。

Mangchangxue (EX-CA) An extra point, seen in *Shuxue xue Gailun* (*An Outline of Acupoints*). 〈Location〉on the right side of the abdomen, on the midpoint of the line connecting the anterior superior iliac spine and the umbilicus. 〈Indications〉acute appendicitis, diarrhea, etc. 〈Method〉Puncture perpendicularly 1.0～1.5 cun. Moxibustion is applicable.

● 毛刺 [máo cì] 《内经》刺法名。出《灵枢·官针》。是九刺之一,指浅刺皮毛以治疗浅部的病症,近代应用的皮肤针即由此发展而来。治疗范围也有了扩大。

Skin Needling A needling technique in *Neijing* (*The Inner Canon of Huangdi*), origianlly from *Lingshu*: *Guanzhen* (*Miraculous Pivot*: *Official Needles*), one of the nine needlings in ancient times, referring to puncturing superficially to treat shallow-sited diseaes. The contemporary cutaneous needle is developed from it, and its applications have also been enlarged.

● 毛茛灸 [máo gèn jiǔ] 天灸的一种。出《本草纲目》卷十七。毛茛又称老虎脚爪草。取其鲜叶捣烂,敷于穴处或患处,初有热辣感,继而所敷皮肤发红、充血,稍时即起水泡。发泡后,局部有色素沉着。以后可自行消失。敷灸时间约1—2小时。如敷于经渠、内关、大椎穴,可治疗疟疾;治疗寒痹可敷于患处,也能与食盐合用制成药丸敷于少商、合谷穴,可治疗急性结膜炎。

Mao Gen (*Herba Ranunculi Japonici*) **Vesiculation** One form of medical vesiculation, originally from Vol. 17 of *Bencao Gangmu* (*Compendium of Materia Medica*), *Mao Gen* (*Herba Ranunculi Japoici*) is also known as tiger's talon grass. 〈Method〉Pound the fresh leaves to pieces, apply to the selected point or diseased area. At first, it has the sensation of heat and numbness, then, the skin covered with butter-cup flushes, congests, and blisters. There local pigmentation may appear after the blisters, and will disappear gradually. The duration of vesiculation is about 1-2 hours. If it is spread on Jingqu (LU 8), Neiguan (PC 6) and Dazhui (DU 14), it is used for treating malarial disease; if it is used for treating cold syndrome, it can be spread on the diseased area. It can also be made into pills after it is mixed with salt. Place the pills on Shaoshang (LU 11) and Hegu (LI 4) points for treating acute conjunctivitis.

● 毛际 [máo jì] 部位名。指下腹部阴毛的边际。如:任脉"上毛际"少阳胆经"绕毛际",均经此处。

Suprapubic Hair Margin A part of the body, referring to the margin of the pubic hair in the lower abdomen. For instance, the Ren Meridian "ascending to the hair margin", the Gallbladder Meridian of Foot-Shaoyang "going around the hair margin", both run through the suprapubic hair margin.

● 卯南卯北 [mǎo nán mǎo běi] 刺法用语。出《席弘赋》。卯之南是午的方位,意指捻针时大指向前(左转)为补;卯之北是子的方位,意指捻针时大指向右(右转)为泻。

South to Mao and North to Mao A needling technique, originally from *Xi Hong Fu*(*Ode to Xi Hong*). South to mao is the direction of wu, referring to the reinforcing method by twirling the needle with the thumb

moving forward (to the left) while north to mao is the direction of zi referring to the reducing method by twirling the needle with the thumb moving backward (to the right).

●卯南酉北[mǎo nán yǒu běi] 刺法用语。出《千金方》卷二十九,十二支配方位:卯是东方,午是南方;酉是西方,子是北方。卯南指的是午,酉北指的是子。后世补泻法中以左转从午,属补;右转从子,属泻。与此说明相类。

South to Mao and North to You A needling technique, originally from Vol. 29 of *Qianjin Fang* (*Presciptions Worth a Thousand Gold*). The coordination of direction in the Twelve Earthly Branches is such that mao means the east, wu the south, you the west, and zi the north. "South to mao" refers to wu and "North to you" refers to zi. In the reinforcing and reducing methods of later ages, leftturn to wu means reinforcing while rightturn to zi means reducing.

●眉本[méi běn] ①经穴别名。见《素问·气穴论》。即攒竹,见该条。②部位名。指眉毛内侧近眶之处,俗称眉头。

1. **Meiben** Another name for Cuanzhu (BL 2) a meridian point originally from *Suwen*: *Qi xue Lun* (*Plain Questions*: *On Loci of Qi*) →攒竹(p.58)
2. **Brow Origin** A part of the body, referring to the medial part of the eyebrow, which is close to the space between the two eyebrows, commonly called brow source.

●眉冲[méi chōng] 经穴名。出《脉经》。属足太阳膀胱经。又名小竹。〈定位〉在头部,当攒竹直上入发际0.5寸,神庭与曲差连线之间(图28)。〈层次解剖〉皮肤→皮下组织→枕额肌额腹。浅层布有滑车上神经和滑车上动、静脉。深层为腱膜下疏松组织和颅骨外膜。〈主治〉痫证、头痛、眩晕、目视不明、鼻塞。平刺0.3—0.5寸;禁灸。

Meichong (BL 3) A meridian point, originally from *Maijing* (*The Classic of Sphygmology*) a point on the Bladder Meridian of Foot-Taiyang also known as Xiaozhu. 〈Location〉 on the head, directly above Cuanzhu (BL 2), 0.5 cun above the anterior hairline, on the line connecting Shenting (DU 24) and Qucha (BL 4) (Fig. 28). 〈Regional anatomy〉 skin → subcutaneous tissue → trontal belly of occipitofrontal muscle. In the superficial layer, there are the supratrochlear nerve and the supratrochlear artery and vein. In the deep layer, there are the subaponeurotic loose connective tissue and the pericarnium. 〈Indications〉 epilepsy, headache, dizziness, blurred vision, stuffy nose. 〈Method〉 Puncture subcutaneously 0.3~0.5 cun. Moxibustion is forbidden.

●眉头[méi tóu] ①经穴别名。见《素问·骨空论》。即攒竹,见该条。②部位名。眉本的俗称。见该条。

1. **Meitou** Another name for Cuanzhu (BL 2), seen in *Suwen*: *Gukong Lun* (*Plain Questions*: *On the Apertures of Bones*). →攒竹(p.58)
2. **Brow Source** A part of the body, popular name of brow origin. →眉本(p.265)

●眉枕线[méi zhěn xiàn] 头针标定线。是从眉中点上缘和枕外粗隆尖端的头侧面连线。

Eyebrow-Occiput Line One of the standard lines for scalp acupuncture, referring to the cephalic line connecting the superior border of the midpoint of the eyebrow and the tip of the external occipital tuberosity.

●梅核气[méi hé qì] 病名。见《赤水玄珠》卷三,多由肝郁气滞,痰凝咽部,痰气互结所致,证见精神抑郁、胸闷、噫气、咽中不适如有物阻、吞之不下、咯之不出、饮食吞咽无障碍、多疑虑、善太息、苔薄白腻、脉弦滑。治宜疏肝解郁,清化痰火。取太冲、内关、丰隆、天突、上星、印堂。

Globus Hyertericus A disease, originally from Vol. 3 of *Chishui Xuanzhu* (*Black Pearl of the Red River*), mostly caused by stagnation of the liver-qi, phlegm accumulated in the throat leading to combination of phlegm and stagnated qi. 〈Manifestations〉 mental depression, suffocation of the chest, eructation, subjective feeling of a foreign body obstructing the throat with inability to or cough it up, but no difficulty in eating and swallowing, easy to have doubts and sighs, pale and greasy tongue with thin coating, wiry and slippery pulse. 〈Treatment principle〉 Relieve depressed liver, clear and remove phlegm-fire. 〈Point selection〉 Taichong (LR 3), Neiguan (PC 6),

Fenglong(ST 40), Tiantu(RN 22), Shangxing(DU 23) and Yintang(EX-HN 3).

●梅花针[méi huā zhēn]　皮肤针的一种,针头由五枚细针组成,用以叩击浅刺皮肤。参见"皮肤针"条。

Plum-Blossom Needle　A kind of dermal needle with a bundle of five short fine needles fixed vertically at one end of the needle, used for superficial percussion with insertion. → 皮肤针(p.292)

●扪法[mén fǎ]　针刺辅助手法名。十四法之一。指起针之后用手指扪按穴位。在《针经指南》、《针灸大成》、《医学入门》中均有论述。

Palpation Method　An auxiliary acupuncture technique, one of the Fourteen Methods, referring to pressing the selected acupoint with the finger after the needle is withdrawn. It was described in *Zhenjing Zhinan* (*A Guide to the Classics of Acupuncture*), *Zhenjiu Dacheng* (*A Great Compendium of Acupuncture and Moxibustion*) and *Yixue Rumen* (*An Introduction to Medicine*).

●梦失精[mèng shī jīng]　见《金匮要略·血痹虚劳病脉证治》。即梦遗。详见该条。

Loss of Essence in Dream　Seen in *Jingui Yaolue: Xuebi Xulao Bing Mai Zheng Zhi* (*Synopsis of the Golden Chamber: Pulse Conditions, Symptoms and Treatments of Blood Bi-Syndrome and Consumptive Diseases*), synonymous with nocturnal emission. → 梦遗(p.266)

●梦遗[mèng yí]　病证名。见《丹溪心法》。又名梦失精。指因梦交而精液遗泄的病证。多因见色思想,相火妄动,或用心过度,心火亢盛所致。证见梦境纷纭,阳事易举,遗精一夜数次或数夜一次,或兼早泄、头晕、心烦少寐、腰酸耳鸣、小便黄、舌质偏红、脉细数。治宜清心降火,滋阴涩精,取心俞、肾俞、关元、神门、中封。

Nocturnal Emission　A disease, seen in *Danxi Xinfa* (*Danxi's Experience*), also known as loss of essence in dream, referring to evacuation of semen due to coition in dream, mostly resulting from hyperactivity of the ministerial fire as a result of emotional irritation, or excesive heart-fire as a result of emotional irritation, or excessive heart-fire because of over-thinking. 〈Manifestations〉a variety of dreams, desirable for male sexuality, discharge of semen several times in one night or once several nights or accompanied by premature ejaculation, dizziness, irritability and insomnia, soreness of the waist and tinnitus, yellowish urine, redish tongue, thready and rapid pulse. 〈Treatment principle〉clear heart-fire, nourish yin and control nocturnal emission. 〈Point selection〉Xinshu(BL 15), Shenshu(BL 23), Guanyuan (RN 4), Shenmen (HT 7), Zhongfeng(LR 4).

●面䪼[miàn jiào]　经穴别名。即承泣。详见该条。

Mianjiao　Another name for the meridian point Chengqi(ST 1). → 承泣(p.44)

●面瘫[miàn tān]　病证名,俗称口眼喎斜。多因脉络空虚,风寒、风热之邪乘虚侵袭面部筋脉,以致气血阻滞,肌肉纵缓不收,一侧面部板滞、麻木、瘫痪,不能作蹙额、皱眉、露齿、鼓颊等动作,口角向健侧歪斜,漱口漏水,进餐时,食物停留于病侧齿颊之间,病侧额纹、鼻唇沟消失,眼睑闭合不全,迎风流泪。治宜祛风络。取风池、翳风、颊车、合谷、地仓、太冲,面部穴位酌予斜针或透穴,初期用泻法,后期用补法加灸。不能抬眉加攒竹,鼻唇沟平坦加迎香,人中歪斜加水沟。

Facial Paralysis　A disease, commonly called deviation of the eye and mouth, mostly caused by deficiency of the meridians and collaterals. Wind-cold, wind-heat pathogens take advantage of the deficiency and attack the muscles and meridians on the face, which leads to stagnation of qi and blood stasis and muscular flaccidity. 〈Manifestations〉facial stiffness, numbness and paralysis on one side, failure to wrinkle forehead and knit brows, exposed teeth, and bulging cheeks, the deviated mouth sloping to the healthy side, water leaks out while brushing teeth, food remains between the teeth and cheeks on the diseased side at the time of eating, disappearance of the wrinkles and nasolabial groove on the ill side, incomplete closure of the eyelid, lacrimation induced by irritation of the wind. 〈Treatment principle〉Dispel wind, dredge the meridians and collaterals. 〈Point selection〉Fengchi(GB 20), Yifeng(SJ 17), Jiache(ST 6), Hegu(LI

4), Dicang (ST 4), Taichong (LR 3). The points on the face should be punctured obliquely or subcutaneously to the other point, reducing method in the initial stage and reinforcing method with moxibustion in the later stage. Add Cuanzhu (BL 2) for the failure of knitting brows, Yingxiang (LI 20) for the disappearance of nasolabial groove, and Shuigou (DU 26) for the deviation of philtrum.

●面痛[miàn tòng] 病证名。指面颊抽掣疼痛而言。可因风寒之邪袭于阳明经脉，或因风热病毒，侵淫面部所致。本病多发于一侧，以面颊上、下颌部为多，呈阵发性放射性电击样剧痛，如撕裂、针刺、火灼一般。疼痛常有一起点，可因吹风、洗脸、说话、吃饭等刺激此点而发作。风寒面痛遇寒则甚，得热则轻，鼻流清涕，苔白脉浮。风热面痛则痛处有灼热感、涎涎、目赤、流泪、苔黄腻、脉浮数，治宜疏通阳明、太阳、少阳筋脉，额部痛取攒竹、阳白、头维、合谷。上颌痛取四白、颧髎、上关、偏历。下颌痛取承浆、颊车、下关、翳风、内庭。寒证加灸。

Facial Pain A disease, referring to spasm and pain on the face, caused by wind-cold pathogen attacking the meridians of yangming or by wind-heat pathogen attacking the face, mostly occurring on one side and seen on the upper part of the face and the lower jaw. Marked by paroxysmal radial, lightning and sharp pain with feelings of tearing, stabbing and scorching. Generally, there is a point of pain, at which the pain is stimulated by wind-attacking, face-washing, speaking and eating. Facial pain due to wind-cold pathogen is manifested as pain getting worse with cold and better with heat, clear and watery nasal discharge, whitish tongue, and superficial pulse. Facial pain due to wind-heat pathogen is manifested as pain with scorching hot feeling; salivation, conjunctive congestion, lacrimation, yellowish and greasy tongue coating, superficial and rapid pulse. 〈Treatment principle〉 Dredge the muscles and Meridians of Yangming, Taiyang and Shaoyang. 〈Point selection〉Cuanzhu(BL 2), Yangbai(GB 14), Touwei(ST 8) and Hegu(LI 4) for pain on the forehead; Sibai(ST 2), Quanliao(SI 18), Shangguan(GB 3) and Pianli(LI 6) for pain on the upper jaw; Chengjiang(RN 24), Jiache (ST 6), Xiaguan(ST 7), Yifeng(SJ 17) and Neiting (ST 44) for pain on the lower jaw. Add moxibustion for cold syndrome.

●面王[miàn wáng] 经穴别名。出《针灸甲乙经》。即素髎。详见该条。

Mianwang Another name for Suliao (DU 25), a meridian point, originally from *Zhenjiu Jia-Yi Jing* (*A-B Classic of Acupuncture and Moxibustion*). →素髎(p. 416)

●面岩[miàn yán] 经外穴名。出《刺疗捷法》。在面部，当鼻翼凸出处平行两侧，上对眶下缘外1/4与内3/4交界处。〈主治〉头面疗疮。直刺0.2—0.3寸。

Mianyan(EX-HN) An extra point, originally from *Ciding Jiefa* (*Simple Acupuncture Method for Boils*). 〈Location〉on the face, level with both sides of the protruding point of the wing of nose; superiorly at the junction of lateral one-fourth of the infraobital margin and medial three-fourths of the infraorbital margin. 〈Indication〉furuncle on the head and face. 〈Method〉Puncture perpendicularly 0.2~0.3 cun.

●面玉[miàn yù] 经穴别名。见《外台秘要》。即素髎。详见该条。

Mianyu Another name for Suliao (DU 25), a meridian point seen in *Waitai Miyao* (*Clandestine Essentials from the Imperial Library*). →素髎(p. 416)

●面针[miàn zhēn] 针刺方法之一。指针刺面部范围内的一些特定穴位，以治疗疾病和针刺麻醉的方法。其穴以《灵枢·五色》面部的视诊部位为主要依据。

Face Acupuncture One of the needling therapies, referring to the method of needling some specific acupoints on the face for therapeutic purposes and acupuncture anesthesia. Selection of these points are mainly based on the visible regions on the face mentioned in *Lingshu*: *Wu Se* (*Miraculous Pivot*: *Five Colors*).

●面正[miàn zhèng] 经穴别名。见《铜人腧穴针灸图经》。即素髎。详见该条。

Mianzheng Another name for Suliao (DU 25), a meridian point seen in *Tongren Shuxue*

Zhenjiu Tujing (*Illustrated Manual of Points for Acupuncture and Moxibustion on a Bronze Statue with Acupoints*). →素髎(p. 416)

●眇[miǎo] 部位名。指腰侧，当胁肋与髂嵴之间的空软处。

Abdomen below Hypochondrium A part of the body, referring to the area of the soft tissues between the hypochondriac region and iliac crest.

●名家灸选[míng jiā jiǔ xuǎn] 书名。日本和气惟亨编著，浅井索皋校阅，平井庸信补正。内容汇集经验灸法。成书于1805年（日文化乙丑年），后又作《续编》及《三篇》。对提倡灸法和记载奇穴影响较大。

Mingjia Jiuxuan (*Moxibustion Collection by Famous Experts*) A book, compiled by a Japanese Waik Kore, proofread by Asai Sakusa, supplemented and revised by Hirai Yoshin, a collection of effective moxibustion method. It was first published in 1805 (Japan Bonka, the year of Yichou), Later, *Xubian* (*Continuation*), and *San Pian* (*Three Chapters*) were written, which had a great impact on abvocating moxibustion method and recording the extra acupoints.

●明光[míng guāng] 经穴别名。出《针灸甲乙经》。即攒竹，详见该条。

Mingguang Another name for Cuanzhu(BL 2), a meridian point originally from *Zhenjiu Jia-Yi Jing* (*A-B Classic of Acupuncture and Moxibustion*). →攒竹(p. 58)

●明灸[míng jiǔ] 为直接灸之别称。见该条。

Visible Moxibustion Another name for direct moxibustion. →直接灸(p. 602)

●明堂[míng táng] ①经穴别名。见《太平圣惠方》。即上星。见该条。②古代帝王宣政之堂。③部位名，指鼻部，也指鼻尖。④指针灸经穴图书及经穴模型。

1. Mingtang Another name for Shangxing (DU 23), a meridian point seen in *Taiping Shenghui Fang* (*Imperial Benevolent Prescriptions*). →上星(p. 354)

2. Bright Hall A hall for emperors declaring regime in ancient times.

3. Obvious Part A part of the body, referring to the nose, also to the apex of nose.

4. Acupuncture Diagram and Model Referring to the diagram of meridians and acupoints and the model with acupoints.

●明堂经[míng táng jīng] 书名。宋代王惟一撰。三卷。已佚。见《宋史·艺文志》。

Mingtang Jing (*Mingtang Classic*) A book, written by Wang Weiyi in the Song Dynasty in 3 volumes, which has been lost. See *Song Shi: Yi Wen Zhi* (*The History of the Song Dynasty: Records of Art and Literature*).

●明堂经络图册[míng táng jīng luò tú cè] 图书名。清画家黄谷据《明堂经脉图》彩绘而成。包括仰人、俯人、及十四经穴图，共十六幅。现存中国历史博物馆。

Mingtang Jingluo Tuce (*Illustrated Manual of Meridians and Collaterals of Mingtang*) An illustrated book drawn in color by Huang Gu, a painter of the Qing Dynasty, based on *Mingtang Jingluo Tu* (*Illustration of Meridian of Mingtang*), in which, looking up figures, looking down figures and diagrams of the Fourteen Meridians were included, 16 paintings in all. Today, it is housed in the Museum of Chinese History.

●明堂经图[míng táng jīng tú] 书名。唐孙思邈撰。图佚。见《千金翼方》。参见"秦承祖"条。

Mingtang Jingtu (*Mingtang Classic with Illustration*) A book, written by Sun Simiao in the Tang Dynasty. The illustrations have been lost. Seen in *Qianjin Yifang* (*A Supplement to Essential Prescriptions Worth a Thousand Gold*). →秦承祖(p. 319)

●明堂孔穴[míng táng kǒng xué] 书名。撰人不详。有一卷本、五卷本两种，均佚。见《隋书·经籍志》。

Mingtang Kongxue (*An Acupoint Atlas*) A book with its author unknown. There are two editions: one in 1 volume and the other in 5 volumes, both of which have been lost. Cf. *Suishu: Jingjizhi* (*The History of the Sui Dynasty: Records of Classics and Books*).

●明堂孔穴图[míng táng kǒng xué tú] 书名。撰人不详。三卷。已佚。见《隋书·经籍志》。

Mingtang Kongxue Tu (*An Atlas of Points for Acupuncture and Moxibustion*) A book in 3 volumes with its author unknown, nonextant. Cf. *Suishu: Jing Ji Zhi* (*The History of the Sui Dynasty: Records of Classics and*

Books.)

●明堂孔穴针灸治要[míng táng kǒng xué zhēn jiǔ zhì yào] 书名。①撰人不详。原书已佚。《针灸甲乙经》中保留其内容。见《针灸甲乙经·序》。②近代孙鼎宜重辑。两卷。1909年成书。其据《针灸甲乙经》原文,除去引自《针经》和《素问》的部分编写而成。卷一述各腧穴的位置;卷二述各病证的主治。此书后编入《孙氏医学丛书》中。

Mingtang Kongxue Zhenjiu Zhiyao (Mingtang Points and Essentials of Acupuncture and Moxibustion Treatment) ① A book with its author unknown. The original book has been lost and the contents are kept in *Zhenjiu Jiayi Jing (A-B Classic of Acupuncture and Moxibustion)*, Cf. *Zhenjiu Jia-yi Jing: Xu (A-B Classic of Acupuncture and Moxibustion: Preface)*. ② A book in 2 volumes, which was recompiled by Sun Dingyi in modern times and completed in 1909, on the basis of the original of *Zhenjiu Jia-yi Jing (A-B Classic of Acupuncture and Moxibustion)* with the exclusion of quotations from *Zhenjing (The Canon of Acupuncture)* and *Su Wen (Plain Questions)* Vol. 1 elaborates the locations of each acupoint, while Vol. 2 expounds the indications of various syndromes. This book is included in *Sunshi Yixue Congshu (Sun's Medical Series)*.

●明堂人形图[míng táng rén xíng tú] 图书名,唐代甄权撰。一卷,已佚。见《新唐书·艺文志》。

Mingtang Renxing Tu (Chart of Acupoints as Shown on a Human Figure) A one-volume book written by Zhen Quan in the Tang Dynasty. It has been lost. Seen in *Xin Tang Shu: Yi Wen Zhi (New History of the Tang Dynasty: Records of Art and Literature)*.

●明堂图[míng táng tú] 古代人体针灸经穴图的通称,唐以前有多种流传,均佚。现存较早的为元代滑寿撰、明代吴崑校、清代魏玉麟重刻的木板刻印挂图,共四幅。

Ming Tang Tu (Mingtang Charts of Acupoints) A general term for the diagrams of acupoints on a human body in ancient times. There were many diagrams spread widely before the Tang Dynasty, but all of them have been lost. The extant ones are the earlier plank cut hanging chart, which were compiled by Hua Shou in the Yuan Dynasty, rectified by Wu Kun in the Ming Dynasty and cut again by Wei Yulin in the Qing Dynasty, 4 paintings in all.

●明堂玄真经诀[míng táng xuán zhēn jīng jué] 书名。撰人不详。一卷,已佚,见《宋史·艺文志》。

Mingtang Xuanzhen Jingjue (Mingtang Miraculous and Quitessential Classic in Verse) A one-volume book with its author unknown. It has been lost. Seen in *Song Shi: Yi Wen Zhi (The History of the Song Dynasty: Records of Art and Literature)*.

●明堂针灸图[míng táng zhēn jiǔ tú] 书名。又称《黄帝明堂针灸图》。撰人不详。三卷。已佚。见宋代《郡斋读书后志》。

Mingtang Zhenjiu Tu (Charts for Acupuncture and Moxibustion) A book in 3 volumes with its author unknown, also known as *Huangdi Mingtang Zhenjiu Tu (The Yellow Emperor's Charts for Acupuncture and Moxibustion)*. It has been lost. Seen in *Junzhai Dushu Houzhi (Records After Reading in the County Study)* in the Song Dynasty.

●命关[mìng guān] ①经外穴名。出《扁鹊心书》。在乳头直下,平脐上4寸处。灸治腹胀、水肿、小便不通、气喘不卧、呕吐翻胃、休息痢、大便失禁、脾疟、胁痛不止、黄黑疸等。②经穴别名。即食窦。见该条。③小儿按摩、诊断用穴,食指末节的掌侧横纹部。见《针灸大成》卷十。

1. **Mingguan (EX-CA)** An extra point, originally from *Bian Que Xinshu (Bian Que's Medical Experiences)*. 〈Location〉directly below the nipples, 4 cun above the umbilicus. 〈Indications〉abdominal distension, edema, dysuria, dyspnea with failure of lying on bed, vomiting and nausea, chronic dysentery with frequent relapse, incontinence of stool, malaris due to spleen deficiency, continuous pain in the hypochondrium, yellowish and darkish cellulitis, etc. 〈Method〉moxibustion.

2. **Mingguan** Another name for the meridian point Shidou. →食窦(p. 386)

3. **Life Pass** The point used for the infantile massage and diagnosis, referring to the transverse crease on the palmar side of the distal

segment of the index finger. Seen in Vol. 10 of *Zhenjiu Dacheng* (*A Great Compendium of Acupuncture and Moxibustion*).

●命门[mìng mén]　①经穴名。出《针灸甲乙经》。属督脉。又名属累、精宫。〈定位〉在腰部，当正中线上，第二腰椎棘突下凹陷中（图12和图7）。〈层次解剖〉针刺经过的层次结构同腰阳关穴。浅层主要布有第二腰神经后支的内侧支和伴行的动、静脉。深层有棘突间的椎外（后）静脉丛。第二腰神经后支的和第二腰动、静脉背侧支的分支或属支。〈主治〉虚损腰痛、脊强反折、遗尿、尿频、泄泻、遗精、白浊、阳萎、早泄、赤白带下、胎屡坠、五带七伤、头晕耳鸣、癫痫、惊恐、手足逆冷。直刺0.5～1寸；可灸。②经穴别名。出《针灸甲乙经》。即石门。见该条。③部位名，指目部。见《灵枢·卫气》。④原气所系的部位。见《难经·三十六难》。

1. **Mingmen** (DU 4)　A meridian point, originally from *Zhenjiu Jia-Yi Jing* (*A-B Classic of Acupuncture and Moxibustion*), a point on the Du Meridian, also known as Shulei and Jinggong. 〈Location〉on the low back and on the posterior midline, in the depression below the spinous process of the 2nd lumbar vertebra (Figs. 12 &.7). 〈Regional anatomy〉The layer structures of the needle insertion are the same as those in Yaoyangguan(DU 3). In the superficial layer, there are the medial branches of the posterior branches of the 2nd lumbar nerve and the accompanying artery and vein. In the deep layer, there are the external (posterior) vertebral venous plexus between the adjacent spinous process, the branches of the posterior branches of the 2nd lumbar nerve and the branches or tributaries of the dorsal branches of the 2nd lumbar artery and vein. 〈Indicatons〉waist pain due to overstrain, stiffness of the spine, opistholonus, enuresis, frequent micturition, emission, sloudyurine, impotence, premature ejaculation, leukorrhea with reddish discharge, repeated abortion, five kinds of strain and seven kinds of impariments, dizziness and tinnitus, epilepsy, terror, cold limbs. 〈Method〉Puncture perpendicularly 0.5～1.0 cun. Moxibustion is applicable.

2. **Mingmen**　Another name for Shimen (RN 5), a meridian point originally from *Zhenjiu Jia-Yi jing A-B Classic of Acupuncture and Moxibustion*). →石门(p. 385)

3. **Life Door**　A part of the body, referring to the ocular region, seen in *Lingshu*: *Wei Qi* (*Miraculous Pivot*: *Defensive Qi*)

4. **Life Gate**　The part to which the source qi is related, seen in *Nanjing*: *Sanshiliu Nan* (*The Classic of Questions*: *Question* 36)

●缪刺[miù cì]　《内经》刺法名。见《灵枢·终始》。《素问·缪刺论》作了具体论述，认为病邪侵犯络脉，应采用"左取右，右取左"的交叉泻络法，如取四肢井穴出血等。缪，是交错的意思。缪刺是交叉取穴泻络，与巨刺的交叉取穴刺经有不同，临床上如对急性扁桃体炎取对侧商阳、少商等穴刺出血等，均属缪刺法，参见"巨刺"条。

Contralateral prick　A needling technique in *Neijing*(*The Canon of Internal Medicine*), seen in *Lingshu*: *Zhong Shi*(*Miraculous Pivot*: *End and Beginning*). It is clearly stated in *Su Wen*: *Miuci Lun* (*Plain Questions*: *On Contralateral Insertion*). It is thought that in the case of pathogenic factors attacking the collaterals, apply the crossing method of dispersing collaterals by way of "right point selection for disorder in the left and left point selection for disease in the right. For instance, select the Jing (Well) points on the four limbs to cause bleeding, etc. Contralateral means crossing. Contralateral prick means dispersing collaterals by contralateral point selection, which is different from contralteral point selection of opposing needling for puncturing meridian. Clinically, selecting Shangyang (LI 1) and Shaoshang (LU 11) on the opposite side pricking and causing bleeding for treating acute tonsillitis is considered contralateral→巨刺(p. 225)

●膜原[mó yuán]　募原的别名。详见该条。

Pleurodiaphragmatic Field　Another name for pleurodiaphragmatic interspace. →募原(p. 274)

●拇指同身寸[mǔ zhǐ tóng shēn cùn]　同身寸的一种。即以患者拇指的指间关节的宽度作为一寸。

Thumb cun　A form of proportional unit of the body, namely, width of the thumb at the interphalangeal skin crease taken as one cun.

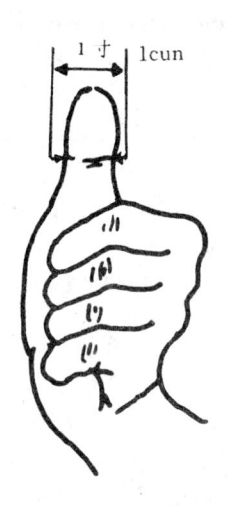

图32 拇指同身寸
Fig 32 Thumb cun

●**跨趾里横纹**[mǔ zhǐ lǐ héng wén] 经外穴名。见《肘后备急方》。在跨趾掌侧, 趾节横纹中点处。〈主治〉疝气。直刺0.2~0.3寸;可灸。

Muzhilihengwen (EX-LE) An extra point, seen in *Zhouhou Beiji Fang* (*A Handbook of Prescriptions for Emergencies*). 〈Location〉on the plantar side of toe, the midpoint of transverse crease of matatarsophlangeal joint. 〈Indication〉hernia. 〈Method〉Puncture perpendicularly 0.2~0.3 cun. Moxibustion is applicable.

●**木香饼**[mù xiāng bǐng] 灸用药饼之一。出《外科证治全书》。取木香末15克, 生地黄30克捣膏, 上两味和匀, 制成饼状, 厚约0.6厘米。可用于间接灸法, 治疗扑损闪挫、气血瘀滞等症。

Mu Xiang (Radix Aucklandiao) Cake A kind of moxibustion cakes used in moxibustion, originally from *Waike Zhengzhi Quanshu* (*A Complete Book of Diagnosis and Treatment of External Diseases*). 〈Method〉Take 15 grams of *Mu Xiang* (*Radix Aucklandiae*) powder and 30 grams of fresh *Di Huang* (*Radix Rehmannias*) smashed like a paste. Mix the two medicines and make them into a cake, about 0.6cm thick. It can be used in indirect moxibustion to treat traumatic injury and sprain, blood stasis and stagnation of qi, etc.

●**目胞**[mù bāo] 部位名, 一名目窠, 一名裹, 俗称眼胞, 现称眼睑, 上面称上眼胞(上眼睑), 下面称下眼胞(下眼睑)。

Palpebral Cyst A part of the body, also known as eye socket, or socket, commonly called as eye cyst, or eyelid cyst at present. The upper part is called upper eye cyst and the lower part lower eye cyst.

●**目本**[mù běn] 部位名。指眼后部。见《灵枢·寒热病》。目本之后脑相连的组织则称目系或眼系, 参见"目系"条。

Eye Source A part of the body, referring to the posterior aspect of the eye, seen in *Ling Shu: Han Re Bing* (*Miraculous Pivot: Cold and Heat Diseases*), the tissue on the posterior aspect of the eye connecting the brain is called ocular connectors or eye system. →目系(p.273)

●**目赤肿痛**[mù chì zhǒng tòng] 病证名。见《世医得效方》。又称风热眼, 风火眼, 天行赤热, 天行赤眼。俗称红眼, 火眼。多因外感风热之邪, 致经气阻滞, 火郁不宣;或因肝胆火盛, 循经上扰, 以致经脉闭阻, 血壅气滞而成, 症见目睛红赤、畏光、流泪、目涩难开, 初起时仅一目, 渐及两侧, 如兼头痛、发热、恶风、脉浮数等为外感风热;如兼有口苦、烦热、舌边尖红、脉弦数等症, 为肝胆火盛。治宜清泄风热, 消肿定痛。取合谷、太冲、睛明、太阳;外感风热者, 加少商、上星;肝胆火盛者, 加行间、侠溪。

Redness, Swelling and Pain of the Eye A disease, seen in *Shiyi Dexiaofang* (*Effective Prescriptions Handed Down for Generations*), also known as eye disease due to wind-heat pathogen, wind-fire eye, epidemic red eye, epidemic red-hot eye, and commonly referred to as red eye or fire eye. Mostly caused by the affection of exopathic wind-heat leading to the stagnation of meridian qi and failure to expel stagnant fire; or by excessive fire in the liver and gallbladder, disturbing the upper along the meridians, leading to the blockage of the meridians and blood stasis and the stagnation of qi. 〈Manifestations〉redness of the eyes, aversion to light, lacrimation, dryness and discomfort feeling of the eyes which are difficult to open, one eye is affected on the onset, and

gradually both eyes. If accmpanied by headache, fever, aversion to wind, superficial and rapid pulse, the case is caused by the affection of the exopathic wind-heat; if accompanied by bitter taste, irritability and fever, redness on the tip and margin of the tongue, wiry and rapid pulse, the case is caused by excessive fire in the liver and gallbladder. 〈Treatment Principle〉Clear wind-heat, relieve swelling and pain. 〈Point selection〉Hegu (LI 4), Taichong (LR 3), Jingming (BL 1), Taiyang(EX-HN 5); add Shaoshang(LU 11) and Shangxing(DU 23) for cases due to affection by exopathic wind-heat; add Xingjian (LR 2), Xiaxi(GB 43) for cases due to excessive fire in the liver and gallbladder.

●目窗[mù chuāng] 经穴名。出《针灸甲乙经》。属足少阳胆经，为少阳、阳维之会。又名至荣、至营、至宫。〈定位〉在头部，当前发际上1.5寸，头正中线旁开2.25寸（图28）。〈层次解剖〉皮肤→皮下组织→帽状腱膜→腱膜下疏松结缔组织。布有眶上神经和颞浅动、静脉的额支。〈主治〉头痛、目眩、目赤肿痛、远视、近视、面浮肿、上齿龋肿、小儿惊痫。平刺0.5～0.8寸；可灸。

Muchuang(GB 16) A meridian point, originally from *Zhenjiu Jia-Yi Jing* (*A-B Classic of Acupuncture and Moxibustion*), a point on the Gallbladder Meridian of Foot-Shaoyang, the Crossing poins of Foot-Shaoyang and Yangwei Meridians, also known Zhirong, Zhiying, or Zhigong. 〈Location〉on the head, 1.5 cun above anterior hairline and 2.25 cun lateral to the midline of the head (Fig. 28). 〈Regional anatomy〉skin→subcutaneous tissue→galea aponeurosis→loose connective below aponeurosis. There are the supraorbital nerve and the frontal branches of the superficial temporal artery and vein in this area. 〈Indications〉headache, vertigo, conjunctival congestion with swelling and pain, myopia and hyperopia, edema of face, swelling of the superior gum, infantile convulsion. 〈Method〉Puncture subcutaneously 05～0.8 cun. Moxibustion is applicable.

●目2[mù er] 耳穴名。位于屏间切迹后下方，用于治疗屈光不正、外眼炎症、假性近视。

Eye 2 (MA) An ear point, its location is in the posterior and interior aspect of the intertragic notch. 〈Indications〉ametropia, infection of outer canthus, and pseudomyopia.

●目纲[mù gāng] 部位名。指上下眼睑部。分称目上纲、目下纲。

Eye Outline A part of the body, referring to the regions of the upper and lower eyelids. It is divided into the upper eye outline and the lower eye outline.

●目窌[mù jiào] 经穴别名，见《外台秘要》。即丝竹空，详见该条。

Mujiao Another name for Sizhukong (SJ 23), a meridian point seen in *Waitai Miyao* (*Clandestine Essentials from the Imperial Library*). →丝竹空(p. 412)

●目临泣[mù lín qì] 经穴别名。见《圣济总录》。即头临泣，详见该条。

Mulinqi Another name for Toulinqi (GB 15), a meridian point seen in *Shengji Zonglu* (*Imperial Medical Encyclopedia*). →头临泣 (p. 444)

●目内眦[mù nèi zì] ①人体部位名。出《灵枢·经脉》。指内眼角，足太阳膀胱之脉，起于目内眦。②经穴别名。即睛明，见该条。

1. Inner Canthus A part of the body, originally from *Lingshu: Jingmai* (*Miraculous Pivot: Meridians*), referring to the medial corner of the eye, the start of the Bladder Meridian of Foot-Taiyang.

2. Muneizi Another name for the meridian point, Jingming→睛明(p. 217)

●目锐眦[mù ruì zì] 部位名。指外眼角。见《灵枢》。又称目外眦，见《医宗金鉴·刺灸心法要诀》。

Lateral Canthus A part of the body, referring to the lateral corner of the eye, seen in *Lingshu* (*Miraculous Pivot*), also known as outer canthus. Seen in *Yizong Jinjian: Cijiu Xinfa Yaojue* (*Golden Mirror of Orthodox Medical Lineage Essentials of Acupuncture and Moxibustion in verse*).

●目上纲[mù shàng gāng] 人体部位名。出《灵枢·经筋》，指上眼睑，又称目上网。纲、网维、约束之意。足太阳膀胱经起于目内眦，其分支的经筋布于上睑，具有司睑开阖的作用。

Upper Eye Outline A part of the body, originally from *Lingshu: Jingjin (Miraculous Pivot: Muscles)*, referring to the upper eyelid, also known as the upper eye net. "Outline" here means netting and restraint. The Bladder Meridian of Foot-Taiyang starts from the inner canthus, its branches are distributed on the upper eyelid, with the function of attending to the open and closure of the eyelid.

●目上网[mù shàng wǎng] 目上纲的别名。见该条。

Upper Eye Net Another name for upper eye outline. →目上纲(p. 272)

●目外眦[mù wài zì] 部位名。指外眼角，参见"目锐眦"条。

Outer Canthus A part of the body, referring to the lateral corner of the eye. →目锐眦(p. 272)

●目外维[mù wài wéi] 部位名。指眼球外侧的联系组织。见《灵枢·经筋》。

Outer Net of the Eye A part of the body, referring to the tissue connected with the lateral side of the eyeball, seen in *Lingshu: Jingjin (Miraculous Pivot: Muscles)*.

●目系[mù xì] 部位名。又称眼系。指眼后与脑相连接的组织。见《灵枢·大惑论》。

Ocular Connectors A part of the body, also known as eye system, referring to the tissue connecting the posterior aspect of the eye with the brain, seen in *Lingshu: Dahuo Lun (Mirculous Pivot: On the Great Puzzlement)*.

●目1[mù yī] 耳穴名。位于屏间切迹前下方，用于治疗青光眼、假性近视。

Eye 1 (MA) An ear point. ⟨Location⟩ on the anterior and posterior side of the intertragic notch. ⟨Indications⟩ glaucoma and pseudomyopia.

●目翳[mù yì] 病证名。见《经验眼科秘书》，是指患黑睛星翳后，遗留大小不等，形状不一的瘢痕而言。本症因瘢痕大小、厚薄形态、色泽不同而又称垂帘障、花翳白陷、凝脂翳、黄液上冲、混睛障、冰瑕翳等，多由毒邪外侵、肝胆火炽、风热壅盛，蒸灼肝胆之络，上攻于黑睛所致；或平素过食辛辣炙煿，热积脾胃，以致三焦之火上燔，毒邪交合，黄仁被灼，脓液内聚而为病，亦有因外伤直接穿破黑睛而发生本证。临床多分两型。风热者，症见眼睛水肿，头痛，眉棱骨痛，畏光羞明，流泪多眵，鼻塞流涕，翳障点状或散或聚，苔薄黄脉浮数，治宜疏风清热明目，取攒竹、睛明、瞳子髎、风池、足临泣。肝肾阴虚者，症见眼睛微红，眼睑无力，常欲垂闭，不得久视，星翳灰白或散或聚，舌红脉细。治宜滋阴明目，取攒竹、睛明、瞳子髎、肝俞、肾俞、大小骨空。

Blurred Vision A disease, seen in *Jingyan Yanke Mishu (Secrets on Experiences in Ophthalmology)*, referring to the vestigal scars in different size and shape left over after pancorned opacity. According to different thickness, shape and color, it is also named fat deposition opacity, hypopyon, interstitial keratitis, thin nedbula causing little visual defect. It is mostly caused by infection of pathogenic factors, flaring-up of fire in the liver and gallbladder, and excessive wind-heat steaming and burning the collaterals of the liver and gallbladder, and then attacking the black of eyes; or by over-eating pungent steamed and baked food, with an accumulation of heat in the spleen and stomach leading to flaring-up of the Sanjiao fire, causing tonins and pathogens to alternately attack and burn the brown cataract, resulting in the inner accumulation of pus. It may be caused by direct penetration of the black of the eye resulting from traumatic injury. Clinically it is generally divided into two types, one due to wind-heat, manifested as edema of the eyes, headache, pain in the supraorbital bone, aversion to light, lacrimation, much eye secretion, nasal obstruction with running nose, spotted nebula either spreading or gathering, thin and yellowish tongue coating, superficial and rapid pulse. ⟨Treatment principle⟩ Dispel wind and clear heat to improve acuity of vision. ⟨Point selection⟩ Cuanzhu (BL 2), Jingming (BL 1), Tongziliao (GB 1), Fengchi (GB 20), Zulinqi (GB 41). The other is due to yin deficiency of the liver and kindney, manifested as slight redness of the eyes, weakness of the eyelid, frequent longing for shutting, difficulty in long time looking, nebula in greyish white spreading or gathering, red tongue and

表10
Table 10

十 二 募 穴 表
Twelve Front-Mu Points

Both Sides 两 侧		Middle 正 中	
脏 腑 Zang or Fu Organ	募 穴 Front-Mu Point	脏 腑 Zang or Fu Organ	募 穴 Front-Mu Point
肺 Lung	中府 Zhongfu(LU 1)	心包 Pericardium	膻中 Danzhong(RN 17)
肝 Liver	期门 Qimen(LR 14)	心 Heart	巨阙 Jüque(RN 14)
胆 Gallbladder	日月 Riyue(GB 24)	胃 Stomach	中脘 Zhongwan(RN 12)
脾 Spleen	章门 Zhangmen(LR 13)	三焦 Sanjiao	石门 Shimen(RN 5)
肾 Kidney	京门 Jingmen(GB 25)	小肠 Small Intestine	关元 Guanyuan(RN 4)
大肠 Large Intestine	天枢 Tianshu(ST 25)	膀胱 Urinary Bladder	中极 Zhongji(RN 3)

thready pulse. 〈Treatment principle〉 Nourish yin to improve acuity of vision. 〈Point selection〉 Cuanzhu (BL 2), Jingming (BL 1), Tongziliao (GB 1), Ganshu (BL 18), Shenshu (BL 23), Dagukong (EX-UE 5) and Xiaogukong (EX-UE 6).

●募腧经[mù shū jīng] 书名，吴吕广撰，已佚。见《针灸甲乙经注》。

Mu Shu Jing (*Classic of Front-Mu and Back-Shu Points*) A book, written by Lü Guang of the Wu Kingdom, no longer extant, seen in *Zhenjiu Jia-Yi Jing Zhu* (*Notes to A-B Classic of Acupuncture and Moxibustion*).

●募穴[mù xué] 经穴分类名。出《素问·奇病论》。指脏腑经气结聚于胸腹部的腧穴。五脏六腑共有十二募穴。脏腑有病时，也可在相关募穴处出现压痛或敏感等异常反应，并可作为诊断和治疗用穴。见表10。

Front-Mu Points A term in the classification of acupoints, originally from *Su Wen: Qibing Lun* (*Plain Questions: On Peculiar Diseases*), referring to the points on the chest and abdomen where the meridian qi of the respective zang-fu organs is infused. There are twelve front-mu points closely related to the zang-fu organs. When a zang or a fu organ is affected, abnormal reactions such as tenderness or sensation may occur in the corresponding front-mu point. These points can be used in diagnosis and treatment. See Table 10.

●募原[mù yuán] 主要指膏（膈）之原、肓之原。出《灵枢·百病始生》。概指病邪蕴结之处。《素问·举痛论》称膜原，王冰注谓：膜，是膈间之膜，即膈膜；原，是指膈（膏）之原鸠尾穴，肓之原气海穴。而《类经》卷十三张介宾注谓：皮里膜外，乃隐藏曲折之所，气血不易流通。如邪气留着于此，则逐渐长大而成积病。如疟痞之类。

Pleurodiaphragmatic Interspace Mainly referring to the origin of diaphragm cardia, originally from *Ling Shu: Baibing Shisheng* (*Miraculous Pivot: Occurrence of Diseases*), generally referring to where the pathogenic factors accumulate. It was named pleurodiaphragmatic interspace in *Su Wen: Jutong Lun* (*Plain Questions: On Acute Pains*). According to Wang Bing's annotation, pleurodiaphragmatic means the memorane of the interdiaphragm, i, e. diaphragmatic, interspace means the origin of diaphragm, Jiuwei (RN 15) and the origin of cardia, Qihai (RN 6). In Zhang Jiebin's annotation in Vol. 13 of *Leijing*

(*Classified Canon*) the interior of the skin and exterior of the diaphragmatic are the hidden and tortuous places where qi and blood are not easy to pass. If the pathogenic factors conceal here, they will develop gradually and lead to the occurence of mass, for instance, malarial mass.

N

●纳干法[nà gān fǎ] 子午流注针法之一。指十二经配合十天干,而天干以甲为首,故又称纳甲法。具体中按日子所属天干开取某经五输穴。见《针灸大全·十二经纳天干歌》:"甲胆乙肝丙小肠,丁心戊胃己脾乡,庚属大肠辛属肺,壬属膀胱癸肾藏,三焦亦向壬中寄,包络同归入癸方"。

Stem-Prescription of Acupoints One of the needling methods of midnight-noon ebb-flow, referring to the Twelve Regular Meridians in combination with the Ten Heavenly Stems. Jia is the first one of the Ten Heavenly Stems, so it is also known as Day-Prescription of Acupoints. In practice, it is to select five-shu points on a certain meridian in accordance with one of the Ten Heavenly Stems in which a day belongs. Seen in *Zhenjiu Daquan*: *Shier Jing Na Tiangan Ge* (*A Complete Work of Acupuncture and Moxibustion*; *Song of the Twelve Regular Meridians Matching the Ten Heavenly Stems*). It reads: Jia gallbladder, Yi liver, Bing small intestine; Ding heart, Wu stomach and Ji spleen position; Geng relating to large intestine and Xin to lung; Ren relating to urinary bladder and Gui kidney staying, Sanjiao also relating to Ren and staying in and peridium also relating to the prescription of Gui.

●纳甲法[nà jiǎ fǎ] 即纳干法。见该条。

Day-Prescription of Acupoints →纳干法(p. 275)

●纳气法[nà qì fǎ] 针刺手法名。见《针灸大全》。又称中气法。纳,指按纳。其法与抽添法类似。先用紧按慢提九数或紧提慢按六数。得气后,将针头斜对病痛处,使气上行,随后将针直起,向下按纳,不使气回流。用于行气、除积。

Qi-Receiving Method A needling technque, seen in *Zhenjiu Daquan*(*A Complete Work of Acupuncture and Moxibustion*), also known as qi-intaking. "纳" means thrusting the needle and accepting qi. This method is similiar to the qi-flowing method of lifting-thrusting the needle. At first, do nine quick thrust and slow lift, or six slow thrust and quick lift, After the needling reaction has been obtained, make the tip of the needle slant to the diseased area, and promote qi to flow upwards, then, straighten the needle and thrust it downwards, so as not to make qi flow back. It is used to promote the flow of qi and remove masses.

●纳支法[nà zhī fǎ] 子午流注针法之一。指十二经配合十二地支,又称纳子法。因地支以子为首,故名。十二经脉按流注顺序挨配十二时辰,当其时针刺其母穴为补,过其时针刺子穴为泻。参见子母补泻法条。

Branch-Prescription of Acupuncture One of the needling methods of midnight-noon ebb-flow, referring to the Twelve Regular Meridians in combination with the Twelve Earthly Branches, also known as hour prescription of acupoints. It is so named because the Twelve Earthly Branches starts with zi, the initial two-hour period. The Twelve Regular Meridians match the hours in a day in the order of their circulations; puncturing the mother point at the exact time is reinforcing, whereas puncturing the son point after to the exact time is reducing. →子母补泻法(p. 625)

●纳子法[nà zǐ fǎ] 即纳支法。见该条。

Hour-Prescription of Acupoints Branch-

prescription of acupoints. →纳支法(p. 275)

●奶积[nǎi jī] 即乳癣。详见该条。

Mass in Breast Wodules in the breast. →乳癣(p. 338)

●奶脾[nǎi pí] 即乳癣。详见该条。

Lump in Breast Wodules in the breast. →乳癣(p. 338)

●奶癣[nǎi xuǎn] 病证名。见《外科正宗》。又名胎癣、乳癣。多为体质过敏,风湿热蕴阻肌肤而成。多发于婴幼儿头,面部。有时可延及其它部位。详见"湿疹"条。

Infantile Eczema A disease, seen in *Waike Zhengzong* (*Orthodox Manual of External Diseases*), also named fetal eczema and eczema in new born. Mostly caused by alergic constitution, accumulation of wind, dampness and heat in muscles and skin, commonly occurring on the head and face of the baby, sometimes extending to other parts of the body. →湿疹(p. 373)

●男阴缝[nán yīn fèng] 经外穴名。见《千金翼方》。在阴茎根部与阴囊相交处正中灸治黄疸、阴卵偏坠等。

Nanyinfeng(EX-CA) An extra point, seen in *Qianjin Yifang* (*A Supplement to Essential Prescriptions Worth a Thousand Gold*). 〈Location〉right in the centre of the juncture of the root of the penis and the scrotum. 〈Indications〉jaundice, orchidoptosis, etc. 〈Method〉moxibustion.

●难产[nán chǎn] 滞产的别名。详见该条。

Difficult Labor Another name for protracted labor. →滞产(p. 607)

●囊底[náng dǐ] 经外穴名。见《太平圣惠方》。在男性阴囊后十字纹中,灸治肾脏风疮、小肠疝气、偏坠、阴囊湿疹、睾丸炎等。

Nangdi(EX-CA) An extra point, seen in *Taiping Shenghui Fang* (*Imperial Benevolent Prescriptions*). 〈Location〉on the midpoint of the posterior crossed crease of the scrotum in male. 〈Indications〉crotal abcess, hernia, orchidoptosis, scrotal eczema, testitis, etc. 〈Method〉moxibustion.

●囊耳[náng ěr] 即聤耳。详见该条。

Ear Cyst Otitis media suppurativa. →聤耳(p. 439)

●囊下缝[náng xià fèng] 经外穴别名。即阴囊缝。详见该条。

Nangxiafeng Another name for the extra point Yingnangfeng(EX-CA). →阴囊缝(p. 557)

●脑崩[nǎo bēng] 即鼻渊之重症,详见该条。

Brain Collapse A serious case of rhinorrhea with turbid discharge. →鼻渊(p. 19)

●脑点[nǎo diǎn] 为缘中之别称。详见该条。

Brain Point(MA) Another name for Central Rim(MA). →缘中(p. 577)

●脑盖[nǎo gài] 经穴别名。出《针灸甲乙经》。即络却。详见该条。

Naogai Another name for Luoque(BL 8), a meridian point originally from *Zhenjiu jia-Yi Jing* (*A-B Classic of Acupuncture and Moxibustion*). →络却(p. 259)

●脑寒[nǎo hán] 即鼻渊之重症,详见该条。

Brain Coldness A serious case of Rhinorrhea with turbid discharge. →鼻渊(p. 19)

●脑户[nǎo hù] 经穴名。出《素问·刺禁论》。属督脉,为督脉、足太阳之会。又名匝会、会额、合颅。〈定位〉在头部,后发际正中直上2.5寸,风府上1.5寸,枕外隆凸陷中(图28和图31)。〈层次解剖〉皮肤→皮下组织→左、右枕额肌枕腹之间→腱膜下疏松组织。布有枕大神经的分支和枕动、静脉的分支或属支。〈主治〉头重、头痛、面赤、目黄、眩晕、面瘤、音哑、项强、癫狂痫证、舌本出血、瘿瘤。平刺0.5～0.8寸;可灸。

Naohu(DU 17) A meridian point, originally from *Su Wen*: *Cijin Lun* (*Plain Questions*: *On Contraindications in Acupuncture*). A point on the Du Meridian, the crossing point of the Du Meridian and Foot-Taiyang, also known as Zahui, Huie, Helu. 〈Location〉on the head, 2.5 cun directly above the midpoint of the posterior hairline, 1.5 cun above Fengfu(DU 16), in the depression on the upper border of the external occipital protuberance (Figs. 28&31). 〈Regional anatomy〉skin→subcutaneous tissue →between occipital belly of left and right occipitofrontal muscles → subaponeurotic loose tissue. There are the branches of the greater occipital nerve and the branches or tributaries of the occipital artery and vein in this area.

●脑空[nǎo kōng] 经穴名。出《针灸甲乙经》。属足少阳胆经,为足少阳、阳维之会。又名颞颥。〈定位〉在头部,当枕外隆凸的上缘外侧,头正中线旁开二寸二分五,平脑户(图28和图31)。〈层次解剖〉皮肤→皮下组织→枕额肌枕腹。布有枕大神经、枕动、静脉、面神经耳后支。〈主治〉头痛、颈项强痛、目眩、目赤肿痛、鼻痛、耳聋、癫痫、惊悸、热病。平刺0.5～0.8寸;可灸。

〈Indications〉heaviness of the head, headache, flushed face, yellowish eyes, vertigo, facial tumor, hoarseness of voice, stiffness of the neck, manic-depressive psychosis, epilepsy, bleeding from the root of the tongue, goiter, 〈Method〉 Puncture subcutaneously 0.5～0.8cun. Moxibustion is applicable.

Naokong (GB 19) A meridian point, originally from *Zhenjiu Jia-Yi Jing* (*A-B Classic of Acupuncture and Moxibustion*). A point on the Gallbladder Meridian of Foot-Shaoyang, the crossing point of Foot-Shaoyang and Yangwei Meridians, also named Nieru. 〈Location〉on the head and on the level of the upper border of the external occipital protuberance or Naohu (DU 17), 2.25 cun lateral to the midline of the head (Figs. 28&31). 〈Regionsl anatomy〉skin→subcutaneous tissue→occipital belly of occipitofrontal muscle. There are the greater occipital nerve, the occipital artery and vein, and the posterior auricular branches of the facial nerve in this area. 〈Indications〉 headache, pain and stiffness of the neck and nape, blurred vision, conjuntival congestion with swelling and pain, pain of the nose, deafness, epilepsy, palpitation due to fright, febrile diseases. 〈Method〉 Puncture subcutaneously 0.5～0.8 cun. Moxibustion is applicable.

●脑漏[nǎo lòu] 即鼻渊之重症,详见该条。

Brain Leakage A serious case of rhinorrhea with turbid discharge. →鼻渊(p.19)

●脑渗[nǎo shèn] 即鼻渊之重症,详见该条。

Oozing of Brain A serious case of rhinorrhea with turbid discharge. →鼻渊(p.19)

●臑[nǎo] 部位名。指上臂,主要指肱二头肌部。

Upper Arm A part of the body, i.e. forearm, mainly referring to the biceps muscle of the arm.

●臑会[nǎo huì] 经穴名,出《针灸甲乙经》。属手少阳三焦经,为手少阳、阳维之会。又名臑髎、臑交。〈定位〉在臂外侧,当肘尖与肩髎的连线上,肩髎下3寸,三角肌的后下缘(图48和图44)。〈层次解剖〉皮肤→皮下组织→肱三头肌长头及外侧头→桡神经→肱三头肌内侧头。浅层有臂后皮神经。深层有桡神经,肱深动、静脉。〈主治〉肩臂痛、瘿气、瘰疬、目疾、肩胛肿痛。直刺0.5～1寸;可灸。

Naohui (SJ 13) A meridian point, originally from *Zhenjiu Jia-Yi Jing* (*A-B Classic of Acupuncture and Moxibustion*), a point on the Sanjiao Meridian of Hand-Shaoyang, the crossing point of the Hand-Shaoyang and Yangwei Meridians, also named Naojiao(交), Naojiao(髎). 〈Location〉on the lateral side of the upper arm and on the line connecting the tip of the olecranon and Jianliao (SJ 14), 3 cun below Jianliao (SJ 14), and on the posterioinferior border of the deltoid muscle (Figs. 48&44). 〈Regional anatomy〉skin→subcutaneous tissue→long head and lateral head of brachial triceps muscle. In the superficial layer, there is the posterior brachial cutaneous nerve. In the deep layer, there are the radial nerve and the deep brachial artery and vein. 〈Indications〉pain in the shoulder and arm, goiter, scrofula, eye disorders, swelling and pain in the scapular area. 〈Method〉Puncture perpendicularly 0.5～1 cun. Moxibustion is applicable.

●臑交[nǎo jiāo] 经穴别名。出《针灸聚英》。即臑会。见该条。

Naojiao(臑交) Another name for Naohui (SJ 13), a meridian point originally from *Zhenjiu Juying* (*Essentials of Acupuncture and Moxibustion*). →臑会(p.277)

●臑髎[nǎo jiāo] 经穴别名。出《针灸甲乙经》。即臑会。见该条。

Naojiao (臑髎) Another name for Naohui (SJ 13), a meridian point originally from *Zhenjiu Jia-Yi Jing* (*A-B Classic of Acupuncture and Moxibustion*). →臑会(p.277)

●臑俞[nǎo shū] 经穴名。出《针灸甲乙经》。属手太阳小肠经,为手太阳、阳维、阳跷脉之会。〈定位〉在肩部,当腋后纹头直上,肩胛冈下缘凹陷中(图48和图

65）。〈层次解剖〉皮肤→皮下组织→三角肌→冈下肌。浅层布有锁骨上外侧神经。深层有肩胛上动、静脉的分支或属支，旋肱后动、静脉的分支或属支等。〈主治〉肩臂痛无力、肩肿，颈项瘰疬。直刺0.6～1寸；可灸。不宜向胸侧深刺，以免损伤肺脏。

Naoshu(SI 10)　A meridian point, originally from *Zhenjiu Jia-Yi Jing* (*A-B Classic of Acupuncture and Moxibustion*), a point on the Small Intestine Meridian of Hand-Taiyang, the crossing point of the Hand-Taiyang, Yangwei and Yangqiao Meridians. 〈Location〉on the shoulder, above the posterior and of the axillary fold, in the depression below the lower border of the scapular spine (Figs. 48&65). 〈Regional anatomy〉skin→subcutaneous tissue→deltoid muscle→infraspinous muscle. In the superficial layer, there is the lateral supraclavicular nerve. In the deep layer, there are the branches or tributaries of the suprascapular artery and vein and posterior circumflex humeral artery and vein. 〈Indications〉aching and weakness in the shoulder and arm, swelling in the shoulder, scrofula on the neck and nape. 〈Method〉Puncture perpendicularly 0.6～1.0 cun. Moxibustion is applicalbe. 〈Cautions〉Deep puncture toward the chest is inapplicable, for fear of damaging the lung.

●内鼻[nèi bí]　耳穴名。位于耳屏内侧面的下二分之一处。具有疏利鼻窍作用。主治鼻炎、副鼻窦炎、鼻衄。

Internal Nose(MA)　An ear point. 〈Location〉on the lower half of the medial aspect of the tragus. 〈Function〉Sooth and dredge the nasal cavity. 〈Indications〉rhinitis, nasosinusitis, epistaxis.

●内侧[nèi cè]　部位名。①指上肢的掌心一侧即屈侧。是手三阴经循行于上肢及其所属穴位分布的部位。②指下肢向正中线的一侧是足三阴经循行于下肢及其所属穴位分布的部位。

Medial Side　A part of the body, referring to ①the palmer side of the upper limbs, i.e. the flexion side, the part where the three yin meridians of the hand circulate along the upper limbs and their acupoints are distributed; ②the side near the anterior median line, the part where the three yin meridians of the foot circulate along the lower limbs and their acupoints are distributed.

●内吹乳痈[nèi chuī rǔ yōng]　病证名。见《寿世保元》。吹乳之一种，指妊娠期乳痈，临床较少见。多由怀孕后期胎气旺，热邪郁蒸而成。溃后难收口。治疗中应注意保胎，详见"乳痈"条。

Acute Mastitis due to Fetus　A disease, seen in *Shoushi Baoyuan* (*Longevity and Life Preservation*), a form of acute mastitis during pregnancy. It is not commonly seen clinically. It is mostly due to the excessive qi of the fetus, and steaming by pathogenic heat, difficulty in healing after ulcer. Take caution for the care of fetus in treatment. →乳痈(p. 339)

●内耳[nèi ěr]　耳穴名。位于6区，参见牙条，用于治疗耳鸣、听力减退、耳性眩晕症。

Internal Ear（MA）　An ear point. 〈Location〉on the 6th section of the ear. 〈Indications〉tinnitus, hypoacusis, auditory vertigo. →牙(p. 533)

●内分泌[nèi fēn mì]　耳穴名。位于耳甲腔底部屏间切迹内。用于治疗痛经、阳痿、月经不调、更年期综合症、内分泌功能紊乱，痤疮、间日疟。

Endocrine(MA IC-3)　An ear point. 〈Location〉at the base of the cavum conchae in the intertragic notch. 〈Indications〉dysmenorrhea, impotence, irregular menstruation (menopausal) climacteric syndrome, abnormality of endocrine function, acne, intermittent malaria.

●内关[nèi guān]　经穴名。出《灵枢·经脉》。属于手厥阴心包经，为本经络穴，八脉交会穴之一，通于阴维脉。〈定位〉在前臂掌侧，当曲泽大陵的连线上，腕横纹上2寸，掌长肌腱与桡侧腕屈肌腱之间（图49和图66）。〈层次解剖〉皮肤→皮下组织→桡侧腕屈肌腱与掌长肌腱之间→指浅屈肌→指深屈肌→旋前方肌。浅层布有前臂内侧皮神经，前臂外侧皮神经的分支和前臂正中静脉。深层在指浅屈肌、拇长屈肌和指深屈肌三者之间有正中神经和正中神经伴行动、静脉。在前臂骨间膜的前方有骨间前运、静脉和间前神经。〈主治〉心痛、心悸、胸痛、胃痛、呕吐、呃逆、失眠、癫狂、痫证、郁证、眩晕、中风、偏瘫、哮喘、偏头痛、热病、产后血晕、肘臂挛痛。直刺0.5～1.0寸；可灸。

Neiguan（PC 6）　A meridian point, originallly from *Lingshu*; *Jingmai* (*Miraculous Pivot*;

Meridians). a point on the Pericardium Meridian of Hand-Jueyin, the Luo(Connecting) Point of the meridian, one of the Eight Confluence Points relating to the Yinwei Meridian. 〈Location〉on the palmar side of the forearm and on the line connecting Quze(PC 3) and Daling(PC 7), 2 cun above the crease of the wrist, between the tendons of the long palmar muscle and radial flexor muscle of the wrist(Figs. 49&66). 〈Regional anatomy〉skin →subcutaneous tissue→between tendons of radial flexor muscle of wrist and long palmar muscle→superficial flexor muscle of fingers→ deep flexor muscle of fingers → quadrate pronate muscle. In the superficial layer, there are the branches of the medial and lateral cutaneous nerves and the median vein of the forearm. In the deep layer, there are the median nerve and the accompanying artery and vein in the superficial flexor muscle of the fingers, the long flexor muscle of the thumb and the deep flexor muscle of the fingers. There are the anterior interosseous artery, vein and nerve on the anterior side of the interosseous membrane of the forearm. 〈 Indications 〉 melancholia, apoplexy, hemiplegia, asthma, migraine, febrile diseases, puerperal faintness, convulsive pain of the elbow and arm. 〈Method〉Puncture perpendicularly 0.5～1.0 cun. Moxibustion is applicable.

●内踝[nèi huái] 部位名。指胫骨下端向外突起处。

Medial Malleolus A part of the body, referring to the process below the inferior end of the tibia.

●内踝尖[nèi huái jiān] 经外穴名。见《备急灸法》又名吕细、踝尖。〈定位〉在足内侧面，内踝的凸起处(图33)。灸治转筋、脚气、牙痛等。

Neihuaijian(EX-LE 8) An extra point, seen in *Beiji Jiufa* (*Moxibustion for Emergencies*), also known as Lüxi, Huaijian. 〈Location〉on the medial side of the foot, at the tip of the medial malleolus (Fig. 33). 〈Indicationis〉 spasm, beriberi, toothache, etc. 〈Method〉 moxibustion.

●内踝前下[nèi huái qián xià] 经外穴名。见《针灸集成》。在内踝下缘中点向前一横指处。灸治翻胃吐食。

Neihuaiqianxia(EX-LE) An extra point, seen in *Zhenjiu Jicheng* (*A Collection of Acupuncture and Moxibustion*). 〈Locations〉one-finger width anterior to the midpoint of the inferior border of the medial malleous. 〈 Indications 〉 egurgitation and vomiting. 〈Method〉 moxibustion.

●内筋[nèi jīn] 经穴别名。出《素问·刺腰痛论》。即交信。见该条。

Neijin Another name for Jiaoxin(KI 8), a meridian point originally from *Suwen*:*Ci Yaotong Lun* (*Plain Questions*:*On Treatment of Lumbago*). →交信(p.198)

●内经[nèi jīng] ①书名。《黄帝内经》的简称。参见该条。②指内行于脏腑部分的经脉，与外行于支么的部分(外经)相对而言。

1. **Neijing**(**The Canon of Internal Medicine**)
Title of a book, short for *Huangdi Neijing* (*The Yellow Emperor's Canon of Internal Medicine*). →黄帝内经(p.174)
2. **Internal Meridians** Refers to the meridiand running interiorly to the zang-fu organs, vs. the meridians running exteriorly along the extremities(external meridians).

●内睛明[nèi jīng míng] 经外穴名。见《针灸学简编》。在目内眦之泪阜上。〈主治〉目赤肿痛、视力模糊，以及视神经萎缩、视网膜出血、结膜炎等。沿眶内侧臂直刺0.5~1寸。勿捻转提插；禁灸。

Neijingming(EX-HN) An extra point, seen in *Zhenjiuxue Jianbian* (*A Concise Book of Acupuncture and Moxibustion*). 〈Location〉on the lacrimal caruncle of the inner canthus. 〈 Indications 〉 conjunctival congestion with swelling and pain, blurred vision, optic atrophy, retina; hemorrhage, conjunctivitis, etc. 〈Method〉Puncture perpendicularly in the medial side of the orbit 0.5-1.0 cun , with no twirling, lifting or thrusting of the needle. Moxibustion is forbidden.

●内灸[nèi jiǔ] 灸法术语。出《本草拾遗》。指吞服生蒜的治病法。

Internal Cauterization A term for cauterization, originally from *Bencao Shiyi* (*Supplement to the Herbal Classic*), referring to the therapy of swallowing fresh garlic.

●内昆仑[nèi kūn lún] ①经穴别名。见《普济方》即太溪。见该条。②经外穴别名。即下昆仑。见该条。

Neikunlun Another name for ①Taixi(KI 3), a meridian point seen in Puji Fang (*Prescriptions for Universal Relief*). →太溪(p. 420)②the extra point Xiakunlun (EX-LE). →下昆仑(p. 489)

●内淋[nèi lìn] 即膏淋。详见该条。

Internal Stranguria →膏淋(p. 133)

●内龙眼[nèi lóng yǎn] 经外穴别名。即内膝眼。见该条。

Neilongyan →内膝眼(p. 281)

●内生殖器[nèi shēng zhí qì] 耳穴名。又称子宫、精宫、天癸。位于三角窝内三分之一。具有扶阳益精、调经和血作用。〈主治〉疼痛、月经不调、白带过多,功能性子宫出血、遗精、早泄、前列腺炎等。

Internal Genitalia (MA) An ear point, also known as Uterus (MA), Seminal Palace (MA), Congenital Essence (MA). 〈Location〉 at the medial 1/3 of the triangular fossa. 〈Functions〉Strengthen yang-qi and replenish vital essence, regulate menstruation by adjusting the flow of qi and blood. 〈Indications〉 pain, irregular menstruation, leukorrhegia, hysfunctional uterine bleeding, seminal emission, premature ejaculation, prostatitis, etc.

●内太冲[nèi tài chōng] 经外穴名。见《针灸集成》。在足背,当踇长伸肌腱侧凹陷中,与太冲平,〈主治〉疝气上冲、呼吸不通。直刺0.1寸;可灸。

Neitaichong (EX-LE) An extra point, originally from *Zhenjiu Jicheng* (*A Collection of Acupuncture and Moxibustion*). 〈Location〉on the dorsum of foot, in the deprssion on tibral side of the long extensor muscle of the great toe, paralel with Taichong (LR 3). 〈Indications〉hernia with stagnated qi rising and difficult breathing. 〈Method〉Puncture perpendicularly 0.1 cun. Moxibustion is applicable.

●内庭[nèi tíng] 经穴名。出《灵枢·本输》。属足阳明胃经,为本经荥穴。〈定位〉在足背,当二、三趾间,趾蹼缘后方赤白肉际处(图60)。〈层次解剖〉皮肤→皮下组织→在第二与第三趾的趾长、短伸肌腱之间→长二、第三跖内头之间。浅层布有足背内侧皮神经和足背静脉网。深层有趾背动、静脉。〈主治〉齿痛、口咽、喉痹、鼻衄、腹痛、腹胀、泄泻、痢疾、足背肿痛、热病。直刺0.3~0.5寸;可灸。

Neiting (ST 44) A meridian point, originally from *Ling Shu: Benshu* (*Miraculous Pivot: Meridian Points*), the Ying (Spring) Point of the Stomach Meridian of Foot-Yangming. 〈Location〉on the instep of the foot, at the junction of the red and white skin proximal to the margin of the web between the 2nd and 3rd toes (Fig. 60). 〈Regional anatomy〉skin→subcutaneous tissue→between tendons of long and short extensor muscles of 2nd and 3rd toes → between heads of 2nd and 3rd metatarsal bones. In the superficial layer, there are the dorsal digital nerve of the medial dorsal pedal cutaneous nerve and the dorsal arteriove nous network of the foot. In the deep layer, there are the dorsal artery and vein. 〈Indications〉 toothache, deviation of the mouth, inflammation of the throat, epistaxis, abdominal distention and pain, diarrhea, dysentery, pain and swelling of the dorsum of foot, febrile diseases. 〈Method〉Puncture perpendicularly 0.3~0.5 cun. Moxibustion is applicable.

●内外二景图[nèi wài èr jǐng tú] 书名,宋代朱肱撰。其以杨保《存真图》,丁德用、石藏用合绘的经穴图为基础,补以针法,编绘而成。刊于1118年,现已佚。见《读书敏求记》。

Neiwai Er Jing Tu (*Two Illustrations on Interior and Exterior of the Body*) A book written by Zhu Hong in the Song Dynasty. He compiled and drew the book on the basis of *Cun Zhen Tu* (*Preserving the True*) by Yang Bao and the diagram of acupoints drawn by Ding Deyong and Shi Cangyong, and supplemented the needling methods. It was published in 1118, already lost. See *Dushu Minqiu Ji* (*Notes from Reading with Keen Sense of Seeking*).

●内外痔[nèi wài zhì] 病证名。见《外科大成》。又名混合痔,指生于肛门齿线上下(肛门内外)的痔。参见"痔疮"、"内痔"、"外痔"各条。

Internal-External Hemorrhoids A disease, originally from *Waike Dacheng* (*A Great Compendium of External Diseases*), also named mixed hemorrhoids, referring to hemorrhoids

seen on the upper and lower dentate line of the anus (in and out of the anus), →痔疮(p. 606)、内痔(p. 282)外痔(p. 456)

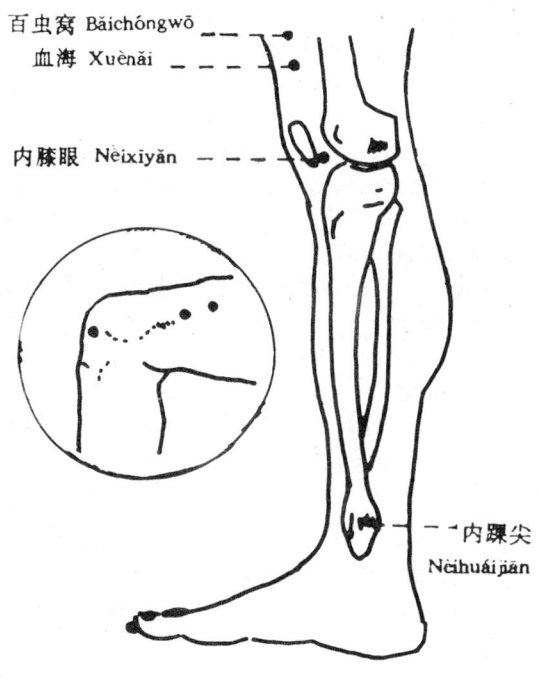

图33 内膝眼、内踝尖穴

Fig 33 Neixiyan and Neihuaijian points

●**内膝眼**[nèi xī yǎn] 经外穴名。见《常用经穴解剖定位》。又名内龙眼。〈定位〉屈膝，在髌韧带内侧凹陷处(图29)。〈层次解剖〉皮肤→皮下组织→髌韧带与髌内侧支持带之间→膝关节囊、翼状皱襞。浅层布有隐神经的髌下支和股神经的前皮支，深层有膝关节的动、静脉网。〈主治〉膝关节炎及其周围软组织炎。从前内向后外与额状面成45度角斜刺0.5～1寸。

Neixiyan(EX-LE 4) An extra point, seen in *Changyong Jingxue Jiepou Dingwei* (*Anatomical Locations of Commonly used Meridian Points*) also known as Neilongyan. 〈Location〉in the depression medial to the patellar ligament when the knee is fixed (Fig. 29). 〈Regional anatomy〉skin→subcutaneous tissue→between patellar ligament and medial parellar retinaculum→articular capsule of knee joint and alar fods. In the superficial layer, there are the infrapatellar branches of the saphenous nerve and the anterior cutaneous branches of the femoral nerve. In the deep layer, there is the arteriovenous. 〈Indication〉gonitis with peripheral soft tissue inflammation. 〈Method〉Puncture obliquely 0.5～1 cun from the anterior of the medial side to the posterior of the lateral side, at a 45° angle with frontal section.

●**内阳池**[nèi yáng chí] 经外穴名。见《经外奇穴治疗诀》。在掌后横纹，大陵上1寸,〈主治〉口腔炎、咽喉痛、鹅掌风、小儿惊风等。直刺0.3～0.5寸；可灸。

Neiyangchi(EX-UE) An extra point, originally from *Jingwai Qixue Zhiliao Jue* (*Pithy Formulas for Treatment with Extra Points*). 〈Location〉on the palmar side of the forearm, 1 cun above Daling (PC 7) which is on the crease of the wrist. 〈Indications〉tomatitis, sore throat, tinea unguium, infantile convulsion, etc. 〈Method〉Puncture perpendicularly 0.3～0.5 cun. Moxibustion is applicable.

●**内迎香**[nèi yíng xiāng] 经外穴名。出《扁鹊神应针灸玉龙经》。〈定位〉在鼻孔内，当鼻翼软骨与鼻甲交界的粘膜处(图34)。〈层次解剖〉鼻粘膜→粘膜下疏松组织。布有面动、静脉的鼻背支之动、静脉网和筛前神经的鼻外支。〈主治〉目赤肿痛、鼻痒、鼻塞、咽喉肿痛、中暑、头痛等。点刺出血。

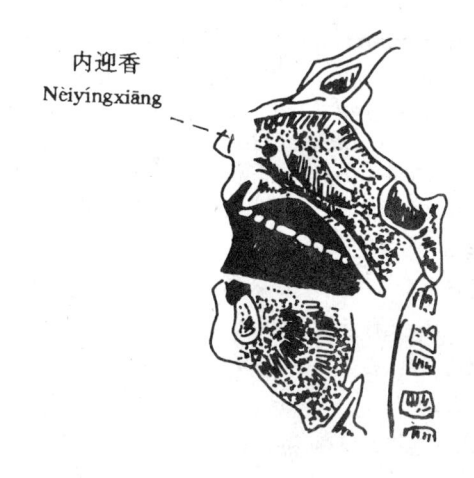

图34 内迎香穴

Fig 34 Neiyingxiang point

Neiyingxiang (EX-HN 9)　An extra point, originally from *Bian Que Shenying Zhenjiu Yulong Jing* (*Bian Que's Jade Dragon Classics of Acupuncture and Moxibustion*). 〈Location〉 in the nostril, at the junction between the mucosa of the alar cartilage of the nose and the nasal concla (Fig. 34). 〈Regional anatomy〉 nasal mucosa → submucous loose connective tissue. There are the arteriovenous network of the dorsal nasal branches of the facial artery and vein and the lateral nasal branches of the anterior ethmoidal nerve in this area. 〈Indications〉 conjunctival congestion with swelling and pain, nasal itching, nasal obstruction, sorethroat, headstroke, headache, etc. 〈Method〉 Prick to cause bleeding.

●内至阴[nèi zhī yīn]　经外穴名。见《针灸学》。在足小趾内侧，趾甲根角旁约0.1寸。〈主治〉小儿惊风，晕厥、脏躁等。直刺0.1～0.2寸；或点刺出血。

Neizhiyin (EX-LE)　An extra point, seen in *Zhenjiuxue* (*Study on Acupuncture and Moxibustion*). 〈Location〉 on the medial side of the little toe, about 0.1 cun lateral to the corner of the toe nail. 〈Indications〉 infantile convulsion, syncope, hysteria, etc. 〈Method〉 Puncture perpendicularly 0.1～0.2 cun or prick to cause bleeding.

●内痔[nèi zhì]　病证名。出《外台秘要》。指生于肛门齿线以上的痔疮。临床多见便血，痔核突出，伴有肛门部不适。参见"痔疮"条。

Internal Hemorrhoid　A disease, originally from *Waitai Miyao* (*Clandestine Essential from the Imperial Library*) referring to hemorrhoids above the dentate line of the anus. Clinically, it is mostly manifested by hemafecia, prolapce of hemorrhoids and discomfort of the anus. →痔疮(p.606)

●能近怯远症[néng jìn qiè yuǎn zhèng]　病证名。见《审视瑶函》。又称近视。多因阅读、书写、近距离工作时的照明不足，姿势不正，持续时间过久所致，若久视伤血，目失所养，亦可为病，此外，也有因禀赋不足而致者，证见视物模糊，视力减退。其病在进展期，可见目痛。若肝肾阴虚者，可兼有失眠，健忘、眼涩痛、腰酸、舌红脉强。治宜滋补肝肾，益气明目，取睛明、攒竹、承泣、光明、风池、肝俞、肾俞。

Near Sighted Disease　A disease, seen in *Shen Shi Yao Han* (*A Precious Book of Ophthalmology*), also known as myopia, mostly due to reading, writing or short-distance work in dim light or with incorrect posture, or overtime. Some cases due to over straining the eyes lead to the consumption of blood and manutrition of the eyes. In addition, it can also be caused by congenital deficiency. 〈Manifestations〉 blurred vision, hypopsia. Eye pain may occur in cases in the progrssive stage; cases of yin-deficiency of the liver and kidney, may be accompanied by insomnia, forgetfulness, dryness and discomfort of the eyes, soreness of the waist, red tongue and thready pulse. 〈Treatment principle〉 Nourish and reinforce the liver and kidney, replenish qi to improve eyesight, 〈Point selection〉 Jingming (BL 1), Cuanzhu (BL 2), Chengqi (ST 1), Guangming (GB 37), Fengchi (GB 20), Ganshu (BL 18) and Shenshu (BL 23).

●泥钱[ní qián]　灸具名。出《针灸易学》。以泥土制成，制如针状而较厚，中有圆孔，上放艾炷以施灸。

Clay Coin　A moxibustion instrument, originally from *Zhenjiu Yixue* (*Acupuncture and Moxibustion Are Easy to Learn*). It was made of clay with a round hole in its centre, like a coin but a bit thicker. 〈Method〉 Place a moxa-cone on the coin for moxibustion.

●泥土灸[ní tǔ jiǔ]　即黄土饼灸。见该条。

Clay Moxibustion　→黄土饼灸(p.176)

●泥丸宫[ní wán gōng]　①经穴别名。见《普济方》。即百会。见该条。②部位名。见《黄庭内景经》。即脑部。

1. **Niwangong**　Another name for Baihui (DU 20), a meridian point originally from *Puji Fang* (*Prescriptions for Universal Relief*). →百会(p.11)

2. **Slurry Pill Palace**　The brain part, a part of the body seen in *Huangting Neijing Jing* (*Canon of Interior View of the Yellow Yard*).

●逆而夺之[nì ér duó zhī]　即迎而夺之。见该条。

Reducing by Puncturing Abversely to Meridian-Qi.　→迎而夺之(p.566)

●逆灸[nì jiǔ]　灸法用语。见《范汪方》指无病而灸，

以期增强人体的抗病能力。

Reverse Moxibustion A term in moxibustion, seen in *Fan Wang Fang* (*Fan Wang's Prescriptions*), referring to the use of moxibustion before the onset of disease for strengthening body resistance.

●逆针灸 [nì zhēn jiǔ] 指对健康人施用针灸。见《千金要方》。没有病而施行针灸曰逆。

Reverse Acupuncture and Moxibustion Performance of acupuncture and moxibustion on a healthy person. It is seen in *Qianjin Yaofang* (*Essential Prescriptions Worth a Thousand Gold*). To perform acupuncture and moxibustion on a healthy person is referred to as "reverse."

●逆注 [nì zhù] 经穴别名。出《针灸甲乙经》。即温溜。见该条。

Nizhu Another name for Wenliu (LI 7), a meridian point originally from *Zhenjiu Jia-Yi Jing* (*A-B Classic of Acupuncture and Moxibustion*). →温溜 (p. 470)

●溺血 [nì xuè] 即尿血。见该条。

Urine with Blood →尿血 (p. 284)

●捻 [niǎn] 针刺基本手法之一。即将针入一定深度后,用拇、食两指一前、一后交替转动的动作,也就是拇、食指向内、外来回捻转的操作过程。捻转时须在既定深度来回捻转,其角度以不超过360度为宜。《内经》中谓之"转"与"旋"。可用于取得针感,或使针感传导,或施行补泻。

Twisting One of the basic needling manipulations. After the needle is inserted to a certain depth, rotate the needle with the thumb and the index finger forward and backward in turn. In other words, it is the manipulation process of twisting the needle with the thumb and the index finger repeatedly moving interiorly and exteriorly. Twist the needle to and fro at a certain depth while manipulating, the degree of twsting should be less than 360°. In *Neijing* (*The Canon of Internal Medicine*), it was called "turning" and "revolving". It is used to obtain a needling reaction, or make the needling reaction conduct, or employ the reinforcing and reducing method.

●捻法 [niǎn fǎ] 针刺手法名。见《针经指南》。为十四法之一。捻同撚,用手指一前一后转动的意思。在《针灸大成》列为下手八法之一,与十二手法中的指撚法相同。参见"左右转"条。

Twirling A needling manipulation, seen in *Zhenjing Zhinan* (*A Guide to Acupuncture and Moxibustion*). One of the Fourteen Methods. Twirling means rotating, referring to turning forward and backward with the fingers. It was taken as one of the Eight Methods in *Zhenjiu Dacheng* (*A Great Compendium of Acupuncture and Moxibustion*), and is the same as the finger-rotating of the Twelve Manipulations. →左右转 (p. 649)

●捻转补泻 [niǎn zhuǎn bǔ xiè] 针刺补泻方法之一。见《灵枢·官能》。原称子午补泻。其法:右手持针,将拇指向前,食指向后捻左转,称为补法;拇指向后,食指向前捻转右转,称为泻法。

Twirling Reinforcing-Reducing One of the reinforcing-reducing methods in acupuncture, seen in *Ling Shu: Guan Neng* (*Miraculous Pivot: Functions and Abilities*), previously called midnight-noon reinforcing and reducing. 〈Method〉Hold the needle with the right hand, twirl it left with the thumb moving forward and index finger backward, which is referred to as reinforcing; twirl the needle right with the thumb moving backward and index finger forward, which is referred to as reducing.

●捻转法 [niǎn zhuǎn fǎ] 针刺手法名。为针刺基本手法之一。针刺入所刺部位一定的深度后,施行以针身为纵轴,顺时针或逆时针方向反复来回转动的行针手法。捻转的角度和频率也因病情和腧穴而异。捻转角度大,频率快,刺激量就大;捻转的角度小,频率慢,刺激量就小。捻转角度一般应在360度以下。另外必须注意捻转时,不可单向捻动,避免针身缠绕肌纤维,造成疼痛和出针困难。

Twirling the Acupuncture Needle A needling manipulation, one of the basic techniques of acupuncture, referring to the manipulation in which the body of needle is taken as a longitudinal axle. Twirl the needle clockwise and counter clockwise repeatedly after the needle is inserted to a certain depth. The angle and frequency of twirling vary on the condition of the disease and acupoints. The

stimulation amount will be larger with more twirling degrees and faster frequency and smaller with fewer twirling degees and slower frequency. The degree of twirling is generally no more than 360. Be sure not to twist the needle in only one direction when twirling, so as to prevent the body of the needle from winding the muscle fiber, and avoid pain and difficulty in withdrawing the needle.

●捻转进针[niǎn zhuǎn jìn zhēn] 进针法之一。毫针进针一般以快速直刺为主,以减少透皮时的疼痛,当针身柔软(如金银质毫针)或局部皮肤坚韧不能快速进针时,则用捻转法。捻转幅度要小,保持针身的挺直,并两手配合动作,以利于进针。

Inserting the Needle by Twirling One of the methods of needle insertion. Fast and perpendicular insertion of the filiform needle is usually used as the main method so as to reduce pain when the needle penetrates through the skin. Inserting the needle by twirling is applied when the needle fails to be inserted quickly because of the soft body of the needle (e. g. one made of gold or silver) or of the tough and tensile skin around the selected point. Twirl the needle in small degrees and keep the body of needle straight with a harmonious movement of the two hands to make the insertion easy.

●念盈药条[niàn yíng yào tiáo] 药艾条之一种。所含药物以桂枝、川乌、雄黄、广皮、檀香、丹参、香附、白芷、藿香、降香、良姜为主。用于风寒湿痹,寒性腹痛,痛经等。

Nian Ying Medicinal Moxa Roll A form of medicinal moxa roll. 〈Constitution〉 *Gui Zhi* (*Ramulus Cinnamomi*), *Chuan Wu* (*Redix Aeoniti*), *Xiong Huang* (*Realgar*), *Guang Pi* (*Pertcarpium*), *Tan Xiang* (*Lignum Santali*), *Dan Shen* (*Radix Salviae Miltiorrhizae*), *Xiang Fu* (*Rhizoma Cyperi*), *Bai Zhi* (*Redix Angelicae Dahuricae*), *Huo Xiang* (*Herba Agastacehis*), *Jiang Xiang* (*Lignum Dalbergiae Odoriferae*), *Liang Jiang* (*Rhizoma Alpiniae Officinarum*). 〈Indications〉 arthralgia due to wind, cold dampness, abdominal pain with coldness, dysmenorrhea, etc.

●尿胞[niào bāo] 经外穴别名。即屈骨端。见该条。

Niaobao Another name for the extra point Quguduan(EX-CA). →屈骨端(p. 326)

●尿床[niào chuáng] 小儿遗尿的别名。详见该条。

Bed-Wetting. →小儿遗尿(p. 502)

●尿道[niào dào] 耳穴名。位于与对耳轮下脚下缘同水平的耳轮处。用于治疗遗尿、尿频、尿急、尿痛、尿潴留。

Urethra(MA) An ear point. 〈Location〉 on the helix and on the level of the lower border of the inferior antinhelix. 〈Indications〉 nuresis, frequent urine, urgency of urination, urodynia, retention of urine.

●尿来[niào lái] 小儿遗尿的别名。详见该条。

Urine Going Out →小儿遗尿(p. 502)

●尿血[niào xuě] ①病证名。出《金匮要略·五脏风寒积聚病脉证并治》。又名溲血、溺血,指小便中混有血液或夹杂血块而言。本证与血淋相似,其区别点为:茎中无明显疼痛者,为尿血;小便时涩痛难忍者,为血淋。多因肾阴不足和心火炽盛所致。临床分为阴虚火旺尿血和心火亢盛尿血。详见各条。②经外穴名。见《千金要方》。在背部,当第7胸椎两旁各5寸,灸治小儿尿血。

1. Hematuria A disease, originally from *Jingui Yaolüe: Wu Zang Feng Han Jiju Bing Mai Zheng Bing Zhi*(*Synopsis of the Golden Chamber: Pulse Conditions, Symptoms and Treatments of Wind and Cold Syndromes of the Five Zang Organs and Abdominal Masses*), also named as bloody urine or urine with blood, referring to urine mixed with blood or blood stasis. This disease is similar to stranguria complicated by hematuria, the differentiation is: Cases without obvious pain in the penis are considered hematuria diseases, some cases with unbearable astringent pain during urination are considered stranguria complicated by hematuria. Hematuria is mostly caused by deficiency of kindney-yin and flaming of heart-fire. It is clinically divided into hematuria due to fire-hyperactivity resulting from yin deficiency and hematuia due to the flaring of heart fire. →阴虚火旺尿血(p. 561)、心火亢盛尿血(p. 509)

2. Niaoxue (EX-B) An extra point, seen in *Qianjin Yaofang*(*Essential Prescriptions Worth*

a Thousand Gold). ⟨Location⟩on the back, 5 cun lateral to the 7th thoracic vertebra. ⟨Indication⟩hematuria in children. ⟨Method⟩moxibustion.

●捏起进针[niē qǐ jìn zhēn]　进针法之一。其法两手配合,用左手拇、食两指将穴位处的肌肤捏起,右手持针在其捏起处沿皮刺入。适用皮肉浅薄而不能深刺的部位。

Inserting the Needle While Pinching Skin　One of the methods of needle insertion. ⟨Method⟩Pinch the skin at point with the thumb and index finger of the left hand, insert the needle into the skin horizontally. This method is suitable for puncturing where soft tissue is too thin to be punctured deeply.

●聂莹[niè yíng]　人名。明针灸家。精于针术,为明针灸家凌云(字汉章)的弟子。事见《浙江通志》。

Nie Ying　An acupuncture-moxibustion expert in the Ming Dynasty, skillful in acupuncture techniques, the disciple of Ling Yun (who styled himself Hanzhang), an expert of acupuncture and moxibustion in the Ming Dynasty. Cf. *Zhejiang Tongzhi* (*General Annals of Zhejiang Province*).

●颞[niè]　耳穴名。又称太阳,位于对耳屏外侧的中部。⟨主治⟩偏头痛。

Temple (MA)　An ear point, also known as Sun (MA). ⟨Location⟩in the middle of the lateral aspect of the antitragus. ⟨Indication⟩migraine.

●颞颥[niè rú]　①经穴别名。出《针灸甲乙经》。即脑空。见该条。②经外穴名。出《脉经》。在眉毛外端与目外眦角连线的中点。⟨主治⟩时邪温病、头痛、眩晕、眼部疾患以及面神经麻痹等。沿皮刺0.3～0.5寸。③部位名。在眉棱骨(眉弓)外侧,耳前动处,俗称太阳,现称翼点。

1. Nieru　Another name for Naokong (GB 19), a meridian point originally from *Zhenjiu Jia Yi-Jing* (*A-B Classic of Acupuncture and Moxibustion*). →脑空(p. 277)

2. Nieru(EX-HN)　An extra point, originally from *Maijing* (*Pulse Classic*). ⟨Location⟩on the midpoint of the line connecting the lateral end of the eyebrow and the corner of the outer canthus. ⟨Indications⟩epidemic febrile disease, headache, vertigo, eye disorders and facial paralysis, etc. ⟨Method⟩Puncture subcutaneously 0.3～0.5 cun.

3. Temple　A part of the body. ⟨Location⟩at the lateral side of the supraorbital bone (Superciliary arch), the leaping part anterior to auricle. Its popular name is Taiyang, now called pterion.

●凝脂翳[níng zhī yì]　即目翳。见该条。

Fat Deposition Opacity　→目翳(p. 273)

●牛皮癣[niú pí xuǎn]　病证名。见《世医得效方》。因患处皮肤如牛领之皮,厚而且坚,故名。由风湿热毒蕴郁肌肤,或因营血不足,血虚风燥,肌肤失养而成。本病好发于项部、肘弯、腘窝、上眼睑及大腿内侧等部。一般表现为局部皮肤受损逐渐变厚,呈淡褐色或深褐色。自觉阵发奇痒,入夜更甚,郁闷烦躁时瘙痒更剧。因搔抓可在病变的周围出现抓痛和血痂,临床可分为风湿化热牛皮癣和血虚风燥牛皮癣。详见各条。

Ox's Skin Tinea (**Neurodermatitis**)　A disease seen in *Shiyi De Xiao-fang* (*Effective Prescriptions Handed Down for Generations*). It is so named because of the thick and solid diseased skin which resembles that of an ox's nape. It is mostly caused by wind, dampness and heat pathogens accumulating in the muscle and skin, or insufficiency of ying blood, blood deficiency and wind-dryness leading to poor nourishment of the skin. The disease frequently occurs on the nape, elbow, politeal fossa, upper eyelid and the medial side of the thigh, etc. It is commonly manifested by local impairment of the skin, with the skin gradually thickening, becoming a light or dark-brown color. There is a subjective feeling of paroxysmal itching, which is more serious at night. The itch is more severe when depression or irritability occurs in the patient. Because scratching an itch may cause scratch marks or blood, or a scab around the diseased skin, the disease is clinically divided into neurodermatitis of heat-transformation due to wind-dampness and neurodermatitis due to blood-deficiency and wind-dryness. →风湿化热牛皮癣(p. 114)、血虚风燥牛皮癣(p. 528)

●扭伤[niǔ shāng]　病证名。指四肢关节或躯体的软组织损伤,如肌肉、肌腱、韧带、血管等扭伤,而无骨折、脱臼、皮肉破损的证候。临床主要表现为受伤部肿胀疼痛,关节活动障碍等,新伤局部有微肿,按压疼痛,表示伤势较轻;如红肿高大,关节屈伸不利,表示伤势轻重,陈伤一般肿胀不明显。本病多由剧烈运动或负重不慎、跌仆、牵拉以及过度扭转等原因,致使筋脉及关节损伤,气血壅滞局部而成。治以行气活血,通络止痛法。以受伤局部取穴为主,肩部取肩髃、肩髎、肩贞;肘部取曲池、小海、天井;腕部取阳池、阳溪、阳谷;腰部取肾俞、腰阳关、委中;髀部取环跳、秩边、承扶;膝部取膝眼、梁丘、膝阳关;踝部取解溪、昆仑、丘墟;颈部取风池、天柱、大杼、后溪。

Sprain　A disease, referring to soft tissue injury of the body or the joints of the four limbs, such as muscle, tendon, ligament or blood vessel sprain, without fracture, dislocation of joints and injury. Clinically, it is mainly manifested by swelling and pain in the affected area and obstruction of the joint movement. New sprains are characterized by local swelling and tenderness, indicating a mild sprain or local redness and severe sprain. Old sprains are usually marked by no obvious local swelling. Sprain is mostly caused by the injury of muscle, tendons, vessels and joints, stagnation of qi and blood in the local area resulting from strenuous exercise or overloading, fall, traction and oversprain. 〈Treatment principle〉 Promote the circulation of qi and blood, dredge the collaterals and arrest pain. 〈Point selection〉 Mainly select local acupoints of the injured area. Shoulder area: Jianyu(LI 15), Jianliao(SJ 14), Jianzhen(SI 9). Elbow area: Quchi(LI 11), Xiaohai(SI 8), Tianjing(SJ 10). Wrist area: Yangchi(SJ 4), Yangxi(LI 5), Yanggu(SI 5). Lumbar area: Shenshu(BL 23), Yaoyangguan(DU 3), Weizhong(BL 40), Thigh area: Huantiao(GB 30), Zhibian(BL 54), Chengfu(BL 36), Knee area: Xiyan(EX-LE 5), Liangqiu(ST 34), Xiyangguan(GB 33). Ankle area: Jiexi(ST 41), Kunlun(BL 60), Qiuxu(GB 40). Neck area: Fengchi(GB 20), Tianzhu(BL 10); Dazhu(BL 11), Houxi(SI 3).

●努法[nǔ fǎ]　针刺手法名,见《针灸问对》。列为十四法之一。①指地行针之前,用手指弹动穴部促使气血充盛。②于行针时用中指侧压针身称为努。具有行气作用,在龙虎升降法中用之。

1. Flicking　A needling manipulation, seen in *Zhenjiu Wendui* (*Catechism of Acupuncture and Moxibustion*). One of the Fourteen Methods. It refers to flicking the selected point with the fingers to make qi and blood sufficient in the local area before needling.

2. Nu　Pressing the body of the needle with one side of the middle finger while inserting the needle is referred to as nu. This method has the function of promoting the flow of qi. It is used in the method of dragon-tiger ascending-descending.

●女膝[nǚ xī]　经外穴名。出《癸辛杂识》。又名女须。位于足后跟,当跟骨中点处。〈主治〉吐泻转筋、骨槽风、齿龈炎、惊悸、精神病等。直刺0.2～0.3寸;可灸。

Nǔxi（EX-LE）　An extra point, originally from *Guixin Zashi*(*Random Thoughts in Guixin Period*), also named Nüxu. 〈Location〉 on the heel and in the center of the calcaneus. 〈Indications〉 vomiting, diarrhea, spasm, osteomyelitis of the maxillary bone, gingival infection, palpitation, mental disorders, etc. 〈Method〉 Puncture perpendicularly 0.2～0.3 cun. Moxibustion is applicable.

●女须[nǚ xū]　经外穴别名。即女膝。见该条。

Nüxu　Another name for the extra point Nüxi(EX-LE). →女膝(p. 286)

●女阴缝[nǚ yīn fèng]　经外穴别名。即玉门头。见该条。

Nüyinfeng　Another name for the extra point Yumentou→玉门头(p. 573)

●疟[nüè]　病证名。出《素问·疟论》等。即疟疾。详见该条。

Malarial Disease　Malaria, a dissease originally from *Suwen*: *Nüe Lun*(*Plain Questions*: *On Malaria*). →疟疾(p. 287)

●疟病[nüè bìng]　病证名。出《金匮要略》。即疟疾。详见该条。

Malarial Illness　Malaria, a disease originally from *Jingui Yaolüe*(*Synopsis of the Golden Chamber*). →疟疾(p. 287)

● 疟疾 [nüè jī] 病证名。见《太平圣惠方》卷七十四。又称痎疟、疟病。是由疟原虫所引起的传染病。多发于夏秋季节。中医学认为本病多由病邪蕴伏半表半里，阴阳分争而致。临床分正疟、温疟、寒疟、瘅疟、劳疟五种类型。详见各条。

Malaria A disease, seen in Vol. 74 of *Taiping Shenghui Fang* (*Imperial Benevolent Prescriptions*), also named malarial disease, malaria tertiand or malarial illness. It is an infectious disease caused by malarial parasites, mostly occurring in summer and autumn. In traditional Chinese medicine it is thought that this disease is commonly due to pathogenic factors accumulating in the half-exterior and half-interior, and combat between yin and yang. Clinically, malaria is divided into five types: lingering malaria, warm malaria, cold malaria, maligment malaria and malaria with general debility→正疟(p. 600)、温疟(p. 470)、寒疟(p. 156)、瘅疟、(p. 586)、劳疟(p. 238)

O

● 呕吐 [ǒu tù] 症状名。见《金匮要略》。指饮食、痰涎从胃中上涌，自口而出。古代文献多以有物有声谓之呕，有物无声谓之吐，无物有声之干呕。因呕与吐常常同时发生，故并称为呕吐。本病多因饮食伤胃、痰饮内扰、肝气犯胃、感受外邪、脾胃虚弱，使胃失和降、气逆于上所致。临床分为伤食呕吐、痰饮呕吐、肝气呕吐、外感呕吐、虚寒呕吐、阴虚呕吐。详见各条。

Vomiting A disease, seen in *Jingui Yaolüe* (*Synopsis of the Golden Chamber*), referring to casting up food and fluid from the stomach by the mouth. According to ancient documents, vomiting with discharge and sound is called gagging, vomiting with discharge but no sound is termed spitting and vomiting with sound but no dischargs is named retching. Because gagging and spitting often occur simutaneously, they are called vomiting. Vomiting is due to the failure of stomach-qi resulting from impairment of the stomach by improper diet, disturbance of phlegm retention, hyperactive liver-qi attacking the stomach or affection by the exopathogen and deficiency of the spleen and stomach. It is clinically divided into vomiting due to improper diet, vomiting due to phlegm retention, vomiting due to hyperactive liver-qi, vomiting due to affection by exopathogen, vomiting due to cold of insufficiency type and vomiting due to yin-deficiency. →伤食呕吐(p. 349)、痰饮呕吐(p. 425)、肝气呕吐(p. 125)、外感呕吐(p. 453)、虚寒呕吐(p. 514)、阴虚呕吐(p. 561)

● 呕血 [ǒu xuè] 病证名。出《素问·举痛论》等。指血随呕吐而出，血出有声。参见"吐血"条。

Hematemesis A disease, originally from *Su Wen*: *Ju Tonglun* (*Plain Quetions*: *On Acute Pains*), referring to spitting blood with sound. →吐血(p. 449)

● 偶刺 [ǒu cì] 《内经》刺法名。出《灵枢·官针》，是十二刺之一，内脏病痛，可当其前(胸、腹)、后(背)选穴针刺。因其前后相对，故称偶刺。然必斜刺，以防伤及内脏。临床上对内脏病痛取胸腹部募穴与背部俞穴同用之俞募配穴，即属此类。

Mated Needling A form of needling in *Neijing* (*The Canon of Internal Medicine*), originally from *Lingshu*: *Guanzhen* (*Miraculous Pivot*: *Official Needles*), one of the Twelve Needling Methods. For treating diseases of the internal organs, the acupoints on the anterior (chest, abdomen) and those on the posterior (back) can be selected. It is so called because these points are located on the front and back oppositely. Be sure to puncture these points obliquely so as not to damage the internal organs. Clinically, selection of the Front-Mu points on the chest and abdomen in combination with the Back-Shu points for treating diseases and pain of internal organs belongs to

this kind.

●偶经取穴[ǒu jīng qǔ xué] 取穴法之一。又称表里经取穴。根据经脉的表里相合关系,选取与其相为表里的另一条经脉上的穴位。如感冒咳嗽属于手太阴肺经病证,而取手阳明大肠经的合谷;胃病属足阳明胃经病证,而取足太阴脾经的公孙等。

Point Selection on the Mated Meridian One of the methods of point selection, also known as point selection on the exterior-interior meridian. Select an acupoint in another meridian which is exteriorly or interiorly related to the main meridian according to the exterior-interior relationship between the meridians. For instance, cough due to common cold pertains to disease of the Lung Meridian of Hand-Taiyin. Yet, Hegu(LI 4) on the Large Intestine Meridian of Hand-Yangming is selected; gastric disorder pertains to diseases of the Stomach Meridian of Foot-Yangming. Yet, Gongsun(SP 4) on the Spleen Meridian of Foot-Taiyin is selcted, and so on.

P

●拍蟹毒[pāi xiè dú] 即虎口疔,详见该条。

Clapping-Crab Poison →虎口疔(p.168)

●排罐法[pái guàn fǎ] 拔罐法的一种。在拔罐治疗时,如属某一肌束劳损时可按肌束的位置成行排列吸拔多个火罐,即为排罐法。

Cupping with Glasses in Alignment One of the methods for cupping in cupping treatment. Many glasses for cupping are arranged in alignment along the muscle bundle for treating the muscle bundle strain, which is called cupping with glasses in alignment.

●排针[pái zhēn] 针刺手法名。①为出针法之别称。见《素问·八正神明论》。详见该条。②指较为密集而排成行的多针刺法。

1. Removing the Needle A term for needling manipulation, another term for the method of withdrawing the needle, seen in *Su Wen: Bazheng Shenming Lun (Plain Questions: On Eight Natural Qi and Divinity)*. →出针法(p.51)

2. Puncturing with Needles in Alignment The method of puncturing densely with many meedles in aligment.

●盘法[pán fǎ] 针刺手法名。见《针经指南》。为十四法之一。针浅刺入皮下后,斜倒针身,将针柄作圆圈形盘转。左按针为补,右盘提针为泻。主要用于腹部,对加强刺激有一定作用,在"龙虎升腾法"中用此法。

Circling A needling manipulation, seen in *Zhenjing Zhinan (A Guide to the classics of Acupuncture)*, one of the Fourteen Methods. After inserting the needle shallowly, slope the body of the needle and make the handle of the needle circle around. Left circling with thrusting of the needle is considered reinforcing while right circling with lifting of the needle is reducing. This method is mainly used on the abdomen, and has the function of strengthening the stimulation of the needling. It is used in the method of "dragon-tiger ascending and prancing".

●旁廷[páng tíng] 经外穴名。见《千金要方》。在胸部,当胸部第四肋间隙,乳头外开2寸,举腋取之。与天溪同位。又名注市。〈主治〉中恶、飞尸遁注、胸胁支满、呕吐喘逆等。斜刺0.5寸,可灸。

Pangting(EX-CA) An extra point, seen in *Qianjin Yaofang (Essential Prescriptions Worth a Thousand Gold)*, also named Zhushi. 〈Location〉on the chest and in the 4th intercostal space, 2 cun lateral to the nipple, selecting the point by raising the arm in the same location as Tianxi(SP 18). 〈Indictions〉attack by pestilent factors, pulmonary tuberculosis, hydrothrax, fullness sensation in the chest and hypochondriac region, vomiting and dyspnea. 〈Method〉Puncture obliquely 0.5 cun. Moxi-

● 膀胱[páng guāng] 耳穴名。位于对耳轮下脚的前下方。用于治疗腰痛、坐骨神经痛、膀胱炎、遗尿、尿潴留、后头痛。

Bladder (MA) An ear point.〈Location〉on the anterior and inferior border of the inferior antihelix crus.〈Indications〉lumbago, sciatica, cystitis, enuresis, uroschesis and occipital headache.

● 膀胱经[páng guāng jīng] 足太阳膀胱经之简称。见该条。

The Bladder Meridian The short form for the Bladder Meridian of Foot-Taiyang. →足太阳膀胱经(p. 640)

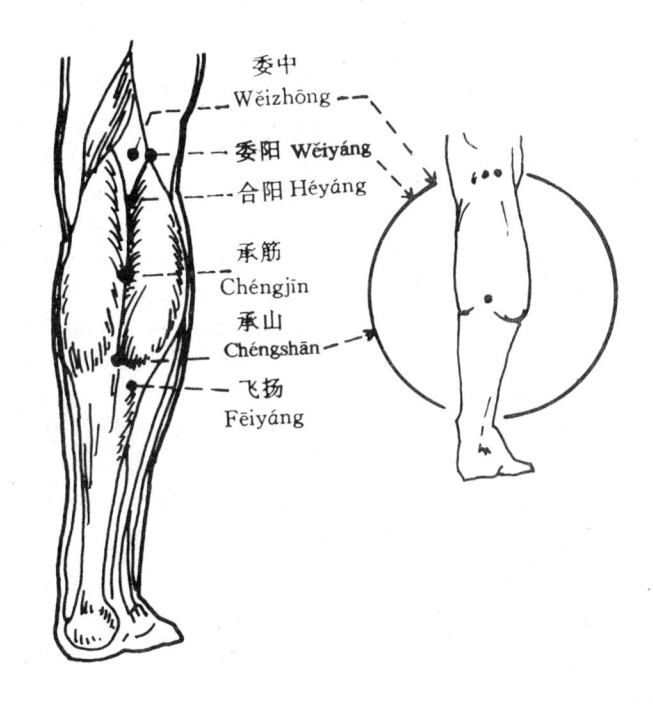

图35.1 膀胱经穴(小腿部)
Fig 35.1 Points of Bladder Meridian(Leg)

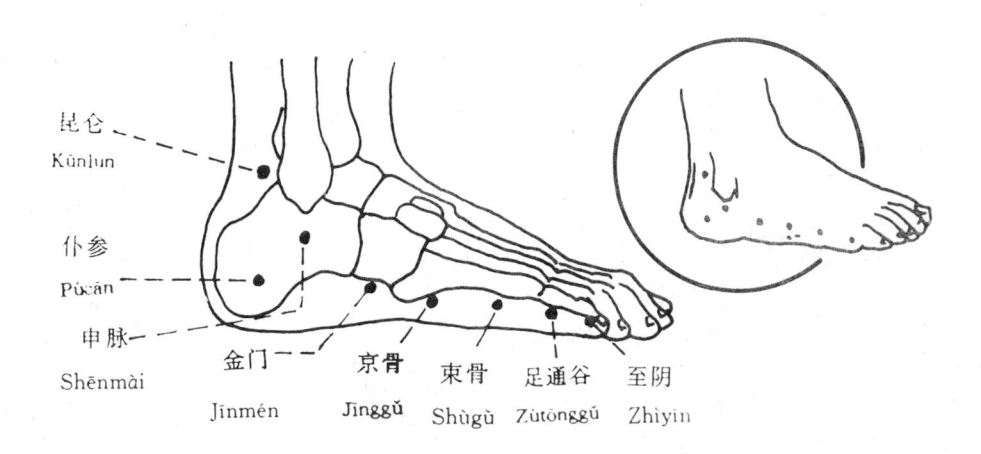

图35.2 膀胱经穴(足部)
Fig 35.2 Points of Bladder Meridian(Foot)

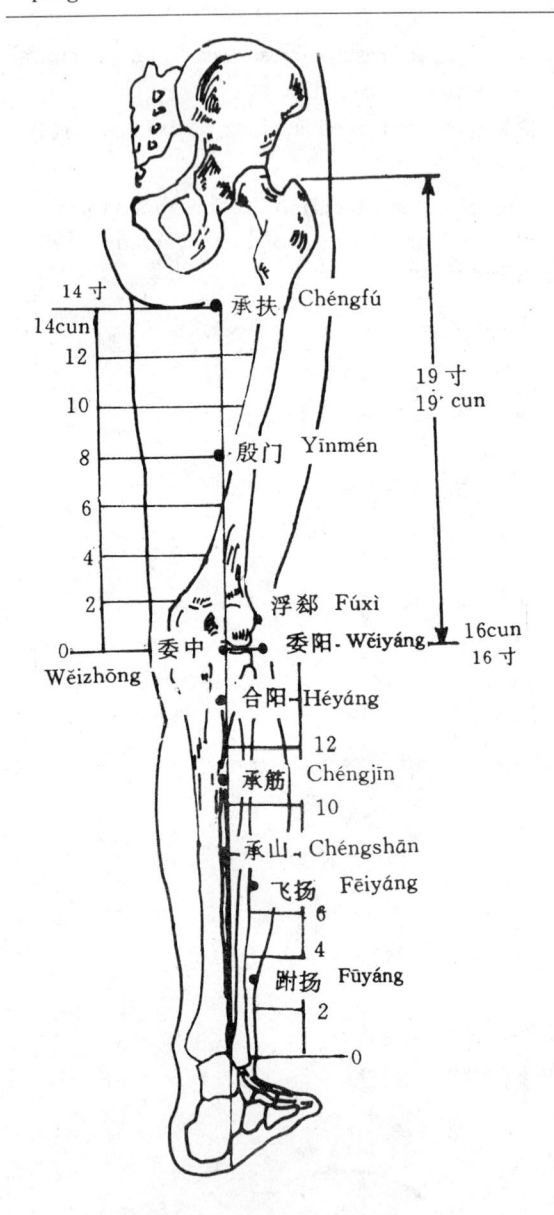

图35.3 膀胱经穴（下肢部）

Fig 35.3 Points of Bladder Meridian (Lower limb)

●膀胱俞[páng guāng shū] 经穴名，见《针灸甲乙经》。属足太阳膀胱经，为膀胱的背俞穴。〈定位〉骶部，当骶正中嵴旁1.5寸，平第二骶后孔(图7)。〈层次解剖〉皮肤→皮下组织→臀大肌→竖脊肌腱。浅层布有臀中皮神经。深层布有臀下的神经的属支和相应脊神经后支的肌支。〈主治〉小便赤涩、遗精、遗尿、腹痛、泄泻、便秘、腰脊强痛、膝足寒冷无力、女子瘕聚、阴部肿痛生疮、淋浊。直刺0.8至1寸；可灸。

Panguangshu (BL 28) A meridian point, seen in *Zhenjiu Jia-Yi Jing* (*A-B Classic of Acupuncture and Moxibustion*), the Back-Shu Point of the Bladder Meridian of Foot-Taiyang. 〈Location〉on the sacrum and on the level of the 2nd posterior sacral foramen, 1.5 cun lateral to the meridian sacral crest (Fig. 7). 〈Regional anatomy〉 skin→subcutaneous tissue → greates gluteal muscle → tendon of erector spinal muscle. In the superficial layer, there are the middle clunial nerves. In the deep layer, there are the branches of the inferior gluteal nerve and the muscular branches of the posterior branches of the related spinal nerves. 〈Indications〉scanty dark urine, seminal emission, enuresis, abdominal pain, diarrhea, constipation, pain and stiffness of the lumbar erea and spine, cold and weakness of the knee and foot, abdominal mass in women, swelling, pain and soreness of the vulva, and stranguria with turbid urine. 〈Method〉Puncture perpendicularly 0.8~1.0 cun. Moxibustion is applicable.

●膀胱足太阳之脉[páng guāng zhú tài yáng zhī mài] 足太阳膀胱经原名。见该条。

The Bladder Vessel of Foot-Taiyang The original name of the Bladder Meridian of Foot-Taiyang. →足太阳膀胱经(p.640)

●配穴法[pèi xuú fǎ] 穴位配伍方法。见《针灸大成》卷五。临床可分表里配穴，阴阳配穴，上下配穴，前后配穴，左右配穴，远近配穴等。古代文献中还有主客原络配穴，八脉八穴配穴，子母补泻，泻南补北等法。此外还有子午流注，灵龟八法等特殊的按时配穴法。参见各条。

Point Prescription Method of selecting related points, seen in Vol. 5 of *Zhenjiu Dacheng* (*A Great Compendium of Acupuncture and Moxibustion*). It is clinically divided into the combination of exterior-interior points, the combination of points on the yin-yang meridians, the combination of superior-inferior points, the combination of anterior-posterior points, the combination of left-right points, the combination of distant-local points and so on. Also, in ancient documents, there were the combination of the host-guest points, the combination of the primary-con-

necting points, the combination of the eight confluent points, the combination of the mother-son points for reinforcing and reducing, the combination of reducing south and reinforcing north. Besides, there were some special point presctiptions given according to the time, such as midnight-noon ebb-flow method and the eight methods of the intelligent turtle. → 表里配穴(p. 24)、阴阳配穴(p. 562)、上下配穴(p. 354)、前后配穴(p. 317)、左右配穴(p. 648)、远近配穴(p. 578)、主客原络配穴(p. 621)、八脉八穴配穴(p. 6)、子母补泻(p. 625)、泻南补北(p. 506)、子午流注(p. 626)、灵龟八法(p. 248)

●贲门[pēn mén] 耳穴名。位于耳轮脚下方外三分之一。用于治疗贲门痉挛、神经性呕吐。

Cardiac Orifice(MA-IC 7) An ear point. 〈Location〉at the lateral 1/3 of the inferior aspect of the helix crus. 〈Indications〉cardiac spasm, neurogenic vomiting.

●盆腔[pén qiāng] 耳穴名。位于与耳轮前缘之弧相平行划两条弧线,将三角窝划为三等份,外三分之一的下二分之一为盆腔。〈主治〉盆腔炎、附件炎、月经不调、下腹疼痛、腹胀等。

Relvic Cavity(MA) An ear point. 〈Location〉Divide the triangular fosse into three equal parts by drawing two lines parallel to the arc of the anterior border of the helix, the lower half of the lateral 1/3 is the Pelvic Cavity(MA). 〈Indications〉pelvic inflammation, annexitis, irregular menstruation, lower abdominal pain, abdominal distension, etc.

●彭九思[péng jiǔ sī] 人名。明针灸家,为徐凤之师。参见"徐凤"条。

Peng Jiusi An expert of acupuncture and moxibustion in the Ming Dynasty, the teacher of Xu Feng. →徐凤(p. 517)

●彭用光[péng yòng guāng] 人名。明代针灸家,江西庐陵(吉安)人。见"痈疽神妙灸经"条。

Peng Yongguang An expert of acupuncture and moxibustion in the Ming Dynasty, a native of Luling(Ji'an), Jiangxi Province. →痈疽神妙灸经(p. 568)

●蓬莱火[péng lái huǒ] 药捻灸之一。见《本草纲目拾遗》卷二。药用西黄、雄黄、乳香、没药、丁香、麝香、火硝得等分;或去西黄,加硼砂、草乌皆可。以棉纸包裹药末,捻成条状。须紧实。用时取其二、三分长一段,以棕黏肉上,点燃施灸。治风痹瘰疬,按患处灸;治水胀,膈气,胃气,按穴灸。

Penglai Fire One form of medicinal thread moxibustion, seen in Vol. 2 of *Bencao Gangmu Shiyi* (*A Supplement to the Compendium of Materia Medica*).〈Constitution〉an equal portion of *Niu Huang* (Calculus bovis), *Xiong Huang* (Realgar), *Ru Xiang* (Resina Olibani, *Mo Yao* (Resina Commiphorae Myrrhea), *Ding Xiang* (Flos Syzygii Aromatici), *She Xiang* (Moschus), *Mang Xiao* (Natrii Sulfa); or , remove *Niu Huang* (Clculus Bovis), add *Peng Sha* (Borax) and *Cao Wu* (Radix Aconiti Kusnezoffii). Wrap the herbal powder with a piece of cotton-made paper, twist it into a moxa roll. Take a piece of the roll, 0.2 or 0.3 cun in length, fix it on the skin with glutinous rice, then ignite it for moxibustion. Give moxibustion on the diseased area if it is used for treating migratory arthralgia and scrofula; give moxibustion on acupoints if it is used for treating distension with edema, hiccup and belching.

●铍针[pī zhēn] 古针具名。出《灵枢·九针论》。九针之一。又名剑针。其形如剑,针尖如剑锋,两面有刃,长四寸,宽二分半。〈主治〉痈疽脓疡,可以切开排脓放血。

Stiletto Needle One of the nine needles used in ancient times, originally from *Ling Shu*: *Jiu zhen Lun* (*Miraculous Pivot*: *On Nine Needles*), also named sword-shaped needle. The needle is shaped like a sword, the tip of the needle like the sharp point of a sword with two edges. The total length is 4 cun and its width is 2.5 fen. 〈Indications〉carbuncle, cellulitis pus and sore. It can be used for discharging pus and blood-letting.

●皮部[pí bù] 部位名。出《素问·皮部论》。经脉在体表皮肤的分布。十二经脉循行在体表的相应区域,称为十二皮部。参见"六经皮部"条。

Cutaneous Regions A part of the body, originally from *Suwen*: *Pibu Lun* (*Plain Questions*: *On Cutaneous Regions*), referring to the distribution of the meridians on the skin areas of the body surface. The skin areas corresponding to the Twelve Regular Meridians a-

long the body surface are named the Twelve Cutaneous Regions. →六经皮部(p.253)

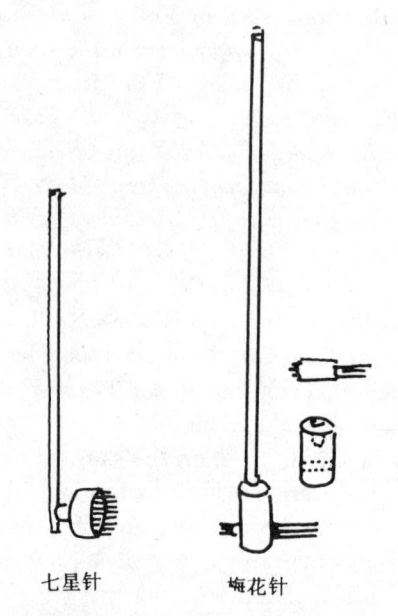

七星针　梅花针
Seven-star steel needle　Plum-blossom needle

图36 皮 肤 针
Fig 36 Dermal needles

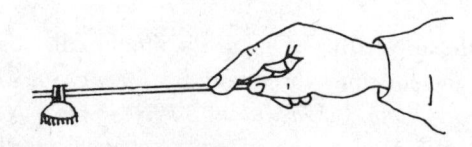

图37 皮肤针持针法
Fig 37 Manipulation of a dermal needle

●皮肤针[pí fū zhēn] 针具名。在古代镵针的基础上发展而来,分小锤式,刷帚式和滚筒式等几种。又按其针数多少,分别称为梅花针(五枚)、七星针(七枚)、罗汉针(十八枚)和丛针(针数不限)等。具有刺激面广,刺激量均匀的优点。因其刺激轻微,适用于小儿,又称为小儿针。

Dermal Needle A needling instrument, developed from shear needles used in ancient times, divided into small-hammer-shaped, brush-shaped and roller-shaped, etc, and also divided according to the number of small needles into plum-blossom needle (5 PS), seven-star needle (7 PS), temple-guard needle (18 PS) and clustered needle (unlimited needles), etc. These needles have the advantage of a broad stimulation area and even stimulation. They are suitable for childern for the mild stimulation, so it is also named infantile needle.

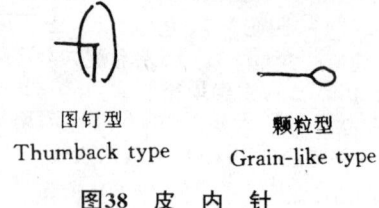

图钉型　颗粒型
Thumback type　Grain-like type

图38 皮 内 针
Fig 38 Intradermal needles

●皮内针[pí nèi zhēn] 针具名。专供皮内埋针使用,分颗粒式皮内针和揿钉式皮内针两种。详见各条。

Intradermal Needle A needling instrument, embedded beneath the skin, and divided into granular intradermal needle and intradermal needle of thumb-tack shape. →颗粒式皮内针(p.231)、揿针式皮内针(p.319)

●皮质下[pí zhì xià] 耳穴名。位于对耳屏内侧面。具有补髓益脑,止痛安神作用,〈主治〉智能发育不全、失眠多梦、肾虚耳鸣、假性近视、神经衰弱。

Subcortex (MA) An ear point. 〈Location〉on the medial side of antitragus. 〈Functions〉Replenish marrow and benefit the brain, arrest pain and tranquilize. 〈Indications〉hypoplasia in intelligence, insomnia and dream-disturbed sleep, tinnitus due to the kidney deficiency, pseudomyopia, neurasthenia.

●琵琶[pí pá] 经外穴名。见《厘正按摩要术》。位于锁骨外侧段前缘。喙突上缘之凹陷中。〈主治〉肩部疼痛、上肢不举等。直刺0.3至0.5寸;可灸。

Pipa (EX-CA) An extra point, seen in *Lizheng Anmo Yaoshu* (*Revised Synopsis of Massage*). 〈Location〉on the anterior border of the lateral side of the clavicle in the depression of the superior border of the coracoid process. 〈Indications〉pain in the shoulder, failure to raise the upper limbs. 〈Method〉Puncture perpendicularly 0.3~0.5 cun. Moxibustion is applicable.

●脾[pí] 耳穴名。①位于耳甲腔的外上方,〈主治〉

腹胀、慢性腹泻、便秘、消化不良、口腔炎、功能性子宫出血、白带过多、内耳眩晕症、食欲不振。②位于耳背中部。主治腹胀腹泻、消化不良。

Spleen (MA) An ear point. ①⟨Location⟩at the lateral and superior aspect of the cavity of concha. ⟨Indications⟩ abdominal distension, chronic diarrhea, constipation, indigestion, stomatitis, dysfunctional uterine bleeding, leukorrhagia, auditory vertigo, anorexia. ②⟨Location⟩in the centre of the back of the ear.⟨Indications⟩abdominal distension and diarrhea, anorexia.

●脾横[pí héng] 经外穴名。见《千金要方》。在第十一胸椎上及左右各1.5寸处。灸治四肢寒热、腰痛不得俯仰、身黄、腹满、食呕、舌根直。

Piheng (EX-CA) An extra point, seen in *Qianjin Yaofang* (*Essential Presriptions Worth a Thousand Gold*). ⟨Location⟩ on the 11th thoracic vertebra, 1.5 cun lateral to each side of the vertebra. ⟨Indications⟩cold and heat of the four limbs, lower back pain and difficulty in flexing and stretching, yellowish body, fullness in the abdomen, vomiting while eating, stiffness of the tongue root. ⟨Method⟩ moxibustion.

●脾经[pí jīng] 足太阴脾经之简称。见该条。

Spleen Meridian The short form for the Spleen Meridian of Foot-Taiyin. →足太阴脾经 (p.643)

●脾舍[pí shè] 经穴别名。出《针灸甲乙经》。即地机。详见该条。

Pishe Another name for Diji (SP 8), a meridian point originally from *Zhenjiu Jia-Yi Jing*(*A-B Classic of Acupuncture and Moxibustion*). →地机(p.78)

●脾俞[pí shū] 经穴名。出《灵枢·背输》。属足太阳膀胱经，为脾的背俞穴。⟨定位⟩在背部，当第十一胸椎棘突下，旁开1.5寸(图7)。⟨层次解剖⟩皮肤→皮下组织→背阔肌→下后锯肌→竖脊肌。浅层布有第十一、十二胸神经后支的皮支的伴行的动、静脉。深层有第十一、十二胸神经后支的肌支和相应肋间、肋下动、静脉的分支或属支。⟨主治⟩胁痛、腹胀、黄疸、呕吐、泄泻、痢疾、便血、完谷不化、水肿、背痛。斜刺0.5至0.8寸；可灸。

Pishu (BL 20) A meridian point, originally from *Ling Shu: Beishu* (*Miraculous Pivot: Back-Shu Points*), a point on the Bladder Meridian of Foot-Taiyang, the Back-Shu point of the spleen. ⟨Location⟩on the back, below the spinous process of the 11th thoracic vertebra, 1.5 cun lateral to the posterior midline (Fig.7). ⟨Regional anatomy⟩skin→subcuta-

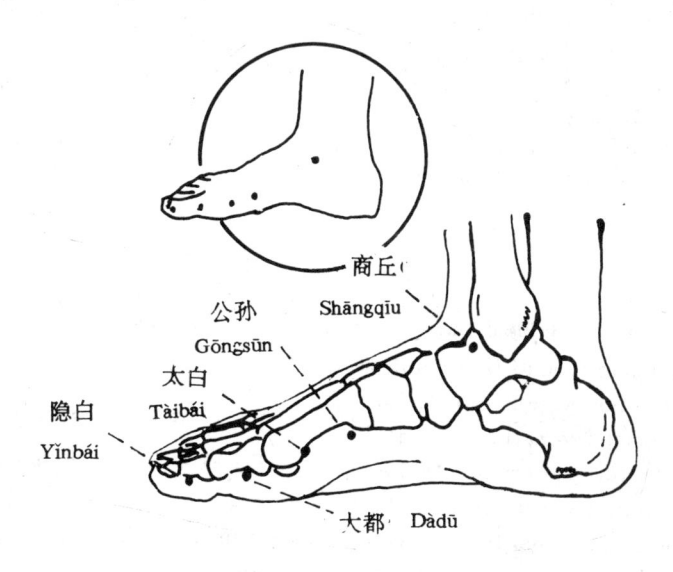

图39.1 脾经穴(足部)

Fig 39.1 Points of Spleen Meridian(Foot)

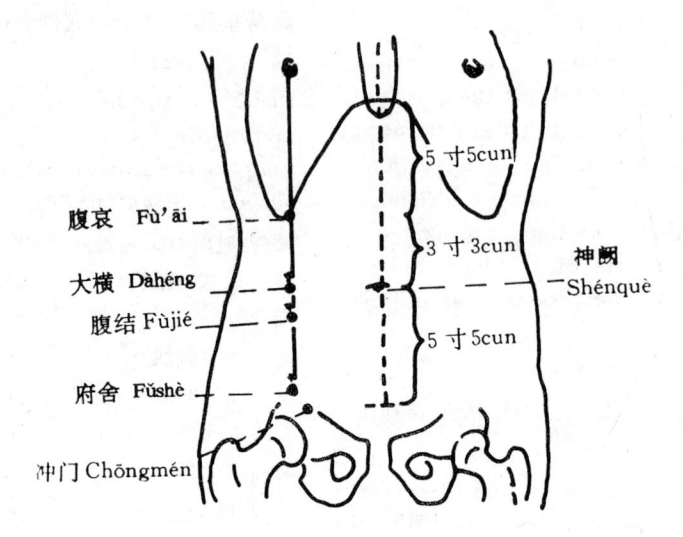

图39.2 脾经穴（腹部）
Fig 39.2 Points of Spleen Meridian (Abdomen)

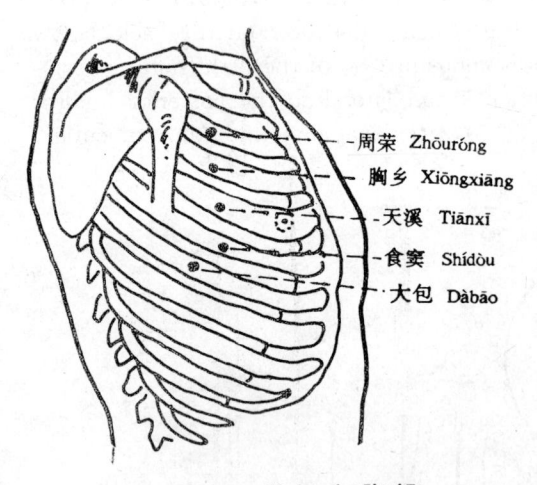

图39.3 脾经穴（胸部）
Fig 39.3 Points of Spleen Meridian (Chest)

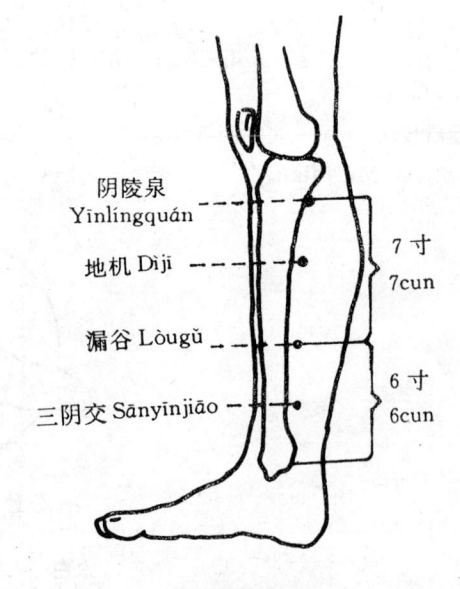

图39.4 脾经穴（小腿部）
Fig 39.4 Points of Spleen Meridian (Leg)

neous tissue→latissimus muscle of back→inferior posterior serratus muscle→erector spinal muscle. In the superficial layer, there are the cutaneous branches of the posterior branches of the 11th and 12th thoracic nerve and the accompanying arteries and veins. In the deep layer, there are the muscular branches of the posterior branches or the 11th and 12th thoracic nerve and the branches or tributaries of the related intercostal and infracostal arteries and veins. 〈Indications〉hypochondriac pain, abdominal distension, jaundice, vomiting, diarrhea, dysentery, hemafecia, stool with undigested food, edema, pain in the back.

⟨Method⟩ Puncture obliquely 0.5～0.8 cun. Moxibustion is applicable.

●**脾胃虚弱经闭**[pí wèi xū ruò jīng bì] 经闭证型之一。多因素体脾胃虚弱，或饮食劳倦，损及脾胃，化源不足，血海空虚，冲任失养所致。证见超龄月经未至，月经闭止。兼见心悸怔忡、气短懒言、神倦肢软、纳少便溏、舌质淡、脉细弱。治宜健脾补胃。取脾俞、胃俞、建里、中脘、足三里、膈俞。

Amenorrhea due to Weakness of the Spleen and Stomach A type of amenorrhea, mostly due to constitutional weakness of the spleen and stomach, or improper diet and overworking which impair the spleen and stomach, leading to a subsequent insufficiency of acquired energy, emptiness of the blood sea and poor nourishment of the Chong and Ren Meridians. ⟨Manifestations⟩ absence of menses over the age of menarche, amenorrhea accompanied by severe palpitations, shortness of breath and lazy in speaking, fatigue, flaccid limbs, poor appetite, watery stools, pale tongue, thready and weak pulse. ⟨Treatment principle⟩ Invigorate the spleen and tonify the stomach. ⟨Point selection⟩ Pishu (BL 20), Weishu (BL 21), Jianli (RN 11), Zhongwan (RN 12), Zusanli (ST 36) and Geshu (BL 17).

●**脾虚便血**[pí xū biàn xuè] 便血证型之一。多因脾气虚弱，脾不统血所致。证见先便后血、血色黯黑、腹痛隐隐、面色不华、神倦懒言、饮食减少、舌淡、脉弱。治宜健脾摄血。取关元、足三里、太白、会阳、脾俞、胃俞。

Hemafecia due to Deficiency of the Spleen A type of hemafecia, mostly caused by deficiency of spleen-qi and the failure of the spleen to keep blood flowing within the vessels. ⟨Manifestations⟩ discharge of stool followed by blood, dull abdominal pain, pale complexion, fatigue, laziness in speaking, anorexia, pale tongue and weak pulse. ⟨Treatment principle⟩ Invigorate the spleen to control the blood. ⟨Point selction⟩ Guanyuan (RN 4), Zusanli (ST 36), Taibai (SP 3), Huiyang (BL 35), Pishu (BL 20) and Weishu (BL 21).

●**脾虚带下**[pí xū dài xià] 带下病证型之一。多因脾失健运，聚湿下注，伤及任、带二脉所致。证见带下色白或淡黄，无臭味，质粘稠，连绵不绝，面色萎黄，纳少便溏，精神疲倦，四肢倦怠，舌质淡，苔白腻。脉缓而弱。治宜健脾益气、利湿止带。取气海、带脉、白环俞、三阴交、足三里、中极。

Leukorrhagia due to Deficiency of the Spleen A type of leukorrhagia, commonly caused by dysfunction of the spleen in transportation, a downward flow of accumulated dampness which impairs the Ren and Dai Meridians. ⟨Manifestations⟩ white or light-yellow leukorrhea without foul smell, sticky and continous vaginel discharg, yellowish complexion, poor appetite and watery stools, lassitude, tiredness of the four limbs, pale tongue with whitish and greasy coating, leisurely and weak pulse. ⟨Treatment principle⟩ Strengthen the spleen and replenish qi, remove dampness and stop leukorrhagia. ⟨Point selection⟩ Qihai (RN 6), Daimai (GB 26), Baihuanshu (BL 30) Sanyinjiao (SP 6), Zusanli (ST 36) and Zhongji (RN 3).

●**脾虚吐血**[pí xū tù xuè] 吐血证型之一。多因脾胃虚弱，不能统血所致。证见吐血较多，血色紫黯，兼见面色㿠白，气怯神疲饮食减少，舌淡苔白，脉沉细。治宜益气摄血。取中脘、脾俞、足三里、隐白。

Hemoptysis due to Deficiency of the Spleen A type of hemoptysis, mostly caused by weakness of the spleen and stomach and failure to keep the blood flowing within the vessels. ⟨Manifestations⟩ severe spitting of blood with a dim-purple color accompanied by a pale compexion, timid breath and lassitude, loss of appetite, pale tongue with whitish coating, deep and thready pulse. ⟨Treatment principle⟩ Replenish qi to control blood. ⟨Point selection⟩ Zhongwan (RN 12), Pishu (BL 20), Zusanli (ST 36) and Yinbai (SP 1).

●**脾虚哮喘**[pí xū xiāo chuǎn] 哮喘证型之一。由于脾虚健运无权，水饮停聚，痰浊内生，壅阻肺气，升降不利所致。证见气短不足以息，语言无力，面色少华，食少，脘痞，痰多，倦怠，大便溏薄，舌胖苔薄腻或白滑，脉细软或濡缓。治宜健脾益气、祛痰平喘。取肺俞、太渊、脾俞、足三里、太白、丰隆、内关、公孙。

Asthma due to Deficiency of the Spleen A type of asthma, mostly caused by dysfunction of the spleen in transportation leading to re-

tention of water-dampness and the formation of phlegm and turbidness which obstruct the lung-qi, resulting in difficulty of the lung-qi to ascend and descend. ⟨Manifestations⟩ weak in speaking, pale compexion, poor appetite, gastric mass, excessive sputum, lassitude, watery stools, enlarged tongue with thin and greasy or whitsh and smooth coating, thready and soft or soft and leisurely pulse. ⟨Treatment principle⟩ Strengthen the spleen and replenish qi, remove phlegm to stop asthma. ⟨Point selection⟩ Feishu (BL 13), Taiyuan (LU 9), Pishu (BL 20), Zusanli (ST 36), Taibai (SP 3) Fenglong (ST 40), Neiguan (PC 6) and Gongsun (SP 4).

●脾虚泻[pí xū xiè] 泄泻证型之一。因脾虚弱,运化无权,水谷不化,清浊不分所致。证见大便时溏、时泻,稍进油腻之品,则大便次数增多,饮食减少,脘腹胀闷不舒,面色萎黄,肢倦乏力,舌淡苔白,脉细弱。治宜健脾益气、升阳止泻。取中脘、章门、胃俞、脾俞、足三里、太阳、商丘。

Diarrhea due to Deficiency of the Spleen A type of diarrhea, mostly due to weakness of the spleen and stomach, dysfunction of the spleen in transportation and production, confusion of nutrition and turbidness. ⟨Manifestations⟩ intermittent watery stool discharge after taking a little greasy food, loss of appetite, distension, fullness and discomfort in the epigastrium and abdomen, yellow complexion, listlessness of the limbs, and acratia, pale tongue with whitish coating, thready and weak pulse. ⟨Treatment principle⟩ Strengthen the spleen and replenish qi, elevate the spleen to arrest diarrhea. ⟨Point selection⟩ Zhongwan (RN 12), Zhangmen (LR 13), Weishu (BL 21), Pishu (BL 20), Zusanli (ST 36), Taiyang (EX-HN 5) and Shangqiu (SP 5).

●脾之大络[pí zhī dà luò] 十五络脉之一。出《灵枢·经脉》。络从渊腋穴(胆经)下三寸的大包穴处分出。散布于胸胁。

The Large Collateral of the Spleen One of the Fifteen Main Collaterals, originally from *Ling Shu*: *Jing Mai* (*Miraculous Pivot*: *Meridians*). The Collateral branches from Dabao (SP 21), 3 cun below Yuanye (GB 22) and spreads over the chest and hypochondrium.

●脾之大络病[pí zhī dà luò bìng] 十五络脉病候之一。出《灵枢·经脉》。本络发生病变,实证可见全身疼痛,虚证可见周身关节弛缓无力。

Diseases of The Large Collateral of the Spleen One of the diseases of the Fifteen Main Collaterals, originally from *Lingshu*: *Jing Mai* (*Miraculous Pivot*: *Meridians*). If pathogenic changes occur in this collateral, excess syndrome may be manifested as pantolgia, deficiency syndrome as flaccidness and weakness of the joints throughout the body.

●脾足太阴之脉[pí zú tài yīn zhī mài] 足太阴脾经的原名。见该条。

The Spleen Vessel of Foot-Taiyin The original name of the Spleen Meridian of Foot-Taiyin. →足太阴脾经 (p. 643)

●痞根[pǐ gēn] 经外穴名。见《医学入门》。⟨定位⟩ 在腰部,当第一腰椎棘突下,旁开3.5寸(图61)。⟨层次解剖⟩ 皮肤→皮下组织→背阔肌→下后锯肌→髂肋肌。浅层主要有第十二胸神经后支的外侧支和伴行的动、静脉。深层主要有第十二胸神经后支的肌支。⟨主治⟩ 痞块、腰痛、胃痛,以及肝脾肿大、肝炎、胃炎、肠炎、肾下垂等。直刺0.5至1寸;可灸。

Pigen (EX-B 4) An extra point, seen in *Yixue Rumen* (*An Introduction to Medicine*). ⟨Location⟩ on the lower back, below the spinous process of the lst lumbar vertebra, 3.5 cun lateral to the posterior midline (Fig. 61). ⟨Regional anatomy⟩ skin → subcutaneous tissue → latissimus muscle of back → inferior posterior serratus muscle → iliocostal muscle. In the superficial layer, there are the lateral cutaneous branches of the posterior branch of the 12th thoracic nerve and the accompanying artery and vein. In the deep layer, there are the muscular branches of the posteror branch of the 12th thoracic nerve. ⟨Indications⟩ mass in the epigastrium and abdomen, lower back pain, gastric pain, hepatomegly and splenomgaly, hepatitis, gastritis, enteritis, nephroptosia, etc. ⟨Method⟩ Puncture perpendicularly 0.5-1.0 cun. Moxibustion is applicable.

●偏骨[piān gǔ] 经穴别名。见《循经考穴编》。即肩髃。见该条。

Piangu Another name for Jianyu(LI 15), a meridian point seen in *Xunjing Kaoxue Bian (Studies on Acupoints along Meridians)*. →肩髃①(p.191)

●偏肩[piān jiān] 经穴别名。见《针灸大成》。即肩髃①。见该条。

Pianjian Another name for Jianyu(LI 15), a meridian point seen in *Zhenjiu Dacheng (A Great Compendium of Acupuncture and Moxibustion)*. →肩髃1.(p.191)

●偏历[piān lì] 经穴名。出《灵枢·经脉》。属手阳明大肠经,为本经络穴。〈定位〉屈肘,在前臂背面桡侧,当阳溪与曲池的连线上,腕横纹上3寸(图48和图6)。〈层次解剖〉皮肤→皮下组织→拇短伸肌→桡侧腕长伸肌腱→拇长展肌腱。浅层布有头静脉的属支,前臂外侧皮神经和桡神经浅支等结构。深层有桡神经的骨间后神经分支。〈主治〉鼻衄、目赤、耳聋、耳鸣、口眼歪斜、喉痛、癫疾、水肿、肩膊肘腕酸痛。斜刺0.3至0.5寸;可灸。

Pianli(LI 6) A meridian point, originally from *Ling Shu: Jing Mai (Miraculous Pivot: Meridians)*, the Luo(Connecting)Point of the Large Intestine Meridian of Hand-Yangming. 〈Location〉with the elbow slightly flexed, on the redial side of the dorsal surface of the forearm on the line connecting Yangxi(LI 5) and Quchi(LI 11), 3 cun above the crease of the wrist (Figs. 48&6). 〈Regional anatomy〉skin →subcutaneous tissue→short extensor muscle of thumb→long radial extensor muscle tendon of wrist → long abductor muscle tendon of thumb. In the superficial layer, there are the tributaries of the cephalic vein, the lateral cutaneous nerve of the forearm and the superficial branches of the radial nerve. In the deep layer, there are the branches of the posterior interosseous nerve of the radial nerve. 〈Indications〉epistaxis, redness of the eyes, deafness, tinnitus, deviation of the mouth and eye, sore throat, epilepsy and disorder of the head, edema, aching of the shoulder, arm, elbow and wrist. 〈Method〉Puncture obliquely 0.3~0.5 cun. Moxibustion is applicable.

●骈指押手[pián zhǐ yā shǒu] 押手方式之一。又称并指押手。四指并拢,以掌面平压于穴位上,另一手(刺手)持针,使针尖部穿过两指间的缝隙而刺入穴内。

Side-by-Side Finger Pressing One of the finger pressing methods, also named abreast finger pressing. Press the selected acupoint with the palmar side of the four fingers side by side, hold the needle with the other hand (needle-holding hand) and let the tip of the needle puncture the acupoint by passing through the space between the two fingers.

●平补平泻法[píng bǔ píng xiè fǎ] 针刺手法名。又称平针法、导气法。①指不分补泻的针刺方法。②与大补大泻相对,指手法较轻,刺激量较小的补泻法。

Uniform Reinforcing-Reducing A form of needling manipulation, also known as even needling method, qi-inducing method. ① Referring to needling manipulations which make no distinction between reinforcing and reducing. ② Opposite to strong reinforcing and strong reducing, referring to the reinforcing-reducing with mild needling manipulation and less stimulation.

●平喘[píng chuǎn] 为对屏尖之别称。详见该条。

Relieving Asthma(MA) Another name for Antitragic Apex(MA). →对屏尖(p.89)

●平衡区[píng héng qū] 头针刺激区。在前后正中线的后点旁开3.5厘米处的枕外粗隆水平线上,向下引平行于前正中线的4厘米长直线。〈主治〉小脑疾病引起的共济失调、平衡障碍、头晕、脑干功能障碍引起的肢体麻木瘫痪等病证。

Equilibrium Area One of the areas of stimulation by scalp acupuncture. 〈Location〉3.5 cun lateral to the posterior point of the anterior and posterior midline, a straight line of 4 cm in length from the external occipital tuberosity downward, which is parallel to the anterior and posterior midline. 〈Indications〉ataxia caused by carabellum disorders, dysequilibrium, dizziness, numbness and paralysis of the limbs resulting from dysfunction of the brain stem, etc.

●平翳[píng yì] 经穴别名。见《医宗金鉴·刺灸心法要诀》。即会阴。见该条。

Pingyi Another name for Huiyin(RN 1), a meridian point seen in *Yizong Jinjian: Cijiu Xinfa Yaojue (The Golden Mirror of Ortho-*

dox Medical Lineage: Essentials of Acupuncture and Moxibustion in Verse). →会阴(p.178)

●平针法[píng zhēn fǎ] 针刺手法名。出《医经小学·针法歌》卷五。指进针后只要求得气，而不分补泻的法。近人有换之为平补平泻法。见该条。

Even Needling A needling method, originally from Vol. 5 of *Yijing Xiaoxue: Zhenfa Ge (Elementary Collections of Medical Classics: Verse on Needling Techniques)*. There is only requirement for the needling reaction after the insertion of the needle, but no requirement for a certain reinforcing and reducing method. It is recently called uniform reinforcing and reducing. →平补平泻法(p.297)

●屏尖[píng jiān] 耳穴名。又称珠顶。位于耳屏上部隆起的尖端。具有清热止痛作用。〈主治〉发热、疼痛。

Tragic Apex (MA) An ear point, also known as Pearl Top(MA). 〈Location〉at the tip of the upper prominence on the border of the tragus. 〈Functions〉Clear heat and arrest pain. 〈Indications〉fever and pain.

●屏间切迹后窝[píng jiān qiē jì hòu wō] 耳廓解剖名称。耳垂背面下方，耳甲腔后隆起的下方凹窝，屏间切迹的背面。

Posterior Fossa of the Intertragic Notch A term of auricular anatomy. 〈Location〉in the superior part of the back of the ear lobe, the inferior depressed forssa of the posterior prominence of the cavum conchae, and the back of the intertragic notch.

●屏轮切迹[píng lún qiē jì] 耳廓解剖名称。对耳屏与对耳轮之间的凹陷。

Notch between the Tragus and the Anthelix A term of auricular anatomy. 〈Location〉in the depression between the tragus and anthelix.

●屏上切迹[píng shàng qiē jì] 耳廓解剖名称。耳屏上缘与耳轮脚之间的凹陷。

Upper Tragic Notch A term of auricular anatomy. 〈Location〉in the depression between the superior border of the tragus and crus of the helix.

●屏翳[píng yì] ①经穴别名。出《针灸甲乙经》。即会阴。见该条。②部位名。即平翳。详见该条。

1. **Pingyi** Another name for Huiyin(RN 1), a meridian point originally from *Zhenjiu Jia-Yi Jing (A-B Classic of Acupuncture and Moxibustion)*. →会阴(p.178)
2. **Perineum** A part of the body. →平翳(p.297)

●迫咳[pò ké] 即顿咳。详见该条。

Pressed Cough Another name for cough at a draught. →顿咳(p.90)

●破伤风[pò shāng fēng] 病证名。见《仙授理伤续断秘方》。又名伤痉、金疮痉。本病先由跌仆、金刃及竹木等造成肢体破伤，风邪由创口侵入而发病。本病在体表受伤一段时间后，出现牙关紧闭，四肢抽搐，角弓反张，颈项强直，面现苦笑之状，脉沉数或弦数。若病不解，正气大虚，邪毒内陷，则见神昏，呼吸急促，语声难出，多汗，脉沉弱等虚象。治宜解毒熄风。取百会、大椎、水沟、三间、后溪、委中、丰隆、申脉。

Tetanus A disease, seen in *Xianshou Lishang Xuduan Mifang (Secret Recipes from a Celestial for Treating Traumatological and Orthopedic Diseases)* also known as convulsion due to trauma, convulsion due to wound produced by metallic tool. This disease is first caused by trauma to the body and limbs produced by a fall, metallic tools or woody material, wind pathogens thus invade the body through the wound. 〈Manifestations〉convulsion of the limbs, opisthotonos, neck and nape rigidity and anguished grinning expression occurs some time after the body is injured. Deep and rapid or wiry and rapid pulse. In cases of persistent tetanus, severe deficiency of vital-qi and invasion of pathogens into the body may appear. Manifasted as crises such as coma, urgent, breath, difficlty in speaking, hyperhidrosis, deep and weak pulse. 〈Treatment principle〉Remove toxic substances and calm the endopathic wind. 〈Point selection〉Baihui (DU 20), Dazhui(DU 14), Shuigou(DU 26), Sanjian(LI 3), Houxi(SI 3), Weizhong(BL 40), Fenglong(ST 40) and Shenmai(BL 62).

●魄户[pò hù] 经穴名。出《针灸甲乙经》。属足太阳膀胱经。又名魂户。〈定位〉在背部，当第三胸椎棘突下，旁开3寸(图7)。〈层次解剖〉皮肤→皮下组织→斜方肌→菱形肌→上后锯肌→竖脊肌。浅层布有第三、四胸神经分支的皮支和伴行的动、静脉。深层有肩胛

背神经,肩胛背动、静脉。第三、四胸神经后支的肌支和相应的肋间后动、静脉背侧的分支或属支。〈主治〉肺痨、咳嗽、气喘、项强、肩背痛,斜刺0.5至0.8寸;可灸。

Pohu(BL 42)   A meridian point, originally from *Zhenjiu Jia-Yi Jing* (*A-B Classic of Acupuncture and Moxibustion*), a point on the Bladder Meridian of Foot-Taiyang, also named Hunhu. 〈Location〉on the back, below the spinous process of the 3rd thoracic vertebra, 3 cun lateral to the posterior midline (Fig. 7). 〈Regional anatomy〉skin→subcutaneous tissue →trapezius muscle→rhomboid muscle→superior posterior serratus muscle→erector spinal muscle. In the superficial layer, there are the cutaneous branches of the posterior branches of the 3rd and 4th thoracic nerves and the accompanying arteries and veins. In the deep layer, there are the dorsal scapular nerve, the dorsal scapular artery and vein, the muscular branches of the posterior branches of the 3rd and 4th thoracic nerves and the branches or tributaries of the dorsal branches of the related posterior intercostal arteries and veins. 〈Indications〉pulmonary tuberculosis, cough, dyspnea, neck rigidity, pain in the shoulder and back. 〈Method〉Puncture obliquely 0.5～0.8 cun. Moxibustion is applicable.

●铺灸[pū jiǔ]   灸法的一种。即长蛇灸。见该条。

Extending Moxibustion   Long-snake-like moxibustion, a form of moxibustion. →长蛇灸 (p. 40)

●仆参[pú cān]   经穴名。出《针灸甲乙经》。属足太阳膀胱经,为足太阳、阳跷之会。又名安邪。〈定位〉在足外侧部,外踝后下方,昆仑直下,跟骨外侧,赤白肉际处(图35)。〈层次解剖〉皮肤→皮下组织→跟骨。布有小隐静脉的属支、腓肠神经跟外侧到和腓动、静脉跟支。〈主治〉下肢痿弱、足跟痛、霍乱转筋、癫痫、脚气、膝肿。直刺0.3至0.5寸;可灸。

Pucan(BL 61)   A meridian point, originally from *Zhenjiu Jia-Yi Jing* (*A-B Classic of Acupuncture and Moxibustion*), a point on the Bladder Meridian of Foot-Taiyang, the Crossing Point of Foot-Taiyang and Yangqiao Meridians, also named Anxie. 〈Location〉on the lateral side of the foot, posterior and inferior to the external malleolus, directly below Kunlun (BL 60), lateral to the calcaneum, at the junction of the red and white skin (Fig. 35). 〈Regional anatomy〉skin→subcutaneous tissue→calcaneus. There are the tributaries of the small saphenous , vein, the lateral calcaneal branches of the sural nerve and the calcaneal branches of the peroneal artery and vein in this area. 〈Indications〉muscular atrophy and flaccidity of the lower limbs, pain in the heel, cramp in cholera morbus, epilepsy, beriberi, swelling of the knee. 〈Method〉Puncture perpendicularly 0.3～0.5 cun. Moxibustion is applicable.

●普济方[pǔ jì fāng]   书名。为明初编修的一部大型医学方书,朱橚等主编,原书一百六十八卷,清《四库全书》将其改订为四百二十六卷,为我国现存最大的方书。其中卷四百零九至四百二十四为针灸门,收录了许多针灸著作的内容。

Puji Fang (**Prescriptions for Universal Relief**)   A book compiled by Zhu Su in the early Ming Dynasty, originally in 168 volumes, revised later into 426 volumes in *SiKu Quanshu*(*Complete Works of Four Treasures*) in the Qing Dynasty, the largest voluminous medical formulary extant in our country. Vols 409-424 are of the acupuncture and moxibustion section and include contents of many works on acpuncture and moxibustion.

Q

● 七次脉 [qī cì mài] 指通过颈部有任督脉及手足三阳经,各有一主要穴。出《灵枢·本输》。(见表11)其中,天容穴在《灵枢》中属足少阳,后人归入手太阳。以上各穴,除天突、风府外,均是阳经在颈部有"入"穴。参见"根溜注入"条。

Seven-Line Points The principal points, located respectively on the Ren, Du and three Hand-Foot Yang Meridians, which pass through the neck, originally from *Ling Shu: Benshu (Miraculous Pivot: Acupoints)* (See Table 11). Among these points, Tianrong (SI 17) pertained to Foot-Shaoyang in *Lingshu (Miraculos Pivot)*, and was classified into Hand-Taiyang by later generations. All these acupoints except Tiantu (RN 22) and Fengfu (DU 16) are the entrance points of the neck on the yang meridian. →根溜注入(p. 141)

表11 七次脉
Table 11 Seven-line points

经脉名 Meridian	颈部穴 Point on the Neck
任 脉 Ren Meridian	天突 Tiantu (RN 22)
督 脉 Du Meridian	风府 Fengfu (DU 16)
手太阳 Hand Taiyang	天窗 Tianchuang (SI 16)
足太阳 Foot Taiyang	天柱 Tianzhu (BL 10)
手阳明 Hand Yangming	扶突 Futu (LI 18)
足阳明 Foot Yangming	人迎 Renying (ST 9)
手少阳 Hand Shaoyang	天牖 Tianyou (ST 16)
足少阳 Foot Shaoyang	天容 Tianrong (SI 17)

● 七星针 [qī xīng zhēn] 针具名。皮肤针的一种,形如小锤,由7枚细针组成,用以叩击浅刺皮肤,参见"皮肤针"条。(图36)

Seven-Star Needle A needling instrument, a form of dermal needle, shaped like a small hammer, composed of seven small needles fixed vertically at the end of a handle, used for superficial insertion. →皮肤针(p. 292)(Fig. 36)

● 期门 [qī mén] 经穴名。见《伤寒论》。属足厥阴肝经,为肝之募穴,足太阴、厥阴、阴维之会。〈定位〉在胸部,当乳头直下,第六肋间隙,前正中线旁开4寸(图40和图73)。〈层次解剖〉皮肤→皮下组织→胸大肌下缘→腹外斜肌→肋间外肌→肋间内肌。浅层布有第六肋间神经的外侧皮支,胸腹壁静脉的属支。深层有第六肋间神经和第六肋间后动、静脉的分支或属支。〈主治〉胸胁胀满疼痛,呕吐,呃逆,吞酸,腹胀,泄泻,饥不欲食,胸中热,咳嗽,奔豚,疟疾,伤寒热入血室。斜刺0.5~0.8寸;可灸。

Qimen (LR 14) A meridian point, seen in *Shanghan Lun (Treatise on Cold-Induced Diseases)*, a point on the Liver Meridian of Foot-Jueyin, the Front-Mu Point of the liver, and the crossing point of Foot-Taiyin, Foot-Jueyin and Yinwei Meridians. 〈Location〉 on the chest, directly below the nipple, in the 6th intercostal space, 4 cun lateral to the anterior midline (Figs. 40&73). 〈Regional anatomy〉 skin→subcutaneous tissue→inferior border of greater pectoral muscle → external oblique muscle of abdomen→external intercostal muscle-internal intercostal muscle. In the superficial layer, there are the lateral cutaneous branches of the 6th intercostal nerve and the tributaries of thoracoepigastric vein. In the deep layer, there are the 6th intercostal nerve and the branches or tributaries of the 6th posterior intercostal artey and vien. 〈Indications〉 pain, distention and fullness in the chest and hypochondriac region, vomiting, hiccup and regurgitation, abdominal distention, diarrhea, hunger with anorexia, irritability in the chest, cough, sensation of gas rushing, malaria, invasion of heat in the blood chamber due to febrile disease. 〈Method〉 Puncture obliquely 0.5~0.8 cun. Moxibustion is applicable.

● 齐刺 [qí cì] 《内经》刺法名。见《灵枢·官针》。又

称三刺、集合刺。为十二刺之一。是三针同用的一种刺法,正中刺一针,旁边夹刺二针。因其三针齐用,故名。以治疗范围较小而深的痹痛等症。

Assembling Puncture   A needling method in *Neijing* (*The Canon of Internal Medicine*), seen in *Lingshu: Guanzhen* (*Miraclous Pivot: Official Needles*), also named triple puncture, gathering puncture. One of the Twelve Needling Techniques, with three needles punctured together, one in the center of the affected part, the two others on both lateral sides. It is so named because the three needles are used togther. It is used for treating deep-rooted othralgia in small areas.

●岐伯[qí bó]   人名。传说中上古时医学家,为黄帝之师,后人又称岐天师。名见《内经》中。《内经》中多以黄帝,岐伯问答的形式来讨论医学理论问题。故后人常岐、黄并称,以代表医学。

Qi Bo   A legendary physician of ancient times, the teacher of Huang Di. Later generations called him Qi, the Heavenly Master, which can be seen in *Neijing* (*The Inner Canon of Huangdi*). In the book theoretical problems on medicine are mostly discussed in the form of questions and answers between Haung Di and Qi Bo. Therefore, Qi and Huang were often mentioned together by later generations as representing medicine.

●岐伯灸[qí bó jiǔ]   经外穴名。见《圣惠方》。又称脐下六一。位于脐下六寸处两旁各一寸六分(《神应经》作一寸)。灸治膀胱气冲两胁时,脐下鸣,阴卵入腹。

Qibojiu   An extra points, seen in *Shenghui Fang* (*Benevolent Prescriptions*), also named Qixialiuyi. 〈Location〉 on the lower abdomen, 6 cun below the centre of the umbilicus and 1.6 cun [1 cun, as stated in *Shen Ying Jing* (*Classic of God Merit*)] lateral to the anterior midline. 〈Indications〉 rushing-up of the bladder-qi to the hypochondrium, borborygmus, undescended testicle. 〈Method〉 moxibustion.

●岐伯灸经[qí bó jiǔ jīng]   书名。一作《黄帝问岐伯灸经》,撰人不详。见于《新唐书·艺文志》一卷。已佚。

Qi Bo Jiujing (**Qi Bo's Moxibustion Classic**)   A book, also known as *Huangdi Wen Qi Bo Jiujing* (*The Yellow Emperor's Questions on Qi Bo's Moxibustion Classic*) with its author unknown, seen in Vol. 1 of *Xin Tangshu: Yi Wen Zhi* (*The New History Book of the Tang Dynasty: Records of Art and Literature*), already lost.

●岐伯针经[qí bó zhēn jīng]   书名。一卷,已佚。见《宋史·艺文志》。

Qi Bo Zhenjing (**Qi Bo's Acupuncture Classic**)   Title of a book, no longer extant, seen in *Songshi: Yi Wen Zhi* (*The Song History Book: Records of Art and Literature*).

●岐骨[qí gǔ]   骨名。指相交成角的两骨。

Bone Juncture   A bone, referring to two bones which intersect and form an angle.

●奇经[qí jīng]   奇经八脉之简称。详见该条。

Extra Meridians   Short for the Eight Extra Meridians. →奇经八脉(p. 301)

●奇经八脉[qí jīng bā mài]   经络名。出《难经·二十七难》。简称奇经,八脉。指十二经脉之外具有不同作用的八条经脉,"奇"有奇零和奇异的含义。奇经八脉具有内不隶属脏腑,外无本经腧穴(任、督两脉除外)和无表里相配的特点,它错综于十二经脉之间,起着调节溢蓄十二正经脉气的作用,其内容包括督脉、任脉、冲脉、带脉、阳跷脉、阴跷脉、阳维脉、阴维脉。详见各条。

Eight Extra Meridians   A category of Meridians and collaterls, originally from *Nan Jing: Ershiqi Nan* (*The Classic of Questions: Question 27*), shortened as Extra Meridians or Eight Meridians, referring to the eight meridians with different functions from those of the Twelve Regular Meridians. "奇" means odd or peculiar. The Eight Extra Meridians have the following characteristics: None of them pertain interiorly to zang-fu organs, none have points exteriorly on its own meridians, with the exception of Du and Ren Meridians and none have external and internal matching relations. They intricately interlock the Twelve Regular Meridians, play a role in regulating and replenishing and storing the qi of the Twelve Regular Meridians, They include Du Meridian, Ren Meridian, Chong Meridian Dai Meridian, Yangqiao Meridian, Yinqiao Meridian, Yangwei Meridian, and Yinwei Meridian. See

these related entries.

●奇经八脉考 [qí jīng bā mài kǎo] 书名。明代李时珍著,一卷,刊于1578年。本书对奇经八脉的循行、主病、所属穴位进行考证,并提出个人见解,是一部研究奇经的重要著作。现有与《濒湖脉学》的合印本。

Qijing Ba Mai Kao (*A Study on the Eight Extra Meridians*)　A one-volume book, written by Li Shizhen in the Ming Dynasty, and published in 1578. In the book, he made textual research on the courses, major disorders and the related acupoints of the eight extra meridians, and put forward his personal views as well. It is an important work for the study of the Eight Extra Meridians. Extant is a co-edition of it with *Pinhu Maixue* (*Pinhu's Sphygmology*).

●奇经纳卦法 [qí jīng nà guà fǎ] 灵龟八法的别称。详见该条。

Method of Associating Extra Meridians with Eight Diagrams　Another name for Eight Methods of the Intelligent Turtle. →灵龟八法 (p. 248)

●奇经纳甲法 [qí jīng nà jiǎ fǎ] ①按时配穴法的一种,又称飞腾八法。见《玉龙经》。系以八脉八穴配八卦,按每日每个时辰的天干推算开穴。具体方法是:逢壬、甲时,开公孙(属乾);逢丙时,开内关(属艮);逢戊时,开临泣(属坎);逢庚时,开外关(属震);逢辛时,开后溪(属巽);逢乙、癸时,开申脉(属坤);逢己时,开列缺(属离);逢丁时,开照海(属兑)。例如甲子日,戊辰时,取临泣;乙巳时,取列缺;庚午时,取外关。②书名,一作《飞腾八法神针》。撰人不详。见明《医藏目录》。书佚。

1. Day-Prescriptions of Extra Meridians　A method for selecting acupoints in accordance with time, also known as Eight Soaring Methods, seen in *Yulong Jing* (*Jade Dragon Classic*), referring to matching the Eight Diagrams with the eight points of the Eight Extra Meridians to calculate the opening point in accordance with the heavenly stems of each period of time in a day. The detailed method is as follows: Select the opening point Gongsun (SP 4) (belonging to Qian diagram) in Ren and Jia; Neiguan (PC 6) (Gen diagram) in Bing; Linqi (Zu linqi, GB 41) (Kan diagrm) in Wu; Waiguan (SJ 5) (Zhen diagram) in Geng; Houxi (SI 3) (Xun diagram) in Xin; Shenmai (BL 62) (Kun diagram) in Yi and Gui; Lieque (LU 7) (Li diagram) in Ji, and Zhaohai (KI 6) (Dui diagram) in Ding. For instance, in the day of Jia-Zi, select Linqi (Zulinqi GB 41) in the Wu-Chen period of time (7a. m. -9a. m.); select Lieque (LU 7) in the Yi-Si period (9a. m. -11a. m.); and select Waiguan (SJ 5) in the Geng-Wu period (11a. m. -1p. m.).

2. Qijing Najia Fa (Day-Prescription of Acupoints of Extra Meridians)　A book also named *Feiteng Bafa Shenzhen* (*Miraculous Acupuncture of Soaring Eight Methods*), its author unmentioned, seen in *Yi Cang Mu Lu* (*Stored Catalogue of Medicine*) of the Ming Dynasty, no longer extant.

●奇输 [qí shū] 指经外奇穴。《类经图翼》有《奇俞类集》。

Peculiar Transmissive Points　Referring to extra points, *Qishu Lei Ji* (*A Collection for Classified Extra Points*) was once mentioned in *Leijing Tu Yi* (*Illustrated Supplements to Classified Canon of Internal Medicine of the Yellow Emperor*). →经外穴 (p. 214)

●奇穴 [qí xué] 指经外穴。详见该条。

Peculiar Points　Another name for extra points. →经外穴 (p. 214)

●脐 [qí] 经穴别名。即神阙。详见该条。

Qi　Another name for the meridian point Shenque (RN 8). →神阙 (p. 363)

●脐旁穴 [qí páng xué] 经外穴别名。出《针灸集成》。即疝气穴。详见该条。

Qipangxue　Another name for Shanqi-xue Point (EX-CA), an extra point originally from *Zhenjiu Jicheng* (*A Collection of Acupuncture and Moxibustion*). →疝气穴 (p. 349)

●脐上下五分穴 [qí shàng xià wǔ fēn xué] 经外穴名。见《千金要方》。在腹部,当脐上下各半寸。〈主治〉小儿囟陷、肠炎、下痢、水肿、疝痛、肠雷鸣、腹直肌痉挛胀、妇科病等。直刺0.5～1寸;可灸。

Qishangxiawufen Points (EX-CA)　Extra points, seen in *Qianjin Yaofang* (*Essential Prescriptions Worth a Thousand Gold*). 〈Location〉on the abdomen, 0.5 cun above and be-

low the umbilicus.〈Indications〉infantile fontanel sinking, entertis, dysentery, edema, pain due to hernia, borborygmus, spasm of straight muscle of abdomen, abdominal distention and tympanites, gynecological diseases, etc.〈Method〉Puncture perpendicularly 0.5～1 cun. Moxibustion is applicable.

●脐下六一[qí xià liù yī] 经外穴别名。即岐伯灸。详见该条。

Qixialiuyi Another name for the extra point, Qibojiu(EX-CA). →岐伯灸(p.301)

●脐中[qí zhōng] ①经穴别名。出《针灸甲乙经》。即神阙。详见该条。②耳穴艇中的别名，参见该条。

1. Qizhong Another name for Shenque(RN 8), a meridian point, originally from *Zhenjiu Jia-Yi Jing(A-B Classic of Acupuncture and Moxibustion)*. →神阙 (p.363)

2. Navel Center (MA) Another name for the ear point, middle cymba conchae. →艇中 Middle Cymba Conchae(MA) (p.440)

●脐中四边穴[qí zhōng sì biān xué] 经外穴名。见《千金要方》。在腹部，当脐中及其上下左右各1寸处。〈主治〉慢性肠炎、小儿一切痉挛、腹部疼痛、胃痉挛、水肿病、肠鸣、疝痛、胃扩张、消化不良等。直刺(脐中不针)0.5～1寸；可灸。

Qizhongsibian Points（EX-CA） Extra points, seen in *Qianjin Yaofang (Essential Prescriptions Worth a Thousand Gold)*〈Location〉on the abdomen, at the centre of and 1 cun superior, inferior and lateral to the umbilicus.〈Indications〉chronic enteritis, all kinds of spasm in childen, abdominal pain, gastric spasm, edema, borborygmus, pain due to hernia, gastric dilatation, indigestion, etc.〈Method〉Puncture perpendicularly 0.5～1 cun. Moxibustion is applicable.

●骑竹马穴[qí zhú mǎ xué] 经外穴名。出《备急灸法》。在背部，约当第10胸椎之两侧各旁开1寸处。灸治发背脑疽、肠痈、牙痛、风瘫肿痛、恶核瘰疬、四肢下部痈疽疔疮等。

Qizhuma Points(EX-B) Extra points, originally from *Beiji Jiufa (Moxibustion Method for Emergencies)*.〈Location〉on the back, about 1 cun lateral to the 10th thoracic vertebra.〈Indications〉carbuncle of the nape, acute appendicitis, toothache, tumor, jaundice due to wind pathogen, obstinate module and scrofula, carbuncle, cellulitis furuncle and sore on the lower part of the limbs.〈Method〉moxibustion.

●蛴螬灸[qí cáo jiǔ] 为隔蛴螬灸之别称。详见该条。

Grub Moxibustion Another name for grub-separated moxibustion. →隔蛴螬灸(p.137)

●綦针[qí zhēn] 古代生活用针具。见《灵枢·九针论》。此针为缝制衣帛的长针。九针中的长针，即仿自此针。

Extreme Needle A needle used in daily life in ancient times, seen in *Lingshu: Jiu Zhen Lun (Miraculous Pivot: On Nine Needles)*. It was a long needle used for sewing clothes and silk. The long needle among the nine needles is an imitation of this.

●气秘[qì bì] 便秘证型之一。见《济生方》。多因情志不畅，气机郁滞，疏泄失职所致。证见大便秘而不甚干结，腹胀痛连及两胁，口苦，目眩，嗳气，舌偏红，苔薄白，脉弦。治宜疏肝理气。取中脘、阳陵泉、气海、行间。

Constipation due to the Disorder of Qi A type of constipation, seen in *Jisheng Fang (Recipes for Saving Lives)*, mostly caused by the stagnation of qi and failure in dispersing the stagnated qi resulting from emotional disturbance.〈Manifestations〉constipation, defection without dry stool, abdominal distention and pain involving the two hypochondriums, bitter taste, blurring of vision, belching, reddish tongue with thin and whitish coating, wiry pulse.〈Treatment principle〉Soothe the liver and regulate the circulation of qi.〈Point selection〉Zhongwan (RN 12), Yanglingquan (GB 34), Qihai(RN 6) and Xingjian(LR 2).

●气冲[qì chōng] ①经穴名。出《针灸甲乙经》。属足阳明胃经，又名气街。〈定位〉在腹股沟稍上方，当脐中下5寸，距前正中线2寸(图40)。〈层次解剖〉皮肤→皮下组织→腹外斜肌腱膜→腹内斜肌→腹横肌。浅层布有腹壁浅动、静脉，第十二胸神经前支和第一腰神经前支的外侧皮支及前皮支。深层：下外侧在腹股沟管内有精索(或子宫圆韧带)、髂腹股沟神经和生殖股神经生殖支。〈主治〉外阴肿痛、腹痛、疝气、月

经不调、不孕、胎产诸疾、阳萎、阴茎中痛。直刺0.8~1.2寸；可灸。②经外穴名。出《千金要方》，又名气堂。详见该条。③经外穴别名。出《医学纲目》。即气中。详见该条。

1. Qichong (ST 30) A meridian point, originally from *Zhenjiu Jia-Yi Jing* (*A-B Classic of Acupuncture and Moxibustion*), a point on the Stomach Meridian of Foot-Yangming, also known as Qijie. ⟨Location⟩ slightly above the inguinal groove, 5 cun below the centre of the umbilicus and 2 cun lateral to the anterior midline (Fig. 40). ⟨Regional anatomy⟩ skin→subcutaneous tissue → aponeurosis of externaloblique muscle of abdomen → internal oblique muscle of abdomen→transverse muscle of abdmen. In the superficial layer, there are the superficial epigastric artery and vein, the lateral and anterior cutaneous branches of the anterior branches of the 12th thoracic nerve and the 1st lumbar nerve. In the deep layer, there are the spermatic cord (or round ligament of the uterus), the ilioinguinal nerve, and the genital branch of the genitofemoral nerve in the inguinal canal at the inferior laterior side of this point. ⟨Indications⟩ pain and swelling of the external genitalia, abdominal pain, hernia, irregular menstruation, sterility, diseases during pregnancy and delivery, impotence, pain in penis. ⟨Method⟩ Puncture perpendicularly 0.8~1.2 cun. Moxibustion is applicable.

2. Qichong (EX) An extra point, originally from *Qianjin Yaofang* (*Essential Prescriptions Worth a Thousand Gold*), also named Qitang. →气堂(p. 310)

3. Qichong Another name for Qizhong (EX-CA), an extra point originally from *Yixue Gangmu* (*An Outline of Medicine*). → 气中 (p. 315)

●气端 [qì duān] 经外穴名。见《千金要方》。⟨定位⟩在足十趾尖端，距趾甲游离缘0.1寸(指寸)，左右共十穴(图3)。⟨层次解剖⟩皮肤→皮下组织。神经支配是：拇趾和第二趾由来自腓浅神经的趾背神经、腓深神经的趾背神经和胫神经的趾足底固有神经支配；第三、第四趾由来自腓浅神经的趾背神经和胫神经的趾足底固有神经支配；小趾由来自腓肠神经的趾背神经、腓浅神经的趾背神经和胫神经的趾足底固有神经支配，血管供应是来源于足底内、外动脉的趾底固有动脉和足背动脉的趾动脉。⟨主治⟩脚气、足趾麻痹、足背红肿，并用于急救等。直刺0.1~0.2寸，或点刺出血；可灸。

Qiduan (EX-LE 12) An extra point, seen in *Qianjin Yaofang* (*Essential Prsceiptions Worth a Thousand Gold*). ⟨Location⟩ ten points at the tips of the 10 toes of both feet, 0.1 cun from the free margin of each toenail (Fig. 3). ⟨Regional anatomy⟩ skin→subcutaneous tissue. ⟨Innervation⟩ The point on the great and 2nd toes is innervated by the dorsal digital nerves from the superficial peroneal and deep peroneal nerves, and the proper digital plantar nerve from the tibial nerve. The point on the 3rd and 4th toes is innervated by the dorsal digital nerve from the superficial peroneal nerve and the proper digital plantar nerve from the tibial nerve. The point on the little toe is innervated by the dorsal digital nerve from the sural nerve and from the superficial peroneal nerve, and the proper digital plantar nerve from the tibial nerve. ⟨Vasculature⟩ The points are supplied by the proper digital plantar artery from the medial and lateral planter arteries of the foot and the dorsal digital artery from the dorsal artery of the foot. ⟨Indications⟩ beriberi, paralysis and numbness of the toes, pain and swelling of the dorsum, and also for emergencies. ⟨Method⟩ Puncture perpendicularly 0.1 ~ 0.2 cun or prick to cause bleeding. Moxibustion is applicable.

●气反 [qì fǎn] 《内经》取穴法别名，指取穴与病所相反。参见"上病下取"、"下病上取"、"中病旁取"各条。

Opposite Qi A form of point selection in *Neijing* (*The Canon of Internal Medicine*) referring to the point selection opposite to the diseased area. → 上病下取 (p. 351)、下病上取 (p. 486)、中病旁取 (p. 608)

●气府 [qì fǔ] 经穴别名。出《针灸甲乙经》。即京门。详见该条。

Qifu Another name for Jingmen (GB 25), a meridian point originally from *Zhenjiu Jia-Yi*

Jing(*A-B Classic of Acupuncture and Moxibustion*). →京门(p. 207)

●**气鼓**[qì gǔ]　鼓胀证型之一。见《杂病源流犀烛》肿胀源流。多因七情郁结,肝郁气滞,气病及血,肝病及脾,输布失职,水湿内停所致。证见腹部膨隆,四肢消瘦,皮色不变,按之陷而即起,恼怒后胀势更甚,嗳气或矢气则舒,大便不爽,苔薄白,脉弦细,治宜疏肝理气,调中消胀。取膻中、中脘、气海、足三里、太冲。

Tympanites due to the Stagnation of Qi　A type of tympanites, seen in *Za Bing Yuanliu Xizhu*(*Bright Candle to Pathology of Miscellaneous Diseases*), mostly due to the stagnation of seven emotions, stagnation of liver-qi, qi-disease affecting blood, pathological changes of the liver affecting the spleen, inability to transport water which leads to the retention of water within the body. ⟨Manifestations⟩ abdominal distention, thin limbs, normal color of skin when depressed, immediate retention of the original state, more serious distention after a rage, or comfort after eructation of wind from bowels, constipation, thin and white coating, taut and thready pulse. ⟨Treatment principle⟩ Relieve the deperessed liver, regulate the Middle Jiao to relieve flatulence. ⟨Point selection⟩ Danzhong (RN 17), Zhongwan (RN 12), Qihai (RN 6), Zusanli (ST 36) and Taichong (LR 3).

●**气管**[qì guǎn]　耳穴名。位于外耳道口与心穴之间。用于治疗咳喘。

Tachea(MA-IC 2)　An otopoint. ⟨Location⟩ between the orifice of the external auditory meatus and Heart (MA). ⟨Indications⟩ cough and dyspnea.

●**气海**[qì hǎi]　①经穴名。见《针灸甲乙经》。属任脉。又名脖胦、下肓、下气海。⟨定位⟩在下腹部,前正中线上,当脐中下1.5寸(图40)。⟨层次解剖⟩皮肤→皮下组织→腹白线→腹横筋膜→腹膜外脂肪→壁腹膜。浅层主要布有第十一胸神经前支的前皮支和脐周静脉网。深层主要有第十一胸神前支的分支。⟨主治⟩绕脐腹痛、水肿鼓胀、脘腹胀满、水谷不化、大便不通、泄痢不禁、癃淋、遗尿、遗精、阳萎、疝气、月经不调、痛经、经闭、崩漏、带下、阴挺、产后恶露不止、胞衣不下、脏气虚惫、形体羸瘦、四肢乏力。直刺0.5～1寸;可灸。孕妇慎用。②四海之一,指膻中。见《灵枢·海论》。详见该条。

Qihai(RN 6)　①A meridian point, seen in *Zhenjiu Jia-Yi Jing*(*A-B Classic of Acupuncture and Moxibustion*), a point of the Ren Meridian, also named Boyang, Xiahuang or Xiaqihai. ⟨Location⟩ on the lower abdomen on the anterior midline, 1.5 cun below the center of the umbilicus (Fig. 40). ⟨Regional anatomy⟩ skin→subcutaneous tissue→linea alba→transverse fascia→extraperitoneal fat tissue → parietal peritoneum. In the superficial layer, there are the anterior cutaneous branches of the anterior branches of the 11th thoracic nerve and the periumbilical venous network. In the deep layer, there are the branches of the anterior branch of the 11th thoracic nerve. ⟨Indications⟩ abdominal pain around the navel, edema and tympanites, distention and fullness in the stomach and abdmen, poor food digestion, constipation, diarrhea, dysuria and stronguria, enuresis, emission, impotence, hernia, irregular menstruation, dysmenorrhea, amenorrhea, metrorrhagia and metrostaxis, leukorrhea, prolapse of uterus, lochiorrhea after delivery, retained placenta, deficiency of zang-qi, thinness, myasthenia of limbs. ⟨Method⟩ Puncture perpendicularly 0.5～1.0 cun. Moxibustion is applicable. Use caution with pregnant women. ②One of the Four Seas, referring to Danzhong (RN 17), seen in *Lingshu: Hai Lun* (*Miraculous Pivot: On Seas*). →膻中(p. 75)

●**气海俞**[qì hǎi shù]　经穴名。出《太平圣惠方》。属足太阳膀胱经。⟨定位⟩在腰部,当第三腰椎棘突下,旁开1.5寸(图7)。⟨层次解剖⟩皮肤→皮下组织→背阔肌腱膜和胸腰筋膜浅层→竖脊肌。浅层布有第三、四腰神经后支的皮支和伴行的动、静脉。深层有第三、四腰神经后支的皮支和伴行的动、静脉。深层有第三、四神经后支的肌支和相应腰动、静脉的分支或属支。⟨主治⟩腰痛,腿膝不利,痛经,痔漏。直刺0.8～1.0寸;可灸。

Qihaishu(BL 24)　A meridian point, originally seen in *Taiping Shenghui Fang*(*Imperial Benevolent Prescriptions*), a point on the Bladder Meridian of Foot-Taiyang. ⟨Location⟩ on the low back, below the spinous

process of the 3rd lumbar vertebra, 1.5 cun lateral to the posterior midline (Fig. 7). 〈Regional anatomy〉 skin → subcutaneous tissue → aponeurosis of latissimus muscle of back and superficial layer of thoracolumbar fascia → erector spinal muscle. In the superficial layer, there are the cutaneous branches of the posterior branches of the 3rd and 4th lumbar nerves and the accompanying arteries and veins. In the deep layer, there are the muscular branches of the posterior branches of the 3rd and 4th lumbar nerves and the branches or tributaries of the related lumbar arteries and veins. 〈Indications〉 lumbago, difficulty in the movement of legs and knees, dysmenorrhea and hemorrhoids complicated by anal fistula. 〈Method〉 Puncture perpendicularly 0.8～1.0 cun. Moxibustion is applicable.

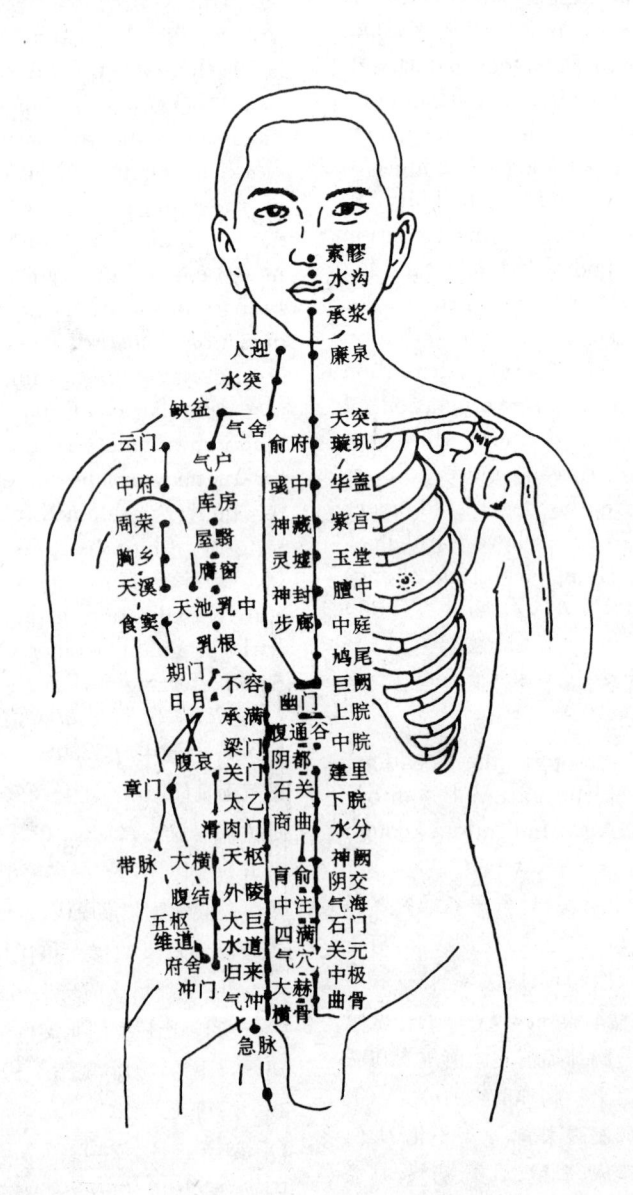

图40 气户等胸腹部穴

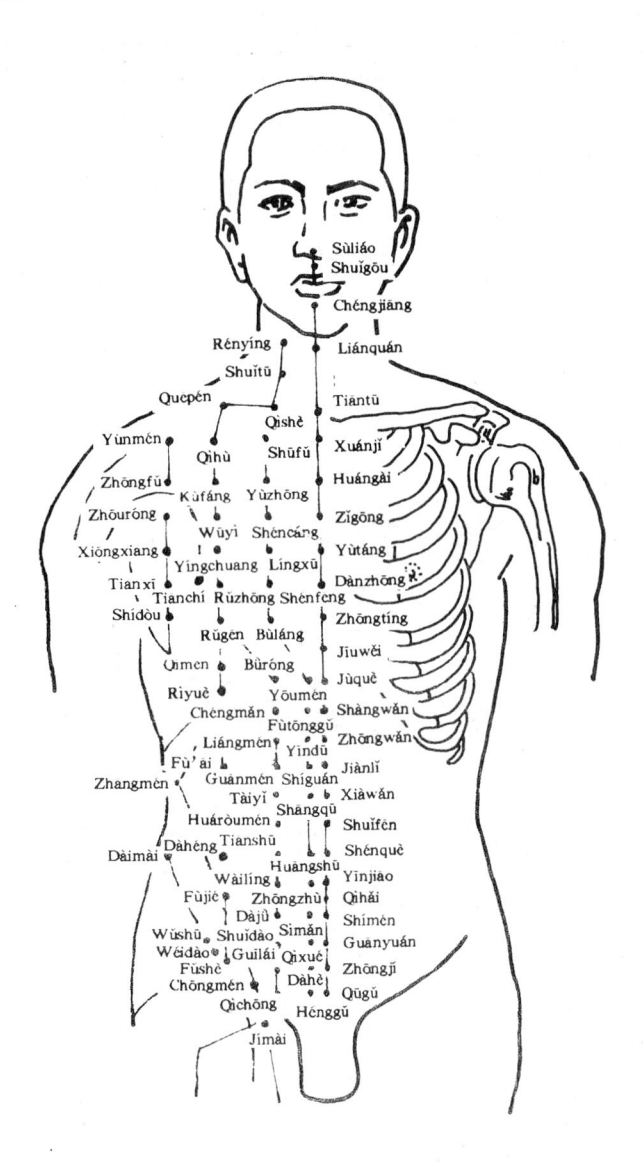

Fig 40 Qihu and other points of chest and abdomen

● 气合 [qì hé] 经穴别名。见《铜人腧穴针灸图经》。即神阙，详见该条。

Qihe Another name for Shenque (RN 8), a meridian point seen in *Tongren Shuxue Zhenjiu Tu-jing* (*Illustrated Manual of Points for Acupuncture and Moxibustion on a Bronze Statue with Acupoints*). → 神阙 (p. 363)

● 气户 [qì hù] 经穴名。出《针灸甲乙经》。属足阳明胃经。〈定位〉在胸部，当锁骨中点下缘，距前正中线4寸（图75）。〈层次解剖〉皮肤→皮下组织→胸大肌。浅层布有锁骨上中间神经。深层有腋动脉和它的分支胸肩峰动脉。〈主治〉气喘、咳嗽、胸胁胀满、吐血、呃逆、胸背、胁肋疼痛。直刺0.2～0.4寸；可灸。

Qihu (ST 13) A meridian point, originally from *Zhenjiu Jia-Yi Jing* (*A-B Classic of Acupuncture and Moxibustion*), a point on the Stomach Meridian of Foot-Yangming. 〈Location〉on the chest, below the midpoint of the lower border of the clavicle, 4 cun lateral to the anterior midline (Fig. 75). 〈Regional anatomy〉skin→subcutaneous tissue→greater pectoral muscle. In the superficial layer, there is the intermediate supraclavicular nerve, in

307

the deep layer, there are the exillary artery and the thoracoacromial artery. 〈Indication〉 asthma, cough, distention and fullness in the chest and hypochondrium, hematemesis, hiccup, pain in the chest, back and hypochondrium. 〈Method〉 Puncture perpendicularly 0.2~0.4 cun. Moxibustion is applicable.

●气街[qì jiē] ①指经气聚集通行的共同道路。出《灵枢·动输》等篇。其范围超出经脉主干之外,分四气街,又称四街,即头气街、胸气街、腹气街、胫气街,手足三阳经都通于头,故脑为头气之街;手三阴经皆通于胸,故胸前和肺俞、心俞等背俞为胸气之街;足三阴经又均通于腹,故肝俞、脾俞、肾俞等及腹旁的冲脉交会穴为腹气之街;足部之经通于气冲穴;故髋骶部及承山、踝上下部为胫气之街。气街的理论说明了经络在头、胸、腹、胫的分段联系。意义与标本、根结相通。②指腹股沟动脉处,如足阳明胃经循行,入气街中。该处有气冲穴。③气冲穴别名。详见该条。

1. Qi-Streets The common way along which the qi of meridians (and collaterals) gathers and passes, originally from *Lingshu: Dongshu (Miraculous Pivot: Continuous Motion of Transportation)*, etc. There are four streets of qi (also named four streets for short) beyond the mainstay of the meridians, i.e. the head street, the chest street, the abdomen street, and the leg street. Because three yang meridians of hand and foot pass through the head, the brain is the street of head qi; because all three yin meridians of the hand pass through the chest, the anterior chest and some back-shu points such as Feishu(BL 13) and Xinshu (BL 15) are the street of chest qi; because all three yin meridins of the foot pass through the abdomen, Ganshu (BL 18), Pishu (BL 20), Shenshu(BL 23), and the crossing points of the Chong Meridian are the street of abdomen qi; because all the meridians of the foot pass through Qichong(ST 30), the hip-sacral region, Chengshan(BL 57), the parts inferior and superior to the ankle are the street of leg qi. The theory of the qi-streets shows the sectional connections of meridians and collaterals in the head, chest, abdomen and leg. Its meaning is that the superficiality and origin, gen (root) and jie (tip) are all connected.

2. Qi-street The area in the groin where pulsation of the femoral artery can be felt. e. g. the Stomach Meridian of Foot-Yangming finds its way in the pathway of qi, and located here is Qichong(ST 30).

3. Qijie Another name for Qichong (ST 30). →气冲(p. 303)

●气厥[qì jué] 厥证证型之一。见《丹溪心法·厥》。指因气机逆乱而引起的昏厥。气厥有虚实之分。如素体健壮,偶因恼怒,突然昏倒,口噤握拳,呼吸急粗,四肢厥冷,舌苔薄白,脉沉弦者为实证,治宜苏厥开窍,取水沟、内关、太冲。若素体虚弱,疲劳惊恐导致的眩晕昏仆,面色苍白,呼吸微弱,汗出肢冷,舌质淡,脉沉微者为虚证,治宜回阳救逆。取百会、气海、足三里。

Syncope Resulting from Disorder of Qi A type of syncope from *Danxi Xinfa: Jue (Danxi's Experience: Jue-Syndromes)*, due to the disorder of qi. It is divided into two types: excess and deficiency. The former due to occasional anger is manifested by sudden fainting in strong people accompanied by lockjaw, fists, shortness of breath, cold limbs, thin and whitish coating, deep and taut pulse. 〈Treatment principle〉Wake the faint by inducing resuscitation. 〈Point selection〉 Shuigou (DU 26), Neiguan(PC 6) and Taichong(LR 3). The latter is manifested by dizziness and fainting due to weakness of the body and is accompanied by pale complexion, fatigue and terror, shallow breathing, sweating, cold limbs, pale tongue, deep and feeble pulse. 〈Treatment principle〉Recuperate depleted yang and rescue the patient form collapse. 〈Point selection〉 Baihui(DU 20), Qihai(RN 6) and Zusanli(ST 36).

●气淋[qì lín] 淋证证型之一。出《脉经》。又名气癃。多因老年肾气衰惫,州都气化不利所致。证见少腹及会阴部胀痛不适,排尿乏力,小便断续,甚则点滴而下,尿意频仍,少气,腰酸,神疲,舌质淡,脉细弱。治宜健脾利湿,益肾固涩。取肾俞、膀胱俞、脾俞、气海、水道、足三里、三阴交。

Stranguria Caused by the Disorder of Qi A type of stranguria, originally from *Maijing (The Classic of Sphygmology)*, also named dysuria due to the disorder of qi. Mostly due

to the deficiency of kidney-qi in the aged, causing disturbance of qi transformation in the bladder. ⟨Manifestations⟩ distending pain in the lower abdomen and the perineum, ascheturesis, short breath, soreness of the waist, mental fatigue. pale tongue, thready and weak pulse. ⟨Treatment principle⟩ Strengthen the spleen and remove dampness by diuresis, tonify the kindney and induce astringency. ⟨Point selection⟩ Shenshu (BL 23), Pangguangshu(BL 28), Pishu(BL 20), Qihai(RN 6), Shuidao (ST 28), Zusanli (ST 36) and Sanyinjiao(SP 6).

●气癃[qì lóng] 见《诸病源候论·淋病诸候》。即气淋。详见该条。

Dysuria due to the Disorder of Qi stranguria, seen in *Zhubing Yuanhou Lun: Lin Bing Zhu Hou*(*General Treatise on the Etiology and Symptomatology of Diseases: Causes and Symptoms of Stranguria*). →气淋(p. 308)

●气门[qì mén] 经外穴名。见《千金要方》。在下腹部,关元旁3寸。⟨主治⟩不孕、崩漏、阴挺、淋症、尿闭、疝气、睾丸炎等。直刺1~1.5寸;可灸。

Qimen (EX-CA) An extra point, seen in *Qianjin Yaofang* (*Essential Prescriptions Wroth a Thousand Gold*). ⟨Location⟩on the lower abdomen, 3 cun lateral to Guanyuan (RN 4). ⟨Indications⟩ sterility, metrorrhagia and metrostaxis, prolapse of uterus, stranguria, anuresis, hernia, orchitis. ⟨Method⟩ Puncture perpendicularly 1.0~1.5 cun. Moxibustion is applcicable.

●气纳三焦[qì nà sān jiāo] 子午流注针法用语,与血纳包络相对。《针灸大全》谓:阳干注腑,甲、丙、戊、庚、壬而重见者,气纳于三焦。即指当阳干重见时,分别按生成的关系取三焦经的五输穴。如甲日于甲戌时开胆经井穴,丙子时取小肠经荥穴,戊寅时取胃经输穴,庚辰时取大肠经经穴,壬午时取膀胱经合穴,至甲申时重见甲,取三焦经荥(水)穴。甲属木。为水生木关系。

Qi Entering Sanjiao An acupuncture term of midnight-noon ebb-flow versus blood entering pericardium. According to *Zhenjiu Daquan* (*A Complete Work of Acupuncture and Moxibustion*), the qi enters the Sanjiao when the yang heavenly stems enter the fu-organs and one of the heavenly stems of Jia (甲), Bing(丙), Wu(戊), Geng(庚) and Ren (壬) appears again. In other words, when yang-heavenly stems appear again, select the five-shu points of the meridian of sanjiao according to the relationship of generation. For instance, select the Jing (Well) points of the Gallbladder Meridian in the Jia-Xu(甲戌)period(7 p.m.-9p.m.)of the day of Jia(甲); the Ying (Spring) points of the Small Intestine Meridian in the Bing-Zi(丙子) period (11p.m.-1a.m.); the Shu (Stream) points of the Stomach Meridian in the Wu-Yin(戊寅) period(3a.m.-5a.m.); the Jing (River) points of the Large Intestine Meridian in the Geng-Chen(庚辰)period (7a.m.-9a.m.); the He (River) points of the Bladder Meridian points in the Ren-Wu(壬午) period(11a.m.-1p.m.) and Jia(甲)appear again in the Jia-Shen(甲申) period (3p.m.-5p.m.), so select the Ying (Spring) points of the Sanjiao Meridian. Jia belongs to wood and this is based on the relationship of water promoting wood.

●气舍[qì shè] 经穴名。出《针灸甲乙经》。属足阳明经。⟨定位⟩在颈部,当锁骨内侧端的上缘,胸锁乳突肌的胸骨头与锁骨头之间(图6.4和图40)。⟨层次解剖⟩皮肤→皮下组织和颈阔肌→胸锁乳突肌的胸骨头与锁骨头之间,浅层布有锁骨上内侧神经,颈横神经的分支和面神经颈支。深层有联络两侧颈前静脉和颈前静脉弓和头臂静脉。⟨主治⟩咽喉肿痛、喘息、呃逆、瘿瘤、瘰疬、颈项强痛、肩肿。直刺0.3~0.4寸;可灸。

Qishe(ST 11) A meridian point, originally from *Zhenjiu Jia-Yi Jing* (*A-B Classic of Acupuncture and Moxibustion*), a point on the Stomach Meridian of Foot-Yangming. ⟨Location⟩on the neck at the upper border of the medial end of the clavicle, between the sternal and clavicular heads of the sternocleidomastoid muscle (Figs. 6.4&40). ⟨Regional anatomy⟩ skin→subcutaneous tissue and platysma muscle→between sternal head and clavicular head of sternocleidomastoid muscle. In the superficial layer, there are the branches of the medial supraclavical nerve, the transverse nerve of the neck and the cervical branches of the nerve. In the deep layer, there are the arch connecting

the bilateral anterior jugular veins and the brachiocephalic vein. 〈Indications〉 swelling and pain of throat, dyspnea, hiccup, goiter, scrofula, stiffness and pain of the neck and nape, swollen shoulder. 〈Method〉 Puncture perpendicularly 0.3~0.4 cun Moxibustion is applicable.

●气俞[qì shū] 经穴别名。出《针灸甲乙经》。即京门。详见该条。

Qishu Another name for Jingmen(GB 25), a meridian point originally from *Zhenjiu Jia-Yi Jing* (*A-B Classic of Acupuncture and Moxibustion*). →京门(p.207)

●气堂[qì táng] 经外穴别名。即经外穴气冲。详见该条。

Qitang Another name for an extra point Qichong. →气冲(p.303)

●气虚崩漏[qì xū bēng lòu] 崩漏证型之一。多因素体脾虚,或饮食劳倦。损伤脾气,中气不足,统摄无权,冲任不固所致。证见血崩下血,或淋漓不绝,血色淡红,面色㿠白,身体倦怠,气短懒言,不思饮食,舌质淡,苔薄白,脉细弱,治宜补益中州,固摄经血。取关元、三阴交、肾俞、交信、气海、脾俞、足三里、膏肓。

Metrorrhagia and Metrostaxis due to Qi Deficiency A type of metrorrhagia and metrostaxis, mostly due to the constitutional insufficiency of the spleen, or improper diet and overstrain, impairment of the spleen-qi, deficiency of qi in the Middle-Jiao, inability to control blood, debility of the Chong and Ren Meridians. 〈Manifestations〉 metrorrhagia, or lingering and light red menstruation, pale complexion, tiredness, short breath, tiredness when speaking, lack of appetite, pale tongue with thin and whitish coating, thready and weak pulse. 〈Treatment principle〉 Replenish the middle-jiao to stop menstruation. 〈Point selection〉 Guanyuan (RN 4), Sanyinjiao (SP 6), Shenshu (BL 23), Jiaoxin (KI 8), Qihai (RN 6), Pishu (BL 20), Zusanli (ST 36) and Gaohuang (BL 43).

●气虚经行先期[qì xū jīng xíng xiān qī] 经行先期证型之一。多因素体虚弱,忧思伤脾,或饮食不节,损伤脾胃,以致中气不足,冲任失固,经血妄行所致。证见经期提前,血量较多,色淡红,质清稀,面色㿠白,精神疲倦,心悸气短,纳少便溏,小腹下坠,舌淡苔薄,脉弱无力。治宜补气摄血,健脾固冲。取膻中、关元、血海、足三里、脾俞、隐白。

Precede Menstrual Cycle due to Qi Deficiency A type of preceded menstrual period, mosly due to constitutional deficiency, impairment of the spleen with melancholy or improper diet impairing the spleen and the stomach, deficiency of qi in the middle-jiao, debility of Chong and Ren Meridians, leading to uncontrollable menstruation. 〈Manifestations〉 advanced menstrual period, strong but pale red and thin menstrual flow, pale complexion, mental fatigue, palpitations, short breath, lack of appetite, loose stool, weighty sensation in the lower abdomen, pale tongue with thin coating, weak pulse. 〈Treatment principle〉 Induce hemostasis by invigorating qi, invigorate the spleen and consolidate the Chong Meridian. 〈Point selection〉 Danzhong (RN 17), Guanyuan (RN 4), Xuehai (SP 10), Zusanli (ST 36), Pishu (BL 20) and Yinbai (SP 1).

●气虚心悸[qì xū xīn jì] 心悸证型之一。见《伤寒明理论》。由阳气虚,心失温养所致。证见心脏悸动不宁,难以自主,善惊易恐,短气,手心多汗,神倦,不易入睡,静卧休息症状可自动减轻。舌苔薄白,脉细数。治宜益安神。取心俞、巨阙、间使、神门。

Palpitations due to Qi Deficiency A type of palpitation, seen in *Shanghan Mingli Lun* (*Exposition on Principles of Exogenous Cold-Induced Diseases*), frequently due to Yang-qi deficiency, the heart lacking warmth and nourishment. 〈Manifestations〉 uncontrollable palpitations, susceptibility to the fright, sleeplessness which can be eased with the patient in a peaceful lying position, thin and white coating, thready and rapid pulse. 〈Treatment principle〉 Supplement qi and tranquilize the mind. 〈Point selection〉 Xinshu (BL 15), Juque (RN 14), Jianshi (PC 5) and Shenmen (HT 7).

●气虚月经过多[qì xū yuè jīng guò duō] 月经过多证型之一。多因身体虚弱,忧思伤脾,中气不足,冲任失固,血失约制所致,证见经行血量过多,或行以时间延长,色淡,质稀,面色㿠白,精神疲倦,气短懒言,

或心悸,小腹空坠。治宜补气摄血,健脾固冲。取膻中、脾俞、中脘、建里、足三里。

Menorrhagia due to Qi Deficiency　　A type of menorrhagia, mostly due to a constitutional deficiency and impairment of the spleen with melancholy, deficiency of qi in the middle-Jiao, debility of the Chong and the Ren Meridians and blood lacking control. 〈Manifestations〉menorrhagia, or longer menstrual period, light-colored and thin menstruation, pale complexion, mental fatigue, short breath, tiredness when speaking, palpitations, hollow and weighty sensation in the lower abdomen. 〈Treatment principle〉Induce hemostasis by invigorating qi, strengthening the spleen to consolidate the Chong Meridian. 〈Point selection〉Danzhong (RN 17), Pishu (BL 20), Zhongwan (RN 12), Jianli (RN 11) and Zusanli (ST 36).

●**气虚痔疮**[qì xū zhì chuāng]　　痔疮证型之一。多因泻痢日久,劳倦,胎产。亦有因出血过多,肛肠气血不调所致。证见面色萎黄,痔脱垂于肛门之外而不能回纳,肛门坠胀,短气懒言,食少乏力,舌淡,脉弱。治宜益气升陷,取百会、长强、关元俞、膈关。

Hemorrhoid due to Qi Deficiency　　A type of hemorrhoid, mostly due to lingering dysentery, over exertion, delivery or too much bleeding, derangment of qi and blood in the anus and intestine. 〈Manifestations〉sallow complexion, prolapse of hemorrhoids, tenesmic and distending sensation of the anus, short breath, tiredness when speaking, lack of appetite, weakness, pale tongue, weak pulse. 〈Treatment principle〉Supplement qi and elevate the sinking qi. 〈Point selection〉Baihui (DU 20), Changqiang (DU 1), Guangyuanshu (BL 26) and Geguan (BL 46).

●**气虚子宫脱垂**[qì xū zǐ gōng tuō chuí]　　子宫脱垂证型之一。多因分娩时用力太过,或产后过早劳力劳动,损伤中气致气虚下陷,胞系无力所致。证见阴道中有鹅卵样物脱出,自觉下腹下坠,精神疲惫,四肢乏力;少气懒言,面色㿠白,白带量多,舌淡苔薄,脉虚弱。治宜益气升阳,固摄胞宫。取百会、气海、维道、足三里、三阴交。

Hysteroptosis due to Qi Deficiency　　A type of hysteroptosis, mostly due to over-exertion in delivery, impairment of qi of the middle-jiao, leading to the sinking of qi in the middle-jiao and flaccidity of the uterus. 〈Manifestations〉something like a goose egg coming out of the vagina, tenesmic sensation in the lower abdomen, mental fatigue, lasitude of limbs, short breath, tiredness when speaking, pale complexion, much leukorrhea, pale tongue with thin coating, feeble and weak pulse. 〈Treatment principle〉Supplement qi, elevate Yang and consolidate the uterus. 〈Point selection〉Baihui (DU 20), Qihai (RN 6) Weidao (GB 28), Zusanli (ST 36) and Sanyinjiao (SP 6).

●**气穴**[qì xué]　　①经穴名。出《针灸甲乙经》。属足少阴肾经。为冲脉、足少阴之会。又名胞门、子户。〈定位〉在下腹部,当脐中下3寸,前正中线旁0.5寸(图40)。〈层次解剖〉皮肤→皮下组织→腹直肌鞘前壁→腹直肌。浅层布有腹壁浅动、静脉的分支或属支,第十一、十二胸神经前支和第一腰前支的前皮支及伴行的动、静脉。深层有腹壁下动、静脉的分支或属支。第十一、十二胸神经前支的肌支和相应的肋间动、静脉。〈主治〉月经不调、白带、小便不通、泄泻、痢疾、腰脊痛、阳萎。直刺或斜刺0.8～1.2寸;可灸。②出《素问•气穴论》。指腧穴。详见该条。

1. **Qixue** (KI 13)　　A meridian point, originally from *Zhenjiu Jia-Yi Jing* (*A-B Classic of Acupuncture and Moxibustion*), a point on the Kidney Meridian of Foot-Shaoyin, the crossing point of the Chong Meridian and the Meridian of Foot-Shaoyin, also named Baomen and Zihu. 〈Location〉on the lower abdomen, 3 cun below the centre of the umbilicus and 0.5 cun lateral to the anterior midline (Fig. 40). 〈Regional anatomy〉skin→subcutaneous tissue→anterior of rectus muscle of abdomen→rectus muscle of abdomen. In the superficial layer, there are the branches or tributaries of the superficial epigastric artery and vein, the anterior cutaneous branches of the anterior branches of the 11th and 12th thoracic and 1st lumbar nerve and the accompanying arteries and veins. In the deep layer, there are the branches or tributaries of the inferior epigastric artery and vein, the muscular branches of the anterior branches of the 11th and 12th thoracic nerve and the related inter-

costal arteries and vein. 〈Indications〉irregular menstruation, leukorrhea, anurresis, diarrhea, dysentery, pain along spinal column, impotence. 〈Method〉Puncture perpendicularly or obliquely 0.8~1.2 cun. Moxibustion is applicable.

2. Acupoints Originally from *Suwen*:*Qi Xue Lun*(*Plain Questions*:*On Loci of Qi*). →腧穴 (p. 407)

●气血不足痿证[qì xuè bù zú wěi zhèng] 痿证证型之一。由脾胃亏虚,精微不输,无以濡养五脏,气血失盈,筋脉肌肉失养,关节不利所致,证见肢体痿软无力,逐渐加重,食少便溏,腹胀,面浮而色不华,气短,神疲乏力,苔薄白,脉细。治宜通经活络,补脾益气。取肩髃、合谷、阳溪、髀关、梁丘、足三里、解溪、中脘、气海、三阴交、大包。

Flaccidity Syndrome due to Deficiency of Qi and Blood A type of flaccidity syndrome due to insufficiency of both the spleen and the stomach, the disorder of food essence transportation, failing to nourish the five zang organs, deficiency of both qi and blood, lack of nourishment in tendon, meridians and muscles, difficulty in the movement of joints. 〈Manifestations〉flaccidity and weakness of the body, which gradually becomes serious, lack of appetite, loose stool, abdominal distention, edema of the face and dim complexion, short breath, lassitude and spiritual tiredness, thin and whitish tongue coating, thready pulse.〈Treatment principle〉Clear and activate the meridians and collaterals; invigorate the spleen and replenish qi. 〈 Point selection 〉 Jianyu(LI 15), Hegu(LI 4), Yangxi(LI 5), Biguan (ST 31), Liangqiu (ST 34), Zusanli (ST 36), Jiexi(ST 41), Zhongwan(RN 12), Qihai(RN 6), Sanyinjiao(SP 6) and Dabao (SP 21).

●气血虚弱乳少[qì xuè xū ruò rǔ shǎo] 乳少证型之一。多因脾胃虚弱,化源不足,或临产失血过多,气血耗损所致。证见乳汁不行,或行亦甚少,乳房无胀感,面色苍白,唇爪无华,或精神倦怠,食少便溏,舌淡无苔,脉虚细。治宜益气补血,佐以通乳。取膻中、乳根、脾俞、足三里。

Hypogalactia due to Deficiency of Qi and Blood A type of hypogalactia, mostly caused by weakness of the spleen and the stomach, lack of formation of qi and blood, or much blood loss with parturient, which leads to the deficiency of qi and blood. 〈Manifestations〉galactostasis, or little milk, without distending sensation in the breasts, pale complexion, pale lips and nails, spiritual tiredness, lack of appetite, loose stool, pale tongue without coating, feeble and thready pulse. 〈Treatment principle〉 Supplement qi and enrich the blood and promote lactation. 〈 Point selection 〉 Danzhong(RN 17), Rugen(ST 18), Pishu(BL 20) and Zusanli(ST 36).

●气血虚弱痛经[qì xuè xū ruò tòng jīng] 痛经的证型之一,多因体质素虚,气血不足,经行之后气血更虚,以致冲任胞脉失养所致。证见经后小腹绵绵作痛,喜温喜按,经血量少,色淡质稀,面色无华,舌淡脉细弱。治宜补气养血,扶脾止痛。取脾俞、胃俞、足三里、关元、三阴交。

Dysmenorrhea due to Deficiency of Qi and Blood A type of dysmenorrhea frequently due to constitutional deficiency, or a deficiency of qi and blood, which becomes more serious after the menstrual period, lack of nourishment of the Chong, Ren and Uterus Meridians. 〈Manifestations〉lingering light pain in the lower abdomen, preference for warmth and pressing, light flow, light-colored and thin menstruation, dim complexion, pale tongue, thready and weak pulse. 〈 Treatment principle〉Invigorate qi and nourish the blood; support the spleen and alleviate pain. 〈Point selection〉 Pishu (BL 20), Weishu (BL 21), Zusanli(ST 36), Guanyuan(RN 4) and Sanyinjiao(SP 6).

●气阴两伤脱疽[qì yīn liǎng shāng tuō jū] 脱疽证型之一。见于疾病的后期,证见患肢皮肤暗红,肉枯筋萎,溃破腐烂,疼痛剧烈,彻夜不安,趺阳脉消失。腐肉脱落,面色萎黄,形瘦神疲,舌淡苔薄白,脉缓。治宜益气养阴。取关元、太溪、足三里、太渊、血海、少府。

Gangrene of Finger or Toe due to Deficiency of Both Qi and Yin A type of gangrene of the finger or toe which occurs at the anaphase of a disease. 〈Manifestations〉dark red skin of the affected part, muscular atrophy, diabrosis,

putrefaction, serious pain, sleeplessness all night, disappearance of fuyang pulse, exfoliation of slough, sallow complexion, thinness, listlessness, pale tongue with thin and whitish coating, leisurely pulse. 〈Treatment principle〉 Supplement qi and nourish yin. 〈Point selection〉Guanyuan (RN 4), Taixi (KI 3), Zusanli (ST 36), Taiyuan (LU 9), Xuehai (SP 10) and Shaofu (HT 8).

●气瘿[qì yǐng] 病证名。出《千金要方》。多因情志抑郁或水土因素，进而气、痰、瘀三者互结于颈部而成。证见颈部粗大，温肿或结块，皮宽而不紧，皮色不变，缠绵难消不溃破，初起全身症状明显，其后可出现咽干口燥，急躁易怒，心悸多汗，五心烦热等证，若阴虚火旺者，可兼见形体消瘦，易饥多食，失眠，潮湿多汗，舌红少苔，脉细数。治宜滋阴降火。取臑会、气舍、间使、太冲、太溪，若气阴两虚者，可兼见气短乏力，便溏纳少，面色萎黄，自汗，舌淡少津，脉细弱。治宜益气养阴。取合谷、天鼎、天突、关元、照海。

Qi Goiter A disease, originally from *Qianjin Yaofang* (*Essential Prescriptions Worth a Thousand Gold*), mostly due to feelings of depression, or the climate and other environmental factors of a place, with the stagnation of qi, phlegm and blood stasis in the cervicle part. 〈Manifestations〉 thick neck, chronic swelling or caking, loose skin with normal color, which linger but do not ulcerate. Obvious symptoms all over the body at the initial stage, developing into dry throat and mouth, dysphoria, irritability, palpitations, hyperhidrosis, dysphoria with feverish sensation in the chest, palms and soles. If the case is one of hyperactivity of fire due to yin deficiency, such manifestations as thinness, frequent sense of hunger, overeating, insomnia, moisture, hyperhidrosis, red tongue with little coating, thready and rapid pulse can also be seen. 〈Treatment principle〉 Nourish yin to reduce pathogenic fire. 〈Point selection〉Naohui (SJ 13), Qishe (ST 11), Jianshi (PC 5), Taichong (LR 3), and Taixi (KI 3); if the case is one with deficiency of both qi and yin, manifestations are as such: short breath, weakness, loose stool, sallow complexion, lack of appetite, spontaneous perspiration, pale tongue with little fluid, thready and weak pulse. 〈Treatment principle〉 Supplement qi and nourish yin. 〈Point selection〉Hegu (LI 4), Tianding (LI 17), Tiantu (RN 22), Guanyuan (RN 4) and Zhaohai (KI 6).

●气郁崩漏[qì yù bēng lòu] 崩漏证型之一。多因肝气郁结，气郁化火，木火炽盛，藏血失职所致。证见崩漏下血，兼见胸胁胀痛，心烦易怒，时欲叹息、脉弦数。治宜疏肝理气止血。取气海、三阴交、隐白、太冲、支沟、大敦。

Metrorrhagia and Metrostaxis due to Qi Stagnation A type of metrorrhagia and metrostaxis, mostly due to the stagnation of the liver-qi, fire transmitted from qi stagnation, excessive wood-fire, the disorder of storing blood. 〈Manifestations〉 metrorrhagia and metrostaxis, accompanied by distending pain in the hypochondrium, vexation, irritability, occasional longing to sigh, taut and rapid pulse. 〈Treatment principle〉Stop bleeding by relieving the depressed liver. 〈Point selection〉Qihai (RN 6), Sanyinjiao (SP 6), Yinbai (SP 1), Taichong (LR 3), Zhigou (SJ 6) and Dadun (LR 1).

●气郁呃逆[qì yù ènì] 呃逆证型之一。因情志抑郁，肝气上乘肺胃，胃气上冲所致。证见呃逆连声，常因情志不畅而加重，伴胸闷、纳减、脘胁胀闷、肠鸣矢气，舌苔薄白，脉弦，治宜顺气解郁，降逆止呃，取天突、膈俞、内关、足三里、行间、侠溪、太溪、期门。

Hiccup due to Qi Stagnation A type of hiccup due to depressed emotions, hyperactive liver-qi attacking the lung and the stomach, adverse rising of the stomach-qi. 〈Manifestations〉 constant hiccup, worsened by low spirit, accompanied by oppressed feeling in the chest, lack of appetite, distention and oppressive feeling in the stomach, and hypochondrium, borborygmus, wind from bowels, thin and whitish tongue coating, taut pulse, 〈Treatment principle〉Lower the adverse flow of qi to alleviate mental depression. 〈Point selection〉Tiantu (RN 22), Geshu (BL 17), Neiguan (PC 6), Zusanli (ST 36), Xingjian (LR 2), Xiaxi (GB 43), Taixi (KI 3) and Qimen (LR 14).

●气郁胃痛[qì yù wèi tòng] 胃痛证型之一。多因气

郁伤肝，肝气犯胃，气机阻滞所致。证见胃脘胀闷，攻撑作痛，痛连两胁，嗳气频繁，大便不畅，每因情志刺激而痛发，舌苔薄白，脉沉弦，治宜疏肝理气止痛，取中脘、足三里、内关、期门、太冲、阳陵泉。

Stomachache due to Qi Stagnation　A type of stomachache, mostly caused by impairment of the liver due to qi stagnation, hyperactive liver-qi attack upon the stomach, resulting in the qi stagnation. ⟨Manifestations⟩ distention and fullness in the stomach, distending pain in the hypochobdria, frequent eructation, constipation, pain due to stimulation of emotions, thin and whitish tongue coating, deep and taut pulse. ⟨Treatment principle⟩ Disperse the depressed liver-qi and alleviate pain. ⟨Point selection⟩ Zhongwan (RN 12), Zusanli (ST 36), Neiguan (PC 6), Qimen (LR 14), Taichong (LR 3) and Yanglingquan (GB 34).

●气原 [qì yuán]　经穴别名。出《针灸甲乙经》。即中极。详见该条。

Qiyuan　Another name for Zhongji (RN 3), a meridian point originally from *Zhenjiu Jia-Yi Jing (A-B C lassic of Acupuncture and Moxibustion)*. →中极 (p. 611)

●气针 [qì zhēn]　①针具名。出《针灸聚英》。指毫针，与火针相对而言。②针刺法。指用注射器将消毒过的空气或氧气，注入穴位的方法，适用于治疗急阳性软组织损伤和落枕等症。

Qi Needle　① A type of needle, originaly from *Zhenjiu Juying (Essentials of Acupuncture and Moxibustion)*; referring to filiform needle, vs. fire needle. ② An acupuncture therapy, the method of injecting sterilized air or oxygen into an acupoint with an injector. ⟨Indications⟩ acute of chronic soft tissue injury and stiffness, etc.

●气之阴郄 [qì zhī yīn xì]　经穴别名。出《针灸甲乙经》。即长强。详见该条。

Qizhiyinxi　Another name for Changqiang (DU 1), a meridian point originally from *Zhenjiu Jia-Yi Jing (A-B Classic of Acupuncture and Moxibustion)*. →长强 (p. 39)

●气至病所 [qì zhì bìng suǒ]　针刺术语。出《针经指南》。气是指针下得气的感应，这种得气感应通过一定的手法，使它到达病变部位，故称，由此可获得更好的疗效。

Arrival of Qi at the Affected Area　A term in acupuncture, originally from *Zhenjing Zhinan (A Guide to the Classic of Acupuncture)*. Qi here refers to the needling sensation, which reaches the affected part by means of manipulations, hence the name. As a result, better curative effect can be achieved.

●气滞经行后期 [qì zhì jīng xíng hòu qī]　经行后期证型之一，多因郁怒伤肝，气机不畅，冲任胞脉血行受阻，以致经血不能按时下达胞宫，证见经期错后，血量较少，经色黯红，夹有瘀块，小腹胀痛，胸胁乳房作胀，舌苔薄白，脉弦。治宜疏肝解郁，理气行血，取气海、气穴、三阴交、太冲、行间、蠡沟。

Delayed Menstrual Period due to Qi Stagnation　A type of delayed menstrual period, mostly caused by impairment of the liver by stagnated anger, impeded circulation of qi, blocked blood circulation of the meridians of Chong, Ren and uterus, inability of menstruation to get to the uterus on time. ⟨Manifestations⟩ delayed menstrual period, light flow and dark red menstruation with blood clots, distending pain in the lower abdomen, distention in the chest, hypochondrium and breasts, thin and whitish coating, taut pulse. ⟨Treatment principle⟩ Relieve the depressed liver, regulate the flow of qi and promote circulation of blood. ⟨Point selection⟩ Qihai (RN 6), Qixue (KI 13), Sanyinjiao (SP 6), Taichong (LR 3), Xingjian (LR 2) and Ligou (LR 5).

●气滞痛经 [qì zhì tòng jīng]　痛经证型之一。多因肝郁气滞，血行受阻，冲任运行不畅，经血滞于胞宫所致。证见经前或经期小便胀痛，胀甚于痛，经行不畅，月经量少，常伴有血块，兼见胸胁乳房胀痛，舌质黯或有瘀斑，苔薄红，脉沉弦。治宜疏肝解郁，理气调整经。取气海、太冲、三阴交、阳陵泉、天枢、内关。

Dysmenorrhea due to Qi Stagnation　A type of dysmenorrhea, mostly due to the stagnation of liver-qi, impeded blood circulation, blocked Chong and Ren Meridians, the stagnation of menstruation in uterus. ⟨Manifestations⟩ distending pain in the lower abdomen before or during menstrual period, with distention more serious than pain, blocked menstruation, light menstruation accompanied by blood clots, dis-

tending pain in hypochondria and breasts, dark tongue with ecchymosis, thin and reddish coating, deep and taut pulse. 〈Treatment principle〉Relieve the depressed liver and regulate the flow of qi to promote menstrual discharge. 〈Point selection〉Qihai(RN 6), Taichong(LR 3), Sanyinjiao (SP 6), Yanglingquan(GB 34), Tianshu(ST 25) Neiguan (PC 6).

●气滞血瘀经闭[qì zhì xuè yū jīng bì] 经闭证型之一。多因肝气郁结,气机不畅,血滞不行所致,证见经闭不行,精神抑郁,烦躁易怒,胸胁胀满,小腹胀痛拒按,舌质紫黯有瘀点,脉沉弦。治宜疏肝理气,活血化瘀,取中极、地机、三阴交、太冲、合谷、期门、支沟。

Amenorrhea due to Stagnancy of Qi and Blood Stasis　A type of amenorrhea, mostly caused by the stagnation of liver-qi, impeded circulation of qi and the stagnation of blood. 〈Manifestations〉amenorrhea, mental depression, dysphoria, distention and fullness of the chest and hypochondrium, distending pain and tenderness in the lower abdomen, dark purple tongue with ecchymosis, deep and taut pulse. 〈Treatment principle〉Relieve the depressed liver and promote blood circulation by removing blood stasis. 〈Point selections〉Zhongji(RN 3), Diji(SP 8), Sanyinjiao (SP 6), Taichong (LR 3), Hegu (LI 4), Qimen (LR 14) and Zhigou(SJ 6).

●气滞血瘀脱疽[qì zhì xuè yū tuō jū] 脱疽证型之一。由气滞血瘀所致。疾病初、中期阶段,患肢畏寒麻木,刺痛,开始出现间歇性跛行,趺阳脉搏动无力,病程日久,则见局部皮肤发冷,持续疼痛,肌肉萎缩,行走困难,足背皮肤颜色变紫、汗毛脱落,趾甲变厚,趺阳脉消失或减弱,脉沉细而迟。治宜活血通络,取膈俞、关元俞、气海、足三里、三阴交、昆仑、冲阳。

Gangrene due to Stagnation of Qi and Blood Stasis　A type of gangrene of the finger or the toe, caused by the stagnation of qi and blood stasis. 〈Manifestations〉intolerance of cold, numbness and aching, pain of limbs, intermittent claudication, weak fuyang pulse in the initial and middle stages; cold sensation and constant pain of local skin, syophagism, difficulty in walking, purple skin of dorsum of the foot, trichomadesis, thickening of toenail, disappearing and weakening of fuyang pulse, deep, thready and slow pulse in the lingering stage. 〈Treatment principle〉Promote blood circulation to remove obstruction in the meridians. 〈Point selection〉Geshu (BL 17), Guanyuanshu(BL 26), Qihai(RN 6), Zusanli (ST 36), Sanyinjiao(SP 6), Kunlun(BL 60) and Chongyang(ST 42).

●气中[qì zhōng] 经外穴名。见《医学纲目》。又名气冲。在下腹部,气海旁1寸,〈主治〉妇人血弱气喘。直刺2寸。

Qizhong(EX-CA)　An extra point, from *Yinxue Gangmu*(*An Outline of Medicine*), also named Qichong. 〈Location〉on the lower abdomen, 1 cun lateral to Qihai(RN 6). 〈Indication〉asthma due to blood deficiency in women. 〈Method〉Puncture perpendicularly 2 cun.

●掐法[qiā fǎ] 针刺手法名。见《奇效良方·针灸门》。以指甲进行按压。

Finger-Nail Pressing　A needling method, seen in *Qixiao Liangfang: Zhenjiu Men* (*Prescriptions of Wonderful Efficacy: Field of Acupunture and Moxibustion*), referring to the manipulation by pressing at an acupoint with a finger-nail.

●千金方　[qiān jīn fāng] 书名。为《千金要方》和《千金翼方》的统称。详见各条。

Qianjin Fang (Prescriptions Worth a Thousand Gold)　A joint title of *Qianjin Yaofang* (*Essential Prescriptions Worth a Thousand Gold*) and *Qianjin Yifang* (*Supplement to Essential Prescriptions Worth a Thousand Gold*).
→千金要方(p.316)、千金翼方(p.316)

●千金十穴歌[qiān jīn shí xué gē] 针灸歌赋名。见《针灸大全》。其将十个常用效穴的主治部位概括为歌诀。即:三里内庭穴,肚腹中妙诀,曲池与合谷,头面恙可彻,腰背痛相连,委中昆仑穴,胸项如有痛,后溪并列缺,环跳与阳陵,膝前兼腋胁。可补即留久,当泻即疏泄。三百六十名,十为千金穴。

Qianjin Shi Xue Ge (A Verse of Ten Acupoints Worth a Thousand Gold)　A verse about acupuncture and moxibustion, seen in *Zhenjiu Daquan* (*A Complete Work of Acupuncture and Mocxibustion*). It summa-

rizes 10 effective acupoints and the locations of its indications into a verse, which reads: Select Sanli (ST 36) and Neiting (ST 44) to treat diseases of the abdomen; puncture Quchi (LI 11)and Hegu (LI 4)to treat diseases in the head and face; select Weizhong (BL 40) and Kunlun (BL 60) to treat pain both in the loin and back; Houxi (SI 3)and Lieque (LU 7) are selected when there is pain in the chest and nape; use Huantiao(GB 30) and Yanglingquan (GB 34), to treat diseases in the axilla and hypochondrum, as well as in the anterior of the knee; retain the needle for a long period of time to reinforce, or reduce if appropriate, Amongst the 360 acupoints, these ten are the most important.

●**千金要方**[qiān jīn yào fāng] 书名。全名《备急千金要方》。唐代孙思邈著。三十卷,成书于652年。全书较系统地总结了唐以前的医学成就,取材丰富,有较高的参考价值,其搜集了大量针灸学文献,除散见于各病证主治项下的针灸处方外,二十九、三十两卷专论针灸。该书对经穴作了认真的考订,首次绘制出彩色针灸图三幅,收载穴位349个,并记载了大量的经外穴;最先提出"阿是穴"的名称及几种指寸取穴法,至今仍被临床应用。

Qianjin Yaofang（Essential Prescriptions Worth a Thousand Gold） A 30-volume book, compiled by Sun Simiao of the Tang Dynasty and finished in A.D. 652. Its full name is *Beiji Qianjin Yaofang（Essential Prescriptions for Emergencies Worth a Thousand Gold）*. It summarizes the medical achievements prior to the Tang Dynasty. Drawing materials from a wide range, the book is of great reference value. In it are collected a large number of works on acupuncture and moxibustion. The 29th and the 30th volumes mainly involve monographs on acupuncture and moxibution in addition to the prescriptions of acupuncture and moxibustion of separate diseases. Careful textual research was made on meridian points, 3-color diagrams of acupuncture and moxibustion were drawn for the first time. 349 acupoints along with many extra points were included in it. The book was the first to present the name of "Ashi point" and several finger-length measuements, which are still adopted in clinic today.

●**千金翼方**[qiān jīn yì fāng] 书名,唐代孙思邈著。为《千金要方》的续编,共三十卷。成书于682年。内容包括药灵、妇人、伤寒、小儿、养性、辟谷、退居、补益、杂病、疱痈、色脉、针灸、禁经等。其中二十六至二十八卷专论针灸,介绍了取穴法,汇集了二十七种病证的针灸治疗方法,其中灸法尤多,论述了针灸适应证和禁忌证,补充了《千金要方》的缺漏。

Qianjin Yifang（Supplement to Essential Prescriptions Worth a Thousand Gold） A 30-volume book, compiled by Sun Simiao of the Tang Dynasty and finished in A.D. 682, the continuation of *Qianjin Yaofang（Essential Prescriptions Worth a Thousand Gold）*, including "Criteria of Medicine", "Women's Diseases", "Exogenous Febrile Diseases", "Infants", "Health Preserving", "Keeping Away Grain", "Living in Seclusion", "Restoration", "Miscellaneous Diseases", "Sore and Carbuncle", "Complexion and Pulse Condition", "Acupuncture and Moxibustion", "Forbidden Meridians," etc. Vols. 26-28 are monographs on acupuncture and moxibustion which introduce the methods of selecting points, compile the acupuncture and moxibustion therapies of 27 diseases, of which the moxibustion therapy makes up its most part, expound indications and contraindications of acupuncture and moxibustion and replenish the gaps and omissions of *Qianjin Yaofang（Essential Prescriptions Worth a Thousand Gold）*.

●**牵正**[qiān zhèng] 经外穴名。见《常用新医疗法手册》。在耳垂前0.5寸,与耳垂中点相平处。〈主治〉面神经麻痹、腮腺炎、口腔溃疡等。斜刺或沿皮刺0.5～1寸;可灸。

Qianzheng（EX-HN） An extra point, seen in *Chang Yong Xinyi Liaofa Shouce（A Manual of New Therapies in Frequent Use）*.〈Location〉0.5 cun anterior to the ear lobe, on the level of the midpoint of the ear lobe.〈Indications〉facial paralysis, parotitis, stomachache.〈Method〉Puncture obliquely or subcutaneously 0.5～1 cun. Moxibustion is applicable.

●**前顶**[qián dǐng] 经穴名。出《针灸甲乙经》。属督脉。〈定位〉在头部,当前发际正中直上3.5寸(百会

前1.5寸)(图28)。〈层次解剖〉皮肤→皮下组织→帽状腱膜→腱膜下疏松组织。布有额神经左、右颞浅动、静脉和额动、静脉的吻合网。〈主治〉癫痫,头晕,目眩,头顶痛,鼻渊,目赤肿痛,小儿惊风。平刺0.3～0.5寸;可灸。

Qianding (DU 21)　A meridian point, originally from *Zhenjiu Jia-Yi Jing* (*A-B Classic of Acupuncture and Moxibustion*), a point on the Du Meridian. 〈Location〉on the head, 3.5 cun directly above the midpoint of the anterior hairline and 1.5 cun anterior to Baihui (DU 20)(Fig. 28). 〈Regionsl anatomy〉skin →subcutaneous tissue→epicranial aponeurosis →subaponeurotic loose tissue. There are the frontal nerve, the anastomotic network of the left and right superficial temporal arteries and veins with the left and right frontal arteries and veins in this area. 〈Indications〉epilepsy, vertigo, dizziness, pain in the vertex, rhinorrhea with turbid discharge, redness, swelling and pain of the eyes, infantile convulsion. 〈Method〉Puncture subcutaneously 0.3～0.5 cun. Moxibustion is applicable.

●前发际穴[qián fà jì xué]　①经外穴名。出《刺疗捷法》。在太阳穴直上3寸,当发际处。〈主治〉颜面疔疮。沿皮刺0.3～0.5寸;可灸。②即发际穴。详见该条3。

1. Qianfaji Point(EX-HN)　An extra point, originally from *Ciding Jiefa* (*Simple Acupuncture Method for Boils*).〈Location〉3 cun directly above Taiyang (EX-HN 5), on the hairline. 〈Indication〉facial furuncle. 〈Method〉Puncture subcutaneously 0.3～0.5 cun. Moxibustion is applicable.

2. Qianfaji　→发际 3. (p. 103)

●前谷[qián gǔ]　经穴名。出《灵枢·本输》。属手太阳小肠经,为本经荥穴。〈定位〉在手尺侧,微握拳,当小指本节(第五掌指关节)前的掌指横纹头赤白肉际(图48和图65)。〈层次解剖〉皮肤→皮下组织→小指近节指骨基底部。有尺神经的指背神经,尺神经的指掌侧固有神经和小指尺掌侧动、静脉等结构。主治热病汗不出、疟疾、癫狂、痫证、耳鸣、目痛、目翳、头顶急痛、颊肿、鼻塞、咽喉肿痛、产后无乳、臂痛、肘挛、手指麻木。直刺0.2～0.3寸;可灸。

Qiangu (SI 2)　A meridian point, originally from *Lingshu*: *Benshu* (*Miraculous Piovt*: *Meridian Points*), the Ying (Spring) point of the Small Intestine Meridian of Hand-Taiyang. 〈Location〉at the junction of the red and white skin along the ulnar border of the hand, at the ulnar end of the crease of the 5th metacarpophalangeal joint when a loose fist is made (Figs. 48&65). 〈Regional anatomy〉skin →subcutaneous tissue→base of proximal phalanx of 5th finger. There are the dorsal digital nerve and the proper palmar digital nerve of the ulnar nerve and the ulnar palmar artery and vein of the 5th finger in this area. 〈Indications〉febrile diseases without sweat, malarial disease, manic-depressive disorder, epilepsy, tinnitus, pain in the eyes, nebula in eyes, sudden pain in the head and the nape, swollen cheek, stuffy nose, swelling and pain of the throat, agalactia after delivery, brachialgia, contracture of the elbow, numbness of the fingers. 〈Method〉Puncture perpendicularly 0.2～0.3 cun. Moxibustion is applicable.

●前关[qián guān]　①经穴别名。出《千金要方》。即瞳子髎。详见该条。②经外穴别名。出《太平圣惠方》。即太阳穴。详见该条。

Qianguan　Another name for ① Tongziliao (GB 1), a meridian point originally from *Qianjin Yaofang* (*Essential Prescriptions Worth a Thousand Gold*).→瞳子髎(p. 443) ② Taiyang (EX-HN 5), an extra point from *Taiping Shenghui Fang* (*Imperial Benevolent Prescriptions*).→太阳(p. 420)

●前后配穴法[qián hòu pèi xué fǎ]　配穴法之一。前,指头面、胸腹。后,指枕顶、腰背。前后部穴位配合使用,多用于五官及内脏疾病的治疗。例如眼病取睛明、风池。舌强不语取廉泉、哑门。胃病取中脘、胃俞等均是。偶刺法及俞募配穴法,也可归属此类。参见各条。

Combination of the Anterior-Posterior Points

A type of point prescription. Anterior refers to the face, head, chest and abdomen; posterior refers to occipitoparietal and lumbodorsal regions. Points in the anterior and posterior are used coordinately for the treatment of diseases of the five sense organs and

internal organs. For example, Jingming (BL 1) and Fengchi (GB 20) for ophthalmopathy; Lianquan (RN 23) and Yamen (DU 15) for inability to speak due to stiff tongue; Zhongwan (RN 12) and Weishu (BL 21) for gastropathy, etc. Both the paired needling and the combination of the Back-Shu points with the Front-Mu points belong to this method.
→偶刺(p. 287)、俞募配穴法(p. 406)

●前后正中线[qián hòu zhèng zhōng xiàn] 头针算定线,是从两眉间中点(正中线前点)至枕外粗隆尖锐下缘(正中线后点)经过头顶的连线。

Anterior-Posterior Midline Marking line for scalp acupuncture connecting the ophryon (the anterior point) with the inferior border of the inion (the posterior point).

●前列腺[qián liè xiàn] 耳穴别名。即艇角,详见该条。

Prostate (MA) Another name for the otopoint, Angle of Cymba Conchae (MA). →艇角(p. 440)

●前神聪[qián shén cōng] 经外穴名。出《类经图翼》。在头部,当前发际正中上4寸。主治中风、头痛、眩晕、癫痫等。沿皮刺0.3～0.5寸;可灸。

Qianshencong (EX-HN) An extra point, originally from *Leijing Tuyi* (*Illustrated Supplements to Classified Canon of Internal Medicine of the Yellow Emperor*). 〈Location〉 on the head, 4 cun above the midpoint of the anterior hairline. 〈Indications〉 apoplexy, headache, dizziness, epilepsy. 〈Method〉 Puncture subcutaneously 0.3～0.5 cun. Moxibustion is applicable.

●荨麻疹[qián má zhěn] 即风疹。详见该条。

Urticaria →风疹(p. 116)

●荨麻疹点[qián má zhěn diǎn] 耳穴名。风溪穴之别称。详见该条。

Urticaria Point (MA) Another name for the otopoint, Fengxi (Wind-Stream) (MA). →风溪(p. 115)

●钱镜湖[qián jìng hú] 人名。清针灸家,里籍不详。于1819年绘成《脏腑正伏侧人明堂图》四幅,遗有刻本。

Qian Jinghu An acupuncture-moxibustion expert of the Qing Dynasty, whose native place is unknown. He completed the four pictures of *Zang-Fu Zheng Fu Ce Ren Mingtang Tu* (*Charts of Acupoints and Zang-Fu Organs at Anteroir, Posterior and Lateral Views*) in 1819 and left its blockprinted edition.

●强刺激[qiáng cì jī] 针灸术语。指刺激强度较大的针灸方法。针刺一般以粗针、高频率、大幅度、长时间的捻转提插,病人针感较为强烈,并向四周或远端扩散。艾灸则以大炷、多壮,或长时间熏灸。适用于体质强壮,起病急骤的患者。

Strong Stimulation An acupuncture and moxibustion term, a needling method with strong stimulation. Generally, when puncture is applied with thick needles and high frequency, great amplitude and long-time twirling, lifting and thrusting, the patient gains a stronger needling sensation which then spreads in all directions or extends distally while moxibustion is characterized by large or multi-shape moxa cones or by long-time fumigation. It is used for acute diseases.

●强间[qiáng jiān] 经穴名。出《针灸甲乙经》,属督脉,又名大羽。〈定位〉在头部。当后发际正中直上4寸(脑户上1.5寸)(图28和图31)。〈层次解剖〉皮肤→皮下组织→帽状腱膜→腱膜下疏松组织。布有枕大神经及左、右枕动、静脉的吻合网。主治头痛、目眩、颈项强痛、癫狂痫证、烦心、失眠、口渴。平刺0.5～0.8寸;可灸。

Qiangjian (DU 18) A meridian point of Du Meridian, originally from *Zhenjiu Jia-Yi Jing* (*A-B Classic of Acupuncture and Moxibustion*), also named *Dayu*. 〈Location〉 on the head, 4 cun directly above the midpoint of the posterior hairline and 1.5 cun above Naohu (DU 17) (Figs. 28&31). 〈Regional anatomy〉 skin→subcutaneous tissue→epicranial aponeurosis→subaponeurotic loose tissue. There are the greater occipital nerve and anastomotic network of the left and right occipital arteries and veins in this area. 〈Indications〉 headache, dizziness, stiffness and pain of the neck and nape, manic-depressive disorder, epilepsy, dysphoria, insomnia, thirst 〈Method〉 Puncture subcutaneously 0.5～0.8 cun. Moxibustion is applicable.

● **强阳**[qiáng yáng] 经穴别名。出《针灸甲乙经》。即络却。详见该条。

Qiangyang Another name for Luoque (BL 8), a meridian point originally from *Zhenjiu Jia-Yi Jing* (*A-B Classic of Acupuncture and Moxibustion*). →络却(p.259)

● **窍阴**[qiào yīn] 经穴名。有二：一在头，一在足。同属足少阳胆经。为便于区分，《圣济总录》称前者为首窍阴，后者为足窍阴。《针灸资生经》改首窍阴为头窍阴。详见各条。

Qiaoyin A pair of meridian points of the Gallbladder Meridian of Foot-Shaoyang. One is on the head and the other on the foot. In order to distinguish them, the former is named Shouqiaoyin (GB 11), while the latter Zuqiaoyin (GB 44) in *Shengji Zonglu* (*Imperial Medical Encyclopaedia*). In *Zhenjiu Zisheng Jing* (*Acupuncture-Moxibustion Classic for Saving Life*) Shouqiaoyin was changed into its present-day name Touqiaoyin (GB 11). →首窍阴(p.405)、足窍阴(p.631)、头窍阴(p.444)

● **切法**[qiē fǎ] 针刺辅助手法名。出《金针赋》。为下针十四法之一，指进针前用手指爪甲于穴位部作切按动作，令气血宣散，便于进行。

Pressure Method An auxiliary manipulation of acupuncture, originally from *Jin Zhen Fu* (*Ode to Gold Needle*), one of the 14 forms of insertion, referring to pressing an acupoint with a finger nail before insertion to facilitate both qi and blood and make the insertion easy.

● **茄病**[qié bìng]即阴挺的别名。见该条，参见子宫脱垂条。

Eggplant-Like Prolapse Another name for prolapse of uterus. →阴挺(p.559)、子宫脱垂(p.625)

● **秦承祖**[qín chéng zǔ]人名。南北朝时期刘宋医学家，精通医药及针灸，著有《偃侧杂针灸经》、《偃侧人经》、《明堂图》等针灸书籍，均已佚。且其为较早绘制经络穴位图的医家之一。

Qin Chengzu A physician of the Liu Song Dynasty (A.D. 420-479) of the Northern and Southern Dynasties, proficient in medicine and acupuncture and moxbustion, and the compiler of *Yance Zazhen Jiujing* (*Canon of Acupuncture at Supine and Lateral Positions*), *Yance Renjing* (*Classic of Human Figure at Anterior and Lateral Views*) and *Mingtang Tu* (*Chart of Acupoints*), etc, monographs on acupuncture and moxibustion. All are lost. He was also one of the earliest physicians who drew diagrams of meridians, collaterals and acupoints.

● **秦越人**[qín yuè rén] 人名。战国时著名医学家，号扁鹊，渤海郡鄚（今河北任丘）人。学医于长桑君，精于脉学，被推为我国脉学的倡导者。除汤药外，善用针灸、按摩等法，疗效明显。《汉书·艺文志》载有《扁鹊内经》、《扁鹊外经》，已佚。《韩非子》、《战国策》等书，载有其事迹。现在《难经》一书系汉代人托名秦越人撰作。

Qin Yueren A famous physician of the Warring States Period, whose assumed name was Bian Que. A native of Mo County, Bohai Jun (Now Renqiu County, Hebei Province). He learned medicine from Chang Sangjun, was proficient in pulse study and was regarded as the initiator of pulse study in China. Besides decoction, he was good at acupuncture, moxibustion, and massage and achieved obvious curative effects. *Hanshu*: *Yi Wen Zhi* (*The History of the Han Dynasty*: *Records of Art and Literature*) includes *Bian Que Neijing* (*Bian Que's Canon of Internal Medicine*) and *Bian Que Waijing* (*Biqn Que's Canon of External Medicine*), which are no longer extant. His deeds are recorded in *Han Feizi* (*The Book of Han Feizi*) and *Zhanguo Ce* (*Intrigues of the Warring States*). The present version of *Nanjing* (*The Classic of Questions*) was compiled in Qin Yueren's name in the Han Dynasty.

● **揿针式皮内针**[qìn zhēn shì pí nèi zhēn] 针具名。皮内针的一种，又名"揿针"，针身绕成圆圈，露出针尖，状如图钉。使用时用镊子夹住针圈，针尖对准穴位，稍捻转一下后揿入，再用胶布固定。留针时间长短视具体情况而定。

Thumb-Back Intradermal Needle A type of intradermal needle, also named thumb-back needle, a thumb-back-shaped needle with the body wound and the tip exposed. Grip the

round part with a pair of tweezers, twirl, and insert it into the point, and then fix it with adhesive plaster. How long the needle is retained is decided according to concrete cases.

●青带[qīng dài] 病证名。见《傅青主女科》。又称带下青候。多因经产之后胞脉正虚,湿浊秽邪乘虚侵袭,或肝经湿热下注,伤及任脉所致。症见阴道流出青绿色粘腻、气味臭秽的液体,连绵不断。治宜调肝清热利湿。取带脉、中极、阴陵泉、下髎、行间、三阴交。

Leukorrhea with Greenish Discharge A disease, seen in *Fu Qingzhu Nüke* (*Fu Qingzhu's Obstetrics and Gynecology*), also named greenish leukorrhen, mostly caused by underfilling of uterine collaterals after delivery, affection of pathogenic damp-evil, or downward flow of damp-heat of the liver meridian impairing the Ren Meridian. 〈Manifestations〉 constant smell, dark green mucus coming out of the vagina. 〈Treatment principle〉Regulate the function of the liver, clear heat and promote diuresis. 〈Point selection〉 Daimai (GB 26), Zhongji (RN 3), Yinlingquan (SP 9), Xialiao (BL 34), Xingjian (LR 2), and Sanyinjiao (SP 6).

●青昊[qīng hào] 经穴别名。出《西方子明堂灸经》。即清冷渊。详见该条。

Qinghao Another name for Qinglengyuan (SJ 11), a meridian point originally from *Xi Fang Zi Ming Tang Jiujing* (*Xi Fang Zi Classic of Moxibustion*).→清冷渊(p. 321)

●青灵[qīng líng] 经穴名。出《太平圣惠方》。属手少阴心经,又名青灵泉。〈定位〉在臂内侧,当极泉与少海的连线上,肘横纹上3寸,肱二头肌的内侧沟中(图49)。〈层次解剖〉皮肤→皮下组织→臂内侧肌间隔与肱肌。浅层布有臂内侧皮神经、前臂内侧皮神经,贵要静脉等结构。深层有肱动、静脉,正中神经、尺神经,尺侧上副动、静脉和肱三头肌等结构。〈主治〉目黄、头痛、振寒、胁痛、肩臂痛。直刺0.3~0.5寸;可灸。

Qingling (HT 2) A meridian point, originally from *Taiping Shenghui Fang* (*Imperial Benevolent Prescriptions*). A point on the Heart Meridian of Hand-Shaoyin, also named Qinglingquan. 〈Location〉 on the medial side of the arm and on the line connecting Jiquan (HT 1) and Shaohai (HT 3), 3 cun above the cubital crease, in the groove medial to the biceps muscle of the arm (Fig. 49). 〈Regional anatomy〉 skin→subcutaneous tissue→medial intermuscular septum of arm and brachial muscle. In the superficial layer, there are the medial cutaneous nerve of the arm, the medial cutaneous nerve of the forearm and the basilic vein. In the deep layer, there are the brachial artery and vein, the median nerve, the ulnar nerve, the superior ulnar collateral artery and vein and the brachial triceps muscle. 〈Indications〉 yellow eyes, headache, shivering, pain in hypochondrium, pain in the shoulder and the arm. 〈Method〉 Puncture perpendicularly 0.3~0.5 cun. Moxbistion is applicable.

●青灵泉[qīng líng quán] 即青灵。出《医学入门》。见"青灵"条。

Qinglingquan Originally from *Yixue Rumen* (*An Introduction to Medicine*). →青灵(p. 320)

●青龙摆尾[qīng lóng bǎi wěi] 针刺手法名。出《金针赋》,又称苍龙摆尾,为飞经走气四法之一。〈方法〉针斜向浅刺,或先深后浅,得气后,将针尖朝向病所,然后将针柄缓缓摆动,好似手扶船舵或左或右以正航向之势。可以达到推动浅部经气运行的目的。

Green Dragon Wagging Its Tail A needling method, originally from *Jinzhen Fu* (*Ode to Gold Needle*), also named verdant green dragon wagging its tail, one of the 4 methods of promoting the circulation of meridian qi. 〈Method〉 Puncture obliquely and superficially, or first deeply and then shallowly. Following needle sensation, the tip of the needle is aimed in the direction of the affected region. The handle of the needle is gently moved left and right like a rudder adjusting its course to impel the flow of superficial meridian qi.

●青盲[qīng máng] 病证名。见《诸病源候论》。多因肝肾阴亏,精血耗损,精气不能上荣,目失涵养;或心营亏损,神气虚耗,以致神光耗散,视力缓降。其证眼外观如常,无翳障气色,唯患者自觉视力逐渐减退。初期自觉视物昏渺,蒙昧不清;或眼前阴影一片,呈现青绿蓝碧或赤黄之色。日久失治,而不辨人物,

不分明暗。肝肾阴亏者，多见眼中干涩、头晕、耳鸣、遗精、腰痠、舌质红、脉细。治宜补益肝肾明目。取承泣、睛明、球后、肝俞、肾俞、光明。心营亏损者，多见眩晕、心烦、怔忡、健忘、梦扰难寐、舌质红、脉虚弱。治宜补益气血，通络明目。取承泣、睛明、球后、心俞、血海、足三里。

Optic Artrophy A disease, seen in *Zhubing Yuanhou Lun* (*General Treatise on the Etiology and Symptomatology of Diseases*), mostly due to the deficiency of liver-yin and kidney-yin, consumption of essence and blood, inability of vital essence and energy to rise to nourish the eyes; or to the consumption of the Ying fluid of the heart, and vitality, leading to the pathologic state of lusterless and spiritless eyes and gradual weakening of vision. ⟨Manifestations⟩ normal appearence of the eyes; without nebula, except for the patient's own sensation of gradual weakening of vision. At the initial stage, blurring of vision or just a shadow in dark green, dark blue or reddish yellow before the eyes; failure to identify people and objects, inabilty to light from shade due to long-time lack of appropriate treatment. ⟨Manifestations⟩ cases with deficiency of liver-yin and kidney-yin: dryness and dizzy sensation in the eyes, tinnitus, emission, soreness of the waist, red tongue, thready pulse. ⟨Treatment principle⟩ Tonify the liver and kidney to improve acuity of vision. ⟨Point selection⟩ Chengqi (ST 1), Jingming (BL 1), Qiuhou (EX-HN 7), Ganshu (BL 18), Shenshu (BL 23) and Guangming (GB 37). Cases with the consumption of the Ying fluid of the heart: dizziness vexation, severe palpitation, amnesia, insomnia due to dreamness, red tougue, feeble and weak pulse. ⟨Treatment principle⟩ Tonify and nourish both qi and blood, remove obstruction in the meridians to improve acuity of vision. ⟨Point selection⟩ Chengqi (ST 1), Jingming (BL 1), Qiuhou (EX-HN 7), Xinshu (BL 15), Xuehai (SP 10) and Zusanli (ST 36).

●清冷泉[qīng lěng quán] 经穴别名。见《备急千金要方》。即清冷渊。详见该条。

Qinglengquan Another name for Qinglengyuan (SJ 11), a meridian point seen in *Beiji Qianjin Yaofang* (*Essential Prescriptions for Emergencies Worth a Thousand Gold*). → 清冷渊 (p. 321)

●清冷渊[qīng lěng yuān] 经穴名。出《针灸甲乙经》。属手少阳三焦经，又名清冷泉、青昊。定位：在臂外侧，屈肘，当肘尖直上2寸，即天井上1寸（图48和图44.2）。〈层次解剖〉皮肤→皮下组织→肱三头肌。浅层布有臂后皮神经。深层有中副动、静脉，桡神经肌支等。〈主治〉头痛、目黄、肩臂痛不能举。直刺0.5～1寸；可灸。

Qinglengyuan (SJ 11) A meridian point, originally from *Zhenjiu Jia-Yi Jing* (*A-B Classic of Acupuncture and Moxibustion*), a point on the Sanjiao Meridian of Hand-Shaoyang, also named Qinglengquan or Qinghao. ⟨Location⟩ with the elbow flexed, on the lateral side of the upper arm, 2 cun above the tip of the olecranon and 1 cun above Tianjing (SJ 10) (Figs. 48&44.2). ⟨Regional anatomy⟩ skin → subcutaneous tissue → brachial triceps muscle. In the superficial layer, there is the posterior brachial cutaneous nerve. In the deep layer, there are the median collateral artery and vein and the muscular branches of the radial nerve. ⟨Indications⟩ headache, yellow eyes, inability to raise the arms due to pain in shoulder joint and arms. ⟨Method⟩ Puncture perpendicularly 0.5～1 cun. Moxibustion is applicable.

●琼瑶发明神书[qióng yáo fā míng shén shū] 书名。又名《琼瑶神书》、《琼瑶捷经灸疾疗病神书》、《针灸神书大成》、《琼瑶真人针经》。旧题宋代刘真人（又作刘党或琼瑶真人）撰，撰年不详。明、清有数种不同的传本。重在论述针手法及诸病的针灸治疗。

Qiong Yao Faming Shenshu (*Miraculous Book of the Pretty Jade's Invention*). Also entitled *Qiongyao Shenshu* (*Miraculous Book of the Pretty Jade*), *Qiongyao Jiejing Jiuji Liaobing Shenshu* (*Pretty Jade's Miraculous Book for Taking Shortcut on the Treatment of Diseases with Moxibustion*), *Zhenjiu Shenshu Dacheng* (*Miraculous Book of Great Compendium of Acupuncture and Moxibustion*) and *Qiongyao Zhenren Zhenjing* (*Canon of Acupuncture of the Pretty Jade Taoist*), said to have been compiled by Liu Zhenren (*or Liu*

Dang or Qiongyao Zhenren) with its compiling time unknown. There were various versions in the Ming and Qing Dynasties. It mainly stated needling manipulations and acupuncture and moxibustion therapy.

● 琼瑶真人八法神针 [qióng yáo zhēn rén bā fǎ shén zhēn] 书名。又称《琼瑶真人八法神针紫芝春谷全书》，题作峨嵋山人黄士真序传。见清《读书敏求记》。参见"黄士真"条。

Qiongyaozhenren Ba Fa Shenzhen (*Miraculous Book of the Pretty Jade's Inventions*) Also entitled *Qiongyaozhenren Ba Fa Shenzhen Zizhi Chungu Quanshu* (*A Divine Book on the Eight Methods of Miraculous Needling of the Pretty Jade Taoist Like Ganoderma Japonicum in Spring Valley*). Its preface was autographed by Huang Shizhen, whose assumed name is Ermeishanren. Seen in *Dushu Minqiu Ji* (*Notes from Reading with Keen Sense of Seeking*) compiled in the Qing Dynasty. →黄士真(p.176)

● 丘经历 [qiū jīng lì] 人名。宋代针灸家，山东益都人。善于针术，曾以针刺治愈患牙槽风而日久颌穿脓血不止的患者。见周密《癸辛杂识》。

Qiu Jingli An expert of acupuncture and moxibustion in the Song Dynasty, a native of Yidu, Shandong Province. He was proficient in acupuncture techniques and had once cured patients suffering from lingering wind of dental alvedi which led to the appearence of holes through the jaw and constant bleeding. Cf. Zhou Mi's *Guixin Zashi* (*Random Thoughts at Guixin Period*).

● 丘珏 [qiū jué] 人名。明代针灸家，字廷美，邵武（属福建）人。见《邵武县志》曾治人中头风，口噤，不踰刻，吐痰数升而愈。

Qiu Jue An acupuncture-moxibustion specialist in the Ming Dynasty who styled himself Tingmei, a native of Shaowu (now in Fujian). It was recorded in *Shaowu Xian Zhi* (*Annals of Shaowu County*) that he could cure patients suffering from wind syndrome of the head and lockjaw. The patients would not recover until he spat much phlegm.

● 丘虚 [qiū xū] 经穴别名。出《太平圣惠方》。即丘墟。详见该条。

Qiuxu Another name for Qiuxu (GB 40), a meridian point originally from *Taiping Shenghui Fang* (*Imperial Benevolent Prescriptions*). →丘墟(p.322)

● 丘墟 [qiū xū] 经穴名。出《灵枢·本输》。属足少阳胆经，为本经原穴，又作丘虚。〈定位〉在足外踝的前下方，当趾长伸肌腱的外侧凹陷处（图8）。〈层次解剖〉皮肤→皮下组织→趾短伸肌→距跟外侧韧带→跗骨窦。布有足背浅静脉，足背外侧皮神经，足背中间皮神经，外踝前动、静脉。〈主治〉颈项痛，腋下肿，胸胁痛，下肢痿痹，外踝肿痛，疟疾，疝气，目赤肿痛，目生翳膜，中风偏瘫。直刺0.5～0.8寸；可灸。

Qiuxu (GB 40) A meridian point, originally from *Ling Shu: Benshu* (*Miraculous Pivot: Meridian Points*). The Yuan (Primary) point of the Gallbladder Meridian of Foot-Shaoyang, also named Qiuxu. 〈Location〉anterior and inferior to the external malleolus, in the depression lateral to the tendon of the long extensor muscle of the toes (Fig. 8). 〈Regional anatomy〉skin→subcutaneous tissue→short extensor muscle of toes→lateral talocalcaneal ligament→tarsal sinus. There are the superficial vein of the dorsum of the foot, the lateral dorsal cutaneous nerve of the foot, the intermediate dorsal cutaneous nerve of the foot, and the lateral anterior malleolar artery and vein in this area. 〈Indications〉pain in the neck and nape, subaxillary swelling, pain in the chest and hypochondriac region, flaccidity and numbness of the lower extremities, swelling and pain of the lateral malleolus, malarial disease, hernia, redness, swelling and pain of the eyes, nebula in the eyes, hemiparalysis due to apoplexy. 〈Method〉Puncture perpendicularly 0.5～0.8 cun. Moxibustion is applicable.

● 球后 [qiú hòu] 经外穴名，见《眼科针灸疗法》。〈定位〉在面部，当眶下缘外1/4与内3/4交界处（图10）。〈主治〉目疾，如视神经炎、视神经萎缩、视网膜色素变性、青光眼、早期白内障、近视、斜视。〈针法〉沿眶下缘从外下向内上，向视神经管方向缓慢直刺0.5～0.8寸，不提插。

Qiuhou (EX-HN 7) An extra point, seen in *Yanke Zhenjiu Liaofa* (*Ophthalmic Acupuncture Therapy*). 〈Location〉on the face, at the

junction of the lateral 1/4 and medial 3/4 of the infraorbital margin (Fig. 10). ⟨Indications⟩ eye diseases, such as optic atrophy, optic neuritis, pigmentazy degeneration of the retina, glaucoma early cataract, myapia, and amblyopia. ⟨Method⟩ From the lateral and inferior part to the medial and superior part, puncture slowly and perpendicularly 0.5 to 0.8 cun toward the opitic canal, without lifting and thrusting manipulations.

●曲鬓[qū bìn] 经穴名。出《针灸甲乙经》。属足少阳胆经,为足太阳、少阳之会。又名曲发。⟨定位⟩在头部,当耳前鬓角发际后缘的垂线与耳尖水平线交点处(图28)。⟨层次解剖⟩同颔厌穴。⟨主治⟩偏头痛、颔颊肿、牙关紧闭、呕吐、齿痛、目赤肿痛、项强不得顾。向后平刺0.5~0.8寸;可灸。

Qubin (GB 7) A merdian point, from *Zhenjiu Jia-Yi Jing* (*A-B Classic of Acupuncture and Moxibustion*), a point on the Gallbladder Merdian of Foot-Shaoyang, the crossing point of Foot-Taiyang and Foot-Shaoyang, also named Qufa. ⟨Location⟩ on the head, at the crossing point of the vertical posterior border of the temples and horizontal line through the ear apex (Fig. 28). ⟨Regional anatomy⟩ skin→subcutaneous tissue→superior auricular muscle→temporal fascia→temporal muscle. In the superficial layer, there are the auriculotemporal nerve and the parietal branches of the superficial temporal artery and vein. In the deep layer, there are the branches of the anterior and posterior deep temporal nerves. ⟨Indications⟩ migraine, swelling of the jaw and cheek, trismus, vomiting, toothache, redness, swelling and pain of the eyes, inability to look around due to stiffneck. ⟨Method⟩ Puncture subcutaneously backwards 0.5~0.8 cun. Moxibustion is applicable.

●曲差[qū chā] 经穴名。出《针灸甲乙经》。属足太阳膀胱经,又名鼻冲。⟨定位⟩在头部,当前发际正中直上0.5寸,旁开1.5寸。即神庭与头维连线的内1/3与中1/3交点上(图28)。⟨层次解剖⟩皮肤→皮下组织→枕额肌额腹。浅层布有滑车上神经和滑车上动、静脉。深层为腱膜下疏松组织和颅骨外膜。⟨主治⟩头痛、目眩、目痛、目视不明、鼻塞、鼻衄。平刺0.3~0.5寸;禁灸。

Qucha (BL 4) A meridian point, from *Zhenjiu Jia-Yi Jing* (*A-B Classic of Acupuncture and Moxibustion*), a point on the Bladder Meridian of Foot-Taiyang, also named Bichong. ⟨Location⟩ on the head, 0.5 cun directly above the midpoint of the anterior hairline and 1.5 cun lateral to the midline, at the junction of the medial third and middle third of the line connecting Shenting (DU 24) and Touwei (ST 8) (Fig. 28). ⟨Regional anatomy⟩ skin→subcutaneous tissue→frontal belly of occipitofrontal muscle. In the superficial layer, there are the supratrochlear nerve and the supratrochlear artery and vein. In the deep layer, there are the subaponeurotic loose connective tissue and the pericranium. ⟨Indications⟩ headache, dizziness, pain of the eye, blurred vision, stuffy nose, apistaxis. ⟨Method⟩ Puncture subcutaneously 0.3~0.5 cun. Moxibustion is forbidden.

●曲池[qū chí] 经穴名。出《灵枢·本输》。属手阳明大肠经,为本经合穴。又名阳泽、鬼臣、鬼腿。⟨定位⟩在肘横纹外侧端,屈肘,当尺泽与肱骨外上髁连线中点(图48和图6)。⟨层次解剖⟩皮肤→皮下组织→桡侧腕长伸肌和桡侧腕短伸肌→肱桡肌。浅层布有头静脉的属支和前臂后皮神经。深层有桡神经,桡侧返动、静脉和桡侧副动、静脉间的吻合支。⟨主治⟩热病、咽喉肿痛、手臂肿痛、上肢不遂、手肘无力、月经不调、瘰疬、疮、疥、瘾疹、丹毒、腹痛吐泻、痢疾、齿痛、目赤痛、目不明、高血压、胸中烦满、瘦疟、癫、狂、疟疾、善惊。直刺0.8~1.2寸;可灸。

Quchi (LI 11) A meridian point, from *Lingshu: Benshu* (*Miraculous Pivot: Meridian Points*) the He-sea point of the Large-Intestine meridian of Hand-Yangming, also named Yangze, Guichen or Guitui. ⟨Location⟩ with the elbow flexed, at the lateral end of the cubital crease, at the midpoint of the line connecting Chize (LU 5) and the external humeral epicondyle (Figs. 48&6). ⟨Regional anatomy⟩ skin→subcutaneous tissue→long radial extensor muscle of wrist and short radial extensor muscle of wrist→brachioradial muscle. In the superficial layer, there are the tributaries of the cephalic vein and the posterior cutaneous nerve of the forearm. In the deep

layer, there are the radial nerve and the anastomotic branches of the radial recurrent artery and vein and the radial collateral artery and vein. 〈Indications〉febrile disease, sore throat, swelling and pain of the arm, paralysis of the upper limbs, weakness of the hand and elbow, irregular menstruation, scrofula, sore, sarcoptdiosis urticaria, erysipelas, abdominal pain with vomiting and diarrhea, dysentery, toothache, redness and pain of the eye, blurred vision, hypertension, vexation and fullness in the chest, clonic convulsion, depressive psychosis, mania, malarial disease, susceptible to fright. 〈Method〉Puncture perpendicularly 0.8～1.2 cun. Moxibustion is applicable.

●曲尺[qū chǐ] 经外穴名。见《医心方》。在足背内侧，内踝前下方，当胫骨前肌腱与蹰长伸肌腱之间凹陷中。〈主治〉少腹疼痛、遗精、疝气等。直刺0.3～0.5寸；可灸。

Quchi (EX-LE) An extra point, seen in *Yixin Fang* (*The Heart of Medical Prescriptions*). 〈Location〉on the medial side of dorsum of foot, anterior and inferior to the medial malleolus, in the depression between the tendons of the long extensor muscle of the great toe and the anterior tibial muscle. 〈Indications〉pain in the sides of lower abdomen, emission, hernia. 〈Method〉Puncture perpendicularly 0.3～0.5 cun. Moxibustion is applicable.

●曲发[qū fà] 经穴别名。出《太平圣惠方》。即曲鬓。详见该条。

Qufa Another name for Qubin (GB 7), a meridian point from *Taiping Shenghui Fang* (*Imperial Benevolent Prescroptions*). →曲鬓 (p.323)

●曲骨[qū gǔ] ①经穴名。出《针灸甲乙经》。属任脉，为任脉、足厥阴之会。又名屈骨、耳骨、回骨。〈定位〉在下腹部，当前正中线上，耻骨联合上缘的中点处（图40）。〈层次解剖〉皮肤→皮下组织→腹白线→腹横筋膜→腹膜外脂肪→壁腹膜。浅层主要布有髂腹下神经前皮支和腹壁浅静脉的属支。深层主要有髂腹下神经的分支。〈主治〉少腹胀满、小便淋沥、遗尿、疝气、遗精、阳萎、阴囊湿痒、月经不调、赤白带下、痛经。直刺0.5～1寸；可灸。内为膀胱，应在排尿后进行针刺。②骨骼部位名。指耻骨联合部。

1. **Qugu** (RN 2) A meridian point, from *Zhenjiu Jia-Yi Jing* (*A-B Classic of Acupuncture and Moxibustion*), a point on the Ren meridian and the meridian of Foot-Jueyin, also named Qugu (屈骨), Ergu or Huigu. 〈Location〉on the lower abdomen, on the anterior midline, at the midpoint of the upper border of the pubic symphysis (Fig. 40). 〈Regional anatomy〉skin→subcutaneous tissue→linea alba→transverse fascia→extraperitoneal fat tissue→parietal peritoneum. In the superficial layer, there are the anterior cutaneous branches of the iliohypogastric nerve and the tributaries of the superficial epigastric vein. In the deep layer, there are the branches of the iliohypogastric nerve. 〈Indications〉distention and fullness in the lower abdomen, dripping urination, enuresis, hernia, emission, impotence, eczema of scrotum, irregular menstruation, leukorrhea with reddish discharge, dysmenorrhea. 〈Method〉Puncture perpendicularly 0.5～1.0 cun. Moxibustion is applicable. Acupuncture should be applied after discharge of urine because of the gallbladder inside.

2. Part of a bone referring to pubic symphysis.

●曲颊[qū jiá] 部位名。见《灵枢·经筋》。指下颌角部。

Angulus Mandibulae A part of the body, seen in *Lingshu*: *Jingjin* (*Miraculous Pivot*: *Muscles along Meridians*), referring to the angles of the jaw.

●曲甲[qū jiǎ] 部位名。为肩胛骨上三分之一，弯曲突出之处，现称肩胛冈。

Qujia A body part, referring to the protrusion part of the superior 1/3 of scapula. It is named spine of scapula now.

●曲角[qū jiǎo] 部位名。见《素问·气府论》。指鬓发上部向前方突出的部分，当颔厌、悬颅、悬厘所在。

Qujiao A part of the body, seen in *Suwen*: *Qifu Lun* (*Plain Questions*: *On Houses of Qi*), referring to the protruding parts of the superior hair on the temple, where Hanyan (GB 4), Xuanlu (GB 5) and Xuanli (GB 6)

●曲节[qū jié] 经穴别名。出《针灸甲乙经》。即少海。详见该条。

Qujie Another name for Shaohai (HT 3), a meridian point originally from *Zhenjiu Jia-Yi Jing* (*A-B Classic of Acupuncture and Moxibustion*). → 少海(p. 357)

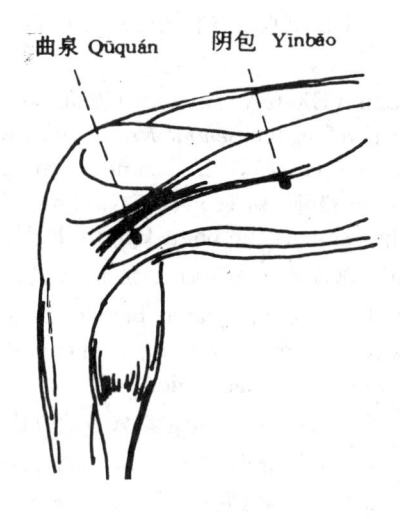

图41 曲泉、阴包穴
Fig 41 Ququan and Yinbao points

●曲泉[qū quán] 经穴名。出《灵枢·本输》。属足厥阴肝经,为本经合穴。〈定位〉在膝内侧,屈膝,当膝关节内侧面横纹内侧端,股骨内侧髁的后缘,半腱肌、半膜肌止端的前缘凹陷处(图81)。〈层次解剖〉皮肤→皮下组织→缝匠肌后缘→股薄肌腱后缘→半膜肌腱→腓肠肌内侧头。浅层布有隐神经,大隐静脉。深层有膝上内侧动、静脉的分支或属支。〈主治〉月经不调、痛经、白带、阴挺、阴痒、产后腹痛、遗精、阳萎、疝气、小便不利、头痛、目眩、癫狂、膝膑肿痛、下肢痿痹。直刺1~1.5寸;可灸。

Ququan (LR 8) A meridian point, from *Lingshu: Benshu* (*Miraculous Pivot: Meridian Points*), a point on the Liver Meridian of Foot-Jueyin, its He (sea) point. 〈Location〉 on the medial side of the knee, at the medial end of the popliteal crease when the knee is flexed, posterior to the medial epicondyle of the tibia, in the depression of the anterior border of the insertions of the semimembranous and semitendinous muscles (Fig. 81). 〈Regional anatomy〉 skin→subcuaneous tissue→posterior border of sartorius muscle→posterior border of tendon of gracilis muscle→tendon of semimembranous muscle→medial head of gastrocnemius muscle. In the superficial layer, there are the saphenous nerve and the great saphenous vein. In the deep layer, there are the branches or tributaries of the medial superior genicular artery and vein. 〈Indications〉 irregular menstruation, dysmenorrhea, leukorrhea, prolapse of uterus, pruritus vulvae, postpartum tormina, emission, impotence, hernia, difficulty in urination, headache, dizziness, manic-depressive disorders, swelling and pain of the front of the knee, flaccidity and numbness of the lower limbs. 〈Method〉 Puncture perpendicularly 1.0~1.5 cun. Moxibustion is applicable.

●曲牙[qū yá] ①部位名。指下颌角的上方。②经穴别名。见《针灸聚英》。即颊车。详见该条。

Quya ①A body part, referring to the superior part of the angle of mandible. ②Another name for Jiache (ST 6), a meridian point seen in *Zhenjiu Juying* (*Essentials of Acupuncture and Moxibustion*). → 颊车. (p. 187)

●曲垣[qū yuán] 经穴名。出《针灸甲乙经》。属手太阳小肠经。〈定位〉在肩胛部,冈上窝内侧端,当臑俞与第二胸椎棘突连线的中点处(图48和图65)。〈层次解剖〉皮肤→皮下组织→斜方肌→冈上肌。浅层有第二、三胸神经后支的皮支和伴行的动、静脉。深层布有肩胛上神经的肌支和肩胛上动、静脉,肩胛背动、静脉的分支或属支。〈主治〉肩胛拘挛疼痛。直刺0.3~0.5寸;可灸。不宜向锁骨上窝上方刺,以免损伤肺脏。

Quyuan (SI 13) A meridian point, from *Zhenjiu Jia-Yi Jing* (*A-B Classic of Acupuncture and Moxibustion*), a point on the Small Intestine Meridian of Hand-Taiyang. 〈Location〉 on the scapula, at the medial end of the suprascapular fossa, at the midpoint of the line connecting Naoshu (SI 10) and the spinous process of the 2nd thoracic vertebra (Figs. 48&65). 〈Regional anatomy〉 skin → subcutaneous tissue → trapezius muscle →

suprapinous muscle. In the superficial layer, there are the cutaneous branches of the posterior branches of the 2nd and 3rd thoracic nerves and their accompanying arteries and veins. In the deep layer, there are the muscular branches of the suprascapular nerve, the branches or tributaries of the suprascapular artery and vein and the dorsal scapular artery and vein. ⟨Indications⟩ muscular contracture and pain of the scapula. ⟨Method⟩ Puncture perpendicularly 0.3～0.5 cun. Moxibustion is applicable. Oblique needling in the direction of the superior part of greater supraclavicular fossa should be avoided for fear of injuring the lung.

●曲泽[qū zé]　经穴名。出《灵枢·本输》。属手厥阴心包经,为本经合穴。⟨定位⟩在肘横纹中,当肱二头肌腱的尺侧缘(图49和图66)。⟨层次解剖⟩皮肤→皮下组织→正中神经→肱肌。浅层有肘正中静脉、前臂内侧皮神经等结构。深层有肱动、静脉,尺侧返动、静脉的掌侧支与尺侧下副动、静脉前支构成的动、静脉网,正中神经的本干。⟨主治⟩心痛、善惊、心悸、胃疼、吐、转筋、热病、烦躁、肘臂痛、上肢颤动、咳嗽。直刺0.8～1寸,或点刺出血;可灸。

Quze (PC 3) A meridian point, originally from *Ling Shu: Benshu* (*Miraculous Pivot: Meridian Points*), a point on the Pericardium Meridian of Hand-Jueyin, its He-sea point. ⟨Location⟩ at the midpoint of the cubital crease, on the ulnar side of the tendon of the biceps muscle of the arm (Figs. 49&66). ⟨Regional anatomy⟩ skin-subcutaneous tissue → medial nerve→brachial muscle. In the superficial layer, there are the medial vein of the elbow and the medial cutaneous nerve of the forearm. In the deep layer, there are the brachial artery and veins, the arteriovenous network formed by the palmar branches of the ulnar recurrent artery and vein with the anterior branches of the inferior ulnar collateral artery and vein, and the trunk of the median nerve. ⟨Indications⟩ precordial pain, susceptible to fright palpitation, stomachache, vomiting, spasm, febrile disease, dysphoria, pain of elbow and arm, tremor of the upper limbs, cough. ⟨Method⟩ Puncture perpendicularly 0.8～1.0 cun, or prick for letting blood. Moxibustion is applicable.

●屈骨[qū gǔ]　经穴别名。出《千金要方》。即曲骨。详见该条。

Qugu Another name for Qugu (曲骨)(RN 2), a meridian point originally from *Qianjin Yaofang* (*Essential Prescriptions Worth a Thousand Gold*). →曲骨1. (p. 324)

●屈骨端[qū gǔ duān]　经外穴名。见《千金要方》。又名横骨、尿胞。在耻骨联合之中点处上缘,位同曲骨穴。参见该条。

Quguduan (EX-CA) An extra point, seen in *Qianjin Yaofang* (*Essential Prescription Worth a Thousand Gold*), also named Henggu or Niaobao. →横骨. (p. 163)、尿胞(p. 284) ⟨Location⟩ the same as the point Qugu(RN 2).

●胠[qū]　部位名。在腋下胁上,是胁肋的总称。

Qu A body part, located below the armpit and above the hypochondrium, a general term for the hypochondriac region.

●取穴法[qǔ xué fǎ]　①指定取穴位的方法。详见"骨度法","拇指同身寸"等条。②指针灸治疗时的取穴方法。临床上分远道取穴,近道取穴,随症取穴等多种。

Methods of Point Selection Referring to ① the location of acupuncture points by measurement. Such as "bone proportional measurement", "thumb cun", etc. ② the methods of point selection in acupuncture and moxibustion. It is clinically divided into distant point seletion, proximal point selection and symptomatologic point selection etc.

●去爪[qù zhǎo]　《内经》刺法名。出《灵枢·刺节真邪》。为刺法五节之一。指饮食不知节慎,喜怒七情过度,影响津液不能正常运行内溢致睾丸、阴囊日渐肿大,俯仰活动受限病证,应用铍针放水以治疗。

Hydrops Discharge by the Stiletto Needle A needling method from *Lingshu: Cijie Zhenxie* (*Miraculous Pivot: Acupuncture Principles and Diseases*), part of *Neijing* (*The Canon of Internal Medicine*). One of the 5 restraints on needling, referring to the use of the stiletto needle to release fluid in order to treat swollen testicles and serotum leading to inability to move forward and backward freely. Generally due to immoderation of drink and food, or ex-

cess emotions, which cause abnormal circulation and overflowing of body fluids resulting in the gradual swelling of the testicles and scrotum.

●**权髎**[quán liáo] 经穴别名。见《千金要方》。即颧髎。详见该条。

Quanliao Another name for Quanliao (SI 18), a meridian point seen in *Qianjin Yaofang* (*Essential Prescriptions Worth a Thousand Gold*). →**颧髎**(p.327)

●**全不产**[quán bù chǎn] 不孕的别名。详见该条。

Issuelessness Another name for sterility. →**不孕**(p.29)

●**全循义**[quán xún yì] 人名。明代针灸家。见"针灸择日编集"条。

Quan Xunyi An expert of acupuncture and moxibustion in the Ming Dynasty. →**针灸择日编集**(p.595)

●**泉门**[quán mén] 经外穴名。见《千金要方》。在女性耻骨联合下缘，阴唇前联合上缘处。灸治妇人不孕、漏赤白。

Quanmen (EX-CA) An extra meridian, seen in *Qianjin Yaofang* (*Essential Prescriptions Worth a Thousand Gold*). 〈Location〉in the inferior border of pubic symphysis, superior to the anterior commissure of labia. 〈Indications〉sterility, leukorrhea with reddish discharge. 〈Method〉moxibustion.

●**泉液**[quán yè] 经穴别名。出《千金要方》。即渊液。详见该条。

Quanye Another name for Yuanye (GB 22), a meridian point originally from *Qianjin Yaofang* (*Essential Prescriptions Worth a Thousand Gold*). →**渊液**(p.575)

●**泉阴**[quán yīn] 经外穴名。出《千金翼方》。在下腹部，当耻骨联合上缘曲骨旁开3寸处。〈主治〉偏坠、睾丸炎等。直刺0.3～1寸；可灸。

Quanyin (EX-CA) An extra point, originally from *Qianjin Yifang* (*Supplement to Essential Prescriptions Worth a Thousand Gold*). 〈Location〉on the lower abdomen, 3 cun lateral to the point Qugu (RN 2) on the upper border of the pubic symphysis. 〈Indications〉swelling with bearing-down pain of one testis, orchitis. 〈Method〉Puncture perpendicularly 0.3～1.0 cun. Moxibustion is applicable.

●**拳尖穴**[quán jiān xué] 经外穴名。见《千金要方》。在手背侧第3掌骨小头之高点，握拳取之。灸治目痛、目翳、癜风、赘疣等。

Quanjianxue (EX-UE) An extra point, seen in *Qianjin Yaofang* (*Essential Prescriptions Worth a Thousand Gold*). 〈Location〉on the dorsum of the hand, at the high point of the small head of the third metacarpal bone, fixing the point when a fist is made. 〈Indications〉pain of eyes, nebula, vitiligo, wart. 〈Method〉moxibustion.

●**颧**[quán] 部位名。亦称頄，亦称面頄骨，眼眶外下侧之高骨，现称颧骨。

Zygomatic Region A body part, the protrusive bone, lateral-inferior to the orbit, also named zygoma and zygomatic bone in the face. It is named zygomatic bone now.

●**颧髎**[quán liáo] 经穴名。出《针灸甲乙经》。属手太阳小肠经，为手少阳、太阳之会。又名兑骨。〈定位〉在面部，当目外眦直下，颧骨下缘凹陷处（图65和图28）。〈层次解剖〉皮肤→皮下组织→颧肌→咬肌→颞肌。浅层布有上颌神经的眶下神经分支，面神经的颧支、颊支，面横动、静脉的分支或属支。深层有三叉神经的下颌神经分支分布。〈主治〉口眼歪斜、眼睑瞤动、齿痛、颊肿、目赤、目黄、面赤、唇肿。直刺0.5～0.8寸。

Quanliao (SI 18) A meridian point originally from *Zhenjiu Jia-Yi Jing* (*A-B Classic of Acupuncture and Moxibustion*), a point on the Small Intestine Meridian of Hand-Taiyang, the crossing point of the Meridian of Hand-Shaoyang and the Meridian of Hand-Taiyang, also named Duigu. 〈Location〉on the face, directly below the outer canthus, in the depression below the zygomatic bone (Figs. 65&28). 〈Regional anatomy〉skin → subcutaneous tissue → zygomatic muscle → masseter muscles → temporal muscle. In the superficial layer, there are the branches of the infraorbital nerve from the maxillary nerve, the zygomatic and buccal branches of the facial nerve, and the branches or tributaries of the transverse facial artery and vein. In the deep layer, there are the branches of the

mandibular nerve from the trigeminal nerve. 〈Indications〉 deviation of the eye and the mouth, twitching of eyelid, toothache, swelling of the inferior part of orbit, conjunctival congestion, yellow eyes, flushed face, swollen lips. 〈Method〉Puncture perpendicularly 0.5～0.8 cun.

●缺盆[quē pén] ①部位名。出《灵枢·经脉》。指锁骨上窝部。②经穴名。出《素问·气府论》。属足阳明胃经。又名天盖。〈定位〉在锁骨上窝中央，距前正中线4寸(图60和图40)。〈层次解剖〉皮肤→皮下组织和颈阔肌→锁骨与斜方肌之间→肩胛舌骨肌(下腹)与锁骨下肌之间→臂丛。浅层布有锁骨上中间神经。深层有颈横动、静脉、臂丛的锁骨上部等重要结构。〈主治〉咳嗽气喘、咽喉肿痛、缺盆中痛、瘰疬。直刺0.2～0.4寸；可灸。不可深刺。

1. Que Pen A body part, originally from *Lingshu*: *Jingmai* (*Miraculous Pivot*: *Meridians*), referring to the supraclavicular fossa.

2. Quepen (ST 12) A meridian point, originally from *Suwen*: *Qifu Lun* (*Plain Questions*: *On Houses of Qi*), a point on the Stomach Meridian of Foot-Yangming, also named Tiangai. 〈Location〉at the centre of the supraclavciular fossa, 4 cun larteral to the anterior midline (Figs. 60&40). 〈Regional anatomy〉 skin → subcutaneous tissue and platysma muscle → between clavicle and trapezius muscle→between inferior belly of omohyoid muscle and subclavicular muscle--brachial plexus. In the superficial layer, there is the intermediate supraclavicular nerve. In the deep layer, there are the transverse cervical artery and vein and the supraclavicular portion of the brachial plexus. 〈Indications〉 cough, asthma, swelling and pain of throat, pain in the supraclavicular fossa, scrofula. 〈Method〉 Puncture perpendicularly 0.2～0.4 cun. Moxibustion is applicable. Deep needling is forbidden.

●缺乳[quē rǔ] 乳少的别名。详见该条。

Lactation Another name for lack of Hypogalactia. →乳少(p. 339)

●雀啄法[què zhuó fǎ] 刺法名。进针后作浅而频数的垂直点刺，类似捣法而较轻。参见"捣法"条。

Bird-Pecking Needling The manipulation of needling by vertical pricking with a small amplitude and high frequency, similar to the pounding method but with a lighter force. →捣法(p. 77)

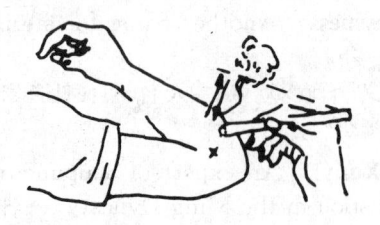

图42 雀啄灸
Fig 42 Sparrow-pecking moxibustion

●雀啄灸[què zhuó jiǔ] 艾条灸的一种。将艾条燃着一端，与施灸部位并不固定在一定的距离，而是象鸟雀啄食一样，一上一下地移动，给以较强的断续的热刺激。

Bird-Pecking Moxibustion A form of moxa-stick moxibustion. Burn one end of a moxastick and move it up and down in a way similar to the pecking of a bird to give the part for moxibustion a stronger intermittent hot stimulation. There is no fixed distance between the moxa stick and the part to be moxibusted.

●阙俞[què shū] 经穴别名。出《千金要方》。即厥阴俞。详见该条。

Queshu Another name for Jueyinshu (BL 14), a meridian point originally from *Qianjin Yaofang* (*Essential Prescriptions Worth a Thousand Gold*). →厥阴俞(p. 230)

R

●**然谷**[rán gǔ] 经穴名。出《灵枢·本输》。属足少阴肾经,为本经荥穴。又名龙渊、龙泉、然骨。〈定位〉在足内侧缘,足舟骨粗隆下方,赤白肉际(图81和图46.1)。〈层次解剖〉皮肤→皮下组织→拇展肌→趾长屈肌腱。浅层布有隐神经的小腿内侧皮支。足底内侧神经皮支和足背静脉网的属支。深层有足底内侧神经和足底内侧动、静脉。主治月经不调、阴挺、阴痒、白浊、遗精、阳萎、小便不利、泄泻、胸胁胀痛、咳血、小儿脐风、口噤不开、消渴、黄疸、下肢痿痹、足跗痛。直刺0.5~1.0寸;可灸。

Rangu (KI 2) A meridian point, originally from *Ling Shu*: *Benshu* (*Miraculous Pivot*: *Meridian Points*), the Ying (Spring) point of the Kidney Meridian of Foot-Shaoyin, also named Longyuan, Longquan or Rangu (然骨). 〈Location〉 on the medial border of the foot, below the tuberosity of the navicular bone, and at the junction of the red and white skin (Figs. 81 & 46.1). 〈Regional anatomy〉 skin → subcutaneous tissue → abductor muscle of great toe → tendon of long flexor muscle of toes. In the superficial layer, there are the medial cutaneous branches of the saphenous nerve to the leg, the cutaneous branches of the medial plantar nerve and the tributaries of the dorsal venous network of the foot. In the deep layer, there are the medial planter nerve and the medial plantar artery and vein. 〈Indication〉 irregular menstruation, prolapse of uterus, pruritus vulvae, cloudy urine, emission, impotence, difficulty in urination, diarrhea, distending pain in the chest and hypochondrium, hemoptysis, tantanus neonatorium in children, lockjaw, diabetes, jaundice, flaccidity and numbness of the lower limbs, pain in the dorsum of the foot. 〈Method〉 Puncture perpendicularly 0.5~1.0 cun. Moxibustion is applicable.

●**然骨**[rán gǔ] ①经穴别名。见《类经图翼》。即然谷。见该条。②骨胳部位名,指内踝前突起的舟骨粗隆部。

1. **Rangu** Another name for Rangu (然谷) (KI 2), a meridian point seen in *Leijing Tuyi* (*Illustrated Supplement to the Classified Canon of Internal Medicine of the Yellow Emperor*). →然谷(p.329)

2. **Rangu** A bone, referring to the protrusive tuberisttas ossis naricutaris anterior to the medal malleolus.

●**然后**[rán hòu] 经外穴名。见《经外奇穴治疗诀》。在足部然谷后0.4寸处。〈主治〉消化不良。直刺0.3~0.5寸;可灸。

Ranhou (EX-LE) An extra point, seen in *Jingwai Qixue Zhiliao Jue* (*Pithy Formulas for Treatment with Extra Points*). 〈Location〉 on the foot, 0.4 cun posterior to Rangu (KI 2). 〈Indication〉 dyspepsia. 〈Method〉 Puncture perpendicularly 0.3~0.5 cun. Moxibustion is applicable.

●**瀼泄**[ráng xiè] 见《杂病源流犀烛》。即五更泄。见该条。

Diarrhea Before Dawn Seen in *Zabing Yuanliu Xizhu* (*Bright Candle to Pathology of Miscellaneous Diseases*), synonymous with morning diarrhea. →五更泄(p.475)

●**热秘**[rè bì] 便秘证型之一。见《济生方》。因热结大肠所致。证见腹部痞满、大便干燥、按之有块作痛、矢气频转、终难排出、烦热口渴、面赤,伴有头痛、小便短黄、口臭、舌苔黄燥、脉滑实。治宜清热保津。泻合谷、曲池、腹结、上巨虚、承山。

Constipation due to Heat A type of constipation, seen in *Jisheng Fang* (*Recipes for Saving Lives*), resulting from accumulation of heat in the large intestine. 〈Manifestations〉 fullness in the abdomen, constipation, pressing pain with mass in the abdomen, frequent wind from bowels, dysphoria with smother-

329

ing sensation, thirst, flushed face, accompanied by headache, scanty yellow urine, foul breath, yellowish and dry coating, slippery and excessive pulse. 〈Treatment principle〉 Save the body fluid by clearing heat. 〈Method〉 Puncture Hegu (LI 4), Quchi (LI 11), Fujie (SP 14), Shangjuxu (ST 37) and Chengshan (BL 57) with reducing method.

●热痹[rè bì] 痹证证型之一。出《素问·四时刺逆从论》。由风湿化热，邪热壅于经络、关节，气血郁滞不通所致。可见四肢关节酸痛、肿大、痛不可近、活动受限，伴有咽痛、发热、多汗而热不退、小便短赤、舌苔厚腻而黄、脉濡数。治宜祛湿清热，活络止痛。取大椎、曲池、合谷、阴陵泉、三阴交。局部取穴参见"行痹"条。

Arthralgia of Heat Type A type of arthralgia, originally from *Suwen*: *Sishi Cini Conglun* (*Plain Questions*: *Acupuncture in Accordance with the Four Seasons*), a result of heat transmitted from pathogenic wind-dampness, accumulation of pathogenic heat in meridians and collaterals and joints, stagnation of qi and blood. 〈Manifestations〉 aching pain and swelling of limb joints, tenderness, inability to move freely, accompanied by sore-throat, fever, lingering fever with hyperhidrosis, scanty and dark urine, thick, greasy and yellowish coating, soft and rapid pulse. 〈Treatment principle〉 Eliminate dampness, clear heat, and invigorate collaterals to relieve pain. 〈Point selection〉 Dazhui (DU 14), Quchi (LI 11), Hegu (LI 4), Yinlingquan (SP 9) and Sanyinjiao (SP 6). For local point selection. →行痹(p. 511)

●热病五十九俞[rè bìng wǔ shí jiǔ shū] 治疗热病的五十九穴。见《素问·水热穴论》。王冰注：即上星、囟会、前顶、百会、后顶、五处、通天、承光、络却、玉枕、头临泣、目窗、正营、承灵、脑空、大杼、中府、缺盆、风门、气冲、足三里、上巨虚、云门、肩髃、委中、魄户、神堂、魂门、意舍、志室、腰俞，共五十九穴。

59 Acupoints for Febrile Diseases The 59 acupoints selected to treat febrile disease, seen in *Suwen*: *Shui Re Xue Lun* (*Plain Questions*: *On Acupoints for Edema and Febrile Diseases*). Wang Bing explained with a note, i.e., Shangxing (DU 23), Xinhui (DU 22), Qianding (DU 21), Baihui (DU 20), Houding (DU 19), Wuchu (BL 5), Tongtian (BL 7), Chengguang (BL 6), Luoque (BL 8), Yuzhen (BL 9), Toulinqi (GB 15), Muchuang (GB 16), Zhengying (GB 17), Chengling (GB 18), Naokong (GB 19), Dazhu (BL 11), Zhongfu (LU 1), Quepen (ST 12), Fengmen (BL 12), Qichong (ST 30), Zusanli (ST 36), Shangjuxu (ST 37), Yunmen (LU 2), Jianyu (LI 15), Weizhong (BL 40), Pohu (BL 42), Shentang (BL 44), Hunmen (BL 47), Yishe (BL 49), Zhishi (BL 52), Yaoshu (DU 2), 59 points in all.

●热府[rè fǔ] 经穴别名。出《千金要方》。即风门。见该条。

Refu Another name for Fengmen (BL 12), a meridian point from *Qianjin Yaofang* (*Essential Prescriptions Worth a Thousand Gold*). →风门(p. 113)

●热霍乱[rè huò luàn] 病证名。霍乱证型之一。见《霍乱论》。又称热气霍乱。多因内伤饮食厚味，或外感暑热、湿热、郁遏中焦所致。证见吐泻骤作、呕吐如喷、暴注下迫、臭秽难闻、头痛发热、口渴而干、腹中绞痛、转筋拘挛、舌红、苔黄腻、脉濡数。治宜疏通中焦，清热除湿。取中脘、天枢、关元、十宣。

Summer Cholera A type of cholera, seen in *Huoluan Lun* (*Treatise on Cholera Morbus*), also known as cholera morbus, mostly due to internal impairment resulting from a fatty diet or exposure to summer-heat and damp-heat leading to stagnation in the Middle-Jiao. 〈Manifestations〉 sudden vomiting and diarrhea, projectile vomiting, spouting diarrhea with offensive smell, headache and fever, thirst and dry mouth, abdominal colic, muscular constricture with spasm, red tongue with yellowish and greasy coating, soft and rapid pulse. 〈Treatment principle〉 Dredge the middle jiao, clear heat and eliminate dampness. 〈Point selection〉 Zhongwan (RN 12), Tianshu (ST 25), Guanyuan (RN 4) and Shixuan (EX-UE 11).

●热灸[rè jiǔ] 灸法的一种。与冷灸相对而言，泛指各种利用热能进行灸治的方法。如艾灸、灯草灸、桑枝灸、油捻灸、阳燧锭灸、电热灸等。参见"冷灸"条。

Hot Moxibustion A kind of moxibustion, as

opposed to crude herb moxibustion, generally referring to all kinds of moxibustion with heat energy, such as moxa-cone and moxa-stick moxibustion, burning rush moxibustion, mulberry twig moxibustion, wick moxibustion, electric heating moxibustion, etc. →冷灸 (p. 241)

●热厥[rè jué]　厥证证型之一。见《素问·厥论》等篇。指邪热过盛，阳郁于里不能外达所致的厥证，证见初病身热头痛、胸腹灼热、渴欲饮水、便秘尿赤、烦躁不安，继则神志昏愦、手足厥冷、脉沉伏而数。治宜苏厥开窍。取水沟、大椎、曲池、内关、十二井穴。

Syncope due to Excess of Heat　A type of syncope, seen in *Suwen: Jue Lun (Plain Questions: Treatise on Cold Limbs)*, etc., due to excessive pathogenic heat and stagnation of yang-heat inside the body. 〈Manifestations〉 fever with headache, burning sensation in the chest and abdomen, thirst with fondness of drink, constipation and dark urine, dysphoria at the initial stage, then unconsciousness, cold limbs, deep, floating and rapid pulse. 〈Treatment principle〉Revive the faint by inducing resuscitation. 〈Point selection〉 Shuigou (DU 26), Dazhui (DU 14), Quchi (LI 11), Neiguan (PC 6) and 12 Jing (Well) points.

●热淋[rè lìn]　淋证证型之一。见《诸病源候论·淋病诸候》。多因湿热蕴结下焦，膀胱气化不利而成。证见小便频急不爽、量少、色黄浑浊、尿路灼热刺痛、小腹坠胀；或有恶寒发热、口苦、便秘、舌质红、苔黄腻、脉数。治宜清利湿热，通淋止痛。取膀胱俞、中极、阴陵泉、合阳、蠡沟、行间。

Stranguria due to Heat　A type of stranguria, seen in *Zhubing Yuanhou Lun: Linbing Zhuhou (General Treatise on the Etiology and Symptomatology of Diseases: Causes and Symptoms of Stranguria)*, mostly due to accumulation of damp-heat in the lower-jiao, and disturbance in qi transformation of the urinary bladder. 〈Manifestations〉 frequent and urgent micturition, difficulty in urination, oliguria, yellowish and turbid urine, burning pain in the urethra, weight and distension sensation in the lower abdomen aversion to cold, fever, bitter taste, constipation, red tongue with yellowish and greasy coating, rapid pulse. 〈Treatment principle〉Eliminate dampness and heat, dredge stranguria and alleviate pain. 〈Point selection〉 Pangguangshu (BL 28), Zhongji (RN 3), Yinlingquan (SP 9), Heyang (BL 55), Ligou (LR 5) and Xingjian (LR 2).

●热气霍乱[rè qì huò luàn]　见《症因脉治》。即热霍乱。见该条。

Cholera Morbus　Originally seen in *Zheng Yin Mai Zhi (Symptoms, Causes, Pulse Conditions and Treatments)*. →热霍乱(p. 330)

●热入营血痉证[rè rù yíng xuè jìng zhèng]　痉证证型之一。由邪热内传营血，热动肝风所致。证见壮热神昏、头晕胀痛、口噤、抽搐、角弓反张；或心烦躁扰、舌红绛、苔黄燥、脉弦数。治宜清泄营血，熄风止痉。取曲泽、劳宫、委中、行间、十宣穴。

Convulsion due to Pathogenic Heat Entering the Ying-Blood　A type of convulsive disease, due to pathogenic heat invading the ying-blood, with occurrence of liver wind resulting from the extreme heat. 〈Manifestations〉unconsciousness with high fever, dizziness, distending headache, lockjaw, clonic convulsion, opisthotonos, or vexation and irritability, deep-red tongue with yellowish and dry coating, wiry and rapid pulse. 〈Treatment principle〉 Clear pathogenic heat in the Ying-blood, calm the endopathic wind to stop convulsion. 〈Point selection〉Quze (PC 3), Laogong (PC 8), Weizhong (BL 40), Xingjian (LR 2) and Shixuan (EX-UE 11).

●热疝[rè shàn]　疝气证型之一。因寒湿之邪蕴结化热，或肝脾二经湿热下注所致。证见睾丸胀痛、阴囊红肿灼热、患部拒按，伴有恶寒发热、头痛肢酸、小便短赤、口中粘腻、舌苔腐厚粘腻、脉濡数。治宜清热化湿、消肿散结。取大敦、照海、阴陵泉、急脉、侠溪。

Hernia Qi due to Heat　A type of hernia, due to accumulation of pathogenic cold-dampness transmitting into heat or the downward flow of damp-heat in the liver and spleen meridians. 〈Manifestations〉 pain in the testis, redness and swelling of scrotum with burning sensation, pain in the affected part when pressed, headache and soreness in the limbs, scanty dark urine, greasy and slimy sensation

in the mouth, beancurdy, thick, sticky and granular coating, soft and rapid pulse. 〈Treatment principle〉 Clear heat and eliminate dampness, subdue swelling and disperse accumulation of the pathogen. 〈Point selection〉 Dadun (LR 1), Zhaohai (KI 6) Yinlingquan (SP 9), Jimai (LR 12) and Xiaxi (GB 43).

● **热吐**[rè tǔ] 小儿呕吐证型之一。见《幼科全书》。又名胃热呕吐。多因乳食停积化热；或夏秋暑热侵袭于胃，以致胃气上逆所致。证见小儿呕吐、吐出物臭秽、身热口渴、面赤烦躁、手足心热、舌红苔黄、脉滑数。治宜清热消食。取曲池、合谷、内庭、下脘、金津、玉液。

Vomiting due to Heat A type of infantile vomiting, seen in *Youke Quanshu* (*A Complete Work of Pediatrics*), mostly due to infantile dyspepsia transforming into heat, or summer-heat affecting the stomach in summer and autumn, adverse rising of the stomach-qi. 〈Manifestations〉 infantile vomiting with foul smell, fever, thirst, flushed face and dysphoria, feverish sensation in the palms and soles, red tongue with yellowish coating, slippery and rapid pulse. 〈Treatment principle〉 Clear pathogenic heat to promote digestion. 〈Point selection〉 Quchi (LI 11), Hegu (LI 4), Neiting (ST 44), Xiawan (RN 10), Jinjin (EX-HN 12), and Yuye (EX-HN 13).

● **热则疾之**[rè zé jí zhī] 针灸治疗原则之一。语出《灵枢·经脉》。与："寒则留之"相对，指对热证可用浅刺而快出针的方法以泻热。参见"寒则留之"条。

Quick Needling for Heat One of the treatment principles of acupuncture and moxibustion, from *Lingshu: Jingmai* (*Miraculous Pivot: Merdians*), in opposition to retaining the needle for cold; referring to shallow puncture and quick withdrawal of the needle, which is used to treat heat-syndromes by purging away pathogenic heat. →寒则留之(p. 158)

● **热瘴**[rè zhàng] 瘴疟之一。因瘴毒疟邪侵入阳盛之体，以致热毒内闭，心神被扰所致。证见热甚寒微、或壮热不寒、头痛、肢体烦痛、面红目赤、胸闷呕吐、烦渴饮冷、大便秘结、小便热赤，甚则神昏谵语、舌质红绛、苔黄腻或垢黑、脉洪数或弦数。治宜解毒除瘴、清热保津、兼清心开窍。取大椎、后溪、间使、液门、曲池、丰隆、内庭、水沟、十二井。

Malignant Malaria due to Heat A type of malignant malaria, due to the invasion of mountainous evil air and malarial pathogens into the body with excessive yang leading to interior stagnation of noxious heat and mental disturbance. 〈Manifestations〉 high fever with slight chills, or high fever without cold, headache, irritability and pain of the limbs, flushed face and redness of the eye, oppressive feeling in the chest and vomiting, polydipsia with preference for cold drinks, constipation, dark urine and burning sensation during urination, even unconsciousness and delirium, deep red tongue with yellowish and greasy or darkish coating, full and rapid or wiry and rapid pulse. 〈Treatment principle〉 Detoxicate and remove mountainous evil air, reduce heat and save body fluids accompanied by removing heat from the heart to restore consciousness. 〈Point selection〉 Dazhui (DU 14), Houxi (SI 3), Jianshi (PC 5), Yemen (SJ 2), Quchi (LI 11), Fenglong (ST 40), Neiting (ST 44), Shuigou (DU 26), and the 12 Jing (Well) points.

● **人部**[rén bù] 穴位浅深分部名。又称人才。指中层，当肌肉之中。参见"三部"条。

Human Portion A layer of an acupoint, also known as human layer, referring to the middle layer within the muscle. →三部(p. 341)

● **人才**[rén cái] 人部的别名。见该条。

Human Layer Another name for human portion. →人部(p. 332)

● **人横**[rén héng] 经穴别名。出《西方子明堂灸经》。即大横，见该条。

Renheng Another name for Daheng (SP 15), a meridian point, originally from *Xi Fang Zi Mingtang Jiujing* (*Xi Fang Zi's Classic of Moxibustion*). →大横(p. 63)

● **人镜经**[rén jìng jīng] 书名。全名《脏腑证治图说人镜经》。明代王宗泉原编，共八卷。内容按十四经编排，汇集古代文献，兼列有关方药及附图。后钱雷加《附录》，张俊英又增《续录》。提出系络、缠络、孙络等新概念。

Renjing Jing (Classic of Mirror for Human Being) A book in 8 volumes, of which the

full name is *Zangfu Zhengzhi Tushuo Renjing Jing* (*Illustrated Classic of Zang-Fu Organs, Diagnosis and Treatment on Human Body*), compiled by Wang Zongquan in the Ming Dynasty. A compilation according to the Fourteen Meridians, a collection of ancient literature, accompanied by a list of related prescriptions and attached drawings. Qian Lei added the appendix later, and Zhang Junying the continuation of the appendix, which put forward some new concepts such as tying collaterals, winding collaterals and minute collaterals, etc.

●**人神**[rén shén] 古代针灸宜忌说之一。出《黄帝蛤蟆经》。意指人神按时巡行各部,其所在部位,忌用针灸。有九部(旁通)人神、十二部人神、行年人神、六十甲子日人神、月内逐日人神、十(天干)日人神、十二(地支)日人神、十二时人神、四季人神、五脏人神等说。见《千金翼方》卷二十八、《普济方》卷四百十一、《针灸大成》卷四。

Renshen (**The Vitality**) One of the theories of do's and don'ts of acupuncture and moxibustion, originally from *Huangdi Hama Jing* (*The Yellow Emperor's Frog Classic*), meaning that both acupuncture and moxibustion are forbidden in the place where the vitality of a human being arrives at a regular time. There is a variety of Renshen, such as Renshen of the nine parts, of the twelve parts, of the certain year, of the cycle of sixty years, of everyday in a month, of the ten heavenly stems, of the twelve Earthly Branches, of the twelve two-hour periods of the four seasons, of the five zang organs, etc. cf. Vol. 28 of *Qianjin Yifang* (*A Supplement to the Prescriptions Worth a Thousand Gold*), Vol. 411 of *Puji Fang* (*Prescriptions for Universal Relief*) and Vol. 4 of *Zhenjiu Dacheng* (*A Great Compendium of Acupuncture and Moxibustion*).

●**人体经穴模型**[rén tǐ jīng xué mó xíng] 针灸教学用具。多用塑料或石膏制成,外形按人体比例缩小,表面标出十四经脉及腧穴位置和名称。

Mannikin with Meridian Points A teaching aid for acupuncture and moxibustion, mostly made of plastic or gypsum and miniatured according to human body scale, on which the fourteen meridians and the location and names of their points are marked.

●**人迎**[rén yíng] 经穴名。出《灵枢·本输》。属足阳明胃经。又名天五会、五会。〈定位〉在颈部,结喉旁,当胸锁乳突肌的前缘,颈总动搏脉动处(图60和图40)。〈层次解剖〉皮肤→皮下组织和颈阔肌→颈固有筋膜浅层及胸锁乳突肌前缘→颈固有筋膜深层和肩胛舌骨肌后缘→咽缩肌。浅层布有颈横神经,面神经颈支。深层有甲状腺上动、静脉的分支或属支,舌下神经祥的分支等结构。主治胸满喘息、咽喉肿痛、头痛、高血压、瘰疬、瘿气、吐逆、霍乱、饮食难下,避开动脉直刺0.2～0.4寸;禁灸。

Renying(ST 9) A meridian point, originally from *Ling Shu*: *Benshu* (*Miraculous Pivot*: *Meridian Points*), a point on the Stomach Meridian of Foot-Yangming, also named Tianwuhui or Wuhui. 〈Location〉on the neck, beside the laryngeal protuberance, and on the anterior border of the sternocleidomastoid muscle where the pulsation of the common carotid artery is palpable(Figs. 60 & 40).〈Regional anatomy〉 skin→subcutaneous tissue and platysma muscle→superficial layer of cervical proper fascia and anterior border of sternocleidomastoid muscle → deep layer of cervical proper fascia and posterior border of omohyoid muscle→constrictor muscle of pharynx. In the superficial layer, there are the transverse nerve of the neck and the cervical branches of the facial nerve. In the deep layer, there are the branches or tributaries of the superior thyroid artery and vein and the branches of the loop of the hypoglossal nerve. 〈Indications〉full sensation in the chest, dyspnea, swelling and pain of the throat, headache, hypertension, scrofula, goiter, vomiting, cholera morbus, dyspepsia. 〈Method〉Avoid artery and puncture perpendicularly 0.2～0.4 cun. Moxibustion is forbidden.

●**人中疔**[rén zhōng dīng] 颜面部疔疮的一种,又名龙泉疔。生于人中部位,易发走黄,切忌挤压。参见"疔疮"条。

Boil on Philtrum A kind of facial boil, also called Longquan (dragon spring) boil, occur

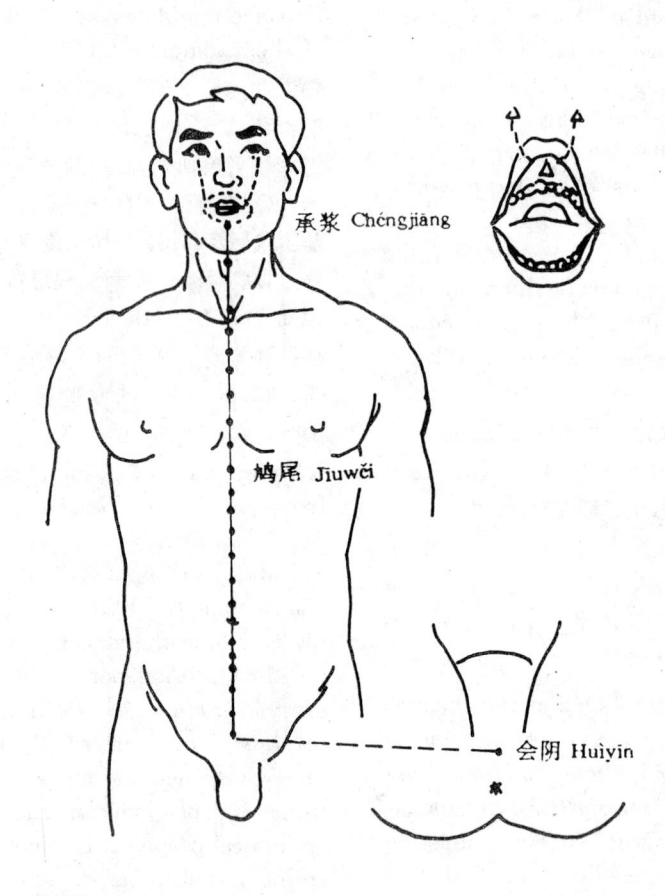

图43.1 任 脉
Fig 43.1 Ren Meridian

ring on the philtrum region and an early development of carbuncle complicated by spticemia, extrusion forbidden. →疔疮(p. 82)

●任脉[rén mài] 奇经八脉之一。见《素问·骨空论》。其循行起于小腹内,从会阴部沿腹部正中上行,经咽喉,下颌,络口唇,沿面部进入目下。

Ren Meridian One of the eight extra meridians, seen in *Suwen*: *Gukong Lun* (*Plain Questions*: *On the Apertures of Bones*). It starts from the inside of the lower abdomen, goes upwards along the abdominal midline from the perineum, then as ends through the throat and mandible, winds the lips and enters along the face into the part inferior to the eyes.

●任脉病[rén mài bìng] 奇经八脉病候之一。出《素问·骨空论》。其主要病症:小腹痛、疝气、带下、癥瘕积聚、不育、月经不调、小便不利、遗尿、遗精、阴中痛等。

Diseases of the Ren Meridian One of the pathogenic manifestations of the Eight Extra Meridians, originally from *Suwen*: *Gukong Lun* (*Plain Questions*: *On the Apertures of Bones*). 〈Manifestations〉pain in the lower abdomen, hernia, leukorrhea, mass in the abdomen, sterility, irregular menstruation, difficulty in urination, enuresis, emission, pain in the pudendum, etc.

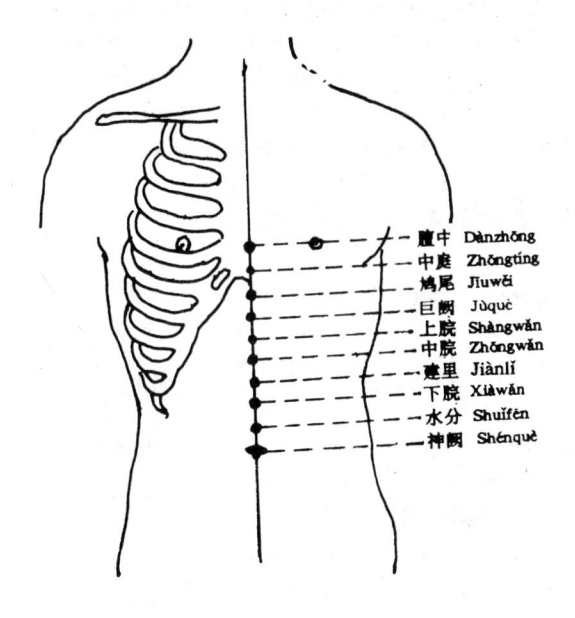

图43.2 任脉穴（腹部）
Fig 43.2 Point of Ren Meridian

● 任脉络脉 [rén mài luò mài] 十五络脉之一。出《灵枢·经脉》。任脉之络名曰鸠尾，其络从鸠尾穴向下散布于腹部。

Collateral of the Ren Meridian One of the Fifteen Main Collaterals, originally from *Lingshu: Jingmai (Miraculous Pivot: Meridians)*, also named Jiuwei, for it spreads down to the abdomen from Jiuwei (RN 15).

● 任脉络脉病 [rén mài luò mài bìng] 十五络脉病之一。出《灵枢·经脉》。实证可见腹皮痛，虚证可见瘙痒。取任脉络穴鸠尾治疗。

Diseases of the Collateral of the Ren Meridian One of the pathogenic manifestations of the Fifteen Main Collaterals, originally from *Lingshu: Jingmai (Miraculous Pivot: Meridians)*. 〈Manifestations〉 pain in the abdominal skin of excess syndrome and itch of the deficiency syndrome. 〈Point selection〉 Jiuwei (RN 15), the Luo (Connecting) points of the Ren Meridian.

● 任脉之别 [rén mài zhī bié] 即任脉络脉。见该条。

Branch of the Ren Meridian →任脉络脉 (p. 335)

● 妊娠耳鸣 [rèn shēn ěr míng] 病证名。见《叶氏女科证治》。多因肾虚，或肝胆火盛所致。肾虚耳鸣者，证见耳鸣头晕、目眩、腰酸。治宜滋阴补肾。取肾俞、志室、三阴交、太溪。肝胆火盛耳鸣者，证见耳鸣、头痛目眩、口苦咽干、心烦不宁。治宜清泻肝胆。取耳门、听宫、听会、阳陵泉、太冲、行间。

Tinnitus During Pregnancy A disease, seen in *Yeshi Nuke Zhengzhi (Ye's Book on Diagnosis and Treatment of Female Diseases)* mostly caused by deficiency of the kidney, or excessive fire of the liver and gallbladder. Manifestations of the syndrome due to deficiency of the kidney: tinnitus and dizziness, vertigo, soreness of the waist. 〈Treatment principle〉 Nourish yin and tonify the kidney. 〈Point selection〉 Shenshu (BL 23), Zhishi (BL 52), Sanyinjiao (SP 6) and Taixi (KI 3). Manifestations of the syndrome due to excessive fire of the liver and gallbladder: tinnitus, dizziness with headache, bitter taste in the mouth and dry throat, irritability. 〈Treatment principle〉 Clear pathogenic heat of the liver and gallbladder. 〈Point selection〉 Ermen (SJ 21), Tinggong (SI 19) Tinghui (GB 2), Yanglingquan (GB 34), Taichong (LR 3) and Xingjian (LR 2).

● 妊娠风痉 [rèn shēn fēng jìng] 子痫的别名。见该条。

Wind-Type Convulsion during Pregnancy Another name for eclampsia gravidarum. →子痫 (p. 627)

● 妊娠腹痛 [rèn shēn fù tòng] 病证名。出《金匮要略·妇人妊娠病脉证并治》。又称胞阻、妊娠小腹痛、子痛。指孕妇发生小腹部疼痛的病证。多因虚寒、血虚、气郁，气血运行失畅，胞脉失养所致。虚寒者，小腹冷痛、得热痛减。治宜温经散寒。取足三里、地机、曲泉，用灸法。血虚者，小腹绵绵作痛、喜按、头痛目眩。治宜养血止痛安胎。取脾俞、胃俞、足三里、血海。气郁者，小腹胀痛、胸脘满闷、烦躁易怒。治宜舒肝解郁。取肝俞、阳陵泉、太溪、太冲。

Abdominal Pain during Pregnancy A disease, originally from *Jingui Yaolüe: Furen Renshen Bing Mai Zheng Bing Zhi (Synopsis of the Golden Chamber: Pulse Conditions, Symptoms and Treatments of the Diseases*

During Pregnancy), also named embarrassment of the fetus, pain in the lower abdomen during pregnancy, or pain due to fetus, mostly caused by cold of insufficiency type, deficiency of blood, stagnation of qi, disorder of qi and blood circulation, which leads to lack of nourishment of the uterine collaterals. Manifestations of the syndrome due to cold of insufficiency type: cold pain in the lower abdomen, which is relieved by warmth. 〈Treatment principle〉Expel pathogenic cold from the meridian. 〈Point selection〉Zusanli (ST 36), Diji (SP 8), and Ququan (LR 8). 〈Method〉 moxibustion. Manifestations of the syndrome due to deficiency of blood: dull and continuous pain in the lower abdomen, which prefers pressing, dizziness with headache. 〈Treatment principle〉Prevent miscarriage by nourishing the blood and alleviating pain. 〈Point selection〉Pishu (BL 20), Weishu (BL 21), Zusanli (ST 36) and Xuehai (SP 10). Manifestations of the syndrome due to stagnation of qi: distending pain in the lower abdomen, distension and fullness in the chest and stomach, dysphoria and irritability. 〈Treatment principle〉Relieve the depressed liver. 〈Point selection〉Ganshu (BL 18), Yanglingquan (GB 34), Taixi (KI 3) and Taichong (LR 3).

●妊娠痉[rèn shēn jìng] 子痫的别名。详见该条。

Convulsion during Pregnancy Another name for eclampsia gravidarum. →子痫(p. 627)

●妊娠呕吐[rèn shēn ǒu tù] 恶阻的别名。详见该条。

Vomiting during Pregnancy Another name for morning sickness. →恶阻(p. 93)

●妊娠伤食[rèn shēn shāng shí] 病证名。见《胤产全书》。多因孕妇脾胃虚弱，饮食不节，伤及脾胃，食水停滞所致。证见脘腹胀满，或呕吐泄泻。治宜健脾消食。取脾俞、胃俞、足三里、内关、公孙。

Dyspepsia during Pregnancy A disease, seen in *Yinchan Quanshu* (*A Complete Book of Obstetrics*), mostly caused by weakness of the spleen and stomach, and improper diet impairing the spleen and stomach, which leads to the retention of food and water. 〈Manifestations〉distension and fullness in the stomach and abdomen, or vomiting and diarrhea. 〈Treatment principle〉Reinforce the spleen to promote digestion. 〈Point selection〉Pishu (BL 20), Weishu (BL 21), Zusanli (ST 36), Neiguan (PC 6) and Gongsun (SP 4).

●妊娠痫证[rèn shēn xián zhèng] 子痫的别名。详见该条。

Epilepsy during Pregnancy Another name for eclampsia gravidarum. →子痫(p. 627)

●妊娠小腹痛[rèn shēn xiǎo fù tòng] 妊娠腹痛的别名。详见该条。

Lower Abdominal Pain during Pregnancy Another name for embarrassment of the fetus. → 妊娠腹痛(p. 335)

●妊娠中风[rèn shēn zhòng fēng] 病名。出《诸病源候论》。多因孕后血虚，经络脏腑失荣，中于风邪，阴阳失调所致。中经络者，证见肌肤不仁、手足麻木、口眼歪斜、甚则半身不遂。治宜养血安胎熄风。取脾俞、胃俞、足三里、风池、阳陵泉。中脏腑者，证见卒然昏倒、痰涎壅盛、不省人事。治宜搜风开窍祛痰。取风池、百会、水沟、丰隆、足三里、阳陵泉、十宣。

Apoplexy in Pregnancy A disease, originally from *Zhubing Yuanhou Lun* (*General Treatise on the Causes and Symptoms*), mostly caused by blood deficiency in pregnancy, lack of nourishment of the meridians and zang-fu organs, and invasion of pathogenic wind leading to imbalance of yin and yang. Manifestations of apoplexy involving the meridians and collaterals: numbness of skin and muscle, numbness of limbs, deviation of the eye and mouth, even hemiplegia. 〈Treatment principle〉Nourish the blood, prevent miscarriage and calm the endopathic wind. 〈Point selection〉Pishu (BL 20), Weishu (BL 21), Zusanli (ST 36), Fengchi (GB 20) and Yanglingquan (GB 34). Manifestations of apoplexy involving zang-fu organs: sudden coma, accumulation of excessive phlegm and saliva in the throat, unconsciousness. 〈Treatment principle〉Expel wind, cause resuscitation and remove phlegm. 〈Point selection〉Fengchi (GB 20), Baihui (DU 20), Shuigou (DU 26), Fenglong (ST 40), Zusanli (ST

36), Yanglingquan (GB 34) and Shixuan (EX-UE 11).

● 日干重见 [rì gān chóng jiàn] 重见时的别称。见该条。

Meeting-Once-Again of the Heavenly Stems Another name for the meeting-once-again period. →重见时 (p. 50)

● 日光灸 [rì guāng jiǔ] 灸法的一种。出《夷坚志》。将艾绒平铺腹部，在日光下曝晒，以达治病目的；或借助聚光镜聚焦而施灸（以患者有温热感为度）。每次10-20分钟。适用于风寒湿痹及慢性虚弱疾病。

Sunlight Moxibustion A form of moxibustion, originally from *Yi Jian Zhi* (*Records of Storming the Strongholds*). 〈Method〉 Expose the mugwort floss spread on the abdomen to sunlight for the treatment of disease, or apply moxibustion with a convex lens (until the patient feels warm). Do this for 10-20 minutes each time. 〈Indications〉 arthralgia due to wind-cold-dampness, and chronic asthenia.

● 日月 [rì yuè] 经穴名。见《针灸甲乙经》。属足少阳胆经，为胆之募穴，为足太阴、足少阳、阳维之会。又名神光。〈定位〉在上腹部，当乳头直下，第七肋间隙，前正中线旁开4寸（图40和图23）。〈层次解剖〉皮肤→皮下组织→腹外斜肌→肋间外肌。浅层布有第六、七、八肋间神经外侧皮支和伴行的动、静脉。深层有第七肋间神经和第七肋间后动、静脉。〈主治〉胁肋疼痛、胀满、呕吐、吞酸、呃逆、黄疸。斜刺0.5～0.8寸；可灸。

Riyue (GB 24) A meridian point, seen in *Zhenjiu Jia-Yi Jing* (*A-B Classic of Acupuncture and Moxibustion*), a point of the Gallbladder Meridian of Foot-Shaoyang, the Front-Mu point of the gallbladder, and the crossing point of the Foot-Taiyin and Foot-Shaoyang and the Yangwei Meridians, also named Shenguang. 〈Location〉 on the upper abdomn, directly below the nipple, in the 7th intercostal space, 4 cun lateral to the anterior midline (Figs. 40 & 23). 〈Regional anatomy〉 skin → subcutaneous tissue → external oblique muscle of abdomen → external intercostal muscle. In the superficial layer, there are the lateral cutaneous branches of the 6th to 8th intercostal nerves and the accompanying arteries and veins. In the deep layer, there are the 7th intercostal nerve and the 7th posterior intercostal artery and vein. 〈Indications〉 distending pain and full sensation in the hypochondrium, vomiting, acid regurgitation, hiccup, jaundice. 〈Method〉 Puncture obliquely 0.5～0.8 cun. Moxibustion is applicable.

● 荣备回避八法 [róng bèi huí bì bā fǎ] 针刺前须注意的八条事项。见明代方贤的《奇效良方·针灸门》。风：天气风盛，令病人避风之处刺之。寒：天气寒冷，令病人向温暖处，先饮汤液醴。暑：夏月热盛，以新水洗其面，于风凉处坐，然后刺。湿：令病人致于高原之处，先服辛燥之物，然后刺。阴：遇阴气重，先服温补之药，然后刺。燥：遇夏月烦躁，令病人于风凉处，先服宣通气血之药，然后刺。车：若病人乘车而来，待气血定再刺。马：若病人乘马而来，候气定再刺。

Eight Evading-Items of Puncturing The eight points for attention before puncturing, seen in *Qixiao Liangfang: Zhenjiu Men* (*Prescriptions of Wonderful Efficacy: Field of Acupuncture and Moxibustion*), compiled by Fang Xian in the Ming Dynasty. Ask the patient to take shelter from wind while acupuncture is applied if it is windy. Apply acupuncture in a warm place with the patient drinking hot water first if it is cold. Have the patient wash his face with fresh water and then sit in a cool place before acupuncture is done if it is too hot. Have the patient stay in high land, have some hot drink or eat some pungent food before he is needled if it is damp. Have the patient take some drugs warm in nature before needling in cloudy weather. Have the patient stay in a cool place, and take some drugs promoting the circulation of both qi and blood before needling if it is dry and hot in summer. Let the patient rest until his qi and blood are calm before he is punctured if he comes by vehicle. Let the patient take a rest until his qi is calm before needling if he comes by horse.

● 肉里之脉 [ròu lǐ zhī mài] 经脉名，出《素问·刺腰痛篇》。指足少阳经在小腿部的支脉。

Meridian in Muscle A meridian, originally

from *Suwen*: *Ci Yaotong Pian* (*Plain Questions*: *On Treatment of Lumbago with Acupuncture*), referring to the branch of the Meridian of Foot-Shaoyang in the leg.

●肉郄[ròu xì] 经穴别名。出《针灸甲乙经》。即承扶。见该条。

Rouxi Another name for Chengfu (BL 36), a meridian point originally from *Zhenjiu Jia-Yi Jing* (*A-B Classic of Acupuncture and Moxibustion*). →承扶(p. 42)

●肉柱[ròu zhù] 经穴别名。出《针灸甲乙经》。即承山。见该条。

Rouzhu Another name for Chengshan (BL 57), a meridian point originally from *Zhenjiu Jia-Yi Jing* (*A-B Classic of Acupuncture and Moxibustion*). →承山(p. 45)

●乳吹[rǔ chuī] 即吹乳。见该条。

Ru Chui (Breast Blowing) →吹乳(p. 52)

●乳蛾[rǔ é] 病证名。见清代屠燮臣《喉科秘旨》。又名蛾子、喉蛾、乳鹅。以其形似乳头,状如蚕蛾而得名。参见"咽喉肿痛"条。

Nipple-Moth (Tonsillitis) A disease, seen in *Houke Mi Zhi* (*The Mysterious Gist of Laryngology*), compiled by Tu Xiechen in the Qing Dynasty, also called moth, moth-like throat or nipple-goose. It looks like a nipple and a sick moth, hence the name. →咽喉肿痛(p. 534)

●乳鹅[rǔ é] 即乳蛾。见该条。

Nipple Goose →乳蛾(p. 338)

●乳根[rǔ gēn] 经穴名。出《针灸甲乙经》。属足阳明胃经,又名薛息、胸薛。〈定位〉在胸部,当乳头直下,乳房根部,第五肋间隙,距前正中线4寸(图60和图40)。〈层次解剖〉皮肤→皮下组织→胸大肌。浅层布有第五肋间神经的外侧皮支,胸腹壁静脉的属支。深层有胸外侧动、静脉的分支或属支,胸内、外侧神经的分支,第五肋间神经,第五肋间后动、静脉。〈主治〉咳喘、胸闷胸痛、乳痈、乳汁少、噎膈。斜刺0.5~0.8寸;可灸。

Rugen (ST 18) A meridian point, originally from *Zhenjiu Jia-Yi Jing* (*A-B Classic of Acupuncture and Moxibustion*), a point on the Stomach Meridian of Foot-yangming, also named Bixi or Xiongbi. 〈Location〉 on the chest, directly below the nipple, on the lower border of the breast, in the 5th intercostal space, 4 cun lateral to the anterior midline (Figs. 60 & 40). 〈Regional anatomy〉 skin→subcutaneous tissue→greater pectoral muscle. In the superficial layer, there are the lateral cutaneous branches of the 5th intercostal nerve and the tributaries of the thoracoepigastric vein. In the deep layer, there are the branches or tributaries of the lateral pectoral artery and vein, the branches of the medial and lateral pectoral nerves, the 5th intercostal nerve and 5th posterior intercostal artery and vein. 〈Indications〉 cough, asthma, fullness and pain in the chest, pain in the breast, lack of lactation, dysphagia. 〈Method〉 Puncture obliquely 0.5~0.8 cun. Moxibustion is applicable.

●乳癖[rǔ pǐ] 病证名。见《中藏经》。又名奶脾、奶积。多由思虑伤脾,郁怒伤肝,以致气滞痰凝;或由肝肾阴虚,互络失养所致。证见乳房中生肿块,形如梅李、鸡卵或呈结节状,质硬无痛,推之可移,不发寒热,皮色不变,可随喜怒消长。临床又可分为肝郁乳癖、阴虚乳癖和痰浊乳癖。详见各条。

Nodules of Breast A disease, seen in *Zhong Cang Jing* (*Canon of the Stored Treasures*), also named stagnation of milk or infantile dyspesia, mostly caused by anxiety impairing the spleen and anger impairing the liver leading to the stagnation of qi and phlegm or by deficiency of the liver and kindey which leads to lack of nourishment of meridians and collaterals of breast. 〈Manifestations〉 nodular masses in the breast resembling a plum or an egg, painless and movable, without change in colour of the skin, fever, disappearance or enlargement along with joy or anger. It is clinically divided into 3 types: nodules of breast due to the stagnation of liver-qi, nodules of breast due to yin-deficiency and nodules of breast due to phlegm turbidity. →肝郁乳癖(p. 129)、阴虚乳癖(p. 561)、痰浊乳癖(p. 425)

●乳上[rǔ shàng] 经外穴名。见《类经图翼》。在胸部当乳头直上1寸处。〈主治〉乳痛、少乳,以及肋间神经痛等。用灸法。

Rushang (EX-CA) An extra point, seen in

Leijing Tuyi (*Illustrated Supplements to Classified Canon of Internal Medicine of the Yellow Emperor*). 〈Location〉 on the chest, 1 cun directly above the nipple. 〈Indications〉 pain of breast, lack of lactation, intercostal neuralgia, etc. 〈Method〉 moxibustion.

●乳少[rǔ shǎo] 病证名。见《保产要旨》。又称缺乳。产后乳汁分泌甚少，不能满足婴儿需要者，称为乳少。多因产后气血亏虚，乳汁化源不足，或肝郁气滞，气血运行不畅，乳汁壅滞不行所致。临床分气血虚弱乳少和肝郁气滞乳少两型。

Hypogalactia A disease, seen in *Baochan Yaozhi* (*The Gist of the Methods for Normal Labor*), also named lack of lactation, referring to very little or no milk secreted from the puerpem breasts, thus not meeting the baby's need. Mostly caused by the deficiency of both qi and blood, lack of resources for milk, or the stagnation of the liver-qi, and abnormal flow of both qi and blood, leading to stagnation of milk. It is clinically divided into two types: lack of lactation due to deficiency of both qi and blood, and lack of lactation due to stagnation of liver-qi.

●乳下[rǔ xià] 经外穴名。见《针灸集成》。在胸部，当乳头直下1寸处。〈主治〉腹痛腹胀、胸胁疼痛、乳肿乳少、小儿癖积、久嗽、反胃、干呕、吐逆、胃脘痛、闭经等。用灸法。

Ruxia (EX-CA) An extra point, seen in *Zhenjiu Jicheng* (*A Collection of Acupuncture and Moxibustion*). 〈Location〉 on the chest, 1 cun below the nipple. 〈Indications〉 abdominal distention and pain, pain in the chest and hypochondrium, swelling of breast and lack of lactation, infantile hypochondriac lump, prolonged cough, regurgitation, retching, vomiting epigastralgia, amenorrhea. 〈Method〉 moxibustion.

●乳癣[rǔ xuǎn] 即奶癣。见该条。

Eczema of Breast Another name for infantile eczema. →奶癣(p.276)

●乳痈[rǔ yōng] 病证名。出《肘后方》。又名吹乳、妒乳、吹奶。是乳房部急性化脓性疾病。发于妊娠期的称"内吹乳痈"，发于哺乳期的称"外吹乳痈"。多由肝气郁结，胃热壅滞而成。临床可分为胃热乳痈和肝郁乳痈。详见各条。

Acute Mastitis A disease, originally from *Zhouhou Fang* (*Handbook of Prescriptions*), also named Chuiru, Duru and Chuinai, a kind of acute and pyogenic disease of the breast. There is interior mastitis during pregnancy and exterior mastitis after delivery. Mostly due to the stagnation of liver-qi and excessive heat in the stomach. It is clinically divided into two types: acute mastitis due to stomach-heat and acute mastitis due to stagnation of liver-qi. →胃热乳痈(p.466)、肝郁乳痈(p.129)

●乳中[rǔ zhōng] 经穴名。出《针灸甲乙经》。属足阳明胃经。〈定位〉在胸部，当第四肋间隙，乳头中央，距前正中线4寸；(图40)。〈层次解剖〉乳头皮肤→皮下组织→胸大肌。浅层布有第四肋间神经外侧皮支，皮下组织内男性主要由结缔组织构成，只有腺组织的迹象，而无腺组织的实质。深层有胸内、外侧神经的分支，胸外侧动、静脉的分支或属支。只作胸腹部腧穴的定位标志—两乳头之间作8寸。不针灸。

Ruzhong (ST 17) A meridian point, originally from *Zhenjiu Jia-Yi Jing* (*A-B Classic of Acupucture and Moxibustion*), a point on the Stomach Meridian of Foot-Yangming. 〈Location〉on the chest, in the 4th intercostal space, at the center of the nipple, 4 cun lateral to the anterior midline (Fig. 40). 〈Regional anatomy〉 skin of mammary nipple→subcutaneous tissue→greater pectoral muscle. In the superficial layer, there are the lateral cutaneous branches of the fourth intercostal nerve. In males, the subcutaneous tissue is mainly composd of the connective tissue and trace, but not parenchyma, of the mammary gland. In the deep layer, there are the branches of the medial and lateral pectoral nerves and the branches or tributaries of the lateral pectoral artery and vein. It only serves as the locative mark for the points on the chest and abdomen, that is 8 cun between the two nipples. Neither acupuncture nor moxibustion is applicable.

●锐针[ruì zhēn] 针具名。见《灵枢·四时气》。又称镵针。指锐利的针。参见"镵针"条。

Sharp Needle A kind of acupuncture needle, seen in *Lingshu: Si Shi Qi* (*Miraculous Pivot:*

Qi of Four Seasons), also known as shear needle, referring to the needle with a very sharp tip. →鑱针(p. 31)

● 锐中[ruì zhōng] 经穴别名。出《针灸聚英》。即神门。见该条。

Ruizhong Another name for Shenmen (HT 7), a merdian point originally from *Zhenjiu Juying* (*Essentials of Acupuncture and Moxibustion*). →神门(p. 362)

● 爇[ruò] 灸法用语。见《周礼·春官·菙氏》。与焫同,灸灼之意。

Stimulation Therapy with Warm Needle A moxibustion term, seen in *Zhou Li*：*Chun Guan*：*Chui Shi* (*The Zhou Rituals*：*the Spring Official*：*the Bamboo Stick and Its Like*), interchangable with *ruo* (焫), meaning burning.

S

● 腮腺[sāi xiàn] 对屏尖之别称。详见该条。

Parotid Gland (MA) Another name for Antofragic Apex (MA). →对屏尖(p. 89)

● 三百六十五会[sān bǎi liù shí wǔ huì] 全身经穴的约数。出《素问·气穴论》、《灵枢·九针十二原》。会,指穴位。意为人体有365个穴位,是经络气血出入会合的地方。

Three Hundred and Sixty-Five Huis The approximate number of all acupoints of the human body, originally from *Suwen*：*Qixue Lun* (*Plain Questions*：*On Loci of Qi*) and *Lingshu*：*Jiu Zhen Shier Yuan* [*Miraculous Pivot*：*Nine Needles and Twelve Yuan* (*Primary*) *Points*]. "会" refers to acupoints, meaning there are 365 acupoints on the human body and they are the places where the qi and blood in meridians flow in and out and join together.

● 三百六十五节[sān bǎi liù shí wǔ jié] 三百六十五是约数,出《素问·调经论》。节,是指经络气血流注出入的部位。意指人体有365个穴位,实际当时不足此数。参见"三百六十五会"条。

Three Hundred and Sixty-Five Sections An approximate number, originally from *Suwen*：*Tiaojing Lun* (*Plain Questions*：*On the Regulation of Meridians*). "Section" is the place where qi and blood in meridians flow in and out, meaning that there were 365 acupoints, but actually there were not as many as 365 acupoints as estimated at that time. → 三百六十五会(p. 340)

● 三百六十五络[sān bǎi liù shí wǔ luò] 是全身络脉的约数。出《灵枢·邪气藏腑病形》。

Three Hundred and Sixty-Five Collaterals The approximate number of all collaterals of the human body, originally from *Lingshu*：*Xieqi Zangfu Bingxing* (*Pathogenic Evils, Zang-fu Organs and Manifestations*).

● 三百六十五穴[sān bǎi liù shí wǔ xué] 全身经穴的约数。

Three Hundred and Sixty-Five Acupoints The approximate number of acupoints of the human body.

● 三变刺[sān biàn cì] 《内经》刺法分类名。出《灵枢·寿夭刚柔》。指针刺出血、出气和针后纳热三法。即对病在营分者,针刺时使其出血;对病在卫分者,针刺时浅刺使邪气得以宣散;针病为寒甚痹痛者,可以采用灸法来治疗。

Three Different Ways of Needling A category of needling in *Neijing* (*The Inner canon of Huangdi*), originally from *Ling shu*：*Shouyao Gangrou* (*Miraculous Pivot*：*Life-Span and Body Constitution*), referring to the three methods of puncturing: to cause bleeding, to discharge qi and to apply moxibustion after needling. Puncture to cause bleeding for treating diseases in ying fen; puncture superficially to dispel pathogenic factors for treating

diseases in wei fen and apply moxibustion for treating numbness and pain due to severe cold evil.

●三部[sān bù]　刺法用语。指穴位的浅、中、深分部。浅部称天部,中部称人部,深部称地部。又总称三才,分称天才、人才、地才。

Three Portions　A term of needling, referring to the superficial, middle and deep layers of a point, which are named respectively the heaven, the human and the earth portions or generally called three Layers—sky layer, human layer and earth layer.

●三才[sān cái]　①原意指天、人、地。针灸中作上、中、下或浅、中、深的分部名。②指三才穴。由百会、璇玑、涌泉组成。〈主治〉癫狂、脏躁、头昏。针一至五分,灸二至五壮。此三穴,百会在顶,应天,主气;涌泉在足底,应地,主精;璇玑在胸,应人,主神。

1. Three Layers　Originally referring to the heaven, human and earth and defined as the upper, middle and low, or the superficial, middle and deep layers of an acupoint in acupuncture.

2. Sancai Points　Referring to the set of acupoints, composed of Baihui (DU 20), Xuanji (RN 21) and Yongquan (KI 1). 〈Indications〉 manic-depressive psychosis, hysteria, dizziness. 〈Method〉 Puncture 0.1～0.5 cun. Apply moxibustion with 2～5 moxa cones. Baihui(DU 20) lies on the top of head corresponding to heaven and taking charge of qi; Yongquan (KI 1) on the sole corresponding to the earth and taking charge of essence of life and Xuanji (RN 21) on the chest corresponding to human being and taking charge of vitality.

●三才解[sān cái jiě]　书名。清代刘润堂著。《沧县志·文献志》载:该书"前五册言针法,将《针灸大全》尽行批驳,独辟新说。后一册言砭法,按穴以小石擦磨。"

Sancai Jie (Explanation of the Three "Geniuses")　A book, compiled by Liu Runtang in the Qing Dynasty. *Cangxian Zhi*: *Wenxian Zhi* (*Annals of Cangxian County*: *Records of Documents*) points out the first 5 volumes of the book are mainly concerned with needling manufacture, give a complete refutation to *Zhenjiu Daquan* (*A Complete Work of Acupuncture and Moxibustion*) and develop original ideas of its own. The last volume deals with stone needling, pressing the acupoint while needling it with a small sharp stone.

●三池[sān chí]　经外穴名。见《经外奇穴汇编》。位于肘部桡侧,曲池及其上、下各开1寸处,共三穴。〈主治〉热病、鼻渊、肘臂酸痛、上肢不遂等。各直刺1-1.5寸;可灸。

Sanchi (EX-UE)　3 extra points seen in *Jingwai Qixue Huibian* (*An Expository Manual of Extra Acupoints*). 〈Location〉 on the radial aspect and near the elbow, three points are located at Quchi (LI 11), 1 cun above or below Quchi (LI 11). 〈Indications〉 febrile disease, rhinorrhea with turbid discharge, aching of the elbow and arm, paralysis of upper extremities. 〈Method〉 Puncture 1～1.5 cun. Moxibustion is applicable.

●三刺[sān cì]　①刺法用语。指分浅、中、深三层进行针刺,在《灵枢·官针》、《灵枢·终始》、《类经》中均有论述。②《内经》刺法名。为齐刺之别称。详见该条。

Triple Needling　① A term of needling, referring to puncturing the superficial, middle and deep layers. It is discussed in *Lingshu*: *Guanzhen* (*Miraculous Pivot*: *Official Needles*), *Lingshu*: *Zhong Shi* (*Miraculous Pivot*: *End and Beginning*) and *Leijing* (*Classified Canon of Internal Medicine of the Yellow Emperor*). ② Another name for assembly puncture, a needling method in *Neijing* (*The Canon of Internal Medicine*). →齐刺(p. 300)

●三管[sān guǎn]　穴位名。出《脉经》。管与脘通,即任脉的上脘、中脘、下脘三穴合称三管。

Sanguan　An acupoint, originally from *Maijing* (*The Classic of Sphygmology*). Here, "guan" is interchangeable with "wan" (脘). "Sanguan" refers to Shangwan (RN 13), Zhongwan (RN 12) and Xiawan (RN 10) of the Ren Meridian.

●三间[sān jiān]　经穴名。出《灵枢·本输》。属于手阳明大肠经,为本经输穴。又名少谷、小谷。〈定位〉微握拳,在手食指本节(第2掌指关节)后,桡侧凹陷处(图48和图6)。〈层次解剖〉皮肤→皮下组织→第一骨

341

间背侧肌→第一蚓状肌与第二掌骨之间→示指的指浅、深屈肌腱与第一骨间掌侧肌之间。浅层：神经由桡神经的指背神经与正中神经的指掌侧固有神经双重分布。血管有手背静脉网，第一掌背动、静脉和示指桡侧动、静脉的分支。深层布有尺神经深支和正中神经肌支。主治目痛、齿痛、咽喉肿痛、手指及手背肿痛、鼽衄、唇焦口干、嗜眠、腹满、肠鸣洞泄。直刺0.3-0.5寸；可灸。

Sanjian (LI 3) A meridian point, originally from *Lingshu: Benshu* (*Miraculous Pivot: Meridian Points*), the Shu (Stream) point of the Large Intestine Meridian of Hand-Yangming, also named Shaogu and Xiaogu. 〈Location〉 In the depression of the radial side, proximal to the 2nd metacarpophalangeal joint when a loose fist is made (Figs. 48 & 6). 〈Regional anatomy〉 skin→subcutaneous tissue→first dorsal interosseous muscle→between first lumbrical muscle and second metacarpal bone →between tendons of superficial and deep flexor muscles of index finger and first palmar interosseous muscle. In the superficial layer, there are the dorsal digital nerve of the radial nerve and the proper palmar digital nerve of the median nerve, the dorsal venous network of the hand, the branches of the first dorsal metacarpal artery and vein and the branches of the radial artery and vein of the index finger. In the deep layer, there are the deep branches of the ulnar nerve and the muscular branches of the median nerve. 〈Indications〉 pain of the eye, toothache, sore throat, swelling and pain of the finger and dorsum of hand, apistaxia, parched lips and dry mouth, drowsiness, abdominal fullness, borborygmus and diarrhea. 〈Method〉 Puncture perpendicularly 0.3～0.5 cun. Moxibustion is applicable.

●三焦[sān jiāo] 耳穴名。位于耳甲腔底部，屏间切迹上方。用于治疗便秘、浮肿、腹胀、手臂外侧疼痛、单纯性肥胖症。

Sanjiao (MA) An auricular point. 〈Location〉 at the base of the cavum conchae, superior to the intertragic notch. 〈Indications〉 constipation, general edema, abdominal distention, pain in the lateral aspect of the arm and obesity.

●三焦经[sān jiāo jīng] 手少阳三焦经之简称。见该条。

Sanjiao Meridian The simple form of the Sanjiao Meridian of Hand-Shaoyang. →手少阳三焦经 (p.393)

●三焦手少阳之脉[sān jiāo shǒu shào yáng zhī mài] 手少阳三焦经原名。详见该条。

The Sanjiao Vessel of Hand-Shaoyang The original name of the Sanjiao Meridian of Hand-Shaoyang. →手少阳三焦经。(p.393)

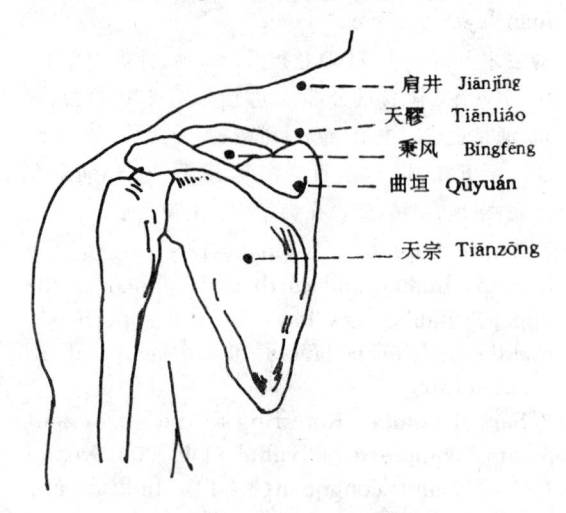

图44.1 三焦经穴（肩部）

Fig 44.1 Points of Sanjiao Meridian (Shouider)

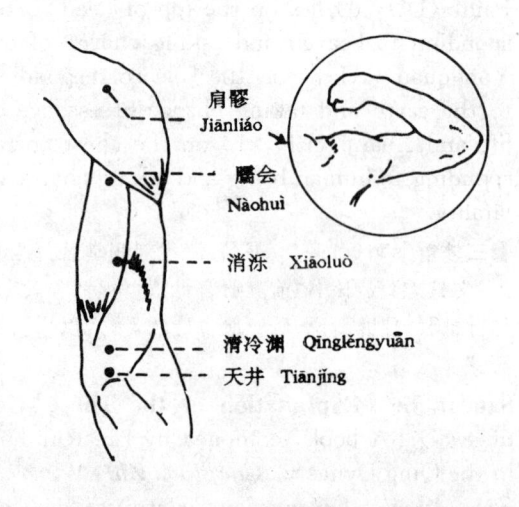

图44.2 三焦经穴（臂部）

Fig 44.2 Points of Sanjiao Meridian (Arm)

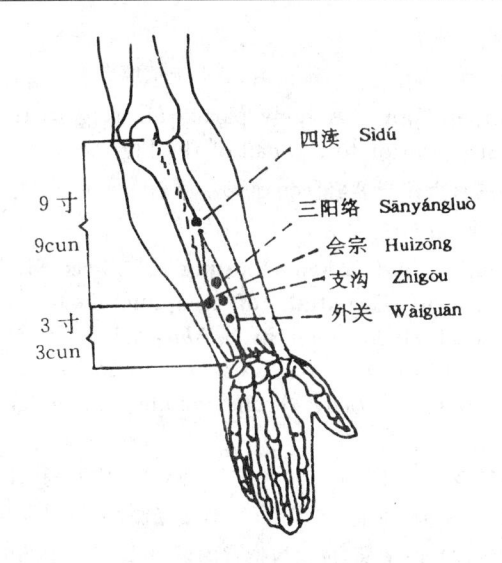

图44.3 三焦经穴(前臂部)
Fig 44.3 Points of Sanjiao Meridian (Forearm)

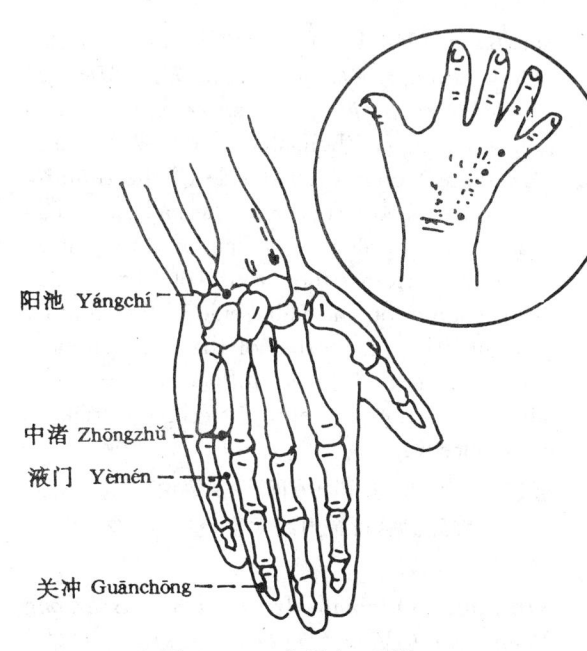

图44.4 三焦经穴(手部)
Fig 44.4 Points of Sanjiao Meridian (Hand)

●三焦俞[sān jiāo shū] 经穴名。出《针灸甲乙经》。属足太阳膀胱经,为三焦的背俞穴。〈定位〉在腰部,当第一腰椎棘突下,旁开1.5寸(图7)。〈层次解剖〉皮肤→皮下组织→背阔肌腱膜和胸腰筋膜浅层→竖脊肌。浅层布有第一、二腰神经后支的皮支和伴行的动、静脉。深层有第一、二腰神经后支的肌支和相应腰动、静脉背侧支的分支或属支。〈主治〉腹胀、肠鸣、完谷不化、呕吐、腹泻、痢疾、小便不利、水肿、肩背拘急、腰脊强痛。直刺0.8-1寸;可灸。

Sanjiaoshu (BL 22) A meridian point, originally from *Zhenjiu Jia-Yi Jing* (*A-B Classic of Acupuncture and Moxibustion*), a point on the Bladder Meridian of Foot-Taiyang, the Back-Shu point of the Sanjiao. 〈Location〉 on the low back, below the spinous process of the lst lumbar vertebra, 1.5 cun lateral to the posterior midline (Fig. 7). 〈Regional anatomy〉 skin → subcutaneous tissue → aponeurosis of latissimus muscle of back and superficial layer of thoracolumbar fascia → erector spinal muscle. In the superficial layer, there are the cutaneous branches of the posterior branches of the lst and 2nd lumbar nerves and the accompanying arteries and veins. In the deep layer there are the muscular branches of the posterior branches of the 1st and 2nd lumbar nerves and the branches or tributaries of the dorsal branches of the related lumbar arteries and veins. 〈Indications〉 fullness or abdominal distention, borborygmus, indigestion, vomiting, diarrhea, dysentery, difficulty in urination, edema, contracture and pain of the shoulder and back, stiffness and pain of the back. 〈Method〉 Puncture perpendicularly 0.8~1 cun. Moxibustion is applicable.

●三角灸[sān jiǎo jiǔ] 经外穴别名,即疝气穴。见该条。

Sanjiaojiu Another name for the extra point Shanqixue (EX-CA). →疝气穴(p. 349)

●三角窝[sān jiǎo wō] 耳廓解剖名称。对耳轮上下脚之间构成的三角形凹窝。

Triangular Fossa An anatomic term of the auricular surface, referring to the triangular depression between the upper and lower cruras of the antihelix.

●三角窝后隆起[sān jiǎo wō hòu lóng qǐ] 耳廓解剖名称。三角窝背面的隆起处。

Tubercle Posterior to the Triangular Fossa An anatomic auricular surface, referring to the protruding part behind the triangular fossa.

●三结交[sān jié jiāo] 经穴别名。出《灵枢·寒热病》。即关元。详见该条。

343

Sanjiejiao Another name for Guanyuan (RN 4), a meridian point originally from *Lingshu: Han Re Bing* (*Miraculous Pivot: Cold and Heat Diseases*). →关元(p. 148)

●三进一退[sān jìn yī tuì] 刺法用语。烧山火手法中用此，其法与一进三退的泻法相对。分三层进针，逐步由浅层、中层，进到深层，一次退针直到浅层。可反复施行。三次进，一次退，体现了徐入疾出，从卫取气的补法原则。

Three Insertions and One Lifting A needling manipulation, generally used in heat-producing needling, the opposite of forward once and backward three times. Needle the 3 layers one after another, from the superficial through the middle to the deep layer little by little and lift the needle from the deep to the superficial layer all at one time. Do this repeatedly. This manipulation embodies the reinforcement principle of slow inserting and quick withdrawing to get qi from weifen.

●三棱针[sān léng zhēn] 针具名。出自古代的锋针。近代用不锈钢制成，针柄较粗为圆柱形，针身呈三棱形，尖端三面有刃，针尖锋利。临床上用它刺破患者身体上一定穴位或浅表血络，放出少量血液来治病。多用于热病、炎症、中暑、昏迷等。对体弱、贫血、低血压及孕妇等应慎用。有出血倾向和血管瘤、血友病患者不宜使用。

Three-Edged Needle A kind of needle developed from the ancient lance needle, now made of stainless steel with a thicker cylinder-shape needle handle and a triangular prism body, whose end has 3 sharp blades. 〈Function〉Puncture certain points or superficial blood vessels to let out a little blood for therapeutic purposes. 〈Indications〉 febrile disease, inflammation, heat stroke, coma. Be careful when applying it to those who are weak, with anemia, hypotension, or pregnant women. Contraindicated for those with hemorrhagic tendency, angioma, hemophilia.

●三里[sān lǐ] ①经穴别名。即足三里，详见该条。②经穴别名。即手三里。详见该条。

Sanli Another name for ① the meridian point Zusanli (ST 36). →足三里(p. 632) ② the meridian point Shousanli (LI 10). →手三里(p. 390)

●三毛[sān máo] 部位名。足大趾爪甲后为三毛。

Dorsal Hair A body part, referring to the part posterior to the nail of the big toe.

●三奇六仪针要经[sān qí liù yí zhēn yào jīng] 书名。见《隋书·经籍志》一卷，书佚。

Sanqi Liuyi Zhen Yaojing ("Three-Six" Canon of Essentials of Acupuncture) A medical book, seen in *Suishu: Jing Ji Zhi* (*The History of the Sui Dynasty: Records of Classics and Books*) one volume, no longer extant.

●三商[sān shāng] 经外穴名。见《江西中医药》。即老商、中商、少商。老商，位于拇指尺侧，距指甲根角旁约0.1寸；中商，位于拇指背侧正中，距指甲根约0.1寸；少商，在拇指桡侧指甲根角旁约0.1寸。〈主治〉昏迷、高热、流行性感冒、急性扁桃体炎、腮腺炎等。点刺出血。

Sanshang (EX-UE) Set of extra points, seen in *Jiangxi Zhongyiyao* (*Jiangxi Journal of Traditional Chinese Medicine and Herbs*), i.e. Laoshang, Zhongshang and Shaoshang. 〈Laoshang〉on the ulnar side of the thumb, 0.1 cun from the corner of the nail. 〈Zhongshang〉on the dorsal median of the thumb, 0.1 cun from the root of the nail. 〈Shaoshang〉on the radial side of the thumb, 0.1 cun from the corner of the nail. 〈Indications〉coma, high fever, influenza, acute tonsillitis and mumps, etc. 〈Method〉Prick to cause bleeding.

●三水[sān shuǐ] 出《素问·示从容论》。①指三阴，即太阴脾经。见《黄帝内经太素》卷十六。②指三阴脏，即肝、脾、肾。

San Shui Originally from *Suwen: Shi Cong Rong Lun* (*Plain Questions: Display in Unhurried Manner*), referring to ① the 3rd yin, i.e. the Spleen Meridian of Foot-Taiyin, seen in *Huang Di Neijing Taisu* (*Comprehensive Notes to the Yellow Emperor's Canon of Internal Classic*). ② the three yin organs, i.e. the liver, spleen and kidney.

●三退一进[sān tuì yī jìn] 刺法用语，为一进三退的别称。详见该条。

Three Liftings and One Insertion A term

for needling manipulation, another name for one insertion and three liftings. → 一进三退 (p. 550)

● 三消[sān xiāo] 病证名。见《丹溪心法·消渴》。上消、中消、下消的合称。详见各条。

Three Types of Diabetes A disease, seen in *Danxi Xinfa: Xiao Ke (Danxi' s Experience: Diabetes)*, i. e. a collective term for diabetes involving the upper, middle and lower jiao. → 上消(p. 354)、中消(p. 615)、下消(p. 491)

● 三阳[sān yáng] ① 经络名。(1)太阳、阳明、少阳的总称。(2)指太阳。参见"三阳三阴"条。② 经穴别名。出《针灸大全》。即百会。详见该条。

1. Three Yang's A category of meridians. Referring to ① the three yang meridians, the collective term for the Meridians of Taiyang, Yangming and Shaoyang. ② the Taiyang Meridian. → 三阳三阴(p. 345)

2. Sanyang Another name for Baihui (DU 20), a meridian point originally from *Zhenjui Daquan (A Complete Work of Acupuncture and Moxibustion)*. → 百会(p. 11)

● 三阳络[sān yáng luò] 经穴名。出《针灸甲乙经》。属手少阳三焦经。又名通间、通门、过门。〈定位〉在前臂背侧，桡尺骨之间，阳池穴上4寸(图48和图44)。〈层次解剖〉在指总伸肌和拇长展肌起端之间；有前臂间背侧动、静脉；布有前臂背侧皮神经，深层为前臂骨间背侧神经。〈主治〉暴喑、耳聋、手臂痛、龋齿痛。直刺0.5～1.0寸；可灸。

Sanyangluo (SJ 8) A meridian point, originally from *Zhenjui Jia-Yi Jing (A-B Classic of Acupuncture and Moxinbustion)*, A point on the Sanjiao Meridian of Hand-Shaoyang, also called Tongjian, Tongmen, Guomen. 〈Location〉on the dorsal side of the forearm, 4 cun above yangchi (SJ 4) between the radius and ulna (Figs. 48 & 44). 〈Regional anatomy〉skin → subcutaneous tissue → extensor muscle of fingers → long abductor muscle of thumb → short extansor muscle of thumb → interosseous membrane of forearm. In the superficial layer, there are the posterior cutaneous nerve of the forearm and the tributaries of the cephalic and basilic veins. In the deep layer, there are the branches or tributaries of the posterior interosseous artery and vein of the forearm and the branches of the posterior interosseous nerve of the forearm. 〈Indications〉sudden loss of voice, deafness, pain in the hand and arm, dental caries and toothache. 〈Method〉 Puncture perpendicularly 0.5～1.0 cun. Moxibustion is applicable.

● 三阳三阴[sān yáng sān yīn] ①经络的命名。三阳三阴的名称广泛应用于经络的命名，包括经脉、经别、络脉、经筋都是如此。阳分太阳、阳明、少阳，总称三阳。阴分太阴、少阴、厥阴，总称三阴。②经络名。出《素问·阴阳类论》、《素问·阴阳别论》。三阳三阴是依阴阳气的盛衰(多少)来分。阳气最盛为阳明，其次为太阳，再次为少阳。阴气最盛为太阴，其次为少阴，再次为厥阴。又可称太阳为三阳，阳明为二阳，少阳为一阳。太阴为三阴，少阴为二阴，厥阴为一阴。分一、二、三，是指六气的次序。参见"六经"条。

Three Yang's and Three Yin's ① A name given to meridians and collaterals. The term is widely used in naming channels, such as meridians, the branches of the twelve meridians, collaterals, and muscular regions of the twelve meridians. Three yang's is a collective term for Taiyang, Yangming and Shaoyang, and three yin's for Taiyin, Shaoyin and Jueyin ② A name for meridians and collaterals, originally from *Suwen: Yin Yang Lei Lun (Plain Questions: On Categories of Yin and Yang)* and *Su Wen: Yin Yang Bie Lun (Plain Questions: Supplementary Exposition of Yin and Yang)*. Three yang's and three yin's are divided according to the excess and deficiency amount of yin-qi and yang-qi. The most excessive of yang-qi is Taiyang, less excessive is Yangming, and the least excessive is Shaoyang. The most excessive of yin-qi is Taiyin, less excessive is Shaoyin, and the least excessive Jueyin. Taiyang is also called the 3rd yang, yangming the 2nd yang, and Shaoyang the 1st yang. Taiyin is also called the 3rd yin, Shaoyin the 2nd yin, and Jueyin the 1st yin. They are so classified in reference to the order of the six types of qi. → 六经(p. 253)

● 三阳五会[sān yáng wǔ huì] 经穴别名。出《史记·

扁鹊传》。《针灸甲乙经》作百会别名。详见"百会"条。

Sanyangwuhui Another name for Baihui (DU 20), as is seen in *Zhenjiu Jia-Yi Jing* (*A-B Classic of Acupuncture and Moxibustion*), a meridian point originally from *Shi Ji: Bian Que Zhuan* (*The Historical Records: Biography of Bian Que*). →百会 (p.11)

●三阴[sān yīn] 经络名。①一说为太阴、少阴、厥阴的总称。② 一说指太阴,包括手太阴肺经与足太阴脾经。出《素问·阴阳类论》等篇。参见"三阳三阴"条。

Three Yin A name of meridians, ① the collective term for the meridians of Taiyin, Shaoyin and Jueyin. ② referring to the Taiyin Meridians, including the lung meridian of Hand-Taiyin and the Spleen Meridian of Foot-Taiyin, originally from *Suwen: Yinyang Leilun*(*Plain Questions: On Categories of Yin and Yang*), etc. →三阳三阴(p.345)

●三阴交[sān yīn jiāo] 经穴名。出《针灸甲乙经》。属足太阴脾经,为足太阴、厥阴、少阴之会。〈定位〉在小腿内侧,当足内踝尖上3寸,胫骨内侧缘后方(图39)。〈层次解剖〉皮肤→皮下组织→趾长屈肌→胫骨后肌→长屈肌。浅层布有隐神经的小腿内侧皮支,大隐静脉的属支。深层有胫神经和胫后动、静脉。〈主治〉脾胃虚弱、肠鸣腹胀、飧泄、消化不良、月经不调、崩漏、赤白带下、阴挺、经闭、癥瘕、难产、产后血晕、恶露不行、遗精、阳萎、阴茎痛、疝气、水肿、小便不利、遗尿、足痿痹痛、脚气、失眠、神经性皮炎、湿疹、荨麻疹、高血压等。直刺0.5～1寸;可灸。孕妇禁刺。

Sanyinjiao (SP 6) A meridian point, originally from *Zhenjiu Jia-Yi Jing* (*A-B Classic of Acupuncture and Moxibustion*), a point on the Spleen Meridian of Foot-Taiyin, the crossing point of the three yin meridians of the foot. 〈Location〉on the medial side of the leg, 3 cun above the tip of the medial malleolus, posterior to the medial border of the tibia (Fig. 39). 〈Regional anatomy〉 skin→subcutaneous tissue→long flexor muscle of toes→posterior tibial muscle→long flexor muscle of great toe. In the superficial layer, there are the medial cutaneous branches of the leg from the saphenous nerve and the tributaries of the great saphenous vein. In the deep layer, there are the tibial nerve and the posterior tibial artery and vein. 〈Indications〉 deficiency of the spleen and stomach, borborygmus and abdominal distension, lienteric diarrhea, dyspepsia, irregular menstruation, metrorrhagia and metrostaxis, leukorrhea with reddish discharge, prolapse of uterus, anemia, mass in the abdomen, difficult labour, postpartum shock, lochiostasis, emission, impotence, pain in penis, hernia, edema, oliguria, enuresis, flaccidity, numbness, and pain in foot, beriberi, insomnia, neurodermatitis, eczema, prurigo and hypertension, etc. 〈Method〉 Puncture perpendicularly 0.5～1 cun. Moxibustion is applicable. Acupuncture is forbidden in pregnant women.

●三阴三阳[sān yīn sān yáng] ①经络名。阳分为太阳、阳明、少阳,合称三阳;阴分为太阴、少阴、厥阴,合称三阴。又可称太阳为三阳,阳明为二阳,少阳为一阳;太阴为三阴,少阴为二阴,厥阴为一阴。参见"六经"条。② 经外穴名。出《针灸孔穴及其疗法便览》。位于耳廓前,近耳廓之发际边缘,颧弓之上缘,左右计二穴。〈主治〉耳聋、耳鸣、上齿痛、咀嚼肌痉挛。可灸。

1. **Three Yin's and Three Yang's** A name for meridians. Three yang's is a collective term for Taiyang, Yangming and Shaoyang; three yin's is a collective term for Taiyin, Shaoyin and Jueyin. Taiyang is also called the 3rd yang, Yangming the 2nd yang, Shaoyang the 1st yang; Taiyin is also called the 3rd yin, Shaoyin the 2nd yin, Jueyin the 1st yin. →六经(p.253)

2. **Sanyinsanyang** (EX-HN) An extra point, originally from *Zhenjui Kongxue Ji Qi Liaofa Bianlan* (*Guide to Acupoints and Acupuncture Theapeutics*). 〈Location〉on the anterior part of the auricle, near the border of the hairline, and at the upper border of the zygomatic arch. 〈Indications〉 deafness, tinnitus, upper toothache, and masticatory spasm. 〈Method〉Moxibustion is applicable in addition to acupuncture.

●散刺[sǎn cì] 刺法之一。见《素问·诊要经终论》。在穴位及周围进行散在的多点浅刺,多用于三棱针

刺法。

Clumpy Pricking A term for needling manipulations, seen in *Suwen: Zhen Yao Jing Luo Lun* (*Plain Questions: On the Essentials of Diagnosis and Exhaustion of Meridians*), referring to shallow and scattered pricking around the acupoints, mostly used in needling with three-edged needles.

●散脉[sǎn mài] ①足太阴之别络。出《素问·刺腰痛篇》。以其散行而上,故称。② 脉象之一。

1. Scattered Vessel A collateral of the meridian of Foot-Taiyin, originally from *Suwen: Ci Yao Tong Pian* (*Plain Questrions: On Treatment of Lumbago with Acupuncture*). It was so named because the meridian runs upward in a scattered manner.

2. Scattered Pulse One type of the manifestations of the pulse condition.

●散笑[sǎn xiào] 经外穴名。出《刺疗捷法》。在面部,当迎香穴下方,鼻唇沟之中点处。〈主治〉鼻塞、面瘫、疔疮等。沿皮刺0.3-0.5寸。

Sanxiao (EX-HN) An extra point, originally from *Ciding Jiefa* (*Simple Acupuncture Method for Boils*). 〈Location〉 on the face, at the inferior aspect of Yingxiang (LI 20), at the midpoint of the nasolabial groove. 〈Indications〉 stuffy nose, facial paralysis and furuncle, etc. 〈Method〉 Puncture subcutaneously 0.3～0.5 cun.

●散针法[sǎn zhēn fǎ] 指在病痛部位选穴针刺。

Scattering Needling A method of puncturing in the diseased area.

●桑木灸[sāng mù jiǔ] 灸法的一种。见《外科正宗》。将桑木条点燃后薰灸患处。可治疗疮毒。

Mulberry Moxibustion A form of moxibustion, seen in *Waike Zhengzong* (*Orthodox Manual of External Diseases*). Fumigate the affected part with a burning mulberry stick. 〈Indications〉 furunculosis.

●桑枝灸[sāng zhī jiǔ] 灸法的一种。见《本草纲目》。其法与神针火类似。参见该条。

Mublerry Twigs Moxibustion A form of moxibustion, seen in *Bencao Gangmu* (*Compendium of Materia Medica*), Similar to miraculous fire needle. →神针火(p. 364)

●颡大[sǎng dà] 经穴别名。见《灵枢·根结》。即头维。详见该条。

Sangda Another name for Touwei (ST 8), a meridian point seen in *Lingshu: Genjie* (*Miraculous Pivot: Root and Branch*). →头维 (p. 445)

●色盲[sè máng] 病证名。见《证治准绳》。又称视物异色,视赤如白。多因先天发育不良,肝肾亏虚,目络气血不和,影响元府功能,以致五色不能辨别。如丧失红色辨色力,为红色盲;丧失绿色辨色力,为绿色盲;红绿均不能辨议者,为全色盲。治宜补益肝肾,调和元府。取睛明、攒竹、瞳子髎、风池、四白、光明、行间。

Color Blindness A disease, seen in *Zhengzhi Zhunsheng* (*Standards for Diagnosis and Treatment*), also called Shiwuyise (seeing an object in a color quite different from its original one), or Shichirubai (seeing red as if seeing white), mostly caused by an innate maldevelopment, deficiency of the liver and kidney, and the derangement of qi and blood of the eye's collaterals, leading to the dysfunction of the brain and failure to distinguish the five colors. For instance, loss of red discrimination is called red blindness; loss of green discrimination green blindness; and loss of both red and green discrimination complete color blindness. 〈Treatment principle〉 Tonify the liver and kidney and regulate the function of the brain. 〈Point selection〉 Jingming (BL 1), Cuanzhu (BL 2), Tongziliao (GB 1), Fengchi (GB 20), Sibai (ST 2), Guangming (GB 37) And Xingjian (LR 2).

●僧坦然[sēng tǎn rán] 人名。明代针灸家,住太平箬村(今属安徽)。善针灸,针细且短,治多验。见《太平府志》。

Seng Tanran An acupuncture moxibustion expert in the Ming Dynasty, living in Taipingzhi village (now in Anhui Province), proficient in acupuncture and moxibustion, especially in puncturing with small and short needles, which was usually effective. Cf. *Taipingfu Zhi* (*Annals of Taipingfu*).

●莎刀[shā dāo] 针具名,小眉刀之别称。详见该条。

Sha Knife A kind of needling instrument, another name for small eyebrow-like kinfe. →小眉刀(p. 504)

●砂淋[shā lìn] 淋证证型之一,即石淋。详见该条。

Sand Stranguria One type of stranguria, i.e. stranguria caused by the passage of urinary stone. →石淋(p. 385)

●砂石淋[shā shí lìn] 淋证证型之一,即石淋,详见该条。

Sand-Stone Stranguria One type of stranguria. →石淋(p. 385)

●山根[shān gēn] 部位名。指鼻根部,约与两眼内眦相平。古代称"頞",又称"下极"。是中医望诊的重要部位。

Hill Foot A part of the body, referring to the radix nasi which is paralel with the two inner canthus, called "*E*" or "*Xiaji*" in ancient times, an important part for observation in traditional Chinese Medicine.

●山眺针灸经[shān tiào zhēn jiǔ jīng] 书名。见宋《崇文总目》一卷。书佚。

Shantiao Zhenjiu Jing (Shantiao Classic of Acupuncture and Moxibustion) A book originally mentioned in the 1st volume of *Chongwen Zongmu* (*Chongwen General Catalogue*) of the Song Dynasty, lost.

●山栀生姜灸[shān zhī shēng jiāng jiǔ] 间接灸的一种。出《灸治经验集》。用黄栀子打碎,水煎成浓汁,加入一些生姜汁,混以面粉和石灰各一份,调成糊状,涂于穴位上。再放一薄生姜片,上置艾炷施灸。

Shan Zhi (Capejasmine) and Fresh Ginger-Separated Moxibustion A kind of indirect moxibustion, originally from *Jiuzhi Jingyan Ji* (*A Collection Experiences of Moxibustion*). 〈Method〉Break shanzhi (Capejasmine) into pieces, boil to a thick juice, then mix with ginger juice, wheat flour and lime into a paste, put the paste and a ginger slice on the selected acupoint, on which, moxa-cone moxibustion is applied.

●闪罐[shǎn guàn] 拨罐法的一种,又称闪罐法。其法将罐子拔上后,立即起下,反复吸拔多次,至皮肤潮红为止。多用于局部皮肤麻木或机能减退的虚证病例。

Quick Cupping A kind of cupping, also called successive flash cupping. 〈Method〉Apply the cup on the affected area and remove it at once. Do the same thing many times over the same area until the skin becomes hypermic red. It is mostly used for local skin numbness and miopragia of deficiency type.

●闪罐法[shǎn guàn fǎ] 为闪罐之别称。详见该条。

Successive Flash Cupping. →闪罐(p. 348)

●闪火法[shǎn huǒ fǎ] 火罐操作的一种方法。其法用长纸条或用镊子夹酒精棉球点燃后,在罐内绕一圈再抽出,迅将罐子罩在应拔的部位上,即可吸住。

Flash-Fire Cupping A kind of cupping. 〈Method〉with a long burning slip of paper or a burning ball of alcohol-cotton held with forceps, go full circle inside the cup and then, take the flame away and cover the part to be cupped immediately with the cup upside-down, the cup can thus be attracted to the skin.

●疝[shàn] 病名。出《素问·大奇论》等。即疝气。详见该条。

Hernia A disease, originally from *Suwen: Daqi Lun* (*Plain Questions: On Extremely Strange Diseases*). i. e. hernial qi. →疝气(p. 348)

●疝气[shàn qì] 病名。又称疝。泛指睾丸、阴囊、少腹肿大疼痛而言。多因坐卧湿地,或淋雨风冷,感受寒湿之邪,循任脉和足厥阴肝经,凝滞于少腹睾丸、阴囊所致。或寒湿之邪蕴结化热,肝脾二经湿热下注,或强力负重,脉络损伤,气虚下陷均可引起。分寒疝、热疝、狐疝等。详见各条。

Hernial Qi A disease, also called hernia, referring to swelling pain in the testicle, scrotum or lower abdomen. Mostly due to sitting and lying on wet land or an attack of cold-dampness pathogen resulting from getting wet in the rain and wind-cold, leading to the stagnation of cold-dampness in the lower abdomen, testicle, and scrotum along the Ren and the Liver Meridian; or to the downward flow of damp-heat of the liver and spleen meridians resulting from the accumulation of cold-dampness; or to the damage of the meridians and collaterals and collapse of qi resulting from overstrain. It is divided into her-

nia due to heat, hernia due to cold and inguinal hernia. →寒疝(p. 156)、热疝(p. 331)、狐疝(p. 167)

●疝气穴[shàn qì xué] 经外穴名。见《医宗金鉴》。又名脐旁穴,三角灸。以两口角间长度为一边作一等边三角形,顶角置脐心,底边呈水平,下两角是穴。主治疝气偏坠。用灸法。

Shanqixue(EX-CA) A pair of extra points, seen in *Yizong Jinjian* (*Golden Mirror of Orthodox Medical Lineage*), also called Qipangxue or Sanjiaojiu. Take the distance between the two angles of the patient's mouth as one side to make an equilateral triangle with the vertex angle on the acromphalus. The lower side being horizontal, the two lower angles are the points. 〈Indications〉hernia and collapse of testicles. 〈Method〉moxibustion.

●伤痓[shāng jìng] 即破伤风。详见该条。

Tetanus due to Injury →破伤风(p. 298)

●伤乳吐[shāng rǔ tù] 小儿呕吐证型之一。见《证治准绳·幼科》。又名嗌乳。哺乳儿常见病。多因乳饮无度,脾气弱不能运化所致。症见乳哺后即吐,或少停而吐。治宜健脾消乳,节制乳食,取脾俞、胃俞、足三里。

Milk Vomiting in Infants A type of vomiting in children, seen in *Zhengzhi Zhunsheng*: *Youke* (*Standards for Diagnosis and Treatment*: *Pediatrics*) also called milk vomiting, one of the common diseases of lactated infants, mostly caused by overeating of milk and dysfunction of the spleen in transportation. 〈Manifestations〉vomiting immediately after drinking. 〈Treatment principles〉Invigorate the spleen, promote digestion and control milk-feeding. 〈Point selection〉Pishu (BL 20), Weishu (BL 21) and Zusanli (ST 36).

●伤食呕吐[shāng shí ǒu tù] 呕吐证型之一。因食滞停积,胃气上逆所致。证见呕吐酸腐,脘腹胀满,嗳气厌食,得食愈甚吐后反快,大便秽臭或溏薄或秘结,苔厚腻,脉滑实。治宜行气导滞。取璇玑、下脘、腹结、足三里、行间。

Vomiting due to Improper Diet A type of vomiting, due to the accumulation of food leading to the adverse-rising of the stomach-qi. 〈Manifestations〉vomiting with sour and rotten discharge, abdominal distention, eructation and anorexia. The case gets worse after eating and better after vomiting, loose stool or constipation with foul smell, thick and greasy tongue coating, slippery and excessive pulse. 〈Treatment principles〉Promote the circulation of qi, remove stagnancy and obstruction of undigested food. 〈Point selection〉Xuanji (RN 21), Xiawan (RN 10), Fujie (SP 14), Zusanli (ST 36) and Xingjian (LR 2).

●伤食吐[shāng shí tù] 小儿呕吐证型之一。见《古今医统》。多因饮食不节,脾胃受损所致。证见频吐酸馊粘液,或吐黄水,或吐清涎,腹胀嗳气,厌食等。治宜健脾和胃,消食导滞。取脾俞、胃俞、建里、中脘、内关、公孙。

Infantile Vomiting due to Improper Diet A type of vomiting in childern, seen in *Gu Jin Yitong* (*The General Medicine of the Past and Present*), mostly caused by improper diet damaging the spleen and stomach. 〈Manifestations〉frequent vomiting with sour mucus, yellowish juice or clear saliva, abdominal distension and eructation, anorexia, etc. 〈Treatment principle〉Strengthen the spleen and stomach, eliminate undigested food by means of stomachics. 〈Point selection〉Pishu (BL 20), Weishu (BL 21), Jianli (RN 11), Zhongwan (RN 12), Neiguan (PC 6) and Gongsun (SP 4).

●伤食泻[shāng shí xiè] 泄泻证型之一。见《丹溪心法·泄泻》。由饮食不节,宿食内停,阻滞肠胃,传导失常所致。证见腹痛肠鸣,泻下粪便臭如败卵,伴有不消化之物,泻后痛减,脘腹痞满,嗳腐酸臭,不思饮食,舌苔垢浊或厚腻,脉滑。治宜消导调中。取中脘、章门、胃俞、脾俞、足三里、隐白、内关、建里、公孙。

Diarrhea due to Improper Diet A type of diarrhea, seen in *Danxi Xinfa*: *Xiexie* (*Danxi's Experience*: *Diarrhea*), due to improper diet and food retention blocking the stomach and intestines leading to abnormal transportation. 〈Manifestations〉abdominal pain and borborygmus, smelly stools with dyspeptic things, pain abated after diarrhea, abdominal distention, sour and rotten eructation, anorexia, curdy coating or thick and greasy coating,

rolling pulse. 〈Treatment principle〉 Remove food retention, promote digestion and regulate the function of the spleen and stomach. 〈Point selection〉 Zhongwan (RN 12), Zhangmen (LR 13), Weishu (BL 21), Pishu (BL 20), Zusanli (ST 36), Yinbai (SP 1), Neiguan (PC 6), Jianli (RN 11) and Gongsun (SP 4).

●商盖[shāng gài] 经穴别名。见《循经考穴编》。即督俞。详见该条。

Shanggai Another name for Dushu (BL 16), a meridian point seen in *Xunjing Kaoxue Bian* (*Studies on Acupoints along the Meridians*). →督俞 (p. 86)

●商陆饼灸[shāng lù bǐng jiǔ] 隔物灸的一种。见《千金翼方》卷二十三。又称隔商陆灸。详见该条。

Pokeberry Root-Cake-Separated Moxibustion A form of material-insulated moxibustion, seen in Vol. 23 of *Qianjin Yifang* (*Supplement to Essential Prescriptions Worth a Thousand Gold*), also called pokeberry root-separated moxibustion. →隔商陆灸 (p. 137)

●商丘[shāng qiū] 经穴名。出《灵枢·本输》。属足太阴脾经，为本经经穴。〈定位〉在足内踝前下方凹陷中，当舟骨结节与内踝尖连线的中点处（图81和图39）。〈层次解剖〉皮肤→皮下组织→内侧（三角）韧带→胫骨内踝。浅层布有隐神经，大隐静脉。深层有内踝前动、静脉的分支或属支。〈主治〉腹胀、肠鸣、泄泻、便秘、食不化、舌本强痛、黄疸、怠惰嗜卧、癫狂、善笑、梦魇、善太息、咳嗽、小儿痫瘛、痔疾、足踝痛。直刺0.3～0.5寸；可灸。

Shangqiu (SP 5) A meridian point, originally from *Lingshu: Benshu* (*Miraculous Pivot: Meridian Points*), the Jing (River) point of the Spleen Meridian of Foot-Taiyin. 〈Location〉 in the depression, anterior and inferior to the medial malleolus, at the midpoint of the line connecting the tuberosity of the navicular bone and the tip of the medial malleous (Figs. 81 & 39). 〈Regional anatomy〉 skin→subcutaneous tissue→medial (triangular) ligament→medial malleolus of tibia. In the superficial layer, there are the saphenous nerve and the great saphenous vein. In the deep layer, there are the branches or tributaries of the medial anterior malleolar artery and vein. 〈Indications〉 abdominal distension, borborygmus, diarrhea, constipation, dyspepsia, pain in the root of the tongue, jaundice, lassitude and drowsiness, manic-depressive psychosis, susceptibility to laughter, susceptibility to sighs, cough, epilepsy in children, hemorrhoids, pain in the foot-ankle. 〈Method〉 Puncture perpendicularly 0.3～0.5 cun. Moxibustion is applicable.

●商曲[shāng qū] 经穴名。出《针灸甲乙经》。属足少阴肾经，为冲脉、足少阴之会。又名高曲。〈定位〉在上腹部，当脐中上2寸，前正中线旁开0.5寸（图40）。〈层次解剖〉皮肤→皮下组织→腹直肌鞘前壁→腹直肌。浅层布有腹壁浅静脉，第八、九、十胸神经前支的前皮支及伴行的动、静脉。深层有腹壁上动、静脉的分支或属支，第八、九、十胸神经前支的肌支和相应的肋间动、静脉。〈主治〉腹痛、泄泻、便秘、腹中积聚。直刺0.5～0.8寸；可灸。

Shangqu (KI 17) A meridian point, originally from *Zhenjiu Jia-Yi Jing* (*A-B Classic of Acupuncture and Moxibustion*), a point on the Kidney Meridian of Foot-Shaoyin, the crossing point of Chong and Foot-Shaoyin Meridians, also called Gaoqu. 〈Location〉 on the upper abdomen, 2 cun above the centre of the umbilicus, and 0.5 cun lateral to the anterior midline (Fig. 40). 〈Regional anatomy〉 skin→subcutaneous tissue→anterior sheath of rectus muscle of abdomen→rectus muscle of abdomen. In the superficial layer, there are the superficial epigasteric vein, the anterior cutaneous branches of the anterior branches of the 8th to 10th thoracic nerves and the accompanying artery and vein, the muscular branches of the anterior branches or tributaries of the superior epigastric artery and vein, the muscular branches of the anterior branches of the 8th to 10th thoracic nerves and the related intercostal arteries and veins. 〈Indications〉 abdominal pain, diarrhea, constipation, and abdominal mass. 〈Method〉 Puncture perpendicularly 0.5～0.8 cun. Moxibustion is applicable.

●商阳[shāng yáng] 经穴名。出《灵枢·本输》。属手阳明大肠经，为本经井穴。又名绝阳。〈定位〉在手食指末节桡侧，距指甲角0.1寸（指寸）（图48和图6）。

〈层次解剖〉皮肤→皮下组织→指甲根。有正中神经的指掌侧固有神经之指背支和示指桡侧动、静脉与第一掌背动、静脉分支所形成的动、静脉网。〈主治〉咽喉肿痛、颐颌肿、下齿痛、耳聋、耳鸣、青盲、热病汗不出、昏厥、中风昏迷、喘咳、肩痛引缺盆。向上斜刺0.2~0.3寸,或点刺出血;可灸。

Shangyang (LI 1) A meridian point, originally from *Lingshu: Benshu* (*Miraculous Pivot: Acupoints*), the Jing (Well) point of the Large Intestine Meridian of Hand-Yangming, also called Jueyang. 〈Location〉on the radial side of the distal segment of the index finger, 0.1 cun from the corner of the nail (Figs. 48 &6). 〈Regional anatomy〉 skin→subcutaneous tissue→root of nail. There are the dorsal digital branches of the proper palmar digital nerve of the median nerve the arteriovenous network formed by the anteries and veins in the radial side of the index finger, and the branches of the first dordal metacarpal artery and vein in this drea. 〈Indications〉 swelling and pain in the throat, mumps, lower toothache, deafness, tinnitus, optic atrophy, febrile diseases but anhidrosis, syncope, apoplectic coma, dyspnea and cough, shoulder pain radiating to the supraclavicular fossa. 〈Method〉 Puncture upward and obliquely 0.2~0.3 cun or prick to cause bleeding. Moxibustion is applicable.

●上胞下垂[shàng bāo xià chuí] 即眼睑下垂的别名。详见该条。

Ptosis Another name for blepharoptosis. →眼睑下垂(p. 535)

●上病下取[shàng bìng xià qǔ] 《内经》取穴法则之一,简称下取。指上部的病证取用下部穴。如牙痛取内庭。

Selection of Lower Points for Upper Diseases A principle of point selection in Neijing (*The Yellow Emperor's Inner Canon*), called selection of lower points lower part point selection for short, referring to treating diseases in the upper part of the body by needling the points of the lower, e.g. treating toothache by needling Neiting (ST 44).

●上慈宫[shàng cí gōng] 经穴别名。出《针灸聚英》。即冲门。详见该条。

Shangcigong Another name for Chongmen (SP 12), a meridian point originally from *Zhenjiu Juying* (*Essentials of Acupuncture and Moxibustion*). →冲门(p. 49)

●上都[shàng dū] 经外穴名。八邪之一。见《奇效良方》。详见"八邪"条。

Shangdu An extra point, one of Baxie (EX-UE 9), seen in *Qixiao Liangfang* (*Prescription of Wonderful Efficiency*). →八邪(p. 8)

●上腭穴[shàng è xué] 经外穴名。见《千金要方》。在口腔内,当上腭缝际前端,齿龈上缘中点处。〈主治〉黄疸等病。斜刺0.1-0.2寸;或点刺出血。

Shang'exue (EX-HN) An extra point, seen in *Qianjin Yaofang* (*Essential Prescriptions Worth a Thousand Gold*). 〈Location〉in the mouth, at the inferior aspect of the palate raphe, at the midpoint of the superior border of the gum. 〈Indications〉 jaundice, etc. 〈Method〉 Puncture obliquely 0.1~0.2 cun or prick to cause bleeding.

●上耳根[shàng ěr gēn] ①耳廓解剖名称。耳廓上缘与头皮附着处。②耳穴名。又名郁中、脊髓1。位于耳根最上缘。用于治疗头痛、腹痛、哮喘、鼻衄。

1. **Upper Ear Root** A term for auricular anatomy, referring to the union part of the superior border of the ear and scalp.
2. **Upper Root of Auricle** (MA) An ear point, also called Yuzhong (MA), Spinal Cord 1 (MA). 〈Location〉at the extreme superior border of the ear root. 〈Indications〉 headache, abdominal pain, asthma and epistaxis.

●上骨[shàng gǔ] 骨骼名,指桡骨。手太阴肺经的循行有"循臂内上骨下廉"。意指沿桡骨的下边。参见《太素》卷八。

The Upper Bone Part of a skeleton, i.e. radius. The distribution of the Lung Meridian of Hand-Taiyin is "along the inferior border of the upper bone in the medial aspect of the upper extremity", i.e. travelling along the inferior border of the radius. Cf. Vol. 8 of *Huangdi Neijing Taisu* (*Comprehensive Notes to the Yellow Emperor's Canon of Internal Medicine*).

●上关[shàng guān] 经穴名。出《灵枢·本输》。属足少阳胆经，为手足少阳、足阳明之会。又名客主人。〈定位〉在耳前，下关直上，当颧弓的上缘凹陷处(图28)。〈层次解剖〉皮肤→皮下组织→颞浅筋膜→颞深筋膜→颞筋膜下疏松结缔组织→颞肌。浅层布有耳颞神经，面神经颞支和颞浅动、静脉。深层有颞深前、后神经的分支。〈主治〉头痛、耳鸣、耳聋、聤耳、口眼㖞斜、面痛、齿痛、惊痫、瘈疭。直刺0.5～0.8寸；可灸。

Shangguan (GB 3) A meridian point originally from *Lingshu: Benshu* (*Miraculous Pivot: Meridian Points*), a point on the Gallbladder Meridian of Foot-Shaoyang, the crossing point of the Hand-and Foot-Shaoyang and Foot-Yangming, also called Kezhuren. 〈Location〉 anterior to the ear, directly above Xiaguan (ST 7), in the depression above the upper border of the zygomatic arch (Fig. 28). 〈Regional anatomy〉skin→subcutaneous tissue→superficial temporal fascia→deep temporal fascia → loose connective tissue → temporal muscle. In the superficial layer, there are the auriculotemporal nerve, the temporal branch of the facial nerve and the superficial temporal artery and vein. In the deep layer, there are the branches of the anterior and posterior deep temporal nerves. 〈Indications〉headache, tinnitus, deafness, ceruminosis, facial paralysis, facial pain, toothache, epilepsy due to terror, and clonic convulsion. 〈Method〉Puncture perpendicularly 0.5～0.8 cun. Moxibustion is applicable.

●上管[shàng guǎn] 经穴别名。出《脉经》。即上脘。详见该条。

Shangguan Another name for Shangwan (RN 13), a meridian point originally from *Maijing*(*The Pulse Classic*). →上脘(p. 353)

●上纪[shàng jì] ①经穴别名。出《素问·气穴论》王冰注。即中脘。详见该条。②经穴别名。见《针灸大全》。即上脘。详见该条。

Shangji Another name for ① Zhongwan (RN 12), a meridian point originally from the Wang Bing' s annotation for *Su Wen: Qixue Lun*(*Plain Questions: On Loci of Qi*). →中脘(p. 614) ② Shangwan (RN 13), a meridian point seen in *Zhenjiu Daquan* (*A Complete Work of Acupuncture and Moxibustion*). →上脘(p. 353)

●上巨虚[shàng jù xū] 经穴名。见《千金翼方》。《灵枢·本输》名巨虚上廉。属足阳明胃经，为大肠的下合穴。又名上林、巨虚、上廉、足上廉。〈定位〉在小腿前外侧，当犊鼻下6寸，距胫骨前缘一横指(中指)(图60)。〈层次解剖〉皮肤→皮下组织→胫骨前肌→小腿骨间膜→胫骨后肌。浅层布有腓肠外侧皮神经。深层有胫前动、静脉和腓深神经。如深刺可能刺中胫后动、静脉和胫神经。〈主治〉腹痛、痢疾、肠鸣、腹胀、便秘、泄泻、肠痈、中风瘫痪、脚气。直刺0.5～1.2寸；可灸。

Shangjuxu (ST 37) A meridian point, seen in *Qianjin Yifang* (*Supplement to Essential Prescriptions Worth a Thousand Gold*), called Juxushanglian in *Ling Shu: Benshu* (*Miraculous Pivot: Meridian Points*), a point on the Stomach Meridian of Foot-Yangming, the lower confluent point of the large intestine, also called Shanglin, Juxu, Shanglian and Zushanglian. 〈Location〉on the anteriolateral side of the leg, 6 cun below Dubi(ST 35), one finger breadth (middle finger) from the anterior crest of the tibia(Fig. 60). 〈Regional anatomy〉skin→subcutaneous tissue→anterior tibial muscle→interosseous membrane of leg→posterior tibial muscle. In the superficial layer, there is the lateral cutaneous nerve of the calf. In the deep layer, there are the anterior tibia artery and vein and the deep peroneal nerve. If the needle is inserted too deep, it may injure the posterior tibial artery and vein and the tibial nerve. 〈Indications〉 abdominal pain, dysentery, borborygmus, abdominal distension, constipation, diarrhea, acute appendicitis, paralysis after apoplexy, and beriberi. 〈Method〉Puncture perpendicularly 0.5～1.2 cun. Moxibustion is applicable.

●上昆仑[shàng kūn lún] 经穴别名。出《太平圣惠方》。即昆仑。详见该条。

Shangkunlun Another name for Kunlun (BL 60), a meridian point originally from *Taiping Shenghui Fang* (*Imperial Benevolent Prescriptions*). →昆仑(p. 236)

●上廉[shàng lián] ①经穴名。出《针灸甲乙经》。属手阳明大肠经，又名手上廉。〈定位〉在前臂背面桡

侧,当阳溪与曲池连线上,肘横纹下3寸(图48和图6)。〈层次解剖〉皮肤→皮下组织→桡侧腕长伸肌腱后方→桡侧腕短伸肌→旋后肌→拇长展肌。浅层有前臂外侧皮神经、前臂后皮神经和浅静脉等分布。深层有桡神经深支穿旋后肌。〈主治〉头痛、偏瘫、手臂肩膊酸痛麻木、腹痛、肠鸣、泄泻。直刺0.5~0.8寸;可灸。②经穴别名,即上巨虚。详见该条。

1. Shanglian(LI 9) A meridian point, originally from *Zhenjui Jia-Yi Jing* (*A-B Classic of Acupuncture and Moxibustion*), a point on the large Intestine Meridian of Hand-Yangming, also called Shoushanglian. 〈Location〉 on the radial side of the dorsal surface of the forearm and on the line connecting Yangxi (LI 5) and Quchi (LI 11), 3 cun below the cubital crease (Figs. 48 & 6). 〈Regional anatomy〉 skin → subcutaneous tissue → posterior part of long radial exensor mulscle of wrist → short radial extensor muscle of wrist → supinator muscle → long abductor muscle of thumb. In the superficial layer, there are the lateral and posterior cutaneous nerves of the forearm and the superficial vein. In the deep layer, there is the supinator muscle perforated by the deep branches of the radial nerve. 〈Indications〉 headache, hemiparalysis, aching pain and numbness of the arm and shoulder, abdominal pain, borborygmus, and diarrhea. 〈Metrhod〉 Puncture perpendicularly 0.5~0.8 cun. Moxibustion is applicable.

2. Shanglian Another name for the meridian point, Shangjuxu (ST 37). →上巨虚(p. 352)

●上髎[shàng liáo] 经穴名。出《针灸甲乙经》。属足太阳膀胱经,为足太阳、少阳之会。〈定位〉在骶部,当髂后上棘与后正中线之间,适对第一骶后孔处(图7)。〈层次解剖〉皮肤→皮下组织→胸腰筋膜浅层→竖脊肌→第一骶后孔。浅层布有臀中皮神经。深层有第一骶神经和骶外侧动、静脉的后支。〈主治〉腰疼、月经不调、阴挺、带下、遗精、阳萎、大小便不利。直刺0.8~1寸;可灸。

Shangliao (BL 31) A meridian point, originally from *Zhenjiu Jia-Yi Jing* (*A-B Classic of Acupuncture and Moxibustion*), a point on the Bladder Meridian of Foot-Taiyang, the crossing point of Foot-Taiyang and Foot-Shaoyang. 〈Location〉 on the sacrum, at the midpoint between the posterio-superior iliac spine and the posterior midline, just at the 1st posterior sacral foramen (Fig. 7). 〈Regional anatomy〉 skin → subcutaneous tissue → superficial layer of thoracolumbar fascia → erector spinal muscle → 1st posterior sacral foramen. In the superficial layer, there is the middle clunial nerve. In the deep layer, there are the posterior branches of the 1st sacral nerve and the lateral sacral artery and vein. 〈Indications〉 lumbar pain, irregular menstruation, prolapse of uterus, leukorrhea, emission, impotence, dyschesia and oliguria. 〈Method〉 Puncture perpendicularly 0.8~1 cun. Moxibustion is applicable.

●上林[shàng lín] 经穴别名。出《圣济总录》。"林"系"廉"字之误。即上巨虚。详见该条。

Shanglin Another name for Shangjuxu (ST 37), a meridian point originally from *Shengji Zonglu* (*Imperial Medical Encyclopedia*). "林" was mistaken for "廉". →上巨虚(p. 352)

●上门[shàng mén] 经穴别名。出《针灸甲乙经》。即幽门。详见该条。

Shangmen Another name for Youmen (KI 21), a meridian point originally from *Zhenjiu Jia-Yi Jing* (*A-B Classic of Acupuncture and Moxibustion*. →幽门(p. 569)

●上气海[shàng qì hǎi] 经穴别名。出《类经图翼》。即膻中。详见该条。

Shangqihai Another name for Danzhong (RN 17), a meridian point originally from *Leijing Tuyi* (*Supplements to Illustrated Classified Canon of Internal Medicine of the Yellow Emperor*). →膻中(p. 75)

●上取[shàng qǔ] 下病上取的简称。详见该条。

Selection of Upper Points The shortened term for the selection of upper points for lower diseases. →下病上取(p. 486)

●上三里[shàng sān lǐ] 经穴别名。即手三里。详见该条。

Shangsanli Another name for the meridian point, Shousanli (LI 10). →手三里(p. 390)

●上脘[shàng wǎn] 经穴名。出《灵枢·四时气》。属任脉,为任脉、足阳明、手太阴之会。又名胃脘、上纪、上管。〈定位〉在上腹部,前正中线上,当脐中上5寸

(图43和图40)。〈层次解剖〉皮肤→皮下组织→腹白线→腹横筋膜→腹膜外脂肪→壁腹膜。浅层主要布有第七胸神经前支的前皮支和腹壁浅静脉的属支。深层主要有第七胸神经前支的分支。〈主治〉胃脘疼痛、腹胀、呕吐、呃逆、纳呆、食不化、黄疸、泄利、虚劳吐血、咳嗽痰多、癫痫。直刺0.5-1寸;可灸。

Shangwan (RN 13) A meridian point, originally from *Lingshu*: *Si Shi Qi* (*Miraculous Pivot*: *Qi of Four Seasons*), a point on the Ren Meridian, the crossing point of the Ren meridian, Foot-Yangming and Hand-Taiyang Meridians, also named Weiwan, Shangji, Shangguan. 〈Location〉 on the upper abdomen, on the anterior midline, 5 cun above the centre of the umbilicus (Figs. 43 &40). 〈Regional anatomy〉 skin→subcutaneous tissue→linea alba→transwerse fascia→extrapenitioneal fat tissue---parietal peritoneum. In the superficial layer, there are the anterior cutaneous branches of the anterior branch of the 7th thoracic nerve and the tributaries of the superficial epigastric vein. In the deep layer, there are the branches of the anterior branch of the 7th thoracic nerve. 〈Indications〉 epigastralgia, abdominal distension, vomiting, hiccup, anorexia, duspepsia, jaundice, diarrhea, spitting blood due to consumption, cough with profuse sputum, and epilepsy. 〈Method〉 Puncture perpendicularly 0.5～1 cun. Moxibustion is applicable.

●上下配穴法[shàng xià pèi xué fǎ] 配穴法之一。指腰部以上与腰部以下的穴配合应用。例如胃病,上肢取内关,下肢取足三里。咽喉痛,上肢取合谷,下肢取内庭等。*八脉交会配穴法的应用,也属于本法范围。

Combination of the Superior-Inferior Points One of the point prescriptions, referring to the coordinated use of the acupoints above and below the lumbar region. For instance, select Neiguan (PC 6) on the upper extremity and Zusanli (ST 36) on the lower for treating gastropathy; Hegu (LI 4) on the upper extremity and Neiting (ST 44) on the lower for treating sorethroat, etc. The Eight confluent points also belong to the application of this method.

●上消[shàng xiāo] 消渴证型之一。出《丹溪心法·消渴》。由心肺火盛,上焦燥热所致。证见以烦渴多饮,口干舌燥为主。兼见尿多,食多,舌尖红,苔薄黄,脉洪数。治宜清肺泻热,生津止渴。取肺俞、鱼际、太渊、心俞、少府、廉泉、胰俞。

Diabetes of the Upper-Jiao One type of diabetes, originally from *Danxi Xinfa*: *Xiao Ke* (*Danxi' s Experience*: *Diabetes*), due to excessive fire of the heart and lung and dry heat of the upper-jiao. 〈Manifestations〉 polydipsia and dry mouth and tongue are the main symptoms, accompanied by polyuria, kolyphagia, redness of the tip of tongue, thin and yellowish tongue coating, surging and rapid pulse. 〈Treatment principle〉 Clear lung-heat, promote the production of body fluid to quench thirst. 〈Point selection〉 Feishu (BL 13), Yuji (LU 10), Taiyuan (LU 9), Xinshu (BL 15), Shaofu (HT 8), Lianquan (RN 23) and Yishu (EX-B).

●上星[shàng xīng] 经穴名。属督脉。又名神堂、鬼堂、明堂。〈定位〉在头部,当前发际正中直上1寸(图28和图5)。〈层次解剖〉皮肤→皮下组织→帽状腱膜→腱膜下疏松组织。布有额神经的分支和额动、静脉的分支或属支。〈主治〉头痛、眩晕、目赤肿痛、迎风流泪、面赤肿、鼻渊、鼻衄、鼻痔、鼻痈、癫狂、痫证、小儿惊风、疟疾、热病。平刺0.5-0.8寸;可灸。

Shangxing (DU 23) A meridian point, on the Du Meridian, also named Shentang, Guitang and Mingtang. 〈Location〉 on the head, 1 cun directly above the midpoint of the anterior hairline (Figs. 28 &5). 〈 Regional anatomy〉 skin→subcutaneous tissue→epicranial aponeurosis→subaponeurotic loose tissue. There are the branches of the frontal nerve and the branches or tributaries of the frontal artery and vein in this area. 〈Indications〉 headache, dizziness, redness and pain of the eye, epiphora induced by wind, flushed and swollen face, nasal sinusitis, epistaxis, nasal polyp, furuncle of the nose, manic-depressive psychosis, epilepsy, infantile convulsion, malaria, and febrile disease. 〈Method〉 Puncture subcutaneously 0.5～0.8 cun. Moxibustion is applicable.

●上龈里[shàng yín lǐ] 经外穴名。见《千金要方》。

在口腔,当上唇粘膜正中处,外与水沟相对。〈主治〉黄疸等。直刺0.1-0.2寸;或点刺出血。

Shangyinli (EX-HN) An extra point, seen in *Qianjin Yaofang* (*Essential Prescriptions Worth a Thousand Gold*). 〈Location〉in the mouth, at the middle of labial frenum, opposite exteriorly to Shuigou (DU 26). 〈Indications〉jaundice, etc. 〈Method〉Puncture perpendicularly 0.1～0.2 cun or prick to cause bleeding.

●上迎香[shàng yíng xiāng] 经外穴名。出《银海精微》。又名鼻通、鼻穿、穿鼻。〈定位〉在面部,当鼻翼软骨与鼻甲的交界处,近鼻唇沟上端处(图10)。〈层次解剖〉皮肤→皮下组织→提上唇鼻翼肌。该处布有眶下神经,滑车下神经的分支,面神经的颊支和内眦动、静脉。〈主治〉鼻炎、鼻旁窦炎、久流冷泪、烂弦火眼等。沿皮刺0.3-0.5寸。

Shangyingxiang (EX-HN 8) An extra point, originally from *Yinhai Jingwei* (*Essentials of Ophthalmology*), also named Bitong, Bichuan or Chuanbi. 〈Location〉on the face, at the junction of the nasal cartilage and concha, near the upper end of the nasolabial groove (Fig. 10). 〈Reginal anatomy〉skin→subcutaneous tissue→levator muscle of upper lip nasal ala. There are the branches of the infraorbital and infratrochlear nerves, the buccal branches of the facial nerve, and the angular artery and vein in this area. 〈Indications〉rhinitis, nasosinusitis, dacryorrhea, marginal blepharitis, etc. 〈Method〉Puncture subcutaneously 0.3～0.5 cun.

●上杼[shàng zhù] 经穴别名。见《循经考穴编》。即大椎。详见该条。

Shangzhu Another name for Dazhui (DU 14), a meridian point seen in *Xunjing Kaoxue Bian*(*Studies on Acupoints Along Meridians*). →大椎(p. 69)

●尚骨[shàng gǔ] 经穴别名。见《循经考穴编》。即肩髃。

Shanggu Another name for Jianyu (LI 15), a meridian point seen in *Xunjing Kaoxue Bian* (*Studies on Acupoints Along Meridians*). →肩髃(p. 191)

●烧山火[shāo shān huǒ] 针刺手法名。见《针灸大全》。其法将预定针刺深度分为浅(天部)、中(人部)、深(地部)三层。操作时由浅至深,将针先刺至天部,以紧按慢提九次,再将针刺入人部,依上法紧按慢提九次。最后将针刺入地部,又紧按慢提九次,然后将针一次退到天部,再如前法操作,自浅层到深层三进三退(实际上是九进三退),此为一度。如此反复几遍(称几度)至病人自觉全身有温热感时为止。出针时快速揉闭其孔,也可结合呼吸补泻之补法,即在患者呼气时进针,吸气时出针,有引经通气,益阳补虚的作用。适用于一切顽麻冷痹及虚寒之证。

Setting the Mountain on Fire A needling technique, seen in *Zhenjiu Daquan* (*A Complete Work of Acupuncture and Moxibustion*). 〈Method〉Divide the predetermined depth into three layers: superficial (heaven part), middle (human part) and deep (earth part). Puncture from the superficial layer (heaven part) to the deep (earth part). Do nine times of quick pressing and slow lifting successively, first in the heaven part, then in the human, and finally in the earth. After that, lift the needle directly to the heaven part and repeat the above from the superficial layer to the deep 3 times inwards and 3 times outwards (Actually it is 9 times inwards and 3 times outwards), and this is one degree. Do all this several times (called several degrees) until the patient feels warm all over his or her body. When withdrawing the needle, rub the hole quickly. It can also be used with the reinforcing and reducing methods by means of respiration. Insert the needle when the patient exhales, and withdraw it when the patient inhales. 〈Functions〉Dredge the meridian qi and invigorate yang. 〈Indications〉stubborn numbness, arthralgia syndromes due to cold, and cold diseases of insufficiency type.

●烧针[shāo zhēn] 古代针法之一。见《伤寒论》。又称火针,燔针,参见"火针"条。

Puncturing with Heated Needle One of the ancient needling methods, seen in *Shanghan Lun* (*Treatise on Cold-Induced Diseases*), also called puncturing with a red-hot needle, or fire needling. →火针(p. 180)

●烧针尾[shāo zhēn wěi] 为温针灸之别称。详见该条。

Puncturing with Heated Needle End →温针灸(p. 471)

●烧灼灸[shāo zhuó jiǔ] 灸法之一种。指直接灸灼穴位皮肤,使之发泡或化脓的灸法。分发泡灸和化脓灸两种。详见各条。

Burning Moxibustion A form of moxibustion, referring to burning the skin at the acupoint directly, causing vesiculation and suppuration. It is divided into vesiculation moxibustion and suppuration moxibustion. →发泡灸(p. 103)、化脓灸(p. 169)

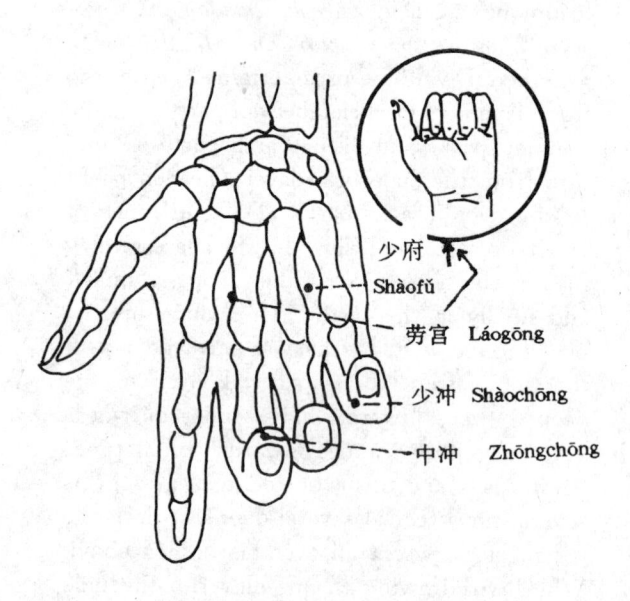

图 45 少府、少冲、劳宫和中冲穴
Fig. 45 Shaofu, Shaochong, Laogong and Zhongchong points

●少冲[shào chōng] 经穴名。出《针灸甲乙经》。属手少阴心经,为本经井穴。又名经始。〈定位〉在手小指末节桡侧,距指甲角0.1寸(指寸)(图45)。〈层次解剖〉皮肤→皮下组织→指甲根。布有尺神经的指掌侧固有神经指背支和指掌侧固有动、静脉指背支形成的动、静脉网。〈主治〉心悸、心痛、胸胁痛、癫狂、热病、中风昏迷、大便脓血、吐血、臑、臂内后廉痛。斜刺0.1寸,或点刺出血;可灸。

Shaochong (HT 9) A meridian point, originally from *Zhenjiu Jia-Yi Jing* (*A-B Classic of Acupuncture and Moxibustion*), the Jing (Well) point of the Heart Meridian of Hand-Shaoyin, also named Jingshi. 〈Location〉 on the radial side of the distal segment of the little finger, 0.1 cun from the corner of the nail (Fig. 45). 〈Regional anatomy〉 skin→subcutaneous tissue→root of nail. There are the dorsal digital branches of the proper palmar digital nerve of the ulnar nerve and the anteriovenous network formed by the dorsal digital arteries and veins in this area. 〈Indications〉 palpitation, precardial pain, pain in the chest and hypochondrium, manic-depressive psychosis, febrile disease, apoplectic coma, pus and bloody stool, spitting blood, pain in the medial posterior border of the upper limbs. 〈Method〉 Puncture obliquely 0.1 cun or prick to cause bleeding. Moxibustion is applicable.

●少府[shào fǔ] 经穴名。出《针灸甲乙经》。属手少阴心经,为本经荥穴。〈定位〉在手掌面,第四、五掌骨之间,握拳时,当小指尖处(图49)。〈层次解剖〉皮肤→皮下组织→掌腱膜→环指的浅、深屈肌腱与小指的浅、深屈肌腱之间→第四蚓状肌→第四骨间背侧肌。浅层有尺神经掌支分布。深层有指掌侧总动、静脉,指掌侧固有神经(尺神经分支)。〈主治〉心悸、胸痛、皮肤瘙痒、阴痒、阴挺、阴痛、小便不利、遗尿、手小指拘挛、掌中热、善笑、悲恐善惊。直刺0.2-0.3寸;可灸。

Shaofu (HT 8) A meridian point, originally from *Zhenjiu Jia-Yi Jing* (*A-B Classic of Acupuincture and Moxibustion*), the Ying (Spring) point of the Heart Meridian of Hand-Shaoyin. 〈Location〉 in the palm, between the 4th and 5th metacarpal bones, at the part of the palm touching the tip of the little finger when a fist is made (Fig. 49). 〈Regional anatomy〉 skin→subcutaneous tissue→palmar aponeurosis→between tendons of superficial and deep flexor muscle of the 4th and 5th fingers→4th lumbrical muscle→4th dorsal interosseous muncle. In the superficial layer, there are the palmar branches of the ulnar nerve. In the deep layer, there are the common palmar digital artery and vein and the proper palmar digital nerve from the ulnar nerve. 〈Indications〉 palpitation, chest pain, skin itching, pruritus vulvae prolapse of uterus, pudendal pain, oliguria, enuresis, lit-

tle finger contracture, feverish sensation in the palm, susceptibility to laughter, susceptibility to sorrow and fear. 〈Method〉 Punture perpendicularly 0.2~0.3 cun. Moxibustion is applicable.

●少谷[shào gǔ] 经穴别名。出《针灸甲乙经》。即三间。详见该条。

Shaogu Another name for Sanjian (LI 3), a meridian point originally from *Zhenjiu Jia-Yi Jing* (*A-B Classic of Acupuncture and Moxibustion*). →三间 (p. 341)

●少关[shào guān] 经穴别名。出《针灸甲乙经》。即阴交。详见该条。

Shaoguan Another name for Yinjiao (RN 7), a meridian point originally from *Zhenjiu Jia-Yi Jing* (*A-B Classic of Acupuncture and Moxibustion*). →阴交 (p. 556)

●少海[shào hǎi] 经穴名。出《灵枢·根结》。属手少阴心经，为本经合穴。又名曲节。〈定位〉屈肘，在肘横纹内侧端与肱骨内上髁连线的中点处（图49和图67）。〈层次解剖〉皮肤→皮下组织→旋前圆肌→肱肌。浅层有前臂内侧皮神经，贵要静脉等分布。深层有正中神经、尺侧返动、静脉和尺侧下副动、静脉的吻合支。〈主治〉心痛、臂麻、手颤、健忘、暴喑、手挛、腋胁痛、瘰疬、颈痛、癫狂善笑、痫证、头痛、目眩、齿龋痛。直刺0.5~0.8寸；可灸。

Shaohai (HT 3) A meridian point, originally from *Lingshu: Gen Jie* (*Miraculous Pivot: Root and Branch*), the He (Sea) point of the Heart Meridian of Hand-Shaoyin, also called Qujie. 〈Location〉 with the elbow flexed, at the midpoint of the line connecting the medial end of the cubital crease and the medial epicondyle of the humerus (Figs. 49 & 67). 〈Regional anatomy〉 skin→subcutaneous tissue→round pronator muscle→brachial muscle. In the superficial layer, there are the medial cutaneous nerve of the forearm and the basilic vein. In the deep layer, there are the median nerve, the anastomotic branches of the ulnar recurrent artery and vein and the inferior ulnar collateral artery and vein. 〈Indications〉 precardial pain, numbness of the arm, hand twitching, amnesia, sudden loss of voice, cheirospasm, axilla and hypochondriac pain, scrofula, neck pain, manic-depressive psychosis, susceptibility to laughter, epilepsy, headache, dizziness, dental caries and toothache. 〈Method〉 Puncture perpendicularly 0.5~0.8 cun. Moxibustion is applicable.

●少吉[shào jí] 经穴别名。见《外台秘要》。即少泽。详见该条。

Shaoji Another name for Shaoze (SI 1), a meridian point seen in *Waitai Miyao* (*Clandestine Essentials from the Imperial Library*). →少泽 (p. 358)

●少商[shào shāng] 经穴名。出《灵枢·本输》。属手太阴肺经，为本经井穴。又名鬼信，为十三鬼穴之一。〈定位〉在手拇指末节桡侧，距指甲角0.1寸（指寸）（图49和图16）。〈层次解剖〉皮肤→皮下组织→指甲根。有正中神经的指掌侧固有神经之指背支和拇主要动、静脉与第一掌背动、静脉分支所形成的动、静脉网。〈主治〉喉痹、咳嗽、气喘、重舌、鼻衄、心下满、中风昏迷、癫、狂、中暑呕吐、热病、小儿惊风、指腕挛急，向腕平刺0.2~0.3寸，或点刺出血；可灸。

Shaoshang (LU 11) A meridian point, originally from *Lingshu: Benshu* (*Miraculous Pivot: Meridian Points*), the Jing (Well) point of the Lung Meridian of Hand-Taiyin, also named Guixin, one of the 13 Ghost Points. 〈Location〉 on the radial side of the distal segment of the thumb, 0.1 cun from the corner of the fingernail (Figs. 49 &16). 〈Regional anatomy〉 skin→subcutaneous tissue→root of nail. There are the dorsal digital branches of the proper palmar digital nerve of the median nerve, the arteriovenous network formed by the principal arteries and veins of the thumb and the 1st dorsal metacarpal arteries and veins in this area. 〈Indications〉 inflammation of the throat, cough, asthma, double tongue, epistaxis, fullness in the epigastrium, apoplectic coma, manic-depressive psychosis, vomiting due to heatstroke, febrile disease, infantile convulsim, finger and wrist contracture. 〈Method〉 Puncture subcutaneously 0.2~0.3 cun to the wrist, or prick to cause bleeding. Moxibustion is applicable.

●少阳脉[shào yáng mài] 早期经脉名。出《帛书》。与足少阳经类似。

●少阳维[shào yáng wéi] 经外穴名。见《外台秘要》。在太溪与复溜穴连线的中点。〈主治〉脚气、慢性湿疹、狼疮、下肢麻痹等。直刺0.3-0.5寸；可灸。

Shaoyangwei (EX-LE) An extra point, seen in *Waitai Miyao* (*Clandestine Essentials from the Imperial Library*). 〈Location〉at the midpoint of the line connecting Taixi (KI 3) and Fuliu (KI 7). 〈Indications〉beriberi, chronic eczema, lupus, numbness and paralysis of the lower limbs, etc. 〈Method〉Puncture perpendicularly 0.3～0.5 cun. Moxibustion is applicable.

●少阴脉[shào yīn mài] 早期经脉名。出《帛书》。与足少阴经类似。

Shaoyin Vessel The early name of a meridian, originally from *Boshu* (*Silk Book*), similar to the Meridian of Foot-Shaoyin.

●少阴俞[shào yīn shū] 经穴别名。出《素问·通评虚实论》。即肾俞。详见该条。

Shaoyinshu Another name for Shenshu (BL 23), a meridian point, originally from *Suwen: Tongping Xushi Lun* (*A Thorough Discussion on Deficiency and Excess*). →肾俞 (p.365)

●少阴郄[shào yīn xì] 经穴别名。出《外台秘要》。即阴郄。详见该条。

Shaoyinxi Another name for Yinxi (HT 6), a meridian point originally from *Waitai Miyao* (*Clandestine Essentials from the Imperial Library*). →阴郄 (p.559)

●少泽[shào zé] 经穴名。出《灵枢·本输》。属手太阳小肠经，为本经井穴。又名小吉、少吉。〈定位〉在手小指末节尺侧，距指甲角0.1寸(指寸)(图48和图65)。〈层次解剖〉皮肤→皮下组织→指甲根。有尺神经指掌侧固有神经的指背支和小指尺掌侧、动静脉指背支形成的动、静脉网。〈主治〉热病、中风昏迷、乳少、乳痈、咽喉肿痛、目翳、疟疾、头痛、耳聋、耳鸣、肩臂外后侧痛。直刺0.1寸，或点刺放血；可灸。

Shaoze (SI 1) A meridian point originally from *Lingshu: Benshu* (*Miraculous Pivot: Meridian Points*), the Jing (River) point of the Small Intestine Meridian of Hand-Taiyang, also named Xiaoji or Shaoji. 〈Location〉on the ulnar side of the distal segment of the little finger, 0.1 cun from the corner of the nail (Figs. 48 & 65). 〈Regional anatomy〉 skin → subcutaneous tissue → root of nail. There are the dorsal digital branches of the proper digital nerve of the ulnar nerve and the anteriovenous network formed by the dorsal digital branches of the ulnar arteries and veins of the little finger in this area. 〈Indications〉 febrile diseases, coma due to apoplexy, hypoglactia, acute mastitis, sore throat, corneal opacity, malaria, headache, deafness, tinnitus, pain in the posterior-lateral aspect of the shoulder and upper limbs. 〈Method〉Puncture perpendicularly 0.1 cun, or prick to cause bleeding. Moxibustion is applicable.

●舌[shé] 耳穴名。位于2区，参见牙条。用于治疗舌炎、口腔炎。

Tongue (MA) An auricular point. 〈Location〉in the 2nd area. 〈Indications〉glossitis, stomatitis. →牙 (p.533)

●舌本[shé běn] ①经穴别名。出《针灸甲乙经》。即风府。详见该条。②经穴别名。出《铜人腧穴针灸图经》。即廉泉。详见该条。③指舌根部。

1. **Sheben** Another name for Fengfu (DU 16), a meridian point originally from *Zhenjiu Jia-Yi Jing* (*A-B Classic of Acupuncture and Moxibustion*). →风府 (p.111)

2. **Sheben** Another name for Lianquan (RN 24), a meridian point originally from *Tongren Shuxue Zhenjiu Tujing* (*Illustrated Manual of Points for Acupuncture and Moxibustion on a Bronze Statue with Acupoints*). →廉泉 (p.244)

3. **Root of the Tongue**

●舌横[shé héng] 经穴别名。出《针灸甲乙经》。即哑门。详见该条。

Sheheng Another name for Yamen (DU 15), a meridian point originally from *Zhenjiu Jia-Yi Jing* (*A-B Classic of Acupuncture and Moxibustion*). →哑门 (p.533)

●舌下穴[shé xià xué] 经外穴名。出《千金要方》。在舌两侧缘，当舌伸出口外，正对口角处。〈主治〉黄疸、急喉风、喉蛾痧等。直刺0.1～0.2寸；或点刺出血。

Shexiaxue(EX-HN) An extra point, originally from *Qianjin Yaofang* (*Essential Prescriptions Worth a Thousand Gold*). 〈Location〉on the lateral borders of lingual surface against the mouth angles when the tongue stretches out. 〈Indications〉jaundice, acute laryngeal infection, tonsillitis. 〈Method〉Puncture perpendicularly 0.1～0.2 cun or prick to cause bleeding.

●舌厌[shé yàn] 经穴别名。出《针灸甲乙经》。即哑门。详见该条。

Sheyan Another name for Yamen(DU 15), a meridian point originally from *Zhenjiu Jia-Yi Jing* (*A-B Classic of Acupuncture and Moxibustion*). →哑门(p.533)

●蛇串疮[shé chuàn chuāng] 即缠腰火丹。见该条。

Snake-Like Blisters →缠腰火丹(p.31)

●蛇丹[shé dān] 病证名。是指在皮肤上出现簇集成群、累累如串球的疱疹，疼痛剧烈的一种皮肤病。又名缠腰火丹。本病多由风火之邪客于少阳、厥阴经脉；或感染湿毒，留滞于太阴、阳明经脉，引起肌肤之营卫壅滞所致。蛇丹初起皮肤发热灼痛，继则出现密集成簇的绿豆至黄豆大小的丘状疱疹，很快变成小泡，三五成群，集聚一处或数处，排列成带状，疱疹之间皮肤正常。严重时，可出现出血点、血疱，患部刺痛呈带索状。临床可分为风火蛇丹，和湿热蛇丹两型。详见各条。

Snake-Like Herpes Zoister A disease, one kind of dermatosis marked by clustered blisters like a string of beads appearing on the skin with sharp pain, also called burning sores around waist. It is mostly due to an invasion of wind-fire pathogen upon the Shaoyang and Jueyin meridians or to infection with noxious dampness, lingering in the Taiyin and Yangming Meridians, resulting in stagnation of Ying and Wei in the skin or muscles. 〈Manifestations〉at the beginning, scorching pain and hot sensation occurring in the skin followed by dense appearance of clustered papules of various sizes from mung bean to soybean, which soon develop into blisters groups of three to five gathering in one or several parts in line. The skin between the blisters is normal. In severe cases, hemorrhagic spots and bloody bullae may appear in the affected part accompanied by circinate stabbing pain. Clinically, it can be divided into two types—— snake-like herpes zoister due to wind-fire pathogen and snake-like herpes zoister due to damp-heat pathogen. →风火蛇丹(p.112)、湿热蛇丹(p.372)

●蛇头[shé tóu] 经穴别名。出《针灸甲乙经》。即温溜。详见该条。

Shetou Another name for Wenliu(LI 7), a meridian point originally from *Zhenjiu Jia-Yi Jing* (*A-B Classic of Acupuncture and Moxibustion*). →温溜(p.470)

●蛇头疔[shé tóu dīng] 病证名。出《证治准绳》。指常见指疔，生于手指尖，肿似蛇头，故名。参见"疔疮"条。

Snake's Head-Like Furuncle A disease, originally from *Zhengzhi Zhunsheng* (*Standards for Diagnosis and Treatment*), a felon commonly seen in clinic, so named because a furuncle with swelling appears in the tip of a finger which looks like the head of a snake. →疔疮(p.82)

●摄法[shè fǎ] 针刺辅助手法名。见《针经指南》。为十四法之一，指用手指甲掐、切、抓、捏经络部位，以利进针。

Assisting A term for an auxiliary acupuncture manipulation, seen in *Zhenjing Zhinan* (*Guide To the Classics of Acupuncture*), one of the Fourteen Manipulations, referring to nipping, pressing, snatching, and pinching the region with finger-nails where the meridians distribute in order to insert the needle easily.

●摄领疮[shè lǐng chuāng] 即牛皮癣。详见该条。

Sores Around the Nape →牛皮癣(p.285)

●申脉[shēn mài] 经穴名。出《针灸甲乙经》。属足太阳膀胱经，八脉交会穴之一。通于阳跷脉。又名鬼路。〈定位〉在足外侧部，外踝直下方凹陷中(图35)。〈层次解剖〉皮肤→皮下组织→腓骨长肌腱→腓骨短肌腱→距跟外侧韧带。布有小隐静脉，腓肠神经的分支和外踝前动、静脉。〈主治〉痫证、癫狂、头痛、眩晕、失眠、腰痛、足胫寒、不能久立坐、目赤痛、项强。直刺0.2～0.3寸；可灸。

Shenmai(BL 62) A meridian point, originally from *Zhenjiu Jia-Yi Jing* (*A-B Classic of Acupuncture and Moxibustion*), a point on the

Bladder Meridian of Foot-Taiyang, one of the Eight Confluence points, connecting with the Yangqiao Meridian, also named Guilu. ⟨Location⟩ on the lateral side of the foot, in the depression directly below the external malleolus (Fig. 35). ⟨Regional anatomy⟩ skin→subcutaneous tissue→tendon of long peroneal muscle→tendon of short peroneal muscle→lateral talocalcaneal ligament. There are the branches of the small saphenous vein, the sural nerve and the lateral anterior malleolus artery and vein in this area. ⟨Indications⟩ epilepsy, manic-depressive psychosis, headache, dizziness, insomnia, lumbago, cold shank and foot, difficulty in long standing and sitting, redness and pain of the eye, stiffness of the nape. ⟨Method⟩ Puncture perpendicularly 0.2~0.3 cun. Moxibustion is applicable.

●身交 [shēn jiāo]　经外穴名。见《千金要方》。在腹部,当脐下0.3寸处。〈主治〉便秘、尿闭、遗尿、白带等。直刺0.5～1寸;可灸。

Shenjiao (EX-CA)　An extra point, seen in *Qianjin Yaofang* (*Essential Prescriptions Worth a Thousand Gold*). ⟨Location⟩ on the abdomen, 0.3 cun below the centre of the umbilicus. ⟨Indications⟩ constipation, anuresis, enuresis, morbid leukorrhea, etc. ⟨Method⟩ Puncture perpendicularly 0.5~1.0 cun. Moxibustion is applicable.

●身柱 [shēn zhù]　经穴名。出《针灸甲乙经》。属督脉。〈定位〉在背部,当后正中线上,第三胸椎棘突下凹陷中(图12和图7)。〈层次解剖〉针刺穿过的层次结构同脊中穴。浅层主要布有第三胸神经后支的内侧皮支和伴行的动、静脉。深层有棘突间的椎外(后)静脉丛,第三胸神经后支的分支和第三肋间后动、静脉侧支的分支或属支。〈主治〉身热头痛、咳嗽、气喘、惊厥、癫狂痫证、腰脊强痛、疔疮发背。斜刺0.5～1寸;可灸。

Shenzhu (DU 12)　A meridian point, on the Du Meridian, originally from *Zhenjiu Jia-Yi Jing* (*A-B Classic of Acupuncture and Moxibustion*). ⟨Location⟩ on the back, on the posterior midline, in the depression below the spinous process of the 3rd thoracic vertebra (Figs. 12 & 7). ⟨Regional anatomy⟩ The layer structures of the needle insertion are the same as those in Jizhong (DU 6). In the superficial layer, there are the medial cutaneous branches of the posterior branches of the 3rd thoracic nerve and the accompanying artery and vein. In the deep layer, there are the external (posterior) vertebral venous plexus between the adjacent spinous proceses, the branches of the posterior branches of the 3rd thoracic nerve and the branches or tributaries of the dorsal branches of the 3rd posterior intercostal artery and vein. ⟨Indications⟩ fever with headache, cough, dyspnea, infantile convulsion, manic-depressive psychosis, epilepsy, stiffness and pain along the spinal column, furuncle, lumbodorsal carbuncle. ⟨Method⟩ Puncture obliquely 0.5~1.0 cun. Moxibustion is applicable.

●神藏 [shén cáng]　经穴名。出《针灸甲乙经》。属足少阴肾经。〈定位〉在胸部,当第二肋间隙,前正中线旁开2寸(图40)。〈层次解剖〉皮肤→皮下组织→胸大肌。浅层布有第二肋间神经的前皮支、胸廓内动、静脉的穿支。深层有胸内、外神经的分支。主治咳嗽、气喘、胸痛、烦满、呕吐、不嗜食。斜刺或平刺0.5～0.8寸;可灸。

Shencang (KI 25)　A meridian point, on the Kidney Meridian of Foot-Shaoyin, originally from *Zhenjiu Jia-Yi Jing* (*A-B Classic of Acupuncture and Moxibustion*). ⟨Location⟩ on the chest, in the 2nd intercostal space, 2 cun lateral to the anterior midline (Fig. 40). ⟨Regional anatomy⟩ skin→subcutaneous tissue→greater pectoral muscle. In the superficial layer, there are the anterior cutaneous branches of the 2nd intercostal nerve and the perforating branches of the internal thoracic artery and vein. In the deep layer, there are the branches of the medial and lateral pectoral nerves. ⟨Indications⟩ cough, dyspnea, chest pain, irritability with full sensation in the chest, vomiting and anorexia. ⟨Method⟩ Puncture obliquely or subcutaneously 0.5~0.8 cun. Moxibustion is applicable.

●神聪 [shén cōng]　四神聪的别名。详见该条。

Shencong　Another name for Sishencong (EX-HN 1). →四神聪 (p. 415)

●神道 [shén dào]　经穴名。出《针灸甲乙经》。属督

脉。又名藏俞、冲道、膊俞。〈定位〉在背部,当后正中线上,第5胸椎棘突下凹陷中(图12和图7)。〈层次解剖〉针刺穿过层次结构同脊中穴。浅层主要布有第五胸神经后支的内侧皮支和伴行的动、静脉。深层有棘突间的椎外(后)静脉丛,第五胸神经后支的分支和第五肋间后动、静脉背侧分支或属支。〈主治〉心痛、惊悸、怔忡、失眠、健忘、中风不语、癫痫、瘛疭、腰脊强、肩背痛、咳嗽、气喘。斜刺0.5~1寸;可灸。

Shendao(DU 11) A meridian point originally from *Zhenjiu Jia-Yi Jing*(*A-B Classic of Acupuncture and Moxibsution*), a point on the Du Meridian, also named Zangshu, Chongdao or Zhuangshu. 〈Location〉on the back, on the posterior midline, in the depression below the spinous process of the 5th thoracic vertebra (Figs. 12 &.7). 〈Regional anatomy〉The layer structures of the needle insertion are the same as those in Jizhong(DU 6). In the superficial layer, there are the medial cutaneous branches of the posterior branches of the 5th thoracic nerve and the accompanying artery and vein. In the deep layer, there are the external(posterior) vertebral venous plexus between the adjacent spinous processes, the branches of the posterior branches of the 5th thoracic nerve and the branches or tributaries of the dorsal branches of the 5th posterior intercostal artery and vein. 〈Indications〉precordial pain, palpitation due to fright, severe palpitation, insomnia, amnesia, aphasia due to apoplexy, epilepsy, clonic convulsion, stiffness along the spinal column, pain in the shoulder and back, cough and dyspnea. 〈Method〉Puncture obliquely 0.5~1.0 cun. Moxibustion is applicable.

●神灯火[shén dēng huǒ] 即神灯照法。详见该条。

Magical Light Fire →神灯照法(p. 361)

●神灯照法[shén dēng zhào fǎ] 灸法的一种。见《神灸经纶》。又称神灯火。用朱砂、雄黄、没药各6克,麝香1.2克,共为细末。每次用三分,红绵纸裹药,搓捻长7寸,麻油浸透,用火点着,离疮疡半寸许,自外而内,在疮疡周围慢慢薰照。用以治疗疮疡初起。《本草纲目》卷六载:"用硫黄、艾叶研匀作捻,浸油点灯,于被中薰之,用治疥癣。"方法类似。

Magical Light Illumination A form of moxibustion, seen in *Shenjiu Jinglun*(*Principles of Magic Moxibustion*), also called magical light fire. 〈Method〉Take *Zhu Sha*(*Cinnabaris*) 6g, *Xiong Huang*(*Realgar*) 6g, *Mo Yao*(*Resina Commiphorae Myrrhae*) 6g, *She Xiang*(*Moschus*)1.2g, and grind them into a powder. For each treatment, use one gram of the powder, wrap it with red cotton paper, roll it into a stick 7 cun in length, soak the stick in sesame oil, ignite one end of the stick, fume slowly from the external to the internal, about 0.5 cun off the sore. 〈Indication〉onset of sore. 〈Indication〉onset ot sore. The method of "grinding sulfur and *Ai Ye*(*Folium Artemisiac Argyi*) evenly to make a stick, soaking it in oil, igniting it and fuming the affected part in quilt for the treamment of scabies and tinea," is similar to this, as is recorded in Vol. 6 of *Bencao Gangmu*(*Compendium of Materia Medica*).

●神封[shén fēng] 经穴名。出《针灸甲乙经》。属足少阴肾经。在胸部,当第4肋间隙,前正中线旁开2寸(图40)。〈层次解剖〉皮肤→皮下组织→胸大肌。浅层布有第四肋间神经的前皮支,胸廓内动,静脉的穿支。深层有胸内、外侧神经的分支。〈主治〉咳嗽、气喘、胸胁支满、呕吐、不嗜食、乳痈。斜刺或平刺0.5~0.8寸;可灸。

Shenfeng(KI 23) A meridian point, on the Kidney Meridian of Foot-Shaoyin, originally from *Zhenjiu Jia-Yi Jing*(*A-B Classic of Acupuncture and Moxibustion*). 〈Location〉on the chest, in the 4th intercostal space, 2 cun lateral to the anterior midline(Fig. 40). 〈Regional anatomy〉skin→subcutaneous tissue→greater pectoral muscle. In the superficial layer, there are the anterior cutaneous branches of the 4th intercostal nerve and the perforating branches of the internal thoracic artery and vein. In the deep layer, there are the branches of the medial and lateral pectoral nerves. 〈Indications〉cough, dyspnea, fullness in the chest and hypochondrium, vomiting, anorexia, acute mastitis. 〈Method〉Puncture obliquely or subcutaneously 0.5~0.8 cun. Moxibustion is applicable.

●神府[shén fǔ] 经外穴名。见《千金要方》。在胸骨剑突之中心处。〈主治〉心痛。沿皮刺0.3~0.5寸;用灸法。

Shenfu (EX-CA) An extra point, seen in *Qianjin Yaofang* (*Essential Prescriptions Worth a Thousand Gold*). ⟨Location⟩ at the center of the xiphoid process. ⟨Indication⟩ precardial pain. ⟨Method⟩ Puncture subcutaneously 0.3~0.5 cun. Moxibustion is applicable.

●神光 [shén guāng] 经穴别名。出《备急千金要方》。即日月。详见该条。

Shenguang Another name for Riyue (GB 24), a meridian point originally from *Beiji Qianjin Yaofang* (*Essential Prescriptions for Emergencies Worth a Thousand Gold*). →日月 (p.337)

●神经衰弱点 [shén jīng shuāi ruò diǎn] 耳穴别名。即垂前。详见该条。

Neurasthenia Point (MA) Another name for the auricular point Anterior Ear Lobe (MA). →垂前 (p.52)

●神灸经论 [shén jiǔ jīng lún] 书名。清代吴亦鼎撰，四卷，刊于1851年。为一灸疗专著。阐述了灸疗的部位、方法、禁忌、灸后调养、诸病病候及所用灸法等，较切合实用。

Shenjiu Jinglun (**Principles of Magic Moxibustion**) A 4-volume book written by Wu Yiding in the Qing Dynasty, published in 1851, a monograph on moxibustion treatment, in which the places, methods and contraindications for moxibustion, recuperation after moxibustion, symptoms and signs of various diseases and the relevant moxibustion methods applied are expounded. They are still practical in clinic.

●神门 [shén mén] ①经穴名。出《针灸甲乙经》。属手少阴心经，为本经输穴、原穴。又名兑冲、中都、锐中、兑骨。⟨定位⟩在腕部，腕掌侧横纹尺侧端，尺侧腕屈肌腱的桡侧凹陷处（图49和图67）。⟨层次解剖⟩皮肤→皮下组织→尺侧腕屈肌腱桡侧缘。浅层有前臂内侧皮神经，贵要静脉属支和尺神经掌支等。深层有尺动、静脉和尺神经。⟨主治⟩心痛、心烦、恍惚、健忘、失眠、惊悸、怔忡、痴呆、悲哭、癫狂、痫证、目黄胁痛、掌中热、呕血、吐血、大便脓血、头痛、眩晕、咽干不嗜食、失音、喘岔上气。直刺0.3~0.5寸；可灸。②耳穴名。位于与耳轮前缘之弧相平行划两条弧线，将三角窝划为三等分，外三分之一的上二分之一为神门穴。具有镇静安神，清热止痛的作用。⟨主治⟩失眠、多梦、疼痛、戒断综合症。为耳针麻醉常用穴。

1. **Shenmen** (HT 7) A meridian point, originally from *Zhenjiu Jia-Yi Jing* (*A-B Classic of Acupuncture and Moxibustion*), the Shu (Stream) point and the Yuan (Primary) point of the Heart Meridian of Hand-Shaoyin, also named Duichong, Zhongdu, Ruizhong or Duigu. ⟨Location⟩ on the wrist, at the ulnar end of the crease of the wrist, in the depression of the radial side of the tendon of the ulnar flexor, muscle of the wrist (Figs. 49 & 67). ⟨Regional anatomy⟩ skin→subcutaneous tissue→radial border of tendon of ulnar flexor muscle of wrist. In the superficial layer, there are the medial cutaneous nerve of the forearm, the tributaries of the basilic vein and the palmar branches of the ulnar nerve. In the deep layer, there are the ulnar artery and vein and the ulnar nerve. ⟨Indications⟩ precardial pain, vexation, absent-mindedness, amnesia, insomnia, palpitation due to fright, severe palpitation, dementia, sobbing with sorrow, manic-depressive psychosis, epilepsy, yellow pigmentation of the sclera, hypochondriac pain, feverish sensation in the palms, hematemesis, spitting blood, stool with pus and blood, headache, dizziness, dry throat and anorexia, aphonia, dyspnea. ⟨Method⟩ Puncture perpendicularly 0.3~0.5 cun. Moxibustion is applicable.

2. **Shenmen** (MA) An auricular point. ⟨Location⟩ at the upper half of the lateral 1/3 of the triangular fossa which is divided into three equal parts by two curved lines parallel to the anterior border of the helix. ⟨Functions⟩ tranquilize and allay excitment, clear heat and alleviate pain. ⟨Indications⟩ insomnia, dream-disturbed sleep, pain, menopausal syndrome. It is a commonly used auricular point in auriculo-acupuncture anesthesia.

●神农经 [shén nóng jīng] 书名。撰人不详。《类经图翼》中曾引用。书佚。

Shen Nong Jing (**Shen Nong Classic**) Title of a book. No details are known about its author. It was quoted in *Leijing Tuyi* (*Supple-*

ments to *Illustrated Classified Canon of Internal Medicine of the Yellow Emperor*) and is no longer extant.

● 神阙[shén què] 经穴名。出《针灸甲乙经》。属任脉,又名脐、脐中、气舍、维会、气合、环谷。〈定位〉在腹中部,脐中央(图43.2和图40)。〈层次解剖〉皮肤→结缔组织→壁腹膜。浅层主要布有第十胸神经前支的前皮支和腹壁脐周静脉网。深层有第十胸神经前支的分支。〈主治〉中风虚脱、四肢厥冷、尸厥、风痫、形惫体乏、绕脐腹痛、水肿鼓胀、脱肛、泄利、便秘、小便失禁、五淋、不孕。禁刺;可灸。

Shenque(RN 8) A meridian point, originally from *Zhenjiu Jia-Yi Jing* (*A-B Classic of Acupuncture and Moxibustion*), a point on the Ren Meridian, also named Qi, Qizhong, Qishe, Weihui, Qihe or Huangu. ⟨Location⟩ on the middle abdomen at the centre of the umbilicus. (Figs. 43.2&40). ⟨Regional anatomy⟩ skin→connective tissue→parietal peritoneum. In the superficial layer, there are the anterior cutaneous branches of the anterior branch of the 10th thoracic nerve and the periumbilical venous network on the abdominal wall. In the deep layer, there are the branches of the anterior branch of the 10th thoracic nerve. ⟨Indications⟩ collapse syndrome of apoplexy, cold limbs, corpse-like syncope, epilepsy due to wind pathogen, fatigue and inertia, abdominal pain around the umbilicus, edema and tympanites, prolapse of the rectum, diarrhea, dysentery, constipation, urinary incontinence, five types of stranguria, sterility. ⟨Method⟩ Acupuncture is forbidden. Moxibustion is applicable.

● 神堂[shén táng] ①经穴名。出《针灸甲乙经》。属足太阳膀胱经。〈定位〉在背部,当第5胸椎棘突下,旁开3寸(图7)。〈层次解剖〉皮肤→皮下组织→斜方肌→菱形肌→竖脊肌。浅层布有第五、六胸神经后支的皮支和伴行的动、静脉。深层有肩胛背神经、肩胛背动、静脉,第五、六胸神经后支的肌支和相应的肋间后动、静脉背侧支的分支或属支。〈主治〉咳嗽、气喘、胸腹满、肩痛、脊背急强。斜刺0.5～0.8寸;可灸。②经穴别名。出《针灸聚英》。即上星。详见该条。

1. Shentang(BL 44) A meridian point, originally from *Zhenjiu Jia-Yi Jing* (*A-B Classic of Acupuncture and Moxibustion*), a point on the Bladder Meridian of Foot-Taiyang. ⟨Location⟩ on the back, below the spinous process of the 5th thoracic vertebra, 3 cun lateral to the posterior midline(Fig. 7). ⟨Regional anatomy⟩ skin→subcutaneous tissue→trapezius muscle→rhomboid muscle→erector spinal muscle. In the superficial layer, there are the cutaneous branches of the posterior branches of the 5th and 6th thoracic nerves and the accompanying arteries and veins. In the deep layer, there are the dorsal scapular nerve, the dorsal scapular artery and vein, the muscular branches of the posterior branches of the 5th and 6th thoracic nerves and the branches or tributaries of the dorsal branches of the related posterior intercostal arteries and veins. ⟨Indications⟩ cough, dyspnea, full sensation in the chest and abdomen, pain in the shoulder, rigidity of the back and spinal column. ⟨Method⟩ Puncture obliquely 0.5～0.8 cun. Moxibustion is applicable.

2. Shentang Another name for Shangxing (DU 23), a meridian point originally from *Zhenjiu Juying* (*Essentials of Acupuncture and Moxibustion*). →上星(p. 354)

● 神庭[shén tíng] 经穴名。出《针灸甲乙经》。属督脉,为督脉、足太阳、阳明之会。又名发际。〈定位〉在头部,当前发际正中直上0.5寸(图28和图5)。〈层次解剖〉皮肤→皮下组织→左、右枕额肌额腹之间→腱膜下疏松组织。布有额神经的滑车上神经和额动、静脉的分支或属支。〈主治〉头痛、眩晕、目赤肿痛、泪出、目翳、雀目、鼻渊、鼻衄、癫狂、痫证、角弓反张。平刺0.3～0.5寸;可灸。

Shenting(DU 24) A meridian point, originally from *Zhenjiu Jia-Yi Jing* (*A-B Classic of Acupuncture and Moxibustion*), a point on the Du Meridian and the crossing point of the Du Meridian and the Meridians of Foot-Taiyang and Yangming, also named Faji. ⟨Location⟩ on the head, 0.5 cun directly above the midpoint of the anterior hairline (Figs. 28&5). ⟨Regional anatomy⟩ skin → subcutaneous tissue→between frontal belly of left and right occipitofontal muscles → subaponcurotic loose tissue. There are the supratrochlear nerve from the frontal nerve and the branches

or tributaries of the frontal artery and vein in this area. 〈Indications〉headache, dizziness, the redness, pain and swelling of the eye, dacryorrhea, nephelium, nyctalopia, rhinorrhea with turbid discharge, epistaxis, manic-depressive psychosis, epilepsy, opisthotonus. 〈Method〉Puncture subcutaneously 0.3~0.5 cun. Moxibustion is applicable.

●神应经[shén yìng jīng] 书名。明代陈会撰,刘瑾辑,一卷,刊于1425年。本书由刘瑾从其师陈会的《广爱书》(针灸书,已佚)十卷中撮要而成。取用119穴编歌诀和插图,并附以针刺的基本方法等内容。

Shen Ying Jing(Classic of God Merit) A single volume book, written by Chen Hui and compiled by Liu Jin in the Ming Dynasty, published in 1425. Liu Jin made an abstraction from the 10 volumes of *Guang Ai Shu(A Book of Fraternity)*, a book on acupuncture and moxibustion which is no longer extant and was written by Chen Hui, his teacher. Presented in the book are verses and illustrations about 119 acupoints and appended to them were some contents of basic acupuncture methods.

●神针火[shén zhēn huǒ] 灸法的一种。见《本草纲目》。又称桃枝灸。用桃树枝沾麻油点火后,吹灭乘热垫棉纸熨灸患处。用以治疗心腹冷痛,风寒湿痹。

Magical Fire-Needle A form of moxibustion, seen in *Bencao Gangmu(Compendium of Material Medica)*, also named peach twig moxibustion. 〈Method〉Ignite a peach twig after it is dipped in sesame oil, blow it out and immediately warm and cauterize the affected part covered with cotton paper while the twig is still hot. 〈Indications〉cold sensation and pain in the chest and abdomen, arthralgia due to wind, cold and dampness.

●神宗[shén zōng] 经穴别名。出《太平圣惠方》。即脊中。详见该条。

Shenzong Another name for Jizhong(DU 6), a meridian point originally from *Taiping Shenghui Fang(Imperial Benevolent Prescriptions)*. →脊中(p.185)

●沈好问[shén hào wèn] 人名。元代针灸家,字裕生,号启明。有"沈铁针"之称。见《仁和县志》。

Shen Haowen An expert in acupuncture and moxibution in the Yuan Dynasty, who styled himself Yusheng, and assumed the name of Qiming, in addition, known as "Iron Needle Shen". Cf. *Renhe Xian Zhi(Records of Renhe County)*.

●肾[shèn] ①耳穴名。位于对耳轮上、下脚分叉处下方。用于治疗肾盂肾炎、腰痛、耳鸣、重听、遗精、阳萎、神经衰弱、气喘、遗尿症、青光眼、月经不调。②耳穴名。位于耳背下部。用于治疗头痛、失眠、眩晕、月经不调。

Kidney(MA) ①An auricular point. 〈Location〉below the bifurcating point between the superior and inferior antihelix cruses. 〈Indications〉pyelonephritis, lumbago, tinnitus, double hearing, emission, impotence, neurasthenia, dyspnea, glaucoma, irregular menstruation. ② An auricular point. 〈Location〉at the lower part of the back auricle. 〈Indications〉headache, insomnia, dizziness, irregular menstruation.

●肾肝之部[shèn gān zhī bù] 针刺的分部。见《难经·七十难》。指肌肉的深层,以肝肾与筋骨相应,故名。

Layer of Kidney and Liver A layer of acupuncture, originally from *Nanjing:Qishi Nan(The Classic of Questions:Question 70)*, referring to the deep layer of muscles corresponding to the liver and kidney, and tendons and bones.

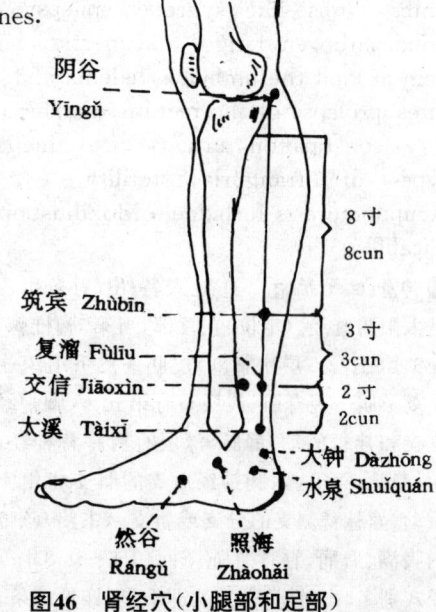

阴谷 Yīngǔ
8寸 8cun
筑宾 Zhùbīn
复溜 Fùliū — 3寸 3cun
交信 Jiāoxìn — 2寸 2cun
太溪 Tàixī
大钟 Dàzhōng
水泉 Shuǐquán
然谷 Rángǔ
照海 Zhàohǎi

图46 肾经穴(小腿部和足部)

Fig. 46 Points of Kidney Meridian(Leg&Foot)

●肾经[shèn jīng] 足少阴肾经之简称。详见该条。

Kidney Meridian Short form for the Kidney Meridian of Foot-Shaoyin. →足少阴肾经 (p. 638)

●**肾囊风**[shèn náng fēng] 病名。见《外科正宗》。又名绣球风。由肝经湿热下注,风邪外袭而成。初起阴囊干燥作痒,喜浴热汤。甚则起疙瘩,形如粟米,色红,搔破浸淫脂水;或热痛如火燎,经久不愈,即阴囊湿疹。详见"湿疹"条。

Scrotal Eczema A disease, originally from *Waike Zhengzong* (*Orthodox Manual of External Diseases*), also called scrotum wind, mainly due to downward flow of damp-heat in the liver meridian and attack of pathogenic wind. 〈Manifestations〉at the intial stage, dryness and itching in the scrotum which may be relieved by hot water or even worse, the occurrence of a reddish milletlike rash with fatty liquid when scratched, or burning pain. It takes a long time to be cured. Synonymous with eczema scroti. →湿疹(p. 373)

●**肾气**[shèn qì] ①肾精化生之气,指肾脏的功能活动,如生长、发育及性机能活动等。②经穴别名。见《医学纲目》。即大横。详见该条。

1. **Kidney Qi** Referring to qi transformed from the kidney essence and the functional activities of the kidney, such as growth, development and sexual ability, etc.

2. **Shenqi** Another name for Daheng (SP 15), a meridian point originally from *Yixue Gangmu* (*An Outline of Medicine*). →大横(p. 63)

●**肾上腺**[shèn shàng xiàn] 耳穴名。位于耳屏下部隆起的尖端。具有清热止痛、解痉驱风作用。〈主治〉风湿性关节炎、腮腺炎、下颌淋巴结炎、间日疟、无脉症、链霉素中毒所致眩晕、瘙痒、疼痛、听力减退。

Adrenal (MA) An auricular point. 〈Location〉at the tip of the lower protubercle on the border of the tragus. 〈Functions〉Clear heat and alleviate pain, expel endogenous wind and relieve convulsion. 〈Indications〉rheumatic arthritis, mumps, mandibular lymphnoditis, malaria tertiana, pulseless disease, dizziness, pruritus, pain and hypoacusis resulting from streptomycin poisoning.

●**肾俞**[shèn shū] 经穴名。出《灵枢·背输》。属足太阳膀胱经,为肾的背俞穴。又名少阴俞。〈定位〉在腰部,当第二腰棘突下,旁开1.5寸(图7)。〈层次解剖〉皮肤→皮下组织→背阔肌腱膜和胸腰筋膜浅层→竖脊肌。浅层布有第二、三腰神经后支的皮支和伴行的动、静脉。深层有第二、三腰神经后支的肌支和相应腰动、静脉背侧支的分支或属支。〈主治〉遗精、阳痿、遗尿、小便频数、月经不调、白带、腰膝痠软、目昏、耳鸣、耳聋、小便不利、水肿、洞泻不化、喘咳少气。直刺0.8～1寸;可灸。

Shenshu(BL 23) A meridian point, originally from *Lingshu: Beishu* (*Miraculous Pivot: Back-Shu Points*), a point on the Bladder Meridian of Foot-Taiyang and the Back-shu point of the kidney, also called Shaoyinshu. 〈Location〉on the low back, below the spinous process of the 2nd lumbar vertebra, 1.5 cun lateral to the posterior midine (Fig. 7). 〈Regional anatomy〉skin→subcutaneous tissue→aponeurosis of latissimus muscle of back and superficial layer of thoracolumbar fascia→erector spinal muscle. In he superficial layer, there are the cutaneous branches of the posterior branches of the 2nd and 3rd lumbar nerves and the accompanying arteries and veins. In the deep layer, there are the muscular branches of the posterior branches of the 2nd and 3rd lumbar nerves and the branches or tributaries of the dorsal branches of the related lumbar arteries and veins. 〈Indications〉seminal emission, impotence, enuresis, frequent micturition, irregular menstruation, mobid leukorrhea, soreness and weakness of the waist and knees, blurred vision, tinnitus, deafness, difficulty in urination, edema, diarrhea with undigested food, cough and dyspnea. 〈Method〉Puncture perpendicularly 0.8～1 cun. Moxibustion is applicable.

●**肾系**[shèn xì] 经外穴名。见《千金要方》。在伏兔下1寸处。〈主治〉消渴、小便数。用灸法。

Shenxi(EX-LE) An extra point, originally from *Qianjin Yaofang* (*Essential Prescriptions Worth a Thousand Gold*). 〈Location〉at the point 1 cun below Futu(ST 32). 〈Indications〉diabetes and frequent micturition. 〈Method〉moxibustion.

●**肾虚不孕**[shèn xū bù yùn] 是不孕的证型之一。

多因禀赋素弱，肾气不足，或久病房劳，损伤肾气而致精亏血少，肾气虚衰，冲任胞脉失养所致。证见月经失调，量少色淡，精神疲倦，头晕耳鸣，腰酸腿软，舌苔白，脉沉。治宜补益肾气，调理冲任。取肾俞、气穴、然谷。

Sterility due to Kidney Deficiency A type of sterility, mostly due to a debilitated constitution and insufficiency of kidney-qi, or prolonged illness and excess of sexual intercourse leading to deficiency of essence and blood, insufficiency of kidney-qi and failure to nourish the Chong and Ren Meridians and uterine collaterals. 〈Manifestations〉 irregular menstruation, with scanty amount and light color, listlessness, dizziness, tinnitus, lassituse in loin and legs, white tongue coating and deep pulse. 〈Treatment principle〉Tonify the kidney and regulate the Chong and Ren Meridians. 〈Point selection〉Shenshu(BL 23), Qixue(KI 13) and Rangu(KI 2).

●肾虚带下[shèn xū dài xià] 带下病证型之一。多因素体肾气不足，或早婚，或分娩过多，损伤肾气，下元亏损，任带失于固约所致。证见带下色白，量多，质清稀，连绵不断，小腹发凉，腰部痠痛，小便频数而清长，夜间尤甚，大便溏薄，舌质淡苔薄白，脉沉迟。治宜温补肾阳，固摄任带。取关元、带脉、肾俞、次髎、照海。

Morbid Leukorrhea due to Kidney Deficiency
A type of morbid leukorrhea, mostly due to constitutional insufficiency of kidney-qi or marriage at an early age, or multiparity leading to imparment of the kidney, deficiency of the Yuan(Primary) qi and unconsolidation of the Ren and Dai Meridians. 〈Manifestations〉 persistent leukorrhea with profuse, whitish and watery discharge, cold feeling in the lower abdomen, soreness and pain of the waist, frequent, colorless and profuse urine especially at night, loose stools, pale tongue with thin and white coating, deep and slow pulse. 〈Treatment principle〉Warm and recuperate the kidney-yang to consolidate and control the Ren and Dai Meridians. 〈Point selection〉Guanyuan(RN 4), Daimai(GB 26), Shenshu(BL 23), Ciliao(BL 32) and Zhaohai(KI 6)

●肾虚经乱[shèn xū jīng luàn] 即肾虚经行先后无定期。详见该条。

Disorder of Menstruation due to Kidney Deficiency →肾虚经行先后无定期(p.366)

●肾虚经行后期[shèn xū jīng xíng hòu qī] 经行后期的证型之一。多因先天不足，早婚，分娩次数多，或房室不节，损伤肾气，精亏血少，冲任不足，胞宫不能按时满溢所致。证见经期错后，血量较少，头晕耳鸣，腰膝痠软等。治宜补肾养阴。取气海、气穴、足三里、三阴交、肾俞、太溪。

Delayed Menstruation due to Kidney Deficiency A type of delayed menstruation, commonly due to congenital deficiency, premature marriage and multiparity, or intemperance in sexual life leading to impairment of the kidney-qi and insufficiency of the essence and blood resulting in hypofunction of the Chong and Ren Meridians to fill the uterus regularly. 〈Manifestations〉delayed menstrual period with scanty menses, dizziness, tinnitus, soreness and weakness of the waist and knees, etc. 〈Treatment principle〉Tonify the kidney and nourish yin. 〈Point selection〉Qihai(RN 6), Qixue(KI 13), Zusanli(ST 36), Sanyinjiao(SP 6), Shenshu(BL 23) and Taixi(KI 3).

●肾虚经行先后无定期[shèn xū jīng xíng xiān hòu wú dìng qī] 经行先后无定期的证型之一。又称肾虚经乱。多因素体肾气不足，房室不节，或孕育过多，肾失封藏，损伤冲任，胞宫蓄溢失调所致。证见经期先后不定，经血量少，色淡质稀，腰膝酸软，头晕耳鸣，舌淡苔白，脉沉弱。治宜补肾调经。取关元、肾俞、三阴交、太溪、水泉。

Menstruation in an Unfixed(either Preceded or Delayed)Period due to Kidney Deficiency
A type of irregular and timeless menstrual cycle, also called disorder of menstruation due to kidney deficiency, commonly due to constitutional deficiency of kidney-qi and intemperance in sexual life or multiparity resulting in dysfunction of the kindey in storing and impairment of the Chong and Ren Meridians leading to irregular filling and storage of the uterus. 〈Manifestations〉 irregular menstrual cycles with scanty, thin and light-colored menses, soreness and weakness of the waist and knees, dizziness, tinnitus, pale tongue with

white coating, deep and weak pulse. 〈Treatment principle〉Tonify the kidney and regulate menses. 〈Point selection〉 Guanyuan (RN 4), Shenshu(BL 23), Sanyinjiao(SP 6), Taixi (KI 3) and Shuiquan(KI 5)

●肾虚哮喘[shèn xū xiāo chuǎn] 哮喘证型之一。由于肾气亏虚,失于摄纳所致。证见短气息促,动则为甚,呼多吸少,气不得续,耳鸣,腰酸,下肢消冷,头晕,舌淡有皱纹,脉沉细无力。治宜固本培元,纳气平喘。取定喘、膏肓、肺俞、气海俞、肾俞、太溪。

Asthma due to Kidney Deficiency A type of asthma due to deficiency of kidney-qi. 〈Manifestations〉 worsened by physical activities, more exhalation and less inhalation, tinnitus, soreness of the loin, cold lower limbs, dizziness, pale tongue with wrinkles, deep thready and weak pulse. 〈Treatment principle〉 reinforce kidney-qi and help inspiration to relieve asthma. 〈Point selection〉 Dingchuan (EX-B 1), Gaohuang (BL 43), Feishu (BL 13), Qihaishu (BL 24), Shenshu (BL 23) and Taixi (KI 3).

●肾虚泻[shèn xū xiè] 泄泻证型之一。又称五更泄。由肾阳虚衰,真火不足,脾土失于温运,运化失常所致。证见黎明之时,脐腹作痛,肠鸣即泻,泻后则安,形寒肢冷,腰膝酸软,舌淡苔白,脉沉细。治宜温肾健脾,固涩止泻。取肾俞、关元、命门、气海、中脘、脾俞、足三里、天枢。

Diarrhea due to Kidney Deficiency A type of diarrhea, also called diarrhea before dawn, due to deficiency of kidney-yang resulting in failure to warm the spleen leading to dysfunction of the spleen in transporation. 〈Manifestations〉pain of the abdomen and around the umbilicus at dawn, loose bowels or borborygmus, which is relieved after diarrhea, cold body and limbs, soreness and weakness of the waist and knees, pale tongue with white coating, deep and thready pulse. 〈Treatment principle〉Warm the kindey to invigorate yang and strengthen the spleen, control discharge of feces to arrest diarrhea. 〈Point selection〉Shenshu (BL 23), Guanyuan (RN 4), Qihai (RN 6), Zhongwan (RN 12), Pishu (BL 20), Zusanli(ST 36) and Tianshu(ST 25).

●肾虚腰痛[shèn xū yāo tòng] 腰痛证型之一。见《千金要方》。多因肾脏虚衰,精血不足,筋骨失养所致。证见起病缓慢,隐隐作痛,绵绵不已。如兼神倦,肢冷,滑精,舌淡,脉细者,为肾阳虚。伴有虚烦,溲黄,舌红,脉细数者,属肾阴。治宜益肾填精,通络止痛。取命门、志室、太溪、肾俞、委中。肾阴虚加照海、三阴交。肾阳虚加悬钟、百会。

Lumbar Pain due to Kidney Deficiency A type of lumbar pain, originally from *Qian Jin Yao fang* (*Essential Prescriptions Worth a Thousand Gold*), commonly due to deficiency of the kidney and insufficiency of blood and essence, resulting in failure to nourish tendons, muscles and bones. 〈Manifestations〉 slow onset, persistent dull pain in the waist, cases due to defficiency of kidney-yang are accompanied by listlessness, cold limbs, spermatorrhea, pale tongue and thready pulse; cases due to deficiency of kidney-yin, are accompanied by restlessness of deficiency type, dark urine, red tongue and thready and rapid pulse. 〈Treatment principle〉Tonify the kidney and replenish essence, activate collaterals to relieve pain. 〈Point selection〉 Mingmen (DU 4), Zhishi (BL 52), Shenshu (BL 23), and Weizhong (BL 40). Add Zhaohai (KI 6) and Sanyinjao(SP 6) for cases due to deficiency of kidney-yin; and add Xuanzhong (GB 39) and Baihui (DU 20) for cases due to deficiency of kindey-yang.

●肾虚月经过少[shèn xū yuè jīng guò shǎo] 月经过少的证型之一。多因先天不足,早婚,分娩次数多,或房室不节,损伤肾气,精亏血少,冲任胞脉气血不足所致。证见月经量过少,色淡红,质稀,头晕耳鸣,腰膝痠软。治宜补肾养血。取脾俞、肾俞、膈俞、命门、关元、足三里、三阴交。

Scanty Menstruation due to Kidney Deficiency A type of scanty menstruation commonly due to congenital deficiency, premature marriage multiparity, or excessive sexual intercourse, resulting in impairment of kidney-qi and insufficiency of essence and blood, leading to deficiency of qi and blood in the Chong-Ren Meridians and uterine collaterals. 〈Manifestations〉thin, pink and scanty menses, dizziness, tinnitus, soreness and weakness of the waist and knees. 〈Treatement principle〉Tonify the

kidney and nourish blood. ⟨Point selection⟩ Pishu(BL 20), Shenshu(BL 23), Geshu(BL 17), Mingmen(DU 4), Guanyuan(RN 4), Zusanli(ST 36) and Sanyinjiao(SP 6).

●**肾虚子宫脱垂**[shèn xū zǐ gōng tuō chuí] 子宫脱垂的证型之一。多因孕育过多，房劳伤肾，以致带脉失约，冲任不固，不能系胞所致。证见阴道中有鹅卵样物突出，小腹下坠，腰腿痠软，小便频数，无白带，阴道干涩，头晕，耳鸣，舌淡红，脉沉弱。治宜调补肾气，固摄胞宫。取关元、子宫、大赫、照海。

Hysteroptosis due to Kidney Deficiency A type of hysteroptosis, commonly due to impairment of the kidney caused by multiparity and excess of sexual life, resulting in debility of the Chong and Ren Meridians, dysfunction of the Dai Meridian in binding meridians and collaterals, leading to failure to keep the uterus high in its normal position. ⟨Manifestations⟩ prolapse of something like a goose egg out of the vagina, tenesmic sensation in the lower abdomen, soreness and weakness of the waist and legs, frequent micturition, dry vagina without leukorrhea, dizziness, tinnitus, pink tongue, deep and weak pulse. ⟨Treatment pinciple⟩Reinforce kidney-qi and strengthen uterine collaterals to elevate the uterus. ⟨Point slection⟩ Guanyuan(RN 4), Zigong(EX-CA 1), Dahe(KI 12) and Zhaohai(KI 6).

●**肾足少阴之脉**[shèn zú shào yīn zhī mài] 足少阴肾经的原名。详见该条。

Foot-Shaoyin Vessel of the Kindey Original name of the Kidney Meridian of Foot-Shaoyin. →足少阴肾经(p. 638)

●**生成数**[shēng chéng shù] 刺法术语。出《河图》。古代《河图》将一、二、三、四、五称作"生数"，六、七、八、九、十称作"成数"。其中逢单为奇数，属天；逢双为偶数，属地。并配合五行，天一、地六为水；地二、天七为火；天三、地八为木；地四、天九为金；天五、地十为土。金代何若愚将这一理论结合刺法，提出补生泻成学说。参见该条。

Growing and Grown Numbers An acupuncture technique, originally from *He Tu* (*The Chart of River*) in ancient times. According to the book, 1, 2, 3, 4 and 5 were called the growing numbers; 6, 7, 8, 9 and 10 the grown numbers. Among them, odd numbers are of the nature of heaven and the even numbers of the nature of the earth. This theory, coordinated with the theory of the five elements, held that in nature the heavenly one and earthly six belong to water, the earthly two and heavenly seven belong to fire, the heavenly three and earthly eight belong to wood, earthly four and heavenly nine belong to metal and heavenly five and earthly ten belong to earth. He Ruoyu of the Jin Dynasty, linking this theory with acupuncture technique, advanced a theory of reinforcing the growing numbers and reducing the grown numbers. →补生泻成(p. 26)

●**生成息数**[shēng chéng xī shù] 刺法术语。见《针灸聚英》卷三。又称定息寸数。指各经的呼吸次数。详见"接气通经"条。

Measurement of the Meridian Qi Flow by Respiration Times An acupuncture techique, originally from *Zhenjiu Juying*(*Essentials of Acupuncture and Moxibustion*), also called respiration times for measuring the length of the meridian qi flow, referring to respiration times for each meridian. →接气通经(p. 201)

●**生姜灸**[shēng jiāng jiǔ] 天灸的一种。取鲜姜适量，洗净后捣如泥膏状，敷于穴位或患部。如敷于乳房部，治疗急性乳腺炎。也可将生姜、鲜疳积草合用，共捣如膏状，于晚上临睡前敷于涌泉穴，翌日晨取去。治疗小儿营养不良。

Fresh Ginger Moxibustion A form of crude herb moxibustion. Take an appropriate amount of fresh ginger, wash it clean and pound it into a paste, then apply the paste on the selected point or affected area for treatment. For instance, apply it to the breast area to treat acute mastitis. In addition, the fresh ginger may also be used with fresh *Gan Ji Cao* (A kind of herb for malnutrition). Pound these two herbs into a paste, then apply it to Yongquan(KI 1) before sleep and remove it next morning for treatment of infantile malnutrition.

●**生熟**[shēng shú] 灸法用语。见《外台秘要》。生，指少灸和火力较小；熟，指多灸和火力较旺。又分小熟和大熟。

Unripeness and Ripeness A moxibustion term, originally from *Waitai Miyao*(*Clandes-*

tine Essentials from the Imperial Library), unripeness referring to little moxibustion or moxibustion with soft fire, and ripeness referring to much moxibustion or moxibustion with strong fire. It is also subdivided into slight ripeness and great ripeness.

●生殖区 [shēng zhí qū]　头针刺激区。从额角处向上引平行于前后正中线的2厘米长直线。〈主治〉功能性子宫出血,盆腔炎,子宫脱垂等。

Reproduction Area　A stimulation area for scalp acupuncture.〈Location〉Draw a 2-cm straight line from the frontal angle upward, parallel to the anterioposterior midline.〈Indications〉functional uterine bleeding, pelvic inflammation and prolapse of uterus, etc.

●圣饼子 [shèng bǐng zǐ]　灸用垫隔药饼之一。见《杨氏家藏方》卷四。〈其配方〉黄连、巴豆各9克,去壳同捣为膏状,捻搓成饼状,大小薄厚如五分硬币即成。用之施灸,可治疗小便不通。

Holy Medicinal Cake　A kind of medicinal cakes used for indirect moxibustion, in which the cake is used as an insulator for moxibustion, originally from Vol. 4 of *Yangshi Jiacang Fang* (*Yang's Home Collection of Formulas*).〈Method〉Take *Huang Lian* (*Rhizoma Coptidis*) 9g and *Ba Dou* (*Fructus Crotonis*) 9g, pound them into a paste and make it into a small cake, the size of a five-fen coin, for application of moxibustion to treat anuresis.

●圣济总录 [shèng jì zǒng lù]　方书名。又名《政和圣济总录》,二百卷,分六十八门,载方两万余首。宋徽宗时由朝廷组织人员编撰,成书于1111-1117年(政和年间)。内容有运气、叙例、治法及临床各科病证证治。书中第一百九十一卷至一百九十四卷为针灸门,有骨空穴法、骨度统论、经脉统论,并分述十二经、奇经八脉及穴位,次为九针统论、刺节统论、灸刺统论、各病灸刺法及灸刺禁忌论。

Shengji Zonglu (Imperial Medical Encyclopaedia)　A medical formulary, also called *Zhenghe Shengji Zonglu* (*Imperial Medical Encyclopaedia in the Reign of Zheng He*) in 200 volumes with 68 sections and over 20,000 formulas, compiled by a staff of court physicians of the Northern Song Dynasty under the rule of Emperor Hui Zong and completed around 1111-1117. It included doctrine on five elements' motion and six kinds of natural factors, preface, treatment principles, differentiation of syndromes and treatment of various diseases. The section of acupuncture and moxibustion is from Vol. 191-194, which discuss the method of point selection, treatise on proportional measurements, treatise on meridians and also expounds the twelve regular meridians, the eight extra meridians and acupoints, followed by treatises on the nine forms of needles, on acupuncture techniques, on moxibustion and acupuncture, on methods of acupuncture and moxibustion for various diseases and on contraindications of acupuncture and moxibustion.

●胜玉歌 [shèng yù gē]　针灸歌赋名。出《针灸大成》。为七言韵语,主要介绍杨继洲家传治验的取穴。

Sheng Yu Ge (Invaluable Experience in Verse)　A verse on acupuncture and moxibustion, originally from *Zhenjiu Dacheng* (*A Great Compendium of Acupuncture and Moxibustion*), a rhymed verse with seven characters to each line, which mainly introduces the methods of selecting points and experiences handed down from Yang Jizhou's family.

●盛则泻之 [shèng zé xiè zhī]　针灸治疗的原则。见《灵枢·经脉》。又称"满则泻之"。与"虚则补之"相对。意指对实证,宜用泻法使邪气虚。

Treating Excess with Reducing Methods　Treatment principle of acupuncture and moxibustion, originally from *Lingshu : Jingmai* (*Miraculous Pivot : Meridians*), also called treating syndromes of excessive pathogenic factors by reducing methods, which means using reducing methods for excess syndromes to make pathogenic factors weaken.

●尸注 [shī zhù]　古病名。见《肘后方》。即肺痨。详见该条。

Tuberculosis of a Corpse　A disease in ancient times, originally from *Zhouhou Fang* (*Handbook of Prescriptions*), synonymous with pulmonary tuberculosis. →肺痨(p. 107)

●失精 [shī jīng]　见《金匮要略·血痹虚劳病脉证治》。即遗精。详见该条。

Loss of Sperm　Seen in *Jingui Yaolüe : Xuebi Xulao Bing Mai Zheng Zhi* (*Synopsis of the Golden Chamber : Pulse Conditions, Symptoms and Treatments of Blood Bi-Syndrome and Consumptive Diseases*), synonymous with e-

mission. →遗精(p.552)

●失眠[shī mián] 即不寐。详见该条。

Insomnia →不寐(p.28)

●失眠穴[shī mián xué] 经外穴名。见《江苏中医》。在足底跟部,当足底中线与内外踝连线相交处。〈主治〉失眠、肢底痛等。直刺0.3~0.5寸;可灸。

Shimianxue(EX-LE) An extra point, originally from *Jiangsu Zhongyi* (*Jiangsu Journal of Traditional Chinese Medicine*). 〈Location〉on the bottom of the heel, at the crossing point of the midline of sole and the line joining the medial malleolus and lateral malleolus. 〈Indications〉insomnia, and pain in the sole, etc. 〈Method〉Puncture perpendicularly 0.3~0.5 cun. Moxibustion is applicable.

●失气[shī qì] ①针刺异常情况。见《灵枢·终始》。指针刺不得法致损伤了正气。②针刺术语。见《灵枢·小针解》。指针刺得气感消失。

1. **Impairment of Qi** An abnormal condition in acupuncture treatment, seen in *Lingshu: Zhong Shi* (*Miraculous Pivot: End and Beginning*), referring to impairment of the vital-qi by incorrect needling methods.

2. **Loss of qi** An acupuncture term, originally from *Lingshu: Xiaozhen Jie* (*Miraculous Pivot: Explanation of Delicate Needling*), referring to the loss of needling sensation.

●失信[shī xìn] 即月经不调的别名。详见该条。

Failing to Keep Menorrhea Another name for irregular menstruation. →月经不调(p.578)

●失枕[shī zhěn] 病名。出《素问·骨空论》。即落枕。详见该条。

Torticollis A disease, originally from *Suwen: Gu Kong Lun* (*Plain Questions: On the Apertures of Bones*). →落枕(p.239)

●施刮术[shī guā shù] 针刺手法名。即刮法的一种。详见该条。

Scraping Manipulation An acupuncture manipulation, a method of scraping. →刮法(p.146)

●湿毒带下[shī dú dài xià] 带下病证型之一。多因经期、产后、胞脉正虚,湿毒秽浊之邪,乘虚内侵直伤胞脉,损伤冲任之气血,以致带脉失约,任脉不固所致。证见带下状如米泔,或黄绿如脓,或夹有血液,量多而臭,阴中瘙痒,口苦咽干,小腹作痛,小便短赤,舌红苔黄,脉滑数。治宜清热解毒,利湿祛邪。取带脉、中极、阴陵泉、下髎、行间。

Leukorrhea due to Noxious Dampness A type of leukorrhea, commonly due to inward invasion of noxious dampness and other filthy pathogenic factors resulting from deficiency of the uterine collaterals during the menstrual period or after delivery, leading to impairment of uterine collaterals, the Chong and Ren Meridians, resulting in their failure to control. 〈Manifestations〉white or greenish yellow vaginal discharge with foul odor and large quantity, occasionally with blood, itching in vagina, pain in the lower abdomen, scanty dark urine, red tongue with yellow coating, slippery and rapid pulse. 〈Treatment principle〉Clear heat and toxic material, remove dampness by diuresis to expel the pathogenic factors. 〈Point selection〉Daimai (GB 26), Zhongji (RN 3), Yinlingquan (SP 9), Xialiao (BL 34) and Xingjian (LR 2).

●湿脚气[shī jiǎo qì] 脚气证型之一。见《太平圣惠方》卷四十五。指脚气病见足胫浮肿者。多因水湿之邪,从下感受,经络不得宣通所致。证见足胫浮肿,脚趾疼痛麻木,逐渐向上蔓延,腿膝沉重酸软,步行乏力,行动不便。偏于寒湿者,则足胫怯寒喜温。偏于湿热者,则足胫灼热喜凉,或有恶寒发热,小便短少,舌苔白腻或浮黄,脉濡数。治宜疏通经络,清化湿热。取足三里、三阴交、阳陵泉、八风。恶寒发热,加合谷、大椎、外关。小便短少,加阴陵泉、昆仑。

Wet Beriberi A type of beriberi syndromes, originally from Vol. 45 of *Taiping Shenghui Fang* (*Imperial Benevolent Prescriptions*), referring to beriberi characterized by edema of legs, usually due to attack of dampness to the lower limbs leading to blockage of the meridians and collaterals. 〈Manifestations〉edema of feet and shanks, numbness and pain of toes, which gradually develops upwards, heaviness, soreness and weakness of legs, weakness of the footsteps, difficult movement. For cases due to cold-dampness, it is accompanied by aversion to cold in legs, preference for warmth; for cases due to damp-heat, it is accompanied by burning sensation of the legs and preference for cool, or fever with chills, scanty urine, white and greasy or yellow coating, soft and rapid pulse. 〈Treatment princi-

ple) dredge the meridians and collaterals and remove heat and dampness. 〈Point selection〉 Zusanli(ST 36), Sanyinjiao(SP 6), Yanglingquan(GB 34)and Bafeng(EX-LE 10); for cases accompanied by fever with chills, add Hegu(LI 4), Dazhui(DU 14) and Waiguan (SJ 5); for cases with scanty urine, add Yinlingquan(SP 9)and Kunlun(BL 60).

●湿热崩漏[shī rè bēng lòu] 崩漏证型之一。多因湿热蕴结下焦,伤及胞络所致。证见血色黯红,兼见带下如注,色如米泔或黄绿如脓,气味臭秽,阴部痒痛,舌苔黄腻,脉濡数。治宜清热利湿。取气海、三阴交、隐白、中极、阴陵泉。

Metrorrhagia and Metrostaxis due to Damp-Heat A type of metrorrhagia and metrostaxis, usually due to retention and accumulation of damp-heat in the lower-jiao resulting in impairment of the uterine collaterals. 〈Manifestations〉uterine bleeding with dark red color, accompanied by massive leukorrhea with white or yellowish green color and foul odor, itching and pain of the vulva, yellow and greasy coating, soft and rapid pulse. 〈Treatment principle〉Clear heat and promote diuresis. 〈Point selection〉Qihai(RN 6), Sanyinjiao (SP 6), Yinbai(SP 1), Zhongji(RN 3), and Yinlingquan(SP 9).

●湿热便血[shī rè biàn xuè] 便血证型之一。多因湿热蕴结大肠,灼伤血络所致。证见先血后便,血色鲜红,肛门灼痛,舌苔黄腻,脉数。治宜清热利湿,和营止血。取长强、次髎、上巨虚、承山。

Hemafecia due to Damp-Heat A type of hemafecia, mostly due to retention and accumulation of damp-heat in the large intestine, resulting in impairment of superficial venules. 〈Manifestations〉Blood comes first, followed by stool in bright red color, burning pain of anus, yellow greasy coating and rapid pulse. 〈Treatment principle〉Clear heat and promote diuresis, regulate Ying to stop bleeding. 〈Point selection〉Changqiang(DU 1), Ciliao(BL 32), Shangjuxu(ST 37)and Chengshan(BL 57).

●湿热丹毒[shī rè dān dú] 丹毒证型之一。多因湿热之邪,侵犯血分,郁于肌表而发。其证除见丹毒的一般症状外,并多发于下肢,发热、心烦、口渴、胸闷、关节肿痛、小便黄赤,苔黄腻,脉濡数。治宜清热化湿,解毒。取合谷、足三里、血海、阴陵泉、阿是穴。见"丹毒"条。

Erysipelas due to Damp-Heat A type of erysipelas usually due to attack of damp-heat to the Xue stage and depression of damp-heat in muscles and skin. 〈Manifestations〉besides the general symptoms of erysipelas, mostly occurring in the lower limbs, it is also accompanied by fever, vexation, thirst, choking sensation in the chest, swelling and pain in the joints, dark urine, yellow, greasy tongue coating, soft and rapid pulse. 〈Treatment principle〉Clear heat, eliminate dampness and detoxicify. 〈Point selection〉Hegu(LI 4), Zusanli(ST 36), Xuehai(SP 10), Yinlingquan (SP 9)and Ashi point. →丹毒(p.71)

●湿热侵淫痿证[shī rè jìn yín wěi zhèng] 痿证证型之一。多因湿邪浸淫经脉,使营卫运行受阻,郁遏生热,津液耗伤,筋脉肌肉失其濡养所致。证见四肢痿软,身体困重,或麻木,微肿,尤以下肢多见,或足胫热气上腾,或有发热,胸痞脘闷,小便短赤涩痛,苔黄腻,脉濡数。治宜通经活络,清利湿热。取肩髃、曲池、合谷、阳溪、髀关、梁丘、足三里、解溪、阴陵泉、脾俞、三阴交。

Flaccidity due to the Invasion of Damp-Heat Pathogen A type of flaccidity, mostly due to the invasion of dampness in meridians, which leads to the blockage of the circulation of Ying and Wei, stagnation of heat, injury of the body fluids and malnutrition of the tendons and muscles. 〈Manifestations〉flaccidity of limbs, heavy sensation of the body, numbness, mild edema, which mostly occurs in the lower extremities, or upward heat-qi from the feet and legs, fever, feeling of stuffness in the chest and epigastrium, scanty deep colored urine, yellowish greasy coating of the tongue, soft and rapid pulse. 〈Treatment pinciple〉Clear and activate the meridians and collaterals, clear heat and promote diuresis. 〈Point selection〉Jianyu (LI 15), Quchi(LI 11), Hegu(LI 4), Yangxi (LI 5), Biguan(ST 31), Liangqiu(ST 34), Zusanli(ST 36), Jiexi(ST 41), Yinlingquan (SP 9), Pishu(BL 20), Sanyinjiao(SP 6).

●湿热痢[shī rè lì] 痢疾证型之一。见《证因脉治》卷四。由湿热积滞肠中,气血阻滞,传导失职所致。证

见大便次数增多,痢下赤白脓血,腥臭粘稠,腹痛坠胀,里急后重,肛门灼热。初起微恶寒,继则发热,口渴、舌苔黄腻,脉滑数。治宜清热化湿,疏调肠胃。取合谷、天枢、上巨虚、曲池、内庭。

Dysentery due to Damp-heat Pathogen A type of dysentery, from Vol. 4 of *Zheng Yin Mai Zhi*(*Symptoms, Causes, Pulse Conditions and Treatments*), caused by the accumulation of damp-heat pathogen in the intestines which leads to the stagnation of blood and qi and irregular transportation of the large intestine. 〈Manifestations〉frequent discharge of ropy bloody mucous stool with a strong odor, heavy and distending pain of abdomen, tenesus, burning sensation of the anus, aversion to cold at the initial stage, and then, fever; thirst, yellowish greasy tongue coating, slippery and rapid pulse. 〈Treatment principle〉Clear heat and eliminate dampness, regulate the intestines and stomach. 〈Point selection〉Hegu (LI 4), Tianshu (ST 25), Shangjuxu (ST 37), Quchi (LI 11), Neiting(ST 44).

●湿热蛇丹[shī rè shé dān] 蛇丹证型之一。疱疹多发于胸面部,除有蛇丹的一般症状外,兼见水疱溃破淋漓,疲乏无力,胃纳不佳,中脘痞闷,苔黄而腻,脉濡数。治宜清热利湿。取外关、内庭、侠溪、阴陵泉,或局部刺络拔罐。参见"蛇丹"条。

Snake-Like Herpes Zoster due to Damp-Heat Pathogen A type of snake-like herpes zoster, mostly occurring in the chest and face. 〈Manifestations〉In addition to common symptoms of herpes zoster, it also has the symptoms of vesicular ulceration, weakness, poor appetite, fullness in the stomach, yellowish greasy coating of the tongue, soft and rapid pulse. 〈Treatment principle〉Clear heat and promote diuresis. 〈Point selection〉Waiguan (SJ 5), Neiting(ST 44), Xiaxi(GB 43), Yinlingquan(SP 6), or puncture the collaterals in the local area followed by cupping. →蛇丹(p. 359)

●湿热湿疹[shī rè shī zhěn] 湿疹证型之一。多由感受风湿热邪,皮肤经络受阻而成。本病初起局部皮肤焮红作痒,迅速出现丘疹与小疱,搔破之后变成糜烂,流黄水,舌苔薄或黄腻,脉浮数或滑数。治宜清泄湿热。取陶道、肺俞、曲池、神门、血海、阴陵泉。

Eczema due to Damp-Heat Pathogen A type of eczema, mostly caused by attack of the pathogenic factors of wind, dampness and heat, which leads to the blockage of the dermatic meridians. 〈Manifestations〉It begins with inflammation of local skin, then small purple vesicles and there is ulceration with yellowish fluid, thin or yellowish and greasy coating of the tongue, superficial and rapid pulse, or slippery and rapid pulse. 〈Treatment principle〉Eliminate dampness and heat. 〈Point selection〉Taodao(DU 13), Feishu(BL 13), Quchi(LI 11), Shenmen(HT 7), Xuehai(SP 10), Yinlingquan(SP 9).

●湿热胁痛[shī rè xié tòng] 胁痛证型之一。见《丹溪心法附余·火郁门》。多由病邪侵袭,湿热郁蒸,肝胆络脉气滞所致。证见胁痛偏于右侧,如刺如灼,急性发作时伴有恶寒发热,口苦,心烦,恶心呕吐,厌油腻,苔黄腻或厚腻,脉弦数。治宜清热化湿,疏肝利胆。取期门、日月、支沟、阳陵泉、曲泉、太冲。

Hypochondriac Pain due to Damp-Heat A type of hypochondriac pain, from *Danxi Xinfa Fuyu*: *Huo Yu Men*(*Supplement to Danxi's Experience*: *Accumulation of Fire*), mostly due to attack of pathogenic factors, retention of damp-heat pathogen and qi-stagnation of the liver and gallbladder. 〈Manifestations〉pricking or burning pain in the right hypochondriac region, during acute period aversion to cold, fever, bitter taste, nausea and vomiting, aversion to oil, yellowish and greasy coating, or thick and greasy coating of the tongue, string-taut and rapid pulse. 〈Treatment principle〉Clear heat and eliminate dampness, soothe the liver and normalize the function of the gallbladder. 〈Point selection〉Qimen(LR 14), Riyue(GB 24), Zhigou(SJ 6), Yanglingquan (GB 34), Ququan (LR 8) and Taichong(LR 3).

●湿热泻[shī rè xiè] 泄泻证型之一。多由湿热或暑湿,伤及肠胃,传导失常所致。证见泄泻腹痛,泄下急迫或泻而不爽,粪色黄褐而臭,肛门灼热,小便短赤,舌苔厚腻,脉濡数或滑数。治宜清化湿热,生津益气。取中脘、天枢、足三里、合谷、内庭、金津、玉液、委中。

Diarrhea due to Damp-Heat A type of diarrhea, mostly due to the invasion of pathogenic damp-heat or summer-heat in the intestines

and stomach, which leads to irregular transportation of the large intestine. 〈Manifestations〉diarrhea and abdominal pain, acute diarrhea, yellowish-brown foul stools, burning sensation of the anus, scanty deep-colored urine, thick and greasy coating of the tongue, soft and rapid pulse, or slippery and rapid pulse. 〈Treatment principle〉Eliminate dampness and heat, promote the production of the body fluid and facilitate qi. 〈Point selection〉Zhongwan (RN 12), Tianshu (ST 25), Zusanli (ST 36), Hegu (LI 4), Neiting (ST 44), Jinjing(EX-HN 12), Yuye (EX-HN 13)and Weizhong (BL 40).

●湿热痔疮[shī rè zhì chāng] 痔疮证型之一。多因饮食失调,嗜食辛辣肥甘,湿热下注,致使肛肠气血不调,络脉瘀滞所致。证见内痔初起,痔核很小,常因大便时摩擦而出血,或出血如射,或点滴不已。如反复发作,痔核增大,引起大便困难,小便不利。兼见口渴,舌红,脉数。治宜清热化瘀。取次髎、长强、会阳、承山、二白。

Hemorrhoid due to Damp-Heat Pathogen A type of hemorrhoid, mostly due to improper diet, pungent and fat food and the downward flow of damp-heat, which leads to derrangement of qi and blood, and blood stasis in the collaterals. 〈Manifestations〉It begins with small hemorrhoids or drop by drop bleeding due to friction, developing into the enlargement of the hemorrnoids. In cases of frequent occurrence there is dyschesia and dribbling urination, accompanied by thirst, red tongue and rapid pulse. 〈Treatment principle〉Clear heat and resolve stagation. 〈Point selection〉Ciliao(BL 32), Changqiang (DU 1), Huiyang (BL 35), Chengshan (BL 57). Erbai (EX-UE 2).

●湿疹[shī zhěn] 病名,是一种常见的皮肤病。由于患病部位不同,而有种种名称。如有"奶癣"、"旋耳疮"、"肾囊风"、"四弯风"等。本病由于感受风热湿邪,皮肤经络受阻而成。临床可分为湿热湿疹和血虚湿疹两种。详见各条。

Eczema A common dermatosis caused by the attack of pathogenic wind, heat and dampness which leads to the blockage of the dermatic meridians. It has different names according to the different affected parts of the body, e.g. infantile eczema, eczema of the ear, acrotal eczema, atopic eczema occurring in the antecubital and the popliteral fossa, etc. Clinically it is divided into eczema due to damp-heat pathogen and eczema due to blood deficiency. →湿热湿疹(p. 372)、血虚湿疹(p. 529)

●十变[shí biàn] ①古代文献名。《难经·六十三难》及《六十四难》均引《十变》言。原书不详。②指十干配合的变化关系。参见"五门十变"条。

1. Shi Bian(Ten Changes) An ancient document, from which much of *Nanjing*:*Liushisan Nan*;*Liushisi Nan*(*The Classic of Questions*:*Questions* 63 & 64)were taken, details of the document are unknown.

2. Ten Changes The variable relations of the combination of the Ten Heavenly Branches. →五门十变(p. 477)

●十二刺[shí èr cì] 《内经》刺法分类,十二节刺的别称。详见该条。

Twelve Puncturing Methods A category of acupuncture techniques in *Neijing*(*The Inner Canon of Huangdi*), another name for the Twelve Methods of Needling. →十二节刺(p. 374)

●十二从[shí èr cóng] 指十二经脉的顺序、走向。出《素问·阴阳别论》。经气相顺则治,相逆则乱。从,顺从之意。《黄帝内经太素》卷三,作"十二顺"。指十二经脉应行之有序,如手之三阴从脏走手等义。

Twelve Successions Order and distribution of the Twelve Regular Meridians, originally from *Su Wen*:*Yin Yang Bie Lun*(*Plain Questions*:*Supplementary Exposition of Yin and Yang*). The meridian-qi in due succession creates a good order where as the meridian-qi going against the succession result in a mess. "Succession" means obedience, taken as the twelve obediences in the Vol. 3 of *Huangdi Neijing Tai Su*(*Comprehensive Notes to the Yellow Emperor's Inner Canon*), referring to the cyclical orders of the Twelve Regular Meridians, such as the Three Yin Meridians of Hand which go from zang to the hand.

表12　　　　　　十二节气和十二中气
Table 12　　12 solar terms and 12 middle solar terms

月	Month	节气	Solar Terms	中气	Middle Solar Terms
正月	January	立春	the Beginning of Spring	雨水	Rain Water
二月	February	惊蛰	the Waking of Insects	春分	the Spring Equinox
三月	March	清明	Pure Brightness	谷雨	Grain Rain
四月	April	立夏	the Beginning of Summer	小满	Grain Full
五月	May	芒种	Grain in Ear	夏至	the Summer Solstice
六月	June	小暑	Slight Heat	大暑	Great Heat
七月	July	立秋	the Beginning of Autumn	处暑	the Limit of Heat
八月	August	白露	White Dew	秋分	the Autumnal Equinox
九月	September	寒露	Cold Dew	霜降	Frost's Descent
十月	October	立冬	the Beginning of Winter	小雪	Slight Snow
十一月	November	大雪	Great Snow	冬至	the Winter Solstice
十二月	December	小寒	Slight Cold	大寒	Great Cold

●十二节[shí èr jié]　①刺法名。出《灵枢·官针》。参见"十二刺"条。②部位名。出《灵枢·邪客》。《类经》卷三张介宾注谓："四肢各三节,共为十二节。"③时令名。出《灵枢·经别》。《黄帝内经太素》卷九杨上善注："十二节谓四时八节。"指立春、春分、立夏、夏至、立秋、秋分、立冬、冬至。汉代以来,一年分为二十四节气,包括十二节气和十二中气。见表十二。

1. Twelve Needlings　A catagory of acupuncture techniques, originally from *Ling Shu*: *Guanzhen* (*Miraculous Pivot*: *Official Needles*). →十二刺(p. 373)

2. Twelve Sections　Parts of the body, originally from *Ling Shu*: *Xieke* (*Miraculous Pivot*: *Invasion of Pathogens*). As Zhang Jiebin annotated in Vol. 3 of *Leijing* (*Classified Canon of Internal Medicine of the Yellow Emperor*), "There are twelve sections in all, with 3 in each of the four limbs."

3. Twelve Solar Terms　Season terms, originally from *Ling Shu*: *Jingbie* (*Miraculous Pivot*: *Divergent Meridians*). In the annotation of Vol. 9 of *Huangdi Neijing Taisu* (*Comprehensive Notes to the Yellow Emperor's Canon of Internal Medicine*), Yang Shangshan explained, "The twelve solar terms means the 4 seasons and the 8 solar terms in them." The eight solar terms refer to the Beginning of Spring, the Spring Equinox, the Beginning of Summer, the Summer Solstice, the Beginning of Autumn, the Autumnal Equinox, the Beginning of Winter, the Winter Solstice. Since the Han dynasty, a year has been divided into twenty-four solar terms which include twelve solar terms and twelve middle solar terms. See Table 12.

●十二节刺[shí èr jié cì]　《内经》刺法分类。出《灵枢·官针》。又称十二刺。包括偶刺,报刺,恢刺,齐刺,扬刺,直针刺,输刺,短刺,浮刺,傍针刺,阴刺,赞刺。详见各条。

Twelve Methods of Acupuncture　A category of acupuncture techniques in *Neijing* (*The Canon of Internal Medicine*), originally from *Lingshu*: *Guanzhen* (*Miraculous Pivot*: *Official Needles*) also named Twelve Needlings, including mated puncture, trigger puncture, lateral puncture, assembling puncture, centrosquare puncture, straight puncture, shu-point puncture, short-thrust puncture, superficial puncture, adjacent puncture, yin puncture and repeated shallow puncture. →偶刺(p. 287)报刺(p. 15)、恢刺(p. 176)、齐刺(p. 300)、扬刺(p. 542)、直针刺(p. 602)、输刺(p. 406)、短刺(p. 88)、浮刺(p. 118)、傍针刺(p. 13)、阴刺(p. 554)、赞刺(p. 582)

●十二禁[shí èr jìn]　针刺禁忌。出《灵枢·终始》。指针刺前后的一些禁忌,如暂时性的劳累、饥饱、情绪激动、气血不足等情况,不宜立即进行针刺;针刺之后,不宜马上进行剧烈活动,需作适当休息,以使气血调和,有助于治疗。

表13　　　　　　　　　　十二经标本部位

Table 13　Location of the origins and superficialities of the 12 meridians

十二经 Twelve Meridians	本	The Origin	标	The Superficiality
足太阳 Foot-Taiyang	在跟以上5寸中	5 cun above the heel	在两络命门(目)	the eyes
足少阳 Foot-Shaoyang	在窍阴之间	Zuqiaoyin(GB 44)	在窗笼(耳)之前	in front of the ear
足阳明 Foot-Yangming	在厉兑	Lidui(ST 45)	在人迎、颊、挟颃颡	Renying(ST 9), cheek, alongside the nasopharnx
足太阴 Foot-Taiyin	在中封前上4寸之中	4 cun anterior superior Zhongfeng(LR 4)	在背俞与舌本	back-shu point, tongue
足少阴 Foot-Shaoyin	在内踝下上3寸中	3 cun above the lower border of medial malleolus	在背俞与舌下两脉	back-shu point, Lianquan(RN 23)
足厥阴 Foot-Jueyin	在行间上5寸所	5 cun above Xingjian (LR 2)	在背俞	Back-shu point
手太阳 Hand-Taiyang	在外踝之后	Posterior to the lateral malleolus	命门(目)之上1寸	1 cun above the eyes
手少阳 Hand-Shaoyang	在小指次指之间上2寸	2 cun above the combination of the little and ring fingers	在耳后上角下外眦	from the posterior superior angle of the ear to the outer canthus
手阳明 Hand-Yangming	在肘骨中上至别阳	from the elbow upwards to Binao(LI 14)	在颜下合钳上	1 cun below the cheek, posterior to Renying(ST 9) & superior to Futu(LI 18)
手太阴 Hand-Taiyin	在寸口之中	the area of the wrist over the radial artery	腋内动脉	the pulse in the axilla
手少阴 Hand-Shaoyin	在锐骨之端	Shenmen(HT 7)	在背俞	back-shu point
手厥阴 Hand-Jueyin	在掌后两筋之间2寸中	Neiguan(PC 6)	在腋下3寸	Tianchi(PC 1)

Twelve Contraindications　The contraindications of acupuncture, originally from *Lingshu: Zhong Shi* (*Miraculous Pivot: End and Beginning*), referring to some contraindications before or after acupuncture, such as temporary fatigue, hunger or fullness, hypermotivity, deficiency of qi and blood. In the above-mentioned cases, acupuncure treatment should not be applied immediately, and after acupuncture, immediate strenuous exercises should be avoided, take a proper rest to make the relationship between qi and blood in order, and this will be helpful to the treatment.

●十二经标本 [shí èr jīng biāo běn]　出《灵枢·卫气》。又称六经标本，指手足六经的标部与本部。标，如树之末梢，言经气弥散之处；本，如树之根本，言经气本源之处。十二经以四肢肘膝以下的某些部(穴)位为本，头面、胸、背的某些部(穴)位为标。其分布部位与根结基本相仿，但标本的联系更为广泛。标本理论进一步说明经脉四肢(本)与头、面、胸、背(标)之间在生理功能与穴位主治上的联系。标本的具体内容见表十三。

The Superficialities and the Origins of the Twelve Meridians　Seen in *Lingshu: Wei Qi* (*Miraculous Pivot: Defensive Qi*), also named the superficialities and the origins of the Six Meridians, referring to those of the Six Meridians of Hand and Foot. "Superficiality", like the branch ending of a tree, is the place where the meridian-qi permeated while "origin", like the root of a tree, is the place where the meridian-qi originates. Some parts (or points) below the elbow or the knee are the "origin" of the Twelve Regular Meridians and some parts (or points) of the head, the face, the chest and the back are the "superficiality". Their locations are basically similar to those of the root and branch, but the relation between the superficiality and the origin is

more extensive. The theory of the superficiality and the origin reveals further the relation of the four limbs (the origin) with the head, the face, the chest, and the back (the superficiality) in their physiological functions and point indications. The concrete contents of the superficiality and the origin are listed in Table 13. (p. 375)

●十二经别 [shí èr jīng bié] 经别名。出《灵枢·经别》。指从十二经脉另行别出，而循行在体腔、头面的重要支脉。十二经脉有各自的经别，合称十二经别。其循行方式，自正经经脉分出，经躯干、脏腑、头项等处，最后仍归于正经经脉中。在循行的过程中，六阳经的经别复注入原来的阳经，六阴经的经别则注入与其表里相合的阳经，共组成六对，称六合。足太阳、足少阴经别为一合，足少阳、足厥阴经别为二合，足阳明、足太阴经别为三合，手太阳、手少阴经别为四合，手少阳、手厥阴经别为五合，手阳明、手太阴经别为六合。其作用主要是加强表里两经在躯体深部的联系，并能通达某些正经未能循行的器官与形体部位，以补其不足。

The Twelve Divergent Meridians Name of divergent meridians, originally from *Ling Shu*: *Jingbie* (*Miraculous Pivot*: *Divergent Meridians*), referring to the important branches derived from the Twelve Regular Meridians and reaching the deep part of the body, the head and the face. Each of the Twelve Meridians has its own divergent meridian, so they are collectively termed the Twelve Divergent Meridians. They circulate in the following manner: deriving from the regular meridians, passing through the trunk zang and fu, head and neck, and finally returning to the regular meridians. In the course of circulation, the six Yang divergent meridians enter the original yang regular meridians again, and the six yin divergent meridians enter the internally and externally-related yang meridians, constituting six pairs called the Six Confluences, namely, (1) the Meridian of Foot-Taiyang and the Divergent Meridian of Foot-Shaoyin. (2) The meridian of Foot-Shaoyang and the Divergent Meridian of Foot-Jueyin. (3) the Meridian of Foot-Yangming and the Divergent Meridian of Foot-Taiyin. (4) The Meridian of Hand-Taiyang and the Divergent Meridian of Hand-Shaoyin. (5) The Meridian of Hand-Shaoyang and the Divergent Meridian of Hand-Jueyin. (6) The Meridian of Hand-Yangming and the Divergent Meridian of Hand-Taiyin. The main function of the divergent meridians is to strengthen the connections between the external and internal meridians in the deep part of the body, and reach the organs and the parts that some of the regular meridians fail to reach to replenish the deficiency.

●十二经动脉 [shí èr jīng dòng mài] 指十二经各有动脉搏动处。出《难经·一难》。据《针灸甲乙经》所载，各经"在动脉应手处"的穴位如下：

手太阴肺经：中府、云门、天府、侠白、尺泽、经渠；

手少阴心经：极泉，少海；

手厥阴心包经：劳宫；

手阳明大肠经：合谷、阳溪、手五里；

手太阳小肠经：天窗；

手少阳三焦经：和髎；

足阳明胃经：大迎、下关、人迎、气冲、冲阳；

足太阳膀胱经：委中；

足少阳胆经：听会、上关；

足太阴脾经：箕门、冲门；

足少阴肾经：太溪、阴谷；

足厥阴肝经：太冲、行间、足五里、阴廉。

Arteries of the Twelve Meridians The respective arteries with palpable pulsation of the Twelve Regular Meridians, originally from *Nanjing*: *Yi Nan* (*Classic of Question*: *Question 1*). According to the records of *Zhenjiu Jia-Yi Jing* (*A-B Classic of Acupuncture and Moxibustion*), the undulatory points of the meridians are as follows: The Lung Meridian of Hand-Taiyin: Zhongfu (LU 1), Yunmen (LU 2), Tianfu (LU 3), Xiabai (LU 4), Chize (LU 5), Jingqu (LU 8); The heart Meridian of Hand-Shaoyin: Jiquan (HT 1), Shaohai (HT 3); The Pericardium Meridian of Hand-Jueyin: Laogong (PC 8); The Large Intestine Meridian of Hand-Yangming: Hegu (LI 4), Yangxi (LI 5), Shouwuli (LI 13); The Small Intestine Meridian of Hand-Taiyang: Tianchuang (SI 16); The Sanjiao Meridian of

Hand-Shaoyang: Erheliao(SJ 22); The Stomach Meridian of Foot-Yangming: Daying(ST 5), Xiaguan(ST 7), Renying(ST 9), Qichong(ST 30), Chongyang(ST 42); The Bladder Meridian of Foot-Taiyang: Weizhong(BL 40); The Gallbladder Meridian of Foot-Shaoyang: Tinghui(GB 2), Shangguan(GB 3); The Spleen Meridian of Foot-Taiyin: Jimen(SP 11), Chongmen(SP 12); The Kidney Meridian of Foot-Shaoyin: Taixi(KI 3), Yingu(KI 10) and The Liver Meridian of Foot-Jueyin: Taichong(LR 3), Xingjian(LR 2), Zuwuli(LR 10), Yinlian(LR 11).

●十二经筋[shí èr jīng jīn] 经络分类名。出《灵枢·经筋》。是经络系统在人体的连属部分，全身筋肉按部位分为手足三阴三阳，即十二经筋。其分布特点与十二经脉基本一致。阳之筋分布在肢体外侧，阴之筋分布在肢体内侧，但都从四肢末端起始走向躯干，结聚于关节和骨骼附近。阳之筋上走头面，阴之筋进入腹腔，但都不入内脏。十二经筋具有联缀四肢关节、维络周身，主司关节运动的作用，它的病变，多表现为痹痛、拘挛、弛缓、转筋、强直和抽搐等运动障碍的病症。

The Twelve Muscle Regions A category of meridians and collaterals, originally from *Lingshu: Jingjin (Miraculous Pivot: Muscle Regions Along Meridians)*, the connecting part of the meridian system in the human body. The tendons and muscles of the whole body are divided into three yins and three yangs of foot and hand, namely, the Twelve Muscle Regions. The distribution of the muscle regions corresponds basically to the course of the Twelve Regular Meridians. The muscle regions of the yang meridians distribute on the lateral side of the body, upward to the hand and face; the muscle regions of yin-meridians on the medial side, entering the abdominal cavity. All the muscle regions start from the terminals of the limbs and run to the trunk. Instead of entering zang and fu organs, they travel along the body surface, and connect with the joints and bones. The Twelve Muscle Regions have the function of connecting the four limbs, joints and the whole body, and governing the movement of the joints. The manifestations of the diseases of the muscle regions are arthralgia, spasm, relaxation, rigidity, convulsion, and dyscinesia.

●十二经脉[shí èr jīng mài] 经脉名。出《灵枢·海论》。人体十二经脉，即手三阴（手太阴肺经、手少阴心经、手厥阴心包经），手三阳（手阳明大肠经、手太阳小肠经、手少阳三焦经），足三阴（足太阴脾经、足少阴肾经、足厥阴肝经），足三阳（足阳明胃经、足太阳膀胱经、足少阳胆经）的合称。为经络系统的主体，故又称正经或十二正经。每一经脉，均各隶属于一定的脏腑。阴经的属脏络腑，阳经的属腑络脏，且外联于头面、躯干、四肢，将人体内外连贯起来，成为一个有机的整体，又是气血运行的主要通道。

The Twelve Meridians Meridians, originally from *Lingshu: Hai Lun (Miraculous Pivot: On Seas)*, a general term for the Twelve Meridians of the human body, that is, the three yin meridians of hand (the Lung Meridian of Hand-Taiyin, the Heart Meridian of Hand-Shaoyin, the Pericardium Meridian of Hand-Jueyin); the three yang meridians of hand (the Large Intestine Meridian of Hand-Yangming, the Small Intestine Meridian of Hand-Taiyang, the Sanjiao Meridian of Hand Shaoyang); The three yin meridians of foot (the Spleen Meridian of Foot-Taiying, the Kidney Meridian of Foot-Shaoyin, the Liver Meridian of Foot-Jueyin), and three yang meridians of foot (the Stomach Meridian of Foot-Yangming, the Bladder Meridian of Foot-Taiyang, the Gallbladder Meridian of Foot-Shaoyang). These are the major trunks of the system of the meridians and collaterals, thus named the Regular Meridians or the Twelve Regular Meridians. Each meridian pertains to certain zang or fu organs, The yin meridians pertain to zang organs linking up the fu, and the yang meridians pertain to the fu organs linking up the zang, connecting exteriorly the head, face, trunk and limbs, integrating the interior and exterior parts of the body into an organic whole, and becoming the leading transportation passage of qi and blood.

●十二经脉歌[shí èr jīng mài gē] 针灸歌赋之一。见清代栗山痴叟所撰《医学便览》第五卷。其内容是

以歌赋的形式叙述十二经脉的循行分布。

Shier Jingmai Ge（A Verse on the Twelve Regular Meridians） One of the verses on acupuncture and moxibustion, from Vol. 1 of *Yixue Bianlan*（*A Brief Guide to Medicine*）written by Li Shan Chi Sou in the Qing Dynasty, in which the courses and distributions of the Twelve Regular Meridians are explained in verses.

●十二经水[shí èr jīng shuǐ] 出《灵枢·经水》。指当时大地上的泾、渭、海、湖、汝、渑、淮、漯、江、河、济、漳等十二条水流。用以比喻十二经脉气血运行的情况。

The Water-Flow of the Twelve Meridians Originally from *Lingshu*: *qingshui*（*Miraculous Pivot*: *Qi and Blood of Meridians*）, referring to the 12 streams on the earth, that is, jing, wei, sea, lake, ru, sheng, huai, luo, jiang, river, ji and zhang, the analogy of the circulation of qi and blood of the Twelve Regular Meridians.

●十二经之海[shí èr jīng zhī hǎi] 血海的别名。详见该条。

The Sea of the Twelve Meridians Another name for the sea of blood. →血海（p.524）

●十二经子母补泻歌[shí èr jīng zǐ mǔ bǔ xiè gē] 针灸歌赋名。是选用本经子母穴进行治疗的一种取穴方法。也是"虚则补其母，实则泻其子"原则在针灸治疗中的具体应用，对于治疗十二经所生病症有一定的指导意义。其内容为：肺泻尺泽补太渊，大肠二间曲池间，胃泻厉兑解溪补，脾在商丘大都边，心先神门后少冲，小肠小海后溪连，膀胱束骨补至阴，肾泻涌泉复溜焉，包络大陵中冲补，三焦天井中渚痊，胆泻阳辅补侠溪，肝泻行间补曲泉。参见"子母补泻法"条。

Shier Jing Zi-Mu Bu Xie Ge（Verses on the Child-Mother Reinforcing-Reducing Method of the Twelve Meridians） A verse of acupuncture and moxibustion about the method of point selection using the child-mother point to treat diseases, it gives a concrete application of the acupunctue treatment principle reinforcing the mother points according to deficient syndromes and reducing the child points according to excess syndromes, and it is a guide for treating diseases of the twelve meridians. The contents are as follows: Lung: reduce Chize and reinforce Taiyuan; Large Intestine: reduce Erjian（LI 2）and reinforce Quchi（LI 11）; Stomach: reduce Lidui（ST 45）and reinforce Jiexi（ST 41）; Spleen: reduce Shangqiu（SP 5）and reinforce Dadu（SP 2）; Heart: reduce Shenmen（HT 7）and reinforce Shaochong（HT 9）; Small Intestine: Xiaohai（SI 8）and Houxi（SI 3）; Bladder: Shugu（BL 65）and Zhiyin（BL 67）; Kidney: Yongquan（KI 1）and Fuliu（KI 7）; Pericardium: Daling（PC 7）and Zhongchong（PC 9）; Sanjiao: Tianjing（SJ 10）and Zhongzhu（SJ 3）; Gallbladder: Yangfu（GB 38）and Xiaxi（GB 43）; Liver: Xingjian（LR 2）and Ququan（LR 8）. →子母补泻法（p.625）

●十二皮部[shí èr pí bù] 部位名。出《素问·皮部论》。指人体表皮按十二经脉分布，划分为十二个部区。参见"皮部"条。

The Twelve Cutaneous Regions Parts of the body, from *Su Wen*: *Pibu*（*Plain Questions*: *On Cutaneous Regions*）, referring to the twelve divisions of the body surface on the basis of the distribution of the Twelve Regular Meridians. →皮部（p.291）

●十二人图[shí èr rén tú] 书。①作者不详，二卷，已佚。见《隋书·经籍志》。②唐代王焘《外台秘要》，原绘有十二人图，即分十二经脉绘图。将督脉并入足太阳，任脉并入足少阴。原图已佚。

1. Shier Ren Tu（The Twelve Pictures of Man） A book in 2 volumes, from *Sui Shu*: *Jing Ji Zhi*（*The History of the Sui Dynasty*: *Records of Classics and Books*）. The book is no longer extant, the author unkown.

2. The Twelve Pictures of Man The 12 pictures of man in *Waitai Miyao*（*Clandestine Essentials from the Imperial Library*）written by Wang Tao in the Tang Dynasty, namely, the pictures of the twelve meridians, the Du Meridian was merged into Foot-Taiyang, and the Ren Meridian into Foot-Shaoyin. The original pictures have been lost.

●十二手法[shí èr shǒu fǎ] 刺法用语。出《针灸大成·三衢杨氏补泻》。原称十二字分次第手法。杨氏将针法的基本操作步骤总结归纳为十二种，包括爪切、

指持、口温、进针、指循、爪摄、针退、指搓、指捻、指留、针摇、指拨。具体操作,详见各条。

Twelve Needling Methods A term in acupuncture, seen in *Zhenjiu Dacheng: Sanqu Yangshi Bu-Xie* (*A Great Compendium of Acupunsture and Moxibustion: Yang's Reinforcing and Reducing Techniques of Three Branches*), originally named the orderly needling methods with 12 words. Yang Jizhou summed up the elementary steps of the needling methods as the following 12 kinds: nail-pressing, finger-holding, mouth warming, inserting the needle, massaging along the meridian with fingers, nail-pressing along the meridian, lifting the needle, twirling the needle slightly with fingers, finger rotating, finger-retaining, shaking the needle and withdrawing the needle. →爪切(p. 586)、指持(p. 603)、口温(p. 234)、进针(p. 206)、指循(p. 604)、爪摄(p. 586)、针退(p. 597)、指搓(p. 603)、指捻(p. 604)、指留(p. 604)、针摇(p. 597)、指拨(p. 603)

●十二正经[shí èr zhèng jīng] 十二经脉的别名。详见该条。

The Twelve Regular Meridians →十二经脉(p. 377)

●十二指肠[shí èr zhǐ cháng] 耳穴名。位于耳轮脚上方外三分之一。用于治疗十二指肠溃疡、幽门痉挛、胆囊炎、胆石症。

Duodenum (MA-SC 1) An ear point. 〈Location〉at the lateral 1/3 of the superior aspect of the helix crus. 〈Indications〉duodenal ulcer, pylorospasm, cholecystitis, cholelithiasis.

●十二字分次第手法[shí èr zì fēn cì dì shǒu fǎ] 刺法术语,十二手法的原称。详见该条。

The Orderly Needling Methods with 12 Words A term in acupuncture, the original name of Twelve Needling Methods. →十二手法(p. 378)

●十六络脉[shí liù luò mài] 十五络脉之外,又加胃之大络,合称十六络。出《类经》卷五,张介宾注。参见"胃之大络"条。

The Sixteen Collaterals A general term for the Fifteen Main Collaterals with the addition of the main collateral from the stomach, originally from the annotation of Vol. 5 of *Leijing* (*The Classified Canon of Internal Medicine of the Yellow Emperor*), by Zhang Jiebin. →胃之大络(p. 469)

●十七椎[shí qī zhuī] ①经外穴名。见《类经图翼》。〈定位〉在腰部,当后正中线上,第五腰棘突下。〈层次解剖〉皮肤→皮下组织→棘上韧带→棘间韧带。浅层主要布有第五腰椎神经后支的皮支和伴行的动、静脉。深层主要有第五腰神经后支的分支和棘突间的椎外(后)静脉。〈主治〉腰痛、腿痛、下肢瘫痪、转胞、痛经、肛门疾患,以及坐骨神经痛,功能性子宫出血等。直刺0.5～1寸;可灸。②骨骼名。指第5腰椎。

1. **Shiqizhui** (EX-B 8) An extra point, originally from *Lei Jing Tu Yi* (*Supplements to Illustrated Classified Canon of Internal Medicine of the Yellow Emperor*). 〈Location〉on the low back and on the posterior midline, below the spinous process of the 5th lumbar vertebra. 〈Regional anatomy〉skin→subcutaneous tissue → supraspinal ligament → interspinal ligament. In the superficial layer, there are the cutaneous branches of the posterior branch of the 5th lumbar nerve and the accompanying artery and vein. In the deep layer, there are the branches of the posterior branch of the 5th lumbar nerve and the external (posterior) vertebral venous plexus between the adjacent spinous processes. 〈Indications〉lumbago, pain and paralysis of lower extrmities, oliguraia and frequency of micturition due to pregnancy, dysmenorrhea, anal disease, sciatica, dysfunctional uterine bleeding, etc. 〈Method〉Puncture perpendicularly 0.5～1.0 cun. Moxibustion is applicable.

2. **The 17th Vertebra** A bone referring to the 5th lumbar vertebra.

●十三鬼穴[shí sān guǐ xué] 古代用来治疗癫狂等症的十三经验效穴。见《千金要方》。分别称"鬼宫",即人中。"鬼信",即少商。"鬼垒",即隐白。"鬼心",即大陵。"鬼路",即申脉,亦指间使。"鬼枕",即风府。"鬼床"即颊车。"鬼市",即承浆。"鬼窟",即劳宫。"鬼堂",即上星。"鬼藏",男指阴下缝,女指玉门头。"鬼臣",即曲池。"鬼封",即舌下中缝。

The 13 Ghost-Points The 13 effective points from clinical experience which were used to treat manic-depressive disorder in ancient

times, from *Qianjin Yaofang* (*Essential Prescriptions Worth a Thousand Gold*), respectively called Guigong, i.e. Renzhong (DU 26); Guixin, i.e. Shaoshang (LU 11); Guilei, i.e. Yinbai (SP 1); Guixin, i.e. Daling (PC 7); Guilu, Shenmai (BL 62) or Jianshi (PC 5); Guizhen, i.e. Fengfu (Du 16); Guichuang, i.e. Jiache (ST 6); Guishi, i.e. Chengjiang (RN 24); Guiku, i.e. Laogong (PC 8); Guitang, i.e. Shangxing (DU 23); Guicang, i.e. raphe of perineum in male, and posterior comissure of labia in female; Guichen, i.e. Quchi (LI 11); Guifeng, i.e. the frenulum of tongue.

●十三穴 [shí sān xué] 即十三鬼穴。详见该条。

The 13 Points →十三鬼穴 (p. 379)

●十四法 [shí sì fǎ] 针刺手法。出《针经指南》。①原称手指补泻法，即：动、退、搓、进、盘、摇、弹、撚、循、扪、摄、按、爪、切。②《金针赋》所述十四法与《针经指南》基本一致，但将"撚"并入"搓"，另加"提"，与"按"对举。③《针灸问对》所斜述的十四法中，又将"爪"与"切"合并，再补充了"努"法。

The Fourteen Needling Methods Acupuncture techniques from *Zhenjing Zhinan* (*Guide to the Classics of Acupuncture*). ① Originally called the finger reinforcing and reducing methods, namely, moving, backing, twirling the needle slightly, inserting, winding, shaking, plucking, rotating, pressing the needling hole, massaging along the meridian, nail-pressing along the meridian, pressing, nail-pressing while inserting the needle and nail-pressing around the point. ② The Fourteen Methods recorded in *Jinzhen Fu* (*Ode to Gold Needle*) are basically in accordance with those in *Zhenjing Zhinan* (*Guide to the Classics of Acupuncture*), but merged "rotating" into "twirling the needle slightly", and added "lifting" as opposed to "pressing". ③ In the Fourteen Methods in *Zhenjiu Wendui* (*Catechism of Acupuncture and Moxibustion*), "nail-pressing while inserting the needle" was merged into "nail pressing around the point", and the method "bending" was added.

●十四经 [shí sì jīng] 经脉名。出《十四经发挥》。十二经脉和任脉、督脉的合称。奇经八脉中，惟任、督二脉有联属的穴位，和十二经脉相同，并与之关系密切，故与十二经相提并论，合称十四经。是经络系统中主要部分（图47）。

The Fourteen Meridians Meridians, originally from *Shisi Jing Fahui* (*An Elaboration of the Fourteen Meridians*). A general term for the Twelve Regular Meridians, Ren and Du Meridians. Of the extra meridians, only Ren and Du Meridians like the twelve regular meridians, have their own points, and are closely related with the Twelve Regular Meridians. All of the above meridians are comprehensively termed the Fourteen Meridians and are the main parts of the system of the meridians and collaterals (Fig. 47).

●十四经发挥 [shí sì jīng fā huī] 书名。元代滑寿（伯仁）著，分三卷。上卷，手足阴阳流注篇；中卷，十四经脉气所发篇；下卷，奇经八脉篇。对十二经脉及任、督二脉的三百五十七穴（双侧）详加考证，是阐明经络学说的重要著作。

Shisi Jing Fahui (An Elaboration of the Fourteen Meridians) A book in 3 volumes, written by Hua Shou (Boren) in the Yuan Dynasty. The first volume was the treatise on the ebb-flow of foot-yangming and hand-yangming, the second was the treatise on the origin of qi of the Fourteen Meridians, and the third was the treatise on the Eight Extra Meridians. The book tested in detail all of the 357 points (on both sides) of the Twelve Regular Meridians, Ren and Du Meridians, and is an important work on the theory of meridians and collaterals.

●十四经发挥合纂 [shí sì jīng fā huī hé zuǎn] 书名。明代张权撰，十六卷。

Shisi Jing Fahui Hezuan (Joint Edition of An Elaboration of the Fourteen Meridians) A book in 16 volumes, written by Zhang Quan in the Ming Dynasty.

●十四经穴 [shí sì jīng xué] 指分布在十二经脉及任、督二脉上的腧穴。又名经穴。早在《内经》中已分经论穴，至《甲乙》有系统的记载，计正中（任、督脉）

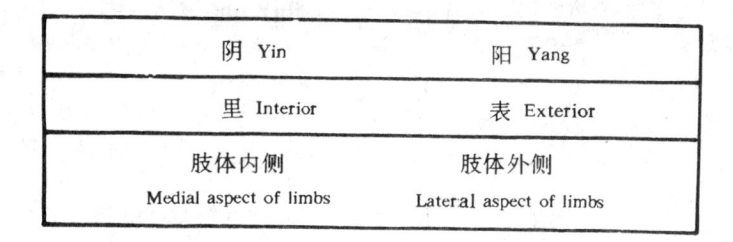

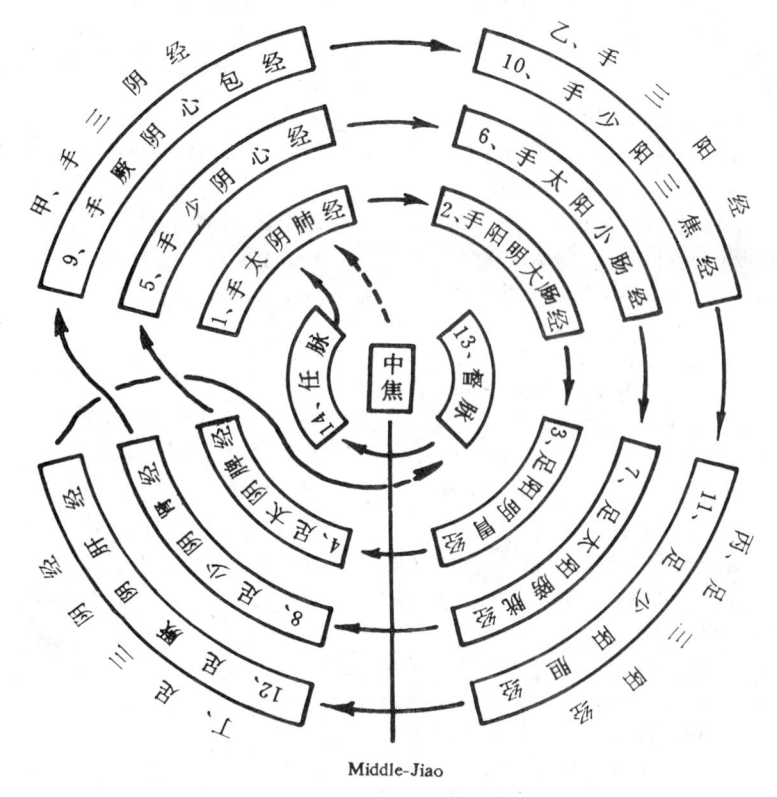

阴 Yin	阳 Yang
里 Interior	表 Exterior
肢体内侧 Medial aspect of limbs	肢体外侧 Lateral aspect of limbs

Middle-Jiao

A. Three Yin Meridians of Hand

1. Lung Meridian of Hand-Taiyin (LU)
5. Heart Meridian of Hand-Shaoyin (HT)
9. Pericardium Meridian of Hand-Jueyin (PC)

B. Three Yang Meridians of Hand

2. Large Intestine Meridian of Hand-Yangming (LI)
6. Small Intestine Meridian of Hand-Taiyang (SI)
10. Sanjiao Meridian of Hand-Shaoyang (SJ)

C. Three Yang Meridians of Foot

3. Stomach Meridian of Foot-Yangming (ST)
7. Bladder Meridian of Foot-Taiyang (BL)
11. Gallbladder Meridian of Foot-Shaoyang (GB)

D. Three Yin Meridians of Foot

4. Spleen Meridian of Foot-TaiYin (SP)
8. Kidney Meridian of Foot-Shaoyin (KI)
12. Liver Meridian of Foot-Jueyin (LR)

13. Du Meridian (DU)
14. Ren Meridian (RN)

图47 十四经循行顺序

Fig. 47 Circulation of the 14 meridians

单穴49穴，两侧（十二经脉）双穴300穴，合计总穴名349穴。以后的针灸著作中续有增加。至清代李学川《针灸逢源》所载，计正中单穴52穴，两则双穴309穴，合计总穴名361个。分别为：督脉28穴，任脉24穴，手太阴肺经11穴，手厥阴心包经9穴，手少阴心经9穴，手阳明大肠经20穴，手少阳三焦经23穴，手太阳小肠经19穴，足阳明胃经45穴，足少阳胆经44穴，足太阳膀胱经67穴，足太阴脾经21穴，足厥阴肝经14穴，足少阴肾经27穴。

Points on the Fourteen Meridians Points on the Twelve Regular Meridians, the Ren and the Du meridians, also named meridian points. Early in *Neijing* (*The Canon of Internal Medicine*), points were dealt with by respective meridians, and recorded systematically in *Jia-Yi* (*A-B Classic of Acupuncture and Moxibustion*). The book stated that there were 49 single points on the midline of the body (Ren and Du Meridians), and 300 double points on both lateral sides (the Twelve Meridians), totally 349 points. In later acupuncture works points were added, until in the Qing Dynasty, *Zhenjiu Fengyuan* (*The Origin of Acupuncture and Moxibustion*) written by Li Xuechuan recorded 32 single points on the midline of the body, 309 double points on both sides, 361 points in all. They were as follows: 28 points on the Du Meridian, 24 on the Ren Meridian, 11 on the Lung Meridian of Hand-Taiyin, 9 on the Pericardium Meridian of Hand-Jueyin, 9 on the Heart Meidian of Hand-Shaoyin, 20 on the Large Intestine Meridian of Hand-Yangming, 23 on the Sanjiao Meridian of Hand-Shaoyang, 19 on the Small Intestine Meridian of Hand-Taiyang, 45 on the Stomach Meridian of Foot-Yangming, 44 on the Gallbladder Meridian of Foot-Shaoyang, 67 on the Bladder Meridian of Foot-Taiyang, 21 on the Spleen Meridian of Foot-Taiyin, 14 on the Liver Meridian of Foot-Jueyin, 27 on the Kidney Meridian of Foot-Shaoyin.

●十王［shí wáng］ 经外穴名。出《针灸经外奇穴治疗诀》。位于十指背侧，沿爪甲根正中点向皮肤部移行约0.1寸处。〈主治〉昏迷、高热、中暑、霍乱、小儿惊厥等。点刺出血。

Shiwang (EX-UE) An extra point, from *Zhenjiu Jingwai Qixue Zhiliao Jue* (*Pithy Acupuncture Formulas for Treatment with Extra Points*). 〈Location〉on the dorsal aspect of the 10 fingers, 0.1 cun directly above the midpoints of the nail roots. 〈Indications〉coma, high fever, heat-strock, cholera, infantile convulsion, etc. 〈Method〉Prick the point to cause bleeding.

●十五别络［shí wǔ bié luò］ 十五络脉的别名。详见该条。

The Fifteen Separating Collaterals →十五络脉(p.382)

●十五络［shí wǔ luò］ 十五络脉的别名。详见该条。

The Fifteen Collaterals →十五络脉(p.382)

●十五络脉［shí wǔ luò mài］ 络脉总称。出《灵枢·经脉》。又称十五络、十五别络。十二经脉各有一支别络，加上任脉络、督脉络和脾之大络，共为十五络脉（见表14）。十二经的络脉都是由表经别入里经，里经别出表经，起着沟通表里两经和加强其在体内联系的作用。任、督脉的络脉和脾之大络，分别位于躯体的前、后、侧部，有通调气血和治疗胸腹、背腰和胁部病症的作用。又《难经·二十六难》以十二经脉之络及阴跷、阳跷之络，与脾之大络，为十五络脉。

The Fifteen Main Collaterals A general term for collaterals, originally from *Lingshu: Jingmai* (*Miraculous Pivot: Meridians*), also named the Fifteen Collaterals and the Fifteen Separating Collaterals. Each of the Twelve Meridians has a collateral, adding the Ren and Du collaterals and the major collateral of the spleen, there are fifteen collaterals in all (See Table 14). The collaterals of the Twelve Meridians enter the internal meridians from the external meridians, or from the internal meridians to the external meridians, playing the role of communicating with the external and internal meridians and strengthening the association of the meridians on the body surface. The Ren and Du collaterals and the major collateral of the spleen are respectively located in the anterior, posterior, and the lateral parts of the body, with the function of regulating qi and blood and treating the diseases of the chest, abdomen, back, loin and hypochondrium. In *Nanjing* (*The Classic of Questions*:

表14
Table 14

十 五 络 脉
The Fifteen Main Collaterls

络脉名 Collateral	穴 名 Point	分布部位 Distribution
手太阴 Hand-Taiyin	列 缺 Lieque(LU 7)	腕上寸半,别(分支)走手阳明 1.5 cun above the wrist,(the branch)entering Hand-Yangming
手厥阴 Hand-Jueyin	内 关 Neiguan(PC 6)	腕上2寸,别走手少阳 2 cun above the wrist,entering Hand-Shaoyang
手少阴 Hand-Shaoyin	通 里 Tongli(HT 5)	腕上一寸半,别走手太阳 1.5 cun above the wrist,entering Hand-Taiyang
手阳明 Hand-Yangming	偏 历 Pianli(LI 16)	腕上3寸,别入手太阴 3 cun above the wrist,entering Hand-Taiyin
手少阳 Hand-Shaoyang	外 关 Waiguan(SJ 5)	腕上2寸,合手厥阴 2 cun above the wrist,entering Hand-Jueyin
手太阳 Hand-Taiyang	支 正 Zhizheng(SJ 7)	腕上5寸,内注手少阴 5 cun above the wrist,entering Hand-Jueyin
足阳明 Foot-Yangming	丰 隆 Fenglong(ST 40)	外踝上8寸,别走足太阴 8 cun above the external malleolus,entering Foot-Taiyin
足少阳 Foot-Shaoyang	光 明 Guangming(GB 37)	外踝上5寸,内注足厥阴 5 cun above the external malleolus,entering Foot-Jueyin
足太阴 Foot-Taiyin	飞 扬 Feiyang(BL 58)	外踝上7寸,别走足少阴 7 cun above the external malleolus,entering Foot-Shaoyin
足太阳 Foot-Taiyang	公 孙 Gongsun(SP 4)	本节后一寸,别走足阳明 1 cun posterior to the base of the lst matatarsal bone, entering Foot-Yangming
足厥阴 Foot-Jueyin	蠡 沟 Ligou(LR 5)	内踝上5寸,别走足少阳 5 cun above the medial malleolus,entering Foot-Shaoyang
足少阴 Foot-Shaoyin	大 钟 Dazhong(KI 4)	内踝后绕跟,别走足太阳 posterior to the medial malleolus,around the heel, entering Foot-Taiyang
任 Ren	鸠 尾 Jiuwei(RN 15)	下鸠尾,散于腹 downwards from Jiuwei(RN 15),distributing in abdomen
督 Du	长 强 Changqiang(DU 1)	挟脊上顶,散于头上 upwards to the back alongside the spine,distributing in the head
脾 Spleen	大 包 Dabao(SP 21)	出渊腋下3寸,布胸胁 emerging from the region 3 cun below Yuanye(GB 22), distributing in chest and hypochondrium

Question 1),the collaterals of the Twelve Regular Meridians, the collaterals of Yinqiao and Yangqiao Meridians and the major collateral of the spleen are taken as the Fifteen Collaterals.

●十五椎[shí wǔ zhuī] ①骨骼名。指第3腰椎。②经外奇穴。在第3腰椎棘突下,即下极俞。详见该条。

1. **The 15th Vertebra** A bone, referring to the 3rd lumbar vertebra.

2. **Shiwuzhui** An extra point below the spinous process of the 3rd lumbar vertebra, synonymous with Xiajishu(EX-B 5). →下极俞 (p. 488)

●十宣[shí xuān]经外穴名。出《奇效良方》。又名鬼城。〈定位〉在手十指尖端,距指甲游离缘0.1寸(指寸),左右共十穴。〈层次解剖〉皮肤→皮下组织。各穴的神经支配:拇指到中指的十宣穴由正中神经分布;环指的十宣穴由桡侧的正中神经和尺侧的尺神经双重分布;小指的十宣穴由尺神经分布。〈主治〉昏迷、晕厥、高热、中暑、癫痫、癔病、小儿惊厥等。针刺出血。

Shixuan(EX-UE 11)　A set of extra point, from *Qixiao Liangfang*(*Prescriptions of Wonderful Efficacy*), also named Guicheng. 〈Location〉ten points on both hands, at the tips of the 10 fingers, 0.1 cun from the free margin of the nails. 〈Regional anatomy〉skin→subcutaneous tissue. The nerves innervating the areas of the points on the thumb, index and middle finger are from the median nerve; on the ring finger is from both the median and ulnar nerves; on the little finger is from the ulnal nerve. 〈Indications〉coma, syncope, high fever, heat-stroke, epilepsy, hysteria, infantile convulsion. 〈Method〉Prick to cause bleeding.

●十一脉[shí yī mài]　指足太阳、足少阳、足阳明、足少阴、足太阴、足厥阴、手太阴、手少阴、手太阳、手少阳、手阳明十一条脉。出马王堆汉墓《帛书》。它的记载较《灵枢·经脉》少一条手厥阴，故称十一脉。在《灵枢·本输》及《灵枢·阴阳系日月》两篇中也未列手厥阴(心主)，与《帛书》类似。参见"帛书经脉"条。

The Eleven Meridians　The 11 meridians of Foot-Taiyang, Foot-Shaoyang, Foot-Yangming, Foot-Shaoyin, Foot-Taiyin, Foot-Jueyin, Hand-Yaiyin, Hand-Shaoyin, Hand-Taiyang, Hand-Shaoyang, Hand-Yangming, from *Boshu*(*Silk Book*) in the Han Tomb at Mawangdui, in which, one meridian less was recorded than the meridians in *Lingshu*: *Jingmai*(*Miraculous Pivot*: *Meridians*), namely, the Meridian of Hand-Jueyin. Thus they were called the eleven meridians. Similar to the meridians recorded in *Boshu*(*Silk Book*), the Pericardium Meridian of Hand-Jueyin was not recorded in *Lingshu*: *Benshu*(*Miraculous Pivot*: *Meridian Points*) and *Lingshu*: *Yinyang Xi Riyue* (*Miraculous Pivot*: *Relation Between Yin-Yang and Sun-Moon*). →帛书经脉(p. 25)

●十一脉灸经[shí yī mài jiǔ jīng]　书名。又名《帛书经脉》，长沙马王堆汉墓(公元前168年)出土帛书之一。分为《阴阳十一脉灸经》和《足臂十一脉灸经》两篇，是论述经脉循行和病候的最早专著。其与《灵枢》所述十二经脉有所不同。手脉称"臂"，不称"手"，缺少"臂厥阴脉"，经脉起止循行方向也与《灵枢》不同。总之，其较《灵枢》叙述简单，但有字迹缺少现象。

Shiyi Mai Jiujing(**Moxibustion Classic of the Eleven Meridians**)　A book, also named *Boshu Jingmai*(*Meridians of the Silk Book*), one of the silk scrolls excavated from the Han tomb at Mawangdui(168 B. C.)in Changsha, divided into *Yinyang Shiyi Mai Jiujing*(*Moxibustion Classic of the Eleven Yin-Yang Meridians*) and *Zu Bi Shiyi Mai Jiujing*(*Moibustion Classic of the Eleven Foot-Arm Meridians*), the earliest monograph on the circulation of the meridians, and the symptoms of diseases. Slightly different from the twelve meridians in *Lingshu*(*Miraculous Pivot*), the meridıns of hand were called in *Ling Shu*(*Miraculous Pivot*), the meridians of hand were called "arm" instead of hand in *Boshu*(*Silk Book.*), the Meridian of Arm-Jueyin was not included, and the origin and end, and the circulating direction of the meridians are also different from those in *Lingshu*(*Miraculous Pivot*). In a word, the explanations were simpler than the explanations in *Lingshu*(*Miraculous Piovt*), but some words were missing.

●石宫[shí gōng]　经穴别名。出《针灸甲乙经》。即阴都。详见该条。

Shigong　Another name for Yindu(KI 19), a meridian point, from *Zhenjiu Jia-Yi Jing*(*A-B Classic of Acupuncture and Moxibustion*). →阴都(p. 554)

●石关[shí guān]　①经穴名。出《针灸甲乙经》。属足少阴肾经，为冲脉、足少阴之会。又名右关、石阙。〈定位〉在上腹部，当脐中上3寸，前正中线旁开0.5寸(图40)。〈层次解剖〉皮肤→皮下组织→腹直肌鞘前壁→腹直肌。浅层布有腹壁浅静脉，第七、八、九胸神经前支及伴行的动、静脉。深层有腹壁上动、静脉的分支或属支，第七、八、九胸神经前支的肌支和相应的肋间动、静脉。〈主治〉呕吐、腹痛、便秘、产后腹痛不孕。直刺0.5～0.8寸；可灸。②经外穴名。见《卫生宝鉴》。位于巨阙旁开五寸。〈主治〉产后两腿急痛不可忍。用灸法。

1. Shiguan(KI 18)　A meridian point, on the Kidney Meridian of Foot-*Shaoyin*, from *Zhenjiu Jia-Yi Jing*(*A-B Classic of Acupuncture and Moxibustion*), the crossing point of the Chong and Foot-Shaoyin Meridians, also named Youguan and Shique. 〈Location〉on the upper abdomen, 3 cun above the centre of the umbilicus, and 0.5 cun lateral to the ante-

rior midline (Fig. 40). 〈Regional anatomy〉 skin→subcutaneous tissue→anterior sheath of rectus muscle of abdomen→recuts muscle of abdomen. In the superficial layer, there are the superficial epigastric vein, the anterior branches of the 7th to 9th thoracic nerves and accompanying arteries and veins. In the deep layer, there are the branches or tributaries of the superior epigastric artery and vein, the muscles of the anterior branches of the 7th to 9th thoracic nerves and the related intercostal arteries and veins. 〈Indications〉 vomiting, abdominal pain, constipation, abdominal pain after delivery. 〈Method〉 Puncture perpendicularly 0.5~0.8 cun. Moxibustion is applicable.

2. **Shiguan** (EX-CA) An extra point, from *Weisheng Baojian* (*Treasured Mirror of Health Protection*). 〈Location〉 5 cun lateral to Juque (RN 14). 〈Indication〉 acute unbearable pain after delivery. 〈Method〉 moxibustion.

●石淋[shí lìn] 淋证证型之一。出《诸病源候论·淋病诸候》。又称砂淋、砂石淋。多因湿热下注，煎熬尿液，结为砂石所致。证见小腹及茎中胀急刺痛，排尿常因砂石而中断，变换体位常能畅通，可伴有腰部、腹部剧烈疼痛。舌苔白或黄腻，脉弦数。治宜清利湿热，通淋止痛。取膀胱俞、中极、阴陵泉、行间、委阳、然谷。

Stranguria Caused by the Passage of Urinary Stone A type of stranguria, originally from *Zhubing Yuanhou Lun*: *Linbing Zhuhou* (*General Treatise on the Etiology and Symptomatology of Diseases*: *Causes and Symptoms of Stranguria*), also named sand stranguria and sand-stone stranguria, mostly due to the downward flow of damp-heat which decocts the urine to form urolithiasis. 〈Manifestations〉 distending and pricking pain in the lower abdomen and penis, dysuria due to the calculi and unblocked by changing posture, severe pain in the loin and abdomen, whitish or yellowish and greasy tongue coating, wiry and rapid pulse. 〈Treatment principle〉 Dispel damp-heat and treat stranguria to stop pain. 〈Point slection〉 Pangguangshu (BL 28). Zhongji (RN 3), Yinlingquan (SP 9), Xingjian (LR 2), Weiyang (BL 39) and Rangu (KI 2).

●石龙芮[shí lóng ruì] 中药名。即毛茛科多年生草本植物毛茛的鲜叶，可用其进行贴敷泡灸，参见"毛茛灸"条。

Shi Long Rui (*Ranunculus Scrleratus*) A Chinese herb, namely, the fresh leaves of the Ranunculaceae perennial herbage *Mao Gen* (*Ranunculus Japonucus*), vesculating moxibustion by applying it to the skin. →毛茛灸 (p. 264)

●石门[shí mén] 经穴名。出《针灸甲乙经》。属任脉，为三焦之募穴。又名利机、精露、丹田、命门。〈定位〉在下腹部，前正中线上，当脐中下2寸(图40)。〈层次解剖〉皮肤→皮下组织→腹白线→腹横筋膜→腹壁外脂肪→壁腹膜。浅层主要布有第十一胸神经前支的前皮支和腹壁浅静脉的属支。深层主要有第十一胸神经前支的分支。〈主治〉腹胀、泄利、绕脐疼痛、奔豚、疝气、水肿、小便不利、遗精、阳萎、经闭、带下、崩漏、产后恶露不止。直刺0.5~1寸；可灸。

Shimen (RN 5) A point on the Ren Meridian, from *Zhenjiu Jia-Yi Jing* (*A-B Classic of Acupuncture and Moxibustion*), the Front-Mu point of the Sanjiao Meridian, also named Liji, Jinglu, Dantian or Mingmen. 〈Location〉 on the lower abdomen, on the anterior midline, 2 cun below the center of the umbilicus (Fig. 40). 〈Regional anatomy〉 skin→subcutaneous tissue → linea alba → transverse fascia → extraperitoneal fat tissue→parietal peritoneurm. In the superficial layer, there are the anterior cutaneous branches of the anterior branches of the 11th thoracic nerve and the tributaries of the superficial epigastric vein. In the deep layer, there are the branches of the anterior branches of the 11th thoracic nerve. 〈Indications〉 abdominal distension, diarrhea, pain near the umbilicus, sensation of gas rushing, hernia, dysuria, nocturnal emission, impotence, amenorrhea, morbid leukorrhagia, methrorrhagia and methrostaxis, postpartum persistent lochia. 〈Method〉 Puncture perpendicularly 0.5~1 cun. Moxibsution is applicable.

●石阙[shí què] 经穴别名。出《备急千金方》。即石关。详见该条。

Shique Another name for Shiguan (KI 18), a

meridian point from *Beiji Qianjin Fang* (*Essential Prescriptions for Emergencies Worth a Thousand Gold*). →石关(p. 384)

●石藏用[shí zàng yòng] 人名。宋代针灸家,字用之,为京师名医。其治疗方术一从古法,常与人灸膏肓穴治病。事见庄绰《灸膏肓穴法》。曾与丁德用合绘经穴图。

Shi Zangyong An expert of acupuncture and moxibustion in th Song Dynasty, also named Yongzhi, a famous physician in the capital. His treatment techniques were based on ancient methods, usually handling diseases with moxibustion on Gaohuang (BL 43), recorded in *Jiu Gaohuangxue Fa* (*Methods of Moxibustion for Gaohuang Point*), written by Zhuang Zhuo. He worked together with Ding Deyong to draw pictures of meridian points.

●石针[shí zhēn] 古针具名。出《礼记内则》。即砭石。参见"砭石"条。

Stone Needle A needling instrument in ancient times, from *Liji Neize* (*The Internal Norms in the Book of Rites*), synonymous with sharp stone. →砭石(p. 22)

●时行顿咳[shí xíng dùn ké] 顿咳的别名。详见该条。

Epidemic Whooping Cough Another name for paroxymal cough. →顿咳(p. 90)

●实按灸[shí àn jiǔ] 灸法名。艾条灸之一种。将艾条(通常用药艾条)点燃一端,隔布或棉纸数层,紧按穴位上施灸。使热气透入皮肉,待火灭热减后,再重新点燃按灸,每穴可按灸几次至几十次。常用于风湿痹症。古代的太乙神针、雷火针灸法属此范畴。

Pressing Moxibsution A kind of moxibustion with moxa-stick. 〈Method〉Light one end of the moxa-stick (usually a medicinal moxastick), press it on the seleted acupoint, separated by cloth or several layers of cotton paper, causing the heat-qi to enter the skin and muscles, relight it and press it again on the point after the fire is out. This method can be applied to each point for several times to treat arthralgia-syndrome due to wind-dampness. The methods of moxibustion with great monad herbal moxastick and moxibustion with thunder-fire herbal moxastick were of this category in ancient times.

●实热牙痛[shí rè yá tòng] 牙痛证型之一。因大肠、胃腑有热,郁久化火,火循经上炎所致。证见牙痛甚剧,兼有口臭、口渴、便秘、舌苔黄、脉弦。治宜清热止痛。取合谷、下关、颊车、内庭、劳宫。

Toothache due to Excess-Heat A type of toothache, due to heat in the large intestine and stomach leading to stagnated fire moving upward along the meridians. 〈Manifestations〉severe toothache, foul breath, thirst, constipation, yellowish tongue coating, wiry pulse. 〈Treatment principle〉Clear heat to stop pain. 〈Point selection〉Hegu (LI 4), Xiaguan (ST 7), Jiache (ST 6), Neiting (ST 44) and Laogong (PC 8).

●实热咽喉肿痛[shí rè yān hóu zhǒng tòng] 咽喉肿痛证型之一。因过食辛辣,引动胃火上蒸,津液受灼,煎炼成痰,痰火蕴结所致。证见咽喉肿痛,高热,口渴引饮,头痛,口臭,痰稠黄,大便结,小便黄,苔黄厚,脉洪数。治宜清胃热,利咽喉。取二间、内庭、天突、丰隆。

Swelling and Pain of the Throat due to Excessive Heat A type of swelling and pain of throat, due to an excessively pungent diet which leads to the upward stomach-fire burning the body fluid to form phlegm, which accumulates to cause fire. 〈Manifestations〉sore throat, high fever, thirst, dark urine, yellowish and greasy tongue coating, surging and rapid pulse. 〈Treatment principle〉Clear stomach heat and relieve sore throat. 〈Point selection〉Erjian (LI 2), Neiting (ST 44), Tiantu (RN 22) and Fenglong (ST 40).

●食道[shí dào] 耳穴名。位于耳轮脚下方中三分之一。具有疏利食道作用。〈主治〉食道炎、食道痉挛、癔球。

Esophagus (MA-IC 6) An ear point. 〈Location〉in the middle 1/3 of the inferior aspect of the helix crus. 〈Function〉Regulate the esophagus. 〈Indications〉esophagitis, spasm of esophagus, globus hystericus.

●食窦[shí dòu] ①经穴名。出《针灸甲乙经》。属足太阴脾经,又名命关。〈定位〉在胸外侧部,当第五肋间隙,距前正中线6寸(图85和图23)。〈层次解剖〉皮肤→皮下组织→前锯肌→肋间外肌。浅层布有第五肋间神经外侧皮支和胸腹壁静脉。深层有胸长神经的分支,第五肋间神经和第五肋间后动、静脉。〈主

治〉胸胁胀痛、腹胀肠鸣、翻胃、食已即止、嗳气、水肿。斜刺0.3~0.5寸，或向外平刺0.5~0.8寸。不可深刺。可灸。

Shidou（SP 17） A point on the Spleen Meridian of Foot-Taiyin, originally from *Zhenjiu Jia-Yi Jing*（*A-B Classic of Acupuncture and Moxibustion*）, also named Mingguan. 〈Location〉on the lateral side of the chest and in the 5th intercostal space, 6 cun lateral to the anterior midline(Figs. 85 & 23). 〈Regional anatomy〉skin→subcutaneous tissue→anterior serratus muscle→external intercostal muscle. In the superficial layer, there are the lateral cutaneous branches of the 5th intercostal nerve and the thoracoepigastric vein. In the deep layer, there are the branches of the long thoracic nerve, the 5th intercostal nerve and the 5th posterior intercostal artery and vein. 〈Indications〉distending pain of the chest and hypochondrium, abdominal distension, borborygmus, vomiting relieved by food, eructation and edema. 〈Method〉Puncture obliquely 0.3~0.5 cun or subcutaneously or 0.5~0.8 cun towads the lateral aspect. Deep needling is forbidden. Moxibustion is applicable.

●食宫[shí gōng] 经穴别名。出《针灸甲乙经》。即阴都。详见该条。

Shigong Another name for Yindu(KI 19), a meridian point originally from *Zhenjiu Jia-Yi Jing*（*A-B Classic of Acupuncture and Moxibustion*）. →阴都(p.554)

●食关[shí guān] 经外穴名。见《医经小学》。在上腹部，当建里旁开1.5寸。〈主治〉噎膈反胃，以及胃炎、肠炎、消化不良等。直刺1~1.5寸；可灸。

Shiguan（EX-CA） An extra point from *Yijing Xiaoxue*（*Elementary Collections of Medical Classics*）. 〈Location〉on the upper abdomen, 0.5 cun lateral to Jianli(RN 11). 〈Indications〉dysphagia, vomiting, gastritis, enteritis, dyspepsia, etc. 〈Method〉Puncture perpendicularly 1~1.5 cun. Moxibustion is applicable.

●食积胃痛[shí jī wèi tòng] 胃痛证型之一。多因暴饮暴食，饮食停滞，胃中气机阻塞所致。证见胃痛，脘腹胀满，嗳腐吞酸，或吐不消化食物，一般在吐食或矢气后痛减，舌苔厚腻，脉滑。治宜消食导滞止痛。取中脘、足三里、内关、梁门、天枢、阴陵泉。

Stomachache due to the Retention of Food A type of gastric pain, due to crapulence and the retention of food, which lead to the blockage of the functional activity of the stomach-qi. 〈Manifestations〉gastric pain which may be relieved by vomiting and wind from bowel, epigastric distension, eructation with fetid odor, acid regurgitation, vomiting with undigested food, thick and greasy tongue coating, slippery pulse. 〈Treatment principle〉Promote digestion and remove stagnancy to stop pain. 〈Point selection〉Zhongwan（RN 12）, Zusanli（ST 36）, Neiguan（PC 6）, Liangmen（ST 21）, Tianshu（ST 25）and Yinglingquan（SP 9）.

●食盐灸[shí yán jiǔ] 敷灸方法之一。取食盐适量，研细炒热，待稍温时纳入脐中（神阙），使与脐平。再将麦麸适量加醋炒热，装入布袋中，置于盐上敷灸。

Moxibustion with Salt A method of applying moxibustion. 〈Method〉Take a suitable amount of salt to grind into a fine powder, heat it and put it into the umbilicus(Shenque RN 8), Level with the abdomen, then heat a suitable amount of wheat barn with vinegar, put it into a bag and place the bag on the salt to apply moxibustion.

●食指[shí zhǐ] 部位名。即次指，古称大指次指。

Index Finger A part of the body, i.e. the 2nd finger, whose archaic name is the finger next to the thumb.

●食滞腹痛[shí zhì fù tòng] 腹痛证型之一。多因宿食停滞肠胃，气机阻滞所致。证见脘腹疼痛拒按，痛则欲泻，泻后痛减，恶食，时时嗳腐吞酸，苔腻，脉滑。治宜化食导滞。取中脘、梁门、天枢、曲池。

Abdominal Pain due to the Retention of Food A type of abdominal pain, mostly caused by the retention of food in the intestines and stomach which lead to the disorder of qi. 〈Manifestations〉epigastric and abdominal pain followed by diarrhea, and relieved after diarrhea, tenderness, poor appetite, eructation with fetid odor, acid regurgitation, greasy tongue coating, slippery pulse. 〈Treatment principle〉Promote digestion and remove the stagnancy of food. 〈Point selection〉Zhongwan（RN 12）, Liangmen（ST 21）, Tianshu（ST

25) and Quchi(LI 11).

●始光[shǐ guāng] 经穴别名。出《针灸甲乙经》。即攒竹。详见该条。

Shiguang Another name for Cuanzhu (BL 2), a meridian point from *Zhenjiu Jia-Yi Jing (A-B Classic of Acupuncture and Moxibustion)*. →攒竹(p. 58)

●始素[shǐ sù] 经外穴名。出《外台秘要》。在侧胸部,当腋窝中线上,渊液穴直上约1寸陷中。〈主治〉胸下支满、腰痛引腹、筋挛、阴气上缩等。斜刺0.3~0.5寸。

Shisu(EX-CA) An extra point, from *Waitai Miyao (Clandestine Essentials from the Imperial Library)*. 〈Location〉on the lateral side of the chest, on the middle axillary line, in the depression about 1 cun above Yuangye (GB 22). 〈Indications〉fullness in the chest and hypochondrium, lumbago radiating to the abdomen, spasm of muscles upward contraction of external genitals. 〈Method〉Puncture obliquely 0.1~0.5 cun.

●视赤如白[shì chì rú bái] 色盲的别名。详见该条。

Seeing Red as if Seeing White Another name for color blindness. →色盲(p. 347)

●视区[shì qū] 头针刺激区。在前后正中线的后点旁开1厘米处的枕外粗隆水平线上,向上引平行于前后正中线的4厘米长直线。〈主治〉皮层性视力障碍。

The Optic Area One stimulated area of scalp acupuncture.〈Location〉Draw a 4-cm straight line upwards, parallel to the anterior-posterior midline, 1 cm evenly beside the external occipital protuberance.〈Indication〉cerebro-cortical visual disturbance.

●视物易色[shì wù yì sè] 即色盲的别名。详见该条。

Monochromatism Another name for color blindness. →色盲(p. 347)

●势头[shì tóu] 阴茎穴的别名。详见该条。

Shitou Another name for Yingjing (EX-CA). →阴茎穴(p. 556)

●是动病[shì dòng bìng] 经络病候用语。出《灵枢·经脉》。即指是动则病。参见"是动、所生病"条。

Meridian Diseases A term for the pathological manifestations of the meridians, from *Lingshu : Jingmai (Miraculous Pivot : Meridians)*. →是动、所生病(p. 388)

●是动、所生病[shì dòng suǒ shēng bìng] 经络病候用语。出《灵枢·经脉》。是动,是指经脉有异常变动时出现的有关病证;所生病,是指此经穴位能主治某方面所发生的病证。

Meridian Diseases and Primary Diseases of Zang and Fu Organs A term for the pathological manifestations of the meridians, from *Ling Shu : Jingmai (Miraculous Pivot : Meridians)*. "Meridian diseases" refer to the diseases caused by the abnormal changes of the meridians while the "primary diseases of Zang and Fu organs" refer to the indications of the meridian points.

●释僧匡[shì sēng kuāng] 人名。隋以前针灸家(宋时为避帝讳,改称僧康)。撰《释僧匡针灸经》。见《隋书·经籍志》,书佚。在《医心方》中有引述。

Shi Sengkuang An acupuncture-moxibustion expert before the Sui Dynasty, (his name was once changed to Shi Sengkang to avoid breaking the Emperor's taboo). His work *Shi Sengkuang Zhenjiu Jing (Shi Sengkuang's Classic of Acupuncture and Moxibustion)* was recorded in *Suishu : Jing Ji Zhi (The History of the Sui Dynasty : Records of Classics and Books)*. The book is no longer extant. Some contents of the book were quoted in *Yi Xin Fang (The Heart of Medical Prescriptions)*.

●释僧匡针灸经[shì sēng kuàng zhēn jiǔ jīng] 书名。释僧匡撰。见"释僧匡"条。

Shi Sengkuang Zhenjiu Jing (Shi Sengkuang's Classic of Acupuncture and Moxibustion) A book, written by Shi Sengkuang. →释僧匡(p. 388)

●释湛池[shì zhàn chí] 人名。明代针灸家,号还无,济宁(今属山东)人。针治疮疡,取效神速。见《济宁府志》。

Shi Zhanchi An acupuncture and moxibustion expert in the Ming Dynasty, who assumed the name of Huanwu, a native of Jining (now in Shandong province). He treated skin and external diseases with acupuncture, and achieved miraculous therapeutic effects. Cf. *Jiningfu Zhi (Annals of Jinjngfu)*.

●手叉发[shǒu chà fā] 即虎口疔。详见该条。

Carbuncle of Hand →虎口疔(p. 168)

●手大指甲后[shǒu dà zhǐ jiǎ hòu] 经外穴名。见《针灸集成》。在手拇指尺侧缘，指关节横纹头赤白肉际处。〈主治〉小儿肠胃病、结膜炎、角膜白翳、雀目等。直刺0.1～0.2寸，或点刺出血；可灸。

Shoudazhijiahou(EX-UE)　An extra point, from *Zhenjiu Jicheng* (*A Collection of Acupuncture and Moxibustion*). 〈Location〉on the ulnar side of the thumb, at the end of the transeverse crease of the digital joints and the junction of the red and white skin. 〈Indications〉diseases of intestines and stomach in children, conjunctivitis, pancorneal opacity, night blindness. 〈Method〉Puncture perpendicularly 0.1～0.2 cun, or prick the point to cause bleeding. Moxibustion is applicable.

●手夫[shǒu fū] 一夫法的别名。详见该条。

Hand Measurement →一夫法(p.550)

●手踝[shǒu huái] 经外穴名。见《针灸孔穴及其疗法便览》。在手腕背侧，桡骨结节之高点处。〈主治〉十指痉挛，上、下齿痛等。用灸法。

Shouhuai(EX-UE)　An extra point, from *Zhenjiu Kongxue Ji Qi Liaofa Bianlan*(*Guide to Acupoints and Acupuncture Therapeutics*). 〈Location〉on the dorsal side of the wrist, at the high point of the styloid process of radius. 〈Indications〉finger spasm, toothache. 〈Method〉moxibustion.

●手厥阴标本[shǒu jué yīn biāo běn] 十二经标本之一。出《灵枢·卫气》。手厥阴之本，在腕上两筋之间二寸中，约当内关穴处；标在腋下三寸天池穴处。参见"十二经标本"条。

The Superficiality and Origin of Hand-Jueyin

One of th superficialities and the origins of the Twelve Meridians, originally from *Lingshu: Wei Qi* (*Miraculous Pivot: Defensive Qi*), the origin of Hand-Jueyin is 2 cun above the wrist, between the tendons of m. palmaris longus and m. flexon madialis, just at Neiguan (PC 6); the superficiality is 3 cun at Tianchi (PC 1), below the axilla. →十二经标本(p.375)

●手厥阴经别[shǒu jué yīn jīng bié] 十二经别之一，原称心主之正。出《灵枢·经别》。在渊腋下三寸处，从手厥阴心包经分出，进入胸腔内，分别归属上、中、下三焦，上达喉咙，浅出于耳后方的完骨部，与手少阳三焦经会合。

The Divergent Meridian of Hand-Jueyin
One of the divergent meridians of the Twelve Meridians, originally named the divergent meridian of the Pericardium from *Lingshu: Jingbie* (*Miraculous Pivot: Divergent Meridians*), deriving from the Pericardium Meridian of Hand-Jueyin, 3 cun below Yuanye (GB 62), pertaining respectively to the upper, middle and lower jiao after entering the thoracic cavity, superiorly reaching the throat, shallowly emerging from Wangu (GB 12) posterior to the ear, and joining the Sanjiao Meridian of Hand-Shaoyang.

●手厥阴经筋[shǒu jué yīn jīng jīn] 十二经脉筋之一。出《灵枢·经筋》。起于中指，与手太阴经筋并行，结于肘内侧，经上臂内侧，结于腋下，向下分散前后，挟脐旁。分支进入腋下，散布胸中，结于膈部。

The Muscles Region of Hand-Jueyin　One of the muscle regions along the Twelve Regular Meridians, from *Lingshu: Jingjin* (*Miraculous Pivot: Muscle Regions Along Meridians*), which starts from the middle finger, moves parallel to the muscle region of Hand-Taiyin, concentrates on the medial side of the elbow, goes along the medial side of the arm, gathers below the axilla, goes downwards to the anterior and posterior part, and along both sides of the umbilicus. Its branches enter the axilla, distribute in the thoracic cavity and join at the diaphragm.

●手厥阴经筋病[shǒu jué yīn jīng jīn bìng] 十二经筋病候之一。出《灵枢·经筋》。手厥阴经筋发病，可见本经筋循行、结聚的部位支撑不适、掣引、转筋、以及胸痛或成息贲病。

Diseases of the Muscle Region of Hand-Jueyin　One of the pathological manifestations of the Twelve Muscle Regions, from *Lingshu: Jingjin* (*Miraculous Pivot: Muscle Regions Along Meridians*). The manifestations of the diseases of the muscle region along the meridian of Hand-Jueyin are disturbance in sustaining the connecting region, contracture, spasm along the course of the meridian and at the site where the muscle concentrates, chest pain or pulmonary mass.

●手厥阴络脉[shǒu jué yīn luò mài] 十五络脉之一，原称手心主之别。出《灵枢·经脉》。其络脉名曰内

关。脉从腕上二寸内关穴分出，出于两筋之间，分支走向手少阳经脉，并沿经向上连系于心包，散络于心系。

The Collateral of the Hand-Jueyin One of the Fifteen Main Collaterals, originally named the branch of Hand-Pericardium, from *Lingshu*: *Jingmai* (*Miraculous Pivot*: *Meridians*), the name of the collateral is Neiguan (PC 6). It derives from Neiguan (PC 6), which is 2 cun above the wrist, goes between the tendons of m. palmaris longus and m. flexon radialis. Its branches join the Meridian of Hand-Shaoyang, go upward along the meridian to connect the pericardium and distribute in the "heart system".

●**手厥阴络脉病** [shǒu jué yīn luò mài bìng] 十五络脉病候之一。出《灵枢·经脉》。实证见心痛；虚证见心中烦乱。可取手厥阴络穴治疗。

Diseases of the Collateral of Hand-Jueyin One of the pathological manifestations of the Fifteen Main Collaterals, from *Lingshu*; *Jingmai* (*Miraculous Pivot*: *Meridians*). 〈Manifestations〉 cardial pain in cases of excess type, dysphoria in cases of deficiency. They can be treated by puncturing the Luo (Connecting) point of Hand-Jueyin.

●**手厥阴心包经** [shǒu jué yīn xīn bāo jīng] 十二经脉之一。原称心主手厥阴心包络之脉。出《灵枢·经脉》。其循行从胸中开始，出而属于心包，通过横膈，经历胸部、上腹和下腹，络于三焦。它外行的主干，沿胸内出胁部，当腋下三寸处向上到腋下，沿上臂内侧行于手太阴经和手少阴经之间，进入肘中，下向前臂，走两筋之间，进入掌中，沿中指桡侧出于末端。它的支脉，从掌中分出，沿无名指出于末端，接手少阳三焦经。

The Pericardium Meridian of Hand-Jueyin One of the Twelve Regular Meridians, originally named the Hand-Jueyin Meridian of Pericardium, from *Lingshu*: *Jingmai* (*Miraculous Pivot*: *Meridians*). 〈The course of the meridian〉 It originates from the chest. Out of the chest, it enters and pertains to the pericardium, then descends through the diaphragm, the chest, the upper and the lower abdomen to connect successively with Sanjiao. The main external stream of the meridian runs inside the chest, emerges from the costal region, and ascends to the axilla from the point 3 cun below it. Along the medial aspect of the upper arm, it runs between the Lung Meridian of Hand-Taiyin and the Heart Meridian of Hand-Shaoyin, to the cubital fossa, and then downwards to the forearm between the tendons of m. palmarus longus and m. flexon canpi radialu, and enters the palm. From there, it runs right to its tip along the radical side of the middle finger. Its branch derives from the palm and runs to its tip along the ring finger, and links with the Sanjiao Meridian of Hand-Shaoyang.

●**手厥阴心包经病** [shǒu jué yīn xīn bāo jīng bìng] 十二经脉病候之一。出《灵枢·经脉》。〈本经主要病候〉掌心发热，臂肘挛急，腋肿，胸胁满闷，心悸，面赤目黄，喜笑不休，或心烦，心痛等症。

Diseases of the Pericardium Meridian of Hand-Jueyin One of the pathological manifestations of the Twelve Meridians, from *Lingshu*: *Jingmai* (*Miraculous Pivot*: *Meridians*). 〈Main pathological manifestations〉 feverish sensation in the centre of the palm, contracture of the elbow and arm, swelling of the axilla, suffocating sensation in the chest and hypochonrium, palpitation, red face and yellow eyes, manic-depressive disorders, dysphoria, cardialgia, etc..

●**手逆注** [shǒu nì zhù] 经外穴名。见《千金要方》。在前臂屈侧，腕横纹上6寸，当掌长肌与桡侧腕屈肌之间。〈主治〉癔病、前臂疼痛、痉挛、麻痹等。直刺0.5～1寸；可灸。

Shounizhu (EX-UE) An extra point, from *Qianjin Yaofang* (*Essential Prescriptions Worth a Thousand Gold*). 〈Location〉 on the flexion side of the forearm, 6 cun above the transeverse crease of the wrist, between the m. palmaris longus and m. flexor radialis. 〈Indications〉 hysteria, pain of the forearm, spasm, numbness and arthralgia, etc. 〈Method〉 Puncture perpendicularly 0.5～1.0 cm. Moxibustion is applicable.

●**手三里** [shǒu sān lǐ] 经穴名。出《针灸甲乙经》。属手阳明大肠经，又名上三里、鬼邪、三里。〈定位〉在前臂背面桡侧，当阳溪与曲池连线上，肘横纹下2寸（图48和图6）。〈层次解剖〉皮肤→皮下组织→桡侧腕

长伸肌→桡侧腕短伸肌→指伸肌的前方→旋后肌。浅层布有前臂外侧皮神经,前臂后皮神经等。深层有桡侧返动、静脉的分支或属支以及桡神经深支。〈主治〉腹胀、吐泻、齿痛、失音、颊肿、瘰疬、偏瘫、手臂麻痛、肘挛不伸、眼目诸疾。直刺0.5～0.8寸;可灸。

Shousanli (LI 10) A meridian point, from *Zhenjiu Jia-Yi Jing* (*A-B Classic of Acupuncture and Moxibustion*), a point on the Large Intestine Meridian of Hand-Yangming, also named Shangsanli, Guixie and Sanli. 〈Location〉on the radial side of the dorsal surface of the forearm and on the line connecting Yangxi (LI 5) and Quchi (LI 11), 2 cun below the cubital crease (Figs. 48 &.6). 〈Regional anatomy〉skin → subcutaneous tissue → long radial extensor muscle of wrist→short radial extensor muscle of wrist → front part of extensor muscle of fingers → supinator muscle. In the superficial layer, there are the lateral and posterior cutaneous nerves of the forearm. In the deep layer, there are the branches or tributaries of the radial recurrent artery and vein and the deep branches of the radial nerve. 〈Indications〉abdominal distension, vomiting and diarrhea, toothache, aphasia, swelling of the cheek, scrofula, paralysis, numbness and pain of the hand and arm, contracture of the elbow and optic diseases. 〈Method〉Puncture perpendicularly 0.5～0.8 cun. Moxibustion is applicable.

●**手三阳经**[shǒu sān yáng jīng] 经络名。出《灵枢·逆顺肥瘦》。手阳明大肠经、手太阳小肠经、手少阳三焦经的总称。手三阳经从手走头,分布在上肢外侧。详见各条。

The Three Yang Meridians of Hand Meridians originally from *Lingshu*: *Nishun Feishou* (*Miraculous Pivot*: *Circulatory Direction of Meridians and Body Constitution*), a general term for the Large Intestine Meridian of Hand-Yangming, the Small Intestine Meridian of Hand-Taiyang and the Sanjiao Meridian of Hand-Shaoyang. They run from hand to head, distributing in the lateral part of the upper extremities. →**手阳明大肠经**(p. 401)、**手太阳小肠经**(p. 398)、**手少阳三焦经**(p. 393).

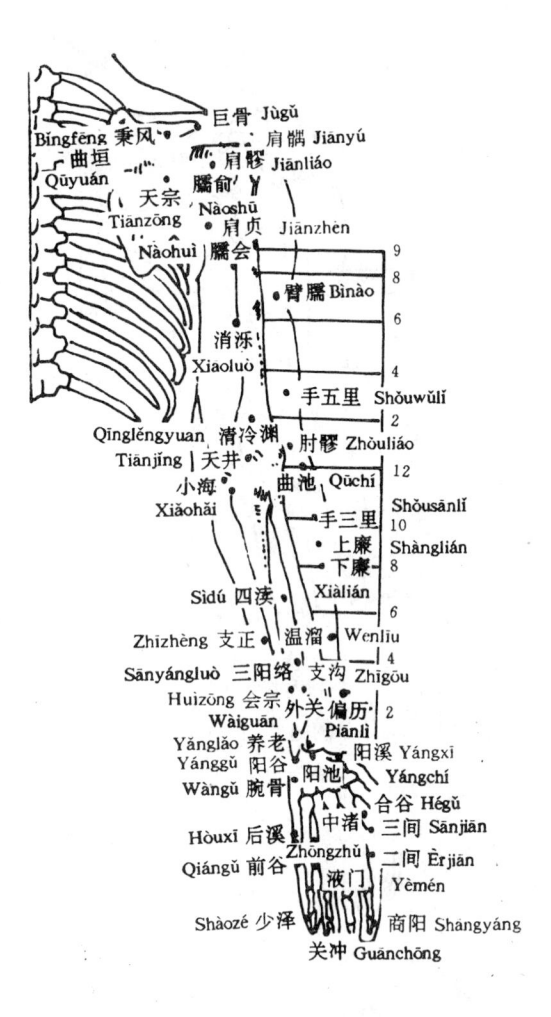

●**手三阴经**[shǒu sān yīn jīng] 经络名。出《灵枢·逆顺肥瘦》。手太阴肺经、手少阴心经、手厥阴心包经的总称。手三阴经从胸走手,分布在上肢内侧。详见各条。

Fig. 48 Points of the three yang meridians of hand

The Three Yin Meridians of Hand Meridians originally from *Lingshu*: *Nishun Feishou* (*Miraculous Pivot*: *Circulatory Direction of Meridians and Body Constitution*), a general term for the Lung Meridian of Hand-Taiyin, the Heart Meridian of Hand-Shaoyin and the Pericardium Meridian of Hand-Jueyin. They run from chest to hand, distributing in the medial part of the upper extremities. →**手太阴肺经**(p. 398)、**手少阴心经**(p. 395)、**手厥阴心包经**(p. 390).

●**手上廉**[shǒu shàng lián] 经穴别名。出《圣济总录》。即上廉。详见该条。

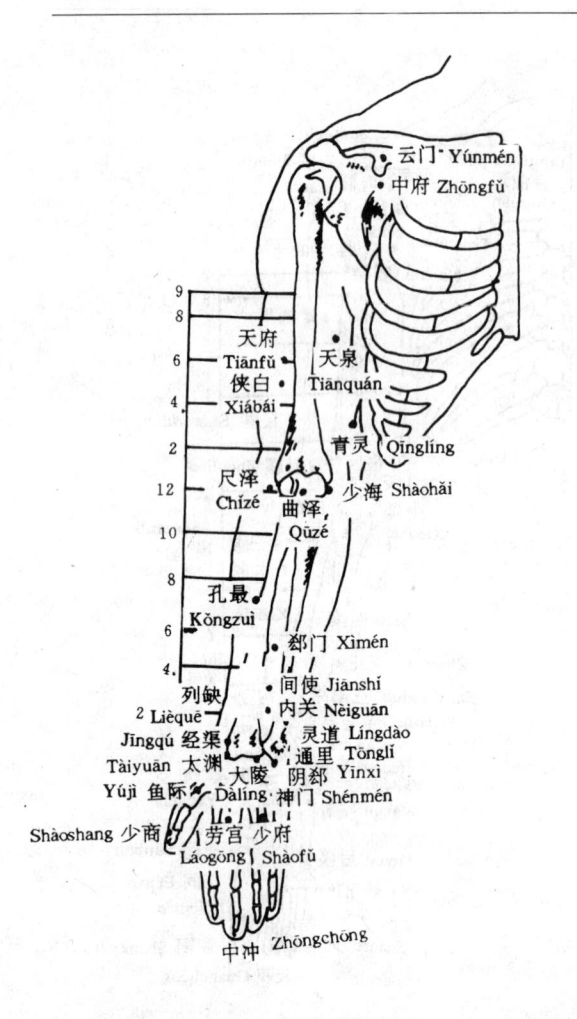

Fig. 49 Points of the three yin meridians of hand

Shoushanglian Another name for Shanglian (LI 9), a meridian point originally from *Shengji Zonglu* (*Imperial Medical Encyclopaedia*). →上廉(p. 352)

●**手少阳标本**[shǒu shào yáng biāo běn] 十二经标本之一。出《灵枢·卫气》。手少阳之本,在小指、次指之间上二寸,约当中渚穴处;标,在耳后上角目下外眦,约当丝竹空穴处。

The Superficiality and Origin of Hand-Shaoyang One of the superficialities and origins of the Twelve Meridians, originally from *Lingshu*: *Weiqi* (*Miraculous Pivot*: *Defensive Qi*), the origin of Hand-Shaoyang is 2 cun above the joint of the small and ring fingers, roughly at the point Zhongzhu(SJ 3), and its superficiality is from the region posterior and superior to the ear to the outer canthus, roughly at Sizhukong(SJ 23).

●**手少阳经别**[shǒu shào yáng jīng bié] 十二经别之一。原名手少阳之正。出《灵枢·经别》。手少阳经别,在头部从本经分出,向下进入缺盆,经过上、中、下三焦,散于胸中。

The Divergent Meridian of Hand-Shaoyang One of the Twelve Divergent Meridians, originally from *Lingshu*:*Jingbie*(*Miraculous Pivot*: *Divergent Meridians*), deriving from its own meridian on the hand, running downwards into the supraclavicular fossa and through the upper, middle and lower jiao, and distributing in the thoracic cavity.

●**手少阳经筋**[shǒu shào yáng jīng jīn] 十二经筋之一。出《灵枢·经筋》。手少阳经筋,起始于第四手指端,结于腕背,走向前臂外侧,结于肘尖部,向上绕行于上臂外侧,上循肩部,走到颈部会合于手太阳经筋。其分支当下颔角部进入,联系于舌根,一支上颔处,沿耳前属目外眦,上达颞部,结于额角。

The Muscle Region of Hand-Shaoyang One of the Twelve Muscle Regions, originally from *Lingshu*: *Jingjin* (*Miraculous Pivot*: *Muscles Regions along Meridians*). Starting from the tip of the ring finger, and concentrating on the dorsal aspect of the wrist, it moves upward along the lateral edge of the forearm, concentrating on the tip of the elbow, reaching the neck after running around the lateral edge of the arm to the shoulder and connecting with the muscle of Hand-Taiyang. One branch reaches the root of the tongue from the angle of the lower jaw and concentrates there. Another branch runs upwards to the lower jaw, reaches the temporal region after running along the outer canthus in front of the ear, and concentrates on the corner of the forehead.

●**手少阳经筋病**[shǒu shào yáng jīng jīn bìng] 十二经筋病候之一。出《灵枢·经筋》。其病可见本经筋循行部位支撑不适,转筋掣引,以及舌卷。

Diseases of the Muscles Region of Hand-Shaoyang One of the pathological manifestations of the Twelve Muscle Regions along Meridians originally from *Lingshu*: *Jingjin* (*Miraculous Pivot*: *Muscle Regions along Meridians*). 〈Manifestations〉 disorder in sus-

taining the circulating parts of the meridian of the regions along the course of the muscles leading to spasm and contracture and curled-up tongue.

●手少阳络脉[shǒu shào yáng luò mài] 十五络脉之一，原名手少阳之别。出《灵枢·经脉》。手少阳络脉名曰外关，其脉从腕关节后二寸处外关穴分出，绕行于臂膊的外侧，进入胸中，会合于心包。

The Collateral of Hand-Shaoyang One of the Fifteen Main Collaterals, originally named the Branch of Hand-Shaoyang, originally from *Lingshu*: *Jingmai* (*Miraculous Pivot*: *Meridians*). The name of the Collateral of Hand-Shaoyang is Waiguan (SJ 5), deriving from this point 2 cun above the transverse crease of the dorsum of the wrist, entering the thoracic cavity after running upwards along the lateral edge of the upper extremities and connecting with pericardium.

●手少阳络脉病[shǒu shào yáng luò mài bìng] 十五络脉病候之一。出《灵枢·经脉》。实证见肘关节拘挛；虚证见肘关节不能收屈运动。可取手少阳络穴治疗。

Diseases of the Collateral of Hand-Shaoyang One of the pathological manifestations of the Fifteen Main Collaterals, originally from *Lingshu*: *Jingmai* (*Miraculous Pivot*: *Meridians*). ⟨Manifestations⟩ contracture of the elbow joint in cases of excess, dyskinesia of the joint in cases of deficiency. Select the Luo (Connecting) point of Hand-Shaoyang to treat such diseases.

●手少阳三焦经[shǒu shào yáng sān jiāo jīng] 十二经脉之一。原名三焦手少阳之脉。出《灵枢·经脉》。其循行起于无名指末端，上行小指与无名指之间，沿着手背，出于前臂外侧尺、桡骨之间，向上通过肘尖，沿上臂外侧，向上通过肩部，交出足少阳经的后面，进入缺盆，分布于膻中，散络于心包，通过膈肌，广泛遍于上、中、下三焦。它的支脉，从膻中上行，出缺盆，上向颈旁，连系耳后，直上出耳上方，弯下向面颊，至眼下部。另一支脉，从耳后进入耳中，出走耳前，经过上关前，交面颊，到外眼角，接足少阳胆经。

The Sanjiao Meridian of Hand-Shaoyang One of the Twelve Regular Meridians, originally named the Hand-Shaoyang Meridian of Sanjiao, originally from *Lingshu*: *Jingmai* (*Miraculous Pivot*: *Meridians*). ⟨The course of the meridian⟩ Originating from the tip of the ring finger, it runs upwards between the 4th and 5th metacapal bones, along the dorsal aspect of the wrist to the lateral aspect of the forearm between the radius and ulna, entering the superaclavicular fossa after ascending through the olecranon along the lateral aspect of the upper arm, past the shoulder region where it goes across and passes behind the Gall Bladder Meridian of Foot-shaoyang, and spreading in the chest Danzhong (RN 17) region to connect with the pericardium. Then, it decends through the diaphragm to distribute extensively in the upper, middle and lower Jiao. One branch originates from chest Danzhong (RN 17), ascending out of the supraclavicular fossa to the neck, running along the posterior border of the ear straight to and out of the region superior to the ear, bending downward to the cheek and terminating in the infraorbital region. Another branch enters the ear from the retroauricular region, running out of it, along the anterior aspect of the ear in front of Shangguan (GB 3), linking with the cheek, and reaching the outer canthus to connect with the Gallbladder Meridians of Foot-Shaoyang.

●手少阳三焦经病[shǒu shào yáng sān jiāo jīng bìng] 十二经脉病候之一。出《灵枢·经脉》。⟨本经主要病候⟩耳聋，耳鸣，咽部肿，喉痹，目外眦痛，颊痛，自汗，耳后及肩部，上臂，肘弯，前臂外侧均可疼痛，无名指活动不利，小腹硬满，气胀，小便不利，遗尿。

Diseases of the Sanjiao Meridian of Hand-Shaoyang One of the pathological manifestations of the Twelve Meridians, originally from *Lingshu*: *Jingmai* (*Miraculous Pivot*: *Meridians*). ⟨Main manifestations⟩ deafness, tinnitus, swelling of the throat, sore throat, pain of the outer canthus, pain of the cheek, spontaneous perspiration, pain of the region posterior to the ear, shoulder, arm, elbow, the lateral aspect of the forearm, dyscinesia of the ring finger, fullness and rigidity of the lower abdomen, flatulence, dysuria, enuresis.

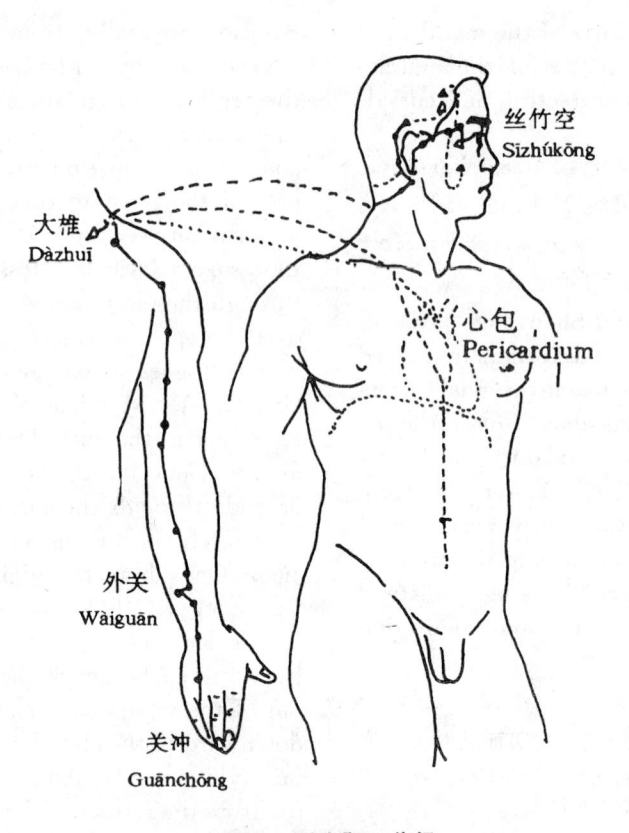

图50 手少阳三焦经
Fig. 50 Sanjiao Meridian of Hand-Shaoyang

●**手少阳、手厥阴经别**[shǒu shào yáng shǒu jué yīn jīng bié] 十二经别中的一合。出《灵枢·经别》。手少阳经别经过离、入、出的循行后，最后合于本经。手厥阴经别经过离、入、出的循行后，合于与其相表里的手少阳经。见"手少阳经别"、"手厥阴经别"条。

The Divergent Meridians of Hand-Shaoyang and Hand-Jueyin One of the confluences of the Twelve Divergent Meridians, originally from *Lingshu*: *Jingmai* (*Miraculous Pivot*: *Meridians*), the divergent meridian of Hand-Shaoyang finally joint its regular meridian after the circulation of deriving, entering and emerging, and the divergent meridian of Hand-Jueyin connects the internally and externally related Meridian of Hand-Shaoyang. →手少阳经别(p.392)、手厥阴经别(p.389)

●**手少阳之正**[shǒu shào yáng zhī zhèng] 手少阳经别的原名。详见该条。

The Divergence of Hand-Shaoyang The original name for the Divergent Meridian of Hand-Shaoyang. →手少阳经别(p.392)

●**手少阴标本**[shǒu shào yīn biāo běn] 十二标本之一。出《灵枢·卫气》。手少阴之本在锐骨之端，约当神门穴处；标在其背俞、心俞穴处。参见"十二经标本"条。

The Superficiality and Origin of Hand-Shaoyin One of the superficialities and origins of the Twelve Meridians, origially from *Lingshu*: *Wei Qi* (*Miraculous Pivot*: *Defensive Qi*), the origin of Hand-Shaoyin is at the end of the caput ulnae, near the point Shenmen (HT 7), and the superficiality is on the Back-Shu point Xinshu (BL 15). →十二经标本(p.375)

●**手少阴经别**[shǒu shào yīn jīng bié] 十二经别之一。原称手少阴之正。出《灵枢·经别》。从手少阴心经分出，在腋下渊液穴处进入胸腔，属于心，向上到喉咙，出于面部，在目内眦处与手太阳小肠经会合。

The Divergent Meridian of Hand-Shaoyin One of the Twelve Divergent Meridians, originally named the Divergence of Hand-Shaoyin, originally from *Lingshu*: *Jingbie* (*Miraculous*

Pivot: *Divergent Meridians*). Deriving from the Heart Meridian of Hand-Shaoyin, it enters the thoracic cavity at the point Yuanye (GB 22) below the axilla to pertain to the heart, from there, ascending to the throat and emerging from the face to join the Small Intestine Meridian of Hand-Taiyang at the inner canthus.

●手少阴经筋[shǒu shào yīn jīng jīn] 十二经筋之一。出《灵枢·经筋》。起于小指内侧，结于锐骨，向上结于肘内侧，向上进入腋内，交于太阴经筋，循行于乳里，结聚于胸中，沿膈向下联系于脐部。

The Muscle Region of Hand-Shaoyin One of the Twelve Muscle Regions Along Meridians, originally from *Lingshu: Jingjin (Miraculous Pivot: Muscle Regions Along Meridians)*. Originating from the medial aspect of the small finger and connecting to the head of ulna, it runs upwards to connect the medial aspect of the elbow, and still upwards, to the axilla to join the Muscle Region of Hand-Taiyin, passing through the breast, concentrating in the thoracic cavity, and descending along the diaphragm to connect with the umbilicus.

●手少阴经筋病[shǒu shào yīn jīng Jīn bìng] 十二经筋病候之一。出《灵枢·经筋》。其病症可见胸内拘急，心下有积块坚伏名为伏梁，上肢筋有病则肘部牵急屈伸不利，本经筋循行部位支撑不适，掣引转筋和疼痛。

Diseases of the Muscle Region of Hand-Shaoyin One of the pathological manifestations of the Twelve Muscle Regions, originating from *Lingshu: Jingjin (Miraculous Pivot: Muscle Regions Along Meridians)*. Manifestations: contracture in the chest, hard and hidden mass located in the upper abdomen called Fuliang, disturbance of flexion and extension of the elbow, disturbance in sustaining the circulating regions; contracture, spasm and pain along the course of the muscles.

●手少阴络脉[shǒu shào yīn luò mài] 十五经脉之一。原称手少阴之别。出《灵枢·经脉》。其络脉名曰通里。脉从腕后一寸通里处分出，和本经并行进入心中，上连舌根，属于目系（眼与脑相连的组织）。分支走向手太阳经。

The Collateral of Hand-Shaoyin One of the Fifteen Collaterals, originally named the branch of Hand-Shaoyin, from *Lingshu: Jingmai (Miraculous Pivot: Meridians)*, the collateral is called Tongli(HT 5), deriving from this point 1 cun above the wrist, parallel to and along with the meridian, entering the heart and winding upwards to connect the root of the tongue, pertaining to the eye-system (tissues connecting the eyes with the brain), its branch runs to the Meridian of Hand-Taiyang.

●手少阴络脉病[shǒu shào yīn luò mài bìng] 十五络脉病候之一。出《灵枢·经脉》。实证见胸膈部支撑胀满；虚证则不能说话。

Diseases of the Colateral of Hand-Shaoyin One of the pathologicial manifestations of the Fifteen Main Collaterals, originally from *Lingshu: Jingmai (Miraculous Pivot: Meridians)*. 〈Manifestations〉distention and fullness in the sustaining region of the chest and diaphragm in cases of excess; aphasia in cases of deficiency.

●手少阴郄[shǒu shào yīn xì] 经穴别名。出《针灸甲乙经》。即阴郄。详见该条。

Shoushaoyinxi Another name for Yinxi(HT 6), a meridian point originally from *Zhenjiu Jia-Yi Jing (A-B Classic of Acupuncture and Moxibustion)*. →阴郄(p. 559)

●手少阴心经[shǒu shào yīn xīn jīng] 十二经脉之一。原称心手少阴之脉。出《灵枢·经脉》。其循行从心中开始，出属于心系（联系心脏的组织），下经横膈，联络小肠。它的一条支脉从心系挟着食道上行，联系目系（指眼球与脑相连的组织）。它外行的主干，从心系上行至肺，出于腋下，沿着上臂内侧，行于手太阳、手厥阴经的后面，下向肘内侧，沿着臂内侧后边，至掌后锐骨部进入掌内后边，沿小指桡侧出于末端，接手太阳小肠经。

The Heart Meridian of Hand-Shaoyin One of the Twelve Regular Meridians, originally named the Hand-Shaoyin Meridian of Heart, originally from *Lingshu: Jingmai (Miraculous Pivot: Meridians)*. 〈The course of the meridian〉Originating from th heart, it emerges from and spreads over the "heart system" (i. e. the tissues connecting the heart), passing downwards through the diaphragm to

connect with the small intestine. One of its branches runs alongside the esophagus from the "heart system" to connect with the "eye system" (i.e. the tissues connecting the eyes with the brain). The exteriorly-running mainstay of the meridian ascends from the "heart system" to the lung, and emerges from the region below the axilla, runs behind the meridians of Hand-Taiyin and Hand-Jueyin along the medial aspect of the upper arm, downwards to the medial aspect of the elbow, along the posterior border of the medial aspect of the forearm to the pisiform region proximal to the palm, enters the posterior part of the palm and emerges, along the radial aspect of the little finger, from its tip to connect the Small Intestine Meridian of Hand-Taiyang.

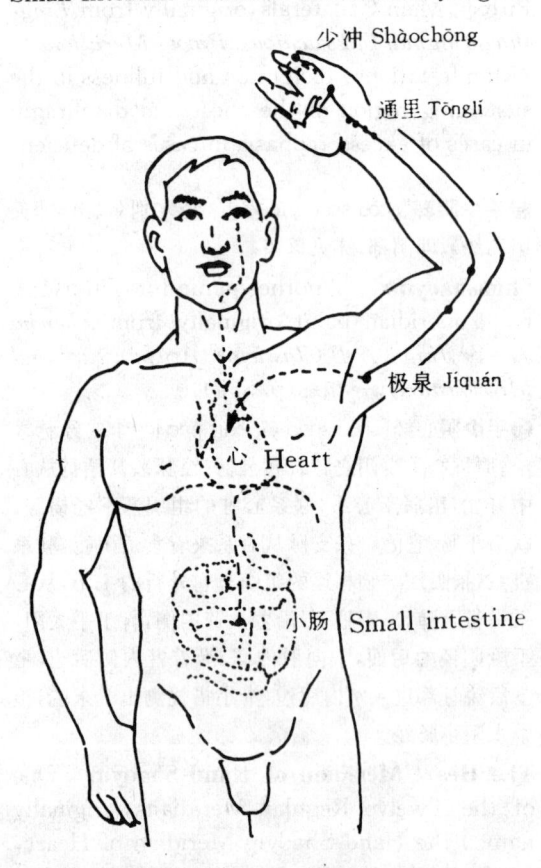

Fig. 51 Heart Meridian of Hand-Shaoyin

● 手少阴心经病 [shǒu shào yīn xīn jīng bìng] 十二经脉病候之一。出《灵枢·经脉》。本经主要病候为：咽干、心痛、渴而欲饮、心烦气短，胸胁痛，目黄，上臂内侧后边厥冷，掌中热痛。

Diseases of the Heart Meridian of Hand-Shaoyin One of the pathological manifestations of the Twelve Regular Meridians, originally from *Ling Shu: Jingmai* (*Miraculous Pivot: Meridians*). 〈Main manifestations〉 dry throat, cardialgia, thirst, vexation, short breath, pain of the chest and hypochondrium, yellow eye, coldness in the posterior region of the medial aspect of the arm, feverish sensation and pain of the palm.

● 手少阴之别 [shǒu shào yīn zhī bié] 即手少阴络脉。详见该条。

The Branch of Hand-Shaoyin →手少阴络脉 (p. 395)

● 手少阴之正 [shǒu shào yīn zhī zhèng] 即手少阴经别。详见该条。

The Divergence of Hand-Shaoyin →手少阴经别。(p. 394)

● 手髓孔 [shǒu suí kǒng] 经外穴名。见"手足髓孔"条。

Shousuikong (EX-UE) An extra point. →手足髓孔 (p. 405)

● 手太阳标本 [shǒu tài yáng biāo běn] 十二经标本之一。出《灵枢·卫气》。手太阳之本，在外踝之后，约当养老穴处。标，在目之上一寸，约当攒竹穴处。

The Superficiality and Origin of Hand-Taiyang One of the superficialities and the origins of the Twelve Meridians, originally from *Lingshu: Wei Qi* (*Miraculous Pivot: Defensive Qi*). The origin of Hand-Taiyang is located in the region posterior to the external malleolus, approximately at Yanglao (SI 6); and the superficiality in the region 1 cun above the eye, approximately at Cuanzhu (BL 2).

● 手太阳经别 [shǒu tài yáng jīng bié] 十二经别之一。原称手太阳之正。出《灵枢·经别》。手太阳经别，在肩关节部从手太阳经分出，向下行入于腋窝部，走向心脏，连系小肠。

The Divergent Meridian of Hand-Taiyang One of the Twelve Divergent Meridians, originally from *Lingshu: Jingbie* (*Miraculous Pivot: Divergent Meridians*). Deriving from the Meridian of Hand-Taiyang in the shoulder

joint, it descends to and enters the axilla and then the heart to connect the small intestine.

●手太阳经筋[shǒu tài yáng jīng jīn] 十二经筋之一。出《灵枢·经筋》。手太阳经筋,起始于手小指的上边,结于腕背,上沿前臂内侧,结于肱骨内上髁后,以手弹该骨处,有感传可及于手小指之上,进入后,结于腋下。其分支走腋后侧,向上绕肩胛部,沿着颈旁出走足太阳经筋的前方,结于耳后乳突部。分支进入耳中,直行的出于耳上,向下结于下颌处,上方的连属于眼外眦。

The Muscle Region of Hand-Taiyang One of the Twelve Muscle Regions along Meridians, originally from *Lingshu: Jingjin (Miraculous Pivot: Muscle Regions Along Meridians)*. The muscle region originates from the dorsal side of the little finger, connects the dorsal aspect of the wrist, and then the poterior region of the medial epicondyle of the humerus along the medial aspect of the forearm. There will be sensation passing downwards to the little finger when it hits this part. It goes upwards to connect the axilla. Its branches run from the posterior axillary side, upwards across the scapular region, emerge from the laterocervical region, pass the region anterior of the muscle region along the Meridian of Foot-Taiyang, connecting the mastoid posterior to the ear. The branches enter the ear. The straight one emerges from the superior of the ear; the downward one connects the cheek; and the upper one connects and pertains to the outer canthus.

●手太阳经筋病[shǒu tài yáng jīng jīn bìng] 十二经筋病候之一。出《灵枢·经筋》。其病可见小指支撑不适,肘内锐骨后缘疼痛,沿臂的内侧,上至腋下,及腋下后侧等处均痛,绕肩胛牵引颈部作痛,并感到耳中鸣响且痛,疼痛牵引颔部,眼睛闭合一会才能看清景物,颈筋拘急,可发生筋痿,颈肿等症。

Diseases of the Muscle Region of Hand-Taiyang One of the pathological manifestations of the Twelve Muscle Regions, originally from *Lingshu: Jingjin (Miraculous Pivot: Muscle Regions of Meridians)*. 〈Manifestations〉 stiffness of the little finger, pain of the posterior border of the alecranon of the ulna, pain along the medial aspect of the arm and upwards to the armpit and its lower posterior side, ache around the scapula radiating to the nape and neck, tinnitus, ear pain radiating to the chin, clear sight only a while after eyes are closed, contractive of the neck tendons and muscles or muscular atrophy, swelling neck, etc.

●手太阳络脉[shǒu tài yáng luò mài] 十五络脉之一。原名手太阳之别。出《灵枢·经脉》。手太阳络脉名曰支正。其络于腕上五寸处支正穴分出,向内侧注入手少阴心经。其支脉上行经肘部,上络于肩髃部。

The Collateral of Hand-Taiyang One of the Fifteen Main Collaterals, originally called the Hand-Taiyang branch, originally from *Lingshu: Jingmai (Miraculous Poivot: Meridians)*. The Hand-Taiyang collateral is named Zhizheng. It derives from Zhizheng (SJ 7), 5 cun above the wrist and goes inward to the Heart Meridian of Hand-Shaoyin. Its branch runs upwards through the elbow to join the Jianyu (LI 15) area.

●手太阳络脉病[shǒu tài yáng luò mài bìng] 十五络脉病候之一。实证见关节弛缓,肘部痿废不用;虚证见皮肤赘生小疣。可取手太阳络穴治疗。

Diseases of the Collateral of Hand-Taiyang
One of the pathological manifestations of the Fifteen Main Collaterals. The disease of excess type is manifested as flaccidity of the elbow and the disease of deficiency type is manifested as verruca appearing on correspondent skin. The Luo (Connecting) point of Hand-Taiyang can be selected for the treatment of these symptoms.

●手太阳、手少阴经别[shǒu tài yáng shǒu shào yīn jīng bié] 十二经别中的一合。出《灵枢·经别》。手太阳经别经过离、入、出的循行后,最后合于本经。手少阴经别经过离、入、出的循行后,合于与其相表里的手太阳经。见"手太阳经别"、"手少阴经别"条。

The Divergent Meridians of Hand-Taiyang and Hand-Shaoyin One confluence of the Twelve Divergent Meridians, originally from *Lingshu: Jingbie (Miraculous Pivot: Divergent Meridians)*. The Hand-Taiyang Divergent Meridian derives from the Hand-Taiyang Meridian, enters it, emerges from it and finally joins the original meridian. The Hand-Shaoyin Divergent Meridian derives from the Hand-Shaoyin meridian, enters it, emerges from it,

and finally joins the Hand-Taiyang Meridian which is internally and externally related with it. →手太阳经别(p. 396)、手少阴经别(p. 394)

●手太阳小肠经[shǒu tài yáng xiǎo cháng jīng] 十二经脉之一。原称小肠手太阳之脉。出《灵枢·经脉》。其循行从小指外侧末端开始,沿手掌尺侧,上向腕部,出尺骨小头部,直上沿尺骨下边,出于肘内侧当肱骨内上髁和尺骨鹰嘴之间,向上沿上臂外后侧,出肩关节部,绕肩胛,交会肩上,进入缺盆,络于心,沿食管,通过膈肌,到胃,属于小肠。它的支脉从缺盆上行沿颈部,上向面颊,到外眼角,回过来进入耳中。另一分支从面颊部分出,上向颧骨,靠鼻旁到内眼角,接足太阳膀胱经。

The Small Intestine Meridian of Hand-Taiyang One of the Twelve Regular Meridians, originally called the Small Intestine Vessel of Hand-Taiyang, originally from *Lingshu: Jingmai* (*Miraculous Pivot: Meridians*). 〈Course of the meridian〉 It starts from the ulnar side of the tip of the little finger, passes along the ulnar side of the dorsum of the hand and reaches upwards to the wrist, emerges from the styloid process of the ulna, ascends along the lower border of the ulna, passes between the olecranon of the ulna and the medial epicondyle of the humerus, and runs along the posterior border of the lateral aspect of the upper arm to the shoulder joint region. Circling around the scapula, it joints the superior aspect of the shoulder and then turns downwards to the supralavicular fossa, connects with the heart, descends from there along the esophagus, passes through the diaphragm, reaches the stomach, and finally enters the small intestine, the organ it pertains to. One branch ascends from the supralavicular fossa along the neck to the cheek. Via the outer canthus, it enters the ear. The other branch from the cheek runs upwards to the infraorbital region and further to the lateral side of the nose. Then, it reaches the inner canthus to link with the Bladder Meridian of Foot-Taiyang.

●手太阳小肠经病[shǒu tài yáng xiǎo cháng jīng bìng] 十二经脉病候之一。本经主要病候为:咽喉痛,腮肿,耳聋,目黄,项强,肩部及上肢外后侧痛,小腹痛、胀,引腰脊,泄泻,大便不利。

Diseases of the Small Intestine Meridian of Hand-Taiyang One of the pathological manifestations of the Twelve Meridians. Its main symptoms and signs are sore throat, acute mumps, deafness, yellow pigmentation of the sclera, stiffness of the nape, pain in the shoulder region and along the posterolateral aspect of the arm, lower abdominal pain and fullness radiating to the waist and spine, diarrhea, loose stool.

●手太阳穴[shǒu tài yáng xué]经外穴别名。即小指尖。详见该条。

Shoutaiyangxue Another name for the extra point, Xiaozhijian (EX-UE). →小指尖(p. 504)

●手太阳之别[shǒu tài yáng zhī bié] 手太阳络脉的原名。详见该条。

Branch of Hand-Taiyang The original name of the Hand Taiyang Collateral. →手太阳络脉(p. 397)

●手太阳之正[shǒu tài yáng zhī zhèng] 手太阳经别的原称。详见该条。

The Hand-Taiyang Divergence The original name for the Hand-Taiyang Divergent Meridian. →手太阳经别(p. 396)

●手太阴标本[shǒu tài yīn biāo běn] 十二经标本之一。见《灵枢·卫气》。手太阴之本,在寸口中;标,在腋内动脉处。参见"十二经标本"条。

The Superficiality and the Origin of Hand-Taiyin One of the superficialities and the origins of the Twelve Meridians, seen in *Lingshu: Weiqi* (*Miraculous Pivot: Defensive Qi*). The origin of Hand-Taiyin is the cun-mouth area (on the wrist over the radial artery) and its superficiality in the region of the axillary artery. →十二经标本(p. 375)

●手太阴肺经[shǒu tài yīn fèi jīng] 十二经脉之一。原称肺手太阴之脉,出《灵枢·经脉》。其循行:起于中焦胃部,向下络于大肠,回绕过来沿着胃的上口,穿过膈肌,属于肺脏,从肺系(肺与喉咙相联系的部位)横行出于腋下,向下沿着上臂内侧,行于手少阴经和手厥阴经的前面,下行至肘窝中,沿着前臂内侧前缘,进入寸口桡动脉搏动处,上向鱼际部,沿着鱼际的边缘,出拇指内侧端。它的支脉,从腕后走向食指内侧,出其端,接手阳明大肠经。

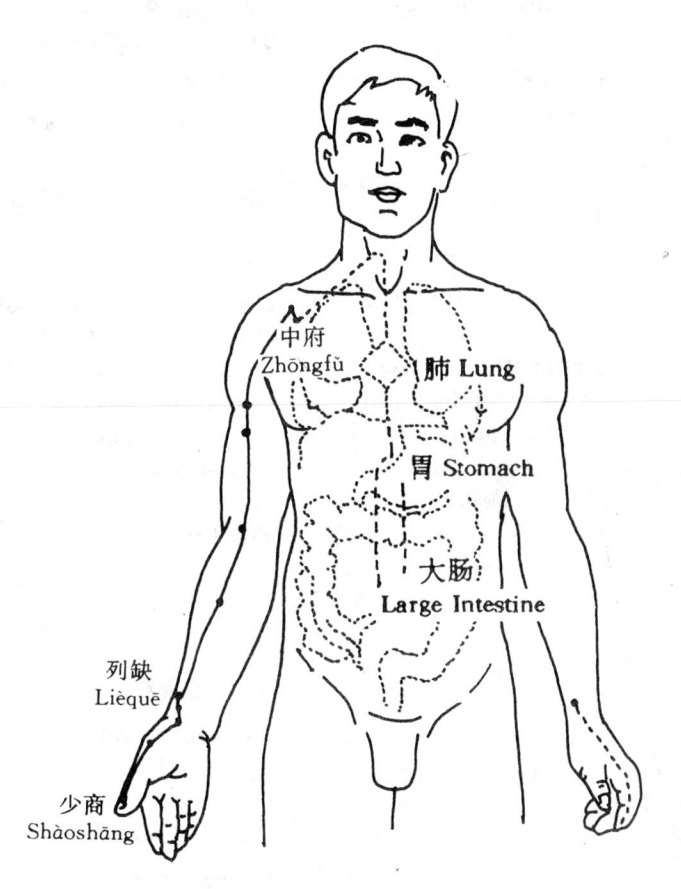

图52 手太阴肺经
Fig. 52 Lung Meridian of Hand-Taiyin

The Lung Meridian of Hand-Taiyin One of the Twelve Regular Meridians, originally known as the Lung Vessel of Hand-Taiyin, originally from *Lingshu: Jingmai* (*Miraculous Pivot: Meridians*). It originates from the middle-jiao (stomach region) and runs downwards to connect with the large intestine. Winding back, it then goes along the upper orifice of the stomach, passes upwards through the diaphragm and enters the lung, its pertaining organ. From the lung system the portion of the lung connecting with the throat, it comes out transversely. It descends along the radial border of the medial aspect of the upper arm, and anterior to the meridians of Hand-Shaoyin and Hand-Jueyin, it reaches the cubital fossa. Then, it goes continuously downwards along the anterior border of the medial aspect of the forearm and enters cun-mouth area where the radial artery pulses. Passing the thenar eminence and going along its radial border, it ends at the medial side of the tip of the thumb. Its branch emerges from the posterior portion of the wrist and runs along the medial aspect of the index finger reaching the tip of the index finger, where it connects with the Large Intestine Meridian of Hand-Yangming.

● 手太阴肺经病 [shǒu tài yīn fèi jīng bìng] 十二经脉病候之一。出《灵枢·经脉》。本经主要病候为：胸部满闷，肺胀，咳嗽，气喘，心烦，气短，锁骨上窝疼痛，肩背痛，上臂内侧上缘疼痛，掌中发热等症。

Diseases of the Lung Meridian of Hand-Taiyin One of the pathological manifestations of the Twelve Meridians, originally from *Lingshu: Jingmai* (*Miraculous Pivot: Meridians*). Its main symptoms and signs are fullness

399

and tightness of the chest, distention of the lung, cough, dyspnea, vexation, shortness of breath, pain in the supraclaviclar fossa, shoulder and back, ache along the superior border of the medial aspect of the forearm, feverish sensation in the palm.

●**手太阴经别**[shǒu tài yīn jīng bié] 十二经别之一,原称手太阴之正。出《灵枢·经别》。在腋前从手太阴肺经分出,行于手少阴经之前,入走肺,向下散于大肠,向上出于缺盆,沿喉咙,复与手阳明大肠经相合。

The Divergent Meridian of Hand-Taiyin One of the Twelve Divergent Meridians, originally known as the Hand-Taiyin divergence, originally from *Lingshu: Jingbie (Miraculous Pivot: Divergent Meridians)*. It derives from the Lung Meridian of Hand-Taiyin at the anteriority of the armpit and goes along the part anterior to the Hand-Shaoyin Meridian. Afterwards, it enters the chest and lung, and then goes downwards and disperses at the large intestine. Winding back, it goes upwards and emerges at the supralavicular fossa, and ascends along the throat joining the Large Intestine Meridian of Hand-Yangming again.

●**手太阴经筋**[shǒu tài yīn jīng jīn] 十二经筋之一。出《灵枢·经筋》。起于大指之上,沿指上行,结于鱼际后,经寸口动脉外侧,沿前臂结于肘中,经上臂内侧,进入腋下,上出缺盆,结于肩髃前。其上方结于缺盆,其下方结于胸里,分散通过膈,与手厥阴经之筋在膈下会合。

The Muscle Region of Hand-Taiyin One of the Twelve Muscle Regions, originally from *Lingshu: Jingjin (Miraculous Pivot: Muscle Regions Along Meridians)*. It starts from the thumb and ascends along it to concentrate at the thenar eminence, passes through the lateral side of the radial artery in the cun-mouth area and goes along the forearm to the elbow fossa. Then, ascending along the medial aspect of the upper arm and entering the armpit, it emerges from the supraclavicular fossa and concentrates at the anteriority of Jianyu (LI 15). Its upper branch concentrates at the supraclavicular fossa, and its lower branch masses in the chest, passes dispersively through the diaphragm to converge in the Hand-Jueyin Muscle Region under the diaphragm.

●**手太阴经筋病**[shǒu tài yīn jīng jīn bìng] 十二经筋病候之一。出《灵枢·经筋》。其病证:在本经筋循行处可出现支撑不适,拘紧掣痛;重者可成息贲病,胁肋拘急,上逆吐血。

Diseases of the Muscle Region of Hand-Taiyin One of the pathological manifestations of the Twelve Muscle Regions, originally from *Lingshu: Jingjin (Miraculous Pivot: Muscle Regions of the Meridians)*. Its main symptoms and signs are stiffness, contracture and pain in the regions of the course of the muscle region; pulmonary mass, contracture of the hypochondiac region, and vomiting. Hematemesis may appear in the severe case.

●**手太阴络脉**[shǒu tài yīn luò mài] 十五络脉之一,原称手太阴之别。出《灵枢·经脉》。其络脉名曰列缺。脉从腕关节桡骨茎突后的分肉之间,腕后一寸半列缺处分出,和本经并行,直入掌中,散布在大鱼际部,走向手阳明经。

The Collareral of Hand-Taiyin One of the Fifteen Main Collaterals, originally called the Branch of Hand-Taiyin, originally from *Lingshu: Jingmai (Miraculous Pivot: Meridians)*. Its collateral is named Lieque and derives from Lieque (LU 7), which locates on the flesh adherent the bone poterior to the styloid process of the radius and 1.5 cun above the crease of the wrist and runs parellel to the Lung Meridian. After directly entering the palm, it distributes in the region of the thenar, and goes to the Hand-Yangming Meridian.

●**手太阴络脉病**[shǒu tài yīn luò mài bìng] 十五络脉病候之一。出《灵枢·经脉》。其病实证可见手掌和手腕部灼热;虚证可见呵欠、尿频、遗尿。可取手太阴络穴治疗。

Diseases of the Collateral of Hand-Taiyin One of the pathological manifestations of the Fifteen Main Collaterals originally from *Lingshu: Jingmai (Mirculous Pivot: Meridians)*. The disease of the excess type is manifested as scorching fever of the palm and the wrist region and disease of the deficiency type is manifested as yawn, frequent micturition and enuresis. The Luo (Connecting) point of Hand-

Taiyin can be used for treating the diseases.

●**手太阴之别**[shǒu tài yīn zhī bié] 即手太阴络脉。详见该条。

The Branch of Hand-Taiyin →手太阴络脉 (p. 400)

●**手太阴之正**[shǒu tài yīn zhī zhèng] 即手太阴经别。详见该条。

The Divergence of Hand-Taiyin →手太阴经别(p. 400)

●**手五里**[shǒu wǔ lǐ] 经穴名。出《灵枢·本输》。属手阳明大肠经，又名五里、臂五里、尺之五里。〈定位〉在臂外侧，当曲池与肩髃连线上，曲池上3寸处(图48和图53)。〈层次解剖〉皮肤→皮下组织→肱肌。浅层有臂外侧下皮神经和前臂后皮神经等结构。深层有桡侧副动、静脉和桡神经。〈主治〉肘臂挛急、疼痛、瘰疬、咳嗽吐血、嗜卧身黄、疟疾。直刺0.5～0.8；可灸。

Shouwuli(LI 13) A meridian point, originally from *Lingshu*: *Benshu* (*Miraculous Pivot*: *Meridian Points*), a point on the Large Intestine Meridian of Hand-Yangming, also called Wuli, Biwuli, or Chizhiwuli. 〈Location〉on the lateral side of the upper arm and on the line connecting Quchi(LI 11) and Jianyu(LI 15), 3 cun above Quchi(LI 11) (Figs. 48 & 53). 〈Regional anatomy〉 skin→subcutaneous tissue→brachial muscle. In the superficial layer, there are the lateral inferior cutaneous nerve of the arm and the posterior cutaneous nerve of the forearm. In the deep layer, there are the radial collateral artery and vein and the radial nerve. 〈Indications〉 muscular stiffness and pain of the elbow and arm, scrofula, cough with spitting blood, somnalence and yellow body, malaria. 〈Method〉 Puncture perpendicularly 0.5～0.8 cun. Moxibustion is applicable.

●**手下廉**[shǒu xià lián] 经穴别名。出《圣济总录》。即下廉。详见该条。

Shouxialian Another name for Xialian (LI 8), a meridian point originally from *Shengji Zonglu* (*Imperial Medical Encyclopaedia*). →下廉(p. 489)

●**手心**[shǒu xīn] 经外穴名。见《千金要方》。在手掌部，当中指指掌横纹中点与大陵穴连线的中处。主治犬痫。用灸法。

Shouxin(EX-UE) An extra point, originally seen in *Qianjin Yaofang* (*Essential Prescriptions Worth a Thousand Gold*). 〈Location〉on the palm, at the midpoint of the line connecting the midpoint on the metacarpophalangeal articulation of the middle finger and Daling(PC 7). 〈Indication〉epilepsy due to the dog bite. 〈Method〉moxibustion.

●**手心主之别**[shǒu xīn zhǔ zhī bié] 即手厥阴络脉。详见该条。

The Branch of Hand-Jueyin →手厥阴络脉 (p. 389)

●**手心主之正**[shǒu xīn zhǔ zhī zhèng] 即手厥阴经别。详见该条。

The Divergence of Hand-Jueyin →手厥阴经别(p. 389)

●**手阳明标本**[shǒu yáng míng biāo běn] 十二经标本之一。出《灵枢·卫气》。手阳明之本，在肘骨中，约当曲池穴处；标，在颈部，在颜下，合钳上。

The Superficiality and Origin of Hand-Yangming One of the superficialities and the origins of the Twlve Meridians, originally from *Lingshu*: *Wei Qi* (*Miraculous Pivot*: *Defensive Qi*). The origin of Hand-Yangming is in the elbow approximately at Quchi (LI 11), and the superficiality in the neck posterior to Renying(ST 9) and superior to Futu(LI 18).

●**手阳明大肠经**[shǒu yáng míng dà cháng jīng] 十二经脉之一，原称大肠手阳明之脉。出《灵枢·经脉》。其循行从食指末端起始，沿食指桡侧缘，行于第一、二掌骨间，进入两筋之间，沿前臂桡侧进入肘外侧，经上臂外侧前边，上肩，出肩峰部前边，向上交会颈部大椎。向下进入缺盆，络于肺，通过横膈，属于大肠。它的支脉，从缺盆，上行颈旁，通过面颊，进入下齿槽，出来挟口旁，交会人中部，左边的向右，右边的向左，上夹鼻孔旁，接足阳明胃经。

The Large Intestine Meridian of Hand-Yangming One of the Twelve Regular Meridians, originally called the Large Intestine Vessel of Hand-Yangming, originally from *Lingshu*: *Jingmai* (*Miraculous Pivot*: *Meridians*). 〈Course〉It starts from the tip of the index finger. Running upwards along the radial side of the index finger and passing through the interspace of the 1st and 2nd metacarpal bones, it enters the depression between the tendons of extensor pollicis longus and brevis.

Then, running along the radial side of the forearm, it reaches the lateral aspect of the elbow. From there, it ascends along the lateral anterior aspect of the upper arm to the shoulder, emerges from the anterior edge of the acromion, and goes up to meet Dazhui (DU 14) on the nape. Then it descends to the supraclavicular fossa to connect with the lung. Passing through the diaphragm, it enters the large intestine, the organ it pertains to. Its branch runs from the supraclavicular fossa upwards to the neck, passes through the cheek and enters the lower gums. Then, it turns back to the side of the mouth and crosses the opposite meridian at the philtrum. From there, the left meridian goes to the right and the right meridian to the left, to the contralateral sides of the nose, where the Large Intestine Meridian links with the Stomach Meridian of Foot-Yangming.

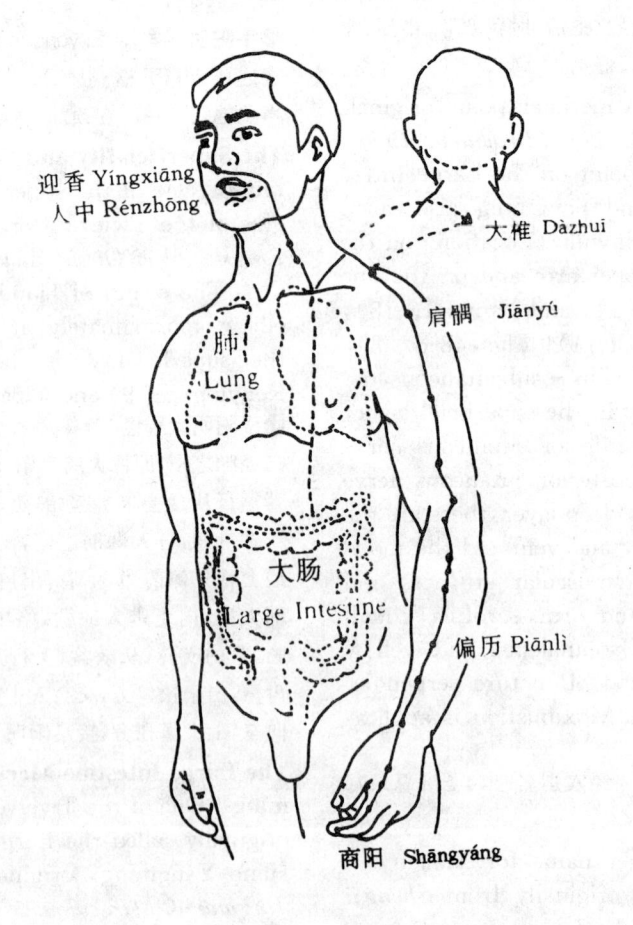

Fig. 53 Large Intestine Meridian of Hand-Yangming

●手阳明大肠经病[shǒu yáng míng dà cháng jīng bìng] 十二经脉病候之一。出《灵枢·经脉》。本经主要病候为：口干，鼻塞，衄血，齿痛，颈肿，喉痹，肩前、上臂部疼痛，食指痛，活动不利，经脉所过之处热肿或寒冷，肠绞痛，肠鸣，泄泻。

Diseases of the Large Intestine Meridian of Hand-Yangming One of the pathological manifestations of the Twelve Meridians, originally from *Lingshu: Jingmai (Miraculous Pivot: Meridians)*. The main symptoms and signs are: dry mouth, stuffy nose, epistaxis, toothache, swelling of the neck, pain and swelling of the throat, pain in the anterior shoulder and the upper arm, ache and stiffness of the index finger, heat and swelling or cold feeling in the region along the course of this meridian, intestinal colic, borborygmus and diarrhea.

●手阳明经别[shǒu yáng míng jīng bié] 十二经别之一，原称手阳明之正。出《灵枢·经别》。手阳明经别，在肩上部肩髃穴处分出，从第七颈椎处进入体腔，下行到达大肠，归属于肺脏，向上沿喉咙，浅出于缺盆部，脉气仍流入手阳明本经。

The Divergent Meridian of Hand-Yangming

One of the Twelve Divergent Meridians, originally known as the Hand-Yangming Divergence, originally from *Lingshu: Jingbie (Miraculous Pivot: Divergent Meridians)*. It derives from Jianyu(LI 15), the superior portion of the shoulder, and enters the body from the 7th cervical vertebra, descends to the large intestine, and goes back to the lung. Running upward along the throat, it emerges superficially from the supraclavicular fossa. Its meridian qi still flows into the Hand-Yangming Meridian.

●手阳明经筋[shǒu yáng míng jīng jīn] 十二经筋之一。出《灵枢·经筋》。手阳明经筋，起于第二手指桡侧端，结于腕背部，向上沿前臂，结于肘外侧，上经上臂外侧，结于肩髃部。分支绕肩胛，挟脊柱两旁，直行的经筋从肩髃部上走颈。分支走向面颊，结于鼻旁颧部，直上行的走向手太阳经筋前方，上左侧额角者，结络于头部向下至右侧下颌。

The Muscle Region of Hand-Yangming One of the Twelve Muscle Regions, originally from *Lingshu: Jingjin (Miraculous Pivot: Muscle Regions Along Meridians)*. It starts from the tip on the radial side of the index finger and concentrates at the dorsum of the wrist. Passing upwards along the forearm, it concentrates at the lateral aspect of the elbow, and then goes upwards along the lateral aspect on the upper arm and masses at the lateral aspect of the elbow. Then, it goes upwards along the lateral side of the upper arm to mass at the region of Jianyu (LI 15). Its branches run around the scapula and link with both sides of the spine; the straight-going muscle region ascends to the neck from Jianyu(LI 15). The branches run to the cheeks and mass at the zygomatic region near the sides of the nose; those going straight upward goes to the anterior portion of the Hand-Taiyang muscle region. The part of the muscle region which ascends to the left corner of the forehead concentrates at the head and descends to the right lower submuntal region.

●手阳明经筋病[shǒu yáng míng jīng jīn bìng] 十二经筋病候之一。出《灵枢·经筋》。其病所过之处可出现支撑不适，拘紧和疼痛，肩关节不能高举，颈不能向两侧顾视。

Diseases of the Muscle Region of Hand-Yangming One of the pathological manifestations of the Twelve Muscle Regions, originally from *Lingshu: Jingjin (Miraculous Pivot: Muscles Along Meridians)*. 〈Manifestations〉stiffness, contracture and pain in the region of the course of this muscle region, failure of the shoulder joint in being raised high and of the neck in turning round.

●手阳明络脉[shǒu yáng míng luò mài] 十五络脉之一，原称手阳明之别。出《灵枢·经脉》。手阳明络脉名曰偏历，其脉在腕关节后三寸处偏历穴分出，走向手太阴经脉。其支脉向上沿着臂膊，经过肩髃部位，上行到下颌角处，遍布于牙齿根部。其支脉入耳中，与耳目所聚集的许多经脉会合。

The Collateral of Hand-Yangming One of the Fifteen Main Collaterals, originally called the Branch of Hand-Yangming, originally from *Lingshu: Jingmai (Miraculous Pivot: Meridians)*. The Hand-Yangming collateral is named Pianli(LI 6). It derives from Pianli(LI

6), which is 3 cun above the crease of the wrist on the dorsal surface, and then goes to the Hand-Taiyin Meridian. One branch runs upwards along the arm and ascends to the angle of the mandible through Jianyu(LI 15)to distribute over the root regions of the teeth. The other branch enters into the ear and meets with the meridians which gather in the eye and ear.

●手阳明络脉病[shǒu yáng míng luò mài bìng] 十五络脉,病候之一。出《灵枢·经脉》。其病实证见龋齿痛,耳聋;虚证齿冷,经气痹阻不通畅。可取手阳明络穴治疗。

Diseases of the Collateral of Hand-Yangming
One of the pathological manifestations of the Fifteen Main Collaterals, originally from *Lingshu: Jingmai (Miraculous Pivot: Meridians)*. The disease of the excess type is manifested as decayed teeth and deafness; that of deficiency type as a cold feeling of the teeth and stagnation of the meridian qi. The Luo (Connecting) point can be selected for the treatment of this disease.

●手阳明、手太阴经别[shǒu yáng míng shǒu tài yīn jīng bié] 十二经别中的一合。出《灵枢·经别》。手阳明经别经过离、入、出的循行后,最后合于本经。手太阴经别经过离、入、出的循行后,合于与其相表里的手阳明经。见"手阳明经别"、"手太阴经别"条。

The Divergent Meridians of Hand-Yangming and Hand-Taiyin One confluence of the Twelve Divergent Meridians, originally from *Ling Shu: Jingbie (Miraculous Pivot: Divergent Meridians)*. The Hand-Yangming Divergent Meridian derives from the Hand-Yangming Meridian, enters it, emerges from it and finally joins the original meridian. The Hand-Shaoyin divergent meridian derives from the Hand-Taiyin meridian, enters it, emerges from it, and finally joins the internally and externally related Hand-Yangming Meridian. →手阳明经别(p.403)、手太阴经别(p.400)

●手阳明之别[shǒu yáng míng zhī bié] 手阳明络脉原称。详见该条。

The Branch of Hand-Yangming The original name of the Hand-Yangming Collateral. →手阳明络脉(p.403)

●手阳明之正[shǒu yáng míng zhī zhèng] 手阳明经别的原称。详见该条。

The Divergence of Hand-Yangming The original name of the Hand-Yangming Divergent Meridian. →手阳明经别(p.403)

●手鱼[shǒu yú] 部位名。为拇指球肌群所形成的隆起,又单称"鱼"。见《灵枢》。参见"鱼际"条。

Hand Fish A part of the body, referring to the eminence formed from the muscle of the thumb, also named "fish" for short, seen in *Lingshu(Miraculous Pivot)*. →鱼际(p.571)

●手掌后白肉际穴[shǒu zhǎng hòu bái ròu jì xué] 经外穴名。见《类经图翼》。在掌后腕横纹中点赤白肉际处。〈主治〉霍乱转筋。用灸法。

Shouzhanghoubairoujixue(EX-UE) An extra point seen in *Leijing Tuyi(Supplements to Illustrated Classified Canon of Internal Medicine of the Yellow Emperor)*. 〈Location〉 at the midpoint of the crease of the wrist, on the junction of the red and white skin. 〈Indication〉 cramp in cholera morbus. 〈Method〉 moxibustion.

●手掌后臂间穴[shǒu zhǎng hòu bì jiān xué] 经外穴名。见《类经图翼》。在前臂屈侧,腕横纹上5横指处,当掌长肌腱与桡侧腕屈肌腱之间。直刺0.5~1.0寸;可灸。

Shouzhanghoubijianxue(EX-UE) An extra point, seen in *Leijing Tuyi(Supplements to Illustrated Classified Canon of Internal Medicine of the Yellow Emperor)*. 〈Location〉 on the palmar side of the forearm and 5 cun above the crease of the wrist, between the tendons of long palmar muscle and radial flexor muscle of the wrist. 〈Method〉Puncture perpendicularly 0.5~1.0 cun. Moxibustion is applicable.

●手针[shǒu zhēn] 指针刺手部穴位的针法。其穴综合手部的经穴,奇穴和按摩用穴。可用治全身各部的病症,属远道取穴法的应用。

Hand Acupuncture An acupuncture therapy for puncturing points on the hand, including meridian points, extra points and massage points. It can be used for the treatment of diseases of any part of the body, and is an application of the method of the distant-proximal point selection.

●手指补泻法[shǒu zhǐ bǔ xiè fǎ] 针刺手法。出《针

经指南》。指针刺操作过程中用以催气、行气补泻的各种手法。窦氏将有关针刺的各种辅助手法总称为手指补泻法,共十四条。后来在《金针赋》、《针灸聚英》、《针灸问对》中均有不同记载。

Finger Reinforcing and Reducing Needling techniques, originally from *Zhenjing Zhinan* (*Guide to the Classics of Acupuncture*), referring to all kinds of manipulations which are used to hasten the arrival of qi and promote the flow of meridian qi to achieve reinforcing and reducing. Mr. Dou generally regarded all the auxiliary acupuncture manipulations as finger reinforcing and reducing, 14 items in all. Later, different records can be seen in *Jinzhen Fu* (*Ode to the Gold Needle*), *Zhenjiu Juying* (*Essentials of Acupuncture and Moxibustion*) and *Zhenjiu Wendui* (*Catechism of Acupuncture and Moxibustion*).

●手中指第一节穴[shǒu zhōng zhǐ dì yī jié xué] 经外穴别名。即中指节。详见该条。

Shouzhongzhidiyijiexue Another name for the extra point, Zhongzhijie (EX-UE). →中指节(p. 615)

●手足大指爪甲[shǒu zú dà zhǐ zhǎo jiǎ] 经外穴别名,即鬼眼。详见该条。

Shouzudazhizhaojia Another name for the extra point, Guiyan (EX-UE/LE). →鬼眼(p. 152)

●手足髓孔[shǒu zú suí kǒng] 经外穴名。见《千金翼方》。手髓孔,疑即经穴腕骨或阳谷。足髓孔,疑即经穴昆仑。详见各条。

Shouzusuikong (EX-UE/LE) A set of extra points, seen in *Qianjin Yifang* (*A Supplement to the Prescriptions Worth a Thousand Gold*). Shouzusuikong (EX-UE) was presumed to be the meridian point Wangu (SI 4) or Yanggu (SI 5), and Zusuikong (EX-LE) was presumed to be the meridian point Kunlun (BL 60). →腕骨(p. 457)、阳谷(p. 537)、昆仑(p. 236)

●守气[shǒu qì] 刺法术语。出《灵枢·小针解》。指针刺得气后须施用适当的手法,不使已得之气消失。

Keeping the Needling Qi A term for a needling technique, originally from *Lingshu: Xiaozhen Jie* (*Miraculous Pivot: Explanation of Delicate Needling*), referring to the application of proper manipulations to make the needling qi retain after the sensation is obtained.

●首窍阴[shǒu qiào yīn] 经穴别名。出《圣济总录》。即头窍阴。详见该条。

Shouqiaoyin Another name for Touqiaoyin (GB 11), a meridian point originally *from Shengji Zonglu* (*Imperial Medical Encyclopaedia*)→头窍阴(p. 444)

●枢持[shū chí] 六经皮部之一,少阳皮部名。出《素问·皮部论》。"枢"是枢纽、枢要的意思;"持"有执持的含义。阳经以少阳为枢,故名"枢持"。

Firm Hinge One of the Cutaneous Regions of the Six Meridians, name of the Shaoyang Cutaneous Region, originally from *Suwen: Pibu Lun* (*Plain Questions: On Cutaneous Regions*). "Hinge" means axis and pivot while "持" means hold. It's so named because Shaoyang is taken as the hinge of all the yang meridians.

●枢儒[shū rú] 六经皮部之一,少阴皮部名。出《素问·皮部论》。"儒"是柔顺的意思。少阴为三阴关阖之枢,其阴气柔顺,故称枢儒。

Gentle Hinge One of the Cutaneous regions of the Six Meridians, name of the Shaoyin Cutaneous region, originally from *Suwen: Pibu Lun* (*Plain Questions: On Cutaneous Regions*). Here, "儒" means gentle, Shaoyin is taken as the hinge of the bolt and door of the three yins, its yin-qi is gentle, so it is named gentle hinge.

●俞府[shū fǔ] 经穴名。出《针灸甲乙经》。属足少阴肾经。〈定位〉在胸部,当锁骨下缘,前正中线旁开2寸(图75和图40)。〈层次解剖〉皮肤→皮下组织→胸大肌。浅层布有锁骨上内侧神经。深层有胸内、外侧神经的分支。〈主治〉咳嗽、气喘、胸痛、呕吐、不嗜食。斜刺或平刺0.5～0.8寸;可灸。

Shufu (KI 27) A meridian point, originally from *Zhenjiu Jia-Yi Jing* (*A-B Classic of Acupuncture and Moxibustion*), a point on the Kindey Meridian of Foot-Shaoyin. 〈Location〉on the chest, below the lower border of the clavicle, 2 cun lateral to the midline (Figs. 75&40). 〈Regional anatomy〉 skin → subcutaneous tissue → great pectoral muscle. In the superficial layer, there are the medial

supraclavicular nerve. In the deep layer, there are the branches of the medial and lateral pectoral nerves. 〈Indications〉 cough, dyspnea, pain in the chest, vomiting, loss of appetite. 〈Method〉 Puncture obliquely or subcutaneously 0.5~0.8 cun. Moxibustion is applicable.

●俞募配穴法[shū mù pèi xué fǎ] 配穴法之一。指以病变脏腑所属的背俞穴与募穴配合应用。如胃病选用胃俞和中脘,膀胱病症选用膀胱俞和中极等。

The Combination of the Back-Shu and the Front-Mu Points One of the methods of point prescription, referring to selecting the Back-Shu and Front-Mu points relating to the affected organs, to be used in combination. For instance, select Weishu (BL 21) and Zhongwan (RN 12) for diseases of the stomach, Pangguangshu (BL 28) and Zhongji (RN 3) for diseases of the urinary bladder, etc.

●舒张押手[shū zhāng yā shǒu] 为撑开进针之别称。详见该条。

Hand Separating and Pressing Another name for tightening skin during insertion. → 撑开进针(p.42)

●输[shū] 腧穴之别名。详见该条。

Transmission Another name for acupoints. → 腧穴(p.407)

●输刺[shū cì] 《内经》刺法名。见《灵枢·官针》。①九刺之一,是一种治疗脏腑病变的针刺方法。如果脏腑有病,可以取相关经脉的荥穴和输穴,及相关的背俞穴,进行针刺。由于这种针刺法突出了本输穴和背俞穴的作用,所以称为输刺。②十二刺之一。此针法是将针垂直刺入较深处候气,得气后慢慢将针垂直提出,而且取穴少,能输通经气泻除邪气,治疗气盛而热的病证。③五刺之一。是一种直进针,直出针,深刺至骨骼的针刺方法。输,有内外输通之义,故称为输刺。因本法要求直刺至骨,肾主骨,所以与肾脏相应。可用于治疗骨痹证。

Shu Needling A needling technique in *Neijing* (*The Canon of Internal Medicine*), seen in *Lingshu*: *Guanzhen* (*Miraculous Pivot*: *Official Needles*). ① One of the Nine Needlings, referring to the needling method of treating pathogenic changes of zang-fu organs. To treat the diseases of zang-fu organs, the Ying (Spring) and Shu (Stream) points of the related meridians and the related Back-Shu points can be punctured. It is so named because the effects of the above points are emphasized. ② One of the Twelve Needlings. Insert the needle perpendicularly to the deep layer and wait for the arrival of qi, then withdraw the needle perpendicularly after getting the needling qi. Only a few acupoints are selected. The technique can dredge the meridian and disperse the pathogen to treat febrile diseases due to excessive pathogens. ③ One of the Five Needlings, referring to the needling method of inserting the needle perpendicularly to the bone and withdrawing it perpendicularly. Here, Shu means transmission between the inner and the outer, so it is named Shu needling. The technique can be used to treat rheumatism involving the bone because the needle is inserted to the bone which is governed by the kidney.

●输脉[shū mài] 经脉名。见《灵枢·百病始生》。又称输之脉。指背部联系脏腑的经脉。足太阳经以总管五脏六腑之背俞穴,故曰输脉。

Back-Shu Meridian A meridian, seen in *Lingshu*: *Baibing Shisheng* (*Miraculous Pivot*: *Occurrence of Diseases*), also known as the Meridian of Back-Shu, referring to the back meridian linking zang-fu organs. The Foot-Taiyang Meridian is called Back-Shu Meridian because it is in charge of the Back-Shu points of the five zang and six fu organs.

●输尿管[shū niào guǎn] 耳穴名。位于肾与膀胱两穴之间。用于治疗输尿管结石及绞痛。

Ureter(MA-SC 7) An auricular point. 〈Location〉 between Kidney (MA) and Bladder (MA-SC 8). 〈Indication〉 colic pain of the ureter calculus.

●输穴[shū xié] 五腧穴之一。输穴多位于掌指或跖趾关节之后,喻脉气较盛,象水流由浅向较深处灌注。用于身体沉重,关节疼痛。

Shu (Stream) Points One of the Five Shu points, mostly located in the part posterior to the metascarpophalongeal or metacarsophalangeal joints. Shu means meridian qi which flows like water, irrigating from the shallow to the deeper layer. It is used for treating heavy

sensations of the body and pain of the joints.

●输之脉[shū zhī mài] 输脉的别名。详见该条。

Meridian of Back-Shu Another name for Back-Shu Meridian. →输脉(p.406)

●属累[shǔ lěi] 经穴别名。出《针灸甲乙经》。即命门。详见该条。

Shulei Another name for Mingmen (DU 4), a meridian point originally from *Zhenjiu Jia-Yi Jing* (*A-B Classic of Acupuncture and Moxibustion*). →命门(p.270)

●暑湿感冒[shǔ shī gǎn mào] 感冒证型之一。由风挟暑湿之邪侵袭肺卫,湿热郁蒸,阻遏清阳所致。证见身热不扬,恶寒少汗,头重如裹,肢体关节酸困重痛,脘痞,呕恶,甚则大便溏,小便短黄,口中淡腻不渴或渴而喜热饮,舌苔厚腻或黄腻,脉缓或浮数。治宜清暑化湿,疏表和里。取列缺、合谷、中脘、足三里、支沟。

Common Cold due to Summer-Heat and Dampness A type of common cold, caused by pathogenic wind with pathogenic summer-heat and dampness attacking the lung and superficial defence, leading to pathogenic heat-dampness sitting up and evaporating to obstruct the luncid yang. ⟨Manifestations⟩ recessive fever, aversion to cold with mild sweating, heavy sensation of the head as if being tied, soreness and heavy pain of joints of the body, fullness of the epigastrium, vomiting, nausea, loose stool, scanty yellow urine, tasteless and greasy sensation in the mouth without feeling thirsty, or with thirst relieved by drinking hot water, thick greasy or yellow greasy tongue coating, superficial rapid or leisurely pulse. ⟨Treatment principles⟩ Clear summer-heat and eliminate dampness, induce diaphoresis and regulate the inner body. ⟨Point selection⟩ Lieque (LU 7), Hegu (LI 4), Zhongwan (RN 12), Zusanli (ST 36), Zhigou (SJ 6).

●鼠粪灸[shǔ fèn jiǔ] 灸法的一种。见《针灸资生经》第三。以干燥鼠粪放于脐部燃着施灸的一种方法。可延年益寿。

Mouse Manure Cauterization One form of cauterization seen in Vol. 3 of *Zhenjiu Zisheng Jing* (*Acupuncture-Moxibustion Classic for Saving Life*). ⟨Method⟩ Put dry mouse manure on the umbilicus, then ignite it for cauterization. It can prolong the life span.

●鼠瘘[shǔ lòu] 病名。出《灵枢·寒热》。即颈腋部淋巴结结核,瘰疬之别名。详见该条。

Mouse-Like Scrofula Another name for scrofula, a disease originally from *Lingshu: Hanre* (*Miraculous Pivot: Cold and Heat*), namely, lymphoid tuberculosis at the neck and armpit. →瘰疬(p.258)

●鼠尾[shǔ wěi] 经外穴名。见《疮疡经验全书》。在足部,当足跟中线,跟骨上缘处。〈主治〉瘰疬。用灸法。

Shuwei (EX-LE) An extra point, seen in *Chuangyang Jingyan Quanshu* (*A Complete Manual of Experiences in the Treatment of Sores*). ⟨Location⟩ on the sole, on the upper edge of the mid line of the heel. ⟨Indication⟩ scrofula. ⟨Method⟩ moxibustion.

●束骨[shù gǔ] 经穴名。出《灵枢·本输》。属足太阳膀胱经,为本经输穴。〈定位〉在足外侧,足小趾本节(第五跖趾关节)的后方,赤白肉际处(图8.2)。〈层次解剖〉皮肤→皮下组织→小趾展肌→小趾对跖肌腱→小趾短屈肌。浅层布有足背外侧皮神经,足背静脉弓的属支。深层有足底固有神经和趾底固有动、静脉。主治癫狂、头痛、项强、目眩、腰背痛、下肢后侧痛。直刺0.3～0.5寸;可灸。

Shugu (BL 64) A meridian point, originally from *Ling Shū: Benshu* (*Miraculous Pivot: Méridian Points*), the Shu (Stream) point of the Bladder Meridian of Foot-Taiyang. ⟨Location⟩ on the lateral side of the foot, below the tuberosity of the 5th metatarsal bone, at the junction of the red and white skin (Fig. 8.2). ⟨Regional anatomy⟩ skin → subcutaneous tissue → abductor muscle of little toe. There are the lateral dorsal cutaneous nerve of the foot and the lateral vein of the foot (the small saphenous vein) in this area. ⟨Indications⟩ manic-depressive disorder, headache, stiffness of the neck, vertigo, pain of the back and loin, pain of the back of the lower limbs. ⟨Method⟩ Puncture perpendicularly 0.3～0.5 cun. Moxibustion is applicable.

●腧穴[shù xué] 指脏腑经络之气输注出入的部位。名见宋代《铜人腧穴针灸图经》。又名节、会、气

穴、气府、砭灸处、骨空、孔穴、输、穴道、穴位，简称穴。腧穴既是针灸治疗的刺激点，又是某些病痛的反应点。人体的腧穴分别归属于经络，而经络又隶属于一定脏腑，这样就使腧穴—经络—脏腑间的相互联系成为不可分割的关系。历代对腧穴的认识不断丰富，一般将腧穴分为三大类：经穴、经外穴、阿是穴。详见各条。

Acupoint Spot, where the qi of zang-fu organs and meridians and collaterals flows in and out, originally from *Tongren Shuxue Zhenjiu Tujing (Illustrated Manual of Points for Acupuncture and Moxibustion on a Bronze Statue with Acupoints)* of the Song Dynasty, also called node, convergence, qi point, qi house, stone needling and moxibustion spot, bone hole, hole, transmission point path, point place, and simply called point. The Acupoint is both the stimulation point of acupuncture and moxibustion treatment and the reaction point of some diseases. Acupoints on the body pertain to the meridians respectively, and the meridians are also related to certain Zang and Fu organs, which makes the connections among acupoints, meridians and Zang-fu organs inseparable. Knowledge about acupoints has unceasingly been enriched in the successive dynasties. Gennerally, Acupoints are divided into 3 kinds: meridian points, extra points and Ashi points. →经穴(p. 215)、经外穴(p. 214)、阿是穴(p. 1)

●腧穴折衷[shù xué zhé zhōng] 书名。日本安井元越撰，两卷，刊于1764年。原书用汉语写成，书中考证《内经》等中国古医书，分记经穴位置并附以"师说"及按语，亦有颇多独到见解。

Shuxue Zhezhong (Acupoint Compromise) A book of 2 volumes written by a Japanese, Yasui Yakikosh, published in 1764. The original book was written in Chinese. In the book, the author did textual research on *Neijing (The Canon of Internal Medicine)* and other ancient Chinese medical books, wrote down the locations of meridian points and attached "the teacher's notes" and his own comments to it, among which, many unique views were put forward.

●率谷[shuài gǔ] 经穴名。出《针灸甲乙经》。属足少阳胆经，为足太阳、少阳之会。又名耳尖。〈定位〉在头部，当耳尖直上入发际1.5寸，角孙直上方（图28和图31）。〈层次解剖〉皮肤→皮下组织→耳上肌→颞筋膜→颞肌。布在耳颞神经和枕大神经会合支及颞浅动、静脉顶支。〈主治〉头痛、呕吐、小儿惊风。平刺0.5～1寸；可灸。

Shuaigu (GB 3) A meridian point, originally from *Zhenjiu Jia-Yi Jing (A-B Classic of Acupuncture and Moxibustion)*, a point on the Gallbladder Meridian of Foot-Shaoyang, the crossing point of Foot-Taiyang and Shaoyang, also named Erjian. 〈Location〉on the head, directly above the ear apex, 1.5 cun above the hairline, directly above Jiaosun (SJ 20) (Figs. 28&31). 〈Regional anatomy〉skin→subcutaneous tissue→superior auricular muscle→temporal fascia→temporal muscle. There are the anastomotic branches of the auriculotemporal and greater occipital nerves and the parietal branches of the superficial temporal artery and vein in this area. 〈Indications〉headache, vomiting, infant convulsion. 〈Method〉Puncture subcutaneously 0.5～1.0 cun. Moxibustion is applicable.

●双目通睛[shuāng mù tōng jīng] 即斜视的别名。详见该条。

Cross-Eye Another name for strabismus. →斜视(p. 506)

●水[shuǐ]。①病证名。出《灵枢·水胀》。即水肿。详见该条。②五行之一。

Water ①Another name for edema, a disease originally from *Ling Shu: Shuizhang (Miraculous Pivot: Edema)*→水肿(p. 411) ②One of the five elements.

●水病[shuǐ bìng] 即水肿。详见该条。

Watery Disease Another name for edema. →水肿(p. 411)

●水道[shuǐ dào] 经穴名。出《针灸甲乙经》。属足阳明胃经。〈定位〉在下腹部，当脐中下3寸；距前正中线2寸（图87和图40）。〈层次解剖〉皮肤→皮下组织→腹直肌鞘前壁外侧缘→腹直肌外侧缘。浅层布有第十一、十二胸神经前支和第一腰神经前支的前皮支及外侧皮支、腹壁浅动、静脉。深层有第十一、十二胸神经前支的肌支。〈主治〉小腹胀满、疝气、痛经、小便不利。直刺0.8～1.2寸；可灸。

Shuidao (ST 28) A meridian point, origi-

nally from *Zhenjiu Jia-Yi Jing* (*A-B Classic of Acupuncture and Moxibustion*), a point on the Stomach Meridian of Foot-Yangming. ⟨Location⟩ on the lower abdomen, 3 cun below the centre of the umbilicus and 2 cun lateral to the anterior midline (Figs. 87&40). ⟨Regional anatomy⟩ skin→subcutaneous tissue→lateral border of anterior sheath of rectus muscle of abdomen→lateral border of rectus muscle of abdomen. In the superficial layer, there are the anterior and lateral cutaneous branches of the anterior branches of the 11th and 12th thoracic nerves and the 1st lumbar nerve, and the superficial epigastric artery and vein. In the deep layer, there are the muscular branches of the anterior branches of the 11th and 12th thoracic nerves. ⟨Indications⟩ distention of the lower abdomen, hernia, dysmenorrhea, dysuria. ⟨Method⟩ Puncture perpendicularly 0.5~1.2 cun. Moxibustion is applicable.

●水分[shuǐ fēn] 经穴名。出《针灸甲乙经》。属任脉,又名中守,分水。⟨定位⟩在上腹部,前正中线上,当脐中上1寸(图43.1和图40)。⟨层次解剖⟩皮肤→皮下组织→腹白线→腹横筋膜→腹膜外脂肪→壁腹膜。浅层主要布有第九胸神经前支的前皮支及腹壁浅静脉的属支。深层有第九胸神经前支的分支。⟨主治⟩腹痛、腹胀、肠鸣、泄泻、翻胃、水肿、小儿陷囟、腰脊强急。直刺0.5~1寸;可灸。

Shuifen (RN 9) A meridian point, originally from *Zhenjiu Jia-Yi Jing* (*A-B Classic of Acupuncture and Moxibustion*), a point on the Ren meridian, also called Zhongshou, Fenshui. ⟨Location⟩ on the upper abdomen on the anterior midline, 1 cun above the centre of the umbilicus (Figs. 43.1&40). ⟨Regional anatomy⟩ skin→subcutaneous tissue→linea alba→transverse fascia→extraperitoneal fat tissue→parietal peritoneum. In the superficial layer, there are the anterior cutaneous branches of the anterior branch of the 9th thoracic nerver and the tributaries of the superficial epigastric vein. In the deep layer, there are the branches of the anterior branch of the 9th thoracic nerve. ⟨Indications⟩ abdominal pain and distention, borborygucus, diarrhea, regurgitation, edema, infantile depressed fontanel, rigidity of the back and spine. ⟨Method⟩ Puncture perpendicularly 0.5~1.0 cun. Moxibustion is applicable.

●水沟[shuǐ gōu] ①经穴名。出《针灸甲乙经》。属督脉,为督脉,手、足阳明之会。又名人中、鬼宫、鬼市。⟨定位⟩在面部,当人中沟的上1/3与中1/3交点处(图40和图5)。⟨层次解剖⟩皮肤→皮下组织→口轮匝肌。该处布有眶下神经的分支和上唇动、静脉。⟨主治⟩昏迷、晕厥、暑病、癫狂、痫证、急慢惊风、鼻塞、鼻衄、风水面肿、㖞僻、齿痛、牙关紧闭、黄疸、消渴、霍乱、瘟疫、脊背强痛、挫闪腰痛。向上斜刺0.3~0.5寸;或用指甲按掐;不灸。②部位名。指鼻下唇上中央之凹陷处。又称人中。

1. **Shuigou** (DU 26) A meridian point, originally from *Zhenjiu Jia-Yi Jing* (*A-B Classic of Acupuncture and Moxibustion*), a point on the Du Meridian, the crossing point of the Du Meridian, Hand-Yangming and Foot-Yangming, also called Renzhong, Guigong or Guishi. ⟨Location⟩ on the face, at the junction of the upper 1/3 and middle 1/3 of the philtrum (Figs. 40&5). ⟨Regional anatomy⟩ skin→subcutaneous tissue→orbicular muscle of mouth. There are the branches of the infraorbital nerve and the superior labial artery and vein in this area. ⟨Indications⟩ coma, syncope, summer-heat diseases, manic-depressive disorder, epilepsy, acute or chronic infantile convulsion, stuffy nose epistaxis, facial edema due to pathogenic wind, facial paralysis, toothache, trismus, jaundice, diabetes, cholera, pestilence, rigidity and pain of the back, lumbago due to contusion. ⟨Method⟩ Puncture obliquely upward 0.3~0.5 cun or press and nip with nails. Moxibustion is not applicable.

2. **Water-Ditch** A part of the body, referring to the middle depression below the nose and above the lip, also called philtrum.

●水鼓[shuǐ gǔ] 鼓胀证型之一。多因嗜酒无度或脾胃不运,水湿内积于腹而外溢于肤。证见腹部胀大如蛙,皮肤光亮,按之凹陷,移时方起,或有下肢水肿,脘腹膜胀,面色滞黄,怯寒,神倦,小便不利,大便溏薄,舌苔白腻,脉沉缓。治宜健脾益肾,调气行水。取脾俞、肾俞、水分、复溜、公孙。

Tympanites due to Fluid Retention One

type of tympanites mainly due to excessive drinking or failure of the spleen and stomach in transportation, leading to body fluid being retained in the abdomen and overflowing to the skin. 〈Manifestations〉 abdominal distension like the belly of a frog, lustroud abdominal color, depression that is shown to rebound or occasional edema in the lower limbs, distention in the epigastrium and abdomen, pallor complexion, chills, lassitude, difficult urination, loose stools, white and greasy tongue coating, deep and slow pulse. 〈Treatment principle〉 Strengthen the spleen and tonify the kidney, promote qi circulation and enhance water discharge. 〈Point selection〉 Pishu (BL 20), Shenshu (BL 23), Shuifen (RN 9), Fuliu (KI 7) and Gongsun (SP 4).

●水罐法[shuǐ guàn fǎ] 拔罐法的一种。见《外台秘要》。利用水蒸气的热力排去空气,使罐内形成负压,以吸着在皮肤上,一般多应用竹罐(吸筒),先放在清水或药液中煮沸3-5分钟,然后用镊子钳出,倒去水液,迅速用毛巾擦去罐口沸水,立即罩在选定部位上即能吸住,参见"拔罐法"条。

Cupping with Boiled Cup One of the cupping therapies, originally from *Waitai Miyao (Clandestine Essentials from the Imperial Library)*, referring to the method which discharges the air inside the cup by the heat of water vapor so as to form a negative pressure in the cup, then make the cup adhere to the skin. In most cases, a bamboo jar (suction-tube) is used. The jar is boiled in clean water or medical solution for 3～5 minutes, then, picked out with tweezers, the liquid is poured out quickly, the water on the jar mouth is quickly wiped off with towel and immediately made to cover and adhere to the selected point. →拔罐法(p.9)

●水灸[shuǐ jiǔ] 天灸的一种。见《理瀹骈文》。指用大蒜涂擦体表以治病的方法。可治疗瘰癧。

Juice Vesiculation A kind of medicinal vesiculation, seen in *Liyue Pianwen (A Rhymed Discourse on External Therapies)*, referring to the method used to treat diseases by rubbing the body surface with garlic. It can be used for treating tuberculosis.

●水门[shuǐ mén] 经穴别名。出《针灸甲乙经》。即水突。详见该条。

Shuimen Another name for Shuitu (ST 10), a meridian point originally from *Zhenjiu Jia-Yi Jing (A-B Classic of Acupuncture and Moxibustion)*. →水突(p.411)

●水气[shuǐ qì] 病症名。①指水肿。详见该条。②指水饮、痰饮。

Retained Fluid A disease, referring to ① edema. →水肿(p.411) ②excessive fluid and phlegm retention.

●水泉[shuǐ quán] ①经穴名。出《针灸甲乙经》。属足少阴肾经,为本经郄穴。又名水原。〈定位〉在足内侧,内踝后下方,当太溪直下1寸(指寸),跟骨结节的内侧凹陷处(图49和图46)。〈层次解剖〉皮肤→皮下组织→跟骨内侧面。浅层布有隐神经的小腿内侧皮支,大隐静脉的属支。深层有胫后动、静脉,足底同、外侧神经和跟内侧支(均是胫神经的分支)。〈主治〉月经不调、痛经、阴挺、小便不利、目昏花、腹痛。直刺0.3～0.5寸;可灸。②经穴别名。见《千金要方》。即大敦穴。详见该条。

1. **Shuiquan** (KI 5) A meridian point, originally from *Zhenjiu Jia-Yi Jing (A-B Classic of Acupuncture and Moxibustion)*, the Xi (Cleft) point of the Kidney Meridian of Foot-Shaoyin, also called Shuiyun. 〈Location〉 on the medial side of the foot, posterior and inferior to the medial malleolus, 1 cun directly below Taixi (KI 3), in the depression of the medial side of the tuberosity of the calcaneum (Figs. 49&46). 〈Regional anatomy〉 skin → subcutaneous tissue → medial side of calcaneus. In the superficial layer, there are the medial cutaneous branches of the saphenous nerve to the leg and the tributaries of the great saphenous vein. In the deep layer, there are the posterior tibial artery and vein, the medial and lateral plantar nerves and the medial calcaneal branches from the tibial nerve. 〈Indications〉 irregular menstruation, dysmonorrhea, prolapse of uterus, difficult urination, blurring of vision, abdominal pain. 〈Method〉 Puncture perpendicularly 0.3～0.5 cun. Moxibustion is applicable.

2. **Shuiquan** Another name for Dadun (LR 1), a meridian point seen in *Qianjin Yaofang*

(*Essential Prescriptions Worth a Thousand Gold*). →大敦(p.62)

●水突[shuǐ tū] 经穴名。出《针灸甲乙经》。属足阳明胃经。又名水门。〈定位〉在颈部,胸锁乳突肌的前缘,当人迎与气舍连线的中点(图40和图28)。〈层次解剖〉皮肤→皮下组织和颈阔肌→颈固有筋膜浅层及胸锁乳突肌→颈固有筋膜深层及肩胛舌骨肌、胸骨甲状肌。浅层布有颈横神经等结构。深层有甲状腺。〈主治〉咳逆上气、喘息不得卧、咽喉肿痛、肩肿、呃逆、瘿瘤、瘰疬。直刺0.3～0.4寸;可灸。

Shuitu (ST 10) A meridian point, originally from *Zhenjiu Jia-Yi Jing* (*A-B Classic of Acupuncture and Moxibustion*), a point on the Stomach Meridian of Foot-Yangming, also named Shuimen. 〈Location〉 on the neck on the anterior border of the sternocleidomastoid muscle, at the midpoint of the line connecting Renying (ST 9) and Qishe (ST 11) (Figs. 40&28). 〈Regional anatomy〉 skin→subcutaneous tissue and platysma muscle→superficial layer of cervical proper fascia and sternocleidomastoid muscle-deep layer of cervical proper fascia, omohyoid muscle and sternothyroid muscle. In the superficial layer, there is the transverse nerve of the neck. In the deep layer, there is the thyroid gland. 〈Indications〉 cough and dyspnea due to reversed flow of lung-qi, inability to lie down due to asthma, sore throat, swelling of the shoulder, hiccup, goiter, scrofula. 〈Method〉 Puncture perpendicularly 0.3～0.4 cun. Moxibustion is applicable.

●水穴[shuǐ xué] 经穴别名。见《外台秘要》。即扶突。详见该条。

Shuixue Another name for Futu (LI 18), a meridian point seen in *Waitai Miyao* (*Clandestine Essentials from the Imperial Library*). →扶突(p.118)

●水原[shuǐ yuán] 经穴别名。出《备急千金要方》。即水泉。详见该条。

Shuiyuan Another name for Shuiquan (KI 5), a meridian point originally from *Beiji Qianjin Yaofang* (*Essential Prescriptions for Emergencies Worth a Thousand Gold*). →水泉(p.410)

●水针[shuǐ zhēn] 针刺疗法的一种,又称穴位注射法,是选用中西药物注入有关穴位以治疗疾病的一种方法。一般选用低浓度的葡萄糖注射液、注射用水、中草药制剂或适于作肌肉注射的药液。用注射器配以细长针头(如5号齿科针头),缓缓注入穴位,不可伤及神经干或将药液注入血管等。注射量,根据药液品种和所选穴位而定,头部约0.1～0.5毫升,耳穴约0.1～0.2毫升,四肢部约0.5～2毫升,腰臂肌肉丰厚处约2～15毫升。如作小剂量穴位注射,剂量约为常规剂量的1/10～1/2。应用本法须熟悉药液性能,有些药物应先作过敏试验(如盐酸普鲁卡因等)。油剂及刺激性过强的药物不宜采用。

Solution-Injected Acupuncture One of the acupuncture therapies, also known as point injection therapy, referring to the method for treating diseases by injecting certain Chinese and Western medicines into relevant acupoints. Usually a low concentration glucose injection, water injection, herbal injection, or other medicaments for muscular injection are used. Inject the solution slowly into the point by using a slender and long syringe needle (e.g. No. 5 dental syringe needle). Be careful not to injure the nerve trunk or inject the solution into blood vessels. The injection dosage is determined according to what the drug is and which point is selected: on the head, about 0.1～0.5 ml; on auricular points, about 0.1～0.2 ml; on the four limbs, about 0.5～2 ml; on the lumbar region with abundant and thick muscles, about 2～15 ml. If the point injection with little dosage is needed, 1/10～1/2 of the routine dosage is recommended. One must be familiar with the effects of the medicament. A hypersensitivity test is required for some medicines (e.g. procaine hycrochloride, etc.). Oily and irritant injections are not suitable for this therapy.

●水肿[shuǐ zhǒng] 病证名。出《素问·水热穴论》。又名水,水气或水病。指人体水液潴留,泛溢肌肤,引起头面,目窠,四肢,腹部,甚至全身水肿而言。本病可因外邪或内伤引起。与肺、脾、肾三脏关系最为密切。临床上多分为阳水、阴水二种,详见各条。

Edema A disease, originally from *Suwen*: *Shui Re Xue Lun* (*Plain Questions*: *On Acupoints for Edema and Febrile Diseases*), also

called water, retained fluid, or watery diseases, referring to fluid retention in the body which overflows to the muscle and skin, leading to edema occurring in the head, face, eyes, limbs and abdomen, or all over the body. It may be caused by exopathogens or internal injury. It is closely related to disfunction of the lung, spleen and kidney. It is clinically divided into two types: yang edema and yin edema. →阳水(p.539)、阴水(p.558)

●睡圣散[shuì shèng sǎn] 古代麻醉药方。其药物组成是：山茄花(即蔓陀罗花，八月收)、火麻花(八月收)。采后研为末，每服三钱，小儿只一钱。见《扁鹊心书》。

Sleep Sage Powder An ancient anesthetic recipe. 〈Constitution〉 the flowers of *Shan Qie* (*Flos Datura*) and *Huo Ma*(*Cannabis Sativa*) (both harvested in August). Grind them into a powder and adminster it, 9 grams each time for an adult, and 3 grams for a child. This recipe was originally seen in *Bianque Xinshu* (*Bian Que's Medical Experience*).

●丝络[sī luò] 络脉名。出《针经指南》。指细小如丝的络脉。

Thready Collateral A category of collaterals, originally from *Zhenjing Zhinan* (*A Guide to the Classics of Acupuncture*), referring to collaterals which are thin as thread.

●丝竹[sī zhú] 经穴别名。见《太平圣惠方》。即丝竹空。详见该条。

Sizhu Another name for Sizhukong (SJ 23), a meridian point seen in *Taiping Shenghui Fang*(*Imperial Benevolent Prescriptions*). →丝竹空(p.412)

●丝竹空[sī zhú kōng] 经穴名。出《针灸甲乙经》。属手少阳三焦经。又名丝竹、目髎、巨髎。〈定位〉在面部，当眉梢凹陷处(图5)。〈层次解剖〉皮肤→皮下组织→眼轮匝肌。布有眶上神经、颧面神经、面神经颞支和颧支、颞浅动、静脉的额支。〈主治〉头痛、目眩、目赤痛、眼睑瞤动、齿痛、癫痫。平刺0.5~1寸；不宜灸。

Sizhukong (SJ 23) A meridian point, originally from *Zhenjiu Jia-Yi Jing* (*A-B Classic of Acupuncture and Moxibustion*), a point on the Sanjiao Meridian of Hand-Shaoyang, also called Sizhu, Mujiao, Jujiao. 〈Location〉 on the face, in the depression of the lateral end of the eyebrow (Fig. 5). 〈Regional anatomy〉 skin→subcutaneous tissue→orbicular muscle of eye. There are the supraorbital nerve, the zygomaticofacial nerve, the temporal and zygomatic branches of the facial nerve, and the frontal branches of the superficial temporal artery and vein in this area. 〈Indications〉 headache, blurred vision, redness and pain of the eye, twitching of the eyelid, toothache, epilepsy. 〈Method〉 Puncture subcutaneously 0.5~1.0 cun. Moxibustion is not applicable.

●四白[sì bái] 经穴名。出《针灸甲乙经》。属足阳明胃经。〈定位〉在面部，瞳孔直下，当眶下孔凹陷处(图28和图5)。〈层次解剖〉皮肤→皮下组织→眼轮匝肌、提上唇肌→眶下孔或上颌骨。浅层布有眶下神经的分支，面神经的颧支。深层在眶下孔内有眶下动、静脉和神经穿出。〈主治〉目赤肿痛、痒、目翳、眼睑瞤动、迎风流泪、头面疼痛、口眼歪斜、眩晕。直刺0.2~0.3寸；禁灸。

Sibai (ST 2) A meridian point, originally from *Zhenjiu Jia-Yi Jing* (*A-B Classic of Acupuncture and Moxibustion*), a point on the Stomach Meridian of Foot-Yangming. 〈Location〉 on the face, directly below the pupil, in the depression of the infraorbital foramen (Figs. 28&5). 〈Regional anatomy〉 skin→subcutaneous tissue→orbicular muscle of eye, levator muscle of upper lip→infraorbital foramen or maxilla. In the superficial layer, there are the branches of the infraorbital nerve and the zygomatic branches of the facial nerve. In the deep layer, the infraorbital artery, vein and nerve pass through the infraorbital foramen. 〈Indications〉 redness, pain and swelling of the eye, itch, corneal opacity, twitching of eyelids, epipgora, ache of the head and face, deviation of the mouth and eye and dizziness. 〈Method〉 Puncture perpendicularly 0.2~0.3 cun. Moxibustion is not applicable.

●四渎[sì dú] 经穴名。出《针灸甲乙经》。属手少阳三焦经。〈定位〉在前臂背侧，当阳池与肘尖的连线上，肘尖下5寸，尺骨与桡骨之间(图44.3和图48)。〈层次解剖〉皮肤→皮下组织→小指伸肌与尺侧腕伸肌→拇长展肌和拇长伸肌。浅层布有前臂后皮神经，

头静脉和贵要静脉的属支。深层有骨间后动、静脉和骨间后神经。〈主治〉暴喑、暴聋、齿痛、气短、咽阻如梗、前臂痛。直刺0.5～1寸；可灸。

Sidu（SJ 9） A meridian point, originally from *Zhenjiu Jia-Yi Jing* (*A-B Classic of Acupuncture and Moxibustion*), a point on the Sanjiao Meridian of Hand-Shaoyang. 〈Location〉on the dorsal side of the forearm and on the line connecting Yangchi(SJ 4) and the tip of the olecranon, 5 cun distal to the tip of the olecranon, between the radius and ulna (Figs. 44.3&48). 〈Regional anatomy〉skin→subcutaneous tissue→extensor muscle of little finger and ulnar extensor muscle of wrist→long abductor and extensor muscle of thumb. In the superficial layer, there are the posterior cutaneous nerve of the forearm and the tributaries of the cephalic and basilic veins. In the deep layer, there are the posterior interosseous artery and vein and the posterior interosseous nerve. 〈Indications〉sudden hoarseness of voice, sudden deafness, toothache, shortness of breath, a subjective sensation as if the throat were compressed, pain in the forearm. 〈Method〉Puncture perpendicularly 0.5～1 cun. Moxibustion is applicable.

● 四缝[sì fèng] 经外穴名。见《奇效良方》。〈定位〉在第二至五指掌侧，近端指关节的中央，一手四穴，左右共八穴。〈层次解剖〉皮肤→皮下组织→指深屈肌腱。分布有指掌侧固有动、静脉的分支或属支和指皮下静脉。食指和中指的四缝穴由正中神经的指掌侧固有神经分布，环指的四缝穴，桡侧的一支来自正中神经的指掌侧固有神经，尺侧的一支来自尺神经的指掌侧固有神经，小指的四缝穴由来自尺神经的指掌侧固有神经分布。主治小儿疳积、小儿消化不良、百日咳、肠蛔虫症、手指关节炎等。点刺，挤出黄白色粘液。

Sifeng（EX-UE 10） A set of extra points, originally seen in *Qixiao Liangfang* (*Prescriptions of Wonderful Efficacy*). 〈Location〉Four points on each hand, on the palmar side of the 2nd to 5th fingers at the centre of the proximal interphalangeal joints. 〈Regional anatomy〉skin→subcutaneous tissue→tendon of deep digital flexor muscle. The blood vessels in the area of each point are the branches or tributaries of the proper palmar digital artery and vein and the subcutaneous digital vein. The nerve in the area of the point between the thumb and index or between the index and middle fingers is the proper palmar digital nerve from the median nerve; between the middle and ring fingers is the proper palmar digital nerve from the median nerve for the radial side and from the ulnar nerve for the ulnar side; between the index and little fingers is the proper palmar digital nerve from the ulnar nerve. 〈Indications〉malnutrition syndrome in children, ascariasis, arthritis of fingers, etc. 〈Method〉Prick with a three-edged needle and squeeze out a small amount of yellowish viscous fluid.

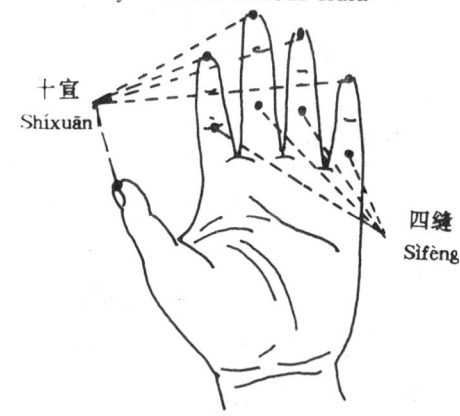

图54 四缝、十宣穴
Fig. 54 Sifeng point

● 四根三结[sì gēn sān jié] 见《标幽赋》、《针灸指南》。指经脉以四肢末端为根，称为"四根"；以头、胸、腹三部的一定部位为结，称为"三结"。说明四肢与头身之间经脉和穴位主治上的相互联系。临床上取四肢穴位治疗头面躯干疾病，与根结之间的相互联系有关。

Four Sources and Three Tubers Originally seen in *Biaoyou Fu* (*Lyrics of Recondite Principles*) and *Zhenjiu Zhinan* (*A Guide to Acupuncture and Moxibustion*). The meridians originate at the ends of the four limbs (the extremities) and concentrate at certain portions of the head, chest and abdomen. Therefore, the ends of the limbs are named the four sources, and the parts of the head, chest and abdomen are named three tubers. They are used to illustrate the relationship of the

meridians and point indications of the four limbs with those of the head and truck. That points on the limbs are clinically selected to treat diseases of the head, face and trunk is relevant to the relationship between sources and tubers.

●四海[sì hǎi] 出《灵枢·海论》。指人身水谷、气、血、髓所汇聚之处。脑为髓海，冲脉为血海，膻中为气海，胃为水谷之海。

Four Seas Originally from *Lingshu*: *Hai Lun* (*Miraculous Pivot*: *On Seas*), referring to the convergent places of food, qi, blood and marrow. The brain is the sea of marrow, the Chong Meridian that of blood, Danzhong (RN 17) that of qi and the stomach that of food stuff.

●四合[sì hé] 出《灵枢·经别》。指手太阳与手少阴经别相合。

Four Confluences Originally from *Lingshu*: *Jingbie* (*Miraculous Pivot*: *Divergent Meridians*), referring to the convergence of the divergent meridians of Hand-Taiyang and Hand-Shaoyin.

●四横纹[sì héng wén] 经外穴名。又称指根、下四缝。见《中国针灸学》。其位于第二、三、四、五指指掌横纹之中点处，左右计八穴。〈主治〉手部疔疮、五指尽痛、腹痛、呕吐，并可解热。点刺出血。

Sihengwen (EX-UE) Set of extra points, also called Zhigen or Xiasifeng, originally seen in *Zhongguo Zhenjiuxue* (*Chinese Acupuncture and Moxibustion*). 〈Location〉four points on each hand, on the palmar side of the 2nd to 5th fingers, at the midpoints of the metacarpophalangeal transversal creases. 〈Indications〉furuncle of hand, pain of fingers, abdominal pain, vomiting, fever. 〈Method〉Prick with a three-edged needle and squeeze out some blood.

●四花[sì huā] 组合穴。见《外台秘要》。又称经门四花。即足太阳膀胱经的胆俞、膈俞四穴。〈主治〉劳瘵、咳嗽、哮喘、虚弱羸瘦等。用灸法。

Sihua Set of points, originally seen in *Waitai Miyao* (*Clandestine Essentials from the Imperial Library*), also called Jingmensihua, referring to the four points on the Bladder Meridian of Foot-Taiyang, i.e. Danshu (BL 19) and Geshu (BL 17). 〈Indications〉consumptive diseases, cough, asthma, asthenia and thinness. 〈Method〉moxibustion.

●四华[sì huá] 即四花穴。详见该条。

Sihua →四花(p. 414)

●四街[sì jiē] 气街的别称。详见该条。

Four Streets →气街(p. 308)

●四经[sì jīng] 指肝、心、肺、肾四条经脉。出《素问·阴阳别论》。因其与春、夏、秋、冬四时相应。故名。

Four Merdians Referring to the four meridians of the Liver, Heart, Lung and Kidney, originally seen in *Suwen*: *Yinyang Bielun* (*Plain Questions*: *Supplementary Exposition of Yin and Yang*). It is so named because the four meridians correspond respectively to the four seasons, i.e. spring, summer, autumn and winter.

●四满[sì mǎn] ①经穴名。出《针灸甲乙经》。属足少阴肾经，为冲脉、足少阴之会。又名髓府、髓中。〈定位〉在下腹部，当脐中下2寸，前正中线旁开0.5寸(图40)。〈层次解剖〉皮肤→皮下组织→腹直肌鞘前壁→腹直肌。浅层布有腹壁浅动、静脉的分支或属支，第十、十一、十二胸神经前支的前皮支和伴行的动、静脉。深层有腹壁下动、静脉的分支或属支，第十、十一、十二胸神经前支的肌支和相应的肋间动、静脉。〈主治〉月经不调、崩漏、带下、不孕、产后恶露不净、小腹痛、遗精、遗尿、疝气、便秘、水肿。直刺0.8～1.2寸；可灸。②经外穴名。出《备急千金要方》。位于脐下2寸旁开1.5寸处。主治月经不调、奔豚、不孕等。用灸法。

1. Siman (KI 14) A meridian point, originally from *Zhenjiu Jia-Yi Jing* (*A-B Classic of Acupuncture and Moxibustion*), a point on the Kidney Meridian of Foot-Shaoyin, a crossing point with the Chong Meridian, also called Suifu or Suizhong. 〈Location〉on the lower abdomen, 2 cun below the centre of the umbilicus and 0.5 cun lateral to the anterior midline (Fig. 40). 〈Regional anatomy〉skin→subcutaneous tissue→anterior sheath of rectus muscle of abdomen→rectus muscle of abdomen. In the superficial layer, there are the branches or tributaries of the superficial epigastric artery and vein, the anterior cutaneous

branches of the anterior branches of the 10th to 12th thoracic nerves and the accompanying arteries and veins. In the deep layer, there are the branches or tributaries of the inferior epigastric artery and vein, the muscular branches of the anterior branches of the 10th to 12th thoracic nerves and the related intercostal arteries and veins. ⟨Indications⟩ menxenia, uterine bleeding, leukorrhagia, sterility, persistent postpartum lochia, lower abdominal pain, emission, neuresis nernia, constipation, edema. ⟨Method⟩ Puncture perpendicularly 0.8~1.2 cun. Moxibustion is applicable.

2. **Siman**(EX-CA) An extra point, originally seen in *Beiji Qianjin Yaofang* (*Essential Prescriptions for Emergencies Worth a Thousand Gold*). ⟨Location⟩ on the lower abdomen, 2 cun below the centre of the umbilicus and 1.5 cun lateral to the anterior midline. ⟨Indications⟩ menoxenia, sensation of gas rushing (like a running pig), sterility, etc. ⟨Method⟩ moxibustion.

●四气街[sì qì jiē] 气街的的别名。详见该条。

Four Qi-Streets →气街(p. 308)

●四神聪[sì shén cōng] 经外穴名。出《银海精微》。又名神聪。〈定位〉在头顶部,当百会前后左右各1寸,共四穴。〈层次解剖〉皮肤→皮下组织→帽状腱膜→腱膜下疏松结缔组织。该处布有枕动、静脉、颞浅动、静脉顶支和眶上动、静脉的吻合网,有枕大神经,耳颞神经及眶上神经的分支。〈主治〉中风、头痛、眩晕、癫痫、狂乱及神经衰弱等。沿皮刺0.3~0.5寸;可灸。

Sishencong (EX-HN 1) A set of extra points, originally seen in *Yinhai Jingwei* (*Essentials of Silvery Sea*), also called Shencong. ⟨Location⟩ four points on the vertex of the head, 1 cun anterior, posterior, and lateral to Baihui (DU 20). ⟨Regional anatomy⟩ skin →subcutaneous tissue→epicranial aponeurosis → subaponeurotic loose connective tissue. There are the network anastomosed by the occipital artery and vein, the parietal branches of the superficial temporal artery and vein with the supraorbital artery and vein, and the branches of the greater occipital, auriculoctemopral nerves in this area. ⟨Indications⟩ apoplexy, headache, dizziness, epilepsy, manic-depressive disorders, and neurasthenia, etc. ⟨Method⟩ Puncture subcutaneously 0.3~0.5 cun. Moxibustion is applicable.

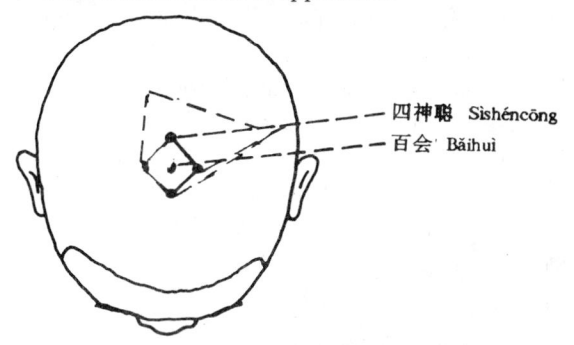

图55 四神聪穴
Fig. 55 Sishencong point

●四弯风[sì wān fēng] 病名。出《医宗金鉴》。由风邪袭入腠理兼挟湿热所致。常见于儿童。好发于对称的肘窝、腘窝、踝侧等处。患处皮肤粗糙肥厚,瘙痒,搔破流水不多。时轻时重,迁延难愈。详见"湿疹"条。

Si Wan Feng (**Atopic Eczema**) A disease, originally from *Yizong Jinjian* (*Gold Mirror of Orthodox Medical Lineage*), due to pathogenic wind accompanied by damp-heat invading the muscular striae, commonly seen in children. It often occurs symmetrically in the antecubital and popliteal fossa, and ankle side, etc. ⟨Manifestations⟩ rough and thick skin with itching, little fluid when soratched and ruptured. Sometimes serious and sometimes light, it is difficult to cure. →湿疹(p. 373)

●四周取穴[sì zhōu qǔ xué] 即邻近取穴。详见该条。

All-Around Point Selection →邻近取穴(p. 247)

●四总穴歌[sì zǒng xué gē] 针灸歌赋名。《针灸大全》首载。即:"肚腹三里留,腰背委中求,头项寻列缺,面口合谷收。"其简要概括了足三里、委中、列缺、合谷这四个常用穴的远道主治作用,为历来针灸学习者传诵。

Si Zongxue Ge (**A Verse about the Four General Acupoints**) An acupuncture and moxibustion verse, originally recorded in *Zhenjiu Daqun* (*A Complete Work of Acupuncture*

and Moxibustion), reading, "Puncture Zusanli(ST 36) to treat diseases in the abdomen; select Weizhong(BL 40) to treat those in the loin or back; search for Lieque(LU 7) if one is affected in the head or neck and take Hegu (LI 4) for the treatment of diseases in the mouth and face." It briefly summarized the distant curative functions of the four commonly used acupoints—Zusanli (ST 36), Weizhong(BL 40), Lieque(LU 7) and Hegu (LI 4). The verse has long been read by students of acupuncture and moxibustion.

●溲血[sōu xuè] 即尿血。详见该条。

Bloody Urine →尿血(p.284)

●嗽血[sòu xuè] 即咳血。详见该条。

Cough with Blood →咳血(p.232)

●素髎[sù liáo] 经穴名。出《针灸甲乙经》。属督脉，又名面王、面玉、面正、鼻准。〈定位〉在面部，当鼻尖的正中央(图40和图28)。〈层次解剖〉皮肤→皮下组织→鼻中隔软骨和鼻外侧软骨，布有筛前神经鼻外支及面动、静脉的鼻背支。〈主治〉鼻塞、鼻衄、鼻流清涕、鼻中瘜肉、鼻渊、酒齄鼻、惊厥、昏迷、新生儿窒息。向上斜刺0.3～0.5寸；或点刺出血；不灸。

Suliao (DU 25) A meridian point, originally seen in *Zhenjiu Jia-Yi Jing (A-B Classic of Acupuncture and Moxibustion)*, a point on the Du meridian, also called Mianwang, Mianyu, Mianzheng or Bizhun. 〈Location〉on the face, at the centre of the nose apex (Figs. 40&28). 〈Regional anatomy〉skin→subcutaneous tissue→septal cartilage of nose and lateral nasal cartilage. There are the lateral nasal branches of the anterior ethmoidal nerve and the dorsal nasal branches of the facial artery and vein in this area. 〈Indcations〉nasal obstruction, epistaxis, watery nasal discharge, nasal polypus, rhinorrhea, ache rosacea, convulsion, loss of consciousness, asphyxia neonatorum. 〈Method〉Puncture obliquely upward 0.3～0.5 cun, or prick to cause bleeding. Moxibustion is forbidden.

●素问[sù wèn] 书名。与《灵枢》合称《内经》，为中医学现存最早的著作。原书九卷，第七卷已遗失。王冰于其中补入七篇大论。该书系统阐述了中医学的基本理论，内有许多有关针灸的重要论述。

Suwen(*Plain Questions*) A book, which, together with *Lingshu (Miraculous Pivot)*, is known as *Neijing* (*The Inner Canon of Huangdi*) and is the earliest extant literature in Traditional Chinese Medicine. It originally had 9 volumes, of which the 7th has already lost. Wang Bing added his seven great chapters into the book. In this book, the fundamental theories were systematically enunciated, and a lot of important discussions on acupuncture and moxibustion were involved.

●蒜钱灸[suàn qián jiǔ] 为隔蒜灸之别称。详见该条。

Moxibustion with Garlic and Coin →隔蒜灸 (p.137)

●随变而调气[suí biàn ěr tiáo qì] 针灸治疗原则之一。语见《灵枢·卫气失常》。意指根据病变部位的深浅和病情的轻重等情况，分别采用适当的针灸治法来调气。

Regulating Qi According to Pathogenic Changes One of the general principles of acupuncture therapy, originally seen in *Lingshu：Wei Qi Shichang (Miraculous Pivot：Abnormalities of Defensive Qi)*, referring to the regulation of qi with appropriate acupuncture methods accoring to the depth of the affected part and the condition of the disease.

●随而济之[suí ěr jì zhī] 刺法用语。见《难经·七十九难》。与"迎而夺之"相对，为迎随补法的原则。补法要顺着经脉循行方向而刺，以补益其经气的不足。

Reinforcing by Puncturing a Point Following its Meridian Course An acupuncture method, originally seen in *Nanjing：Qishijiu Nan (The Classic of Questions：Question 79)*. As opposed to "reducing by puncturing a point against its meridian course", this is a principle of "reinforcing achieved by needling in the direction which the needle tip points to." The reinforcing is done by puncturing a point along its meridian course to make up for the deficiency of the meridian qi.

●随年壮[suí nián zhuàng] 灸法用语。见《千金翼方》卷二十七。指随年龄的大小而决定灸的壮数，即年几岁，灸几壮。

Age Moxa Cones A moxibustion term, orig-

inally seen in Vol. 27 of *Qianjin Yifang* (*Supplement to the Essential Prescriotions Worth a Thousand Gold*), referring to the method of deciding the number of moxa cones to be used by the patient's age, namely, the number of moxa cones equals the age.

●随症取穴[suí zhèng qǔ xué] 取穴法之一。根据疾病的症候而选用有治疗作用的穴位。如发热取大椎，胸闷取内关，痰多取丰隆，腹痛取足三里等。

Symptomatologic Point Selection A method of acupoint selection, referring to the method of choosing curative points according to symptoms, e.g. select Dazhui (DU 14) for fever, Neiguan (PC 4) for choking sensation in the chest, Fenglong (ST 40) for profuse sputum, Zusanli (ST 36) for abdominal pain.

●髓府[suí fǔ] 经穴别名。出《针灸甲乙经》。即四满，详见该条。

Suifu Another name for Siman (KI 14), a meridian point originally seen in *Zhenjiu Jia-Yi Jing* (*A-B Classic of Acupuncture and Moxibustion*). →四满(p. 414)

●髓海[suí hǎi] 四海之一。出《灵枢·海论》。指脑。脑是髓液汇集之处。故称。其气血输注出入的重要穴位，上在头顶中央的百会穴，下在风府。其证候：髓海有余，则轻劲多力，自过其度，髓海不足，则脑转耳鸣，胫酸眩冒，目无所见，懈怠安卧。

Sea of Marrow One of the four seas, originally from *Lingshu*: *Hai Lun* (*Miraculous Pivot: On Seas*), referring to the brain. It is so named because the bone marrow and cerebrospinal fluid converge in the brain. The important points for the entrance and exit of qi and blood of the marrow reservoir are, in the upper portion, Baihui (DU 20) and in the lower portion Fengfu (DU 16). 〈Manifestations〉 excess syndromes which include sensations of light body and strength, activity exceeding the normal limit; asthenia syndrome including dizziness, tinnitus, sore tibiae, vertigo, blindness, lassitude of limbs and addiction to lying.

●髓空[suí kōng] 经穴别名。出《针灸甲乙经》。即腰俞。详见该条。

Suikong Another name for Yaoshu (DU 2), a meridian point originally seen in *Zhenjiu Jia-Yi Jing* (*A-B Classic of Acupuncture and Moxibustion*). →腰俞(p. 545)

●髓孔[suí kǒng] ①经穴别名。出《针灸甲乙经》。即大迎。详见该条。②经穴别名。出《外台秘要》。即腰俞。详见各条。

Suikong Another name for ①Daying (ST 5), a meridian point originally seen in *Zhenjiu Jia-Yi Jing* (*A-B Classic of Acupuncture and Moxibustion*). →大迎(p. 65) ②Yaoshu (DU 2), a meridian point originally seen in *Waitai Miyao* (*Clandestine Essentials from the Imperial Library*). →腰俞(p. 545)

●髓俞[suí shù] 经穴别名。见《针灸大全》。即腰俞。详见该条。

Suishu Another name for Yaoshu (DU 2), a meridian point originally from *Zhenjiu Daquan* (*A Complete Work of Acupuncture and Moxibustion*). →腰俞(p. 545)

●髓中[suí zhōng] 经穴别名。出《针灸聚英》。即四满。详见该条。

Suizhong Another name for Siman (KI 14), a meridian point originally seen in *Zhenjiu Juying* (*Essentials of Acupuncture and Moxibustion*). →四满(p. 414)

●孙鼎宜[sūn dǐng yí] 人名。清代医学家。曾据《针灸甲乙经》所载补辑《明堂孔穴附针灸治要》。参见该条。

Sun Dingyi A medical expert of the Qing Dynasty. He compiled *Mingtang Kongxue Fu Zhenjiu Zhiyao* (*An Outline of Points for Acupuncture and Moxibustion*), on the basis of what is recorded in *Zhenjiu Jia-Yi Jing* (*A-B Classic of Acupuncture and Moxibustion*). →明堂孔穴针灸治要(p. 269)

●孙络[sūn luò] 指络脉的分支。出《素问·气穴论》。又称孙脉。

Minute Collaterals Branches of the collaterals, originally from *Suwen*: *Qixue Lun* (*Plain Questions*: *On Loci of Qi*), also called minute vessels.

●孙脉[sūn mài] 孙络的别名。详见该条。

Minute Vessels Another name for minute collaterals. →孙络(p. 417)

●孙思邈[sūn sī miǎo] 人名。唐代著名医学家，京兆华原(今陕西耀县)人。其精于养生，深研医学，总结了唐以前的医学理论及临床经验，著成《千金要方》和《千金翼方》两书。书内均有针灸专篇。

Sun Simiao A well-known medical expert in the Tang Dynasty, a native from Huayuan, Jingzhao (now Yaoxian County, Shanxi Province). He was conversant in health preservation, made profound research on medicine, summed up the medical theories and the clinical experience prior to the Tang Dynasty, and wrote *Qianjin Yaofang* (*Prescriptions Worth a Thousand Gold*) and *Qianjin Yifang* (*A Supplement to the Prescriptions Worth a Thousand Gold*). There are special chapters on acupuncture and moxibustion in both books.

●孙思邈针经[sūn sī miǎo zhēn jīng] 书名,唐代孙思邈撰。见《宋史·艺文志》,已佚。

Sun Simiao Zhenjing (Sun Simiao's Classic of Acupuncture), A book, written by Sun Simiao of the Tang Dynasty, seen in *Songshi*: *Yiwen Zhi* (*The History of the Song Dynasty*: *Records of Art and Literature*), already lost.

●孙卓三[sūn zhuō sān] 人名。明代针灸家,浮梁(今江西景德镇北)人,精于针灸,治病多用土法,有良效,在当地闻名。事见《饶州府志》。

Sun Zhuosan An acupuncture-moxibustion expert of the Ming Dynasy, a native from Fuliang (now north of the town of Jingde, Jiangxi Province). Proficient in acupuncture, he often applied indigenous methods which were very effective in the treatment of diseases, and was well-known throughout his native place. His deeds were recorded in *Raozhoufu Zhi* (*Annals of Raozhoufu*).

●缩脚肠痈[suō jiǎo cháng yōng] 即肠痈。详见该条。

Acute Appendicitis with Legs Flinching → 肠痈(p.41)

●锁骨[suǒ gǔ] 耳穴名。〈定位〉将耳舟部分为六等分,自上而下,第六等份为锁骨。用于治疗肩关节周围炎,无脉症。

Clavicle (MA-SF 5) An auricular point. 〈Location〉Divide the scapha area into 6 equal parts, of which, from superior to inferior the 6th part is clavicle. 〈Indications〉periarthritis of the shoulder and pulseless disease.

●所生病[suǒ shēng bìng] 经脉病候用语。出《灵枢·经脉》。在每条经脉循行之后,接叙"是动则病……"及"是主某所生病者……"意指这一经脉在异常变动时就会出现有关病症,而这一经脉的穴位即能主治该经脉所发生的病症。

Meridian Diseases due to Related Organs A term for meridian diseases, originally from *Lingshu*: *Jingmai* (*Miraculous Pivot*: *Meridians*). In this chapter, there is a description of each meridian, followed by such sentences as "The pathogenic change of a meridian is manifested as ···", and "The points on the meridian can be used to treat ···", which means a certain disease will occur on account of the abnormal change of a certain meridian, and the points of the meridian can be selected for the treatment of the disease.

T

●他经取穴[tā jīng qǔ xué] 即异经取穴。详见该条。

Selection of Points on Other Meridians → 异经取穴(p.552)

●胎风[tāi fēng] 子痫的别名。详见该条。

Spasm due to Fetus Another name for eclampsia. →子痫(p.627)

●胎位不正[tāi wèi bù zhèng] 胞不正的别名,详见该条。

Malposition of Fetus Another name for abnormal position of fetus. →胞不正(p.13)

●胎癣[tāi xuǎn] 即奶癣。详见该条。

Fetal Eczema →奶癣(p.276)

●胎衣不出[tāi yī bù chū]　即胞衣不下。详见该条。

Retardative Fetus　Another name for retention of placenta. →胞衣不下(p.14)

●胎衣不下[tāi yī bù xià]　即胞衣不下。详见该条。

Lingering Fetus　Another name for retention of placenta. →胞衣不下(p.14)

●太白[tài bái]　经穴名。出《灵枢·本输》。属足太阴脾经，为本经输穴、原穴。〈定位〉在足内侧缘，当足大趾本节(第一跖趾关节)后下方赤白肉际凹陷处(图49和图39.1)。〈层次解剖〉皮肤→皮下组织→展肌→短屈肌。浅层布有隐神经、浅静脉网等。深层有足底内侧动、静脉的分支或属支，足底内侧神经的分支。〈主治〉胃痛、腹胀、腹痛、肠鸣、呕吐、泄泻、痢疾、便秘、痔漏、脚气、饥不欲食、善噫、食不化、心痛脉缓、胸胁胀痛、体重节痛、痿证。直刺0.3~0.5寸；可灸。

Taibai(SP 3)　A meridian point, originally from *Lingshu: Benshu* (*Miraculous Pivot: Meridian Points*), the Shu(Stream) point and Yuan(Primary) point of the Spleen Meridian of Foot-Taiyin. 〈Location〉on the medial border of the foot, in the depression of the junction of the red and white skin, posterior and inferior to the 1st metatarsophalangeal joint(Figs. 49&39.1). 〈Regional Anatomy〉skin→subcutaneous tissue→abductor muscle of geart toe→short flexor muscle of great toe. In the superficial layer, there are the saphenous nerve and the superficial venous network. In the deep layer, there are the branches or tributaries of the medial plantar artery and vein and the branches of the medial plantar nerve. 〈Indications〉stomachache, abdominal distention, abdominal pain, borborygaus, vomiting, diarrhea, dysentery, constipation, anal hemorrhoid, beriberi, hunger with anorexia, frequent eructation, dyspepsia, precordial pain with slow pulse, distention and pain in the chest and hypochondrium, heavy sensation in the body and aching joints, flaccidity syndrome. 〈Method〉Puncture perpendicularly 0.3~0.5 cun. Moxibustion is applicable.

●太仓[tài cāng]　①经穴别名。出《针灸甲乙经》。即中脘。详见该条。②部位名。见《灵枢·胀论》。指胃部。

1. **Taicang**　Another name for Zhongwan (RN 12), a meridian point originally from *Zhenjiu Jia-Yi Jing* (*A-B Classic of Acupuncture and Moxibustion*). →中脘(p.614)

2. **Big Granary**　A part of the body, seen in *Lingshu: Zhang Lun* (*Miraculous Pivot: Treatise on Distention*), referring to the gastric region, the stomach.

●太冲[tài chōng]　经穴名。出《灵枢·本输》。属足厥阴肝经，为本经输穴、原穴。又名大冲。〈定位〉在足背侧，当第一跖骨间隙的后方凹陷处(图17.2)。〈层次解剖〉皮肤→皮下组织→拇长伸肌腱与趾长伸肌腱之间→拇短伸肌腱的外侧→第一骨间背侧肌。浅层布有足背静脉网、足背内侧皮神经等。深层有腓深神经和第一跖背动、静脉。〈主治〉头痛、眩晕、疝气、月经不调、癃闭、遗尿、小儿惊风、癫狂、痫证、胁痛、腹胀、黄疸、呕逆、咽喉嗌干、目赤肿痛、膝股内侧痛、足跗肿、下肢痿痹。直刺0.5~0.8寸；可灸。

Taichong(LR 3)　A meridian point, originally from *Lingshu: Benshu* (*Miraculous Pivot: Meridian Points*), the Shu(Stream) point and Yuan(Primary) point of the Liver Meridian of Foot-Jueyin, also known as Dachong. 〈Location〉on the instep of the foot, in the depression of the posterior end of the 1st interosseous metatarsal space(Fig. 17.2). 〈Regional anatomy〉skin→subcutaneous tissue→between tendons of long extensor muscle of great toe and long extensor muscle of toes→lateral side of short extensor muscle of great toe→1st dorsal interosseous muscle. In the superficial layer, there are the venous network of the dorsum of the foot and the medial dorsal cutaneous nerve of the foot. In the deep layer, there are the deep peroneal nerve and the 1st dorsal metatarsal artery and vein. 〈Indications〉headache, vertigo, hernia, irregular menstruation, dysuria and uroschesis, enuresis, infantile convulsion, manic-depressive psychosis, epilepsy, hypochondriac pain, abdominal distention, jaundice, vomiting, sore throat and dry throat, redness, swelling and pain of the eyes, pain in the medial aspect

of the femur and knee, swelling of the dorsum of the foot, flaccidity and numbness of the lower limbs. ⟨Method⟩ Puncture perpendicularly 0.5~0.8 cun. Moxibustion is applicable.

●太冲脉[tài chōng mài] 经脉名。出《素问·上古天真论》。指冲脉。详见该条。

Great Chong Vessel Another name for the Chong Meridian, a meridian originally from *Suwen: Shanggu Tianzhen Lun (Plain Questions: On Preservation of Congenital Primary Qi of the Ancient People)* →冲脉(p. 48)

●太陵[tài líng] 经穴别名。出《针灸甲乙经》。即大陵。详见该条。

Tailing Another name for Daling (PC 7), a meridian point originally from *Zhenjiu Jia-Yi Jing (A-B Classic of Acupuncture and Moxibustion)*. →大陵(p. 64)

●太泉[tài quán] 经穴别名。见《千金翼方》。即太渊。详见该条。

Taiquan Another name for Taiyuan (LU 9), a meridian point seen in *Qianjin Yifang (A Supplement to the Essential Prescriptions Worth a Thousand Gold)*. →太渊(p. 423)

●太溪[tài xī] 经穴名。出《灵枢·本输》。属足少阴肾经,为本经输穴、原穴。又名吕细、大溪、内昆仑。⟨定位⟩在足内侧,内踝后方,当内踝尖与跟腱之间的凹陷处(图49和图83)。⟨层次解剖⟩皮肤→皮下组织→胫骨后肌腱、趾长屈肌腱与跟腱、跖肌腱之间→拇长屈肌。浅层布有隐神经的小腿内侧皮支,大隐静脉的属支。深层有胫神经和胫后动、静脉。⟨主治⟩头痛、目眩、咽喉肿痛、齿痛、耳聋、耳鸣、咳嗽、气喘、胸痛、咯血、消渴、月经不调、失眠、健忘、遗精、阳萎、小便频数、腰脊痛、下肢厥冷、内踝肿痛。直刺0.5~0.8寸;可灸。

Taixi (KI 3) A meridian point, originally from *Lingshu: Benshu (Miraculous Pivot: Meridian Points)*, the Shu (Stream) point and Yuan (Primary) point of the Kidney Meridian of Foot-Shaoyin, also called Lüxi, Daxi or Neikunlun. ⟨Location⟩ on the medial side of the foot, posterior to the medial malleolus, in the depression between the tip of the medial malleolus and Achilles tendon (Figs. 49&83). ⟨Regional anatomy⟩ skin → subcutaneous tissue → between tendons of posterior tibial muscle and long flexor muscle of toes and tendon of plantar muscle and Achilles tendon → long flexor muscle of great toe. In the superficial layer, there are the medial cutaneous branches of the saphenous nerve to the leg and the tributaries of the great saphenous vein. In the deep layer, there are the tibial nerve and the posterior tibial artery and vein. ⟨Indications⟩ headache, dizziness, swelling and pain of the throat, toothache, deafness, tinnitus, cough, dyspnea, pain in the chest, hemoptysis, diabetes, irregular menstruation, insomnia, amnesia, emission, impotence, frequent micturition, pain in the lower back and along the spinal column, cold lower limbs, swelling and pain of the medial malleolus. ⟨Method⟩ Puncture perpendicularly 0.5~0.8 cun. Moxibustion is applicable.

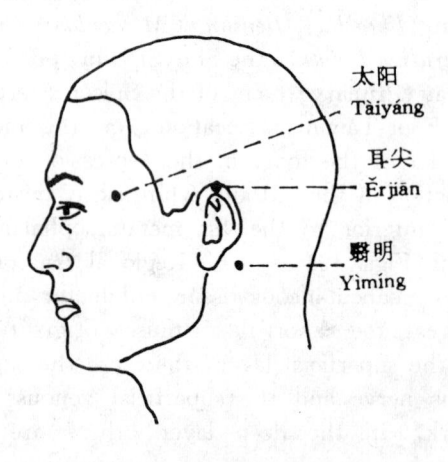

图56 太阳、耳尖、翳明穴
Fig. 56 Taiyang, Erjian, and Yiming points

●太阳[tài yáng] ①经脉名。包括手太阳小肠经和足太阳膀胱经,与少阴经互为表里。②经外穴名。见《银海精微》等。别名前关、当阳。⟨定位⟩在颞部,当眉梢与目外眦之间,向后约一横指的凹陷处。⟨层次解剖⟩皮肤→皮下组织→眼轮匝肌→颞筋膜→颞肌。该处布有颧神经的分支颧面神经,面神经的颞支和颧支,下颌神经的颞神经和颞浅动、静脉的分支或属支。⟨主治⟩头痛、面瘫、目疾、牙痛等。直刺0.3~0.5寸,或沿皮刺0.5~1寸,或三棱针点刺出血。③经穴

别名。出《千金要方》注,即瞳子髎。详见该条。④耳针穴位。现耳穴名称为颞。在对耳屏中区外侧,对耳屏软骨边缘,枕和额二穴之间,常用于治疗偏、正头痛,眩晕,眼痛等。⑤部位名。为颞之别称。详见该条。

1. **Taiyang** Name of meridians, including the small Intestine Meridian of Hand-Taiyang and the Bladder Meridian of Foot-Taiyang. They have an exterior-interior interrelationship with Shaoyin Meridians.

2. **Taiyang**(EX-HN 5) An extra point, seen in *Yinhai Jingwei* (*Essentials of Ophthalmology*), etc., also called Qianguan, Dangyang. 〈Location〉at the temporal part of the head, between the lateral end of the eyebrow and the outer canthus, in the depression one finger breadth behind them. 〈Regional anatomy〉skin → subcutaneous tissue → orbicular muscle of eye → temporal fascia → temporal muscle. There are the zygomaticofacial branch of zygomatic nerve, the temporal and zygomatic branches of the facial nerve, the temporal nerve of the mandibular nerve and the branches or tributaries of the superficial temporal artery and vein in this area. 〈Indications〉headache, facial paralysis, eye diseases, toothache, etc. 〈Method〉Puncture perpendicularly 0.3～0.5 cun or subcutaneously 0.5～1 cun. Prick to cause bleeding with a three-edged needle.

3. **Taiyang** Another name for Tongziliao (GB 1), a meridian point, originally from an annotation on *Qianjin Yaofang*(*Essential Prescriptions Worth a Thousand Gold*). →瞳子髎 (p. 443)

4. **Taiyang** (MA) An auricular point. Its present-day name is Temple (MA). 〈Location〉between Occiput(MA) and Forehead (MA), on the edge of antitragus cartilage, at the lateral aspect of the central part of the antitragus. 〈Indications〉migraine, headache, vertigo, ophthalmalgia, etc.

5. **Taiyang** Another name for the temple, a part of the body. →颞(p. 285)

●太一[tài yī] 经穴别名。出《千金要方》。即太乙。详见该条。

Taiyi Another name for Taiyi(ST 23), a meridian point originally from *Qianjin Yaofang* (*Essential Prescriptions Worth a Thousand Gold*). →太乙(p. 421)

●太乙[tài yǐ] 经穴名。出《针灸甲乙经》。属足阳明胃经。〈定位〉在上腹部,当脐中上2寸,距前正中线2寸(图87和图40)。〈层次解剖〉皮肤→皮下组织→腹直肌鞘前壁→腹直肌。浅层布有第八、九、十胸神经前支的外侧皮支和前支及腹壁浅静脉。深层有腹壁上动、静脉的分支或属支,第八、九、十胸神经前支的肌支。〈主治〉癫狂、心烦不宁、胃痛、消化不良。直刺0.8～1.2寸;可灸。

Taiyi (ST 23) A meridian point, originally from *Zhenjiu Jia-Yi Jing* (*A-B Classic of Acupuncture and Moxibustion*), a point on the Stomach Meridian of Foot-Yangming.〈Location〉on the upper abdomen, 2 cun above the centre of the umbilicus and 2 cun lateral to the anterior midline (Figs. 87&40).〈Regional Anatomy〉skin→subcutaneous tissue→anterior sheath of rectus muscle of abdomen→rectus muscle of abdomen. In the superficial layer, there are the lateral and anterior cutaneous branches of the anterior branches of the 8th to 10th thoracic nerves and the superficial epigastric vein. In the deep layer, there are the branches or tributaries of the superior epigastric artery and vein and the muscular branches of the anterior branches of the 8th to 10th thoracic nerves.〈Indications〉manic-depressive psychosis, vexation and restlessness, stomachache, indigestion.〈Method〉Puncture perpendicularly 0.8～1.2 cun. Moxibustion is applicable.

●太乙神针[tài yǐ shén zhen] ①艾条灸的一种。出《太乙神针心法》。将掺有一定成份药末的艾条一端燃着,用布七层包扎后,按于穴上,冷则易之,每穴约灸5～7次。其艾条中所掺药物,各家所载不一。近代多以檀香、山柰、羌活、桂枝、木香、雄黄、白芷、沉香、独活、硫黄、甘松、香附、丹参、细辛等药末,与艾绒混合制成艾条。②书名。清代邱时敏编,成书于清光绪四年(1878年)。

1. **Taiyi Miraculous Moxa Roll** One of the methods of moxa roll moxibustion, originally from *Taiyi Shenzhen Xinfa* (*Experiences in Moxibustion with Great Monad Herbal Stick*).〈Method〉Ignite one end of the moxa roll con-

taining herbal powder, wrap it in 7 layers of cloth, and put it on the point. Change it when it becomes cool. Moxibustion should be applied 5~7 times for each point. The herbs mixed into moxa rolls vary in different medical books. In modern times, moxa rolls are made from a mixture of moxa wool and powder, commonly made of *Tan Xiang* (*Lignum Santali*), *Shan Nai* (*Rhizoma Kaempferiae*), *Qiang Huo* (*Rhizoma Seu Radix Notopterygii*), *Gui Zhi* (*Ramulus Cinnamomi*), *Mu Xiang* (*Radix Auklandae*), *Xiong Huang* (*Realgar*), *Bai Zhi* (*Radix Angelicae Dahuricae*), *Chen Xiang* (*Lignum Aquilariae Resinatum*), *Du Huo* (*Radix Angelicae Pubescentis*), *Liu Huang* (*Sulfur*), *Gan Song* (*Rhizoma Nardostachyos*), *Xiang Fu* (*Rhizoma Cyperi*), *Dan Shen* (*Radix Salviae Miltiorrhizae*) and *Xi Xin* (*Herba Asari*).

2. **Taiyi Shen Zhen**（Magic Moxibustion with Great Monad Herbal Stick） A medical book compiled by Qiu Shimin of the Qing Dynasty and finished in the 4th year of Guang Xu's reign of the Qing Dynasty (1878)

●太乙神针方[tài yǐ shén zhēn fāng] 书名。清代陈惠畴编,冯卓怀订正。成书于同治年间(1862—1874年)。

Taiyi Shenzhen Fang（Recipes of Great Monad Herbal Moxa Stick） A medical book compiled by Chen Huichou of the Qing Dynasty with revisions made by Feng Zhuohuai. It was completed in the reign of Tongzhi (1862-1874) of the Qing Dynasty.

●太乙神针集解[tài yǐ shén zhēn jí jiě] 书名。清代孔广培撰,刊于1872年。本书是在《太乙神针》基础上增订而成,为讨论药卷灸法的著作。

Taiyi Shenzhen Jijie（Exposition on Methods of Moxibustion with Great Monad Herbal Stick） A medical book by Kong Guangpei of the Qing Dynasty, published in 1872. It was revised and enlarged on the basis of *Taiyi Shenzhen*（*Magic Moxibustion with Great Monad Herbal Stick*）and is a monograph on the discussion of the methods of moxa roll moxibustion with herbal medicine.

●太乙神针心法[tài yǐ shén zhēn xīn fǎ] 书名。清代韩贻丰撰。书分两卷,上卷为证治法,下卷有针治医案,书后附太乙神针传授渊源诚文。成书于康熙五十六年(1717年)。为我国现存最早的太乙针专著。

Taiyi Shenzhen Xinfa（Experiences in Moxibustion with Great Monad Herbal Stick） A two-volume book written by Han Yifeng of the Qing Dynasty. Vol. 1 is about syndromes and therapeutic methods and Vol. 2 is about the medical records of acupuncture. Attached to it is the admonishment on the regin of Taiyi's miraculous moxa roll. This book, completed in the 56th year of Kang Xi's reign, is the earliest extant monograph on Taiyi's miraculous moxa roll.

●太阴[tài yīn] ①经脉名。出《素问·阴阳离合论》。包括手太阴肺经和足太阴脾经,与阳明经互为表里。②经外穴名。出《外台秘要》。位于内踝直上,胫骨内侧缘后凹陷中。左右计二穴。灸治脚气等。③经穴别名。出《千金要方》。即三阴交。详见该条。

1. **Taiyin** Name of meridians, originally from *Suwen*：*Yinyang Lihe Lun* (*Plain Questions*：*On the Parting and Meeting of Yin and Yang*), including the Lung Meridian of Hand-Taiyin and the Spleen Meridian of Foot-Taiyin. They have an exterior-interior interrelationship with Yangming Meridians.

2. **Taiyin**（EX-LE） An extra point, originally from *Waitai Miyao* (*The Medical Secrets of an Official*). ⟨Location⟩ directly above the medial malleolus, in the depression of posterior border of medial aspect of tibia, two points in all in the left and right lower limbs. ⟨Indication⟩ beriberi. ⟨Method⟩ moxibustion.

3. **Taiyin** Another name for Sanyinjiao（SP 6）, a meridian point originally from *Qianjin Yaofang*（*Essential Prescriptions Worth a Thousand Gold*）. →三阴交（p.346）

●太阴络[tài yīn luò] 经穴别名。见《千金要方》。即漏谷。详见该条。

Taiyinluo Another name for Lougu（SP 7）, a meridian point seen in *Qianjin Yaofang* (*Essential Prescriptions Worth a Thousand Gold*). →漏谷（p.256）

●太阴脉[tài yīn mài] 早期经脉名。出马王堆汉墓《帛书》。指足太阴经。

Taiyin Vessel An ancient name for a meridian, originally from *Boshu* (*Silk Book*), which was unearthed in a Han Dynasty tomb near Mawangdui, referring to the Meridian of Foot-Taiyin.

●太阴蹻[tài yīn qiāo] 经穴别名。见《外台秘要》。即照海。详见该条。

Taiyinqiao Another name for Zhaohai (KI 6), a meridian point seen in *Waitai Miyao* (*Clandestine Essentials from the Imperial Library*), →照海(p. 586)

●太渊[tài yuān] 经穴名。出《灵枢·九针十二原》。属手太阴肺经，为本经输穴、原穴、八会穴之脉会。又名太泉、大泉、鬼心。〈定位〉在腕掌侧横纹桡侧，桡动脉搏动处(图49和图16)。〈层次解剖〉皮肤→皮下组织→桡侧腕屈肌腱与拇长展肌腱之间。浅层有前臂外侧皮神经，桡神经浅支和桡动脉浅支等分布。深层有桡动、静脉等。〈主治〉咳嗽、气喘、咳血、呕血、烦满、胸背痛、掌中热、缺盆中痛、喉痹、腹胀、噫气、呕吐、妒乳、无脉症、手腕无力疼痛。直刺0.2～0.3寸；可灸。

Taiyuan (LU 9) A meridian point, originally from *Lingshu*: *Jiu Zhen Shier Yuan* [*Miraculous Pivot*: *The Nine Needles and Twelve Yuan* (*Primary*) *Points*], the Shu (Stream) point and Yuan (Primary) point of the Lung Meridian of Hand-Taiyin, and the influential point of pulse, also known as Taiquan, Daquan or Guixin. 〈Location〉 at the radial end of the crease of the wrist, where the pulsation of the radial artery is palpable (Figs. 49&16). 〈Regional Anatomy〉 skin→subcutaneous tissue→between tendons of radial flexor muscle of wrist and long abductor muscle of thumb. In the superficial layer, there are the lateral cutaneous nerve of the forearm, the superficial branches of the radial nerve and the superficial palmar branches of the radial artery. In the deep layer, there are the radial artery and vein. 〈Indications〉 cough, dyspnea, hemoptysis, hematemesis, vexation, pain in the chest and back, heat sensation in the palms, pain in the supraclavicular forssa, sore throat, abdominal distention, eructation, vomiting, acute mastitis, pulseless disease, wrist weakness with pain. 〈Method〉 Puncture perpendicualry 0.2～0.3 cun. Moxibustion is applicable.

●太钟[tài zhōng] 经穴别名。见《素问·刺腰痛论》王冰注。即大钟。详见该条。

Taizhong Another name for Dazhong (KI 4), a meridian point seen in Wang Bing's annatation on *Su Wen*: *Ci Yaotong Lun* (*Plain Question*: *On Treatment of Lumbago With Acupuncture*). →大钟(p. 66)

●太祖[tài zǔ] 经外穴别名。即崇骨。详见该条。

Taizu Another name for the extra point Chonggu(EX). →崇骨(p. 50)

●弹法[tán fǎ] 针刺辅助手法名。①见《针经指南》。为十四法之一。指针刺后用手指弹动针柄，以加强针感。②指针刺前用手指弹动皮肤，以利得气。

Flicking An auxiliary needling method, ①. seen in *Zhenjing Zhinan* (*A Guide to the Classic of Acupuncture*), one of the Fourteen Methods, referring to flicking the handle of the needle after insertion to strengthen the needling sensation. ② referring to flicking the regional skin with fingers before puncturing to promote the arrival of qi.

●痰火心悸[tán huǒ xīn jì] 心悸证型之一。多因饮食伤脾，湿盛生痰，郁而化热，痰火内扰，神不守舍所致。证见心悸时发时止、烦躁不宁、胸闷、头晕、失眠多梦、容易惊醒、口苦、咳嗽咯痰稠粘、小便黄、大便不爽、舌苔黄腻、脉滑数。治宜清火化痰，取灵道、郄门、肺俞、尺泽、丰隆。

Palpitation due to Phlegm-Fire A type of palpitation, mostly due to impairment of the spleen resulting from improper diet, and the formation of phlegm due to excessive dampness, which stagnates and produces heat, and phlegm-fire which disturbs inside the body leading to mental derangement. 〈Manifestations〉 intermittent palpitations, irritability, restlessness, oppression feeling in the chest, dizziness, insomnia and dreamy sleep, waking up easily with a start, bitter taste, cough with pituitary sputum, dark urine, dyschezia, yellow greasy tongue coating, slippery and rapid pulse. 〈Treatment principle〉 Clear fire and remove phlegm. 〈Point selection〉 Lingdao (HT 4), Ximen (PC 4), Feishu (BL

13), Chize (LU 5), and Fenglong (ST 40).

●痰厥[tán jué] 厥证证型之一。见《世医得效方》。指因痰盛气闭而引起的厥证。证见突然昏厥、喉中痰鸣、或呕吐涎沫、呼吸气粗、舌苔白腻、脉沉滑。治宜苏厥化痰。针水沟、内关、巨阙、丰隆。

Syncope due to Phlegm A type of syncope, seen in *Shiyi De Xiaofang* (*Effective Formulas Handed Down for Generations*), referring to syncope due to the blockage of qi resulting from phlegm. 〈Manifestations〉 sudden syncope, wheezing sound in throat, or vomiting saliva with foam, asthma, white greasy tongue coating, deep and slipery pulse. 〈Treatment principle〉 Restore consciousness and remove phlegm. 〈Point selection〉 Shuigou (DU 26), Neiguan (PC 6), Juque (RN 14), and Fenglong (ST 40). 〈Method〉 acupuncture.

●痰热哮喘[tán rè xiāo chuǎn] 哮喘证型之一。由于风热与痰饮互结,肺失清肃所致。证见咳喘气粗、喉中痰鸣如吼、面红、发热有汗、痰黄质稠、咯痰不爽、口渴、烦躁、咳引胸痛、舌苔黄腻、脉浮洪或滑数。治宜清热化痰平喘。取合谷、大椎、丰隆、尺泽、孔最、内关。

Asthma due to Phlegm-Heat A type of asthma. It is due to the accumulation of wind-heat and phlegm retention and the impairment of the lung in purifying and descending. 〈Manifcstations〉 cough with gasping, loud rale in the throat, flushed complexion, fever with sweating, thick yellow sputum which is difficult to discharge, thirst, dysphoria, cough inducing pain of chest, yellow greasy tongue coating, superficial and surging or slippery and rapid pulse. 〈Treatment principle〉 Clear heat, disperse phlegm and relieve asthma. 〈Point selection〉 Hegu (LI 4), Dazhui (DU 14), Fenglong (ST 40), Chize (LU 5), Kongzui (LU 6), and Neiguan (PC 6).

●痰湿不孕[tán shī bù yùn] 不孕证型之一。多因体质肥盛,恣食厚味,痰湿内生,影响冲任胞络,难以摄精成孕。证见形体肥胖、头晕心悸、白带量多、月经不调、舌苔白腻、脉滑。治宜健脾燥湿化痰。取中极、气冲、四满、丰隆、中髎、太冲。

Sterility due to Phlegm-Dampness A type of sterility, mostly due to phlegm and dampness resulting from obesity and a fatty diet which obstruct the Chong and Ren Meridians and affects uterine fertization. 〈Manifestations〉 obesity, dizziness and palpitation, profuse leukorrhea, irregular menstruation, white greay tongue coating, slippery pulse. 〈Treatment principle〉 Strengthen the spleen, eliminate dampness and reduce phlegm. 〈Point selection〉 Zhongji (RN 3), Qichong (ST 30), Siman (KI 14), Fenglong (ST 40), Zhongliao (BL 33), and Taichong (LR 3).

●痰湿咳嗽[tán shī ké sòu] 咳嗽证型之一。因痰湿壅肺,肺气不得宣降所致。证见咳嗽多痰、痰白而粘、胸脘满闷、身重易倦、舌苔白腻、脉濡滑。治宜健脾化湿、宣肺利气。取太渊、太白、尺泽、丰隆、合谷。

Cough due to Phlegm-Dampness A type of cough, due to the accumulation phlegm-dampness in the lung, and obstruction of the lung-qi. 〈Manifestations〉 cough with profuse phlegm, pituitary and white sputum, oppressive feeling in the chest and stomach, heavy sensation in the limbs, lassitude, white greasy tongue coating, and soft slippery pulse. 〈Treatment principle〉 Invigorate the spleen to eliminate dampness, ventilate the lung to relieve functional disturbance of the lung-qi. 〈Point selection〉 Taiyuan (LU 9), Taibai (SP 3), Chize (LU 5), Fenglong (ST 40) and Hegu (LI 4).

●痰湿月经过少[tán shī yuè jīng guò shǎo] 月经过少证型之一。多因素体肥胖、躯脂过盛,或嗜食厚味,痰湿内生,阻塞经脉,以致冲任血行涩滞。证见月经过少、色淡质稀、兼见白带量多、面色㿠白、头晕心悸、下肢轻度浮肿等。治宜健脾燥湿化痰。取建里、中脘、脾俞、胃俞、足三里、三阴交、丰隆。

Scanty Menstruation due to Phlegm-Dampness A type of scanty menstruation, mostly due to obesity, excessive fat in the body, or a rich fatty diet which produces phlegm-dampness in the interior obstructing the meridians. This leads to stasis of blood in the Chong and Ren Meridians. 〈Manifestations〉 scant, light coloured and thin menses with profuse leukorrhea, pale complexion, dizziness and palpitation, mild edema of the lower limbs, etc. 〈Treatment principle〉 Strengthen the spleen,

eliminate dampness and resolve phlegm. ⟨Point selection⟩ Jianli (RN 11), Zhongwan (RN 12), Pishu (BL 20), Weishu (BL 21), Zusanli (ST 36), Sanyinjiao (SP 6), and Fenglong (ST 40).

●痰湿阻滞经闭[tán shī zǔ zhì jīng bì] 经闭证型之一。多因脾失健运，痰湿内盛，阻于冲任所致。证见经闭不行、形体肥胖、胸胁满闷、神疲倦怠、白带量多、苔腻脉滑。治宜健脾化痰。取中极、地机、合谷、三阴交、丰隆、次髎。

Amenorrhea due to Stagnation of Phlegm-Dampness One type of amenorrhea, mostly due to dysfunction of the spleen in transportation, excessive phlegm-dampness inside the body, which obstructs the Chong and Ren Meridians. ⟨Manifestations⟩ obstruction of menses, obesity, fullness and tightness in the chest and hypochondrium, fatigue and lassitude, profuse leukorrhea, greasy tongue coating and slippery pulse. ⟨Treatment principle⟩ Strengthen the spleen and reduce phlegm. ⟨Point selection⟩ Zhongji (RN 3), Diji (SP 8), Hegu (LI 4), Sanyinjiao (SP 6), Fenglong (ST 40) and Ciliao (BL 32).

●痰饮呕吐[tán yǐn ǒu tù] 呕吐证型之一。见《证因脉治》卷二。因痰饮内停，胃气不降所致。证见呕吐多为清水痰涎、脘闷不食、头眩心悸、苔白腻、脉滑。治宜蠲饮化痰。取章门、公孙、中脘、丰隆、足三里、内关。

Vomiting due to Retention of Phlegm One type of vomiting, seen in *Zheng Yin Mai Zhi* (*Symptoms, Causes, Pulse Conditions and Treatments*). It is due to the retention of phlegm inside the body and failure of the stomach-qi to descend. ⟨Manifestations⟩ vomiting with watery phlegm, fullness in the stomach and anorexia, dizziness and palpitation, white and greasy tongue coating, slippery pulse. ⟨Treatment principle⟩ Remove fluid and resolve phlegm. ⟨Point selection⟩ Zhangmen (LR 13), Gongsun (SP 4), Zhongwan (RN 12), Fenglong (ST 40), Zusanli (ST 36) and Neiguan (PC 6).

●痰滞恶阻[tán zhì è zǔ] 恶阻证型之一。多因脾虚失运，痰湿内生，孕后经血闭阻，冲脉之气上逆，痰饮随逆气上冲所致。证见妊娠初期、呕吐痰涎、胸闷纳呆、心悸气短、口淡乏味、苔白腻、脉滑。治宜健脾化痰，降逆和胃。取阴陵泉、丰隆、足三里、中脘、幽门。

Morning Sickness due to Phlegm Stagnation A type of morning sickness, mostly due to dysfunction of the spleen in transportation, phlegm-dampness produced in the interior, stagnation and stasis of the blood in the meridians during the early days of pregnancy, upward adverse flow of qi of the Chong Meridian accompanied with phlegm fluid. ⟨Manifestations⟩ in the initial period of pregnancy, vomiting with phlegm-salivation, oppressive feeling in the chest and loss of appetite, palpitations and short breath, lack of taste, white greasy tongue coating, slippery pulse. ⟨Treatment principle⟩ Strengthen the spleen and reduce phlegm, lower the adverse flow of qi and regulate the stomach. ⟨Point selection⟩ Yinlingquan (SP 9), Fenglong (ST 40), Zusanli (ST 36), Zhongwan (RN 12) and Youmen (KI 21).

●痰浊乳癖[tán zhuó rǔ pǐ] 乳癖证型之一。多因忧思伤脾，痰湿阻滞乳络而成。其证除见乳癖一般症状外，兼见眩晕、恶心、胸闷脘痞、食少便溏、咳嗽痰涎、苔腻、脉滑。治宜化痰通络。取膺窗、丰隆、膻中、脾俞、中脘。参见"乳癖"条。

Breast Nodules due to Phlegm Turbidity A type of breast nodules, mostly due to melancholy and anxiety impairing the spleen and leading to the stagnation of phlegm in the collaterals of the breast. ⟨Manifestations⟩ apart from the common symptoms of breast-nodules usually accompanied with vertigo, nausea, oppressive feeling in the chest and fullness in the gastric region, poor appetite and diarrhea, cough with sputum and salivation, greasy tongue coating, slippery pulse. ⟨Treatment principle⟩ Resolve phlegm and remove the obstruction in the collaterals. ⟨Point selection⟩ Yingchuang (ST 16), Fenglong (ST 40), Danzhong (RN 17), Pishu (BL 20), Zhongwan (RN 12). →乳癖 (p. 339)

●痰浊头痛[tán zhuó tóu tòng] 头痛证型之一。见《张氏医通》。由痰浊上蒙所致。证见头额昏痛如裹、胸脘痞闷、恶心、呕吐痰涎、便溏、舌苔白腻、脉滑。治

宜化痰降浊,通络止痛。取中脘、丰隆、百会、印堂、丝竹空。

Headache due to Phlegm Turbidity A type of headache, seen in *Zhangshi Yitong* (*Zhang's Treatise on General Medicine*). It is due to the head being confused by phlegm-dampness. 〈Manifestations〉 headache, dizziness with a tightening feeling in the forehead, fullness in the chest and stomach, nausea, vomiting with phlegm-salivation, loose stool, white greasy tongue coating, slippery pulse. 〈Treatment principle〉 Resolve phlegm and lower turbidity, remove the obstruction in the collaterals to relieve pain. 〈Point selection〉 Zhongwan (RN 12), Fenglong (ST 40), Baihui (DU 20), Yintang (EX-HN 3) and Sizhukong (SJ 23).

●痰浊胸痹[tán zhuó xiōng bì] 胸痹证型之一。因痰浊盘踞,胸阳闭阻不通所致。证见胸闷如窒而痛、气短喘促、咳嗽痰多粘腻色白,舌苔白腻、脉濡缓。治宜通阳化浊。取巨阙、膻中、郄门、太渊、丰隆。

Obstruction of Qi in the Chest due to Phlegm Turbidity A type of obstruction to stagnation of phlegm resulting from qi in the chest, due to the retention of phlegm-dampness confusing and obstructing the chest-yang. 〈Manifestations〉 choking pain in the chest, shortness of breath, cough with copious whitish pituitary sputum, white greasy tongue coating, soft and slightly slow pulse. 〈Treatment principle〉 Promote the circulation of yang and resolve turbidity. 〈Point selection〉 Juque (RN 14) Danzhong (RN 17), Ximen (PC 4), Taiyuan (LU 9) and Fenglong (ST 40).

●桃枝灸[táo zhī jiǔ] 即神针火。详见该条。

Peach-Twig Cauteriztion →神针火(p.364)

●陶瓷针[táo cí zhēn] 古代以陶瓷碎片砭刺。参见"陶针"、"瓷针"条。

Pottery and Porcelain Needles In ancient times, pottery and porcelain fragments were used for needling. →陶针(p.426)、瓷针(p.53)

●陶道[táo dào] 经穴名。出《针灸甲乙经》。属督脉,为督脉、足太阳之会。〈定位〉在背部,当后正中线上,第一胸椎棘突下凹陷中(图12.2和图7)。〈层次解剖〉针刺穿过的层次结构同脊中穴。浅层主要布有第一胸神经后支的内侧皮支和伴行的动、静脉。深层有棘突间的椎外(后)静脉丛,第一胸神经后支的分支和第一肋间后动、静脉背侧支的分支或属支。〈主治〉头痛项强、恶寒发热、咳嗽、气喘、骨蒸潮热、胸痛、脊背酸痛、疟疾、癫狂、角弓反张。斜刺0.5~1寸;可灸。

Taodao (DU 13) A meridian point, originally from *Zhenjiu Jia-Yi Jing* (*A-B Classic of Acupuncture and Moxibustion*), a point on the Du Meridian, the crossing point of the Du Meridian and Foot-Taiyang. 〈Location〉 on the back, on the posterior midline, in the depression below the spinous process of the 1st thoracic vertebra (Figs. 12.2&7). 〈Regional anatomy〉 The layer structures of the needle insertion are the same as those in Jizhong (DU 6). In the superficial layer, there are the medial cutaneous branches of the posterior branches of the 1st thoracic nerve and the accompanying artery and vein. In the deep layer, there are the external (posterior) vertebral venous plexus between the adjacent spinous processes, the branches of the posterior branchs of the 1st thoracic nerve and the branches or tributaries of the dorsal branches of the 1st posterior intercostal artery and vein. 〈Indications〉 headache and rigidity of the nape, fever and aversion to cold, cough, dyspnea, hectic fever due to yin-deficiency, pain in the chest, aching pain in the spine and back, malarial disease, manic-depressive psychosis and opisthotonus. 〈Method〉 Puncture obliquely 0.5~1 cun. Moxibustion is applicable.

●陶针[táo zhēn] 古代针具。古代以陶瓦碎片砭刺。现在广西壮族民间还有用陶针治疗疾病的。一般用废旧陶瓷片洗净敲碎制成,并按其锋芒大小分别使用。粗者用于重刺放血,细者可用于小儿,一般多取中者。针刺部位常取背正中线、夹脊穴以及腹正中线、夹脐旁线等。

Pottery Needle An ancient needling apparatus. In ancient times, pottery fragments were used for needling. Today, the people of Zhuang nationality in Guangxi Province still use pottery needles to treat diseases. Usually, the needles are made of fragments of waste or used pottery which have been cleaned. Their

uses vary according to the sizes of cutting edges. The big ones are used for pricking heavily to cause bleeding, the small ones for children, the medium-sized for general use. The needling regions are usually on the posterior midline, Jiaji (EX-B 2) points, the anterior midline and the lines lateral to the umbilcus, etc.

●套管进针[tào guǎn jìn zhēn] 进针法之一。用稍短于所用毫针的空心细管垂直放在穴位上,将平柄的毫针放入管内,快速叩击露出的针柄,使针尖迅速刺入皮下,然后抽去套管。这一方法可减少进针的痛感。

Inserting the Needle Through a Pipe One of the methods of needle insertion. Put a small hollow pipe, which is a bit shorter than the needle, vertically on the point, place a flat-handle filiform needle in the pipe, knock the exposed handle quickly to enable the needle tip to be punctured into the skin, and then take away the pipe. This method can reduce the painful sensation during insertion.

●套管式皮肤针[tào guǎn shì pí fū zhēn] 皮肤针的一种。呈圆柱状,上端有弹簧装置,按压时有细针数枚从底面的小孔中伸出,浅刺皮肤以治病。适用于小儿或畏针者。参见"皮肤针"条。

Casing-Type Dermal Needle A kind of dermal needle, shaped like a cylinder with a spring device installed on the upper end, when the device is pressed, several fine needles, which are used in shallow puncturing to treat skin diseases, come out through the small holes at the bottom. It is suitable for children and patients who fear needling. →皮肤针(p. 292)

●特定穴[tè dìng xué] 经穴分类名。指十四经中具有特殊治疗作用,并有特定称号的腧穴。包括在四肢肘、膝以下的五腧穴、原穴、络穴、郄穴、八脉交会穴、下合穴;在胸腹、背腰部的背俞穴、募穴;在四肢躯干部的八会穴以及全身经脉的交会穴。详见各条。

Specific Points A catalogue of the meridian points, referring to those with special therapeutic effects and having specific names, including the Five Shu Points, Yuan (Primary) Points, Luo (Connecting) Points, Xi (Cleft) Points, Eight Confluence Points and Lower Confluent Points located below the elbow and knee; Back-Shu Points on the back, and Front-Mu Points on the chest and abdomen; Eight Influential Points on the limbs and trunk and Crossing Points of the meridians in the whole body. →五腧穴(p. 479) 原穴(p. 577)、络穴(p. 260)、郄穴(p. 485)、八脉交会穴(p. 7)、下合穴(p. 487)、背俞穴(p. 16)、募穴(p. 274)、八会穴(p. 6)、交会穴(p. 193)

●提插补泻[tí chā bǔ xiè] 针刺补泻法之一。见《黄帝内经》。针刺时以提针和插针的轻重缓急来区分补

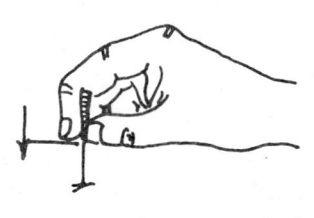

插针法   Thrusting method   提针法   Lifting method

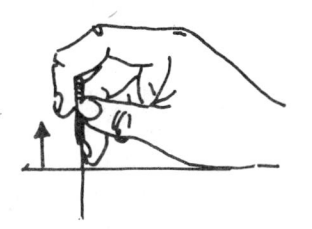

图57 提 插 法
Fig. 57 Lifting and Thrusting

泻。方法：在得气的基础上，将针由浅向深反复地重插轻提为补；反之，将针由深向浅重提轻插为泻。

Reinforcing and Reducing by Lifting and Thrusting the Needle One of the reinforcing and reducing methods, seen in *Huangdi Neijing*(*The Yellow Emperor's Canon of Internal Medicine*). Reinforcing and reducing are distinguished by the strength and speed of lifting and thrusting during needling. 〈Method〉 When qi is obtained, reinforcing is achieved by repeated heavy thrusts and gentle lifting of the needle from shallow to deep, whereas reducing is achieved by repeated heavy lifting and gentle thrusting of the needle from deep to shallow.

●提插法[tí chā fǎ] 针刺基本手法之一。针尖进至所刺部位的一定深度后，做上下、进退针的动作，使针从浅层插至深层，再由深层提到浅层，如此反复地上提下插。这种行针手法，称为提插法。

Lifting and Thrusting One of the basic needling techniques. When the needle is inserted to a given depth at the point, apply lifting and thrusting of the needle, i.e. make the needle go from the shallow layer to the deep layer by thrusting it and from the deep layer to the shallow layer by lifting it. The lifting and thrusting is done repeatedly. This manipulation is called the method of lifting and thrusting.

●提法[tí fǎ] 针刺手法名。见《金针赋》。为十四法之一。与按（插）法对举，指将针上提的动作。其法本于《难经》"动而伸之"。伸，就是提的意思。《针经指南》十四法，将伸、提列作"动"法的内容。《金针赋》则另分出。参见"动而伸之"条。

Lifting A needling method seen in *Jinzhen Fu* (*Ode to Gold Needle*). One of the 14 Methods, as opposed to thrusting, referring to lifting the needle. It is based on "stretching while moving" as is seen in *Nanjing* (*The Classic of Questions*). "Stretching" here means lifting. Both stretching and lifting are included in the contents of the "moving" method in the 14 Methods of *Zhenjing Zhinan* (*A Guide to the Classic of Acupuncture*). Yet, they were separately stated in *Jinzhen Fu* (*Ode to Gold Needle*). →动而伸之(p.84)

●提捏进针[tí niē jìn zhēn] 进针方法之一。以一只手拇指和食指将针刺部位的皮肤捏起，另一只手持针于捏起处刺入。本法多用于皮肉浅薄部位的进针。

Inserting the Needle while Pinching the Skin One of the methods for inserting the needle. While the skin at the point region is pinched by the thumb and the index finger of one hand, the needle held by the other hand is inserted into the pinched skin. It is commonly used for inserting the needle in shallow and thin regions of the skin.

●提气法[tí qì fǎ] 针刺手法名。见《针灸大成》卷四。又称提针法。指先用紧提慢按六数，得气后，稍加捻转并轻轻将针提起，使针感加强。用于治疗局部麻木、发凉等。

Qi-Lifting Method A needling technique, seen in Vol. 4 of *Zhenjiu Dacheng* (*A Great Compendium of Acupuncture and Moxibustion*), also named needle-lifting method. After swiftly lifting and slowly thrusting the needle 6 times and gaining qi (the needling sensation), twirl the needle slightly and then lift it gently to strengthen the needling sensation. This method is used for the treatment of regional numbness and cold feeling.

●提针法[tí zhēn fǎ] 为提气法之别称。详见该条。

Needle-Lifting Method →提气法(p.428)

●体表标志[tǐ biǎo biāo zhì] 即体表解剖标志。详见该条。

Landmarks on Body Surface →体表解剖标志(p.428)

●体表解剖标志[tǐ biǎo jiě pāo biāo zhì] 又名体表标志。指在活体体表可以观察、触摸到的骨性突起和凹陷，肌肉的轮廓以及皮肤皱纹等。可分为固定标志和活动标志。见各条。

Anatomical Landmarks on Body Surface Also named landmarks on body surface, referring to the prominences and depressions of bones, the outline of muscles and the wrinkles of the skin, etc. which can be observed and touched on the surface of a living body. They are divided into fixed landmarks and moving landmarks. →固定标志(p.146)、活动标志(p.179)

●体表解剖标志定位法[tǐ biǎo jiě pāo biāo zhì dìng

wèi fǎ] 腧穴定位的方法之一。指以体表解剖学的各种体表标志为依据来确定腧穴位置的方法。

Location According to Anatomical Landmarks on Body Surface One of the methods for locating points, referring to the method of determining the position of points according to various landmarks on the body surface in surface anatomy.

●体位[tǐ wèi] 为针灸体位之简称。详见该条。

Posture Short for posture for acupuncture and moxibustion. →针灸体位(p.594)

●体针[tǐ zhēn] 针刺术语。泛指取用身体各部位的经穴或奇穴,以治疗疾病的针刺方法。与耳针、头针等局限性取穴的针刺方法相对而言。

Body Acupuncture A term in needling, referring generally to the method of puncturing the meridian or extra points on each part of the body for the treatment of diseases. It is versus auricular and scalp acupuncture, etc.—the needling methods of selecting local points.

●替灸膏[tì jiǔ gāo] 敷贴用药之一。见《杨氏家藏方》卷九。方用附子30克,吴茱萸、马蔺花、蛇床子各少许,木香3克,肉桂(去皮)6克,研为细末。用药末一匙,以姜汁调成糊膏状,摊于纸上,贴于脐部,以脐部觉热为度。可以治疗下焦虚冷、真气衰弱、泄利腹痛、气短等。

Adhesive Plaster Substitute for Moxibustion One of the application methods seen in Vol. 9 of *Yangshi Jiacang Fang* (*Yang's Home Collection of Formulas*). ⟨Composition⟩ *Fu Zi* (*Radix Aconiti Praparata*) 30g, a little *Wu Zhu Yu* (*Fructus Evodae*), *Ma Lin Hua* (*Flos Iridis Pallidae*) and *She Chuang Zi* (*Fructus Cnidii*), *Mu Xiang* (*Radix Aucklandiae*) 3g, *Rou Gui* (*Cortex Cinnamomi*) (peeled) 6g. ⟨Method⟩ Grind all of the above herbs into a fine powder. Take a spoonful of the powder and some *Jiang Zhi* (*succus zingiberis*), mix them into a paste, and spread it on a piece of paper. Apply it to the umbilical region and keep it there until a heat sensation appears in the region. ⟨Indications⟩ cold due to insufficiency in the lower Jiao, weakness of genuine-qi, diarrhea with abdominal pain, shortness of breath, etc.

●天部[tiān bù] 穴位浅深分部名。又称天才。指浅层,当皮下部分。参见"三部"条。

Heaven Portion A term for the depth of points, also called heaven part, referring to the shallow layer, i.e. the subcutaneous part. →三部(p.341)

●天才[tiān cái] 穴位浅深分部名。为天部之别称。详见该条。

Heaven Layer A term for the depth of points, another name for the heaven portion. →天部(p.429)

●天池[tiān chí] ①经穴名。出《灵枢·本输》。属手厥阴心包经,为手厥阴、足少阳之会。又名天会。⟨定位⟩在胸部,当第四肋间隙,乳头外1寸,前正中线旁开5寸(图40)。⟨层次解剖⟩皮肤→皮下组织→胸大肌→胸小肌。浅层有第四肋间神经外侧皮支,胸腹壁静脉的属支。如果是女性,除上述结构之外,皮下组织内还有乳腺等组织。深层 有胸内、外侧神经,胸外侧动、静脉的分支或属支。⟨主治⟩胸闷、心烦、咳嗽、痰多、气喘、胸痛、腋下肿痛、瘰疬、疟疾、乳痈。斜刺或平刺0.5~0.8寸;可灸。②经穴别名。出《针灸甲乙经》。即承浆。详见该条。

1. Tianchi (PC 1) A meridian point, originally from *Lingshu*: *Benshu* (*Miraculous Pivot*: *Meridian Points*), a point on the Pericardium Meridian of Hand-Jueyin, the crossing point of Hand-Jueyin and Foot-Shaoyang Meridians, also called Tianhui. ⟨Location⟩ on the chest, in the 4th intercostal space, 1 cun lateral to the nipple and 5 cun lateral to the anterior midline (Fig. 40). ⟨Regional anatomy⟩ skin→subcutaneous tissue→greater pectoral muscle→smaller pectoral muscle. In the superficial layer, there are the lateral cutaneous branches of the 4th intercostal nerve and the tributaries of the thoracoepigastric vein. In females, besides the above-mentioned vessel and nerve, there are also the glandular tissues in the subcutaneous layer. In the deep layer, there are the medial and lateral pectoral nerves and the branches or tributaries of the lateral thoracic artery and vein. ⟨Indications⟩ oppressive feeling in the chest, vexation, cough with copious sputum, dyspnea pain in the chest, subaxillary swelling and pain, scrofula, malaria, acute mastitis. ⟨Method⟩ Puncture obliquely or subcutaneously 0.5

~0.8 cun. Moxibustion is applicable.

2. **Tianchi** Another name for Chengjiang (RN 24), a meridian point originally from *Zhenjiu Jia-Yi Jing* (*A-B Classic of Acupuncture and Moxibustion*). →承浆(p. 43)

●天冲[tiān chōng] 经穴名。出《针灸甲乙经》。属足少阳胆经,为足太阳、少阳之会。别名天衢。〈定位〉在头部,当耳根后缘直上入发际2寸,率谷后0.5寸处(图28和图31)。〈层次解剖〉皮肤→皮下组织→耳上肌→颞筋膜→颞肌。布有耳颞神经和枕小神经以及枕大神经的会合支,颞浅动、静脉顶支和耳后动、静脉。〈主治〉头痛、齿龈肿痛、癫痫、惊恐、瘿气。平刺0.5~1.0寸;可灸。

Tianchong (GB 9) A meridian point originally from *Zhenjiu Jia-Yi Jing* (*A-B Classic of Acupuncture and Moxibustion*), a point on the Gallbladder Meridian of Foot-Shaoyang, the crossing point of Foot-Shaoyang and Foot-Taiyang, also called Tianqu. 〈Location〉 on the head, directly above the posterior border of the ear root, 2 cun above the hairline and 0.5 cun posterior to Shuaigu (GB 8) (Figs. 28&31). 〈Regional anatomy〉 skin→subcutaneous tissue→superior auricular muscle→temporal fascia→temporal muscle. There are the anastomotic branches of the aurculotemporal nerve and the lesser and greater occipital nerves, the parietal branches of the superficial temporal artery and vein, and the posterior auricular artery and vein in this area. 〈Indications〉 headache, swelling and pain of the gum, epilepsy, diseases due to terror and fear, and goiter. 〈Method〉 Puncture subcutaneously 0.5~1.0 cun. Moxibustion is applicable.

●天窗[tiān chuāng] 经穴名。出《灵枢·本输》。属手太阳小肠经。又名窗笼、天笼。〈定位〉在颈外侧部,胸锁乳突肌的后缘,扶突后,与喉结相平(图28)。〈层次解剖〉皮肤→皮下组织→胸锁乳突肌后缘→肩胛提肌→头、颈夹肌。浅层有耳大神经,枕小神经和颈外静脉。深层布有颈升动、静脉的分支或属支。〈主治〉耳聋、耳鸣、咽喉肿痛、颈项强痛、暴喑、颊肿痛、颈瘿、瘾疹、癫狂、中风。直刺0.3~0.5寸;可灸。

Tianchuang (SI 16) A meridian point, originally from *Lingshu: Benshu* (*Miraculous Pivot: Meridian Points*), a point on the Small Intestine Meridian of Hand-Taiyang, also called Chuanglong or Tianlong. 〈Location〉 on the lateral side of the neck, posterior to the sternocleidomastoid muscle and Futu (LI 18), on the level of the laryngeal protuberance (Fig. 28). 〈Regional anatomy〉 skin→subcutaneous tissue → posterior border of sternocleidomastoid muscle→levator muscle of scapula→splenius muscle of neck and head. In the superficial layer, there are the greater auricular nerve, the lesser occipital nerve and the external jugular vein. In the deep layer, there are the branches or tributaries of the ascending cervical artery and jugular vein. 〈Indications〉 deafness, tinnitus, sore throat, stiffness and pain of the neck and nape, sudden aphasia, swelling and pain of the cheek, goiter, urticaria, manic-depressive psychosis, apoplexy. 〈Method〉 Puncture perpendicularly 0.3~0.5 cun. Moxibustion is applicable.

●天聪[tiān cōng] 经外穴名。见《千金要方》。在头部,当前发际直上,为鼻尖至发际距离的1/2处。〈主治〉头痛、身寒热、腰背强直等。沿皮刺0.3~0.5寸;可灸。

Tiancong (EX-HN) An extra point, seen in *Qianjin Yaofang* (*Essential Prescriptions Worth a Thousand Gold*). 〈Location〉 on the head, directly upward from the anterior hairline, at the half way point of the distance from the nasal apex to the anterior hairline. 〈Indications〉 headache, chills and fever, stiffness of the waist and back, etc. 〈Method〉 Puncture subcutaneously 0.3~0.5 cun. Moxibustion is applicable.

●天吊风[tiān diào fēng] 即慢惊风的别名。详见该条。

Convulsion with Up-Lifted Eyes →慢惊风 (p. 263)

●天顶[tiān dǐng] 经穴别名。出《太平圣惠方》。即天鼎。详见该条。

Tianding Another name for Tianding (LI 17), a meridian point originally from *Taiping Shenghui Fang* (*Imperial Benevolent Precriptions*). →天鼎(p. 431)

●天鼎[tiān dǐng]　　经穴名。出《针灸甲乙经》。属手阳明大肠经。又名天顶。〈定位〉在颈外侧部,胸锁乳突肌后缘,当结喉旁,扶突穴与缺盆连线中点(图6.4和图28)。〈层次解剖〉皮肤→皮下组织→胸锁乳突肌后缘→斜角肌间隙。浅层内有颈横神经、颈外静脉和颈阔肌等结构。深层有颈升动、静脉的分支或属支,在斜角肌间隙内有臂丛等结构。〈主治〉咽喉肿痛、暴喑、气梗、瘿气、瘰疬。直刺0.3～0.5寸;可灸。

Tianding (LI 17) A meridian point, originally from *Zhenjiu Jia-Yi Jing* (*A-B Classic of Acupuncture and Moxibustion*), a point on the Large Intestine Meridian of Hand-Yangming, also named Tianding. (天*顶)〈Location〉on the lateral side of the neck, at the posterior border of the sternocleidomastoid muscle beside the laryngeal protuberance, at the midpoint of the line connecting Futu (LI 18) and Quepen (ST 12) (Figs. 6.4&28).〈Regional anatomy〉skin→subcutaneous tissue→posterior border of sternocleidomastoid muscle→interspace of scalene muscle. In the superficial layer, there are the transverse nerve of the neck, the external jugular vein and the platysma muscle. In the deep layer, there are the branches or tributaries of the ascending cervical artery and vein and the brachial plexus in the interspace of the scalene muscle.〈Indications〉swelling and pain of the throat, sudden aphasia, obstruction of qi, goiter, scrofula.〈Method〉Puncure perpendicularly 0.3～0.5 cun. Moxibusion is applicable.

●天府[tiān fǔ]　　经穴名。出《灵枢·本输》。属手太阴肺经。〈定位〉在臂内侧面,肱二头肌桡侧缘,腋前纹头下3寸处(图49)。〈层次解剖〉皮肤→皮下组织→肱肌。浅层有头静脉,臂外侧皮神经。深层布有肱动、静脉的肌支和肌皮神经的分支。〈主治〉气喘、鼻衄、吐血、瘿气、上臂内侧痛。直刺0.3～0.5寸;可灸。

Tianfu (LU 3) A meridian point, originally from *Lingshu: Benshu* (*Miraculous Pivot: Meridian Points*), a point on the Lung Meridian of Hand-Taiyin.〈Location〉on the medial side of the upper arm and on the radial border of the biceps muscle of the arm, 3 cun below the anterior end of the axillary fold (Fig. 49).〈Regional anatomy〉skin→subcutaneous tissue→brachial muscle. In the superficial layer, there are the cephalic vein and the lateral cutaneous nerve of the arm. In the deep layer, there are the muscular branches of the brachial artery and vein and the branches of the musculocutaneous nerve.〈Indications〉dyspnea, epistaxis, hematemesis, goiter, pain in the medial side of the upper arm.〈Method〉Puncture perpendicularly 0.3～0.5 cun. Moxibustion is applicable.

●天盖[tiān gài]　　经穴别名。出《针灸甲乙经》。即缺盆。详见该条。

Tiangai Another name for Quepen (ST 12), a meridian point originally from *Zhenjiu Jia-Yi Jing* (*A-B Classic of Acupuncture and Moxibustion*).→缺盆(p.328)

●天癸[tiān guǐ]　　耳穴别名。为内生殖器之别称。详见该条。

Tiangui(MA) Another name for the auricular point, Internal Genitalia(MA).→内生殖器(p.280)

●天会[tiān huì]　　经穴别名。出《针灸甲乙经》。即天池。详见该条。

Tianhui Another name for Tianchi(PC 1), a meridian point originally from *Zhenjiu Jia-Yi Jing* (*A-B Classic of Acupuncture and Moxibustion*).→天池(p.429)

●天火[tiān huǒ]　　即丹毒。详见该条。

Heavenly Fire →丹毒(p.71)

●天泾[tiān jīng]　　经穴别名。见《东医宝鉴》。即天泉。详见该条。

Tianjing Another name for Tianquan (PC 2), a meridian point, seen in *Dong Yi Bao Jian* (*Treasured Mirror of Oriental Medicine*).→天泉(p.433)

●天井[tiān jǐng]　　经穴名。出《灵枢·本输》。属手少阳三焦经,为本经合穴。〈定位〉在臂外侧,屈肘时,当肘尖直上1寸凹陷处(图48和图50)。〈层次解剖〉皮肤→皮下组织→肱三头肌。浅层布有臂后皮神经等结构。深层有肘关节动、静脉网,桡神经肌支。〈主治〉偏头痛、胁肋、颈项、肩背痛、耳聋、瘰疬、瘿气、癫痫。直刺0.5～1.0寸;可灸。

Tianjing (SJ 10) A meridian point, seen in

Lingshu: Benshu (*Miraculous Pivot: Meridian Points*), the He (Sea) point of the Sanjiao Meridian of Hand-Shaoyang. ⟨Location⟩ on the lateral side of the upper arm, in the depression 1 cun to the tip of the olecranon when the elbow is fixed (Figs. 48&50). ⟨Regional anatomy⟩ skin→subcutaneous tissue→brachial triceps muscle. In the superficial layer, there is the posterior brachial cutaneous nerve. In the deep layer, there are the arteriovenous network of the elbow joint and the muscular branches of the radial nerve. ⟨Indications⟩ migraine, pain in the hypochondriac region, neck and nape, shoulder and back, deafness, scrofula, goiter, epilspsy. ⟨Method⟩ Puncture perpendicularly 0.5~1.0 cun. Moxibustion is applicable.

●天灸[tiān jiǔ] 灸法种类之一。又称自灸、冷灸、无热灸、药物发疱灸。系利用某些对皮肤有刺激作用的药物外敷于穴位上，使其发疱以起到类似艾条灸法的效果。如用大蒜、毛茛、天南星、蓖麻子、威灵仙捣成糊状外敷。或以白芥子、斑蝥等研末水调外敷。敷药部位初起时感到发烫、灼痛，渐致起疱。发疱作用以斑蝥最强，大蒜等较轻。如敷药时间短，也可以只引起充血发烫而不致起疱。一般关节病痛可局部选穴。哮喘可敷膻中、大椎、肺俞。疟疾可敷内关、大椎。扁桃体炎可敷合谷。滞产可敷涌泉等。敷药发疱后应注意防止感染。

Medicinal Vesiculation A form of moxibustion, also called spontaneous moxibustion, cold moxibustion, non-fire moxibustion and vesiculating moxibustion with herbs, in which irritating drugs are applied to the selected points so as to cause blisters, creating effects similar to that of common moxibustion. For instance, pound *Da Suan* (*Bulbus Allii*), *Mao Gen* (*Ranunculus Japonucus*), *Tian Nan Xing* (*Rhizoma Arisaematis*), *Bi Ma Zi* (*Semen Ricini*), *Wei Ling Xian* (*Radix Clematidis*) into a paste and apply it to the selected points, or mix powder of *Bai Jie Zi* (*Semen Sinapis Albae*), *Ban Mao* (*Mylabris*) etc. with water into a paste and apply it to the selected point. The patient may initially have local hot feelings and scorching pain and then blisters gradually occur on the skin around the point. The vesiculating effect of *Ban Mao* (*Mylabris*) is the strongest and that of *Da Suan* (*Bulbus Allii*) etc. is relatively mild. Only local congestion and scorching pain may be caused without blister if the time for applying drugs is not long. Generally speaking, apply the drug paste to local points for treating arthralgia, apply it to Danzhong (RN 17), Dazhui (DU 14) and Feishu (BL 13) for asthma, apply it to Neiguan (PC 6) and Dazhui (DU 14) for malarial diseases, apply it to Hegu (LI 4) for tonsillitis, apply it to Yongquan (KI 1) for prolonged labor. ⟨Caution⟩ Infection should be prevented after vesiculation.

●天臼[tiān jiù] 经穴别名。出《针灸甲乙经》。即通天。详见该条。

Tianjiu Another name for Tongtian (BL 7), a meridian point originally from *Zhenjiu Jia-Yi Jing* (*A-B Classic of Acupuncture and Moxibustion*). →通天 (p. 441)

●天髎[tiān liáo] 经穴名。出《针灸甲乙经》。属手少阳三焦经。为手少阳、阳维之会。⟨定位⟩在肩胛部，肩井与曲垣的中间，当肩胛骨上角处(图50和图7)。⟨层次解剖⟩皮肤→皮下组织→斜方肌→冈上肌。浅层布有锁骨上神经和第一胸神经后支外侧皮支。深层有肩胛背动、静脉的分支或属支，肩胛上动、静脉的分支和属支，以及肩胛上神经等结构。⟨主治⟩肩臂痛、颈项强痛、胸中烦满。直刺0.5~0.8寸;可灸。

Tianliao (SJ 15) A meridian point, originally from *Zhenjiu Jia-Yi Jing* (*A-B Classic of Acupuncture and Moxibustion*), a point on the Sanjiao Meridian of Hand-Shaoyang, the crossing point of the Meridians of Hand-Shaoyang and Yangwei. ⟨Location⟩ on the scapula, at the midpoint between Jianjing (GB 21) and Quyuan (SI 13), at the superior angle of the scapula (Figs. 50&7). ⟨Regional anatomy⟩ skin→subcutaneous tissue→trapezius muscle→supraspinous muscle. In the superficial layer, there are the supraclavicular nerve and the lateral cutaneous branches of the posterior branches of the 1st thoracic nerve. In the deep layer, there are branches or tributaries of the dorsal scapular artery and vein, the branches or tributaries of the

suprascapular artery and vein, and the suprascapular nerve. 〈Indications〉 pain in the arm and shoulder, stiffness and pain in the neck and nape, irritable full sensation in the chest. 〈Method〉 Puncture perpendicularly 0.5～0.8 cun. Moxibustion is applicable.

●天笼[tiān lóng]　经穴别名。出《循经考穴编》。即天窗。详见该条。

Tianlong　Another name for Tianchuang (SI 16), a meridian point originally from *Xun Jing Kao Xue Bian* (*Studies on Acupoints Along Meridians*)→天窗(p. 430)

●天满[tiān mǎn]　经穴别名。出《针灸资生经》。即百会。详见该条。

Tianman　Another name for Baihui (DU 20), a meridian point, originally from *Zhenjiu Zisheng Jing* (*Acupuncture-Moxibustion Classic for Saving Life*).→百会(p. 11)

●天南星灸[tiān nán xīng jiǔ]　天灸方法之一。将天南星研碎，用醋调成膏状，贴敷一定穴位上，可以治疗口㖞、舌糜、小儿口疮等。

Tian Nan Xing (Rhizoma Arisaematis) Vesiculation　One of the medicinal vesiculation methods. 〈Method〉 Grind tuber of *Tian Nan Xing* (*Rhizoma Arisaematis*) and make it a paste with vinegar, then apply it to the selected points. 〈Indications〉 deviated mouth, erosion of the tongue and infantile aphtha, etc.

●天瞿[tiān qú]　经穴别名。出《千金要方》。即天突。详见该条。

Tianqu　Another name for Tiantu (RN 22), a meridian point originally from *Qianjin Yaofang* (*Essential Prescriptions Worth a Thousand Gold*).→天突(p. 434)

●天衢[tiān qú]　经穴别名。出《千金要方》。即天冲。详见该条。

Tianqu　Another name for Tianchong (GB 9), a meridian point originally from *Qianjin Yaofang* (*Essential Prescriptions Worth a Thousand Gold*).→天冲(p. 430)

●天泉[tiān quán]　经穴名。出《针灸甲乙经》。属手厥阴心包经。又名天温、天湿、天泾。〈定位〉在臂内侧，当腋前纹头下2寸，肱二头肌的长、短头之间(图49)。〈层次解剖〉皮肤→皮下组织→肱二头肌→肱肌→喙肱肌腱。浅层布有臂内侧皮神经的分支。深层

肌皮神经和肱动、静脉的肌支。〈主治〉心痛、胸胁胀满、咳嗽、胸背及上臂内侧痛。直刺0.5～0.8寸；可灸。

Tianquan (PC 2)　A meridian point, originally from *Zhenjiu Jia-Yi Jing* (*A-B Classic of Acupuncture and Moxibustion*), a point on the Pericardium Meridian of Hand-Jueyin, also named Tianwen, Tianshi and Tianjing. 〈Location〉 on the medial side of the arm, 2 cun below the anterior end of the axillary fold, between the long and short heads of the biceps muscle of the arm (Fig. 49). 〈Regional anatomy〉 skin→subcutaneous tissue→brachial biceps muscle→brachial muscle→tendon of coracobrachial muscle. In the superficial layer, there are the branches of the medial brachial cutaneous nerve. In the deep layer, there are the musculocutaneous nerve and the muscular branches of the brachial artery and vein. 〈Indications〉 precardial pain, fullness in the chest and hypochondrium, cough, pain in the chest, back and medial aspect of the upper arm. 〈Method〉 Puncture perpendicularly 0.5～0.8 cun. Moxibustion is applicable.

●天容[tiān róng]　经穴名。出《灵枢·本输》。属手太阳小肠经。又名大容。〈定位〉在颈外侧部，当下颌角的后方，胸锁乳突肌的前缘凹陷中(图28)。〈层次解剖〉皮肤→皮下组织→面动脉后方→二腹肌腱及茎突舌骨肌。浅层有耳大神经和颈外静脉等结构。深层有面动、静脉，颈内静脉，副神经，迷走神经，舌下神经，颈上神经节等重要结构。〈主治〉耳鸣、耳聋、咽喉肿痛、咽中如梗、颊肿、瘿气、头颈痈肿、呕逆吐沫。直刺0.5～0.8寸；可灸。

Tianrong (SI 17)　A meridian point, originally from *Lingshu: Benshu* (*Miraculous Pivot: Meridian Points*), a point on the Small Intestine Meridian of Hand-Taiyang, also named Darong. 〈Location〉 on the lateral side of the neck, posterior to the mandibular angle, in the depression of the anterior border of the sternocleidomastoid muscle (Fig. 28). 〈Regional anatomy〉 skin→subcutaneous tissue→posterior side of facial artery→tendons of digastric muscle and stylohyoid muscle. In the superficial layer, there are the greater auricular nerve and the external jugular vein. In the deep lay-

er, there are the facial artery and vein, the internal jugular vein, the acessory nerve, the vagus nerve, the hypoglossal nerve and the superior cervical ganglion. 〈Indications〉 tinnitus, deafness, swelling and pain of the throat, obstructing feeling in the pharynx, swelling of the check, goiter, carbuncle and swelling on the nape, vomiting with salivation. 〈Method〉 Puncture perpendicularly 0.5～0.8 cun. Moxibustion is applicable.

●天圣针经[tiān shèng zhēn jīng]　书名,指《铜人腧穴针灸图经》。详见该条。

Tiansheng Zhenjing (Imperial Holy Classic of Acupuncture)　Title of a book, referring to *Tongren Shuxue Zhenjiu Tujing* (*Illustrated Manual of Points for Acupuncture and Moxibustion on a Bronze Statue with Acupoints*). →铜人腧穴针灸图经(p. 442)

●天湿[tiān shī]　经穴别名。见《外台秘要》。即天泉。详见该条。

Tianshi　Another name for Tianquan (PC 2), a meridian point seen in *Waitai Miyao* (*Clandestine Essentials from the Imperial Library*). →天泉(p. 433)

●天枢[tiān shū]　经穴名。出《灵枢·骨度》。属足阳明胃经,为大肠之募穴。又名长溪、谷门、循元、补元、循际、循脊。〈定位〉在腹中部,距中2寸(图87和图40)。〈层次解剖〉皮肤→皮下组织→腹直肌鞘前臂→腹直肌。浅层布有第九、十、十一胸神经前支的外侧皮支和前皮支及脐周静脉网。深层有腹壁上、下动、静脉的吻合支、第九、十、十一胸神经前支的肌支。〈主治〉腹痛、呕吐、腹胀、肠鸣、癥瘕、痢疾、泄泻、便秘、肠痈、痛经、月经不调、热甚狂言、疝气、水肿。直刺0.8～1.2寸;可灸。

Tianshu (ST 25)　A meridian point, originally from *Lingshu: Gudu* (*Miraculous Pivot: Bone Measurement*), a point on the Stomach Meridian of Foot-Yangming, and the Front-Mu point of the Large Intestine Meridian, also named Changxi, Gumen, Xunyuan, Buyuan, Xunji and Xunji. 〈Location〉 on the middle abdomen, 2 cun lateral to the centre of the umbilicus (Figs. 87&40). 〈Regional anatomy〉 skin →subcutaneous tissue→anterior sheath of rectus muscle of abdomen→rectus muscle of abdomen. In the superficial layer, there are the lateral and anterior cutaneous branches of the anterior branches of the 9th to 11th thoracic nerves and the periumbilical venous network. In the deep layer, there are the anastomotic branches of the superior and inferior epigastric arteries and veins and the muscular branches of the anterior branches of the 9th to 11th thoracic nerves. 〈Indications〉 abdominal pain and distension, vomiting, borborygmus, mass in the abdomen, dysentery, dirrhea, constipation, acute append mass in the abdomen, dysmenorrhea, irregular menstruation, ravings due to excessive heat, hernia and edema. 〈Method〉 Puncture perpendicularly 0.8～1.2 cun. Moxibustion is applicable.

●天突[tiān tū]　经穴名。出《灵枢·本输》。属任脉,为阴维、任脉之会。又名玉户、天瞿。〈定位〉在颈部,当前正中线上,胸骨上窝中央(图40和图28)。〈层次解剖〉皮肤→皮下组织→左、右胸锁乳突肌腱(两胸骨头)之间→胸骨柄颈静脉切迹上方→左、右胸骨甲状肌→气管前间隙。浅层布有锁骨上内侧神经,皮下组织内有颈阔肌和颈静脉弓。深层有头臂干、左颈总动脉、主动脉弓和头臂静脉等重要结构。〈主治〉咳嗽、哮喘、胸中气逆、咯唾脓血、咽喉肿痛、舌下急、暴喑、瘿气、噎膈、梅核气。先直刺0.2～0.3寸,然后沿胸骨柄后缘、气管前缘缓慢向下刺入0.5～1寸;可灸。

Tiantu (RN 22)　A meridian point, originally from *Lingshu: Benshu* (*Miraculous Pivot: Meridian Points*), a point on the Ren Meridian, also named Yuhu and Tianqu. 〈Location〉 on the neck, at the anterior midline, and the centre of the superasternal fossa (Figs. 40&28). 〈Regional anatomy〉 skin → subcutaneous tissue → between two sternal heads of sternocleidomasoid muscles → superior side of suprasternal notch → between bilateral sternothyroid muscles→anterior space of trachea. In the superficial layer, there are the medial supraclavicular nerve, the platysma and the jugular arch of veins in the subcutaneous tissues. In the deep layer, there are some important structures, including the brachiocephalic trunk, the left common carotid artery, the aortic arch and the brachiocephalic vein. 〈Indica-

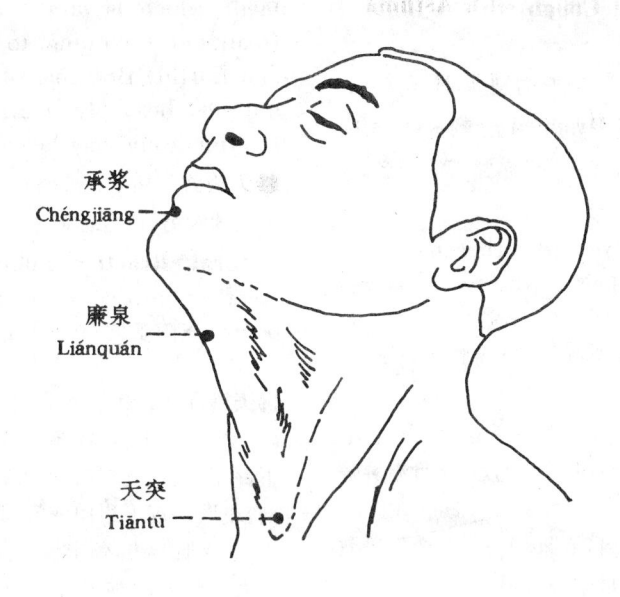

Fig 58 Tiantu, Lianquan and Chengjiang points

tions) cough, asthma, adverse flow of qi in the chest, cough and spitting with blood and pus, swelling and pain of the throat, sublingual contracture, sudden loss of voice, goiter, dysphagia and globus hystericus. 〈Method〉 First, puncture perpendicularly 0.2～0.3 cun, then slowly insert the needle downwards along the posterior aspect of the sternum and the anterior aspect of the trachea 0.5～1 cun. Moxibustion is applicable.

●天温[tiān wēn] 经穴别名。出《针灸甲乙经》。即天泉。详见该条。

Tianwen Another name for Tianquan (PC 2), a meridian point originally from *Zhenjiu Jia-Yi Jing* (*A-B Classic of Acupuncture and Moxibustion*). →天泉(p.433)

●天五会[tiān wǔ huì] 经穴别名。出《针灸甲乙经》。即人迎。详见该条。

Tianwuhui Another name for Renying (ST 9), a meridian point originally from *Zhenjiu Jia-Yi Jing* (*A-B Classic of Acupuncture and Moxibustion*). →人迎(p.333)

●天溪[tiān xī] 经穴名。出《针灸甲乙经》。属足太阴脾经。〈定位〉在胸外侧部,当第四肋间隙,距前正中线6寸(图39.3和图40)。〈层次解剖〉皮肤→皮下组织→胸大肌→胸小肌。浅层布有第四肋间神经外侧皮支和胸腹壁静脉的属支。深层有胸内、外侧神经的分支、胸肩峰动、静脉的胸肌支和胸外侧动、静脉的分支或属支。〈主治〉胸胁疼痛、咳嗽、乳痈、乳汁少。向外平刺或斜刺0.5～0.8寸;可灸。

Tianxi (SP 18) A meridian point, originally from *Zhenjiu Jia-Yi Jing* (*A-B Classic of Acupuncture and Moxibustion*), a point on the Spleen Meridian of Foot-Taiyin. 〈Location〉 on the lateral side of the chest, in the 4th intercostal space, 6 cun lateral to the anterior midline (Figs. 39.3&40). 〈Regional anatomy〉 skin → subcutaneous tissue → greater pectoral muscle → smaller pectoral muscle. In the superficial layer, there are the lateral cutaneous branches of the 4th intercostal nerve and the tributaries of the thoracoepigastric vein. In the deep layer, there are the branches of the medial pectoral nerve and the lateral pectoral nerve, the pectoral branches of the thoracoacromial artery and vein and the branches or tributaries of the lateral thoracic artery and vein. 〈Indication〉 pain in the chest and hypochondrium, cough, acute mastitis and insufficient lactation. 〈Method〉 Outwardly puncture subcutaneously or obliquely 0.5～0.8 cun. Moxibustion is applicable.

●天哮[tiān xiāo] 顿咳的别名。详见该条。

Epidemic Paroxysmal Cough with Asthma →顿咳(p.90)

●天哮呛[tiān xiāo qiàng] 顿咳的别名。详见该条。

Epidemic Cough with Dyspnea →顿咳(p.90)

●天行赤热[tiān xíng chì rè] 目赤肿痛的别名。详见该条。

Epidemic Red-Hot Eye Another name for redness, swelling and pain of the eye. →目赤肿痛(p.271)

●天行赤眼[tiān xíng chì yǎn] 目赤肿痛的别名。详见该条。

Epidemic Red Eye Another name for redness, swelling and pain of the eye. →目赤肿痛(p.271)

●天星十二穴[tiān xīng shí èr xué] 十二个经验效穴。见《针灸大全》。即天星十一穴增太冲一穴。详见该条。

Twelve Heavenly-Star Points The twelve effective points, seen in *Zhenjiu Daquan* (*A Complete Work of Acupuncture and Moxibustion*), formed by adding Taichong (LR 3) to the eleven heavenly-star points. →天星十一穴(p.436)

●天星十一穴[tiān xīng shí yī xué] 十一个经验效穴。见《扁鹊神应针灸玉龙经》。即三里、内庭、曲池、合谷、委中、承山、昆仑、环跳、阳陵泉、通里、列缺。

Eleven Heavenly-Star Points The 11 proven effective points, seen in *Bian Que Shenying Zhenjiu Yulong Jing* (*Bian Que's Jade Dragon Classics of Acupuncture and Moxibustion*), including Zusanli (ST 36), Neiting (ST 44), Quchi (LI 11), Hegu (LI 4), Weizhong (BL 40), Chengshan (BL 57), Kunlun (BL 60), Huantiao (GB 30), Yanglingquan (GB 34), Tongli (HT 5) and Lieque (LU 7).

●天医[tiān yī] 古代针灸宜忌说之一。出《黄帝虾蟆经》。按日时的干支推算天医所在,为治病吉利时日,有行年天医、月天医、日天医等。

Heavenly Treatment One of the theories about compatibility and incompatibility of acupuncture and moxibustion in ancient times, originally from *Huangdi Hama Jing* (*The Yellow Emperor's Frog Classic*), referring to calculating the time for heavenly treatment which is propitious to the patient for treatment according to the Heavenly Stems and Earthly Branches of day and hour, including year heavenly treatment, month heavenly treatment and day heavenly treatment, etc.

●天应穴[tiān yìng xué] 即阿是穴、以痛为输、不定穴的别名。详见各条。

Natural Reactive Point Another name for Ashi Point, pressure pain point and non-fixed point. →阿是穴(p.1)、以痛为输(p.552)、不定穴(p.28)

●天牖[tiān yǒu] 经穴名。出《灵枢·本输》。属手少阳三焦经。〈定位〉在颈侧部,当乳突的后方直下,平下颌角,胸锁乳突肌的后缘(图28和图31)。〈层次解剖〉皮肤→皮下组织→胸锁乳突肌与斜方肌之间→头、颈夹肌→头、颈半棘肌。浅层布有颈外静脉属支、耳大神经和枕神经。深层有枕动、静脉的分支或属支,颈深动、静脉升支。〈主治〉头晕、头痛、面肿、目昏、暴聋、项强。直刺0.5～1寸;可灸。

Tianyou (SJ 16) A meridian point, orignally from *Lingshu: Benshu* (*Miraculous Pivot: Meridian Points*), a point on the Sanjiao Meridian of Hand-Shaoyang. 〈Location〉 on the lateral side of the neck, directly below the posterior border of the mastoid process, at the level of the mandibular angle, and on the posterior border of the sternocleidomastoid muscle (Figs. 28 & 31). 〈Regional anatomy〉 skin→subcutaneous tissue → between sternocleidomastod muscle and trapezial muscle→splenius muscle of head and neck→semispinal muscles of head and neck. In the superficial layer, there are the tributaries of the external jugular vein, the great auricular nerve and the lesser occipital nerve. In the deep layer, there are the branches or tributaries of the lesser occipital atery and vein, and the ascending branches of the deep cervical artery and vein. 〈Indications〉 dizziness, headache, edema of face, blurred vision, sudder loss of hearing and stiffness of the nape. 〈Method〉 Puncture perpendicularly 0.5～1 cun. Moxibustion is applicable.

●天元太乙歌[tiān yuán tài yǐ gē] 针灸歌赋名。见《神应经》。为七言韵语,部分内容取自《席弘赋》。

Tianyuan Taiyi Ge (Verse of Taiyi in Nature)

A verse about acupuncture and moxibustion, seen in *Shenying Jing* (*Classic of God Merit*), using the rhyming style with seven words to each line. Some contents were extracted from *Xihong Fu* (*Ode to Xi Hong*).

●天柱[tiān zhù] 经穴名。出《灵枢·本输》。属足太阳膀胱经。〈定位〉在项部，大筋（斜方肌）外缘之后发际凹陷中，约后发际正中旁开1.3寸（图28和图7）。〈层次解剖〉皮肤→皮下组织→斜方肌→头夹肌的内侧→头半棘肌。浅层布有第三颈神经后支的内侧支和皮下静脉等结构。深层有枕大神经。〈主治〉头痛、项强、眩晕、目赤肿痛、鼻塞、不闻香臭、咽肿、肩背痛、足不任身。直刺0.5～1寸；可灸。

Tianzhu (BL 10) A meridian point, originally from *Lingshu: Benshu* (*Miraculous Pivot: Meridian Points*), a point on the Bladder Meridian of Foot-Taiyang. ⟨Location⟩ on the nape, in the depression of the lateral border of the trapeizal muscle and 1.3 cun lateral to the midpoint of the posterior hairline (Figs. 28&7). ⟨Regional anatomy⟩ skin → subcutaneous tissue → trapeizal muscle → medial border of splenius muscle of head → semispinal muscle of head. In the superficial layer, there are the medial branches of the posterior branches of the 3rd cervial nerve and the subcutaneous veins. In the deep layer, there is the greater occipital nerve. ⟨Indications⟩ headache, stiffness of the nape, dizziness, pain, redness and swelling of the eyes, stuffy nose, anosmia, swelling of the throat, pain in the shoulder and back, flaccid lower limbs. ⟨Method⟩ Puncture perpendicularly 0.5～1 cun. Moxibustion is applicable.

●天柱骨[tiān zhù gǔ] 骨骼部位名。指颈椎。

Tianzhu Bone Part of a skeleton, referring to the cervical vertebra.

●天宗[tiān zōng] 经穴名。出《针灸甲乙经》。属手太阳小肠经。〈定位〉在肩胛部，当冈下窝中央凹陷处，与第四胸椎相平（图48和图65.1）。〈层次解剖〉皮肤→皮下组织→斜方肌→冈下肌。浅层有第四胸神经后支的皮支和伴行的动、静脉。深层布有肩胛上神经的分支和旋肩胛动、静脉的分支或属支。〈主治〉肩胛疼痛、肘臂外后侧痛、气喘、乳痈。直刺0.5～1.5寸；可灸。

Tianzong (SI 11) A meridian point, originally from *Zhenjiu Jia-Yi Jing* (*A-B Classic of Acupuncture and Moxibustion*), a point on the Small Intestine Meridian of Hand-Taiyang. ⟨Location⟩ on the scapula, in the depression of the centre of the subscapula fossa, at the level of the 4th thoracic vertebra (Figs. 48&65.1). ⟨Regional anatomy⟩ skin → subcutaneous tissue → trapezial muscle infraspinous muscle. In the superficial layer, there are the cutaneous branches of the posterior branches of the 4th thoracic nerve and their accompanying arteries and veins. In the deep layer, there are the branches of the suprascapular nerve and the branches or tributaries of the circumflex scapular artery and vein. ⟨Indications⟩ pain in the scapular region and lateral posterior aspect of the elbow and arm, shortness of breath and acute mastitis. ⟨Method⟩ Puncture perpendicularly 0.5～1.5 cun. Moxibustion is applicable.

●条口[tiáo kǒu] 经穴名。出《针灸甲乙经》。属足阳明胃经。〈定位〉在小腿前外侧，当犊鼻下8寸，距胫骨前缘一横指（中指）（图60.5）。〈层次解剖〉皮肤→皮下组织→胫骨前肌→小腿骨间膜→胫骨后肌。浅层布有腓肠外侧皮神经。深层有胫前动、静脉和腓深神经。如深刺可能刺中腓动、静脉。〈主治〉小腿冷痛、麻痹、脘腹疼痛、跗肿、转筋、湿痹、肩臂痛。直刺0.5～1.5寸；可灸。

Tiaokou (ST 38) A meridian point, originally from *Zhenjiu Jia-Yi Jing* (*A-B Classic of Acupuncture and Moxibustion*), a point on the Stomach Meridian of Foot-Yangming. ⟨Location⟩ on the anteriolateral side of the leg, 8 cun below Dubi (ST 35), one finger breadth (middle finger) lateral to the anterior crest of the tibia (Fig. 60.5). ⟨Regional anatomy⟩ skin → subcutaneous tissue → anterior tibial muscle → interosseous membrane of leg → posterior tibial muscle. In the superficial layer, there is the lateral cutaneous nerve of the calf. In the deep layer, there are the anterior tibial artery and vein and the deep peroneal nerve. If the needle is inserted too deep, it may injure the posterior tibial artery and vein. ⟨Indications⟩ cold-pain in the shank, palsy of the shank, abdominal pain, edema of the dorsum of the foot, spasm

of the leg, arthralgia due to dampness and pain in the shoulder and arm. 〈Method〉 Puncture perpendicularly 0.5~1.5 cun. Moxibustion is applicable.

●调气[tiáo qì]　刺法用语。见《灵枢·刺节真邪》。指针刺具有调整经气的作用。调气可以说是在取得感应的基础上适当调节其感应,以起到调整机体功能,增强人体抗病能力的作用。

Regulating Qi　An acupuncture technique, seen in *Lingshu: Cijie Zhenxie (Miraculous Pivot: Acupuncture Principles and Diseases)*, referring to the effect of the needling on regulating the meridian qi. In other words, it means properly regulating the needling reaction based on the arrival of needling reaction in order to regulate the functions of the organism and strengthen the body resistance.

●调气法[tiáo qì fǎ]　指调节针感的各种方法。包括捻转、提插、呼吸配合、手指循按,以及龙虎升腾、纳气、青龙摆尾、白虎摇头、苍龟探穴、赤凤迎源等法。

Qi-Regulating Methods　The various methods for regulating needling reactions, including twirling, lifting and thrusting, cooperation with respiration, pressing and massaging along the meridian with the fingers, dragon-tiger leap and soar, accepting qi, green dragon wagging tail, white tiger shaking head, grey turtle exploring cave and red phoenix greeting source, etc.

●挑草子[tiáo cǎo zǐ]　即挑治法。详见该条。

Pricking out Grass Seed　→挑治法(p.438)

●挑刺[tiáo cì]　刺法名。指用三棱针等刺入穴位皮肤,再将其浅层组织挑断的方法。参见"挑治法"条。

Pricking　An acupuncture technique, referring to the method of pricking the skin around the selected point with a three-edged needle and then pricking and breaking the subcutaneous tissue. →挑治法(p.438)

●挑针疗法[tiáo zhēn liáo fǎ]　即挑治法。详见该条。

Needle Pricking Therapy　→挑治法(p.438)

●挑治法[tiáo zhì fǎ]　又称挑针疗法、挑草子。是指用三棱针等针具于穴位或特殊疹点上,挑出皮下的白色纤维样物,或挤出一些液体以治病的方法。临床挑治多于背部疹点或选穴。疹点稍突出于皮肤,颜色可为灰白、棕褐或淡红色等,压之不褪色(须与毛囊炎、色素斑等相区别)。每次挑1~2点,又可根据病情选取有关穴位挑治。须注意消毒,挑治后局部以灭菌纱布覆盖。挑刺、挑痔法均属此法。

Pricking Therapy　Also called needle pricking therapy or pricking out grass seed. A therapeutic method of pricking certain points or specific papuloid spots with a three-edged needle or other acupuncture instruments and pricking out white fiber-like substance from the subcutaneous tissue, or squeezing out some fluid. Clinically the pricking therapy is often used to prick certain points or papuloid spots on the back. The papula slightly sticks out with greyish, dark brown or pink colors which will not fade by pressing (should be differentiated from pigmented spots and folliculitis). Each treatment is to prick 1-2 spots or relevant points according to the patient's condition. 〈Caution〉 Take care to sterilize and cover the pricked area with sterilized gauze. The pricking and hemorrhoid pricking method are both of this therapy.

●挑痔法[tiáo zhì fǎ]　指用针挑刺腰骶部的特殊疹点(痔点)或穴位,以治痔疾的方法。

Hemorrhoid-Pricking　A method of pricking the specific papuloid spot (hemorrhoid point) on the lumboscral portion or selected acupoints with the needle so as to treat hemorrhoid.

●铁针[tiě zhēn]　古针具名。指以熟铁制成的针具。

Iron Needle　a kind of ancient acupuncture needle, referring to a needle made of wrought iron.

●听呵[tīng hē]　经穴别名。出《针灸资生经》。即听会。详见该条。

Tinghe　Another name for Tinghui(GB 2), a meridian point originally fom *Zhenjiu Zisheng Jing (Acupuncture-Moxibusion Classic for Saving Life)*. →听会(p.439)

●听河[tīng hé]　经穴别名。见《针灸大全》。即听会。详见该条。

Tinghe　Another name for Tinghui(GB 2), a

meridian point seen in *Zhenjiu Daquan* (*A Complete Work of Acupuncture and Moxibustion*). →听会 (p. 439)

●听宫 [tīng gōng] 经穴名。出《灵枢·刺节真邪》。属手太阳小肠经,为手足少阳、手太阳之会。又名多所闻。〈定位〉在面部,耳屏前,下颌骨髁状突的后方,张口时呈凹陷处(图28、图50、图65)。〈层次解剖〉皮肤→皮下组织→外耳道软骨。布有耳颞神经,颞浅动、静脉耳前支的分支或属支等结构。〈主治〉耳聋、耳鸣、聤耳、失音、癫疾、痫证、齿痛。直刺0.5~1.0寸;可灸。

Tinggong (SI 19) A meridian point, from *Lingshu : Ci Jie Zhen Xie* (*Miraculous Pivot : Acunpucture Principles and Diseases*). A point on the Small Intestine Meridian of Hand-Taiyang, and a crossing point of Hand-Shaoyang, Foot-Shaoyang and Hand-Taiyang, also known as Duosuowen. 〈Location〉on the face, anterior to the tragus and posterior to the mandibular condyloid process, in the depression formed by opening the mouth (Figs. 28&50,65). 〈Regional anatomy〉skin → subcutaneous tissue → external meatal cartilage. There are the auriculotemporal nerve and the branches or tributaries of the anterior auricular branches of the superficial temporal artery and vein in this area. 〈Indications〉 deafness, tinnitus, otorrhea, aphasia, manic-depressive disorders, epilepsy and toothache. 〈Method〉 Puncture perpendicularly 0.5~1.0 cun. Moxibustion is applicable.

●听会 [tīng huì] 经穴名。出《针灸甲乙经》。属足少阳胆经。又名听呵、听河、后关。〈定位〉在面部,当耳屏间切迹的前方,下颌骨髁突的后缘,张口有凹陷处(图28)。〈层次解剖〉皮肤→皮下组织→腮腺囊→腮腺。浅层布有耳颞神经和耳大神经。深层布有颞浅动、静脉和面神经丛等结构。〈主治〉耳鸣、耳聋、聤耳流脓、齿痛、下颌脱臼、口眼㖞斜、面痛、头痛。直刺0.5寸;可灸。

Tinghui (GB 2) A meridian point, from *Zhenjiu Jia-Yi Jing* (*A-B Classic of Acupuncture and Moxibustion*). A point on the Gallbladder Meridian of Foot-Shaoyang, also called Tinghe(呵), Tinghe(河) and Houguan. 〈Location〉on the face, anterior to the intertragic notch, in the depression formed by opening the mouth and posterior to the condyloid process of the mandible. (Fig. 28). 〈Regional anatomy〉skin → subcutaneous tissue → capsule of parotid gland→parotid gland. In the superficial layer, there are the auriculotemporal nerve and the great auricular nerve. In the deep layer, there are the superficial temporal artery and vein and the phexus of the facial nerve. 〈Indications〉 tinnitus, deafness, otorrhea with discharge of pus, toothache, dislocation of mandibular joint, facial hemiparalysis, pain in the face, and headache. 〈Method〉 Puncture perpendicularly 0.5 cun. Moxibustion is applicable.

●葶苈饼灸 [tíng lì bǐng jiǔ] 隔葶苈饼灸之别称。详见该条。

Cake-Moxibustion of Tingli (**Semen Lepiddli Seu Desocurainiae**)→隔葶苈饼灸(p. 137)

●聤耳 [tíng ěr] 病证名。见《诸病源候论》。泛指耳窍化脓性疾病。以脓带黄者为聤耳;以脓带青色者为囊耳;脓带红色为风耳;脓带白色为缠耳;脓带黑色为耳疳。多因劳伤气血,热乘虚而入,邪随血气至耳,热聚化火成脓。临床分聤耳实证,聤耳虚证。详见各条。

Otitis Media Suppurative A disease, seen in *Zhubing Yuanhou Lun* (*General Treatise on the Etiology and Symptomatology of Diseases*), referring to suppurative disease of the external acoustic meatus. Clinically, diseases with yellowish purulent discharge are regarded as otitis media suppurative, with greenish purulent discharge as nang ear, with pink purulent discharge as otopyrrhagia, with whitish purulent discharge as chan ear, and with dark purulent discharge as chronic suppurative otitis media. Mostly due to qi and blood being injured by overstrain and to the ear being invaded by pathogenic heat, leading to the accumulation and suppuration of heat and fire evils. Clinically it is divided into excess otitis media suppurative and deficiency otitis media suppurative.

→聤耳实证(p. 439)、聤耳虚证(p. 440)

●聤耳实证 [tíng ěr shí zhèng] 聤耳证型之一。多因肝胆郁火和三焦湿热所致。证见耳底痛、流黄色粘脓、听力减弱、发热头痛、脘闷便秘、舌质红苔黄、脉

弦数。治宜疏风清热,解毒开窍。取风池、翳风、听宫、合谷、外关、足临泣。

Excess Syndrome of Otitis Media Suppurative
A type of otitis media suppurative, mostly due to stagnation of fire in the liver and gallbladder, and damp-heat in the Sanjiao. ⟨Manifestations⟩ earache with yellowish purulent discharge, hypoacucis, fever, headache, abdominal fullness and constipation, reddened tongue with yellowish coating, wiry and rapid pulse. ⟨Treatment principle⟩ Dispel wind and clear damp-heat, detoxify and open the orifices. ⟨Point selection⟩ Fengchi (GB 20), Yifeng (SJ 17), Tinggong (SI 19), Hegu (LI 4), Waiguan (SJ 5), and Zulinqi (GB 41).

●**聤耳虚证** [tíng ěr xū zhèng] 聤耳证型之一。多因脾虚失健,湿浊不化,停聚耳窍所致。证见耳中流脓、终年不愈、脓水清稀不断或如粘丝状、眩晕、四肢倦怠、食少、面色萎黄、舌质淡、苔白、脉濡弱。治宜健脾化湿。取听会、足三里、阳陵泉、太白。

Deficiency Syndrome of Otitis Media Suppurative A type of otitis media suppurative, mostly due to the accumulation of dampness in the ear resulting from deficiency of the spleen. ⟨Manifestations⟩ persistent discharge of watery or sticky and threadlike pus, dizziness, lassitude of limbs, poor appetite, shallow complexion, pale tongue with white coating, soft amd weak pulse. ⟨Treatment principle⟩ Strengthen the spleen to eliminate dampness. ⟨Point selection⟩ Tinghui (GB 2), Zusanli (ST 36), Yanglingquan (GB 34), and Taibai (SP 30).

●**艇角** [tǐng jiǎo] 耳穴名。又名前列腺。位于耳甲艇内上角。用于治疗前列腺炎、尿道炎。

Angle of Cymba Conchae (MA) An auricular point, also called Prostate (MA). ⟨Location⟩ at the medial superior angle of cymba conchae. ⟨Indications⟩ prostatitis, urethritis.

●**艇中** [tǐng zhōng] 耳穴名。又名脐周。位于耳甲艇中央。用于治疗低热、腹胀、胆道蛔虫症、听力减退、腮腺炎。

Middle Cymba Conchae (MA) An auricular point, also called Around Umbilicus (MA). ⟨Location⟩ in the centre of the cymba conchae. ⟨Indications⟩ low fever, abdominal distention, filiary ascariasis, hypoacusis, and parotitis.

●**通谷** [tōng gǔ] ①经穴别名。即腹通谷。详见该条。②经穴别名。即足通谷。详见该条。

Tonggu Another name for ① the meridian point Futonggu (KI 20). →腹通谷 (p. 122); or ② the meridian point Zutonggu (BL 66). →足通谷 (p. 644)

●**通关** [tōng guān] 经穴别名。见《针经摘英集》。即阴都。详见该条。

Tongguan Another name for Yindu (KI 19), a meridian point seen in *Zhenjing Zhaiying Ji* (*A Collection of Gems from Acupuncture Classics*). →阴都 (p. 554)

●**通间** [tōng jiān] 经穴别名。出《素问·骨空论》王冰注。即三阳络。详见该条。

Tongjian Another name for Sanyangluo (SJ 8), a meridian point from Wang Bing's annotation for *Suwen: Gukong Lun* (*Plain Questions: On the Apertures of Bones*). →三阳络 (p. 345)

●**通经接气** [tōng jīng jiē qì] 刺法用语。①指催行经气的一些针刺手法。见"飞经走气法"。②即接气通经。详见该条。

Dredging Meridians to Promote the Qi-Circulation A term in acupuncture. (1) Referring to some of the needling methods which can hasten the circulation of meridian qi. →飞经走气法 (p. 105) (2) Another name for continuing the qi circulation and promoting meridians. →接气通经 (p. 201)

●**通里** [tōng lǐ] 经穴名。出《灵枢·经脉》。属手少阴心经,为本经络穴。⟨定位⟩在前臂掌侧,当尺侧腕屈肌腱的桡侧缘,腕横纹上1寸(图49和图67)。⟨层次解剖⟩皮肤→皮下组织→尺侧腕屈肌与指浅屈肌之间→指深屈肌→旋前方肌。浅层有前臂内侧皮神经,贵要静脉属支等分布。深层有尺动、静脉和尺神经分布。⟨主治⟩暴喑、舌强不语、心悸、悲恐畏人、头痛目眩、妇人经血过多、崩漏、肩、臑、肘、臂内侧后缘痛。直刺0.2~0.5寸;可灸。

Tongli (HT 5) A meridian point, from *Lingshu: Jingmai* (*Miraculous Pivot: Meridians*)

the Luo (Connecting) point of the Heart Meridian of Hand-Shaoyin. ⟨Location⟩ on the palmar side of the forearm and on the radial side of the tendon of the ulnar flexor muscle of the wrist, 1.0 cun proximal to the crease of the wrist(Figs. 49&67). ⟨Regional anatomy⟩ skin → subcutaneous tissue → between ulnar flexor muscle of wrist and superficial flexor muscle of fingers→deep flexor muscle of fingers→quadrate pronator muscle. In the superficial layer, there are the medial cutaneous nerve of the forearm and the tributaries of the basilic vein. In the deep layer, there are the ulnar artery and vein and the ulnar nerve. ⟨Indications⟩ sudden loss of voice, stiffness of tongue and aphasia, palpitation, grief, headache and dizziness, menorrhagia, metrorrhagia and metrostaxis, and shoulder pain, pain along posterior border of the medial aspect of the upper extremities. ⟨Method⟩ Puncture perpendicularly 0.2～0.5 cun. Moxibustion is applicable.

●通理[tōng lǐ] ①经外穴名。出《针灸集成》。在足背部,当第4、5跖骨间,小趾跖趾关节上2寸处。⟨主治⟩崩漏、月经过多。斜刺0.3～0.5寸;可灸。②经穴别名。即通里。详见该条。

1. Tongli(EX-LE) An extra point, originally from *Zhenjiu Jicheng (A Collection of Acupuncture and Moxibustion)*. ⟨Location⟩ on the dorsum between the 4th and 5th metatarsal tones, 2 cun above the joint of the little toe. ⟨Indications⟩ metrorrhagia and metrostaxis menorrhagia. ⟨ Method ⟩ Puncture obliquely 0.3～0.5 cun. Moxibustion is applicable.

2. Tongli Another name for the meridian point Tongli(HT 5). →通里(p. 440)

●通门[tōng mén] 经穴别名。见《针灸聚英》。即三阳络。详见该条。

Tongmen Another name for Sanyangluo(SJ 8), a meridian point seen in *Zhenjiu Juying (Essentials of Acupuncture and Moxibustion)*. →三阳络(p. 345)

●通天[tōng tiān] 经穴名。出《针灸甲乙经》。属足太阳膀胱经。又名天白。⟨定位⟩在头部,当前发际正中直上4寸,旁开1.5寸(图28)。⟨层次解剖⟩皮肤→皮下组织→帽状腱膜。浅层布有眶上神经,眶上动、静脉和枕大神经,枕动、静脉与耳颞神经,颞浅动、静脉的神经间吻合和血管的吻合网。深层为腱膜下疏松结缔组织和颅骨外膜。⟨主治⟩头痛、头重、眩晕、口㖞、鼻塞多清涕、鼻衄、鼻疮、鼻渊、鼻窒、颈项难以转侧、瘿气。平刺0.3～0.5寸;可灸。

Tongtian(BL 7) A meridian point, from *Zhenjiu Jia-Yi Jing(A-B Classic of Acupuncture and Moxibustion)*. A point on the Bladder Meridian of Foot-Taiyang, also called Tianjiu. ⟨Location⟩ on the head, 4 cun directly above the midpoint of the anterior hairlline and 1.5 cun lateral to the midline(Fig. 28). ⟨Regional anatomy⟩ skin→subcutaneous tissue→epicranial aponeurosis. In the superficial layer, there are the supraorbital nerve and the supraorbital artery and vein, the interneural and inttervascular anastomotic network of the greater occipital nerve, the occipital artery and vein, the auriculotemporal nerve and the superficial temporal artery and vein. In the deep layer, there are the subaponeurotic loose connective tissue and the pericranium. ⟨ Indications ⟩ headache, heaviness in the head, dizziness, wry mouth, nasal obstruction with running nose, epistaxis, pyogenic infection of nose, rhinorrhea with turbid discharge, stuffy nose, stuffiness of th neck and nape, and goiter. ⟨Method⟩Puncture subcutaneously 0.3～0.5 cun. Moxibustion is applicable.

●通玄指要赋[tōng xuán zhǐ yào fù] 针灸歌赋名。即《流针指要赋》。窦默作。刊于1332年。初载于罗天益的《卫生宝鉴》。论刺法、配穴等。据载本书内容多源于其师李氏的经验。

Tongxuan Zhiyao Fu(Ode to the Apprehension of Abstruse Essentials of Acupuncture)

One of the verses on acupunmcture and moxibustion. i.e. *Liuzhen Zhiyao Fu (Acupuncture Ode of the Essentials of Flow)*, written by Dou Mo and published in 1332. It was initially included in *Weisheng Baojian(Treasured Mirror of Health Protection)* by Luo Tianyi. The verse dealt with acupuncture manipulation and point prescriptions, etc. It was recorded that the contents of this book mostly originated from the experi-

ence of Mr. Li, the author's teacher.

●**同名经配穴法**[tóng míng jīng pèi xué fǎ] 配穴法之一。指手足同名称的经脉所属穴配合同用。如手、足太阴,手、足阳明等。各经脉均相互衔接,治疗上有协同作用。例如齿痛,取手阳明经的合谷和足阳明经的内庭。本法与接经取穴同出手足同名经相接的理论。接经取穴是指同名经穴可以互相为用,即足经病取手经穴,手经病取足经穴。本法系指手足同名经穴可上下配合应用。参见该条。

Combination of Points on Meridians with the Same Name One of the point prescriptions, referring to the cooperative selection of points on meridians with the same name on the hand and foot, e. g. both Hand- and Foot-Taiyin or Hand- and Foot-Yangming etc., connects with each other, these meridians have a cooperative function in treating diseases, e. g. Hegu (LI 4) of hand-Yangming and Neiting (ST 44) of Foot-Yangming can be used to treat toothache. Both this method and selecting points on connected meridians derive from the theory that meridians of the same name connect with each other. Selecting points on connected meridians means that points on meridians with the same name can be used alternately, i. e. diseases of the Hand Meridians can be treated by selecting points on Foot Meridians, while diseases of Foot meridians can be treated by selecting points on Hand Meridians. But this method means that points of the meridians with the same name on the upper or lower part of the body can cooperatively be selected.

→接经取穴(p. 201)

●**同名经取穴**[tóng míng jīng qǔ xué] 即接经取穴。详见该条。

Selecting Points on the Meridians with the Same Name→接经取穴(p. 201)

●**同身寸**[tóng shēn cùn] 取穴的一种长度标准。均用患者本人体表的某些标志作为测量的单位。包括中指同身寸、拇指同身寸、横指同身寸。详见各条。

Finger Cun A lengthwise unit for locating acupoints, i. e. some anatomical landmarks of the patient's body are used as measurement units, including Middle-Finger Cun, Thumb Cun and Four-Finger Cun. →中指同身寸(p. 615)、拇指同身寸(p. 270)、横指同身寸(p. 164)

●**同阴之脉**[tóng yīn zhī mài] 经络名。出《素问·刺腰痛篇》。指足少阳经在小腿的别络。王冰注:是阳辅穴,当外踝上五寸处走向厥阴,并经下络足跗,故称同阴脉。

Collateral of the Same Yin A collateral from *Suwen: Ci Yao Tong Pian (Plain Questions: On Treatment of Lumbago with Acupuncture)*, i. e. the collateral of the Foot-Shaoyang Meridian in the leg. Wang Bing annotated that it derives from Yangfu(GB 38), travels from the point 5 cun above the external malleolus, to the Meridian of Foot-Jueyin, then goes along the meridian to spread over the dorsum; therefore, it is named the collateral of the same yin.

●**铜人**[tóng rén] ①指供针灸教学所用铜铸的人体经脉腧穴模型。最早铸制铜人的是北宋针灸学家王惟一。②书名。《铜人腧穴针灸图经》的简称。详见该条。

1. Bronze Statue A bronze model used in teaching acupuncture and moxibustion which is marked with meridians and acupoints. The first one was cast by Wang Weiyi, an acupuncture-moxibustion expert in the Northern Song Dynasty.

2. Tongren(A Bronze Statue) A book title, abbreviation for *Tongren Shuxue Zhenjiu Tujing (Illustrated Manual of Points for Acupuncture and Moxibustion on a Bronze Statue with Acupoints)*. →铜人腧穴针灸图经(p. 442)

●**铜人腧穴针灸图经**[tóng rén shù xué zhēn jiǔ tú jīng] 书名。又名《新铸铜人腧穴针灸图经》。简称《铜人经》或《铜人》。宋代王惟一撰,三卷,成书于1026年。书中列述十四经穴,附穴图,并对《灵枢·经脉》原文作了注释。

Tongren Shuxue Zhenjiu Tujing (Illustrated Manual of Points for Acupuncture and Moxibustion on a Bronze Statue with Acupoints) A book, also named *Xin Zhu Tongren Shuxue Zhenjiu Tujing (Illustrated Manual of Points for Acupuncture and Moxibustion on a Newly-Cast Bronze Statue with Acupoints)*. It is abbreviated as *Tongren Jing (Classic on the Bronze Figure)* or *Tongren (A Bronze Statue)*, written by Wang Weiyi in the Song

Dynasty, three volumes in all and completed in 1026. In the book, the author narrated the points of the 14 meridians with illustrations charts, and annotated the original of *Lingshu*: *Jingmai* (*Miraculous Pivot*: *Meridians*).

●铜人针灸方 [tóng rén zhēn jiǔ fāng] 书名。撰人不详,一卷,书佚。见明《绿竹堂书目》。

Tongren Zhenjiu Fang (Prescriptions for Acupuncture and Moxibustion on a Bronze Statue with Acupoints) A single-volume book written by an unknown author, already lost, seen in *Lü Zhu Tang Shumu* (*Lu Zhu Tang Catalogue*) of the Ming Dynasty.

●铜人指要赋 [tóng rén zhǐ yào fù] 针灸歌赋名。见《针灸聚英》。其赋主要是涉及行针的要领,文多采自《素问》。

Tongren Zhiyao Fu (A Prose on the Essentials of a Bronze Statue with Acupoints) One of the verses on acupuncture and moxibustion, seen in *Zhenjiu Juying* (*Essentials of Acupuncture and Moxibustion*). It mainly dealt with the essentials of needling. Most of the contents were extracted from *Su Wen* (*Plain Questions*).

●童玄 [tóng xuán] 经穴别名。见《古今医统》。即列缺。详见该条。

Tongxuan Another name for Lieque (LU 7), a meridian point seen in *Gu Jin Yitong* (*The General Medicine of the Past and Present*). → 列缺 (p. 246)

●瞳子髎 [tóng zǐ liáo] 经穴名。出《针灸甲乙经》。属足少阳胆经,为手太阳、手足少阳之会。又名后曲、太阳、前关、鱼尾。〈定位〉在面部,目外眦旁,当眶外侧缘处 (图28和图5)。〈层次解剖〉皮肤→皮下组织→眼轮匝肌→颞筋膜→颞肌。浅层布有颧神经的颧面支与颧颞支。深层有颞深前、后神经和颞深前、后动脉的分支。〈主治〉头痛、目赤、目痛、怕光羞明、迎风流泪、远视不明、内障、目翳。向后平刺或斜刺0.3~0.5寸;或点刺出血。

Tongziliao (GB 1) A meridian point, from *Zhenjiu Jia-Yi Jing* (*A-B Classic of Acupuncture and Moxibustion*), a point on the Gallbladder Meridian of Foot-Shaoyang, the Crossing Point of Hand-Taiyang and Hand- and Foot-Shaoyang, also called Houqu, Taiyang, Qianguan and Yuwei. 〈Location〉on the face, lateral to the outer canthus, on the lateral border of the orbit. (Figs. 28&5). 〈Regional anatomy〉skin → subcutaneous tissue → orbicular muscle of eye → temporal fascia → temporal muscle. In the superficial layer, there are the zygomaticofacial and zygomaticotemporal branches of the zygomatic nerve. In the deep layer, there are the anterior and posterior deep temporal nerves and the branches of the anterior and posterior deep temporal arteries and veins. 〈Indications〉headache, redness and pain of the eye, photophobia, epiphora induced by wind, myopia, internal oculopathy and nebula. 〈Method〉Puncture subcutaneously or obliquely 0.3～0.5 cun, or prick to bleed.

●筒灸 [tǒng jiǔ] 灸法的一种。见《千金要方》。利用细竹管或苇管塞入耳中,在另一端施灸。用治口眼歪斜、耳病等。

Tube Moxibustion A kind of moxibustion, seen in *Qianjin Yaofang* (*Essential Prescriptions Worth a Thousand Gold*). Put one end of a thin bamboo tube into the ear, then do moxibustion at the other end. 〈Indications〉facial paralysis, ear diseases, etc.

●痛痹 [tòng bì] 痹证证型之一。出《素问·痹论》。由风寒湿邪痹阻经络,以寒邪偏盛所致。证见肌肉关节疼痛,痛势较剧,痛处有冷感,得热痛减,遇寒则甚,常喜按揉击拍以求缓解,舌苔薄白、脉浮紧。治宜疏通经络,祛邪止痛。取阳池、肾俞、关元、足三里,近部与循经取穴,详见"行痹"条。

Arthralgia Aggravated by Pathogenic Cold A type of arthralgia, from *Suwen*: *Bi Lun* (*Plain Questions*: *On Bi-Syndromes*), due to the stagnation of meridians resulting from pathogenic wind, cold and dampness, especially from excess cold-evil. 〈Manifestations〉pain in muscles and joints, severe pain with cold feelings, alleviated by massage, white thin tongue coating, superficial and tense pulse. 〈Treatment principle〉Dredge the meridians and collaterals and eleminate the pathogenic factors to alleviate pain. 〈Point selection〉Yangchi (SJ 4), Shenshu (BL 23), Guangyuan (RN 4), and Zusanli (ST 36), selecting points

in the local area near the affected region and along the meridian, see "migratory arthralgia." →行痹(p. 511)

●痛经[tòng jīng] 病证名。又称经前腹痛、经行腹痛、月水来腹痛、经后腹痛等。指每在月经期，或行经前后，出现小腹及腰部疼痛，甚则剧痛难忍者，称为痛经。临床常见有气滞痛经，血瘀痛经，寒湿凝滞痛经，气血虚弱痛经，肝肾亏损痛经等。详见各条。

Dysmenorrhea A disease, also named abdominal pain before, during, or after menstruation, referring to the gynecological disease with gypogastric and lumbar pain prior to, during, or after the menstual period, even with intolerable pain. Clinically, the diseases are divided into dysmenorrhea due to qi stagnation, dysmenorrhea due to blood stasis, dysmenorrhea due to deficiency of qi and blood, dysmenorrhea due to impairment of liver and kidney. →气滞痛经(p. 314)、血瘀痛经(p. 531)、寒湿凝滞痛经(p. 156)、气血虚弱痛经(p. 312)、肝肾亏损痛经(p. 126)

●偷针[tōu zhēn] 即针眼。详见该条。

Bail of Eye. →针眼(p. 597)

●头冲[tóu chōng] 经外穴名。出《千金要方》。位当上臂肱二头肌的桡侧，伸手直向前，侧头靠臂时，鼻尖所触之处。《针灸资生经》作臂臑别名；《经外奇穴图谱》指天府。

Touchong (EX-UE) An extra point, from *Qianjin Yaofang* (*Essential Prescriptions Worth a Thousand Gold*). ⟨Location⟩near the radial border of the tendon of musculus biceps brachii, at the point the nasal tip touches when the arm stretches anteriorly and the head nods laterally. It was another name for Binao (LI 14) in *Zhenjiu Zisheng Jing* (*Acupuncture-Moxibustion Classic for Saving Life*); or referring to Tianfu (LU 3) in *Jingwai Qixue Tupu* (*An Atlas of Extra Points*).

●头缝[tóu fèng] 经穴别名。见《针灸大全》。即头维。详见该条。

Toufeng Another name for Touwei (ST 8), a meridian poin seen in *Zhenjiu Daquan* (*A Complete Work of Acupuncture and Moxibustion*). →头维(p. 445)

●头横骨[tóu héng gǔ] 部位名。指枕骨。见《素问·骨空论》。

Transverse Bone of Head A part of the body, referring to the occiptial bone, seen in *Su Wen: Gukong Lun* (*Plain Questions: On the Apertures of Bones*).

●头临泣[tóu lín qì] 经穴名。见《针灸资生经》。属足少阳胆经，为足太阳、少阳、阳维之会。又名目临泣、临泣。⟨定位⟩在头部，当瞳孔直上入前发际0.5寸，神庭与头维连线的中点处(图28)。⟨层次解剖⟩皮肤→皮下组织→帽状腱膜→腱膜下疏松结缔组织。布有眶上神经和眶上动、静脉。⟨主治⟩头痛、目眩、目赤痛、流泪、目翳、鼻塞、鼻渊、耳聋、小儿惊痫、热病。平刺0.5~0.8寸；可灸。

Toulinqi (GB 15) A meridian point, seen in *Zhenjiu Zisheng Jing* (*Acupuncture-Moxibustion Classic for Saving Life*). A point on the Gallbladder Meridian of Foot-Shaoyang, the crossing point of Foot-Taiyang, Foot-Shaoyang, and Yangwei Meridians, also called Mulinqi or Linqi. ⟨Location⟩on the head, directly above the pupil and 0.5 cun above the anterior hairline, at the midpoint of the line connecting Shenting (DU 24) and Touwei (ST 8) (Fig. 28). ⟨Regional anatomy⟩ skin→subcutaneous tissue → epicranial aponeurosis → loose connective tissue below aponeurosis. There are the supraorbital nerve and the supraorbital artery and vein in this area. ⟨Indications⟩headache, dizziness, redness and pain of the eye, dacryorrhea, blurred vision, nasal obstruction, sinusitis, deafness, infantile convulsion, febrile diseases. ⟨Method⟩Puncture subcutaneously 0.5~0.8 cun. Moxibustion is applicable.

●头皮针[tóu pí zhēn] 针具名。为头针之别称。详见该条。

Scalp Needle A kind of acupuncture instrument, another name for head needle. →头针1. (p. 446)

●头窍阴[tóu qiào yīn] 经穴名。见《针灸资生经》。《针灸甲乙经》原名窍阴。属足少阳胆经，为足太阳、少阳之会。又名枕骨、首窍阴。⟨定位⟩在头部，当耳后乳突的后上方，天冲与完骨的中1/3与下1/3交点处(图28和图31)。⟨层次解剖⟩皮肤→皮下组织→帽状腱膜。布有枕小神经和耳后动、静脉的分支。⟨主治⟩

头痛、眩晕、颈项强痛、胸胁痛、口苦、耳鸣、耳聋、耳痛。平刺0.5～0.8寸；可灸。

Touqiaoyin (GB 11) A meridian point seen in *Zhenjiu Zisheng Jing* (*Acupuncture-Moxibustion Classic for Saving Life*), orginally named Qiaoyin in *Zhenjiu Jia-Yi Jing* (*A-B Classic of Acupuncture and Moxibustion*), a point of the Gallbladder Meridian of Foot-Shaoyang, the crossing point of Meridians of Foot-Shaoyang and Foot-Taiyang, also called Zhengu, Shouqiaoyin. 〈Location〉on the head, posterior and superior to the mastoid process, at the junction of the middle one third and lower one third of the curved line connecting Tianchong (GB 9) and Wangu (GB 12) (Figs. 28 & 31). 〈Regional anatomy〉 skin→subcutaneous tissue → epicranial aponeurosis. There are the occipital nerve and the branches of the posterior auricular artery and vein in this area. 〈Indications〉headache, dizziness, stiff pain of the neck and nape, pain in the hypochondriac region, bitter taste, deafness and pain in the ear. 〈Method〉Puncture subcutaneously 0.5～0.8 cun. Moxibustion is applicable.

●头疼[tóu téng] 即头痛。详见该条。

Pain in the Head →头痛 (p. 445)

●头痛[tóu tòng] 病证名。出《素问·平人气象论》等。亦称头疼。整个头部以及头的前、后、偏侧部的疼痛，均称头痛。头为诸阳之会，精明之府，五脏六腑之气血皆上会于此。凡六淫外感，脏腑内伤，导致阳气阻塞，浊邪上踞，肝阳上亢，精髓气血亏损，经络运行失常等，均能导致头痛。临床可分为风寒、风热、风湿、肝阳、血虚、痰浊、瘀血头痛。详见各条。

Headache A disease, originally from *Suwen*: *Pingren Qixiang Lun* (*Plain Questions*: *On Normal People's Physiology*), also called head pain. Pain in the whole head, or in the anterior, posterior and lateral part are generally called headache. The head is the confluence of all the yang, it is the residence of intelligence, and the qi and blood of the five zang organs and six fu organs gather there. All factors, such as affection by six external etiological factors, injury of interal organs leading to obstruction of yang-qi, accumulation of turbid pathogenic factor in the upper, hyperactivity of the liver-yang, consumption of qi, blood and essence and marrow, and abnormal circulation of the qi and blood in the meridians, can cause headache. It is clinically divided into headache due to wind-cold pathogen, headache due to wind-heat pathogen, headache due to wind-dampness pathogen, headache due to liver-yang trouble, headache due to blood deficiency, headache due to phlegm-turbidity, and headache due to blood stasis. →风寒头痛(p. 112)、风热头痛(p. 114)、风湿头痛(p. 115)、肝阳头痛(p. 127)、血虚头痛(p. 529)、痰浊头痛(p. 425)、瘀血头痛(p. 570)

●头维[tóu wéi] 经穴名。出《针灸甲乙经》。属足阳明胃经，为足少阳、阳明、阳维之会。又名颡大、头缝。〈定位〉在头侧部，当额角发际上0.5寸，头正中线旁4.5寸（图28和图24）。〈层次解剖〉皮肤→皮下组织→颞肌上缘的帽状腱膜→腱膜下疏松结缔组织→颅骨外膜。布有耳颞神经的分支，面神经的颞支，颞浅动、静脉的额支等结构。〈主治〉眼痛、头痛、目眩、迎风流泪、眼睑眴动、视物不明。针刺向下或向后平刺0.5～0.8寸；禁灸。

Touwei (ST 8) A meridian point, originally from *Zhenjiu Jia-Yi Jing* (*A-B Classic of Acupuncture and Moxibustion*), a point on the Stomach Meridian of Foot-Yangming, the crossing point of the Meridians of Foot-Shaoyang, Foot-Yangming and Yangwei, also called Sangda or Toufeng. 〈Location〉on the lateral side of the head, 0.5 cun above the anterior hairline at the corner of the forehead, and 4.5 cun lateral to the midline of the head (Figs. 28 & 24). 〈Regional anatomy〉 skin → subcutaneous tissue→epicranial aponeurosis→ subaponeurotic loose connective tissue → pericranium. There are the branches of the auriculotemporal nerve, the temporal branches of the facial nerve and the frontal branches of the superficial temporal artery and vein in this area. 〈Indications〉 pain of the eyes, headache, blurred vision, lacrimation, twitching of the eyelids, poor vision. 〈Method〉Puncture downwards or backwards 0.5～0.8 cun subcutaneously. Moxibustion is forbidden.

●头眩[tóu xuàn] 见《金匮要略·中风历节病脉证

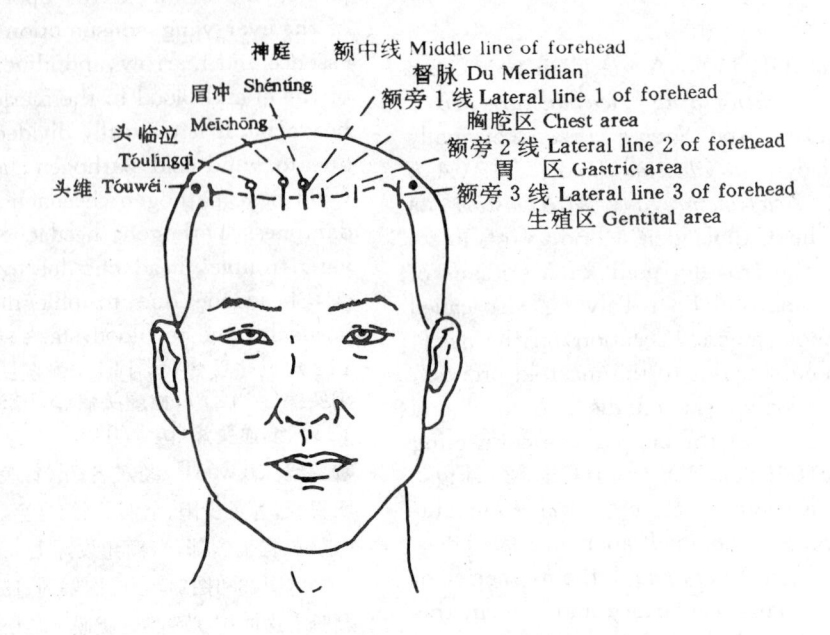

神庭 额中线 Middle line of forehead
眉冲 Shénting
Meichōng 督脉 Du Meridian
头临泣 额旁 1 线 Lateral line 1 of forehead
Tóulíngqì 胸腔区 Chest area
头维 Tóuwéi 额旁 2 线 Lateral line 2 of forehead
胃 区 Gastric area
额旁 3 线 Lateral line 3 of forehead
生殖区 Genital area

图59.1 头针线（前面）
Fig 59.1 Scalp acupuncture lines (Anterior view)

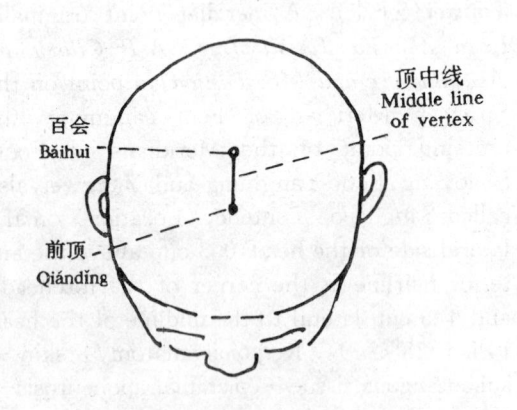

顶中线 Middle line of vertex
百会 Bǎihuì
前顶 Qiándǐng

图59.2 头针线（顶面）
Fig 59.2 Scalp acupuncture lines (Vertex view)

并治》。指头部昏晕。详见"眩晕"条。

Faintness Seen in *Jingui Yaolüe: Zhong Feng Li Jie Bing Mai Zheng Bing Zhi* (*Synopsis of the Golden Chamber: Pulse Conditions, Symptoms and Treatments of Windstroke and Arthralgia*), referring to a faint feeling in the head. →眩晕(p.520)

●头针[tóu zhēn] ①针具名。又称头皮针。针刺头皮部特定刺激区时选用，一般为28～30号，长1.5～2寸的毫针。②指头针疗法。详见该条。

1. Head Needle An acupuncture apparatus, also called scalp needle, it is used for needling specific stimulation areas of the scalp, usually a filiform needle in No. 28～30, 1.5～2.0 cun in length.

2. Scalp Acupuncture →头针疗法(p.446)

●头针疗法[tóu zhēn liáo fǎ] 是针刺头皮部特定刺激区（图1～5）治疗疾病的方法。于1972年报道推广，它是在针刺疗法与现代医学关于大脑皮层功能定位理论相结合的基础上发展起来的。操作时，一般沿皮下缓慢捻转进针，当达到一定深度时，停止进退，切勿提插，再行大幅度快速捻转，出现针感后，再持续捻转3～4分钟，留针10～20分钟，其间再捻转1～2次。本法适用于中风后遗症、震颤性麻痹、舞蹈病、肢体运动障碍等。

Scalp Acupuncture Therapy A therapy for treating diseases by needling specific stimulation areas of the scalp (Figs. 1-5). Reported in

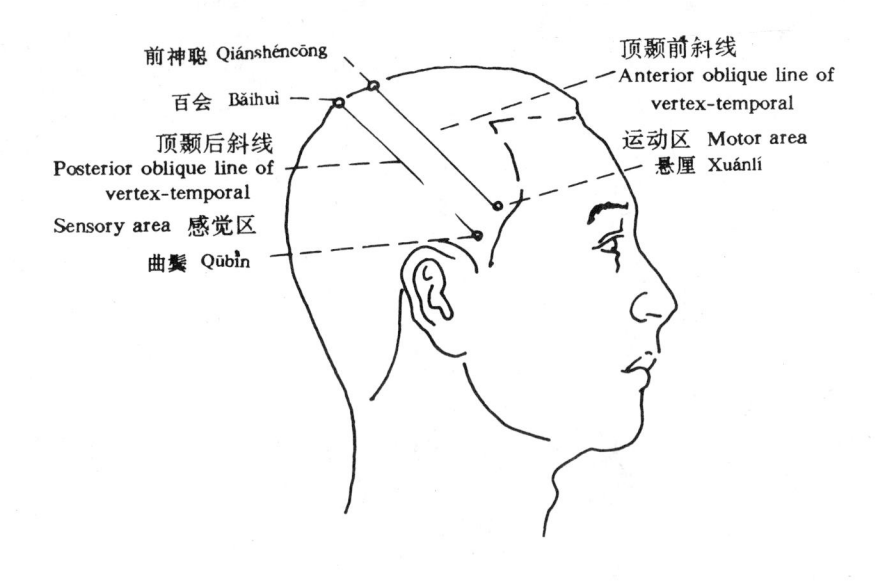

图59.3.1 头针线(侧面)

Fig 59.3.1 Scalp acupuncture lines(Lateral view)

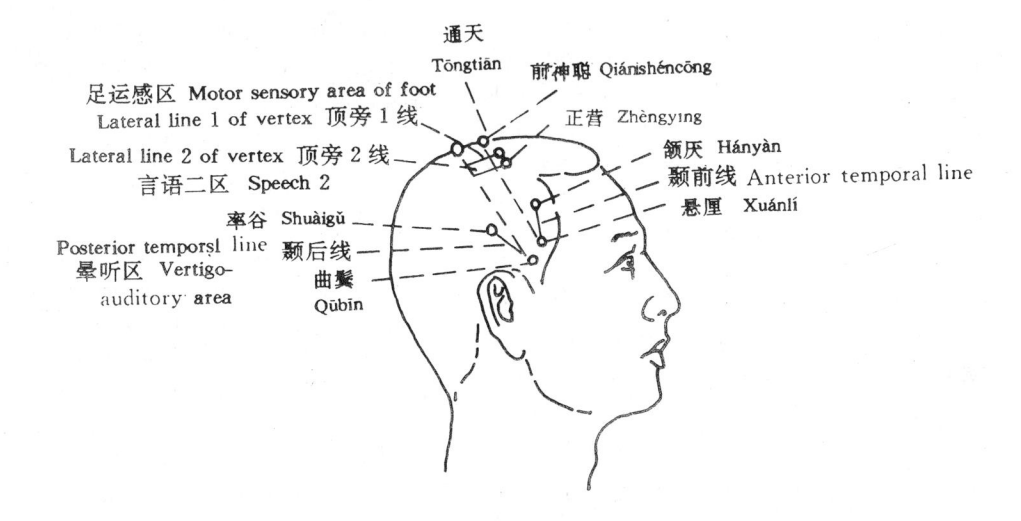

图59.3.2 头针线(侧面)

Fig 59.3.2 Scalp acupuncture lines(Lateral view)

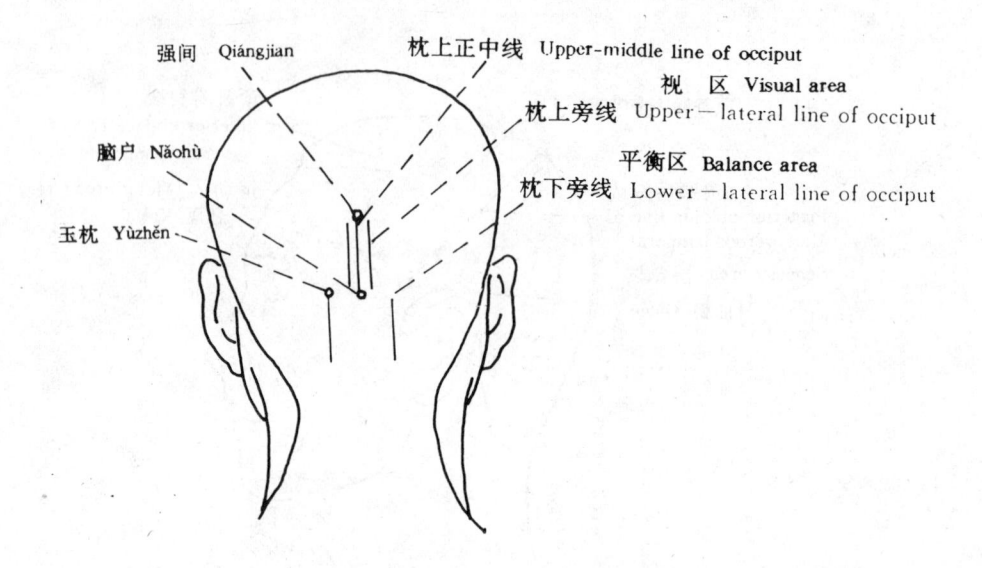

[Diagram: Scalp acupuncture lines (Posterior view) with labels: 强间 Qiángjian, 脑户 Nǎohù, 玉枕 Yùzhěn, 枕上正中线 Upper-middle line of occiput, 视区 Visual area, 枕上旁线 Upper-lateral line of occiput, 平衡区 Balance area, 枕下旁线 Lower-lateral line of occiput]

图59.4 头针线(后面)
Fig 59.4 Scalp acupuncture lines(Posterior view)

1972, this method has been popularized on the basis of the intergration of acupuncture therapy and modern medicine on the functional location of cerebral cortex. 〈Method〉 In the course of manipulation, subcutaneously insert the needle while twisting it slowly to a proper depth, stop inserting the needle, and don't lift and thrust the needle, then twirl the needle rapidly and greatly. After the needling sensation is obtained, twirl the needle continuously for 3~4 minutes, then retain the needle for 10~20 minutes, and repeat the manipulation 1~2 times during the needle-retention. 〈Indications〉 apoplectic sequela, Parkinson's disease, chorea, and dyscinesia of the limbs, etc.

●透刺[tòu cì] 刺法名。将针按一定方向透达某穴或某部。在四肢内外侧或前后侧相对穴位间可直透,各部上下方或前后方相邻穴位间可斜透或沿皮透。

Penetrating Needling A needling technique. 〈Method〉Insert the needle in a certain direction to reach a certain point or part. To corresponding points on the medial and lateral or anterior and posterior of the four limbs, straight penetration can be applied. To neighbouring points on the superior and inferior parts, oblique or subcutaneous penetration can be applied.

●透天凉[tòu tiān liáng] 针刺手法名。出《金针赋》。其法将预定针刺深度分为上(天部)、中(人部)、深(地部)三层。操作时由深至浅,将针直达地部,以紧提慢按六次;再退至人部,以紧提慢按六次;再退至天部,又紧提慢按六次。然后将针一次进到地部,再如前法操作。自深层到浅层三退三进(实际上是九退三进),此为一度。如此反复几度,到病人自觉针下或全身有寒凉感为止,出针时摇大针孔,不揉闭针孔。此法多用于热症、急性痈肿等症。

Thorough Heavenly Cool A needling technique, originally from *Jinzhen Fu*(*Ode to Gold Needle*). 〈Method〉Divide the predetermined puncture depth into three portions, upper (superficial portion), middle (medium portion) and lower (deep portion). In the course of acupuncture manipulation, the needle is inserted from the lower to the upper. First, insert the needle directly into the deep portion, lift it quickly and thrust it slowly for six times, then lift the needle to the medium portion to do the same manipulation six times. Finally lift the needle to the superficial portion to do the same manipulation six times again. After that, insert

the needle directly into the deep portion again to do the above manipulation. Three liftings and three insertions from the deep to the shallow (actually nine liftings and three insertions) are one turn. Repeat the manipulation for several turns till the patient feels cool in the punctured area or in the whole body. On withdrawing the needle, shake it to enlarge the hole, do not press the hole. This method is the most common one to treat febrile diseases, acute carbuncle, etc.

●土疳 [tǔ gān]　即针眼。详见该条。

Disorder of Earth-Orbiculus　→ 针眼 (p. 597)

●吐血 [tù xuè]　病证名。见《金匮要略·惊悸吐衄下血胸满瘀血脉证并治》。其血出自胃腑，从口而出。若血随呕吐而出者，称作呕血。多因郁怒，醇酒，伤食，劳倦等导致脏腑热盛，阴虚火旺，或因脾虚气弱而致。临床可分为胃热吐血，肝火吐血，脾虚吐血。详见各条。

Spitting Blood　A disease, seen in *Jingui Yaolüe: Jingji Tuxue Xiaxue Xiongman Yuxue Mai Zheng Bing Zhi* (*Synopsis of the Golden Chamber: Pulse Conditions, Symptoms and Treatments of Fright, Palpitation, Hematemesis, Epistaxis, Hemafecia, Thoracic Fullness and Blood Stasis*). Blood comes from the stomach and is spat out of the mouth. If blood comes out when vomiting, it is called hematemesis. This is due to emotional depression, improper diet and overworking leading to excessive heat in the zang-fu organs, hyperactivity of fire due to yin deficiency, or to deficiency of the spleen and weakness of qi. Spitting blood can be clinically divided into spitting blood due to the stomach heat, spitting blood due to the liver fire and spitting blood due to deficiency of the spleen. → 胃热吐血 (p. 467)、肝火吐血 (p. 125)、脾虚吐血 (p. 295)

●团岗 [tuán gǎng]　经外穴名。出《千金要方》。又名环岗。在骶部，当小肠俞直下2寸处。灸治大小便不通、腰痛等。

Tuangang (EX-B)　An extra point, originally from *Qianjin Yaofang* (*Essential Prescriptions Worth a Thousand Gold*), also called Huangang. 〈Location〉on the sacral portion, 2.0 cun directly below Xiaochangshu (BL 27). 〈Indications〉constipation, difficulty in urination, pain in the loin, etc.

●推而纳之 [tuī ěr nà zhī]　刺法用语。见《难经·七十八难》。为针刺补法操作的要领，与泻法"动而伸之"相对。指针刺取得感应后，将针推进并向下按纳（插）为补。后世所称的"紧按慢提"的补法操作，即以此为根据。

Thrusting while Pushing the Needle　A needling technique, seen in *Nanjing: Qishiba Nan* (*The Classic of Questions: Question 78*). The key for the reinforcing method of acupuncture, opposite to the reducing method of lifting while pulling. It refers to the manipulation in which, after the needling response is obtained, the needle is pressed down (thrusted) while being pushed. This is a reinforcing method. The reinforcing manipulation of "quick thrusting and slow lifting" of later generations is based on this.

●推罐法 [tuī guàn fǎ]　拨罐法的一种。又称拉罐法、走罐法。于火罐吸着后，将罐推拉移动以扩大其作用面。应用时先在罐口和治疗部位上涂上一些凡士林油膏或石蜡等润滑剂。将杯罐用闪火或投火法等，使吸着皮肤片刻后，再用手捏住罐体慢慢分段来回推移约6~8次，到局部出现红晕为止。本法多用于背腰部。适用于风湿痛和胃肠病等。

Cupping by Pushing the Cup　A kind of cupping, also called cupping by drawing the cup or cupping by moving the cup. 〈Method〉 When the cup is sucked to the skin, push and draw to move the cup so as to enlarge the functioning area. Before cupping, smear some lubricant such as vaseline or paraffin oil, etc. on the affected area and the edge of the cup. When applying the fire-throwing or fire-flashing method to make the cup attach to the skin, hold the cup with the hand and one section after another, push it to and fro slowly about 6-8 times until the skin of the affected area becomes red. The method is usually applied to the lumbodorsal part, suitable for rheumatic pain and gastrointestinal diseases.

●推引 [tuī yǐn]　刺法用语。见《素问·离合真邪论》。推，指进；引，指退。后人用于说明对针感传导的控制。

Pushing and Pulling A term for a needling technique, seen in *Suwen: Lihe Zhenxie Lun (Plain Questions: On the Expelling and Parting of Evil-Qi From Vital-Qi)*. Pushing here means inserting, pulling refers to lifting. In later generations, it is used to indicate the control of radiating needling sensations.

●推针[tuī zhēn] 为鍉针之别称。详见该条。

Pushing Needle Another name for spoon needle. →鍉针(p. 77)

●退[tuì] 针刺基本手法之一。与"进"相对而言，即将针从深部(地部)退至较浅部(人部)或浅部(天部)，向上引退的操作过程。《黄帝内经》中所谓"伸"，即"退"之意。目的是为了减轻针感。

Lifting A basic needling manipulation, the opposite of inserting, referring to the manipulation process in which the neele is lifted from the deep (earth) portion to the less deep (human) portion to the shallow (sky) portion. In the book of *Huangdi Neijing (The Yellow Emperor's Inner Canon)*, it is called "pulling", which is synonymous with "lifting". The purpose of the method is to reduce the needling response.

●退法[tuì fǎ] 针刺手法名。见《针经指南》。为十四法之一。指退针的方法。古出针时，出针豆许，补时出针宜泻三吸，泻时出针宜补三呼，再停少时，方可出针。目前退针的方法，宜从深部缓缓退至皮下，留置片刻以待气缓，当针下不觉沉紧时随即拔出。

Withdrawing An acupuncture manipulation, seen in *Zhenjing Zhinan (A Guide to the Classics of Acupuncture)*, one of the Fourteen Methods, referring to the method of withdrawing the needle. In ancient times, when withdrawing, yet the needle withdrawn a little bit. For reinforcement, do reducing for the period of three inspirations while withdrawing the needle; for reduction, do reinforcing for the period of three expirations while withdrawing the needle. Then retain the needle in the body for a while, and withdraw the needle. At present, the method of withdrawing the needle is to lift the needle slowly from the deep portion to the subcutaneous portion, retain it until qi gets unhurried and withdraw it quickly when the doctor feels no tension and dragging sensation around the needle.

●臀[tún] ①耳穴名。位于对耳轮下脚的外三分之一处。用于治疗臀部疾患、腰骶疼痛、坐骨神经痛、臀筋膜炎。②部位名。指腰以下二股之上，尻旁大肉，即臀大肌的部位。

1. Buttock(MA-AH 5) An auricular point. 〈Location〉at the lateral 1/3 of the inferior antihelixcrus. 〈Indications〉pain at the corresponding area, pain of the lumbosacral region, sciatica, gluteal fasciitis.

2. Buttock A body part, referring to the part below the waist and above the thigh, the muscle beside the sacrum, which refers to greater gluteal muscle.

●臀中[tún zhōng] 经外穴名。见《常用经穴解剖学定位》。在臀部，以大转子和坐骨结节线为底边，向上作一等边三角形，其顶点是穴。〈主治〉坐骨神经痛、下肢偏瘫、荨麻疹等。直刺1.5~2.5寸；可灸。

Tunzhong(EX-B) An extra point, seen in *Changyong Jingxue Jiepouxue Dingwei (Anatomical Locations of Commonly Used Meridian Points)*. 〈Location〉on the buttocks. Draw an equilateral triangle with the line connecting the greater trochanter of the femur and the ischial tuberosity as the base, and the point is at the apex of the triangle. 〈Indications〉sciatica, hemiparalysis of the lower limbs, urticaria, etc. 〈Method〉Puncture perpendicularly 1.5~2.5 cun. Moxibustion is applicable.

●托颐位[tuō yí wèi] 针灸体位名。指两手掌根相对托住下颌的体位。用于针灸头顶部的体位。

Posture for Cupping Chin in Hands An acupuncture posture, referring to the posture in which the two palmar roots jointly cup the chin. It's used for acupuncture and moxibustion on the scalp.

●脱肛[tuō gāng] 病证名。出《诸病源候论》。又名截肠。指直肠下端脱出肛门之外而言。多因气虚下陷或湿热下注大肠而致。临床分为脱肛实证和脱肛虚证两类。详见各条。

Prolapse of Rectum A disease, originally from *Zhubing Yuanhou Lun (General Treatise on the Etiology and Symptomatology of Diseases)*, also called blockage of rectum, refer-

ring to prolapse of the lower portion of the rectum out of the anus, mostly due to qi collapse and deficiency, or downward flow of damp-heat to the large intestine. It is clinically divided into two kinds: prolapse of rectum of excess type and prolapse of rectum of deficiency type→脱肛实证(p.451)、脱肛虚证(p.451)

●脱肛实证[tuō gāng shí zhèng] 脱肛证型之一。因便秘、痔疮,湿热郁于直肠,局部肿胀,排便时过度努责,约束受损所致。证多见于痢疾急性期和痔疮发炎时,自觉肛门坠胀、便意频急、努责不遗余力、迫使直肠脱垂,伴有局部红肿、灼热、痛痒、舌苔黄腻、脉数。治宜清泄湿热。针长强、大肠俞、承山、曲池、支沟、阴陵泉。

Prolapse of Rectum of Excess Type One type of prolapse of rectum, caused by constipation, hemorrhoids, damp-heat accumulated in the rectum leading to local edema and over-exerting in defecation resulting in impairment of restraint. ⟨Manifestations⟩mostly seen in acute dysentery and inflammatory hemorrhoids, distending and prolapse feeling of the anus, frequent and urgent sensation of defecation, over-exerting in defecation leading to prolapse of the rectum, accompanied with local redness and swelling, hot sensation, pain and itch, yellow and greasy tongue coating, rapid pulse. ⟨ Treatment principle ⟩ Remove pathogenic damp-heat. ⟨Point selection⟩ Changqiang (DU 1), Dachangshu (BL 25), Chengshan (BL 57), Quchi (LI 11), Zhigou (SJ 6) and Yinlingquan (SP 9).

●脱肛虚证[tuō gāng xū zhèng] 脱肛证型之一。多因久痢久泻及妇女生育过多,体质虚弱,中气下陷,收摄无权所致。证见发病缓慢,仅在大便时感觉肛门坠胀,肠端经度脱垂,便后能自行还纳,久则不能自行回缩,须推托方能复位。伴有面色萎黄、神疲乏力、头晕、心悸、苔薄白、脉濡细。治宜益气升提。取百会、长强、大肠俞、承山、气海、足三里。

Prolapse of Rectum of Dificiency Type One type of prolapse of rectum, caused by lingering diarrhea and dysentery, overbirth in women, constitutional insufficiency, collapse of the qi in the middle-jiao resulting in failure of control. ⟨Manifestations⟩ slow onset of disease, distending and prolapsed feeling of the anus in defecation, slight prolapse of the lower end of the rectum which may return itself after defecation, but in long-standing cases, no return of itself unless it is pushed back, accompanied by sallow complexion, lassitude, listlessness, dizziness, palpitation, white and thin tongue coating, soft and thready pulse. ⟨Treatment principle⟩Supplement qi to make it rise. ⟨Point selection⟩Baihui(DU 20), Changqiang(DU 1), Dachangshu(BL 25), Chengshan(BL 57)Qihai(RN 6) and Zusanli(ST 36).

●脱骨疔[tuō gǔ dīng] 即脱疽。详见该条。

Bone-Dropping Boil →脱疽(p.451)

●脱骨疽[tuō gǔ jū] 即脱疽。详见该条。

Bone-Dropping Cellulitis →脱疽(p.451)

●脱疽[tuō jū] 病证名。出《刘涓子鬼遗方》。又名脱痈、脱骨疽、脱骨疔。多发于四肢末端,尤其下肢更为多见。指(趾)溃烂不愈,久则(趾)指节脱落,故名。由于寒湿内侵以致经络凝滞,痹阻不通,郁久化热;或因偏嗜烟酒,膏粱厚味,蕴热壅滞经络,热盛肉腐而成坏疽。临床可分气滞血瘀脱疽,气阴两伤脱疽。详见各条。

Gangrene of Finger or Toe A disease, originally from *Liu Juanzi Yifang* (*Liu Juanzi's Bequeathed Prescriptions*), also called dropping carbuncle, bone-dropping boil, bone-dropping cellulitis. Mostly found in the ends of the four limbs, especially in the lower limbs, manifested as ulcers or gangrenes in the fingers or toes. In lingering case, dropping of the bones of the toe (finger), thus it is named. It is due to the invasion of cold-dampness leading to blockage of the meridian, resulting in the production of heat due to prolonged stagnation, or due to over smoking and wine-drinking, overeating a fatty diet, stagnated heat blocking the meridian, excessive heat leading to gangrene of finger or toe. Clinically it is divided into gangrene of the finger or toe due to qi-stagnation and blood stasis and gangrene of finger or toe due to deficiency of qi and blood. →气滞血瘀脱疽(p.315)、气阴两伤脱疽(p.312)

●脱痈[tuō yōng] 见《灵枢·痈疽》。即脱疽。详见该条。

Dropping Carbuncle Seen in *Ling Shu: Yongju* (*Miraculous Pivot: Carbuncle and Oth-*

●脱证[tuō zhèng] 病证名。是以亡阴亡阳为特征的病证。多因高热大汗,剧烈吐泻,失血过多,阴液或阳气暴亡散失所致。由于阴阳互根,阴竭则阳亡,阳亡则阴无以化而告竭,所以亡阴亡阳互为因果,难以截然分开,只是先后主次不同而已。亡阴证见汗出粘而热、兼见肌肤热、手足温、口渴喜饮、甚则昏迷、脉细数、按之无力。亡阳见大汗淋漓、汗清稀而凉、兼见肌肤凉、手足冷、口不渴、喜热饮、倦卧神疲、甚则昏不知人、脉微欲绝。治宜回阳固脱,调节阴阳。取素髎、关元、涌泉、足三里。亡阳加气海。亡阴加太溪。

Prostration Syndrome A disease, characterized by yang depletion and yin depletion, mostly due to high fever, profuse sweating, severe vomiting, diarrhea and over bleeding resulting in sudden exhaustion of yin-fluid or yang-qi. As yin and yang are related to each other, depletion of yin may give rise to that of yang; depletion of yang can not produce yin-fluid, which results in yin exhaustion, so the depletion of yin or yang is a mutual causal connection. They can not be divided absolutely, only differentiated as early or late and primary or secondary. Yin depletion syndrome is manifested as hot and sticky sweating, often accompanied by fever, hot hands and feet, desire for drinks, coma in severe case, thready, feeble and rapid pulse. Yang depletion syndrome is manifested as profuse, cold and light sweating, accompanied by cold body and limbs, no thirst, desire for hot drinks, sleep in bending posture, weariness or coma in severe case, barely palpable pulse. 〈Treatment principle〉 Recuperate depleted yang and rescue the patient from collapse, regulate yin and yang. 〈Point slection〉 Suliao (DU 25), Guanyuan (RN 4), Yongquan (KI 1), Zusanli (ST 36), For depleted yang, Qihai (RN 6) is added, and for depleted yin, Taixi (KI 3) is added.

W

●外鼻[wài bí] 耳穴名。位于耳屏正中。〈主治〉鼻疖、鼻塞、鼻前庭炎、鼻炎、单纯性肥胖症。

External Nose (MA-T 1) An auricular point. 〈Locations〉on the centre of the tragus. 〈Indication〉nasal furuncle, stuffy nose, nasal vestibulitis, rhintis, simple obesity.

●外侧[wài cè] 部位名。①指手背一侧即伸侧,是手三阳经循行于上肢及其所属穴位分布的部位。②指下肢外侧,是足三阳经循行于下肢及其所属穴位分布的部位。

Lateral Aspect A part of the body, referring to ①the aspect of dorsum of the hand, namely, extensive side, which is the part in which three yang meridians of hand and their points are distributed. ②the anterio-lateral aspect of the lower limbs which is the part in which the three yang meridians of foot and their points are distributed.

●外吹乳痈[wài chuī rǔ yōng] 病证名。见《寿世保元》。吹乳之一种。指产后乳痈。旧说因儿吮乳熟睡,鼻孔凉气袭入乳房,与热乳凝结而成。实则由于吮乳熟睡致伤或咬伤乳头后感染所致。详见乳痈条。

Acute Mastitis due to External Blowing A disease, seen in *Shoushi Baoyuan* (*Longevity and Life Preservation*), one kind of blowing breast, referring to acute mastitis after delivery. In the past, it was said that when the baby sucked the breast while sleeping, the cold air from his (her) nose entered the breast and mixed with the warm milk resulting in the disease. But, in fact, the disease is caused by infection due to an injury or biting of the nipple by the baby sucking in sleep. →乳痈(p.339)

●外耳[wài ěr] 耳穴名。又称耳。位于屏上切迹近耳轮部。具有滋肾水、潜肝阳作用。〈主治〉外耳道炎、中耳炎、耳鸣、眩晕。

External Ear (MA) An auricular point, also

called ear(MA). ⟨Location⟩on the supratragic notch close to the helix. ⟨Function⟩ Nourish the yin of the kidney; check hyperactivity of the liver-yang. ⟨Indications⟩ inflammation of the external auditory canal, otitis media, tinnitus, dizziness.

●外耳道口[wài ěr dào kǒu] 耳廓解剖名称。在耳甲腔内，被耳屏遮盖着的孔窍。即外耳道的开口。

Opening of the External Auditory Meatus
A term for auricle anatomy, referring to the exit of the external auditory in the cavum concha covered by the tragus.

●外感风疹[wài gǎn fēng zhěn] 风疹证型之一。多因腠理不固，风邪侵袭，遏于肌肤而成。其证除见风疹的一般症状外，起病急骤、身热口渴、或兼咳嗽、肢体酸楚、苔薄白、脉濡数。治宜疏风和营。取风池、大椎、肩髃、曲池、外关、足三里、三阴交。参见风疹条。

Rubella due to Exopathogen A type of rubella, mostly due to poor function of the skin and muscles and wind pathogen invading the body and accumulating in the skin. Besides the general symptoms of rubella, sudden onest, fever, thirst, cough, sore and pain in the limbs, thin and white tongue coating, rapid and soft pulse are also common symptoms. ⟨Treatment principle⟩ Dispel wind and regulate the nutrients. ⟨Point selection⟩ Fengchi (GB 20), Dazhui (DU 14), Jianyu (LI 15), Quchi (LI 11), Waiguan (SJ 5), Zusanli (ST 36) and Sanyinjiao (SP 6). →风疹 (p. 116)

●外感呕吐[wài gǎn ǒu tù] 呕吐证型之一。由于风、寒、暑、湿之邪以及秽浊之气，侵犯胃腑，以致胃失和降，胃气上逆所致。其证偏寒则呕吐暴急、吐出多为清水稀涎、喜暖畏寒、大便溏薄、伴恶寒发热，头痛，苔白、脉浮等。偏热侧呕吐频繁、饮水进食即吐、吐出酸苦胆汁或热臭、口渴欲饮冷饮而恶热、大便燥结、伴有头痛、发热、舌红、脉数等，治宜解表和中。取大椎、外关、合谷、内庭、中脘、三阴交、太冲。偏寒加脾俞、胃俞；偏热加金津、玉液。

Vomiting due to Exopathogen A type of vomiting, caused by wind, cold, summer-heat and damp pathogens, and filthy and turbid qi invading the stomach leading to failure of the stomach-qi to descend and the adverse flow of stomach-qi. Cases with cold are manifested as the sudden and violent vomiting, vomiting with some clear fluid and thin saliva, desire for warmth and fear of chill, loose stool accompanied by aversion to cold, fever, headache, white tongue coating and superficial pulse. Cases with heat are manifested as frequent vomiting, vomiting right after eating or drinking, eructation with sour-bitter bile or fetid odor due to heat, thirst, desire for cold drinks, aversion to heat, dry stools, accompanied by headache, fever, red togue, rapid pulse. ⟨Treatment principle⟩ Relieve the exterior syndrome and regulate the spleen and stomach. ⟨Point selection⟩ Dazhui (DU 14), Waiguan (SJ 5), Hegu (LI 4), Neiting (ST 44), Zhongwan (RN 12), Sanyinjiao (SP 6) and Taichong (LR 3). For cold, add pishu (BL 20) and Weishu (BL 21) for heat, Jinjin (EX-HN 12) and Yuye (EX-HN 13) can be added.

●外勾[wài gōu] 经穴别名。出《针灸大全》。即伏兔。详见该条。

Waigou Another name for Futu (ST 32), a meridian point originally from *Zhenjiu Daquan* (*A Complete Work of Acupuncture and Moxibustion*). →伏兔 (p. 117)

●外关[wài guān] 经穴名。出《灵枢·经脉》。属手少阳三焦经，为本经络穴，八脉交会穴之一，通于阳维脉。又名阳维穴。⟨定位⟩在前臂背侧，当阳池与肘尖的连线上，腕背横纹上2寸，尺骨与桡骨之间（图48和图50）。⟨层次解剖⟩皮肤→皮下组织→小指伸肌和指伸肌→拇长伸肌和示指伸肌。浅层布有前臂后皮神经，头静脉和贵要静脉的属支。深层有骨间后动、静脉和骨间后神经。⟨主治⟩热病、头痛、颊痛、耳聋、耳鸣、目赤肿痛、胁痛、肩背痛、肘臂屈伸不利、手指疼痛、手颤。直刺0.5～1寸；可灸。

Waiguan (SJ 5) A meridian point, originally from *Lingshu: Jing Mai* (*Miraculous Pivot: Meridians*), the Luo (connecting) point of the Sanjiao meridian of Hand-Shaoyang, one of the eight confluence points, connecting with the Yangwei Meridian, also called Yangwei. ⟨Location⟩on the dorsal side of the forearm, on the line connecting Yangchi (SJ 4) and the tip of the olecranon, 2 cun proximal to the dorsal crease of the wrist, between the radius and ulna (Figs. 48&50). ⟨Regional anatomy⟩ skin→subcutaneous tissue→extensor muscle of little finger and extensor muscle of fingers →long extensor muscle of thumb and exten-

sor muscle of index finger. In the superficial layer, there are the posterior cutaneous nerve of the forearm and the tributaries of the cephalic and basilic veins. In the deep layer, there are the posterior interosseous artery and vein and the posterior interosseous nerve. 〈Indications〉febrile disease, headache, pain in the check, deafness tinnitus, redness, swelling and pain of the eye, pain in the hypochondiac region, pain in the arm and shoulder, motor impairment of the elbow and arm, pain in the fingers, trembling of the hand. 〈Method〉Puncture perpendicularly 0.5~1 cun. Moxibustion is applicable.

●外踝[wài huái]部位名。指腓骨下端向外突起处。

Lateral Malleolus　A body part, referring to the protuberance of the lower end of the fibula.

●外踝尖[wài huái jiān]　经外穴名。见《千金要方》。〈定位〉在足外侧面, 外踝的凸起处(图9)。〈层次解剖〉皮肤→皮下组织→外踝。布有胫前动、静脉的外踝网, 腓动脉的外踝支和腓肠神经及腓浅神经的分支。均灸治转筋、脚气等。

Waihuaijian（EX-LE 9）　An extra point, seen in *Qianjin Yaofang* (*Essential Prescriptions Worth a Thousand Gold*). 〈Location〉on the lateral side of the foot, at the tip of the lateral malleolus (Fig. 9). 〈Regional anatomy〉skin→subcutaneous tissue→lateral malleolus. There are the lateral malleolar network of the anterior tibial artery, the lateral malleolar branches of the peroneal artery, the branches of the sural nerve and the superficial peroneal nerve in this area. 〈Indications〉convulsion, beriberi, etc. 〈Method〉moxibustion.

●外踝前交脉[wài huái qián jiāo mài]　经外穴名。见《针灸孔穴及其疗法便览》。位于足背踝关节部, 当内、外踝高点连线的中、外1/4交点处。灸治风齿疼痛。

Waihuaiqianjiaomai（EX-LE）　An extra point, seen *Zhenjiu Kongxue Jiqi Liaofa Bianlan* (*Guide to Acupoints and Acupuncture Therapeutics*). 〈Location〉on the dorsum of the ankle joint, at the junction of the middle and lateral 1/4 of the line connecting the two tips of the medial and external malleolus. 〈Indication〉toothache due to wind. 〈Method〉moxibustion.

●外踝上[wài huái shàng]　经外穴名。见《千金要方》在外踝尖上3寸。灸治筋急不能行。

Waihuaishang（EX-LE）　An extra point, seen in *Qianjin Yaofang* (*Essential Prescriptions Worth a Thousand Gold*). 〈Location〉3 cun above the tip of the lateral malleolus. 〈Indication〉muscular contracture leading to the inability to move. 〈Method〉moxibustion.

●外金津玉液[wài jīn jīn yù yè]　经外穴名。见《芒针疗法》。在廉泉穴直上1.5寸, 旁开0.3寸处。〈主治〉中风失语、流涎、以及舌面溃疡、舌肌麻痹或痉挛、口腔炎等。向舌根方向斜刺0.5~1寸。

Waijinjinyuye（EX-HN）　A pair of extra points seen in *Mangzhen Liaofa* (*Elongated Needle Therapy*). 〈Location〉1.5 cun straight above Lianquan (RN 23), 0.3 cun external to the point. 〈Indications〉aphasia and salivation due to wind stroke, linguofacial ulcer, muscular paralysis or spasm of tongue. 〈Method〉Puncture obliquely 0.5~1.0 cun in the direction of the tongue root.

●外经[wài jīng]　出《灵枢·邪气脏腑病形》。指经脉的外行部分, 与内行于脏腑部分相对而言。

External Meridians　Originally from *Lingshu*; *Xieqi Zangfu Bingxing* (*Miraculous Pivot: Pathogenic Evils, Zang-Fu Organs and Manifestations*), referring to the externally distributed parts of meridians versus the internally distributed parts of meridians.

●外灸膏[wài jiǔ gāo]　敷贴用方药之一。见《杨氏家藏方》。方用木香、附子(炮去皮脐)、蛇床子、吴茱萸、胡椒、川乌头六味药各6克, 研为细末掺匀。取上药末9克, 面粉6克, 用生姜汁调和成膏状, 摊于纸上, 贴敷于脐部。可治疗虚寒、下痢赤白、时腹隐痛、肠滑不禁等症。

External Moxibustion Adhesive Plaster　One of the moxibustion methods, seen in *Yangshi Jiacang Fang* (*Yang's Home Collection of Formulas*). 〈Ingredients〉*Mu Xiang* (*Radix Aucklandiae*), *Fu Zi* (*Radix Aconiti Praeparata*) (with peel and handle removed), *She Chuang Zi* (*Fructus Chidii*), *Wu Zhu Yu* (*Fructus Euodiae*), *Hu Jiao* (*Pericarpium Zanthoxyli*), *Chuan Wu Tou* (*Radix Aconiti*), 6g of each. Grind the herbs into a powder and mix them evenly. Take 9g of the mixed pow-

er, 6g of wheat flour and mix them into a medicinal extract with ginger juice. Put it on paper and stick the plaster on the navel. 〈Indications〉cold due to deficiency, dysentery with blood and whitish discharge, occasional abdominal dull pain, uncontrolled laxation.

●外科灸法论粹新书[wài kē jiǔ fǎ lùn cuì xīn shū] 书名。宋·徐梦符撰。见《宋史·艺文志》。已佚。
Waike Jiufa Luncui Xinshu(*A New Book on Essentials of Moxibustion for External Diseases*) A book compiled by Xu Mengfu in the Song Dynasty, seen in *Songshi: Yi Wen Zhi* (*The History of the Song Dynasty: Records of Art and Literature*).

●外劳宫[wài láo gōng] 经外穴名。见《小儿推拿方脉活婴秘旨全书》。又名项强穴。〈定位〉在手背侧、第二、三掌骨之间，掌指关节后0.5寸（指寸）（图69）。〈层次解剖〉皮肤→皮下组织→第二骨间背侧肌→第一骨间掌侧肌。布有桡神经浅支的指背神经，手背静脉网和掌背动脉。〈主治〉消化不良、腹泻、便溏、小儿急慢惊风、落枕、指不能伸、指掌麻、痒等。直刺0.3～0.5寸；可灸。
Wailaogong(EX-UE 8) An extra point seen in *Xiaoer Tuina Fangmai Huoying Mizhi Quanshu*(*A Complete Work of Infantile Massotherapy*). Also called Xiangqiang Point. 〈Location〉on the dorsum of the hand, between the 2nd and 3rd metacarpal bones and 0.5 cun proximal to the metacarpophalangeal joint(Fig. 69). 〈Regional anatomy〉skin→subcutaneous tissue → 2nd dorsal interosseous muscles → 1st volar interosseous muscles. There are the dorsal digital nerves of the superficial branch of the radial nerve, and the dorsal manus network of hand and dorsal metacarpel arteries. 〈Indications〉indigestion, diarrhea, loose stool, acute and chronic infantile convulsion, stiff neck, failure of fingers to stretch, numbness of fingers and palm, itching. 〈Method〉Puncture perpendicularly 0.3～0.5 cun. Moxibustion is applicable.

●外陵[wài líng] 经穴名。出《针灸甲乙经》。属足阳明胃经。〈定位〉在下腹部，当脐中下1寸，距前正中线2寸（图60.4和图40）。〈层次解剖〉皮肤→皮下组织→腹直肌鞘前臂→腹直肌。浅层布有第十、十一、十二胸神经前支的外侧皮支和前皮支及腹壁浅静脉。深层有腹壁下动、静脉的分支或属支，第十、十一、十二胸神经前支的肌支。〈主治〉腹痛、疝气、月经痛、心如悬引脐腹痛。直刺0.8～1.2寸；可灸。
Wailing(ST 26) A meridian point, originally from *Zhenjiu Jia-Yi Jing* (*A-B Classic of Acupuncture and Moxibustion*), a point on the Stomach Meridian of Foot-Yangming. 〈Location〉on the lower abdomen, 1 cun below the centre of the umbilicus and 2 cun lateral to the anterior midline (Figs. 60.4&40). 〈Regional anatomy〉skin→subcutaneous tissue→anterior sheath of rectus muscle of abdomen→rectus muscle of abdomen. In the superficial layer, there are the lateral and anterior cutaneous branches of the anterior branches of the 10th to 12th thoracic nerves and the superficial epigastric vein. In the deep layer, there are the branches or tributaries of the inferior epigastric artery and vein and the muscular branches of the anterior branches of the 10th to 12th thoracic nerves. 〈Indications〉abdominal pain, hernia, dysmenorrhea, umbilical and abdominal pain due to hanging feeling of the heart. 〈Method〉Puncture perpendicularly 0.8～1.2 cun. Moxibustion is applicable.

●外丘[wài qiū] 经穴名。出《针灸甲乙经》。属足少阳胆经。本经郄穴。〈定位〉在小腿外侧，当外踝尖上7寸，腓骨前缘，平阳交（图8.4）。〈层次解剖〉皮肤→皮下组织→腓骨长、短肌→前肌间隔→趾长伸肌→拇长伸肌。浅层布有腓肠外侧皮神经。深层有腓浅神经，腓深神经和胫前动、静脉。〈主治〉颈项强痛、胸胁痛、狂犬伤毒不出、下肢痿痹、癫疾、小儿龟胸，直刺0.5～0.8寸；可灸。
Waiqiu(GB 36) A meridian point, originally from *Zhenjiu Jia-Yi Jing* (*A-B Classic of Acupuncture and Moxibustion*), the Xi(Cleft) point of the Gallbladder Meridian of Foot-Shaoyang. 〈Location〉on the lateral side of the leg, 7 cun above the tip of the external malleolus, on the anterior order of the fibula, and on the level of Yangjiao(BG 35)(Fig. 8.4). 〈Regional anatomy〉skin→subcutaneous tissue→long and stort peroneal muscles→anterior intermuscular septum→long extensor muscle of toes→long extensor muscle of great toe. In the superficial layer, there is the lateral sural cutaneous nerve. In the deep layer, there are the superficial and deep peroneal nerves and the

anterior tibial artery and vein. ⟨Indications⟩ stiffness and pain of the neck and nape, pain in the chest and hypochondrium, dog bite with toxin retained inside, flaccidity and numbness in the lower limbs, epilepsy, pigeon breast in children. ⟨Method⟩ Puncture perpendicularly 0.5~0.8 cun. Moxibstion is applicable.

●外生殖器[wài shēng zhí qì] 耳穴名。位于与耳轮下脚上缘同水平的耳轮处。用于治疗外生殖器病症；会阴部皮肤病、阳萎、急性睾丸炎、附睾丸炎。

External Genitalia(MA-H 4) An auricular point. ⟨Location⟩ on the helix, level with the upper border of the inferior antihelix crus. ⟨Indications⟩ external genital diseases, dermatosis of the perineum, impotence, acute orchitis, epididymitis.

●外枢[wài shū] 经外穴别名。出《针灸甲乙经》。即维道。见该条。

Waishu Another name for Weidao(GB 28), a meridan point, originally from *Zhenjiu Jia-Yi Jing* (*A-B Classic of Acupuncture and Moxibustion*). →维道(p. 460)

●外台秘要[wài tái mì yào] 书名。唐·王焘编著。全书四十卷，一千一百零四门，载方六千余首。成书于752年（天宝十一年）。该书汇集了初唐及唐以前的医学著作。书中引录各书均附出处，为研究我国唐以前医学的一部重要参考著作。其中第三十九卷为《明堂灸法》，载述灸法和经穴，原有附图，已不传。王氏尤重灸法，其内容多引自《针灸甲乙经》、《千金要方》等医籍。其它各卷如疟、霍乱、奔豚、瘰疬、疝等均列有灸法。

Waitai Miyao (Clandestine Essentials from the Imperial Library) A book, compiled by Wang Tao in the Tang Dynasty, consisting of 40 volumes in all, with 1104 categories and more than 6,000 prescriptions, finished in 752 (the 11th year in the reign of Tian Bao). In the book, the author collected medical classics prior to and in the early years of the Tang Dynasty. The sources of the classics quoted in the book are attached. It is an important reference in the study of the medicine before the Tang Dynasty. The 39th volume is entitled *Mingtang Jiufa* (*Acupoints for Moxibustion*), in which the methods of moxibustion and acupoints were recorded, originally with charts, but lost. Dr. Wang especially emphasized the methods of moxibustion. Its contents were quoted from *Zhenjiu Jia-Yi Jing* (*A-B Classic of Acupuncture and Moxibustion*), *Qianjin Yaofang* (*Essential Prescriptions Worth a Thousand Gold*), and other medical books. The other volumes, e. g. Malaria, Cholera, Sensation of Gas Rushing, Scrofula and Hernia, etc. all dealt with the methods of moxibustion.

●外膝眼[wài xī yǎn] 经外穴名。与内膝眼相对，合称膝眼。外膝眼与犊鼻同位。参见各条。

Waixiyan(EX-LE) An extra point as compared with Neixiyan (EX-LE 4). Its joint name with Neixiyan(EX-LE 4)is called Xiyan (EX-LE 5). It is in the same position as Dubi (ST 35). →内膝眼(p. 281)、膝眼(p. 483)、犊鼻(p. 88)

●外痔[wài zhì] 病证名。出《千金要方》。指生于肛门齿线以下的痔疮。证见局部皮瓣赘生，一般无疼痛，或肛门部有异物感，或见红肿、疼痛。参见痔疮条。

External Hermorrhoids A disease, originally from *Qianjin Yaofang* (*Essential Prescriptions Worth a Thousand Gold*), referring to hemorrhoids under anal dentate line. ⟨Manifestations⟩ visible swollen veins in local position, generally without pain, but with foreign body sensation around the anus or redness and swelling, pain of the weins in the anus. →痔疮(p. 606)

●完骨[wán gǔ] ①经穴名。出《素问·气穴论》。属足少阳胆经，为足太阳、少阳之会。在头部，当耳后乳突的后下方凹陷处（图28和图31）。⟨层次解剖⟩在胸锁乳突肌附着部上方，在耳后动静脉分支；布有枕小神经本干。⟨主治⟩头痛、颈项强痛、颊肿、喉痹、龋齿、口眼歪斜、癫痫、疟疾。斜刺0.5~0.8寸；可灸。②部位名。指耳后隆起的颞骨乳突。

Wangu(GB 12) A meridian point, originally from *Suwen: Qixue Lun* (*Plain Questions: On Loci of Qi*), a point on the Gallbladder Meridian of Foot-Shaoyang, the crossing point of Foot-Taiyang and Foot-Shaoyang. ⟨Location⟩ on the head, in the depression posterior and inferior to the mastoid process(Figs. 28&31). ⟨Regional anatomy⟩skin→subcutaneous tissue →sternocleidomastoid muscle→splenius mus-

cle of head→longest muscle of head. In the superficial layer, there are the lesser occipital nerve and the branches or tributaries of the posterior auricular artery and vein. In the deep layer, there are the deep cervical artery and vein. If the needle is inserted too deep, the vertebral artery may be injured. 〈Indications〉 headache, stiffness and pain of the neck and nape, swelling cheek, sore throat, dental caries, deviation of the eye and mouth, epilepsy, malaria. 〈Method〉Puncture obliquely 0.5～0.8 cun. Moxibustion is applicable.

2. **Wangu** A part of the body, referring to the mastoid process behind the ear.

●碗灸[wǎn jiǔ] 间接灸的一种。见《串雅外编》。又称隔碗灸。是用碗作间隔物而施灸的一和方法。在碗内置艾绒如五分硬币状,再在艾绒上放灯心草四根,摆成十字形,以火点燃,待艾燃尽再添新艾再灸,灸至碗内有水蒸气,灸处痛止为度。适用于乳腺炎。

Bowl Moxibustion A kind of indirect moxibustion seen in *Chuanya Waibian* (*External Treatise on Folk Medicine*). Also called bowl-separated moxibustion, referring to the method of using a bowl as a separation for moxibustion. 〈Method〉Put argyi wool in the shape of a 5-fen coin in a bowl, then put 4 pieces of rush pith on the argyi wool like a cross and ignite them. As they burn out, add more moxa. The moxibustion is applied until the appearance of water vapor in the bowl and the disappearance of the pain in the affected region. 〈Indication〉mastadenitis.

●腕[wàn] ①耳穴名,位于将耳舟部分为六等分,自上而下,第二等份为腕。可用于治疗腕部疾患、胃痛。②部位名。臂与手相联之关节。

1. **Wrist**（MA-SF 2） An auricular point. 〈Location〉on the 2nd from top to bottom of the six equal parts of the scapha area. 〈Indications〉diseases of the wrist and stomachache.

2. **Wrist** a part of body, the joint connecting the arm and hand.

●腕骨[wàn gǔ] 经穴名。出《灵枢·本输》。属手太阳小肠经。为本经原穴。〈定位〉在手掌尺侧,当第五掌骨基底与钩骨之间的凹陷处,赤白肉际(图48和图65)。〈层次解剖〉皮肤→皮下组织→小指展肌→豆掌韧带。浅层布有前臂内侧皮神经,尺神经掌支,尺神经手背支和浅静脉等。深层有尺动、静脉的分支或属支。〈主治〉头痛、项强、耳鸣、目翳、指挛臂痛、黄疸、热病汗不出、疟疾、胁痛、颈项颔肿、消渴、目流冷泪、惊风、瘛疭。直刺0.3～0.5寸;可灸。

Wangu（SI 4） A meridian point, originally from *Lingshu*:*Benshu* (*Miraculous Pivot*:*Meridian Points*), the Yuan(Primary)Point of the Small Intestine Meridian of Hand-Taiyang. 〈Location〉on the ulnar border of the hand in the depression between the proximal end of the 5th metacarpal bone and hamate bone, and at the junction of the red and white skin (Figs. 48&65). 〈Regional anatomy〉skin →subcutaneous tissue→abductor muscle of 5th finger→pisometacarpal ligament. In the superficial layer, there are the medial cutaneous nerve of the forearm, the palmar branches of the ulnar nerve, the dorsal branches of the ulnar nerve and the superficial vein. In the deep layer, there are the branches or tributaries of the ulnar artery and vein. 〈Indications〉headache, stiffness of the nape, tinnitus, nephelium, finger contracture, pain in the arm, jaundice, febrile disease without sweating, malaria, hypochondriac pain, swelling of the neck, nape and mandible, diabetes, lacrimation with cooling tears, convulsion. 〈Method〉Puncture perpendicularly 0.3～0.5 cun. Moxibustion is applicable.

●腕踝针[wàn huái zhēn] 针刺方法。针刺腕关节或踝关节上方六个特定点以治病的方法。其穴(点),距腕上或踝上两横指处,分别适应全身各部的病证。针刺时沿皮下向上方刺入1.4寸左右,不须出现感应,留针半小时以上,可用于功能性疾病和神经性疼痛。

Wrist-Ankle Needling An acupuncture method, referring to the method of puncturing the six specific points above the joint of wrist or ankle in order to treat diseases. The points are two-finger breadth above the wrist or ankle, and applicable for diseases on every part of the body. 〈Method〉Puncture subcutaneously towards the upper 1.4 cun. It is unnecessary for the needling feeling to appear. Retain the needle in the point for more than half an hour. 〈Indications〉functional diseases and nervous pain.

●腕劳[wàn láo] 经穴别名。即列缺。见该条。

Wanlao →列缺(p.246)

● 腕掌、背侧横纹 [wàn zhǎng bèi cè héng wén] 部位名。指尺、桡骨茎突远端连线上的横纹。其居于掌侧的叫掌横纹,居于背侧的叫背侧横纹。

Palmar Cross Striation of the Wrist, Dorsal Cross Striation of the Wrist Parts of the body, referring to the two cross striations on the line connecting the distal styloid processes of the ulna and radius. The one on the palmar side is called the palmar cross striation; the one on the dorsal side is called the dorsal cross striation.

● 踠 [wàn] 部位名。胫下尽处之曲节,一名脘,现称踝关节。

Ankle A part of body, referring to the joint below the end of the shin, now called ankle joint.

● 王冰 [wáng bīng] 人名。唐代医学家。自号启玄子。曾任太仆令,故亦称"王太仆"。其在《素问》散佚的情况下,进行重新编次、整理、注释,改《素问》原九卷本为二十四卷本。成书于762年。书中亦有对穴位的注释等。

Wang Bing A medical expert of the Tang Dynasty, whose assumed name is Qi Xuanzi. He once held an office, Tai Pu and was called Wang Tai Pu. As *Su Wen* (*Plain Questions*) was lost, he recatalogued, resystematized and annotated it, changing the 9 volumes of the original into 24 volumes. The book was completed in 762. There are also notes to points in the book.

● 王处明 [wáng chù míng] 人名。宋代针灸家。著《玄秘会要针经》,已佚。

Wang Chuming An acupuncture-moxibustion expert in the Song Dynasty, the compiler of *Xuanmi Huiyao Zhenjing* (*Mysterious Canon of the Essentials of Acupuncture*), already lost.

● 王国瑞 [wáng guó ruì] 人名。元代针灸家。兰溪(今属浙江)人。撰《扁鹊神应针灸玉龙经》。

Wang Guorui An acupuncture-moxibustion expert in the Yuan Dynasty. A native of Lanxi (now of Zhejiang Province), the compiler of *Bian Que Shenying Zhenjiu Yulong Jing* (*Bian Que's Jade Dragon Classics of Acupuncture and Moxibustion*).

● 王好古 [wáng hào gǔ] 人名。元代医家。字进之,号海藏。赵州(今河北赵县)人。曾学医于李东垣,著《阴证略例》、《此事难知》、《医垒元戎》。并善用针法,特别注重原穴的应用,称"拔原法"。参见该条。

Wang Haogu A medical expert in the Yuan Dynasty, who styled himself Jinzhi, and assumed the name of Haicang. A native of Zhaozhou (Zhaoxian County, Hebei Province today). He once learned from Li Dongyuan, the compiler of *Yinzheng Lueli* (*Brief Illustration of Internal Yin-Syndromes*), *Cishi Nan Zhi* (*This Matter Is Difficult to Know*) and *Yilei Yuanxu* (*The Chief General of the Medical Rampart*). Proficient at acupuncture, he paid special attention to the use of the Yuan (Primary) Points, called selection of Yuan (Primary) Points. →拔原法(p.9)

● 王怀隐 [wáng huái yǐn] 人名。宋代医官。睢阳(今属河南)人。978年奉命主编《太平圣惠方》。992年完成,共一百卷。其收录了唐以前的医方和部分有关针灸的资料。

Wang Huaiyin A medical official in the Song Dynasty. A native of Suiyang (now of Henan Province). In 978, he was appointed chief editor to compile *Taiping Shenghui Fang* (*Imperial Benevolent Prescriptions*) which was completed in 992, 100 volumes in all. In the book, the author collected prescriptions and parts of acupuncture materials before the Tang Dynasty.

● 王开 [wáng kāi] 人名。元代针灸家。字启元,号镜泽,兰溪(今属浙江)人。撰《重注标幽赋》、《增注针经秘语》、《针灸全书》等,均佚。

Wang Kai An acupuncture-moxibustion expert in the Yuan Dynasty, who styled himself Qi Yuan, and assumed the name of Jing Ze. A native of Lanxi (now of Zhejing Province), the author of *Chongzhu Biaoyou Fu* (*Supplementary Notes to the Lyrics of Recondite Principles*). *Zengzhu Zhenjing Miyu* (*Supplementary Notes to the Acupuncture Canon with Mysterious Expressions*), *Zhenjiu Quanshu* (*A Complete Book of Acupuncture and Moxibustion*), but all are nonextant.

● 王克明 [wáng kè míng] 人名。宋代医学家,字彦昭,饶州乐平(今属江西)人,后迁居湖州乌程(今属

浙江)。自幼潜心医学,尤擅针灸,治风痿、风噤、气秘腹胀等效果明显。参见《宋史》。

Wang Keming A medical expert in the Song Dynasty, who styled himself Yanzhao, a native of Leping of Raozhou (Now of Zhejing Province). Later he moved to Wucheng of Huzhou (now of Zhejiang Province). He devoted himself to medicine with great concentration when he was young, and was especially good at acupuncture. He obtained obvious effects in the treatment of flaccidity due to wind, lockjaw due to wind and abdominal distention due to obstruction of qi. Cf. *Songshi* (*History of the Song Dynasty*).

●王焘[wáng tāo] 人名。唐医学家。郿(今陕西眉县)人。自幼喜好医术,在弘文馆(国家图书馆)供职多年,博览群书,编成《外台秘要》四十卷,其为唐以前集医学大成之作。内有《明堂灸法》一卷。

Wang Tao A medical expert in the Tang Dynasty, a native of Mei (today's Meixian County, Shanxi Province). He was fond of medicine in his childhood. He worked in Hongwen Library (the National Library) for many years, and was extensively read. He compiled *Waitai Miyao* (*Clandestine Essentials from the Imperial Library*) in 40 volumes, the greatest collection of medicine before the Tang Dynasty, including a volume of *Ming Tang Jiufa* (*Acupoints for Moxibustion.*)

●王惟一[wáng wéi yī] 人名。宋代著名针灸学家。又名王惟德。里籍不详。曾在太医局任职。其奉诏于1026年编成《铜人腧穴针灸图经》三卷,并刻文于石碑,1029年主持铸成针灸铜人两具,是针灸学发展史上的创举。对国内外针灸学发展有较大影响。参见《铜人腧穴针灸图经》条。

Wang Weiyi A famous expert of acupuncture and moxibustion in the Song Dynasty, also named Wang Weide. No details are known about his native place. He once held an office in the Imperial Medical Bureau. He compiled the three-volume *Tongren Shuxue Zhenju Tujing* (*Illustrated Manual of Points for Acupuncture and Moxibustion on a Bronze Statue with Acupoints*) under imperial edict in 1026; which was carved on stone tablets. He conducted the casting of two bronze acupuncture statues in 1029—a breakthough in the development of acupuncture-moxibustion history—which bore great influence upon the development of acupuncture-moxibustion both at home and abroad. →铜人腧穴针灸图经(p. 442)

●王禹[wáng yǔ] 人名。汉代医家。师于淳于意,通针灸。见《史记·扁鹊仓公列传》。

Wang Yu A medical expert in the Han Dynasty. Learning from Chunyu Yi, he was proficient in acupuncture and moxibustion. Seen in *Shiji*: *Bian Que Canggong Liezhuan* (*The Historical Record*: *Biographies of Bian Que and Canggong*).

●王执中[wáng zhí zhōng] 人名。宋代针灸学家。字叔权,瑞安(今浙江瑞安)人。著《针灸资生经》七卷。书中记载临证有效穴位和灸法经验并对某些针灸禁穴提出不同意见。事见《温州府志》。参见《针灸资生经》条。

Wang Zhizhong An expert of acupuncture and moxibustion of the Song Dynasty, who styled himself Shuquan. A native of Ruian (today's Ruian, Zhejiang Province), the compiler of *Zhenjiu Zisheng Jing* (*Acupuncture-Moxibustion Classic for Saving Life*) in 7 volumes, in which effective points for clinical problems and experience in moxibustion were recorded and different ideas about some forbidden points were advanced. His deeds can be seen in *Wenzhoufu Zhi* (*Annals of Weizhoufu*) →针灸资生经(p.595)

●王宗泉[wáng zōng quán] 人名。明代医家。杭州人。曾撰《脏腑证治图说人镜经》。其徒钱雷又作"附录"。

Wang Zongquan A medical expert in the Ming Dynasty, a native of Hangzhou. He wrote *Zang-Fu Zhengzhi Tushuo Renjing Jing* (*Illustrated Classic of the Diagnosis and Treatment of Diseases of the Zang-Fu Organs*). His student, Qian Lei, wrote the appendix for the book.

●王纂[wáng zuǎn] 人名。南朝刘宋针灸家。海陵(今江苏泰州)人。深研医药,尤精针石。事见《异苑》。

Wang Zuan An acupuncture-moxibustion expert of Liu Song in the Southern Dynasties. A native of Hailing (today's Taizhou, Jiangsu

Province). He made a thorough research on medicine and was especially proficient in acupuncture and stone needling. His deeds can be seen in *Yi Yuan* (*A Garden of Wonders*).

●微针[wēi zhēn] 针具名。又称小针,意指细小的针具,泛指九针,与砭石相对而言。

Minute Needle A needling instrument, also called the small needle, referring to small and tiny needles. It can also refer to the nine needles in general as compared with bian (stone needle).

●维胞[wéi bāo] 经外穴名。见《经外奇穴汇编》。在侧腹部,当髂前上棘下方之凹陷中。〈主治〉子宫下垂。直刺0.5～1寸;可灸。

Weibao (EX-CA) An extra point, seen in *Jingwai Qixue Huibian* (*An Expository Manual of Extra Points*). 〈Location〉on the lateral abdomen, in the depression inferior to the anterior superior iliac spine. 〈Indication〉hysteroptosis. 〈Method〉Puncture 0.5～1.0 cun. perpendicularly. Moxibustion is applicable.

●维道[wéi dào] 经穴名。出《针灸甲乙经》。属足少阳胆经,为足少阳、带脉之会。又名外枢。〈定位〉在侧腹部,当髂前上棘的前下方,五枢前下0.5寸(图40和图23)。〈层次解剖〉皮肤→皮下组织→腹外斜肌→腹内斜肌→腹横肌→髂腰肌。浅层布有旋髂浅动、静脉,第十一、十二胸神经前支和第一腰神经前支的外侧皮支及伴行的动、静脉。深层有旋髂深动、静脉,股外侧皮神经,第十一、十二胸神经前支和第一腰神经前支的肌支及相应的动、静脉。〈主治〉腰胯痛、少腹痛、阴挺、疝气、带下、月经不调、水肿。向前下方斜刺0.8～1.5寸;可灸。

Weidao (GB 28) A meridian point, originally from *Zhenjiu Jia-Yi Jing* (*A-B Classic of Acupuncture and Moxibustion*), a point on the Gallbladder Meridian of Foot-Shaoyang, the crossing point of Foot-Shaoyang and the Belt Meridian, also called Waishu. 〈Location〉on the lateral side of the abdomen, anterior and inferior to the anteriosuperior iliac spine, 0.5 cun anterior and inferior to Wushu (GB 27) (Figs. 40 & 23). 〈Regional anatomy〉skin → subcutaneous tissue → external oblique muscle of abdomen → internal oblique muscle of abdomen → transverse muscle of abdomen → iliopsoas muscle. In the superficial layer, there are the superficial circumflex iliac artery and vein, the lateral cutaneous branches of the anterior branches of the 11th and 12th thoracic and the 1st lumbar nerves and the accompanying arteries and veins. In the deep layer, there are the deep circumflex iliac artery and vein, the lateral cutaneous nerve of the thigh, the muscular branches of the anterior branches of the 11th and 12th thoracic and 1st lumbar nerves and the related arteries and veins. 〈Indication〉pain in the waist and hip, pain in the side of the lower abdomen, prolapse of the uterus, hernia, morbid leukorrhea, irregular menstruation and edema. 〈Method〉Puncture 0.8～1.5 cun obliquely in the anterior-inferior direction. Moxibustion is applicable.

●维宫[wéi gōng] 经外穴名。见《经外奇穴汇编》。在侧腹部,当髂前上棘下方凹陷斜下1寸处。〈主治〉子宫下垂。直刺0.5～1寸;可灸。

Weigong (EX-CA) An extra point, seen in *Jingwai Qixue Huibian* (*An Expository Manual of Extra Points*). 〈Location〉on the lateral abdomen. 1 cun obliquely below the depression inferior to the anterior superior iliac spine. 〈Indication〉hysteroptosis. 〈Method〉Puncture 0.5～1.0 cun perpendicularly. Moxibustion is applicable.

●维会[wéi huì] ①经穴别名。出《卫生宝鉴》。即百会,见该条。②经穴别名。出《循经考穴编》。即神阙。见该条。

Weihui Another name for ① Baihui (DU 20), a meridian point originally from *Weisheng Baojian* (*A Treasured Mirror of Health Protection*). →百会 (p. 11) ② Shenque (RN 8), a meridian point originally from *Xunjing Kaoxue Bian* (*Studies on Acupoints Along Meridians*). →神阙 (p. 363)

●尾翠[wěi cuì] 经外穴名。见《太平圣惠方》。又名小儿疳痢,小儿疳瘦。〈定位〉正在尾骨尖端直上3寸。〈主治〉小儿疳痨羸瘦、消化不良、腹痛下痢、脱肛等。沿皮刺0.5～1寸;可灸。

Weicui (EX-B) An extra point, seen in *Taiping Shenghui Fang* (*Imperial Benevolent Prescriptions*), also called Xiaoerganli, Xiaoerganshou. 〈Location〉3 cun directly above the

lower tip of the coccyx. 〈Indications〉infantile malnutrition, tuberculosis and emaciation, dyspepsia, abdominal pain, diarrhea and proctoptosis. 〈Method〉Puncture subcutaneously 0.5~1 cun. Moxibustion is applicable.

●尾闾[wěi lǘ] ①经穴别名。见《古今医统》。即长强。见该条。②骨名。即尾骨。

1. **Weilü** Another name for Changqiang(DU 1), a meridian point seen in *Gu Jin Yitong* (*The General Medicine of the Past and Present*). →长强(p. 39)

2. **Weilü** Name of a bone, referring to coccyx.

●尾穷骨[wěi qióng gǔ] 经外穴名。见《针灸集成》。在尾骶部，当尾骨尖上1寸及左右各1寸处，共三穴。灸治腰痛、尾骶痛、淋症、便秘、尿闭、痔疮等。

Weiqionggu(EX-B) An extra point, seen in *Zhenjiu Jicheng* (*A Collection of Acupuncture and Moxibustion*). 〈Location〉on the caudal and sacral region, one point is 1 cun above the lower tip of the coccyx, and the other two are 1 cun on each side of the above point, three points in all. 〈Indications〉lumbago, pain in the caudal and sacral region, stranguria, constipation, enuresis, hemorrhoid, etc. 〈Method〉 moxibustion.

●尾翳[wěi yì] 经穴别名。出《针灸甲乙经》。即鸠尾。见该条。

Weiyi Another name for Jiuwei(RN 15), a meridian point originally from *Zhenjiu Jia-Yi jing* (*A-B Classic of Acupuncture and Moxibustion*). →鸠尾(p. 219)

●委阳[wěi yáng] 经穴名。出《灵枢·本输》。属足太阳膀胱经，为三焦的下合穴，又名郄阳。〈定位〉在腘横纹外侧端，当股二头肌腱的内侧(图35.2和图35.3)。〈层次解剖〉皮肤→皮下组织→股二头肌→腓肠外侧头→腘肌起始腱和腘肌。浅层布有股后皮神经。深层有腓总神经和腓外侧皮神经。〈主治〉腰脊强痛、小腹胀满、小便不利、腿足拘挛疼痛、痿厥不仁。直刺0.5~0.1寸；可灸。

Weiyang(BL 39) A meridian point, originally from *Lingshu*:*Benshu*(*Miraculous Pivot*: *Meridian Points*), a point on the Bladder Meridian of Foot-Taiyang, the lower confluent point of Sanjiao. Also called Xiyang. 〈Location〉at the lateral end of the popliteal crease, medial to the tendon of the biceps muscle of the thigh(Figs. 35.2&35.3). 〈Regional anatomy〉skin → subcutaneous tissue → biceps muscle of thigh → lateral head of gastrocnemius muscle → origin of popliteal muscle and plantar muscle. In the superficial layer, there is the posterior femoral cutaneous nerve. In the deep layer, there are the common peroneal nerve and the lateral cutaneous nerve of the calf. 〈Indications〉stiffness and pain in the waist and along the spine, distension and fullness of the lower abdomen, difficulty in urination, spasm and pain in the legs and feet, flaccidity with cold limbs and numbness. 〈Method〉Puncture 0.5~1.0 cun perpendicularly. Moxibustion is applicable.

●委中[wěi zhōng] 经穴名。出《灵枢·本输》。属足太阳膀胱经，为本经合穴。又名血郄、中郄、郄中、委中央。〈定位〉在腘横纹中点，当股二头肌腱与半腱肌肌腱的中间(图35.2和35.3)。〈层次解剖〉皮肤→皮下组织→腓肠肌内、外侧头之间。浅层布有股后皮神经和小隐静脉。深层有胫神经、腘动、静脉和腓肠动脉等。〈主治〉腰痛、髋关节屈伸不利、腘筋挛急、下肢痿痹、中风昏迷、半身不遂、腹痛、吐泻、疟疾、癫疾、反折、衄血不止、遗尿、小便难、自汗、盗汗、丹毒、疔疮、发背。直刺0.5~1寸，或点刺出血；可灸。

Weizhong(BL 40) A meridian point, originally from *Lingshu*:*Benshu*(*Miraculous Pivot*: *Meridian Points*), the He-sea point of the Bladder Meridian of Foot-Taiyang, also called Xuexi, Zhongxi, Xizhong or Weizhongyang. 〈Location〉at the midpoint of the popliteal crease, between the tendons of the biceps muscle of the thigh and the semitendinous muscle(Figs. 35.2&35.3).〈Regional anatomy〉skink → subcutaneous tissue → between lateral and medial heads of gastrocnermius muscle. In the superficial layer, there are the posterior femoral cutaneous nerve and the small saphenous vein. In the deep layer, there are the tibial nerve, the popliteal artery and vein, and the peroneal artery. 〈Indications〉lumbago, difficulty in bending and stretching the hip joint, contracture of the popliteal tendon, flaccidity and numbness of the lower limbs, un-

consciousness due to apoplexy, hemiplegia, abdominal pain, vomiting and diarrhea, malaria, epilepsy, opisthotomus, apostaxis, enuresis, difficulty in urination, spontaneous perspiration, night sweat, erysipelas, furuncle and lumbodorsal carbuncle. 〈Method〉 Puncture perpendicularly 0.5～1 cun, or prick to cause bleeding. Moxibustion is applicable.

●委中央[wěi zhōng yāng] 经穴别名。出《灵枢·邪气藏府病形》。即委中。详见该条。

Weizhongyang Another name for Weizhong (BL 40), a meridian point originally from *Lingshu: Xieqi Zang-Fu Bingxing* (*Miraculous Pivot: Pathogenic Evils, Zang-Fu Organs and Manifestations*). →委中(p. 461)

●痿躄[wěi bì] 病证名。见《素问·痿论》。即痿证。详见该条。

Flaccidity and Lameness A disease, originally seen in *Suwen: Wei Lun* (*Plain Questions: On Flaccidity Syndromes*). →痿证(p. 462)

●痿证[wěi zhèng] 病证名。出《素问·痿论》等篇。又名痿躄。指肢体萎弱无力，肌肉萎缩，甚至运动功能丧失而成的瘫痪的病证。多由于五脏之热，灼伤津液；或因湿热阻于阳明，胃津不行致使皮毛、肌肉、血脉、筋骨无以营养所致。临床分为肺热伤津、湿热浸淫、气血不足、肝肾阴虚型痿证。详见各条。

Flaccidity Syndrome A disease, originally from *Suwen: Wei Lun* (*Plain Questions: On Flaccidity Syndromes*), also called flaccidity and lameness, referring to the paralytic disease manifested as softness and weakness of the limbs and body, muscular patrophy, and even loss of motor functions, mostly due to pathogenic heat of the five zang organs leading to the impairment of the body fluid, or obstruction of dampness and heat in Yangming, failure of stomach fluid to transport leading to the under nourishment of the skin, hair, flaccidity syndrome due to the impairment of body fluid by lung-heat, flaccidity syndrome due to the invasion of damp-heat pathogen, flaccidity syndrome due to the deficiency of qi and blood and flaccidity syndrome due to the yin-deficiency of the liver and kidney. →肺热伤津痿证(p. 108)、湿热浸淫痿证(p. 371)、气血不足痿证(p. 312)、肝肾阴虚痿证(p. 126)

●卫生针灸玄机秘要[wèi shēng zhēn jiǔ xuán jī mì yào] 书名。明·杨继洲家传医书。详见针灸大成条。

Weisheng Zhenjiu Xuanji Miyao (**Mysterious Clandestine Essentials of Acupuncture and Moxibustion for Health Protection**) A medical book, handed down from the family of Yang Jizhou of the Ming Dynasty. →针灸大成(p. 591)

●卫世杰[wèi shì jié] 人名。宋代针灸家。1220年徐正卿刻印《针灸资生经》曾经其订证。参见针灸资生经条。

Wei Shijie An acupuncture-moxibustion expert in the Song Dynasty, who had once done proofreading and made corrections for the book *Zhenjiu Zisheng Jing* (*Acupuncture-Moxibustion Classic for Saving Life*) before it was carved and printed by Xu Zhengqing in 1220. →针灸资生经(p. 595)

●胃[wèi] 耳穴名。位于耳轮脚上消失处周围。用于治疗胃痉挛、胃炎、胃溃疡及失眠、牙痛、消化不良。

Stomach (MA) An auricular point. 〈Location〉 around the area where the helix crus terminates. 〈Indications〉 gastrospasm, gastritis, gastric ulcer, insomnia, toothache, indigestion.

●胃仓[wèi cāng] 经穴名。出《针灸甲乙经》。属足太阳膀胱经。〈定位〉在背部，当第十二胸椎棘突下，旁开3寸(图7)。〈层次解剖〉皮肤→皮下组织→背阔肌→下后锯肌→竖脊肌→腰方肌。浅层布有第十二胸神经和第一腰神经后支的外侧皮支和伴行的动、静脉。深层有第十二胸神经和第一腰神经后支的肌支和相应的动、静脉侧支的分支或属支。〈主治〉腹胀、胃脘痛、水肿、小儿食积、脊背痛。斜刺0.5～0.8寸；可灸。

Weicang (BL 50) A meridian point, originally from *Zhenjiu Jia-Yi Jing* (*A-B Classic of Acupuncture and Moxibustion*), a point on the Bladder Meridian of Foot-Taoyang. 〈Location〉 on the back, below the spinous process of the 12th thoracic vertebra, 3 cun lateral to the posterior midline (Fig. 7). 〈Regional anatomy〉 skin → subcutaneous tissue → latissimus muscle of back → inferior posterior serratus muscle → erector spinal muscle → lumbar

quadrate muscle. In the superficial layer, there are the lateral cutaneous branches of the posterior branches of the 12th thoracic and 1st lumbar nerves and the accompanying arteries and veins. In the deep layer, there are the muscular branches of the posterior branches of the related arteries and veins. ⟨Indications⟩ abdominal distension, stomachache, edema, infantile indigestion with food retention, spinal and back pain. ⟨Method⟩ Puncture obliquely 0.5~0.8 cun. Moxibustion is applicable.

●胃反[wèi fǎn] 出《金匮要略·呕吐哕下利病脉证治》。即反胃。详该条。

Reversing Movement of Food from the Stomach Originally from *Jingui Yaolüe: Outu Yue Xiali Bing Mai Zheng Zhi* (*Synopsis of the Golden Chamber: Pulse Conditions, Symptoms and Treatments of Vomiting, Hiccup and Diarrhea*). →反胃(p. 104)

●胃腑不和不寐[wèi fǔ bù hé bù mèi] 不寐证型之一。因饮食所伤，脾胃不和，湿盛生痰，郁久化热，痰热上扰心神所致。证见睡眠不实，心中懊恼，脘痞、嗳气、头晕目眩，甚则呕哕痰涎、舌苔黄腻、脉滑或弦。治宜化痰和胃安神。取中脘、丰隆、厉兑、隐白、通里、内关。

Insomnia due to Derangement of the Stomach A type of insomnia, caused by improper diet leading to lack of coordination between the spleen and stomach, excessive accumulation of phlegm and dampness and stagnant phlegm producing heat. The phlegm-heat flares up to disturb the heart and mind. ⟨Manifestations⟩ shallow spleep, feverish sensation in the chest, fullness of the stomach, eructation, dizziness and blurred vision, vomiting and hiccup with phlegm and saliva, yellow and greasy tongue coating, slippery or wiry pulse. ⟨Treatment principle⟩ Resolve phlegm, regulate and tranquilize the stomach. ⟨Point selection⟩ Zhongwan(RN 12), Fenglong(ST 40), Lidui(ST 45), Yinbai(SP 1), Tongli(HT 5), and Neiguan(PC 6).

●胃管[wèi guǎn] 经穴别名。出《千金要方》。即中脘。详见该条。

Weiguan Another name for Zhongwan(RN 12), a meridian point originally from *Qianjin Yaofang* (*Essential Prescriptions Worth a Thousand Gold*). →中脘(p. 614)

●胃寒呃逆[wèi hán è nì] 呃逆证型之一。由寒邪犯胃，胃气失于和降所致。证见呃逆声沉缓有力、胃脘冷胀、喜得热饮、手足冷、口不渴、小便清长、大便溏薄、舌苔白润、脉迟缓。治宜温中祛寒，降逆止呃。取天突、膈俞、中脘、内关、足三里、章门、脾俞。

Hiccup due to Stomach-Cold A type of hiccup, mostly caused by cold evil attacking the stomach resulting in the failure of stomach-qi to descend. ⟨Manifestations⟩ deep-sounding, slow and forceful hiccup, distension with cold sensation of the stomach, preference for hot drink, cold hands and feet, unawareness of thirst, profuse clear utrine, loose stool, white and moist tongue coating, slow and leisurely pulse. ⟨Treatment principle⟩ Warm the middle-jiao to dispel cold; lower the adverse flow of the stomach-qi to stop hiccup. ⟨Point selection⟩ Tiantu(RN 22), Geshu(BL 17), Zhongwan(RN 12) Neiguan(PC 6), Zusanli(ST 36), Zhangmen(LR 13) and Pishu(BL 20).

●胃寒恶阻[wèi hán è zǔ] 恶阻证型之一。多因平素脾胃虚寒，孕后胞门闭塞，脏气内阻，寒饮上逆所致。证见呕吐清水、倦怠畏寒、喜热饮、舌淡苔白、脉沉无力。治宜温胃止呕。取足三里、中脘、上脘、幽门。

Morning Sickness due to Stomach Cold A type of morning sickness, mostly caused by constitutional deficiency and cold of the spleen and stomach, obstruction of the orifice of the uterus during pregnancy, obstruction of the zang-qi resulting in adverse rising of cold fluid. ⟨Manifestations⟩ vomiting of clear fluid, lassitude, aversion to cold, preference for hot water, pale tongue with whitish coating, deep and weak pulse. ⟨Treatment principle⟩ Warm the stomach to stop vomiting. ⟨Point selection⟩ Zusanli(ST 36) Zhongwan(RN 12), Shangwan(RN 13) and Youmen(KI 21).

●胃经[wèi jīng] 足阳明胃经之简称。见该条。

The Stomach Meridian The shortened name of the Stomach Meridian of Foot-Yangming. →足阳明胃经(p. 647)

●胃区[wèi qū] 头针刺激区。从瞳孔直上发际处为起点，向上引平行于前后正中线2厘米长直线。⟨主

治〉胃炎,胃溃疡等引起的胃痛、上腹部不适。

The Gastric Area An area for scalp acupuncture. 〈Location〉Take the hair margin directly above the pupil as a starting point, draw a 2-cm line directly upwards, parallel to the anteriorposterior midline. 〈Indications〉stomachache and epigastric discomfort due to gastritis and gastric ulcer, etc.

●胃热鼻衄[wèi rè bí nǜ] 鼻衄证型之一。因胃热熏蒸所致。证见鼻衄血、血色鲜红、口渴引饮、胸闷烦躁、口臭便秘、舌红苔黄、脉数有力。治宜清胃泄热止因。取内庭、上星、二间、上巨虚、隐白。

Epistaxis due to Stomach-Heat A type of epistaxis, caused by fumigation of the stomach-heat. 〈Manifestations〉nasal bleeding of fresh red color, thirst relieved by drinking, oppressive sensation in the chest and restlessness, smell in the mouth, constipation, red tongue with yellowish coating, rapid and forceful pulse. 〈Treatment principle〉Clear stomach-heat to stop bleeding. 〈Point selection〉Neiting(ST 44), Shangxing(DU 23), Erjian(LI 2), Shangjuxu(ST 37) and Yinbai (SP 1).

●胃热呃逆[wèi rè è nì] 呃逆证型之一。因嗜食辛辣醇酒及温补之品,胃肠蕴积实热,胃火上冲所致。证见呃逆声音洪亮、冲逆而出、口臭烦渴、喜冷饮、小便短赤、大便秘结、舌苔黄、脉滑数。治宜清降泄热,和胃止呃。取天突、膈俞、内关、足三里、曲池、合谷、内庭。

Hiccup due to Stomach-Heat A type of hiccup, caused by excessive eating of spicy food and warm tonics, over drinking of wine leading to the accumulation of excess heat in the stomach and intestine resulting in the ascending of stomach fire. 〈Manifestations〉loud-sounding and forceful hiccup in a hasty manner, smell in the mouth, excessive thirst, preference for cold drink, scanty dark urine, constipation, yellow tongue coating, slippery and rapid pulse. 〈Treatment principle〉Clear heat, regulate the stomach and stop hiccup. 〈Point selection〉Tiantu(RN 22), Geshu(BL 17), Neiguan(PC 6), Zusanli(ST 36), Quchi(LI 11), Hegu(LI 4) and Neiting(ST 44).

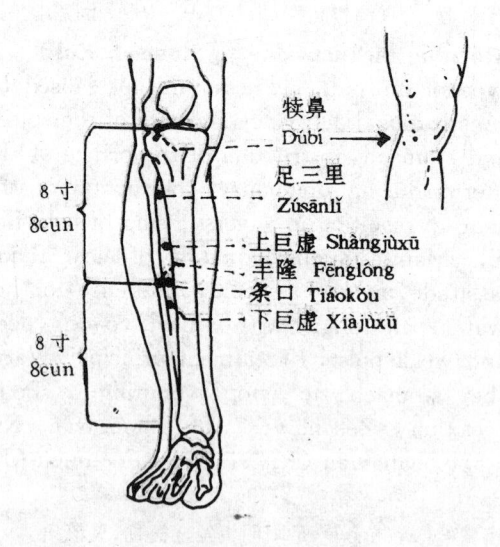

图60.1 胃经穴(小腿部)
Fig. 60.1 Points of Stomach Meridian(Leg)

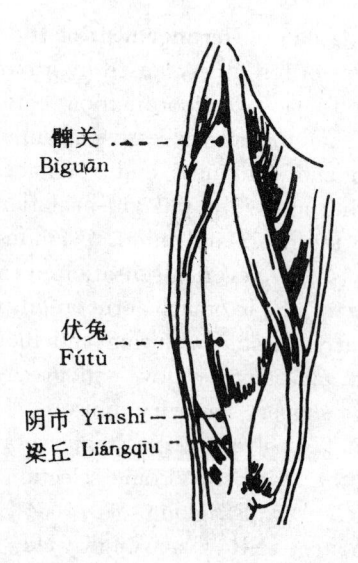

图60.2 胃经穴(大腿部)
Fig. 60.2 Points of Stomach Meridian(Thigh)

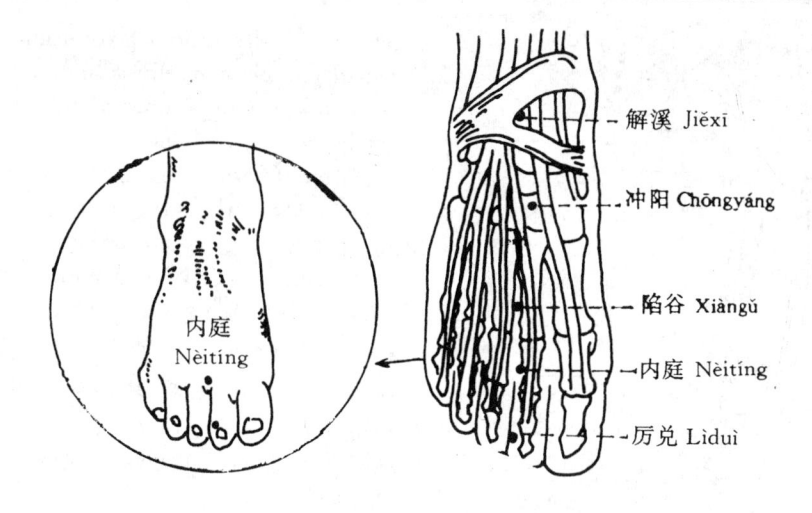

图60.3 胃经穴（足部）

Fig. 60.3 Points of Stomach Meridian (Foot)

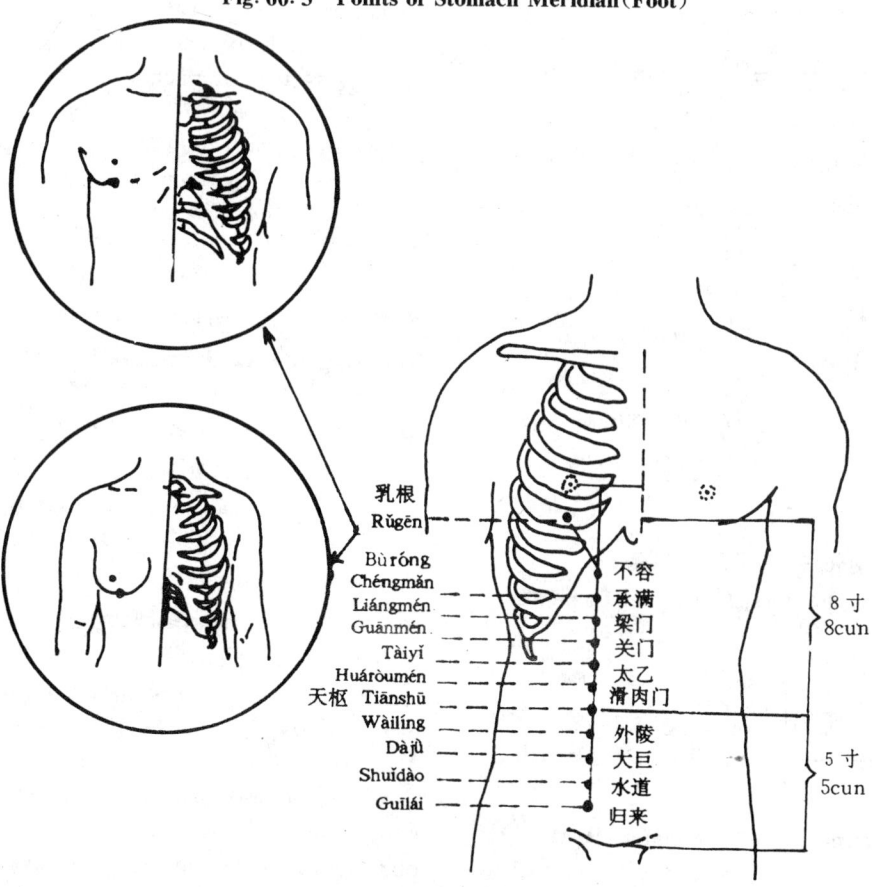

图60.4 胃经穴（腹部）

Fig. 60.4 Points of Stomach Meridian (Abdomen)

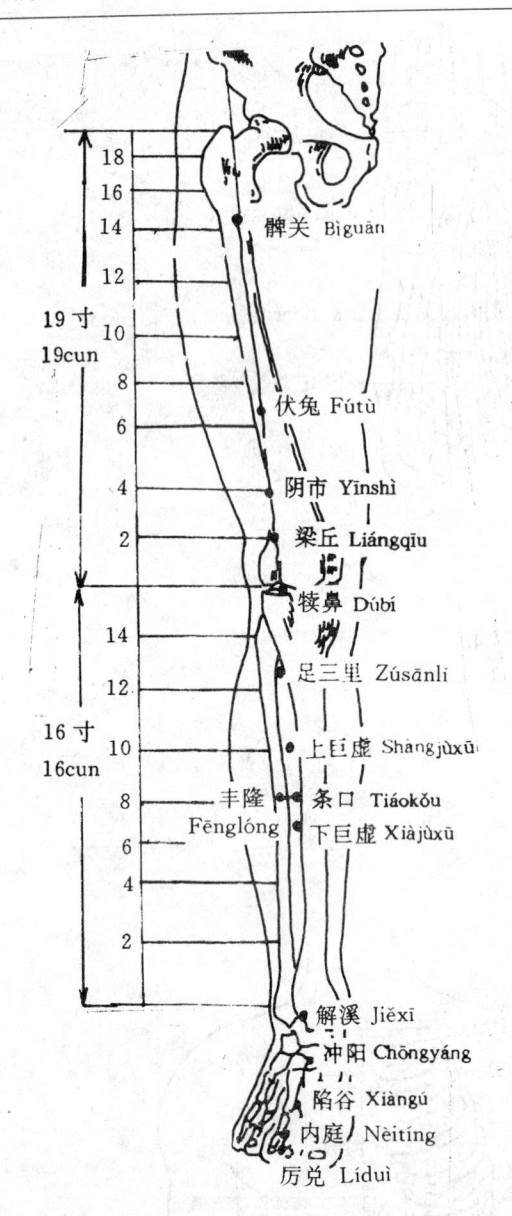

图60.5 胃经穴(下肢部)

Fig. 60.5 Points of Stomach Meridian (Lower limb)

●**胃热恶阻**[wèi rè è zǔ] 恶阻证型之一。多因平素胃热,孕后冲脉气盛,胃气不降所致。证见呕吐心烦、颜面潮红、口渴喜冷饮、便秘、舌红、苔黄、脉滑数。治宜清胃热,降逆止呕。取足三里、上脘、公孙、内关、内庭。

Morning Sickness due to Stomach-Heat One type of morning sickness, mostly caused by constitutional heat in the stomach, excessive qi in the Chong meridian during pregnancy resulting in the failure of the stomach-qi to descend. 〈Manifestations〉vomiting, vexation, flushed complexion, thirst and preference for cold drink, constipation, red tongue with yellowish coating, slippery and rapid pulse. 〈Treatment principle〉Clear heat from the stomach; lower the adverse flow of stomach-qi to stop vomiting. 〈Point selection〉Zusanli(ST 36), Shangwan (RN 13), Gongsun (SP 4), Neiguan(PC 6)and Neiting(ST 44).

●**胃热风疹**[wèi rè fēng zhěn] 风疹证型之一。多因胃肠积热,郁于肌表所致。其证除见风疹的一般症状外,发疹时伴有脘腹疼痛、纳呆、大便秘结或泄泻、苔黄腻、脉滑数。治宜清热和营。取风府、曲池、天枢、足三里、血海。

Rubella due to Stomach-Heat A type of rubella, mostly caused by the accumulation of heat in the stomach resulting in the retention of the heat in the skin portion of the body. 〈Manifestations〉Besides the common symptoms of rubella, it is accompanied, when rubella occurs, by stomachache and abdominal pain, loss of appetite, constipation or diarrhea, yellow and greasy tongue coating, slippery and rapid pulse. 〈Treatment principle〉Clear heat to regulate the Rong-fen. 〈Point selection〉Fengfu(DU 16)Quchi(LI 11), Tianshu(ST 25), Zusanli(ST 36)and Xuehai(SP 10).

●**胃热呕吐**[wèi rè ǒu tù] 即热吐。详见该条。

Vomiting due to Stomach-Heat →热吐(p. 332)

●**胃热乳痈**[wèi rè rǔ yōng] 乳痈证型之一。多因恣食厚味,胃经积热,或乳头破裂,外邪火毒侵入,脉络阻塞,排乳不畅,火毒与积乳互凝,结肿疼痛。证见初起乳房结决、胀肿疼痛、排乳不畅、同时全身不适、寒热往来,兼见口渴欲饮、或恶心呕吐、口臭便秘、苔黄腻、脉弦数。治宜清热散结。取膺窗、下巨虚、丰隆、温溜。乳汁壅胀加膻中、少泽;头痛发热加合谷、风池。

Acute Mastitis due to Stomach-Heat A type of acute mastitis, mostly caused by over indulgence in greasy food, accumulation of heat in the stomach meridian, or broken nipple with exogenous and fire-toxin invasion leading to obstruction in the meridians and collateral difficulty in lactation, coaglation of five-toxin and stagnant lactation, resulting in mastitis. 〈Manifestations〉initially, mass in the breast

with distension, swelling and painful sensation, difficulty in lactation, general discomofort, alternative attacks of chill and fever, thirst longing for drinking, or nausea and vomiting, foul smell in the mouth, constipation, yellow and greasy tongue coating, wiry and rapid pulse. ⟨Treatment principle⟩ Clear heat and resolve masses. ⟨Point selection⟩ Yingchuang(ST 16), Xiajuxu(ST 39), Fenglong(ST 40), Wenliu(LI 7). If breast distension occurs, add Tangzhong (RN 17), and Shaoze(ST 1), if headache and fever occur, add Hegu(LI 4) and Fengchi(GB 20).

●胃热吐血[wèi rè tǔ xuè] 吐血证型之一。多由醇酒厚味、过食辛辣，胃中积热，或情志过极，胃络损伤所致。证见吐血鲜红或紫黯夹有食物残渣、脘腹胀痛、口臭、大便色黑或便秘、舌质红苔黄腻、脉滑数。治宜清泄胃热，降逆止血。取上脘、郄门、内庭。

Spitting Blood due to Stomach-Heat A type of spitting blood, mostly caused by over indulgence of alcohol, greasy and spicy food, leading to the accumulation of the heat in the stomach, or emotional stress leading to injury of the collaterals of the stomach. ⟨Manifestation⟩ spitting blood of fresh or dark purple color with residue of food, epigastric and abdominal distension and pain, foul smell in the mouth, black stool or constipation, red tongue with yellowish and greasy coating, slippery and rapid pulse. ⟨Treatment principle⟩ Clear heat from the stomach, and lower the adverse flow of the stomach-qi to stop bleeding. ⟨Point selection⟩ Shangwan (RN 13), Ximen (PC 4) and Neiting (ST 44).

●胃俞[wèi shū] 经穴名。出《针灸甲乙经》。足太阳膀胱经，为胃的背俞穴。⟨定位⟩在背部，当第十二胸椎棘突下，旁开1.5寸(图7)。⟨层次解剖⟩皮肤→皮下组织→胸腰筋膜浅层和背阔肌腱膜→竖脊肌。浅层布有第十二胸神经和第一腰神经后支的皮支和伴行的动、静脉。深层有第十二胸神经和第一腰神经后支的肌支和相应的动、静脉的分支或属支。⟨主治⟩胸胁痛、胃脘痛、腹胀、翻胃、呕吐、肠鸣、完谷不化。直刺0.5～0.8寸；可灸。

Weishu(BL 21) A meridian point, originally from *Zhenjiu Jia-Yi Jing* (*A-B Classic of Acupuncture and Moxibustion*), a point on the Bladder Meridian of Foot-Taiyang, the Back-Shu point of the stomach. ⟨Location⟩ on the back, below the spinous process of the 12th thoracic vertebra, 1.5 cun lateral to the posterior midline (Fig. 7). ⟨Regional anatomy⟩ skin → subcutaneous tissue → superficial layer of thoracolumbar and aponeurosis of latissimus muscle of back→erector spinal muscle. In the superficial layer, there are the cutaneous branches of the posterior branches of the 12th thoracic and 1st lumbar nerves and the accompanying arteries and veins. In the deep layer, there are the muscular branches of the posterior branches of the 12th thoracic and 1st lumbar nerves and the branches or tributaries of the related arteries and veins. ⟨Indications⟩ pain in the chest and hypochondrium, stomachache, abdominal distension, regurgitation, vomiting, borborygmus and diarrhea with undigested food. ⟨Method⟩ Puncture perpendicularly 0.5～0.8 cun. Moxibustion is applicable.

●胃痛[wèi tòng] 病证名。又名胃心痛、心下痛、胃脘痛、心痛等。指上腹部近剑突下疼痛。多由忧思恼怒，气郁伤肝，使肝气失其条达，横逆犯胃，气机阻塞；或禀赋不足，中阳素虚，脾胃虚寒；或饮食不慎，思虑劳累，或感受寒邪，伤及脾胃所致。临床上分为气郁胃痛、虚寒胃痛、寒积胃痛、食积胃痛和阴虚胃痛等。详见各条。

Stomachache A disease, also called stomach-heart pain, pain below the heart, epigastric pain and cardiac pain, referring to pain of the upper abdomen and below the xiphoid process. Mostly due to melancholy or emotional disturbance leading to the stagnation of qi which may impair the liver, causing dysfunction of the liver in maintaining the free flow of qi. This leads to liver qi attacking the stomach, resulting in the obstruction of stomach qi. Or due to congenital deficiency, constitutional weakness of the middle-yang, cold and deficiency of the spleen and stomach, or improper diet, exhaustion due to excessive worries, or invasion by exogenous cold, leading to the impairment of the spleen and stomach. It is clinically divided into stomachache due to the qi-stagnation, stomachache due to cold of

insufficiency type, stomachache due to cold accumulation, stomachache due to the retention of food and stomachache due to yin-deficiency. → 气郁胃痛(p. 313)、虚寒胃痛(p. 515)、寒积胃痛(p. 155)、食积胃痛(p. 387)、阴虚胃痛(p. 562)

●**胃脘**[wèi wǎn] ①经穴别名。见《针灸聚英》,即上脘。详见该条。②经穴别名。见《类经图翼》。即中脘。详见该条。

Weiwan Another name for ① Shangwan (RN 13), a meridian point seen in *Zhenjiu Juying* (*Essentials of Acupuncture and Moxibustion*). → 上脘(p. 353) ② Zhongwan (RN 12), a meridian point seen in *Leijing Tuyi* (*Illustrated Supplements to Classified Canon of Internal Medicine of Yellow Emperor*) → 中脘(p. 614)

●**胃脘痛**[wèi wǎn tòng]病证名。出《素问·五常政大论》等篇。即胃痛。详见该条。

Epigastric Pain A disease, originally from *Su Wen; Wu Chang Zheng Da Lun* (*Plain Questions; On the Routines and Laws of the Five Evolutive Phases*), etc. → 胃痛(p. 467)

●**胃脘下俞**[wèi wǎn xià shū] 经外穴名。见《千金要方》。又名胰俞。〈定位〉在背部,当第八胸椎棘突下,旁开1.5寸。〈层次解剖〉皮肤→皮下组织→斜方肌→背阔肌→竖脊肌。浅层主要布有第八胸神经后支的皮支和伴行的动、静脉。深层有第八胸神经后支的肌支和第八肋间动、静脉背侧的分支或属支。〈主治〉消渴、咽喉干燥、腹痛、呕吐、肋间神经痛等。斜刺0.3~0.5寸;可灸。

Weiwanxiashu (EX-B 3) An extra point, seen in *Qianjin Yaofang* (*Essential Prescriptions Worth a Thousand Gold*), also called Yishu 〈Location〉on the back, below the 8th thoracic spinous process, 1.5 cun lateral to the posterior midline. 〈Regional anatomy〉skin →

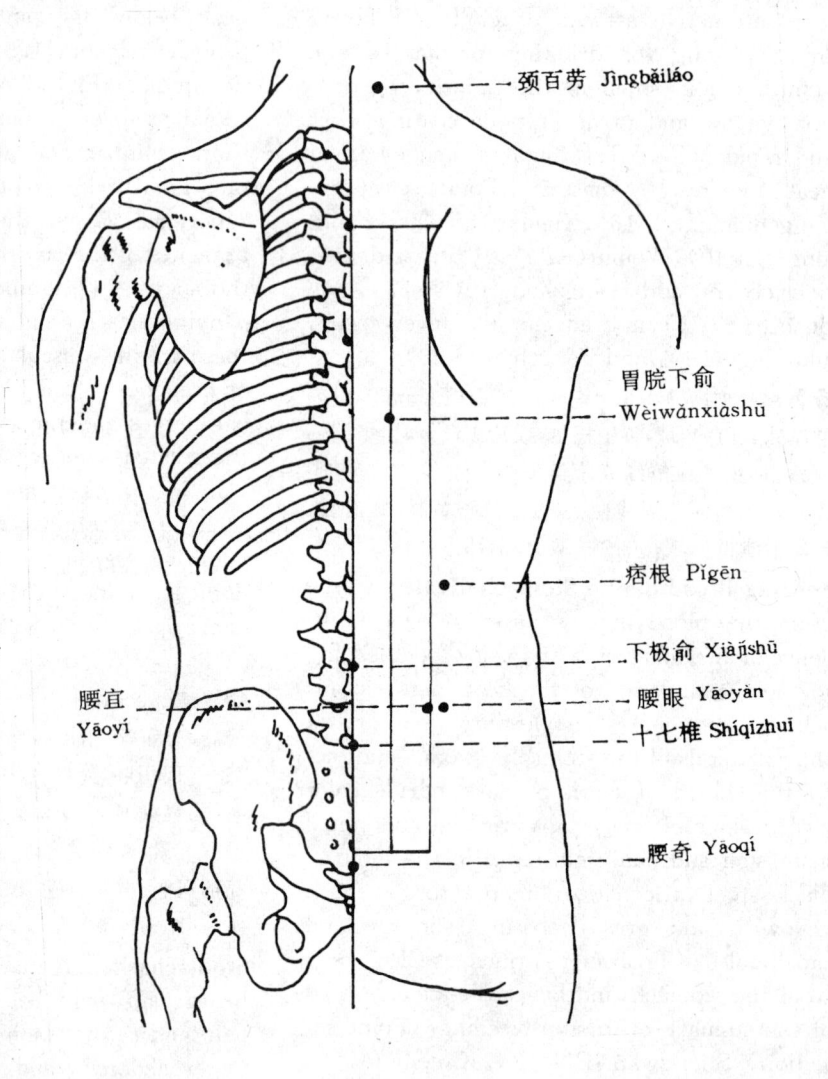

图61 胃脘下俞等经外穴(背面)
Fig. 61 Weiwanxiashu and other extra points (Back view)

subcutaneous tissue → trapezius muscle → broadest muscle of back → erector spinal muscle. In the superficial layer, there are the cutaneous branches of the 8th rami posteriores nervorum thoracalium and accompanying arteries and veins. In the deep layer, there are the muscular branches of the 8th rami posteriores nervorum theracalium and the dorsal branches of tributaries of the 8th posterior intercostal arteries and veins. 〈Indications〉 diabetes, dry throat, abdominal pain, vomiting, intercostal neuralgia. 〈Method〉 Puncture obliquely 0.3～0.5 cun. Moxibustion is applicable.

●胃维 [wèi wéi] 经穴别名。出《外台秘要》。即地仓。详见该条。

Weiwei Another name for *Dicang* (ST 4), a meridian point originally from *Waitai Miyao* (*Clandestine Essentials from the Imperial Library*). →地仓 (p. 78)

●胃心痛 [wèi xīn tòng] 病证名。出《灵枢·厥病》。即胃痛。详见该条。

Stomach-Heart Pain A disease, originally from *Lingshu*: *Juebing* (*Miraculous Pivot*: *On Jue Diseases*). →胃痛 (p. 467)

●胃虚恶阻 [wèi xū è zǔ] 恶阻证型之一。多因脾胃素弱，孕后冲脉气盛，致使胃失和降所致。证见脘腹胀满、恶心呕吐、或食入即吐、神倦思睡、舌淡苔白、脉缓滑无力。治宜健脾和中，调气降逆。取足三里、上脘、中脘、公孙。

Morning Sickness due to Stomach Deficiency
A type of morning sickness, mostly caused by constitutional deficiency of the spleen and stomach, excessive qi in the Chong meridian during pregnancy, leading to the failure of stomach-qi to descend. 〈Manifestations〉 epigastric distension and fullness, nausea, vomiting even instant vomiting upon food intake, lassitude and sluggishness, pale tongue with whitish coating, slow, slippery and weak pulse. 〈Treatment principles〉 Strengthen the spleen and stomach, regulate qi and lower the adverse flow of stomach-qi. 〈Point selection〉 Zusanli (ST 36), Shangwan (RN 13), Zhongwan (RN 12) and Gongsun (SP 4).

●胃之大络 [wèi zhī dà luò] 络脉名。胃之大络名曰虚里。见该条。

The Large Collateral of Stomach A collateral, whose name is Xuli. →虚里 (p. 515)

●胃足阳明之脉 [wèi zú yáng míng zhī mài] 足阳明胃经的原称。见该条。

The Stomach Vessel of Foot-Yangming The original name of the Stomach Meridian of Foot-Yangming. →足阳明胃经 (p. 647)

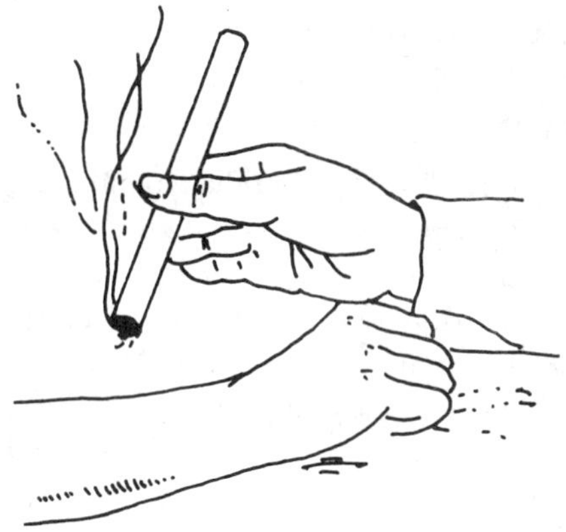

图62 温 和 灸
Fig. 62 Mild warm moxibustion

●温和灸 [wēn hé jiǔ] 为艾条灸的一种。又称温灸。指局部温热而不灼伤皮肤的灸治方法。施灸时将艾条一端点燃，对准施灸部位，约距0.5～1寸左右熏灸，使患者局部有温热感而无灼痛。一般灸3～5分钟，至皮肤稍呈红晕为度。对于昏厥，局部知觉减退的患者和小儿等，医者可将食指或中指，置于施灸部位，掌握施灸热度，防止烫伤。

Mild Moxibustion A kind of moxibustion with a moxa stick, also called warming moxibustion, referring to moxibustion therapy by warming the local place without burning the skin. 〈Method〉 For moxibustion, ignite one end of a moxa stick, put the ignited end directly above the local place to warm it, 0.5～1 cun or so away from the place. It is good for the patient to feel warmth without pain. Usually apply 3～5 minutes each time until the skin around the place becomes flushed. For a child or a patient with syncope and distur-

bance of perception in the local place, the doctor should control the temperature of moxibustion by putting his index finger or middle finger on the place so as to avoid scalding the patient.

●温溜[wēn liū] 经穴名。出《针灸甲乙经》。属手阳明大肠经,为本经郄穴。又名逆注、蛇头、池头。〈定位〉屈肘,在前臂背面桡侧,当阳溪与曲池连线上,腕横纹上5寸(图48和图53)。〈层次解剖〉皮肤→皮下组织→桡侧腕长伸肌腱→桡侧腕短伸肌。浅层布有头静脉,前臂外侧皮神经和前臂后皮神经等。深层:在桡侧腕长伸肌和桡侧腕短伸肌腱之前有桡神经浅支。〈主治〉头痛、面肿、鼻衄、口舌痛、咽喉肿痛、肩背酸痛、肠鸣腹痛、癫、狂、吐舌。直刺0.5～0.8寸;可灸。

Wenliu(LI 7) A meridian point, originally from *Zhenjiu Jia-Yi Jing* (*A-B Classic of Acupuncture and Moxibustion*), the Xi-Cleft point of the Large Intestine Meridian of Hand-Yangming, also called Nizhu, Shetou and Chitou. 〈Location〉with the elbow flexed on the radial side of the dorsal surface of the forearm, on the line connecting Yungxi(LI 5) and Quchi(LI 11), 5 cun above the crease of the wrist (Figs. 48&53). 〈Regional anatomy〉skin→subcutaneous tissue→long radial extensor muscle tendon of wist→short radial extensor muscle of wrist. In the superficial layer, there are the cephalic vein, the lateral cutaneous nerve of the forearm and the posterior cutaneous nerve of the forearm. In the deep layer, there are the superficial branches of the radial nerve before the tendons of the long and short radial extensor muscles of the wrist. 〈Indications〉headache, swelling of the face, epistaxis, swelling and pain in the mouth and tongue, sore throat, soreness and pain of the shoulder and back, borborygmus, abdominal pain, manic-depressive psychosis, wagging tongue. 〈Method〉Puncture perpendicularly 0.5～0.8 cun. Moxibustion is applicable.

●温灸[wēn jiǔ] 温和灸之别称。见该条。

Warming Moxibustion Another name for mild moxibustion. →温和灸(p.469)

●温灸器[wēn jiǔ qì] 灸具名。又称灸疗器。用金属制成圆筒,底部有数十小孔,放艾绒或药末于其内,用时以火点燃,将筒置于灸处,使热力透入肌肤。有调和气血,温中散寒的作用。对妇女、儿童及畏针者尤为适用。

Mild-Moxibustioner A moxibustion apparatus, also called moxibustion treatment apparatus. 〈Method〉Prepare a tube made of metal, with dozens of small holes in the bottom, and a smaller tube with over ten small holes in it, place argyi wool or medical powder in the smaller tube. When the moxibustion is applied, ignite it and put the tube on a certain position to make the heat go through the skin and muscle. 〈Functions〉Regulate qi and blood, warm the middle-jiao to dispel cold. 〈Indications〉especially suitable for women, children and those who are afraid of needles.

●温疟[wēn nüè] 疟疾证型之一。出《素问·疟论》。因素有伏热,复感疟邪所致。证见热多寒少、汗出不畅、头痛、骨节酸痛、口渴引饮、便秘尿赤、舌红苔黄、脉弦数。治宜清热解表,和解少阳。取大椎、后溪、曲池、足临泣、间使。

Pyrexial Malaria A type of malaria, originally from *Suwen: Nüe Lun*(*Plain Questions: On Malaria Diseases*), caused by pathogenic heat retained in the body and the invasion of the pathogenic factor of malaria disease. 〈Manifestations〉high fever with mild chills, hypohidrosis, headache, arthragia, thirst with preference to drink, constipation and turbid urine, red tongue with yellow coating, taut and rapid pulse. 〈Treatment principle〉Clear heat and relieve exterior syndrome, readjust Shaoyang by mediation. 〈Point selection〉Dazhui(DU 14), Houxi(SI 3), Quchi(LI 11), Zulinqi(GB 41) and Jianshi(PC 5).

●温脐法[wēn qí fǎ] 间接灸法的一种。见《医学入门》。药用五灵脂、白芷、青盐各6克,麝香少许研为药末,另用荞麦粉和水作成圆圈,置于脐上,把药末放入脐中,以艾火灸之,灸至患者脐中温暖为止。此法适用于妇科病证。

Umbilical Warming A kind of indirect moxibustion, seen in *Yixue Rumen*(*An Introduction to Medicine*). Take *Wu Ling Zhi*(*Faeces Trogopterorum*) 6g, *Bai Zhi*(*Radix Angelicae Dahuicae*) 6g, salt 6g and a little *She Xiang*(*Moschus*), and grind them into powder, mix some buckwheat flour with water and shape it

into a circle, put the circle on the umbilicus. Place the medical powder in the circle and put the ignited mugwort over the medical powder until the patient feels warm. This method is indicated for gynecopathy.

●温筒灸[wēn tǒng jiǔ] 为温灸器灸之别称。参见温灸器条。

Moxibustion with a Warm Tube Another name for moxibustion with a mild-moxibustioner. →温灸器(p. 470)

●温针[wēn zhēn] 为温针灸之别称。详见该条。

Warm Needling Another name for needle warming through moxibustion. →温针灸(p. 471)

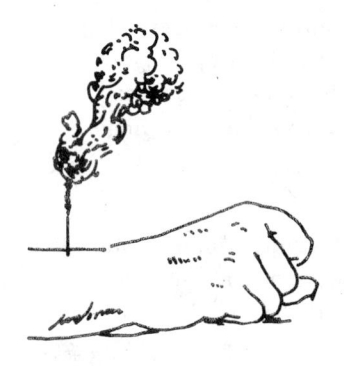

图63 温针灸
Fig. 63 Warm needle moxibustion

●温针灸[wēn zhēn jiǔ] 灸法的一种。见《伤寒论》。又称温针、传热灸、烧针尾。指针刺后以艾绒裹于针尾,点燃加温,使针下温热的一种治疗方法,具有宣通气血,温通经络的作用。适用于寒滞经络,气血痹阻的病证。如腰脊关节痛、肢体冷痛、脘腹冷痛、便溏寒泻、腹胀等。近代之电热针,便由此法发展而来。参见各条。

Warm Needle Moxibustion A form of moxibustion, originally from *Shanghan Lun* (*Treatise on Cold-Induced Diseases*), also called warm needling, heat-conducting moxibustion or burning the needle handle, referring to a therapeutic technique of making the needle warm by burning mugwort on the handle of the needle after inserting it into the body. 〈Functions〉Regulate the flow of qi; promote blood circulation and the flow of qi by warming the meridian.〈Indications〉pain along the spinal column, cold-pain of the extremities and abdomen, loose stool, abdominal distention, all the symptoms caused by the stagnation of pathogenic cold in the meridian and impeded circulation of blood and qi. The modern electrothermal needle is evolved from this method. →温针(p. 471)、传热灸(p. 51)、烧针尾(p. 355)、电热针(p. 80)

●闻人耆年[wén rén qí nián] 人名。宋代针灸家。槜李(今浙江嘉兴)人。善针灸。积四十余年临床经验著《备急灸法》一卷。刊于1226年。

Wenren Qinian An acupuncture-moxibustion expert in the Song Dynasty, born in Zuili (Today's Jiaxing, Zhejiang Province), good at acupuncture and moxibustion, the compiler of *Beiji Jiufa* (*Moxibustion for Emergencies*) on basis of the 40 years of his clinical experiences, published in 1226.

●卧位[wò wèi] 针灸体位名。又分仰卧位、侧卧位、俯卧位。详见各条。

Lying Postures Postures in acupuncture, divided into supine postures, siderecumbent posture and prone posture. →仰卧位(p. 544)、侧卧位(p. 31)、俯卧位(p. 120)

●卧针[wò zhēn] 针刺术语。行针时将针退至皮下使针倾斜如卧,以备再作沿皮刺或留针。

Prone Needling An acupuncture term. While needling, lift the needle to the subcutaneous level, make it oblique as if it were lying, for repuncturing subcutaneously or retaining the needle.

●乌梅灸[wū méi jiǔ] 药物敷贴法的一种。取乌梅肉1克,加醋捣成泥膏,敷于患处。如治疗鸡眼、脚垫,敷灸前患处先用温开水浸泡,用刀刮去表面角质层,取上药贴于患处,每次敷12小时。

Wu Mei (Fructus Mume) Moxibustion A topical application of herbs. Take *Wu Mei* (*Fructus Mume*) 1 g, pound it with vinegar into a paste and apply the paste on the affected area. For the treatment of corn and callosity, soak the affected area with warm water before moxibustion and scrape out the horny layer on the surface and then apply the medical paste topically on the affected area for 12 hours each

time.

●乌梅蒸气灸[wū méi zhēng qì jiǔ] 灸法的一种。取乌梅60克,五味子、石榴皮各10克,水煎后倒入盆或大桶中对准患部用气熏灸。用于子宫脱垂。

Wu Mei(Fructus Mume) Steam Moxibustion
A kind of moxibustion. Take *Wu Mei* (*Fructus mume*) 60 g, *Wu Wei Zi* (*Fructus Schisandrae*) 10 g, *Shi Liu Pi* (*Pericarpium Granatl*) 10 g, decoct them in water, then put the fluid in a tube or pot and steam the affected region with it. 〈Indication〉 prolapse of uterus.

●屋翳[wū yì] 经穴名。出《针灸甲乙经》。属足阳明胃经。〈定位〉在胸部,当第二肋间隙,距前正中线4寸。〈层次解剖〉皮肤→皮下组织→胸大肌→胸小肌。浅层布有第二肋间神经外侧皮支。深层在胸肩峰动、静脉的分支或属支,胸内、外侧神经的分支。〈主治〉咳嗽、气喘、唾脓血痰、胸胁胀痛、乳痛、皮肤疼痛、瘛疭、身肿。直刺0.2~0.3寸,或向内刺0.5~0.8寸;可灸。

Wuyi(ST 15) A meridian point, originally from *Zhenjiu Jia-Yi Jing* (*A-B Classic of Acupuncture and Moxibustion*), a point on the Stomach Meridian of Foot-Yangming. 〈Location〉 on the chest, in the 2nd intercostal space, 4 cun. lateral to the anterior midline. 〈Regional anatomy〉 skin→subcutaneous tissue→greater pectoral muscle→smaller pectoral muscle. In the superficial layer, there are the lateral cutaneous branches of the second intercostal nerve. In the deep layer, there are the branches or tributaries of the thoracoacromial artery and vein and the branches of the medial pectoral and lateral pectoral nerves. 〈Indications〉cough, asthma, coughing out purulent sputum mixed with blood, pain and distention in the chest and hypochondrium, breast abscess, pain in the skin, clonic convulsion, edema of the body. 〈Method〉Puncture perpendicularly 0.2~0.3 cun, or obliquely inward 0.5~0.8 cun. Moxibustion is applicable.

●无瘢痕灸[wú bān hén jiǔ] 艾炷灸的一种。又称非化脓灸。指灸后达到温烫为主,不致形成疮灸,既不化脓,也不留下瘢痕,称为无瘢痕灸。其法可采用小艾炷放在穴位上,点燃后,不等艾火烧到皮肤,当病人感到灼痛时,再更换艾炷继续施灸,以局部皮肤充血、红晕为度。

Non-Scarring Moxibustion A form of moxa cone moxibustion, also called non-festering moxibustion, referring to warmth felt by the patient with no festers or scars left on the skin, so it is called non-scarring moxibustion. 〈Method〉Place a small moxa cone on the point, ignite it until the local skin feels pain, without burning the skin and then remove it for another one until the skin becomes flush.

●无名[wú míng] 经外穴的别名。即二椎下。见该条。

Wuming →二椎下(p. 102)

●无名指[wú míng zhǐ] 部位名。又称环指。即第四指,古称小指次指,即小指侧之次指。

The Anonymous Finger A part of the body, also called the ring finger; in ancient times, called the finger next to the little one, namely, the 2nd from the little finger.

●无热灸[wú rè jiǔ] 灸法之一。为天灸之别称。见该条。

Non-Warming Moxibustion A form of moxibustion, another name for medical vesiculation. →天灸(p. 432)

●无子[wú zǐ] 即不孕。详见该条。

Childlessness →不孕(p. 29)

●吴复桂[wú fù guì] 人名。北宋医家。开宝六年(973年)奉命编修《开宝新详定本草》二十卷。太平兴国七年(982年)又参加编写《太平圣惠方》。淳化年间(990—994年)为太宗侍御医,并著有《金匮指微诀》一卷,已佚。另据《宋史·艺文志》载,其还著《小儿明堂针灸经》一卷,已佚。

Wu Fugui A physician in the Northern Song Dynasty. In the 6th year of Kaibao's reign (A.D. 973), he was instructed to compile *Kaibao Xin Xiangding Bencao*(*Kaibao Newly Revised Book of Material Medica*) in 20 volumes. In the 7th year of Taiping Xingguo(A. D. 982), he participated in writing *Taiping Shenghui Fang*(*Imperial Benevolent Prescriptions*). In the reign of Chunhua (A.D. 990-994), he was the imperial physician of Taizong and wrote the book of *Jingui Zhiwei Jue*(*Subtle Knacks of the Golden Chamber*),

which has beed lost. According to *Songshi:Yi Wen Zhi*(*Song History: Records of Art and Literature*), he also wrote a book of *Xiaoer Mingtang Zhenjiu Jing*(*Classic of Acupuncture and Moxibustion for Children*) in one volume, which is no longer extant.

●吴嘉言[wú jiā yán] 人名。明针灸家。分水(今浙江桐庐)人。世医家庭，曾任太医院吏目，精于针灸，撰《针灸原枢》、《医学会元》，已佚。见《严州府志》。

Wu Jiayan An acupuncture-moxibustion expert of the Ming Dynasty, a native of Fenshui (today's Tonglu of Zhejiang Province), from a hereditary doctors' family. He was once appointed Limu in the Institute of Imperial Physician and was good at acupuncture. His writings include *Zhenjiu Yuanshu* (*A Discussion on the Key Parts of Acupuncture and Moxibustion*) and *Yixue Huiyuan* (*Essentials of Medicine*), both of which have been lost. All of these have been mentioned in *Yanzhoufu Zhi*(*Annals of Yanzhoufu*).

●吴昆[wú kūn] 人名。明医家。字山甫，别号鹤皋，歙县(今属安徽)人。家中多藏书，自幼攻读医学著作，于江、浙一代医名很大。著《医方考》、《脉语》、《吴注黄帝内经素问》、《针方六集》等。后者为针灸文献的分类考证做了大量工作。还撰有《砭碫考》，已佚。

Wu Kun A physician of the Ming Dynasty, who styled himself Shanfu, also named Hegao, born in Shexian County(now in Anhui Province). He assiduously studied medical books in childhood and collected a large number of books. He was very well-known throughout the Jiangsu-Zhejiang areas. His works include *Yifang Kao*(*Textual Studies on Prescriptions*), *Mai Yu* (*Discussion on Sphygmology*), *Wu Zhu Huangdi Neijing Su Wen* (*Wu's Annotations on the Plain Questions of the Yellow Emperor's Canon of Internal Medicine*), *Zhenfang Liu Ji* (*Six Collections of Acupuncture Prescriptions*). He did a lot of work in the classification and test of acupuncture documents. He also wrote the book *Bian Rui Kao*(*Textual Studies on Stone Needling and Cauterization Therapy*), which has been lost.

●吴谦[wú qiān] 人名。清代名医。字六吉。安徽歙县人。曾任太医院判。与刘裕铎主持编纂《医宗金鉴》其中《订正伤寒论注》、《订正金匮要略注》二种为吴氏自编。《医宗金鉴》曾用作太医院教本。

Wu Qian A physician in the Qing Dynasty, who styled himself Liuji, a native of Shexian County, Anhui Province, once the official of the Institute of Imperial Physicians, with Liu Yuduo, he took charge of the compilation of the *Yizong Jinjian*(*Gold Mirror of Orthodox Medical Lineage*) in which *Dingzheng Shanghan Lunzhu*(*Revised Treatise on Cold-Induced Diseases*) and *Dingzheng Jingui Yaolüe Zhu* (*Revised Notes to Synopsis of the Golden Chamber*) were written by him personally. *Yizong Jinjian*(*Gold Mirror of Orthodox Medical Lineage*) was once used as text book in the Imperial Institute of Physicians.

●吴文炳[wú wén bǐng] 人名。明代针灸家。字沼轩，号光甫，建武(今湖北南漳县一带)人。著《神医秘诀遵经奥旨针灸大成》、《食物本草》、《医家赤帜益辨全书》等。

Wu Wenbing An acupuncture-moxibustion expert in the Ming Dynasty, who styled himself Zhaoxuan and assumed the name of Guangfu, a native of Jianwu (today's Nanzhang County, Hubei Province), the writer of *Shenyi Mijue Zunjing Aozhi Zhenjiu Dacheng* (*A Great compendium of Acupuncture and Moxibustion Based on the Secrets of Highly Skilled Doctor and the Profundities of Classics*), *Shiwu Bencao*(*Dietary Materia Materia Media*), *Yijia Chizhi Yibian Quanshu* (*Physician's Complete Book Supplementary Debates by Taking a Clear-Cut Stand*).

●吴亦鼎[wú yì dǐng] 人名。清代针灸家。字砚丞，安徽歙县人。于咸丰元年(1851年)，汇集历代名家灸法，著成《神灸经论》四卷，对灸法理论有所发挥。亦撰《麻疹备要方论》一书。

Wu Yiding An acupuncture-moxibustion expert in the Qing Dynasty, who styled himself Yancheng, a native of Shexian County of Anhui Province. In the first year(1851)of Xianfeng's reign, he collected different moxibustion theories of successive dynasties, and wrote the book *Shenjiu Jinglun*(*Principles of Magic Moxibustion*) in 4 volumes which fur-

ther elaborated moxibustion theories. He also wrote the book *Mazhen Beiyaofang Lun* (*Treatise on Essential Prescriptions for Measles*).

●吴之英[wú zhī yīng] 人名。清代医家。对针灸经络曾进行考释,与罗绍骥合编《经脉分图》,于1900年印行。

Wu Zhiying A physician in the Qing Dynasty, once engaged in textual research of acupuncture and moxibustion and meridians. He wrote *Jingmai Fentu* (*Separate Illustrations of Meridians*) together with Luo Shaoji, which was published in 1900.

●五倍子灸[wǔ bèi zǐ jiǔ] 灸法的一种。用五倍子与醋熬成膏,贴于脐部,用于治疗小儿泻泄、盗汗。

Wu Bei Zi (Galla Chinensis) Moxibustion A form of moxibustion. 〈Method〉Decoct *Wu Bei Zi* (*Galla Chinensis*) and vinegar into a paste, apply the paste on the umbilicus. 〈Indications〉pediatric diarrhea, night sweat.

●五倍子蒸气灸[wǔ bèi zǐ zhēng qì jiǔ] 灸法的一种。取五倍子250克,白矾10克,上药煎沸后倒入木桶内,患者坐于桶上用蒸气熏灸。用于直肠脱垂等症。

Wu Bei Zi (Galla Chinensis) Steaming Moxibustion A form of moxibustion. 〈Method〉 Take *Wu Bei Zi* (*Galla Chinensis*) 250g, *Bai Fan* (*Alum*) 10g, decoct them in water, then put the medicinal fluid in a wooden tub or pot for steaming bath. 〈Indication〉prolapse of rectum.

●五变[wǔ biàn] 指五脏与五行等的对应关系。出《灵枢·顺气一日分为四时》。即指脏、色、时、音、味五个方面的变化,主要是用以说明疾病的表现,是谓之脏有五变。依此说,每种变化都有井、荥、输、经、合五种腧穴与之相应。如脏主冬,冬刺井;色主春,春刺荥;时主夏,夏刺输;音主长夏,长夏刺经;味主秋,秋刺合,是谓五变以主五输。这种按季分刺五输的方法,重点是季节时间与所刺输穴的相应关系。又如,病在脏者取之井;病变于色者,取之荥;病时间时甚者,取之输;病变于音者,取之经;经满而血者,病在胃及以饮食不节得病者,取之合,是指五变所表现的不同特征以及五输相应的针刺方法。上述均谓之刺有五变。参见五行条。

Five Changes Referring to the corresponding relation between five zang-organs and five elements, originally from *Lingshu: Shunqi Yi Ri Fenwei Si Shi* (*Miraculous Pivot: Correspondence between a day and the Qi of Four Seasons*), indicating the changes of five aspects, namely zang-organ, color, time, note and flavor. Mainly used to explain the manifestation of diseases as the zang-organs have five changes. According to this theory, each change includes the Five-Shu points—the Jing (Well) point, Ying (Spring) point, Shu (Stream), Jing (River) and He (Sea), which correspond to it, i.e. the zang-organ in charge of winter, needle Ying (Well) point in winter; the color of spring, needle Ying (Spring) points in spring; the time of summer, needle Shu (Stream) points in summer; the note of the 6th mouth of the lunar year needle Jing (River) points in the mouth; the flavor of autumn, needle He (Sea) points in autumn. This is called "five changes in charge of Five-Shu Points". The method, needling the Five-Shu based on seasons, mainly refers to the corresponding relationship between seasons and points to be needled, To further explain it, Jing (Well) points are selected for zang organ diseases; the Jing (Spring) points for color diseases; the Shu (Stream) point for time diseases; the Jing (River) points for note diseases; the He (Sea) points for stomach and improper diet diseases. All of this refers to different characteristic symptoms of five changes and acupuncture therapy corresponding to Five-Shu points used in acupuncture. What is mentioned above is called five changes of acupuncture. →五行(p. 480)

●五变刺[wǔ biàn cì] 《内经》刺法分类名。出《灵枢·顺气一日分为四时》。指按五类不同病情变化选用五腧穴针刺。参见五变条。

Five-Change Acupunture A category of acupuncture manipulations in *Neijing* (*The Canon of Internal Medicine*), originally from *Lingshu: Shunqi Yi Ri Fen Wei Si Shi* (*Miraculous Pivot: Correspondence between a Day and the Qi of Four Seasons*), referring to selecting Five-Shu Points for acupuncture in accordance with five different changes of

patient's condition. →五变(p.474)

●五处[wǔ chù] 经穴名。出《针灸甲乙经》。属足太阳膀胱经。又名巨处。〈定位〉在头部,当前发际正中直上1寸,旁开1.5寸(图28)。〈层次解剖〉皮肤→皮下组织→枕额肌额腹。浅层布有滑车上神经和滑车上动、静脉。深层为腱膜下疏松组织和颅骨外膜。〈主治〉头痛、目眩、目视不明、痫证、小儿惊风。平刺0.3～0.5寸;禁灸。

Wuchu (BL 5) A meridian point, originally from *Zhenjiu Jia-Yi Jing* (*A-B Classic of Acupuncture and Moxibustion*), a point on the Bladder Meridian of Foot-Taiyang, also called Juchu. 〈Location〉on the head, 1 cun directly above the midpoint of the anterior hairline and 1.5 cun lateral to the midline (Figs. 28). 〈Reginal anatomy〉skin→subcutaneous tissue →frontal belly of occipitofrontal muscle. In the superficial layer, there are the supratrochlear nerve and the supratrochlear artery and vein. In the deep layer, there are the subaponeurotic loose connective tissue and pericranium. 〈Indications〉 headache, dizziness, blurred vision, epilepsy, infantile convulsions 〈Method〉Puncture subcutaneously 0.3～0.5 cun. Moxibustion is forbidden.

●五刺[wǔ cì] 《内经》刺法分类。出《灵枢·官针》。又称五脏刺。是按皮、脉、筋、肉、骨分成五种刺法,以应合五脏。包括半刺、豹文刺、关刺、合谷刺、输刺。详见各条。

Five Ancient Needling Techniques A category of acupuncture manipulations in *Neijing* (*The Canon of Internal Medicine*), originally from *Lingshu: Guan Zhen* (*Miraculous Pivot: Official Needles*), also called needling methods for the five zang-organs. The classification is in accordance with skin, blood circulation, tendons, muscles and bones, including extremely shallow puncture, leopard-spot puncture, joint puncture, Hegu puncture and Shu-point puncture. →半刺(p.12)、豹文刺(p.15)、关刺(p.147)、合谷刺(p.161)、输刺(p.406)

●五夺禁刺[wǔ duó jìn cì] 针刺禁忌。出《灵枢·五禁》。指脱形、亡血、大汗亡阳、大泄亡阴、产后暴崩这五种元气大虚的病情,针刺不能用泻法。

Needling for Five Kinds of Exhaustions Forbidden Contraindications in acupuncture, originally from *Lingshu: Wu Jin* (*Miraculous Pivot: Five Contraindications*), referring to excessive emaciation, severe hemorrhage, depletion of yang due to profuse sweating, depletion of yin due to serious diarrhea and postpartum metrorrhagia, the five conditions of exhausting primordial qi, for which the reducing methods of acupuncture are forbidden.

●五更泄[wǔ gēng xiè] 病证名。见《寿世保元》。又名晨泄、瀼泄。指黎明前作泄。多因肾虚所致。即肾虚泻。详见该条。

Diarrhea Before Dawn A disease, originally from *Shoushi Baoyuan* (*Longevity and Life Preservation*), also called morning diarrhea or diarrhea just before dawn, referring to diarrhea, usually occurring just before dawn, due to deficiency of the kidney. →肾虚泻(p.367)

●五过[wǔ guò] 刺法术语。出《灵枢·五禁》。是指针刺补泻过度。即指补之过度,资其邪气;泻之过度,竭其正气。五脏外合之皮、脉、肉、筋、骨,有邪正虚实,宜平调之,如补泻过度,则谓之五过。

Five Excesses An acupuncture manipulation, originally from *Ling Shu: Wu Jin* (*Miraculous Pivot: Five Contraindications*), referring to over-reinforcing or over-reducing in acupuncture. Over-reinforcing encourages pathogen, and over-reducing exhausts vital qi. The suitable reinforcing-reducing method should be used in relation to: pathogenic factors, vital functions, deficiency or excess syndrome in skin meridians, muscles, tendons and bones and interrelated with the five zang organs. Over-reinforcing and over-reducing are called the five excesses.

●五虎[wǔ hǔ] 经外穴名。见《奇效良方》。在手指背侧当2、4掌骨小头高点处。灸治五指拘挛。

Wuhu (EX-UE) An extra point, originally from *Qixiao Liang Fang* (*Prescriptions of Wonderful Efficacy*). 〈Location〉on the dorsum of the hand, on the high points of the 2nd &4th metacarpal bones at their small ends. 〈Method〉moxibustion for finger muscular constricture.

●五会[wǔ huì] ①经穴别名。出《铜人腧穴针灸图经》。即人迎。见该条。②经穴别名。见《针灸大全》。即百会。见三阳五会条。

Wuhui Another name for ① Renying (ST 9), a meridian point orginally from *Tongren Shuxue Zhenjiu Tujing (Illustrated Manual of Points for Acupuncture and Moxibustion on a Bronze Statue with Acupoints)*. →人迎 (p. 333) ② Baihui, a meridian point originally from *Zhenjiu Daquan (A Complete Work of Acupuncture and Moxibustion)*. →百会 (p. 11) →三阳五会 (p. 345)

●五节刺 [wǔ jié cì] 《内经》刺法分类。出《灵枢·刺节真邪篇》。分别列举五种刺法的应用，即振埃、发矇、去爪、彻衣、解惑。详见各条。

Five Acupuncture Techniques A category of acupuncture manipulations in *Neijing (The Canon of Internal Medicine)*, originally from *Lingshu: Ci Jie Zhen Xie Pain (Acupuncture Principles and Diseases)*, which lists respectively the application of five kinds of acupuncture techniques, including flicking ash, treating poor vision, removing pathogenic factors, taking off clothes and clearing puzzles→振埃 (p. 598), 发矇 (p. 103), 去爪 (p. 326), 彻衣 (p. 41), 解惑 (p. 201)

●五禁 [wǔ jìn] 古代针灸禁忌之一。出《灵枢·五禁》。根据天干而规定不同日期不可刺人体的某一部位。甲乙日不可刺头部；丙丁日不可刺肩喉；戊己日不可刺腹部；庚辛日不可刺股膝关节处；壬癸日不可刺足胫部。

Five Contraindications Set of the contraindications for acupuncture, originally from *Lingshu: Wu Jin (Miraculous Pivot: Five Contraindications)*. According to the Heavenly Stems, some part of the body can not be punctured on specific days, i.e. no needling on the head on the day of Jia or Yi; no needling on the shoulder and larynx on the day of Bing or Ding; no acupuncture on the abdomen on the day of Wu or Ji; no acupuncture on the joints of thigh and knee on the day of Geng or Xin, and no needling on the leg and foot on the day of Ren or Gui.

●五经 [wǔ jīng] 五脏的经脉。出《素问·经脉别论》。即肝经、脾经、心经、肺经、肾经。

Five Meridians The meridians of the five zang-organs, originally from *Suwen: Jingmai Bielun (Plain Questions: Supplementary Exposition of Meridians)*, referring to the Liver Meridian, the Spleen Meridian, the Heart Meridian, the Lung Meridian and the Kidney Meridian.

●五决 [wǔ jué] 指肝、心、脾、肺、肾五脏之脉，在脉诊中有决定意义。出《素问·五藏生成篇》。由五脉按表里相合关系，又分为十脉，即足少阴、巨(太)阳；足少阳、厥阴；足太阴、阳明；手阳明、太阴；手巨(太)阳、少阴。

Five Determinants The pulses of the five zang organs, which play a decisive role in pulse diagnosis, originally from *Suwen: Wu Zang Shengcheng Pian (Plain Questions: Physiology and Pathology of the Five Zang Organs)*. Based on the exterior-interior interrelationship, the five pulses are divided into ten—Foot-Shaoyin and-Ju (Tai) Yang; Foot-Shaoyang and-Jueyin; Foot-Taiyin and-Yangming; Hand-Yangming and-Taiyin; and Hand-Ju(Tai)Yang and-Shaoyin.

●五里 [wǔ lǐ] ①经穴别名。有二：一属阳明大肠经，在上臂；一属足厥阴肝经，在股内侧。为便于区别，《圣济总录》称前者为臂五里，后者为足五里《针灸资生经》称前者为手五里。后者为足五里。详见各条。②经穴别名。出《针灸甲乙经》。即劳宫。见该条。

Wuli Another name for ① a meridian point, which is of two kinds, one belonging to the Large Intestine Meridian of Hand-Yangming on the upper arm, another belonging to the Liver Meridian of Foot-Jueyin, on the inferior border of the thigh. In order to differentiate them from each other, the former was called Biwuli, the latter was called Zuwuli in *Shengji Zonglu (Imperial Medical Encyclopaedia)*. In *Zhengjiu Zi Sheng Jing (Acupuncture-Moxibustion Classic for Saving Life)*, the former was called Shouwuli (LI 13) and Zuwuli (LR 10). →手五里 (p. 401) 足五里 (p. 644) ② Laogong (PC 8), a meridian point originally from *Zhenjiu Jia-Yi Jing (A-B Classic of Acupuncture and Moxibustion)*. →劳宫 (p. 237)

●五门 [wǔ mén] 子午流注针法用语。出《标幽赋》。指十天干隔五相合，即甲与己合，乙与庚合，丙与辛合，丁与壬合，戊与癸合。参见五门十变条。

Five Gates A term of midnight-noon ebb-flow acupuncture, originally from *Biaoyou Fu*

(*Lyrics of Recondite Principles*), referring to the combinations of the ten Heavenly Stems in twos, one with the 5th one from it, i. e Jia with Ji, Yi with Geng, Bing with Xin, Ding with Ren, and Wu with Gui. →五门十变 (p. 477)

●五门十变 [wǔ mén shí biàn] 子午流注针法用语。五门指十天干隔五相合,详见五门条。十变指十天相干合后的变化,即甲己化土,乙庚化金,丙辛化水,丁壬化木,戊癸化火,又称五运。子午流注针法根据这种五门夫妻相配化生五运的理论,当阳日逢阴时或阴日逢阳时而无开穴时,可以"夫妻互用",即甲日与己日通用,乙日与庚日通用等。

Five Gates and Ten Changes An acupuncture technique of midnight-noon ebb-flow. The "Five Gates" refers to the paired every-other-five combinations of the ten Heavenly Stems. →五门 (p. 476). The "ten changes" refers to those following the Heavenly Stems combinations, namely, Jia-Ji changes into earth, Yi-Geng into metal, Bing-Xin into water; Ding-Ren into wood and Wu-Gui into fire. It's also called the five-element evolutions. According to the theory of five gates, the combination of husband and wife will induce five-element evolutions, when the Yang-day meets the Yin-hour and vice versa, and there is no openable point, the "husband" and "wife" are interchangeable, i. e. the Jia-day is interchangeable with the Ji-day and the Yi-day with Geng-day, etc.

●五逆 [wǔ nì] 指五种与证不相符合的重危病症。见《灵枢·五禁》。热性病,脉应洪大,但反见沉静,在出汗之后,脉应沉静,但反见躁动,脉症相反,是逆症之一;患泻下的病,脉宜沉静,而反见洪大之脉,是正虚邪盛,为逆症之二;肢体痹着,久病不愈,高起的肌肉破溃,身体发热,一侧的脉搏难以摸到,为逆症之三;久病遗、泄、淋、浊、汗等致阴血受损,使形体消瘦,若见发热、肤色苍白、枯晦不泽、大便下血块较严重的,为逆症之四;人有久发寒热、身体消瘦、脉坚硬搏指的,是逆症之五。五逆的病证均须慎用针刺。

Five Deteriorating Cases The five kinds of severe and dangerous diseases which their manifestations go disharmonious with, originally from *Lingshu: Wu Jin* (*Miraculous Pivot: Five Contraindications*). In the diseases of febrile nature the pulse should be full and large but exhibits a deep and calm pulse, and after sweating, the pulse should be deep and calm but exhibits restlessly, the pulse being opposite to the syndromes. This is the first deteriorating case. In diarrhea, the pulse should be deep and calm but feels full and large, this is due to weakened body resistance while pathogenic factors prevail. This is the second deteriorating case. The limbs are numb, long-standing and incurable, the portion of muscular bulge is diabrosis with body fever and one side of pulse difficult to feel. This is the third deteriorating case. In long-standing cases, e-mission, dliarrhea, stranguria, turbid urine, sweating leading to the impairment of yin and blood, resulting in emaciation. If it is manifested by fever, pale and dingy complexion, and severe hematochezia, it is then the fourth deterioration case; The one with fever and cold for a long-standing time, emaciation and hard feeling of pulse throbbing, is the fifth deteriorating case. Acupuncture should be used carefully in the treatment of the five deteriorating cases.

●五胠俞 [wǔ qū shù] 经穴别名。见《素问·刺疟篇》。即譩譆,见该条。

Wuqushu Another name for Yixi (BL 45), a meridian point originally from *Suwen: Cinüe Pian* (*Plain Questions: Acupuncture Methods for Malarial Diseases*). →譩譆 (p. 553)

●五色带下 [wǔ sè dài xià] 病证名。见《千金要方》。又称带五色俱下,带下五色。多因湿热蕴结下焦,积瘀成毒,损伤冲任带脉所致。证见五色秽浊之液从阴道流出,或有恶臭气味,绵绵不断。凡见此者,当注意生殖器官有无恶性病变。参见温毒带下条。

Multicolored Vaginal Mucoid Discharge A symptom, originally from *Qianjin Yaofang* (*Essential Prescriptions Worth a Thousand Gold*), also called five-colored leukorrhea or vaginal mucoid discharge of five colors, mostly due to downward flow of damp and heat pathogens into the lower jiao, accumulating to form toxin, and impair the Chong, Ren and Dai Meridians. 〈Manifestations〉 continuous mucoid discharge with filthy and various col-

ors and fetid smell from the vagina. For this kind of patient, be careful to see whether the genitals have a malignant tumor. →湿毒带下 (p. 370)

●**五十九刺**[wǔ shí jiǔ cì] 腧穴归类。出《灵枢·热病》。治疗热病的五十九穴。其为：商阳、关冲、少泽、少商、中冲、少冲、后溪、中渚、三间、少府、束骨、足临泣、陷谷、太白、五处、承光、通天、头临泣、目窗、正营、承灵、脑空、听会、完骨、承浆、哑门、百会、囟会、神庭、风府、廉泉、风池、天柱。其上腧穴除属任、督脉穴外，均为双侧取穴，共计五十九穴。

Fifty-Nine Needlings A category of acupoints, originally from *Lingshu: Rebing* (*Miraculous Pivot: Febrile Diseases*), the fifty-nine acupoints for treating febrile diseases: Shangyang(LI 1), Guanchong(SJ 1), Shaoze(SI 1), Shaoshang(LU 11), Zhongchong(PC 9), Shaochong(HT 9), Houxi(ST 3), Zhongzhu(SJ 3), Sanjian(LI 3), Shaofu(HT 8), Shugu(BL 65), Zulinqi(GB 41), Xiangu(ST 43), Taibai(SP 3), Wuchu(BL 5), Chengguang(BL 6), Tongtian(BL 7), Toulinqi(GB 15), Muchuang(GB 16), Zenyeng(GB 17), Chengling(GB 18), Naokong(GB 19), Tinghui(GB 2) Wanggu(GB 12), Chengjiang(RN 24), Yamen(DU 15), Baihui(DU 20), Xinghui(DU 22), Shenting(DU 24), Fengfu(DU 16), Lianquan(RN 23), Fengchi(GB 20), Tianzhu(BL 10). Except the acupoints of the Du and Ren meridians, all the above-mentioned acupoints are selected bilaterally. The total number of the acupoints is fifty-nine.

●**五枢**[wǔ shū] 经穴名。出《针灸甲乙经》属足少阳胆经，为足少阳、带脉之会。〈定位〉在侧腹部，当髂前上棘的前方，横平脐下3寸处（图40和图23）。〈层次解剖〉皮肤→皮下组织→腹外斜肌→腹内斜肌→腹横肌。浅层布有第十一、十二胸神经前支和第一腰神经前支的外侧皮支及伴行的动、静脉。深层有旋髂深动、静脉，第十一、十二胸神经，第一腰神经前支的肌支及相应的动、静脉。〈主治〉阴挺，赤白带下，月经不调，疝气，少腹痛，便秘，腰胯痛。直刺0.8～1.5寸；可灸。

Wushu(GB 27) A meridian point, originally from *Zhenjiu Jia-Yi Jing* (*A-B Classic of Acupuncture and Moxibustion*), a point on the Gallbladder Meridian of Foot-Shaoyang, the crossing point of the Foot-Shaoyang and Dai Meridians. 〈Location〉on the lateral side of the abdomen, anterior to the anteriosuperior iliac spine, 3 cun below the level of the umbilicus (Figs. 40 & 23). 〈Regional anatomy〉skin → subcutaneous tissue → external oblique muscle of abdomen → internal oblique muscle of abdomen → transvers muscle of abdomen. In the superficial layer, there are the lateral cutaneous branches of the anterior branches of the 11th and 12th thoracic and 1st lumbar nerves and accompanying arteries and vein. In the deep layer, there are the deep circumflex iliac artery and vein, the muscular branches of the anterior branches of the 11th and 12th thoracic and 1st lumbar nerves and the related arteries and veins. 〈Indications〉prolapse of uterus, leukorrhea with reddish discharge, irregular menstruation, hernia, pain in the lower abdomen, constipation, lumbosacral pain. 〈Method〉Puncture perpendicularly 0.8～1.5 cun. Moxibustion is applicable.

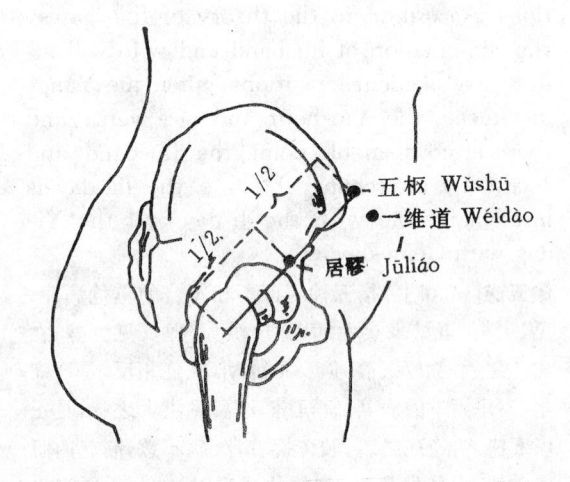

图64 五枢、维道、居髎穴

Fig 64 Wushu, Weidao and Juliao points

●**五腧配穴法**[wǔ shù pèi xué fǎ] 配穴法之一。指特定穴中井、荥、输、经、合五腧穴的配伍应用方法，包括五腧穴主症配穴，子母补泻，泻南补北，大接经法，子午流注法等。

Point Prescription of the Five Shu One of the point prescriptions referring to the application of the combination of the specific points in acupuncture, i.e. Jing (Well), Ying (Spring), Shu (Stream), Jing (River) and He (Sea)—the Five-Shu Points. The methods include selecting points according to the main symptoms, mother-child reinforcing-reducing, the combination of reducing south and reinforcing north, greatly connecting meridian method and midnight-noon ebb-flow.

● 五腧穴 [wǔ shù xué] 经穴分类名。指十二经脉在肘、膝关节以下的井、荥、输、经、合五个特定穴,简称"五腧"。出《灵枢·九针十二原》。这是以水流的大小来比喻各经脉气运行由小到大,由浅入深,由远而近的特点。五腧穴与五行相配属,阳经的五腧穴从井穴开始,依次与金水木火土相配属;阴经的五腧穴从井穴开始,依次与木火土金水相配属。见表16.1 & 16.2。

Five-Shu Points A category of meridian points, referring to the five specific points of twelve meridians. Jing (Well), Ying (Spring), Shu (Stream), Jing (River) and He (Sea), which are located in the limbs distal to the knee and elbow, simply called Five-Shu, originally from *Lingshu: Jiu Zhen Shier Yuan* (*Miraculous Pivot: Nine Needles and Twelve Yuan (Primary) Points*). The size of water flow is an analogy used to describe the characteristics of the qi in meridians moving from the small to the large, from the shallow to the deep and from far to near. The five elements are attached to the five-shu points, attaching to metal, water, wood, fire and earth in order; the Five-Shu point of yin meridians begin from Jing (Well) points attaching to wood, fire, earth, metal and water in order, see Table 16.1 & 16.2.

● 五态之人 [wǔ tài zhī rén] 古代将人分为五种类型,即太阴之人、少阴之人、太阳之人、少阳之人、阴阳平和之人。根据此五类人的筋骨气血即体质的不同,治疗时采用不同的方法。

表16.1　　　　　　阴经五腧穴与五行的配属
Table 16.1 Matching of the five-shu points of the 6 Yin meridians with the five elements

六阴经 Six Yin Meridians	井(木) Jing(Well) Wood	荥(火) Ying(Spring) Fire	输(土) Shu(Stream) Earth	经(金) Jing(River) Metal	合(水) He(Sea) Water
肺(金) Lung (Metal)	少商 Shaoshang (LU 11)	鱼际 Yuji (LU 10)	太渊 Taiyuan (LU 9)	经渠 Jingqu (LU 8)	尺泽 Chize (LU 5)
肾(水) Kidney (Water)	涌泉 Yongquan (KI 1)	然谷 Rangu (KI 2)	太溪 Taixi (KI 3)	复溜 Fuliu (KI 7)	阴谷 Yingu (KI 10)
肝(木) Liver (Wood)	大敦 Dadun (LR 1)	行间 Xinjian (LR 2)	太冲 Taichong (LR 3)	中封 Zhongfeng (LR 4)	曲泉 Ququan (LR 8)
心(火) Heart (Fire)	少冲 Shaochong (HT 9)	少府 Shaofu (HT 8)	神门 Shenmen (HT 7)	灵道 Lingdao (HT 4)	少海 Shaohai (HT 3)
脾(土) Spleen (Eartn)	隐白 Yinbai (SP 1)	大都 Dadu (SP 2)	太白 Taibai (SP 3)	商丘 Shangqiu (SP 5)	阴陵泉 Yinlingquan (SP 9)
心包(相火) Pericarum (Ministerial fire)	中冲 Zhongchong (PC 9)	劳宫 Laogong (PC 8)	大陵 Daling (PC 7)	间使 Jianshi (PC 5)	曲泽 Quze (PC 3)

表16.2　阳经五腧穴与五行的配属
Table 16.2 Matching of the five-shu points of the 6 Yang meridians with the five elements

六阳经 Six Yang Meridians	井(金) Jing(Well) Metal	荥(水) Ying(Spring) Water	输(木) Shu(Stream) Wood	经(火) Jing(River) Fire	合(土) He(Sea) Earth
大肠(金) Large Intestine (Metal)	商阳 Shangyang (LI 1)	二间 Erjian (LI 2)	三间 Sanjian (LI 3)	阳溪 Yangxi (LI 5)	曲池 Quchi (LI 11)
膀胱(水) Bladder (Water)	至阴 Zhiyin (BL 67)	足通谷 Zutonggu (BL 66)	束骨 Shugu (BL 65)	昆仑 Kunlun (BL 60)	委中 Weizhong (BL 40)
胆(木) Gallbladder (Wood)	足窍阴 Zuqiaoyin (GB 44)	侠溪 Xiaxi (GB 43)	足临泣 Zulinqi (GB 41)	阳辅 Yangfu (GB 38)	阳陵泉 Yanglingquan (GB 34)
小肠(火) Small Intestine (Fire)	少泽 Shaoze (SI 1)	前谷 Qiangu (SI 2)	后溪 Houxi (SI 3)	阳谷 Yanggu (SI 5)	小海 Xiaohai (SI 8)
胃(土) Stomach (Earth)	厉兑 Lidui (ST 45)	内庭 Neiting (ST 44)	陷谷 Xiangu (ST 43)	解溪 Jiexi (ST 41)	足三里 Zusanli (ST 36)
三焦(相火) Sanjiao (Ministerial fire)	关冲 Guanchong (SJ 1)	液门 Yemen (SJ 2)	中诸 Zhongzhu (SJ 3)	支沟 Zhigou (SJ 6)	天井 Tianjing (SJ 10)

People of Five Kinds In ancient time humanities were divided into five types, namely, the types of Taiyin, Shaoyin Taiyang, Shaoyang and equilibrium of Yin and Yang. According to the differences in tendons, bones, qi and blood the constitutions of human beings—among the five types, different treatments were adopted.

●五邪刺[wǔ xié cì] 《内经》刺法理论。出《灵枢·刺节真邪》。论述对不同的病情宜用不同的刺法。五邪是指痈邪、盛大的邪、微弱的邪、热邪、寒邪，刺治五邪的方法有五条，即肿聚不散的应使其消散，邪盛有余的须驱除其邪气，体虚邪微者当补益而使其强壮，痹热的病应消灭其痹热，寒痹病应助阳热以温血气。刺五邪的针具是：刺痈疡当用铍针，刺大邪当用锋针，刺小邪当用圆利针，刺热邪当用镵针，刺寒邪当用毫针。

Needling Treating Five Pathogenic Factors
The needling theory of *Neijing*(*The Canon of Internal Medicine*), originally from *Ling Shu*: *Ci Jie Zhen Xie*(*Miraculous Pivot*: *Acupuncture Principles and Diseases*), expounding different needling techniques for treating different diseases. Five pathogenic factors refer to the pathogens of carbuncle, excess, faintness, heat and cold. For the five pathogenic factors there are five needling principles—resolve edemata and sores in the disease due to carbuncle pathogen; eliminate the pathogenic factors in patients with excess pathogen; tonify and strengthen the body of the debility patients with faint pathogen; clear away the bi(stagnant)-heat for the disease due to heat-evil; and invigorate yang-heat to warm qi and blood for treating the five pathogenic factors: stiletto needle for sore and carbuncle, lance needle for excess pathogen, round-sharp needle for faint pathogen, sheer needle for heat pathogen, and filiform needle for cold pathogen.

●五行[wǔ xíng] 见《尚书·洪范》。指水、火、木、金、土五类最基本的物质,后来用于对各种事物现象的归类,并说明其相互关系。木、火、土、金、水,依次为相生,隔一为相克(乘),反克为侮。中医基础理论中主要以五行配合五脏和经脉,从生克乘侮说明其相互依存、相互制约的关系,解释生理、病理和治法的变化。五行归类表见表17。

表17　　　　　　五　行　归　类

Table 17　　The Classification of things according to the theory of five elements

五行 Five Elements	脏 Viscera	色 Color	方 Orientation	时 Season	腧 Five-Shu Points	音 Note	味 Taste	日 Day
木 Wood	肝 Liver	青 Blue	东 East	春 Spring	荥 Ying(Spring)	角 Jiao	酸 Sour	甲乙 Jiayi
火 Fire	心 Heart	赤 Red	南 South	夏 Summer	输 Shu(stream)	徵 Zhi	苦 Bitter	丙丁 Bingding
土 Earth	脾 Spleen	黄 Yellow	中 Middle	长夏 Later Summer	经 Jing(River)	宫 Gong	甘 Sweet	戊己 Wu ji
金 Metal	肺 Lung	白 White	西 West	秋 Autumn	合 He(Sea)	商 Shang	辛 Pungent	庚辛 Gengxin
水 Water	肾 Kidney	黑 Black	北 North	冬 Winter	井 Jing(Well)	羽 Yu	咸 Salty	壬癸 Rengui

Five Elements　Originally from *Shang Shu: Hong Fan(The Book of Documents:The Great Norm)*, referring to the five most fundamental elements—water, fire, wood, metal and earth, later used to classify all kinds of things and phenomona and expound the relationship among them. The relationship among wood, fire, earth, metal and water, in this order, is generation; in the one-interval order is restriction; in the opposite order is reverse restriction. In the theory of Traditional Chinese Medicine, the five elements are attributed respectively to five zang organs and meridians, from the relationship of wood, fire, earth, metal, and water, to explain the interpromotion and interrestraint of the five elements and to expound the changes of physiology, pathology and therapeutic methods. For the classification of things according to the theory of the five elements, see Table 17.

●五脏刺[wǔ zàng cì]　《内经》刺法分类。为五刺之别称。见该条。

Needling Methods for Five Zang Organs　A category of needling methods in *Nei Jing(The Inner Canon of Huangdi)*, another name for five needlings. →五刺(p.475)

●五脏六腑之海[wǔ zàng liù fǔ zhī hǎi]　①指冲脉。出《灵枢·逆顺肥瘦》。因其总领诸经气血，调节五脏六腑都禀受其气血的濡养。②指足阳明经。出《素问·痿论》。阳明为多气多血之经，主润宗筋，束筋骨而利机关。③指胃。出《灵枢·五味》。因其受纳水谷，为各脏腑营养之源，故名。

The Sea of Five Zang Organs and Six Fu Or-gans　Refering to ①the Chong Meridian, originally from *Lingshu: Ni Shun Fei Shou (Miraculous Pivot: Circulatory Direction of Meridians and Body Constitution)*. It controls the qi and blood of all meridians and regulates the qi and blood which nourishes the five zang organs and six fu organs; ② the Stomach Meridian of Foot-Yangming, originally from *Suwen:Wei Lun(Plain Questions:On Flaccidity Syndromes)*. Yangming Meridian is one with an abundance of qi and blood, taking charge of moistening the urogenital region, controlling muscles and bones and relieving the rigidity of joints; ③the stomach, originally from *Lingshu: Wu Wei(Miraculous Pivot: On Five Tastes)*. Being the receiver and container of water and food, it is the source of nutrition of all zang- and fu-organs, and so is called the sea of five zang-organs and six fu-organs.

●舞蹈震颤控制区[wǔ dǎo zhèn chàn kòng zhì qū]　头针刺激区。在运动区向前移1.5厘米的平行线。〈主治〉舞蹈病、震颤麻痹、震颤麻痹综合症。

The Chorea-Trembling Controlled Area　The stimulated area of scalp acupuncture. 〈Location〉the parallel line, 1.5cm in front of the motor area. 〈 Indication 〉 chorea, Parkinson's disease, Parkinsonian syndrome.

●恶食[wù shí]　恶阻的别名。详见该条。

Aversion to Food　→恶阻(p.93)

●恶子[wù zǐ]　恶阻的别名。详见该条。

Aversion to Fetus　→(恶阻)(p.93)

●恶字[wù zì]　恶阻的别名。详见该条。

Wuzi　→恶阻(p.93)

X

●西方子明堂灸经[xī fāng zǐ míng táng jiǔ jīng] 书名。八卷,元初刊行,作者姓氏不详。此为灸法专书,主要论述全身腧穴的灸法与主治。各卷分绘正面、侧背面、侧伏面的腧穴图及其主治和灸法,并于各穴处论可灸与不可灸。见《四库全书》和《中国医学大成》。

Xi Fang Zi Mingtang Jiujing (Xi Fang Zi Classic of Moxibustion) A book with eight volumes, published in the early period of the Yuan Dynasty, its writer unknown. A special book of moxibustion, mainly expounding moxibustion and the indications of acupoints of the body, each volume of which includes the drawings of acupoint illustrations of front, lateral-back and lateral-bend postures, indications for moxibustion and furthermore, marks in each acupoint whether moxibustion is aplicable or not. Seen in *Siku Quanshu* (*Complete Works of Four Treasuries*) and *Zhongguo Yixue Dacheng* (*A Great Collection of the Chinese Medical Books*).

●吸杯法[xī bēi fǎ] 拔罐法的别称。见该条。

Cup-Sucking →拔罐法(p.9)

●吸筒[xī tǒng] 拔罐工具。见《瑞竹堂验方·疮科》。也称竹管疗法。

Sucking Tube The instrument of cupping, originally from *Rui Zhu Tang Yanfang: Chuang Ke* (*Rui Zhu Tang's Experienced Prescriptions: Department for Sores*), also called bamboo jar therapy.

●息胞[xī bāo] 胞衣不下的别名。见该条。

Resting Placenta Another name for retention of placenta. →胞衣不下(p.14)

●息胎[xī tāi] 胞衣不下的别名。见该条。

Delayed Delivery of Placenta Another name for retention of placenta. →胞衣不下(p.14)

●溪谷[xī gǔ] 部位名。谷,形容肌肉呈现的凹陷,溪,形容小的凹陷。参见大谷、小溪条。

Streams and Valleys A part of the body, with valleys referring to the depressions between the muscles and streams the narrow depressions. →大谷(p.62)、小溪(p.504)

●溪穴[xī xué] ①经穴别名。出《针灸甲乙经》。即归来。见该条。②即䪼穴。承泣的别名。出《外台秘要》。见该条。

1. Xixue Another name for Guilai(ST 29), a meridian point originally from *Zhenjiu Jia-Yi Jing* (*A-B Classic of Acupuncture and Moxibustion*). →归来(p.150)

2. Xi(溪)xue Synonymous with Xi(䪼)xue and another name for Chengqi(ST 1), originally from *Waitai Miyao* (*Clandestine Essentials from the Imperial Library*). →䪼穴(p.484)

●膝[xī] 耳穴名。位于对耳轮上脚的中部。用于治疗膝部疾患,膝关节肿痛。

Knee (MA-AH 3) An auricular point. ⟨Location⟩middle portion of the superior autihelix crus. ⟨Indications⟩pain and dysfunction at the corresponding part of the body, swelling and pain of the knee joint.

●膝顶[xī dǐng] 经外穴别名。即鹤顶。见该条。

Xiding Another name for the extra point Heding(EX-LE 2). →鹤顶(p.162)

●膝关[xī guān] 经穴名。出《针灸甲乙经》。属足厥阴肝经。⟨定位⟩在小腿内侧,当胫骨内上髁的后下方,阴陵泉后1寸,腓肠肌内侧头的上部(图81)。⟨层次解剖⟩皮肤→皮下组织→腓肠肌。浅层布有隐神经的小腿内侧皮支,大隐静脉的属支。深层有腘动、静脉,胫神经等结构。⟨主治⟩膝膑肿痛、寒湿走注、历节痛风、下肢痿痹。直刺0.8～1.0寸;可灸。

Xiguan (LR 7) A meridian point, originally from *Zhenjiu Jia-Yi Jing* (*A-B Classic of Acupuncture and Moxibustion*), a point on the Liver Meridian of Foot-Jueyin. ⟨Location⟩on the medial side of the leg, posterior and inferi-

or to the medial epicondyle of the tibia, 1 cun posterior to Yinlingquan(ST 9), at the upper end of the medial head of the gastronemius muscle (Fig. 81). ⟨Regional anatomy⟩ skin→subcutaneous tissue→gastronemius muscle. In the superficial layer, there are the medial cutaneous branches of the leg from the saphenous nerve and the tributaries of the great saphenous vein. In the deep layer, there are the popliteal artery and vein and the tibial nerve. ⟨Indications⟩ swelling and pain of the knee joint, disturbance due to pathogenic cold and dampness, severe and migratory athralgia, flaccidity and numbness of legs. ⟨Method⟩ Puncture perpendicularly 0.8～1.0 cun. Moxibustion is applicable.

●膝目[xī mù] 经外穴别名。出《外台秘要》。即膝眼。见该条。

Ximu Another name for Xiyan(EX-LE 5), an extra point originally from *Waitai Miyao (Clandestine Essentials from the Imperial Library)*. →膝眼(p. 483)

●膝旁[xī páng] 经外穴名。见《太平圣惠方》。在腘窝横纹之两端，每肢二穴，左右计四穴。〈主治〉腰痛不能俯仰、脚酸不能久立。直刺0.5～1寸；可灸。

Xipang(EX-LE) An extra point, originally from *Taiping Shenghui Fang (Imperial Benevolent Prescriptions)*. ⟨Location⟩ at both ends of the popliteal transverse crease, two points on each leg, four points for two legs. ⟨Indications⟩ lumbar pain, inability to bend or lift the head, flaccidity of the foot without being able to stand for a long time. ⟨Method⟩ Puncture perpendicularly 0.5～1.0 cun. Moxibustion is applicable.

●膝上[xī shàng] 经外穴名。见《中国针灸学》。在膝关节上部，当髌骨上缘直股肌腱两侧凹陷中各一穴，左右计四穴。〈主治〉膝关节炎。直刺0.5寸；可灸。

Xishang(EX-LE) An extra point, originally from *Zhongguo Zhenjiuxue (Chinese Acupuncture and Moxibustion)*. ⟨Location⟩ on the upper part of the knee, a pair of points located in the two depressions, lateral to the tendon of m. rectus femoris, superior to the knee-cap, four points in two legs. ⟨Indication⟩ gonitis. ⟨Method⟩ Puncture perpendicularly 0.5 cun. Moxibustion is applicable.

●膝外[xī wài] 经外穴名。见《千金翼方》。在膝部，当膝横纹外侧端，股二头肌前缘处。灸治痈疡。

Xiwai(EX-LE) An extra point, originally from *Qianjin Yifang (Supplement to the Essential Prescriptions Worth a Thousand Gold)*. ⟨Location⟩ in the knee, at the lateral end of the popliteal transverse crease, on the anterior border of the tendon of m. biceps femoris. ⟨Methods⟩ moxibustion for sores.

●膝下[xī xià] 经外穴名。见《千金翼方》。在膝部，当髌骨尖下缘髌韧带处。灸治转筋胫骨痛。

Xixia(EX-LE) An extra point, originally from *Qianjin Yifang (Supplement to the Essential Prescriptions Worth a Thousand Gold)*. ⟨Location⟩ in the knee, on the inferior border of the patellar tip, at the patellar ligament. ⟨Methods⟩ moxibustion for spasm and pain in the tibia.

●膝眼[xī yǎn] 经外穴名。出《千金要方》。又名膝目、鬼眼、屈膝。〈定位〉屈膝，在髌韧带外侧凹隐处。在内侧的称内膝眼，在外侧的称外膝眼(图29)。〈层次解剖〉膝眼之内侧穴，称内膝眼，层次解剖参阅内膝眼穴。膝眼之外侧穴，即足阳明胃经的犊鼻穴，层次解剖参阅犊鼻穴。〈主治〉膝痛、腿脚重痛、脚气、下肢麻痹等。向膝中斜刺0.5～1寸，或向内、外膝眼互透。

Xiyan(EX-LE 5) An extra point, originally from *Qianjin Yaofang (Essential Prescriptions Worth a Thousand Gold)*, also called Ximu, Guiyan, Quxi. ⟨Location⟩ A pair of points in the two depressions lateral to the patellar ligament with the medial one called Neixiyan, and the lateral one Waixiyan(Fig. 29). ⟨Regional anatomy⟩ The medial point of Xiyan(EX-LE 5) is also called Neixiyan (EX-LE 4). For its layer anatomy, refer to Neixiyan (EX-LE 4). The lateral point of Xiyan(EX-LE 5) is exactly the Dubi(ST 35) of the Stomach Meridian of Foot-Yangming. For its layer anatomy, refer to Dubi (ST 35). ⟨Indications⟩ knee pain, pain and heaviness in the leg and foot, beriberi, leg numbness. ⟨Method⟩ Puncture obliquely towards the knee joint 0.5～1.0 cun, or penetrate from Neixiyan to Waixiyan and *vice versa*.

●膝阳关[xī yáng guān]　经穴名。出《针灸甲乙经》。原名阳关,现称膝阳关,属足少阳胆经。又名阳陵、寒府、关陵、关阳。〈定位〉在膝外侧,当阳陵泉上3寸,股骨外上髁上方的凹陷处(图8.1和8.3)。〈层次解剖〉皮肤→皮下组织→髂胫束后缘→腓肠肌外侧头前方。浅层布有股外侧皮神经。深层有膝上外侧动、静脉。〈主治〉膝膑肿痛、腘筋挛急、小腿麻木。直刺0.8～1寸;可灸。

Xiyangguan(GB 33)　A meridian point, originally from *Zhenjiu Jia-Yi Jing* (*A-B Classic of Acupuncture and Moxibustion*), originally called Yangguan, and now called Xiyangguan, a point of the Gallbladder Meridian of Foot-Shaoyang, also called Yangling, Hanfu, Guanling, Guanyang. 〈Location〉on the lateral side of the knee, 3 cun above Yanglingquan (GB 34), in the depression above the external epicondyle of the femur (Figs. 8. 1&8. 3). 〈Regional anatomy〉skin→subcutaneous tissue→posterior border of illiotibial tract→anterior side of lateral head of gastrocnemius muscle. In the superficial layer, there is the lateral cutaneous nerve of the thigh. In the deep layer, there are the lateral superior genicular artery and vein. 〈Indications〉swelling and pain of the knee and joint, spasm of the tendon of popliteal fossa, numbness of leg. 〈Method〉Puncture perpendicularly 0. 8～1. 0 cun. Moxibustion is applicable.

●鼷穴[xī xué]　经穴别名。即承泣。见该条。

Xixue　Another name for the meridian point Chengqi(ST 1). →承泣(p. 44)

●席弘[xí hóng]　人名。宋针灸家。弘或作宏,字弘远,号梓桑君,江西人。家世以针灸相传,针术高超,有许多传人。

Xi Hong　An acupuncture-moxibustion expert in the Song Dynasty, Hong(弘)can also be Hong(宏). He styled himself Hongyuan and assumed the name Zisang Jun, a native of Jiangxi Province. Coming from a long line of doctors of acupuncture and moxibustion, he was skillful in acupuncture and had many students.

●席弘赋[xí hóng fù]　针灸歌赋名。撰人不详,首见于《针灸大全》。其叙述席弘一派的针灸经验,主讲针灸配穴及补泻手法,区分左右捻针。为七言韵语。

Xi Hong Fu(**Ode to Xi Hong**)　A verse of acupuncture and moxibustion with an unknown writer, seen in *Zhenjiu Daquan* (*A Complete Work of Acupuncture and Moxibustion*), expounding the experiences of acupuncture and moxibustion of the school of Xi Hong. The verse mainly introduces point prescription and reinforcing and reducing methods of acupuncture, distinguishing the left rotation from right rotation of the needle. It's a verse with seven characters to each line.

●系络[xì luò]　络脉名。出《经络汇编》。指从十五络脉分出的细小络脉。

Tiny Collaterals　A category of collaterals, originally from *Jingluo Huibian*(*An Expository Manual of Meridians and Collaterals*), referring to the minute collaterals deriving from the Fifteen Main Collaterals.

●郄门[xì mén]　经穴名。出《针灸甲乙经》。属手厥阴心包经,为本经郄穴。〈定位〉在前臂掌侧,当曲泽与大陵的连线上,腕横纹上5寸(图66)。〈层次解剖〉皮肤→皮下组织→桡侧腕屈肌腱与掌长肌腱之间→指浅屈肌→指深屈肌→前臂骨间膜。浅层有前臂外侧皮神经,前臂内侧皮神经分支和前臂正中静脉。深层有正中神经。正中神经伴行动、静脉,骨间前动脉、神经等结构。〈主治〉心痛、心悸、胸痛、心烦、咳血、呕血、衄血、疔疮、癫疾。直刺0.5～1.0寸;可灸。

Ximen(PC 4)　A meridian point, originally from *Zhenjiu Jia-Yi Jing* (*A-B Classic of Acupuncture and Moxibustion*), the *Xi*(Cleft) point of the Pericardium Meridian of Hand-Jueyin. 〈Location〉on the palmar side of the forearm and on the line connecting Quze(PC 3) and Daling(PC 7), 5 cun above the crease of the wrist (Fig. 66). 〈Regional anatomy〉skin→subcutaneous tissue→between tendons of radial flexor muscle of wrist and long palmar muscle→superficial flexor muscle fingers→deep flexor muscle of fingets→interosseous membrane of forearm. In the superficial layer, there are the branches of the lateral and medial cutaneous nerves of the forearm and the median vein of the forearm. In the deep layer, there are the median nerve and the accompa-

表18　　　　　　　十六郄穴
Table 18　　　　　　16 Xi (Cleft) Points

阴经	YIN MERIDIAN	郄穴	XI(Cleft) Point
手太阴肺经	The Lung Meridian of Hand-Taiyin	孔最	Kongzui(LU 6)
手厥阴心包经	The Pericardium Meridian of Hand-Jueyin	郄门	Ximen(PC 4)
手少阴心经	The Heart Meridian of Hand-Shaoyin	阴郄	Yinxi(HT 6)
足太阴脾经	The Spleen Meridian of Foot-Taiyin	地机	Diji(SP 8)
足厥阴肝经	The Liver Meridian of Foot-Jueyin	中都	Zhongdu(LR 6)
足少阴肾经	The Kidney Meridian of Foot-Shaoyin	水泉	Shuiquan(KI 5)
阴维脉	The Yinwei Meridian	筑宾	Zhubin(KI 9)
阴跷脉	The Yinqiao Meridian	交信	Jiaoxin(KI 8)
阳经	YANG MERIDIAN	郄穴	Xi(Cleft) Point
手阳明大肠经	The Large Intestine Meridian of Hand-Yangming	温溜	Wenliu(LI 7)
手少阳三焦经	The Sanjiao Meridian of Hand-Shaoyang	会宗	Huizong(SJ 7)
手太阳小肠经	The Small Intestine Meridian of Hand-Taiyang	养老	Yanglao(SI 6)
足阳明胃经	The Stomach Meridian of Foot-Yangming	梁丘	Liangqiu(ST 34)
足少阳胆经	The Gallbladder Meridian of Foot-Shaoyang	外丘	Waiqiu(GB 36)
足太阳膀胱经	The Bladder Meridian of Foot-Taiyang	金门	Jinmen(BL 63)
阳维脉	Yangwei Meridian	阳交	Yangjiao(GB 35)
阳跷脉	Yangqiao Meridian	跗阳	Fuyang(BL 59)

nying artery and the anterior interosseous artery and nerve. 〈Indications〉cardiac pain, palpitations, pain in chest, vexation, haemophysis, hematemesis, epistaxis, furuncle, epilepsy. 〈Method〉Puncture perpendicularly 0.5～1.0 cun. Moxibustion is applicable.

●郄穴[xì xué]　经穴分类名。见《针灸甲乙经》。指各经经气所深聚的地方，多分布在四肢肘膝以下。十二经脉各有一郄穴，阴阳跷脉及阴阳维脉也各有一个郄穴，合而为十六郄穴。临床多用于治疗急性病症。见表18。

Xi(Cleft) Points　A category of meridian points, seen in *Zhenjiu Jia-Yi Jing*(*A-B Classic of Acupuncture and Moxibustion*), referring to the places where the meridian qi is deeply converged. Most of them are located below the elbow or knee. Each of the Twelve Regular Meridians and the Meridians of Yinqiao, Yangqiao, Yinwei and Yangwei has a Xi (Cleft) point, 16 in all. The Xi (Cleft) points are clinically used for treating acute diseases. See Table 18.

●郄阳[xì yáng]　经穴别名。出《素问·刺腰痛篇》。即委阳。见该条。

Xiyang　Another name for Weiyang (BL 39), a meridian point originally from *Suwen*: *Ci Yaotong Pain* (*Plain Questions*: *On Treatment of Lumbago with Acupuncture*). →委阳 (p.461)

●郄中[xì zhōng]　经穴别名。见《素问·刺腰痛篇》王冰注。即委中。见该条。

Xizhong　Another name for Weizhong (BL 40), a meridian point seen in Wang Bing's annotation on *Su Wen*: *Ci Yaotong Pian* (*Plain Questions On Treatment of Lumbago with Acupuncture*). →委中 (p.461)

●细辛灸[xì xīn jiǔ]　敷灸方法之一。取细辛适量，研为细末，加醋少许，调如糊膏状，敷于穴位上，外覆油纸，胶布固定。如敷涌泉或神阙穴治疗小儿口腔炎。

Xi Xin (Herba Asari) Vesiculation　A method of moxibustion for application. Grind the proper amount of *Xi Xin* (*Herba Asari*) into powder, and make it a paste with a small amount of vinegar, then apply the paste on the selected acupoint, cover it with oilpaper and fix it with adhesive plaster, e.g. apply the paste on Yongquan (KI 1) or Shenque (RN 8) for treating infantile stomatitis.

●侠白[xiá bái]　经穴名。出《针灸甲乙经》。属手太阴肺经，又名夹白。〈定位〉在臂内侧面，肱二头肌桡侧缘，腋前纹头下4寸，或肘横纹上5寸处（图52）。〈层次解剖〉皮肤→皮下组织→肱肌。浅层有头静脉，臂外侧皮神经分布。深层布有肱动、静脉的肌支和肌皮

神经的分支。〈主治〉咳嗽、气短、干呕、烦满、上臂内侧痛。直刺0.3～0.5寸；可灸。

Xiabai（LU 4） A meridian point, originally from *Zhenjiu Jia-Yi Jing*（*A-B Classic of Acupuncture and Moxibustion*）, a point on the Lung Meridian of Hand-Taiyin, also called Jiabai. 〈Location〉on the medial side of the upper arm, on the radial border of the biceps muscle of the arm, 4 cun below the anterior end of the axillary fold, or 5 cun above the cubital crease (Fig. 52). 〈Regional anatomy〉skin→subcutaneous tissue→brachial muscle. In the superficial layer, there are the cephalic vein and the lateral cutaneous nerve of the arm. In the deep layer, there are the muscular branches of the brachial artery and vein and the branches of the musculocutaneous nerve. 〈Indications〉cough, shortness of breath, retching, fullness and irritability, precardial pain, aching in the medial aspect of the upper arm. 〈Method〉Puncture perpendicularly 0.3～0.5 cun. Moxibustion is applicable.

●侠承浆[xiá chéng jiāng] 经外穴名。出《千金要方》。在下颌部，承浆穴外开一寸，当颏孔处。〈主治〉黄疸、面瘫、齿痛、唇疔疮以及齿龈溃烂、三叉神经痛等。直刺0.3～0.5寸。

Xiachengjiang（EX-HN） An extra point, originally from *Qianjin Yaofang*（*Essential Prescriptions Worth a Thousand Gold*）. 〈Location〉on the mandible, 1 cun lateral to Chengjiang (RN 24), at the mental foramen. 〈Indications〉jaundice, facial paralysis, toothache, furuncle on the lips, ulceration of the gums, prosopalgia, etc. 〈Method〉Puncture perpendicularly 0.3～0.5 cun.

●侠上星[xiá shàng xīng] 经外穴名。见《千金要方》。位于鼻直上入发际一寸，旁开三寸处。灸治鼻中瘜肉。

Xiashangxing（EX-HN） An extra point, seen in *Qianjin Yaofang*（*Essential Prescriptions Worth a Thousand Gold*）. 〈Location〉3 cun lateral to the place 1 cun posterior to the anterior hairline of the head. 〈Indication〉nasal polyp. 〈Method〉moxibustion.

●侠溪[xiá xī] 经穴名。出《灵枢·本输》。属足少阳胆经，为本经荥穴。〈定位〉在足背外侧，当第四、五趾间，趾蹼缘后赤白肉际处（图82）。〈层次解剖〉皮肤→皮下组织→第四趾的趾长、短伸肌腱与第五趾的趾长、短伸肌腱之间→第四与第五趾的近节趾骨底之间。布有足背中间皮神经的趾背神经和趾背动、静脉。〈主治〉头痛、眩晕、耳鸣、耳聋、目外眦赤痛、颊肿、胸胁痛、膝股痛、脐酸、足跗肿痛、疟疾。直刺或斜刺0.3～0.5寸；可灸。

Xiaxi（GB 43） A meridian point, originally from *Lingshu*: *Benshu*（*Miraculous Pivot*: *Meridian Points*）, the Ying (Spring) point of the Gallbladder Meridian of Foot-Shaoyang. 〈Location〉on the lateral side of the instep of the foot, between the 4th and 5th toes, at the junction of the red and white skin, proximal to the margin of the web (Fig. 82). 〈Regional anatomy〉skin→subcutaneous tissue→between tendons of 4th long and short extensor muscles of toe and tendons of 5th long and short extensor muscle of toe→between bases of 4th and 5th proximal phalangeal bones. There are the dorsal digital nerve of the intermediate dorsal cutaneous nerve of the foot and the dorsal digital artery and vein in this area. 〈Indications〉headache, dizziness, palpitations due to fright, tinnitus, deafness, redness and pain of the outer canthus, swelling of the cheek, aching in the chest and hypochondrium, pain in the knee and hip, aching of the shank, swelling and pain of the dorsum of foot, malaria. 〈Method〉Puncture perpendicularly or obliquely 0.3～0.5 cun. Moxibustion is applicable.

●侠玉泉[xiá yù quán] 经外穴别名。即子宫穴。见该条。

Xiayuquan Another name for the extra point *Zigong*（EX-CA 1）.→子宫（p. 624）

●下病上取[xià bìng shàng qǔ] 《内经》取穴法则之一。简称上取。指下部的病症取用上部穴。如足跟疼取大杼。

Selecton of Upper Points for Lower-Part Diseases One of the principles of selecting points in *Neijing*（*The Canon of Internal Medicine*）, known as upper selection, referring to treating diseases of the lower part of the body by puncturing acupoints in the upper part, e.g. treating painful heels by needling

Dazhu(BL 11).

●下部冰冷不孕[xià bù bīng lěng bù yùn] 胞寒不孕的别名。详见该条。

Sterility due to Ice-Cold Lower Abdomen Another name for sterility due to retention of cold in uterus. →胞寒不孕(p. 13)

●下唇疔[xià chún dīng] 颜面部疔疮的一种，生于下唇部位。切忌挤压。参见"疔疮"条。

Furuncle on the Lower Lip A kind of furuncle on the face, occurring on the lower lip. Be sure not to press it. →疔疮(p. 82)

●下都[xià dū] ①经穴别名，即中渚。见该条。②经外穴名。八邪之一。见《奇效良方》。位置与"中渚穴"同。

1. **Xiadu** Another name for the meridian point Zhongzhu(SJ 3). →中渚(p. 615)
2. **Xiadu**(EX-UE) An extra point, one of the Baxie (EX-UE 8) points, seen in *Qixiao Liangfang* (*Prescriptions of Wonderful Efficacy*). Its location is the same as that of Zhongzhu(SJ 3).

●下渎[xià dú] 经穴别名。出《医学入门》。即中渎。见该条。

Xiadu(渎) Another name for Zhongdu(GB 32), a meridian point originally from *Yixue Rumen* (*An Introduction to Medicine*) →中渎(p. 609)

●下耳根[xià ěr gēn] ①耳穴名。又名脊髓2。位于耳垂与面颊交界下缘。用于治疗头痛、腹痛、哮喘。②耳廓解剖名称。指耳垂与面部附着处。

1. **Lower Auricle Root**(MA) An auricular point, also known as Spinal Cord 2 (MA). 〈Location〉at the inferior edge of the junction of the earlobe and cheek. 〈Indications〉headache, abdominal pain, asthma.
2. **Lower Auricular Root** An anatomy term for the pinna, referring to the junction of the earlobe and face.

●下番[xià fān] 阴挺的别名。见该条。参见"子宫脱垂"条。

Appearing of the Uterus Another name for prolapse of uterus and vagina. →阴挺(p. 559)、子宫脱垂(p. 625)

●下关[xià guān] 经穴名。出《灵枢·本输》。属足阳明胃经，为足阳明、少阳之会。〈定位〉在面部耳前方，当颧弓与下颌切迹所形成的凹陷中(图24)。〈层次解剖〉皮肤→皮下组织→腮腺→咬肌与颞骨颧突之间→翼外肌。浅层布有耳颞神经的分支，面神经的颧支，面横动、静脉等结构。深层有上颌动、静脉，舌神经，下牙槽神经，脑膜中动脉和翼丛等。〈主治〉齿痛、面疼、耳聋、耳鸣、聤耳、牙关开合不利、口眼歪邪、眩晕。直刺0.3～0.5寸;可灸。闭口取穴。

Xiaguan(ST 7) A meridian point, originally from *Lingshu*: *Benshu* (*Miraculous Pivot*: *Meridian Points*), a point on the Stomach Meridian of Foot-Yangming, the crossing point of Foot-Yangming and Foot-Shaoyang Meridians. 〈Location〉on the face, anterior to the ear, in the depression between the zygomatic arch and mandibular notch (Fig. 24). 〈Regional anatomy〉skin→subcutaneous tissue parotid gland→between masseter muscle and zygomatic process of temporal bone→lateral pterygoid muscle. In the superficial layer, there are the branches of the auriculotemporal nerve, the zygomatic branches of the facial nerve and the transverse facial artery and vein. In the deep layer, there are the maxillary artery and vein, the lingual nerve, the inferior alveolar nerve, the middle meningeal artery and the pterygoid plexus. 〈Indications〉toothache, facial pain, deafness, tinnitus, otorrhea, lockjaw and loosening of temporomandibular joint, deviation of the mouth and eye, dizziness. 〈Method〉Puncture perpendicularly 0.3～0.5 cun. Moxibustion is applicable. Close the mouth while the point is being selected.

●下管[xià guǎn] 经穴别名。出《脉经》即下脘。见该条。

Xiaguan Another name for Xiawan (RN 10), a meridian point originally from *Maijing* (*The Classic of Sphymology*). →下脘(p. 490)

●下合穴[xià hé xué] 经穴分类名。又称六腑下合穴。见《灵枢·邪气脏腑病形》。其中除三焦的下合穴在膀胱经上，大肠、小肠的下合穴在胃经上，其它经的下合穴均在本经上。详见表19。

Lower Confluent Points A category of meridian points also know as the lower confluent points of the six fu organs, seen in *Lingshu*: *Xieqi Zang Fu Bingxing* (*Miraculous*

Table 19 The Lower Confluent Points

手足三阳 Three Yang Meridians of Hand and Foot		六腑 Six Fu Organs	下合穴 Lower Confluent Points
手三阳 Three Yang of the Hand	阳明 Yangming 太阳 Taiyang 少阳 Shaoyang	大肠 Large Intestine 小肠 Small Intestine 三焦 Sanjiao	上巨虚 Shangjuxu(ST 37) 下巨虚 Xiajuxu(ST 39) 委阳 Weiyang(BL 39)
足三阳 Three Yang of the Foot	太阳 Taiyang 阳明 Yangming 少阳 Shaoyang	膀胱 Bladder 胃 Stomach 胆 Gallbladder	委中 Weizhong(BL40) 足三里 Zusanli(ST 36) 阳陵泉 Yanglingquan(GB 34)

Pivot: *Pathogenic Evils, Zang-Fu Organs and Manifestations*). Among them, except the lower confluent point of Sanjiao on the Bladder Meridian, the lower confluent points of the large intestine and small intestine on the Stomach Meridian, the lower confluent points of the other meridians are all on their own meridians. See Table 19.

●下横[xià héng] 经穴别名。见《神灸经纶》。即横骨。见该条。

Xiaheng Another name for Henggu (KI 11), a meridian point seen in *Shenjiu Jinglun (Principles of Magic Moxibustion)*. →横骨 (p. 163)

●下肓[xià huāng] ①经穴别名。出《针灸甲乙经》。即气海。见该条。②即气街。见该条。

Xiahuang ①Another name for Qihai (RN 6), a meridian point originally from *Zhenjiu Jia-Yi Jing (A-B Classic of Acupuncture and Moxibustion)*. →气海 (p. 305) ②→气街 (p. 308)

●下极[xià jí] 〈1〉部位名。①指会阴部。②指鼻根部。见《灵枢·五色》。③指肛门。〈2〉经穴别名。①会阴穴别名。见该条。②横骨别名。见该条。

1. The Lower End A part of the body, referring to ①the perineum; ②the radix nasi, seen in *Lingshu: Wu Se (Miraculous Pivot: Five Colors)*; ③anus.

2. Xiaji Another name for①Huiyin (RN 1). →会阴 (p. 178); ②Henggu (KI 11). →横骨 (p. 163)

●下极俞[xià jí shū] 经外穴名。见《备急千金要方》。〈定位〉在腰部,当后正中线上,第三腰椎棘突下(图61)。〈层次解剖〉皮肤→皮下组织→棘上韧带→棘间韧带。浅层有第四腰神经后支的内侧支和伴行的动、静脉。深层有棘突间的椎外(后)静脉丛,第四腰神经的后支的分支和第四腰动、静脉背侧支的分支和属支。〈主治〉腹痛、腰痛、泄泻、膀胱炎、肠炎等。直刺0.5~1寸;可灸。

Xiajishu (EX-B 5) An extra point, seen in *Beiji Qianjin Yaofang (Essential Prescriptions Worth a Thousand Gold for Emergencies)*. 〈Location〉on the low back and on the posterior midline, below the spinous process of the 3rd lumbar vertebra (Fig. 61). 〈Regional anatomy〉 skin → subcutaneous tissue → supraspinal ligament→interspinal ligament. In the superficial layer, there are the medial branches of the posterior branch of the fourth lumbar nerve and the accompanying artery and vein. In the deep layer, there are the external (posterior) vertebral venous plexus of the spinous process, the posterior branch of the 4th lumbar nerve and the branch of the dorsal branch of the 4th lumbar artery and vein. 〈Indications〉 abdominal pain, lumbago, diarrhea, cystitis and enteritis, etc. 〈Method〉 Puncture perpendicularly 0.5~1.0 cun. Moxibusion is applicable.

●下极之俞[xià jí zhī shū] ①经穴别名。出《难经·二十八难》。即长强。见该条。②经穴别名。出《难经·二十八难》。即会阴。见该条。③经外穴别名。即下极俞。见该条。

Xiajizhishu Another name for①Changqiang (UD 1), a meridian point originally from *Nanjing: Ershiba Nan (The Classic of Questions: Question 28)*. →长强 (p. 39) ② Huiyin (RN 1), a meridian point originally from *Nanjing: Ershiba Nan (The Classic of Questions: Question 28)*. →会阴 (p. 178) ③the extra point Xiajishu (EX-B 5). →下极俞 (p. 488)

●下纪[xià jì] 经穴别名。出《素问·气穴论》。即关元。见该条。

Xiaji Another name for Guanyuan(RN 4), a meridian point originally from *Suwen: Qixue Lun (Plain Questions: On Loci of Qi)*. →关元 (p. 148)

●下巨虚[xià jù xū] 经穴名。见《备急千金要方》。《灵枢·本输》名巨虚下廉。属足阳明胃经,为小肠的下合穴。〈定位〉在小腿前外侧,当犊鼻下9寸,距胫骨前缘一横指(中指)(图60.1)。〈层次解剖〉皮肤→皮下组织→胫骨前肌→小腿骨间膜→胫骨后肌。浅层布有腓肠外侧皮神经。深层有胫前动、静脉和腓深神经。〈主治〉小腹痛、腰脊痛引睾丸、乳痈、下肢痿痹、泄泻、大便脓血。直刺0.5～1.0寸;可灸。

Xiajuxu (ST 39) A meridian point, seen in *Beiji Qianjin Yaofang (Essential Prescriptions for Emergencies Worth a Thousand Gold)*, known as Juxuxialian in *Lingshu: Benshu (Miraclous Pivot: Meridian Points)*, a point on the Stomach Meridian of Foot-Yangming, the lower confluent point of the Small Intestine. 〈Location〉on the anteriolateral side of the leg, 9 cun below Dubi (ST 35), one finger breadth(middle finger) from the anterior crest of the tibia (Fig. 60.1). 〈Regional anatomy〉 skin → subcutaneous tissue → anterior tibial muscle→interosseous membrane of leg→posterior tibial muscle. In the superficial layer, there is the lateral cutaneous nerve of the calf. In the deep layer, there are the anterior tibial artery and vein and the deep peroneal nerve. 〈Indications〉lower abdominal pain, pain in the back and spine radiating to the testicles, breast abscess, impairment pain and paralysis of the lower extremities, diarrhea, bloody and mucous stool. 〈Method〉Puncture perpendicularly 0.5～1.0 cun. Moxibustion is applicable.

●下昆仑[xià kūn lún] ①经穴别名。出《针灸大全》。即昆仑。见该条。②经外穴名。见《太平圣惠方》。又名内昆仑。位于跟腱前缘平外踝尖下一寸处。〈主治〉冷痹、腰痛、偏头风、半身不遂、脚重痛不得履地等。直刺0.3～0.5寸;可灸。

1. **Xiakunlun** Another name for Kunlun(BL 60), a meridian point originally from *Zhenjiu Daquan (A Complete Work of Acupuncture and Moxibustion)*. →昆仑(p. 236)

2. **Xiakunlun** (EX-LE) An extra point, seen in *Taiping Shenghui Fang (Imperial Benevolent Prescriptions)*, also called Neikunlun. 〈Location〉anterior to the achilles tendon, 1 cun inferior to the tip of the exterior malleolus. 〈Indications〉arthralgia due to cold, lumbago, migraine, hemiplegia and motor impairment of the foot, etc. 〈Method〉Puncture perpendicularly 0.3～0.5 cun. Moxibustion is applicable.

●下利[xià lì] 病证名。古代医书对痢疾的别称。出《伤寒杂病论》。参见"痢疾"条。

Frequent Bowel Motions A disease, another name for dysentery in ancient medicinal books, originally from *Shanghan Zabing Lun (Treatise on Cold-Induceed and Miscellaneous Diseases)*. →痢疾(p. 244)

●下廉[xià lián] ①经穴名。出《针灸甲乙经》。属手阳明大肠经,又名手下廉。〈定位〉在前臂背面桡侧,当阳溪与曲池连线上,肘横纹下4寸(图48和图6.1)。〈层次解剖〉皮肤→皮下组织→肱桡肌→桡侧腕短伸肌→旋后肌。浅层布有前臂外侧皮神经和前臂后皮神经等。深层有桡神经深支的分支。〈主治〉头风、眩晕、目痛、肘臂痛、腹痛、食物不化、乳痈。直刺0.5～0.8寸;可灸。②经穴别名。即下巨虚。见该条。

1. **Xialian** (LI 8) A meridian point, originally from *Zhenjiu Jia-Yi Jing (A-B Classic of Acupuncture and Moxibuṣtion)*, a point on the Large Intestine Meridian of Hand-Yangming, also named Shouxialian. 〈Location〉on the radial side of the dorsal surface of the forearm, on the line connecting Yangxi (LI 5) and Quchi (LI 11), 4 cun below the cubital crease (Figs. 48 & 6.1). 〈Regional anatomy〉skin → subcutaneous tissue → brachioradial muscle → short radial excentsor muscle of wrist → supinator muscle. 〈Indications〉 headache, dizziness, pain of the eye, pain in the elbow and arm, abdominal pain, indigestion, breast abscess. 〈Method〉Puncture perpendicularly 0.5～0.8 cun. Moxibustion is applicable.

2. **Xialian** Another name for the meridian point Xiajuxu(ST 39). →下巨虚(p. 489)

●下髎[xià liáo] 经穴名。出《针灸甲乙经》。属足太阳膀胱经。〈定位〉在骶部,当中髎下内方,适对第四骶后孔处(图7)。〈层次解剖〉皮肤→皮下组织→臀

大肌→竖脊肌。浅层布有臀中皮神经。深层有臀上、下动、静脉的分支或属支,臀下神经、第四骶神经和骶外侧动、静脉的后支。〈主治〉小腹痛、肠鸣、泄泻、便秘、小便不利、腰痛。直刺0.8~1.0寸;可灸。

Xialiao(BL 34) A meridian point, originally from *Zhenjiu Jia-Yi Jing* (*A-B Classic of Acupuncture and Moxibustion*), a point on the Bladder Meridian of Foot-Taiyang. 〈Location〉on the sacrum, medial and inferior to Zhongliao(BL 33), just at the 4th posterior sacral foramen (Fig. 7). 〈Regional anatomy〉skin → subcutaneous tissue → greatest gluteal muscle→erector spinal muscle. In the superficial layer, there is the middle clunial nerve. In the deep layer, there are the branches or tributaries of the superior and inferior gluteal arteries and veins, the inferior gluteal nerve of the 4th sacral nerve and the posterior branches of the lateral sacral artery and vein. 〈Indications〉lower abdominal pain, borborygmus, diarrhea, constipation dysuria, and lumbago. 〈Method〉Puncture perpendicularly 0.8~1 cun. Moxibustion is applicable.

●下林[xià lín] 经穴别名。出《圣济总录》。即下巨虚。"林"系"廉"字之误。见该条。

Xialin Another name for Xiajuxu(ST 39), a meridian point originally from *Shengji Zonglu* (*Imperial Medical Encyclopaedia*). Here, "林" was mistaken for "廉". →下巨虚(p.489)

●下陵[xià líng] 经穴别名。出《灵枢·本输》。即足三里。见该条。

Xialing Another name for Zusanli(ST 36), a meridian point originally from *Lingshu: Benshu* (*Miraculous Pivot: Meridian Points*). →足三里(p.632)

●下陵三里[xià líng sān lǐ] 经穴别名。出《灵枢·九针十二原》。即足三里。见该条。

Xialingsanli Another name for Zusanli(ST 36), a meridian point originally from *Lingshu: Jiu Zhen Shier Yuan* (*Miraculous Pivot: Nine Needles and Twelve Yuan(Primary) Points*). →足三里(p.632)

●下气海[xià qì hǎi] 经穴别名。见《类经》卷八,张介宾注。即气海。见该条。

Xiaqihai Another name for Qihai(RN 6), a meridian point seen in Zhang Jiebin's annotation to Vol. 8 of *Leijing* (*Classified Canon of Internal Medicine of the Yellow Emperor*). →气海(p.305)

●下取[xià qǔ] 上病下取的简称。见该条。

Selection of Lower Points The short name for selection of lower points for upper diseases. →上病下取(p.351)

●下三里[xià sān lǐ] 经穴别名。见《针灸集成》。即足三里。见该条。

Xiasanli Another name for Zusanli(ST 36), a meridian point seen in *Zhenjiu Jicheng* (*A Collection of Acupuncture and Moxibustion*). →足三里(p.632)

●下手八法[xià shǒu bā fǎ] 针刺手法。出《针灸大成》。为八法之别称。即是杨氏在"十二字分次第手法"的基础上,精简补充提出的八种手法:揣、爪、搓、弹、摇、扪、循、捻。

Eight Methods for Needling Manipulation A general term for acupuncture manipulations, originally from *Zhenjiu Dacheng* (*A Great Compendium of Acupuncture and Moxibustion*), another name for the Eight Methods—those put forward by Dr. Yang on the basis of the "twelve words for the sequence of acupuncture manipulation" after simplfying and supplementing them—fathoming, clawing, twisting, flicking, shaking, pressing, massaging along meridians, and twirling.

●下四缝[xià sì fèng] 指根的别名。见该条。

Xiasifeng Another name for Zhigen. →指根(p.604)

●下脘[xià wǎn] 经穴名。出《灵枢·四时气》。属任脉,为足太阴、任脉之会。又名下管、幽门。〈定位〉在上腹部,前下中线上,当脐中上2寸(图40和图43.2)。〈层次解剖〉皮肤→皮下组织→腹白线→腹横筋膜→腹膜外脂肪→壁腹膜。浅层主要布有第九胸神经前支的前皮支和腹壁浅静脉的属支。深层有第九胸神经前支的分支。〈主治〉脘痛、腹胀、呕吐、呃逆、食谷不化、肠鸣、泄泻、痞块、虚肿。直刺0.5~1.0寸;可灸。

Xiawan(RN 10) A meridian point, originally from *Lingshu: Si Shi Qi* (*Miraculous Pivot: Qi of Four Seasons*), a point on the Ren Meridians, the crossing point of the Foot-Taiyin and Ren Meridians, also called

Xiaguan and Youmen. ⟨Location⟩on the upper abdomen and on the anterior midline, 2 cun above the centre of the umbilicus (Figs. 40 &43.2). ⟨Regional anatomy⟩ skin→subcutaneous tissue→linea alba→transverse fascia→extraperitoneal fat tissue → parietal peritoneum. In the superficial layer, there are the anterior cutaneous of the anterior branch of the 9th thoracic nerve and the tributaries of the superficial epigastric vein. In the deep layer, there are the branches of the anterior branch of the 9th thoracic nerve. ⟨Indications⟩upper abdominal pain, abdominal distension, vomiting, hiccup, indigestion, borborygmus, diarrhea, abdominal mass, edema due to asthenia. ⟨Method⟩ Puncture perpendicularly 0.5～1.0 cun. Moxibustion is applicable.

●下消[xià xiāo] 消渴证型之一。出《丹溪心法·消渴》。多由肾水亏竭，气化失常所致。证见小便频数，量多而略稠，口干舌燥，渴而多饮，头晕，目糊，颧红，虚烦，善饥而食不甚多，腰膝酸软，舌质红，脉细数。久病阴虚及阳，可兼见面色禾黑，畏寒肢冷，尿量特多，男子阳萎，女子经闭，舌质淡，苔白，脉沉细无力。治宜补肾益阴。针肾俞、肝俞、太溪、太冲、复溜。

Diabetes Involving the Lower Jiao A type of diabetes, originally from *Danxi Xinfa*: *Xiaoke*(*Danxi' s Experience*: *Diabetes*), mostly due to deficiency and consumption of kidney-yin leading to disturbance in qi transformation. ⟨Manifestations⟩ frequent urination in heavy quantity and turbid quality, dry mouth and tongue, desire for profuse drinking, dizziness, blurred vision, flushed zygomatic region, restlessness due to deficiency, easy hunger but not good appetite, soreness and weakness of the lumbus and knees, red tongue, thready and rapid pules. If the chronic yin deficiency affects yang, there will be dark complexion, aversion to cold and cold extremities, profuse urinary discharge, impotence in men, amenorrhea in women, pale tongue with white coating, deep and thready and weak pulse. ⟨Treatment principle⟩Nourish the kidney to replenish yin. ⟨Point selection⟩ Shenshu (BL 23), Ganshu (BL 18), Taixi (KI 3), Taichong (LR 3) and Fuliu (KI 7).

●下血[xià xuè]即便血。见该条。

Loosening the Bowels with Blood →便血(p. 24)

●下腰[xià yāo] 经外穴名。见《千金要方》。在骶部，当第二骶骨嵴与第三骶骨嵴之间处。灸治慢性肠炎、久痢不愈、难产等。

Xiayao(EX-B) An extra point, seen in *Qianjin Yaofang* (*Essential Prescriptions Worth a Thousand Gold*). ⟨Location⟩ on the sacral region, in the depression between the 2nd and 3rd sacral crest. ⟨Indications⟩ chronic enteritis, chronic dysentery, and difficult labor, etc. ⟨Method⟩ moxibustion.

●下针十四法[xià zhēn shí sì fǎ] 针刺手法。十四法的别称。见该条。

Fourteen Methods for Needling Manipulation A term in acupuncture manipulation, another name for the Fourteen Methods. →十四法(p. 380)

●夏英[xià yīng] 人名。明代针灸家。字时彦，杭州人。撰《灵枢经脉翼》，刊于1497年。其内容是以《十四经发挥》注释《灵枢·经脉》原文。

Xia Ying An acupuncture-moxibustion expert in the Ming Dynasty, who styled himself Shiyan, a native of Hangzhou, compiler of " Lingshu" Jingmai Yi (*Supplement to the Meridians of "Miraculous Pivot"*) which was published in 1497. In the book, annotations were made on the original text of *Lingshu*: *Jingmai* (*Miraculous Piovt*: *Meridians*) according to *Shisi Jing Fahui*(*An Elaboration of the Fourteen Meridians*).

●痫证[xián zhèng] 病名。出《素问·大奇论》等篇。是一种发作性神志异常的疾病，亦称"癫痫"，俗称羊痫风。多因风痰挟火过盛，或气血素虚，暴受惊吓所致。或与遗传有关。本病分虚、实两型。详见"痫证虚证"、"痫证实证"条。

Epilepsy Disease A disease, originally from *Suwen*: *Daqi Lun* (*Plain Questions*: *On Extremely Strange Diseases*). A paroxysmal mental disorder, also named epilepsy and commonly called convulsion with screaming like a sheep, mostly due to wind-phlegm accompanied by excessive fire or a constitutional deficiency of qi and blood, and sudden attack by

fear, or due to factors relating to heredity. The disease is divided into excess and deficiency types→. 痫证虚证(p.492)、痫证实证(p.492)

● 痫证实证[xián zhèng shí zhèng] 痫证证型之一。多由心肝气郁或脾虚生湿,以致气郁化火,炼液为痰,气火挟痰横窜经络,上蒙清窍,迫使阴阳发生一时性的逆乱所致。证见发病时猝然昏倒,不省人事,牙关紧闭,角弓反张,口吐白沫,手足抽搐,发作后仅有头晕,体乏,休息后即如常人。治宜熄风化痰,降火宁神。取身柱、本神、鸠尾、丰隆、太冲。发作时加水沟、颊车、神门。夜间发作加照海,白昼发作加申脉。

Excess Type of Epilepsy A type of epilepsy, mostly due to qi-stagnation of the liver and heart or dampness resulting from the deficiency of the spleen; stagnation of qi turns into pathogenic fire which in a long run evaporates the dampness to form phlegm, then the fire carries the phlegm into the channels and preserves there and rushes up to disturb the mind, resulting in an epilepsy attack, a temporary lack of coordination between the yin and yang. ⟨Manifestations⟩sudden fall with loss of consciousness, lockjaw, opisthotonos mouth foaming, convulsion of the limbs after the attack, mere dizziness, inertia, and the patient being normal after a rest. ⟨Treatment principle⟩ Calm the pathogenic wind and reduce phlegm; send down pathogenic fire and relieve mental stress. ⟨Point selection⟩Shengzhu(DU 12), Benshen(GB 13), Jiuwei(RN 15), Fenglong(ST 40), Taichong(LR 3), Shuigou(Du 26), Jiache (ST 6) and Shenmen (HT 7) Should be added for paroxysm; Zhaohai(KI 6) for the attack at night, and Shenmai(BL 62) for the attack in the daytime.

● 痫证虚证[xián zhèng xū zhèng] 痫证证型之一,多因痫证反复发作,以致心血不足,肾气亏虚,脏腑失调,气机逆乱所致。证见癫痫后期,发作次数频繁,抽搐程度减弱,额出冷汗,呼吸困难有鼾声,舌紫,脉细而弦。醒后精神萎靡、眩晕、心悸、食少、腰膝酸软,表情痴呆,智力减退。治宜补益心脾,化痰镇痉,针通里、丰隆、肾俞、中脘、足三里、阳陵泉、三阴交、筋缩。发作时取水沟、合谷、太冲。昏迷不醒者,酌针涌泉,灸气海。

Deficiency Type of Epilepsy A type of epilepsy, mostly due to repeated relapses of epilepsy which lead to deficiency of the heart-blood and kidney-qi, and the imbalance of zang-fu organs and pathogenic changes of qi. ⟨Manifestations⟩seen in the later period of epilepsy: frequent relapses, mild convulsion, sweating with cold feeling of the forehead, dyspneic respiration with snore, purplish tongue, thready and wiry pulse. After the seizure, ease is menifested as listlessness, dizziness, palpitations, poor appetite, lassitude and soreness of the wrist and knee, apathy, mantal deficiency. ⟨Treatment principle⟩ Nourish the heart and spleen, reduce phlegm and relieve spasm. ⟨Point selection⟩Tongli(HT 5), Fenglong(ST 40), Shenshu(BL 23), Zhongwan(RN 12), Zusanli(ST 36), Yanglingquan(GB 34), Sanyinjiao(SP 6) and Jinsuo(DU 8). Shuigou(DU 26), Hegu(LI 4), Taichong(LR 3) should be selected during the seizure. For coma Yongquan (KI 1) should be properly punctured, moxibustion should be done on Qihai(DN 6).

● 陷谷[xiàn gǔ] 经穴名。出《灵枢·本输》。属足阳明胃经,为本经输穴。又名陷骨。⟨定位⟩在足背、当第二、三跖骨结合部前方凹陷处(图60.3)。⟨层次解剖⟩皮肤→皮下组织→趾长伸肌腱→趾短伸肌腱的内侧→第二骨间背侧肌→收肌斜头。浅层布有足背内侧皮神经和足背静脉网。深层有第二跖背动、静脉等结构。⟨主治⟩面目浮肿、水肿、肠鸣、腹痛、足背肿痛,直刺0.3～0.5寸;可灸。

Xiangu(ST 43) A meridian point, originally from *Lingshu: Benshu (Miraculous Pivot: Meridian Points)*, the Shu(Stream) point of the Stomach Meridian of Foot-Yangming, also called Xiangu(陷骨). ⟨Location⟩on the instep of the foot, in the depression distal to the commissure of the 2nd and 3rd metatarsal bones (Fig. 60.3). ⟨Regional anatomy⟩skin→subcutaneous tissue → tendon of long extensor muscle of toes→medial side of tendon of short extensor muscle of toes → 2nd dorsal interosseous muscle→oblique head of adductor of great toe. In the superficial layer, there are the medial dorsal cutaneous nerve and the dorsal venous network of the foot. In the deep layer, there are the 2nd dorsal metatarsal

artery and vein. 〈Indications〉edema of the face and eye, edema, borborygmus, abdominal pain, swelling and pain of the dorsum pedis. 〈Method〉Puncture 0.3～0.5 cun perpendicularly. Moxibustion is applicable.

●陷骨[xiàn gǔ] 经穴别名。见《普济方》。即陷谷。见该条。

Xiangu（陷骨） Another name for Xiangu(ST 43),（陷谷）, a meridian point, seen in *Puji Fang*(*Prescriptions for Universal Relief*).→陷谷(p.492)

●陷下则灸之[xiàn xià zé jiǔ zhī] 针灸治则之一。出《灵枢·经脉》。指虚寒病证，脉陷下不起者，是气虚血滞，宜用灸法以温经散寒。

Treating Subsidence with Moxibustion One of the treatment principles of acupuncture and moxibustion, originally from *Lingshu*: *Jingmai*(*Miraculous Pivot*: *Meridians*), referring to asthenia-cold diseases with subsident pulse, which are caused by deficiency of qi and stagnation of blood, and should be treated with moxibustion to warm the meridians and dispel pathogenic cold.

●香附饼[xiāng fù bǐng] 灸用药饼的一种。见《外科证治全书》。将生香附研为细末，用生姜汁调和为饼，敷患处，用艾灸治。临床上多用于治疗瘰疬痰毒、皮肤红肿。

Xiang Fu（Rhizoma Cyperi）Cake One of the medicinal cakes for moxibustion, seen in *Waike Zhengzhi Quanshu*(*Complete Book of Diagnosis and Treatment of External Diseases*). Grind the raw *Xiang Fu*(*Rhizoma cyperi*) into a powder, and make a cake by mixing it with ginger juice. Apply the cake on the affected region, then, apply moxibustion on it for treatment. It is generally used for treating scrofula, subcutaneous nodule due to phlegm, and swelling and redness of skin.

●香硫饼[xiāng liú bǐng] 灸用药饼的一种。见《种福堂公选良方》卷二。麝香6克，辰砂12克，硼砂6克，细辛12克，具为细末；角刺6克，川乌尖6克，二味俱用黄酒250克煮干为末；硫磺192克。先用硫磺、角刺、川乌入铜构内，火上化开，再入前四味末搅匀，候冷打碎成黄豆大。用时用干面捏成钱大，先放在患处，置药一块在上，连灸三壮，主治寒湿气。

Xiang Liu（Moschussulfur）Cake A kind of medicinal cakes for moxibustion, seen in Vol. 2 of *Zhongfutang Gongxuan Liangfang*(*Zhong Fu Tang Effective Prescriptions*). 〈Constitution〉*She Xiang*(*Moschus*)(6g), *Chen Sha*(*Cinnabar*)(12g), *Peng Sha*(*Borax*)(6g), *Xi Xin*(*Herba Asari*)(12g). Ground into powder separately; *Jiao Ci*(*Spina Gleditsiae*)(6g), *Chuan Wu Jian*(*Redix Aconitic*)(6g) boiled in yellow rice wine(250g) and then ground into powder; *Liu Huang*(*Sulfur*)(192g). First, put *Liu Huang*(*Sulfur*), *Jiao ci*(*Spina Gleditsiae*) and *Chuan Wu*(*Radix Aconitis*)into a copper mug, melt them on the fire, then, add the above-mentioned powder of the four herbs, and stir evenly. After it cools, break it into pieces as big as soybeans. When doing the treatment, make a cake of flour as big as a coin. Put it on the affected region and then put a piece of the medicine on top of it to achieve moxibustion. Generally, three medicinal cones are burnt one after another for treating diseases due to pathogenic cold and dampness.

●香砂灸[xiāng shā jiǔ] 即硫朱灸。见该条。

Xiang Sha（Moschus Chinnabaris）Moxibustion →硫朱灸(p.252)

●项强穴[xiàng qiáng xué] ①经外穴名。见《经外奇穴汇编》。在手背，当第二、三掌骨小头向后方之凹陷处。主治项强。直刺0.5～0.8寸。②经外穴别名。即落枕。见该条。③经外穴别名。即外劳宫。见该条。

1. **Xiangqiangxue**（EX-UE） An extra point, originally from *Jingwai Qixue Huibian*(*An Expository Manual of Extra Acupoints*).〈Location〉on the dorsal aspect of the hand, in the depression posterior to the 2nd and 3rd metacarpophalangeal articulations.〈Indication〉stiffness of the nape.〈Method〉Puncture 0.5～0.8 cun perpendicularly.

2. **Xiangqiangxue** Another name for the extra point Laozhen(EX-UE).→落枕(p.239)

3. **Xiangqiangxue** Another name for the extra point Wailaogong(EX-UE 8).→外劳宫(p.455)

●消瘅[xiāo dàn] 病证名。出《素问·评热病论》等篇。①即消渴。见该条。②指肝、心、肾三经阴虚内热，

而外消肌肉的病证。

Depletive Heat Diseases originally from *Suwen: Ping Rebing Lun (Plain Questions: Detailed Discussion on Febrile Diseases)*, etc., referring to ①diabetes. →消渴(p. 494) ②diseases marked by emaciation, due to the endogenous pathogenic heat resulting from yin deficiency of the liver, heart and kidney.

●消渴[xiāo kě]　病名。出《素问·奇病论》。又名鬲痟、消瘅。宋元以后又有称三消者，泛指以多饮、多食、多尿症状为特点的病证。多由①思虑过度，情绪不安；②过食膏粱厚味，饮酒过度；③恣情纵欲，以致心火偏亢，胃中积热，肾精亏耗，封藏失职所致。临床分为上、中、下三消。详见各条。

Diabetes A disease, originally from *Suwen: Qibing Lun (Plain Questiona: On Peculiar Diseases)*, also known as consumptive heat, or depletive heat. After the Song and Yuan Dynasties, it was also called three consumptions, referring to the disease characterized by polydipsia, polyphagia and polyuria. Mostly due to ① emotional stress and irritability, ② excessive rich fatty diet, overdrinking and ③sexual indulgence, which leads to hyperactive fire retention of heat in the stomach and deficiency of kidney resulting in dysfunction of the kidney in controlling and storing. The disease is clinically divided into three types—upper consumption, middle consumption and lower consumption. →上消(p. 354)、中消(p. 615)、下消(p. 491)

●消疬[xiāo lì]　经外穴名。见《针灸集成》。位于背部，以平结喉之颈项周长，自大椎穴直下尽处左右旁开0.5寸处。灸治瘰疬。

Xiaoli（EX-B） An extra point, seen in *Zhenjiu Jicheng (A Collection of Acupuncture and Moxibustion)*. Take the perimeter of the neck at the position level to the Adam's Apple, measure from Dazhui (DU 14) straight down to the point at the further end of the length and 0.5 cun lateral to it. 〈Indication〉scrofula. 〈Method〉moxibustion.

●消泺[xiāo luò]　经穴名。出《针灸甲乙经》。属手少阳三焦经。〈定位〉在臂外侧，当清冷渊与臑会连线的中点处(图48和44.2)。〈层次解剖〉皮肤→皮下组织→肱三头肌长头→肱三头肌内侧头。浅层由臂后皮神经分布。深层布有副动、静脉和桡神经的肌支。〈主治〉头痛、颈项强痛、臂痛、齿痛、癫疾。直刺0.8～1.2寸；可灸。

Xiaoluo（SJ 12） A meridian point, originally from *Zhenjiu Jia-Yi Jing (A-B Classic of Acupuncture and Moxibustion)*, a point on the Sanjiao Meridian of Hand-Shaoyang. 〈Location〉on the lateral side of the upper arm, at the midpoint of the line connecting Qinglengyuan (SJ 11) and Naohui (SJ 13) (Figs. 48 &44.2). 〈Regional anatomy〉skin → subcutaneous tissue→long head of brachial triceps muscle→medial head of brachial triceps muscle. In the superficial layer, there is the posterior brachial cutaneous nerve. In the deep layer, there are the median collateral artery and vein and the muscular branches of the radial nerve. 〈Indications〉headache, stiffness of the neck and nape, aching of the arm, toothache, depressive psychosis. 〈Method〉Puncture perpendicularly 0.8～1.2 cun. Moxibustion is applicable.

●消癖神火针[xiāo pǐ shén huǒ zhēn]　见《种福堂公选良方》。艾卷灸的一种。用蜈蚣一条、木鳖、五灵脂、雄黄、乳香、没药、阿魏、三棱、蓬术、甘草、皮硝各一钱，闹羊花、硫磺、山甲、牙皂各二钱，麝香三钱，甘遂五分，艾绒二两，制作如雷火针，以灸治痞块。

Mass-Disintegrating Miraculous-Fire Needle
Originally from *Zhong Fu Tang Gongxuan Liangfang (Zhong Fu Tang Effective Prescriptions)*. A type of moxa roll for moxibustion including *Wu Gong (Scalopexdra)* (1 strip), *Mu Bie (Semen Momerdicae)* (3g), *Wu Ling Zhi (Faeces Tragopterorum)* (3g), *Xiong Huang (Realgar)* (3g), *Ru Xiang (Resina Boswelliae Carterii)* (3g), *Mo Yao (Resina Commiphorae Myrrhea)* (3g), *A Wei (Resina Ferulae)* (3g), *San Ling (Rhizoma Sparganii)* (3g), *Peng Zhu (Rhizoma zedoariae)* (3g), *Gan Cao (Radix glycyrrhizae)* (3g), *Pi Xiao (Natrii Sulfas)* (3g), *Nao Yang Hua (Rhododendron molle)* (6g), *Liu Huang (Sulfur)* (6g), *Shan Jia (Squanma manitis)* (6g), *Ya Zao (Spina Gleditsiae)* (6g), *She Xiang (Moschus)* (9g) *Gan Sui (Radix Euphorbiae Kansui)* (1.5g) and *Argyi wool* (60g). Its manufacture is the same as that of the thun-

●哮喘[xiāo chuǎn] 病证名。为哮证与喘证的合称。哮,指呼吸急促而喉间有痰鸣声;喘,指呼吸迫促,甚则可见张口抬肩,不能平卧。二者多同时并见,不易区分。其基本病因是痰饮内伏。临床分为寒饮哮喘,痰热哮喘,脾虚哮喘,肺虚哮喘,肾虚哮喘等证型。详见各条。

Asthma A disease, a joint name for wheezing syndrome and dyspnea syndrome. "Wheezing" refers asthmatic breathing with phlegm-caused sound in the throat. "Dyspnea" refers to hasty shallow breathing, with the mouth open and shoulders raised, and failure to lie down on back. Very often both syndromes occur at the same time, and it is not easy to tell them apart. The basic pathogenic factor is the retention of phlegm and fluid in the body. This disease is clinically divided into asthma due to cold fluid retention, asthma due to phlegm-heat, asthma due to deficiency of the spleen, asthma due to deficiency of the lung, and asthma due to deficiency of the kidney. →寒饮哮喘(p.158)、痰热哮喘(p.424)、脾虚哮喘(p.295)、肺虚哮喘(p.109)、肾虚哮喘(p.367)

●痟渴[xiāo kě] 病证名。见元代危亦林《世医得效方》卷七。即消渴。见该条。

Thirst due to Consumptive Heat A disease, seen in Vol. 7 of *Shiyi De Xiaofang*(*Effective Prescriptions Handed Down for Generations*) written by Wei Yilin in the Yuan Dynasty. →消渴(p.494)

●小肠[xiāo cháng] 耳穴名。位于耳轮脚上方中三分之一。用于治疗消化不良、心悸等。

Small Intestine(MA-SC) An auricular point. 〈Location〉at the middle 1/3 of the superior aspect of the helix crus. 〈Indications〉indigestion, palitations, etc.

●小肠经[xiǎo cháng jīng] 手太阳小肠经之简称。见该条。

Small Intestine Meridian The shortened name for the Small Intestine Meridian of Hand-Taiyang. →手太阳小肠经(p.398)

●小肠气[xiǎo cháng qì] 狐疝的又名。见该条。

Pathogenic Qi of the Small Intestine Another name for inguinal hernia. →狐疝(p.167)

●小肠手太阳之脉[xiǎo cháng shǒu tài yáng zhī mài] 手太阳小肠经的原名。见该条。

The Small Intestine Vessel of Hand-Taiyang
  The original name of the Small Intestine Meridian of Hang-Taiyang. →手太阳小肠经(p.398)

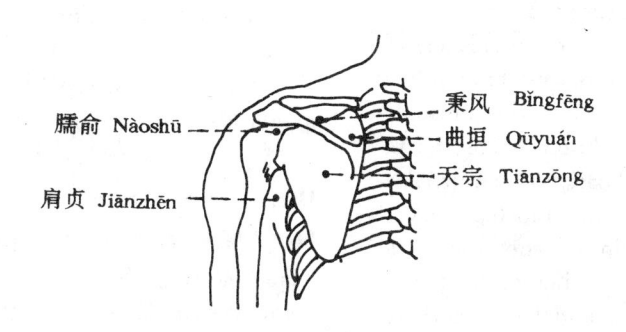

图65.1 小肠经穴(肩部)
Fig 65.1 Points of Small Intestine Meridian(Shoulder)

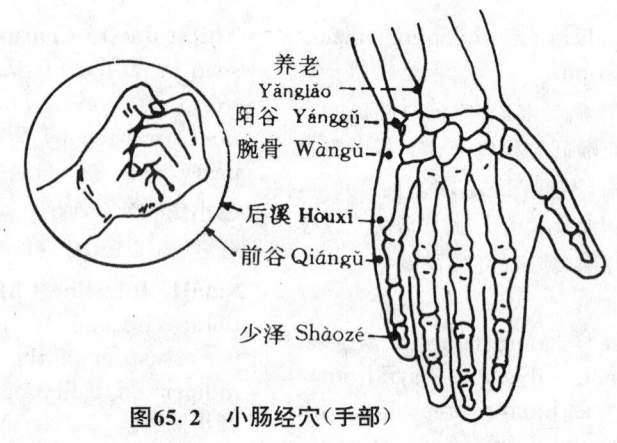

养老 Yǎnglǎo
阳谷 Yánggǔ
腕骨 Wàngǔ
后溪 Hòuxī
前谷 Qiángǔ
少泽 Shàozé

Fig 65.2 Points of Small Intestine Meridian (Hand)

●小肠俞[xiǎo cháng shū] 经穴名。出《脉经》。属足太阳膀胱经,为小肠的背俞穴。〈定位〉在骶部,当骶正中嵴旁1.5寸,平第一骶后孔(图7)。〈层次解剖〉皮肤→皮下组织→臀大肌内侧缘→竖脊肌腱。浅层布有臀中皮神经。深层布有臀下神经的属支和相应脊神经后支的肌支。〈主治〉遗精、遗尿、尿血、白带、小腹胀痛、泄泻、痢疾、痔疾、疝气、腰腿疼。直刺0.8~1.0寸;可灸。

Xiaochangshu(BL 27) A meridian point, originally from *Maijing*(*The Classic of Sphygmology*), a point on the Bladder Meridian of Foot-Taiyang, the back-shu point of the small intestine. 〈Location〉on the sacrum and on the level of the 1st posterior sacral foramen, 1.5 cun lateral to the median sacral crest(Fig. 7). 〈Regional anatomy〉skin→subcutaneous tissue→medial border of greatest gluteal muscle→tendon of erector spinal muscle. In the superficial layer, there are the middle clunial nerves. In the deep layer, there are the branches of the inferior gluteal nerve and the muscular branches of the posterior branches of the related spinal nerves. 〈Indications〉nocturnal emission, enuresis, hematuria, morbid leukorrhea, distention and pain of the lower abdomen, diarrhea, dysentery, hemorrhoid, hernia, aching of the lumbar and leg. 〈Method〉Puncture 0.3~0.5 cun perpendicularly. Moxibustion is applicable.

●小儿半身不遂[xiǎo ér bàn shēn bù suí] 病证名。见《医林改错》。指小儿一侧运动障碍或完全丧失。多因伤寒、瘟疫、痘疹、吐泻等病后元气亏损,筋脉失养所致。症见小儿肢体一侧运动障碍或完全丧失,面色苍白,甚则手足筋挛。治宜舒筋活络,扶正祛邪。取肩髃、曲池、列缺、少商、合谷、手三里、环跳、足三里、阳陵泉、风市、解溪。

Hemiplegia in Children A disease, originally seen in *Yilin Gaicuo*(*Corrections on the Errors of Medical Works*), referring to infantile dyscinesia or akinesis of the limbs on one side, mostly due to the weakness of the primordial qi and failure to nourish muscles caused by febrile diseases pestilence, smallpox, vomiting and diarrhea, etc. 〈Manifestations〉infantile dyscinesia, or even akinesis of one side extremities, pale complexion, even clonic spasm of hand and foot. 〈Treatment principle〉Relax muscles and activate collaterals, strengthen the body resistance to eliminate pathogenic factors. 〈Point selection〉Jianyu (LI 15), Quchi (LI 11), Lieque(LU 7), Shaoshang(LU 11), Hegu(LI 4), Shousanli(LI 10), Huantiao(GB 30), Zusanli(ST 36), Yanglingquan(GB 34), Fengshi(GB 31), Jiexi(ST 41).

●小儿呃逆[xiǎo ér è nì] 即小儿哕的别名。见该条。

Hiccup in Children →小儿哕(p.502)

●小儿疳痢[xiǎo ér gān lì] 尾翠的别名。见该条。

Xiaoerganli Another name for the extra point, Weicui(EX-B). →尾翠(p.460)

●小儿疳瘦[xiǎo ér gān shòu] 尾翠的别名。见该条。

Xiaoerganshou Another name for the extra point, Weicui(EX-B). →尾翠(p.460)

●小儿肛痒[xiǎo ér gāng yǎng] 病证名。指小儿肛门瘙痒,多因嗜食甘肥,大肠湿热积滞,日久生虫蚀

于肛门所致。症见小儿肛门瘙痒,以夜间尤甚,并有啼哭不眠等症,见于蛲虫病等,治宜清热燥湿,杀虫止痒。取大肠俞、三阴交、阴陵泉、曲池、百虫窝。

Anal Itching in Children A disease, referring to the itching in a child's anus, mostly due to parasites corroding at the anus resulting from over-eating of a fatty diet and the stagnation of damp-heat in the large intestine. ⟨Manifestations⟩ infantile anal itching that worsens at night with morbid night crying and insomnia, etc. This disease is generally seen in oxyuriasis. ⟨Treatment principle⟩ Clear away heat and eliminate dampness, destroy parasites and relieve itching. ⟨Point selection⟩ Dachangshu(BL 25), Sanyinjiao(SP 6), Yinlingquan(SP 9), Quchi(LI 11), Baichongwo(EX-LE 3).

●小儿龟胸穴[xiǎo ér guī xiōng xué] 小儿鸡胸穴的别名。见该条。

Xiaoerjixiongxue →小儿鸡胸穴(p. 497)

●小儿寒厥[xiǎo ér hán jué] 小儿厥证之一。见《寿世保元》。又称小儿阴厥。多因阳气衰于下,阴寒过盛所致。症见四肢厥冷、身冷脉沉、口唇色青、小便色白,治宜回阳救逆。取关元,重灸,以鼻尖有汗为度。

Cold Limbs in Children due to Pathogenic Cold One of the jue syndromes in children, seen in *Shoushi Baoyuan* (*Longevity and Life Preservation*), also called cold limbs trouble due to yin due to yin trouble in children, mostly due to exhaustion of yang at the lower-jiao and excess of yin-cold. ⟨Manifestations⟩ deadly cold extremities, cold body and deep pulse, cyanatic and white urine. ⟨Treatment principle⟩ Recuperate depleted yang and rescue the patient from collapse. ⟨Point selection⟩ Guanyuan(RN 4). ⟨Method⟩ Apply moxibustion until sweat appears at the nasal tip of the infant.

●小儿昏迷[xiǎo ér hūn mí] 病证名。指小儿突然或逐渐对周围环境意识完全消失,对外界刺激无反应的证候。此由痰热内闭所致。症见小儿昏迷,不省人事,面红气粗,喉中鸣,舌尖红,脉细滑数。治宜清热、化痰、开窍。取大椎、间使、内关、尺泽、合谷、少商、丰隆、水沟。

Coma in Children A disease referring to the syndrome of sudden or gradual onset of unconsciousness with no reaction upon external irritation, caused by internal stagnation of phlegm, heat. ⟨Manifestations⟩ coma in children, loss of consciousness, flushed face and gasping for breath, wheezing sound in the throat, red tip of the tongue, rapid and slippery thready pulse. ⟨Treatment principle⟩ Clear pathogenic heat, eliminate phlegm and induce resuscitation. ⟨Point selection⟩ Dazhui(DU 14), Jianshi(PC 5), Neiguan(PC 6), Chize(LU 5), Hegu(LI 4), Shaoshang(LU 11), Fenglong(ST 40) and Shuigou(DU 26).

●小儿鸡胸穴[xiǎo ér jī xiōng xué] 经外穴名。见《太平圣惠方》。又名小儿龟胸穴。位于第二、三、四肋间隙,距前正中线2.5寸处,左右共六穴。灸治小儿鸡胸。

Xiaoerjixiongxue(EX-CA) An extra point, originally seen in *Taiping Shenghui Fang* (*Imperial Benevolent Prescriptions*), also called Xiaoerguixiongxue. ⟨Location⟩ on the intercostal depressions between each two ribs of the 2nd, 3rd and 4th ribs, 2.5 cun lateral to the anterior midline, six points in all on both sides. ⟨Indication⟩ pectus carinatum in children. ⟨Method⟩ Moxibustion.

●小儿厥证[xiǎo ér jué zhèng] 病证名。见《杂病源流犀烛》。指小儿真元虚,手足厥冷的症候。临床有寒厥和热厥之分。见"小儿寒厥"、"小儿热厥"条。

Cold Limbs in Children A disease seen in *Zabing Yuanliu Xizhu* (*Bright Candle to Pathology of Miscelloneous Diseases*), referring to deadly cold extremities in children due to the insufficiency of vital qi. This disease is clinically divided into cold limbs in children due to pathogenic cold & cold limbs in children due to excess of heat. →小儿寒厥(p. 497)、小儿热厥(p. 498)

●小儿咳嗽[xiǎo ér ké sòu] 病证名。①小儿腠理不密,容易感冒,表邪侵入,首先犯肺,因而在冬、春气候多变的季节,最易引起咳嗽。②小儿如消化不良,以致脾为湿困,容易生痰,痰湿内蕴,则肺气失宣,亦致咳嗽。③体质素弱,久咳伤津,导致虚火上炎而使津气亏虚,肾不纳气,则肺气更虚而咳嗽加剧。因此小儿咳嗽,可分为外感咳嗽、痰湿咳嗽、肺虚咳嗽三类。①外感咳嗽。症见恶寒发热,咳嗽有力,咽痛,头

痛,舌苔薄白或薄黄,脉浮紧或浮数。治宜疏风解表,宣肺止咳。取肺俞、风门、尺泽、列缺、合谷,毫针浅刺,用泻法。②痰湿咳嗽,症见小儿咳声重浊,喉中痰鸣,食少倦怠,舌苔白腻,脉滑或濡。治宜健脾化湿,祛痰止咳。取肺俞、脾俞、太渊、太白、丰隆、合谷。③肺虚咳嗽,症见咳嗽阵作,少气无力,痰少质粘,面颊略红,舌尖偏红,苔薄黄,脉濡或滑。治宜滋阴益气止咳。取肺俞、经渠、太溪、太渊、太冲。

Cough in Children A disease mostly caused by pathogenic changes: ①Failure of superficial-qi to protect the body against the invasion of pathogenic factors; the exogenous evils first attack the lung, which leads to the onset of common cold mostly in winter and spring. ②The obstruction of lung-qi, resulting from indigestion leading to the retention of dampness in the spleen, which produces phlegm and stagnation of damp-phlegm in the lung. ③The dysfunction of the lung resulting from the constitutional deficiency of the body and the damage of body fluid which lead to the flaring-up of fire of deficient type causing body fluid deficiency and failure of the kidney to relieve air. This disease is clinically divided into the following types: ①Cough due to exopathy. 〈Manifestations〉fever, chills, forceful cough, sore throat, headache, white or yellow thin tongue coating, superficial tight or rapid pulse. 〈Treatment principle〉Expel wind to relieve superficial syndrome, ventilate the lung to relieve cough. 〈Point selection〉Feishu(BL 13), Fengmen(BL 12), Chize(LU 5), Lieque(LU 7) and Hegu(LI 4). 〈Method〉 Puncture superficially with reducing method. ②Cough due to phlegm and dampness. 〈Manifestations〉cough with unclear sound, wheezing sound in the throat, poor appetite and weary feeling, white and greasy tongue coating, slippery or soft pulse. 〈Treatment principle〉Invigorate the spleen to remove dampness; expel phlegm to relieve cough. 〈Point selection〉Feishu(BL 13), Pishu(BL 20), Taiyuan(LU 9), Taibai(SP 3), Fenglong(ST 40) and Hegu(LI 4). ③Cough due to deficiency of the lung. 〈Manifestations〉paroxysmal cough, listlessness and inertia, little but mucoid sputum, flushed face and cheek, reddish tip of the tongue, thin yellow tongue coating, soft or slippery pulse. 〈Treatment principle〉Enrich yin and invigorate qi to relieve cough. 〈Point selection〉Feishu(BL 13) Jingqu(LU 8), Taixi(KI 3), Taiyuan(LU 9) and Taichong(LR 3).

●小儿麻痹证[xiǎo ér má bì zhèng] 即小儿痿证。见该条。

Infantile paralysis Another name for infantile flaccidity syndrome. →小儿痿证(p. 500)

●小儿明堂针灸经[xiǎo ér míng táng zhēn jiǔ jīng] 书名。宋代吴复珪著,一卷,书佚。见《宋史·艺文志》。

Xiaoer Ming Tang Zhenjiu Jing(Ming Tang Classic of Acupuncture and Moxibustion on Children) A book written by Wu Fugui in the Song Dynasty, single volume, lost. It is seen in *Songshi: Yi Wen Zhi(The History of the Song Dynasty: Records of Art and Literature)*.

●小儿呕吐[xiǎo ér ǒu tù] 病证名。见《圣济总录》。多由饮食不节,损伤胃气,不能运化所致,由于病因各异,临床分寒吐、热吐、伤食吐、伤乳吐、积吐、虫吐、惊吐等。详见各条。

Infantile Vomiting A syndrome seen in *Shengji Zonglu(Imperial Medical Encyclopedia)*, mostly caused by the impairment of stomach-qi and failure in transportation resulting from improper diet. Due to the different causes of the disease, it is clinically divided into vomiting due to pathogenic clod, vomiting due to pathogenic heat, vomiting due to improper diet, milk vomiting in infancy, vomiting due to the retention of food, vomiting caused by intestinal parasitosis and vomiting in infancy induced by fright. →寒吐(p. 157)热吐(p. 332)、伤食吐(p. 349)、伤乳吐(p. 349)、积吐(p. 182)、虫吐(p. 49)、惊吐(p. 217)

●小儿热厥[xiǎo ér rè jué] 病证名。见《张氏医通》。是小儿厥证之一。又称小儿阳厥,多因邪热过盛。阳气内郁,不能透达四肢所致。症见四肢厥冷而胸腹灼热,舌干,苔黄燥或焦黑起刺,伴恶热,口渴,烦躁不得眠,小便赤涩或便秘,甚至神昏谵语等,治宜清热、解郁,开窍。取水沟、内关、合谷、大椎、陷谷、足三里、太冲。不留针。

Cold Limbs in Children due to Excess of Heat A syndrome, seen in *Zhangshi Yitong* (*Zhang's Treatise on General Medicine*), a type of infantile syncope, also known as clod limbs in children due to yang trouble, mostly caused by excess pathogenic heat and stagnation of yang-qi leading to failure to warm the four limbs. ⟨Manifestations⟩deadly cold limbs with high fever and a feeling of burning in the chest and abdomen, dryness of the tongue, dry and yellowish or black and thorny tongue coating accompanied by aversion to heat, thirst, irritability leading to sleeplessness, dark urine with difficulty and pain or constipation, and coma or delirium. ⟨Treatment principle⟩ Clear heat, regulate qi by alleviation of mental depression and induce resusatation. ⟨Point selection⟩Shuigou (DU 26), Neiguan (PC 6), Hegu (LI 4), Dazhui (DU 14), Xiangu (ST 43), Zusanli (ST 36), Taichong (LR 3). ⟨Method⟩Puncture the acupoints without retainning the needle.

●小儿热泻[xiǎo ér rè xiè] 病证名。小儿为纯阳之体,感受暑热。邪热入里,热迫大肠而成腹泻。症见小儿腹泻伴有阵阵肠鸣腹痛。烦躁啼哭,肛门灼热,小便短赤,治宜泄热止泻。取合谷、曲池、内庭、天枢。

Diarrhea in Children due to Pathogenic Heat A syndrome. Children are of pure-yang constitution, if they are attacked by summer-heat, the pathogenic heat may go to the interior and invade the large intestine, then abdominal diarrhea will occur. ⟨Manifestations⟩ infantile diarrhea acompanied by intermittent borborygmus and abdominal pain, irritability and crying, burning sensation of the anus, scanty dark urine. ⟨Treatment principle⟩ Expel pathogenic heat to stop diarrhea. ⟨Point selection⟩ Hegu(LI 4), Quchi(LI 11), Neiting (ST 44) and Tianshu(ST 25).

●小儿身热吐泻[xiǎo ér shēn rè tù xiè] 病证名。见《儒门事亲》。多因外感六淫,内伤乳食所致,临床证见小儿身热,呕吐,泄泻,伴有腹满不能进食,嗜睡、烦躁、口热等,治宜解表和胃,止吐泻。取曲池、合谷建里、天枢、内关、公孙。

Infantile Vomiting with Diarrhea and Fever A syndrome, seen in *Ru Men Shi Qin* (*Confucian's Duties to Their Parents*), mostly caused by the affection of the six exopathogens and improper feeding. ⟨Manifestations⟩ fever, vomiting, diarrhea, accompanied by abdominal fullness with the failure of food intake, somnolence, irrtability, hot mouth, etc. ⟨Treatment principle⟩ Relieve exopathogens and regulate stomach to relieve vomiting and diarrhea. ⟨Point selection⟩Quchi (LI 11), Hegu (LI 4), Jianli (RN 11), Tianshu (ST 25), Neiguan(PC 6) and Gongsun(SP 4).

●小儿食痫[xiǎo ér shí xián] 经外穴名。见《经外奇穴图谱》。在上腹部,前正中线上,脐上7.5寸处。灸治小儿癫痫。

Xiaoershixian（EX-CA） An extra point, seen in *Jingwai Qixue Tupu*(*An Atlas of Extra Points of Acupuncture and Moxibustion*). ⟨Location⟩on the upper abdomen, 7.5 cun above the umblilcus, on the anterior midline. ⟨Indication⟩ infantile epilepsy. ⟨Method⟩ Moxibustion.

●小儿睡惊[xiǎo ér shuì jīng] 经外穴名。见《经外奇穴图谱》。在肘横纹桡侧端直上0.3寸。灸治小儿睡惊、肘臂疼痛等。

Xiaoershuijing（EX-UE） An extra point, seen in *Jingwai Qixue Tupu*(*An Atlas of Extra Points for Acupuncture and Moxibustion*). ⟨Location⟩0.3 cun directly above the radial end of the transverse crease of the elbow. ⟨Indications⟩sleep fright in children, pain in the elbow and arm, etc. ⟨Method⟩Moxibustion.

●小儿痰泻[xiǎo ér tán xiè] 病证名。见《慈幼便览》。多由脾虚不振,运化失常,水湿不化,聚而生痰,痰湿下注,并走肠间所致,症见泻无定时,质粘而稠,神疲乏力。治宜健脾化痰。取脾俞、建里、足三里、丰隆。不留针。

Diarrhea in Children due to Phlegm A syndrome, seen in *Ciyou Bianlan*(*A Brief Guide for Care of Infants*). Mostly due to spleen deficiency and dysfunction of the spleen in transportation and transformation leading to the retention of water within the body which causes phlegm. Then, the phlegm-dampness attacks the lower jiao and intestine causing diarrhea. ⟨Manifestations⟩diarrhea with sticky and thick stool and without definite time, and

lassitude. 〈Treatment principle〉Invigorate the spleen to resolve phlegm. 〈Point selection〉 Pishu (BL 20), Jianli (RN 11), Zusanli (ST 36), Fenglong (ST 40). 〈Method〉Puncture these acupoints without retaining the needles.

●小儿头痛[xiǎo ér tóu tòng] 病证名。见《医宗金鉴·幼科杂病心法要诀》。临床多见风寒头痛与内热头痛两类。①风寒风袭。因风寒侵袭，上犯巅顶经脉，气血不和，经络阻遏所致。症见恶寒发热，巅顶额角部作痛。治宜疏散风寒。取风池、百会、风府、列缺、合谷，毫针浅刺，用泻法。②内热头痛。因小儿脾胃脆嫩，过食肥甘厚腻食物，引起脾胃消化功能失调，积滞化热、热极生火，火性上炎，循足阳明经上行所致。症见鼻干目痛，上至头额，下至齿颊，痛无定时。治宜清泄阳明经热。取上星、头维、合谷、商阳。商阳穴点刺出血。

Infantile Headache A syndrome, seen in *Yizong Jinjian: Youke Zabing Xinfa Yaojue (Gold Mirror of Orthodox Medical Lingeage: Essential of Personal Experience for Miscellaneous Diseases of Pediatrics)*. It is clinically divided into two types: headache due to wind cold and headache due to internal heat. ①Headache due to wind cold, caused by the the derangement of qi and blood and the blockage of the meridians resulting from wind-cold attacking the collaterals of vertex. 〈Manifestations〉aversion to cold and fever, pain in the vertex and temple. 〈Treatment principle〉Expel wind-cold. 〈Point selection〉 Fengchi (GB 20), Baihui (DU 20), Fengfu (DU 16), Lieque (LU 7), Hegu (LI 4). 〈Method〉Filiform needles are used to puncture the points with the reducing method. ② Headache due to internal heat, caused by overeating fleshy and greasy food leading to disorder of the digestive function of the spleen and stomach, which causes accumulated food to grow into heat, the excessive heat transforms into fire, and the fire flames up along the Meridian of Foot-Yangming. 〈Manifestations〉dry nose, pain in the eyes radiating to the vertex and teeth, pain without definite time. 〈Treatment principle〉 Clear heat from the Meridian of Foot-Yangming. 〈Point selection〉 Shangxing (DU 23), Touwei (ST 8), Hegu (LI 4), Shangyang (LI 1). Prick Shangyang (LI 1) to cause bleeding.

●小儿脱肛[xiǎo ér tuō gāng] 病证名。见《诸病源候论》。指肛管直肠甚至部分结肠移位下降外脱的证象。多因小儿血气未充，或因久泄久痢等，以致中气下陷，不能摄纳而致。治宜补中益气，升阳举陷。取百会、足三里、长强、承山。用补法，可灸百会穴。

Prolapse of Rectum in Children A syndrome, seen in *Zhubing Yuanhou Lun (General Treatise on the Etiology and Symptomatology of Diseases)*, referring to the displacement, descent and external prolapse of the anal canal rectum and occasionally part of the colon, mostly caused by insufficiency of blood and qi in children or by prolonged diarrhea and dysentery leading to the sinking of middle-jiao qi and failure to receive qi. 〈Treatment principle〉Reinforce the middle-jiao and invigorate qi, elevate the spleen-yang to relieve the sinking of qi. 〈Point selection〉 Baihui (DU 20), Zusanli (ST 36), Changqiang (DU 1) and Chengshan (BL 57). 〈Method〉Puncture the points with the reinforcing method. Moxibustion is applicable on Baihui (DU 20).

●小儿痿证[xiǎo ér wěi zhèng] 病证名。见《医碥》。又称小儿麻痹症。指小儿四肢软弱，无力运动的病证，多由于感受风、湿、热邪引起。临床分肺热证、湿热证、肝肾两亏证。①肺热证。多因风热袭肺，耗伤肺之津液，肺朝百脉而输布津液，肺热叶焦则筋脉失养所致。症见发热、咳嗽、咽红、呕吐腹泻、肢体疼痛，继而萎软无力，苔薄白，脉细数。治宜宣肺解表，散风清热。取合谷、列缺、风池、曲池。毫针浅刺，用泻法。②湿热证。多因湿热蕴蒸阳明，阳明受病而宗筋弛缓，不能束筋骨利关节所致。症见发热，肢体疼痛而沉重，不敢触动，继而肢体萎软，烦躁，嗜睡，汗多，苔黄腻，舌红，脉濡数。治宜清热利湿。取曲池、足三里、阴陵泉、三阴交。③肝肾两亏证。多因病久不愈，肝肾两虚，精血亏损，筋骨关节失养所致。症见筋软骨萎，肌肉萎缩，关节畸形，舌淡，脉沉细。治宜补益肝肾，调理阳明。取肝俞、肾俞、腰阳关、阳陵泉、绝骨、太溪、足三里、曲池。可加灸。

Flaccidity Syndrome in Children A syndrome from *Yi Bian (A Book on Medicine)*, also known as infantile paralysis, referring to softness and weakness of the limbs in children and a failure to be able to exercise, mostly

caused by attack of pathogenic wind, dampness and heat. Clinically, it is divided into flaccidity due to lung-heat, flaccidity due damp-heat and flaccidity due to the impairment of both the liver and the kindney. ①Flaccidity due to lung-heat. Mostly due to wind-heat attacking the lung and consuming the fluid of the lung. Because "the lung transports body fluid to all the meridians", lung-heat and its burnt lobes lead to failure to nourish tendons and muscles. ⟨Manifestations⟩ fever, cough, redness of the throat, vomiting and diarrhea, pain of the limbs gradually transforming into lethargy, thin and whitish tognue coating, thready and rapid pulse. ⟨Treatment principle⟩ Promote the dispersing function of the lung and relieve the exterior syndrome, expel wind and clear heat. ⟨Point selection⟩ Hegu(LI 4), Lieque(LU 7), Fengchi(GB 20) and Quchi(LI 11). ⟨Method⟩Filiform needles are used to puncture subcutaneously with the reducing method. ② Flaccidity due to damp-heat. Mostly due to damp-heat steaming the Yangming Meridian and leading to a softness and weakness of the muscles and failure to strengthen the bones and benefit the joints. ⟨Manifestations⟩ fever, pain and heaviness of the limbs, fear of being touched and a gradual softening and weakening of the limbs, irritability, desired to sleep, excess sweating of the limbs, red tongue with yellowish and greasy coating, soft and rapid pulse. ⟨Treatment principle⟩ Clear heat and promote diuresis. ⟨Point selection⟩ Quchi(LI 11), Zusanli(ST 36), Yinlingquan(SP 9) and Sanyinjiao(SP 6). ③ Flaccidity due to impairment of both the liver and kidney. Mostly due to prolonged illness, deficiency of the liver and kidney, consumption of the nourishment of the muscles and bones. ⟨Manifestations⟩ softness of the muscles and bones, muscular atrophy, deformity of the joints, pale tongue with deep and thready pulse. ⟨Treatment principle⟩ Reinforce the liver and kidney, regulate the Yangming Meridian. ⟨Point selection⟩ Ganshu(BL 18), Shenshu(BL 23), Yaoyangguan(DU 3), Yanglingquan(GB 34), Juegu(GB 39), Taixi(KI 3), Zusanli(ST 36) and Quchi(LI 11). ⟨Method⟩ Besides puncturing, moxibustion is also applicable.

●小儿泄泻[xiǎo ér xiè xiè] 病证名。是以大便次数增多，便下稀薄，或水样便为特征的一种病证，临床多见湿热泻、伤食泻、阳虚泻。①湿热泻。多因小儿外感暑湿，困扰脾胃，以致运化失常，清浊不分，形成泄泻。症见泻下稀薄，色黄而秽臭，身热口渴，肛门灼热，小便短赤，舌苔黄腻，脉滑数。治宜清热利湿。取中脘、天枢、足三里、曲池、内庭。②伤食泻。多因饮食不节，乳食停滞，损伤肠胃，消化不良，水谷不分，并走肠间，形成泄泻。症见腹部胀痛，痛则欲泻，泻后痛减，大便腐臭，状如败卵，嗳啰腐食，或呕吐不消化食物，舌苔垢腻，脉滑而实。治宜消食导滞。取中脘、建里、天枢、气海、足三里、内庭。③阳虚泻。多因久病脾胃虚弱，肾阳不足，命门火衰，不能温运水谷，下注于肠，形成泄泻。症见时泻时止或久泻不愈，大便溏或完谷不化，每于食后作泻，纳呆，神疲肢倦，面色萎黄，甚则四肢厥冷，舌淡苔白，脉细缓。治宜健脾温肾。取脾俞、肾俞、足三里、章门。用补法，加灸。

Infantile Diarrhea A syndrome, marked by an increasing amount of discharge of watery stool, damp-heat diarrhea, diarrhea due to improper diet and diarrhea due to yang-deficiency are often seen in clinic. ①Diarrhea due to damp-heat. Mostly due to attack of exogenous summer dampness, which disturbs the spleen and stomach and leads to dysfunction of the spleen, a failure to distinguish clarity from turbidity and to the occurrence of diarrhea. ⟨Manifestations⟩ thin or watery stool with yellow color and foul smell, fever and thirst, burning sensation of the anus, scanty and dark urine, yellowish and greasy tongue coating, and slippery and rapid pulse. ⟨Treatment principle⟩ Clear heat and promote diuresis. ⟨Point selection⟩ Zhongwan(RN 12), Tianshu(ST 25), Zusanli(ST 36), Quchi(LI 11) and Neiting(ST 44). ②Diarrhea due to improper diet. Mostly due to improper diet; retention of the undigested food damages the intestine and stomach, which leads to indigestion and failure to distinguish water from food and to the occurrence of diarrhea. ⟨Manifestations⟩ abdominal distension and pain, diarrhea when abdomen feels pain, pains relief after diarrhea, foul smell of the stools, like a rotten egg, eruc-

tation with fetid odor, or vomiting of undigested food, thich and greasy tongue coating, and slippery and solid pulse. ⟨Treatment principle⟩ Promote digestion to remove stagnation of undigested food. ⟨Point selection⟩ Zhongwan (RN 12), Jianli (RN 11), Tianshu (ST 25), Qihai (RN 6), Zusanli (ST 36) and Neiting (ST 44). ③Diarrhea due to yang-deficiency. Mostly due to prolonged illness leading to deficiency of the spleen and stomach, insuficiency of kiney-yang, the decline of the Ming Men Huo (The fire of the life gate) and failure to warm and transport food which causes diarrhea. ⟨Manifestations⟩ intermittent diarrhea or prolonged diarrhea, watery stools or stools with undigested food, diarrhea occurring after eating, poor appetite, lassitude and fatigue, shallow complexion, dead coldness of the limbs, pale tongue with white coating, thready and slow pulse. ⟨Treatment principle⟩ Invigorate the spleen and warm the kidney. ⟨Point selection⟩ Pishu (BL 20), Shenshu (BL 23), Zusanli (ST 36), and Zhangmen (LR 13). ⟨Method⟩ Puncture with reinforcing method. Moxibustion is applicable.

●小儿阳厥[xiǎo ér yáng jué] 小儿热厥的别名。见该条。

Cold Limbs in Children due to Yang Trouble
Another name for cold limbs in children due to excess of heat. →小儿热厥(p. 498)

●小儿遗尿[xiǎo ér yí niào] 病证名。见《诸病源候论》。又称尿来、尿床。是指三岁以上的小儿，睡眠中小便经常自遗，醒后方觉的一种病症。临床分两型。①肾阳不足型。多由肾气不足，下元不固，膀胱约束无权而发生遗尿。症见睡中遗尿，醒后方觉，一夜可发生1～2次或更多，兼见面色㿠白，小便清长而频数，甚则肢冷恶寒，舌质淡，脉沉迟无力。治宜温补肾阳。取关元、中极、肾俞、膀胱俞、太溪。用补法，多灸。②脾肺气虚型。多因脾虚不能制水，肺虚不能通调水道，故脾肺气虚，上虚不能制下，膀胱约束无力而发生遗尿。症见睡中遗尿，尿频而量少，兼见面色㿠白，精神倦怠，四肢乏力，食欲不振，大便稀溏，舌质淡，脉沉细。治宜补益脾肺。取气海、太渊、足三里、三阴交、百会、脾俞、肺俞。用补法，加灸。

Enuresis in Children A syndrome, originally from *Zhubing Yuanhou Lun* (*General Treatise on the Etiology and Symptomatolgy of Diseases*), also known as nocturnal enuresis in children or bed-wetting, referring to children of more than 3 years old unconsciously urinating during sleep. It is divided into the following two types: ① Kidney-yang deficiency type. Mostly due to deficiency of the kidney-qi, unconsolidation of the lower vital organs and failure of the urinary bladder to control urination. ⟨Manifestations⟩ enuresis during sleep, 1-2 times or more within one night, being conscious of what has happened after waking up. Accompanied by pale complexion, clear and frequent urine, cold limbs and aversion to cold, pale tongue with deep, slow and weak pulse. ⟨Treatment principle⟩ Warm and reinforce kidney-yang. ⟨Point selection⟩ Guanyuan (RN 4), Zhongji (RN 3), Shenshu (BL 23), Pangguangshu (BL 28) and Taixi (KI 3). ⟨Method⟩ Puncture the points with reinforcing method. Heavy moxibustion is applicable. ② Spleen-qi and lung-qi deficiency type. Mostly due to inability to control water because of the deficient spleen and the inability to regulate water of the deficient lung. Therefore, the qi deficiency of the spleen and lung lead to the failure of the urinary bladder to control urination. ⟨Manifestations⟩ enuresis, frequent micturition with a small amount of urine, accompanied by pale complexion, lassitude, weakness of the limbs, poor appetite, watery stools, pale tongue, and a deep and thready pulse. ⟨Treatment principle⟩ Invigorate the spleen and benefit the lung. ⟨Point selection⟩ Qihai (RN 6), Taiyuan (LU 9), Zusanli (ST 36), Sanyinjiao (SP 6), Baihui (DU 20), Pishu (BL 20) and Feishu (BL 13). ⟨Method⟩ Puncture with the reinforcing method in combination with moxibustion.

●小儿阴厥[xiǎo ér yīn jué] 小儿寒厥的别名。见该条。

Cold Limbs in Children due to Yin Trouble
Another name for cold limbs in children due to pathogenic cold. →小儿寒厥(p. 497)

●小儿哕[xiǎo ér yuě] 病证名。见《诸病源候论》。又称小儿呃逆。多因脾胃运化失调，食滞胃脘，胃气

上逆所致。症见呃逆声音响亮，连续有力，口渴，面赤。治宜和胃降逆。取中脘、内关、足三里、膈俞。毫针浅刺，用泻法，不留针。

Hiccough in Children　A syndrome, from *Zhubing Yuanhou Lun* (*General Treatise on the Etiology and Symptomatology of Diseases*), also known as infantile hiccup, mostly caused by the disorder of the transportation and transformation function of the spleen and stomach and the retention of food in the stomach which causes the stomach-qi adversly rise. 〈Manifestations〉Continous hiccup with loud and clear sound, thirst and flushed face. 〈Treatment principle〉Regulate the stomach to lower the adverse flow of the stomach-qi. 〈Point selection〉Zhongwan (RN 12), Neiguan (PC 6), Zusanli (ST 36) and Geshu (BL 17). 〈Method〉filiform needle are used to puncture the points with the reducing method and without retaining the needles.

●小儿针[xiǎo ér zhēn]　针具名。即皮肤针。因其适用于小儿患者。故名。参见该条。

Infantile Needle　A needling instrument, synonymous with dermal needle. It is so named because it is suitable for children. →皮肤针(p.292)

●小骨空[xiǎo gǔ kōng]　经外穴名。见《扁鹊神应针灸玉龙经》。〈定位〉在小指背侧近侧指间关节的中点处(图76)。〈层次解剖〉皮肤→皮下组织→指背腱膜。布有指背动、静脉的分支及属支和尺神经的指背神经的分支。灸治目疾、耳聋、喉痛、指痛等。

Xiaogukong(EX-UE 6)　An extra point, from *Bianque Shenying Zhenjiu Yulong Jing* (*Bian Que's Jade Dragon Classics of Acupuncture and Moxibustion*). 〈Location〉on the dorsal side of the little finger, at the center of the proximal interphalangeal joint (Fig. 76). 〈Regional anatomy〉skin→subcutaneous tissue→dorsal digital aponeurosis. There are the branches or tributaries of the dorsal digital artery and vein and the branches of the dorsal digital nerve of the ulnar nerve in this area. 〈Indications〉eye disorders, deafness, inflammation of the throat and pain in the finger. 〈Method〉moxibustion.

●小骨孔[xiǎo gǔ kǒng]　即小骨空。见该条。

Xiaogukong(孔)　→小骨空(p.503)

●小谷[xiǎo gǔ]　经穴别名。即三间，见该条。

Xiaogu　Another name for the meridian point, Sanjian(LI 3). →三间(p.341)

●小海[xiǎo hǎi]　经穴名。出《灵枢·本输》。属手太阳小肠经，为本经合穴。〈定位〉在肘内侧，当尺骨鹰嘴与肱骨内上髁之间凹陷处(图48)。〈层次解剖〉皮肤→皮下组织→尺神经沟内。浅层有前臂内侧皮神经尺侧支，臂内侧皮神经，贵要静脉属支等结构，深层：在尺神经沟内有尺神经，尺神经的后外侧有尺侧上副动、静脉与尺动、静脉的尺侧返动、静脉后支吻合成的动、静脉网。〈主治〉颊肿、颈项肩背外后侧痛、头痛目眩、耳聋、耳鸣、癫、狂、痫证、疡肿。直刺0.2～0.3寸；可灸。

Xiaohai(SI 8)　A meridian point, from *Ling Shu*: *Ben Shu* (*Miraculous Pivot*: *Meridian Points*), the *He-sea* point of the Small Intestine Meridian of Hand-Taiyang. 〈Location〉on the medial side of the elbow, in the depression between the olecranon of the ulna and the medial epicondyle of the humerus (Fig. 48). 〈Regional anatomy〉skin→subcutaneous tissue→groove of ulnar nerve. In the superficial layer, there are the ulnar branches of the medial cutaneous nerve of the forearm, the medial cutaneous nerve of the arm and the tirbutaries of the basilic vein. In the deep layer, there are the ulnar nerve, the arteriovenous network formed by the superior ulnar collateral arteries and veins and the posterior branches of the ulnar recurrent artery and vein on the posterior lateral side of the ulnar nerve. 〈Indications〉swelling of the cheek, pain in the nape and the latero-posterior aspect of the shoulder and arm, headache and blurring of vision, deafness, tinnitus, manic-depressive disorder, epilepsy, swelling sores 〈Method〉Puncture perpendicularly 0.2～0.3 cun. Moxibustion is applicable.

●小茴香灸[xiǎo huí xiāng jiǔ]　间接灸法之一。取小茴香100克，干姜末50克，醋糟500克。将上药炒热，装入布袋中，敷于穴位或患处施灸。每次5～10分钟。适于脘腹疼痛、寒痹等证。

Moxibustion with Xiao Hui Xiang(*Fructus Foeniculi*)　A form of indirect moxibustion,

composed of *Xiao Hui Xiang* (*Fructus Foeniculi*)100g, powder of dried ginger 50g, vinegar dross 500g. Fry the herbs before putting them into a cloth-bag, then place the bag on the diseased area for moxibustion, 5~10 minutes per time. Used for treating gastric and abdominal pain, arthralgia due to cold, etc.

●小吉[xiǎo jí] 经穴别名。出《针灸甲乙经》。即少泽。见该条。

Xiaoji Another name for Shaoze (SI 1), a meridian point from *Zhenjiu Jia-Yi Jing* (*A-B Classic of Acupuncture and Moxibustion*). →少泽(p.358)

●小眉刀[xiǎo méi dāo] 针具名。又名痧刀。以钢质制成,柄长1~2寸,刀口倾斜似眉,故名。用于割治、挑刺、泻血。

Knife with an Eye-Brow-Shaped Edge A kind of needling instrument, also called a measles knife, made of steel with a handle of 1~2 cun long. So named because the edge of the knife is shaped like eye-brows. It is used for cutting, picking a thorn, and causing bleeding.

●小天心[xiǎo tiān xīn] 经外穴名。出《针灸大成》。在手掌侧,当大鱼际与小鱼际交接处之中点。〈主治〉惊风抽搐,高热神昏,小便不通,心绞痛,风湿性心脏病等。直刺0.3~0.5寸。

Xiaotianxin (EX-UE) An extra point, from *Zhenjiu Dacheng* (*A Great Compendium of Acupuncture and Moxibustion*). 〈Location〉on the palmar side, on the midpoint of the junction between the big thenar eminence and small thenar eminence. 〈Indications〉Infantile convulsion and spasm, high fever and coma, difficulty in discharging urine, angina pactoris, and rheumatic heart disease, etc. 〈Method〉Puncture perpendicularly 0.3~0.5 cun.

●小溪[xiǎo xī] 部位名。出《素问·五脏生成篇》。参见"溪谷"条。

Small Streams A part of the body, from *Suwen*: *Wu Zang Shengcheng Pian* (*Plain Questions*: *Physiology and Pathology of the Five Zang Organs*). →溪谷(p.482)

●小针[xiǎo zhēn] 针具名。出《灵枢·九针十二原》和《灵枢·小针解》。为微针的别称。见该条。

Small Needle A needling instrument, from *Lingshu*: *Jiu Zhen Shier Yuan* (*Miraculous Pivot*: *Nine Needles and Twelve Yuan* (*Primary Points*) and *Ling Shu*: *Xiaozhen Jie* (*Miraculous Pivot*: *Explanation of Delicate Needling*), another name for minute needle. →微针(p.460)

●小指(趾)次指(趾)[xiǎo zhǐ(zhǐ) cì zhǐ(zhǐ)] 部位名。出《灵枢·经脉》。指无名指或足第四趾。

Finger (Toe) Next to the Little One A part of the body, from *Lingshu*: *Jingmai* (*Miraculous Pivot*: *Meridians*), referring to the ring finger or the fourth toe.

●小指尖[xiǎo zhǐ jiān] 经外穴名。见《千金要方》。又名小指头、手太阳穴、盐哮。在手小指尖端,左右计二穴。〈主治〉黄疸、癫疝、消渴、百日咳。直刺0.1~0.2寸;可灸。

Xiaozhijian (EX-UE) An extra point, seen in *Qianjin Yaofang* (*Essential Prescriptions Worth a Thousand Gold*), also named Xiaozhitou, Shoutaiyangxue or Yanxiao. 〈Location〉at the tip of the little finger, two points on both hands. 〈Indications〉jaundice, swelling of the scrotum, diabetes and whooping cough. 〈Method〉Puncture perpendicularly 0.1~0.2 cun. Moxibustion is applicable.

●小趾尖[xiǎo zhǐ jiān] 经外穴名。出《针灸孔穴及其疗法便览》,位于足小趾尖端,左右计二穴。〈主治〉难产、头痛、眩晕、消渴。毫针刺0.1~0.2寸;可灸。

Xiaozhijian (EX-LE) An extra point, from *Zhenjiu Kongxue Jiqi Liaofa Bianlan* (*Guide to Acupoints and Acupuncture Therapeutics*). 〈Location〉at the tip of the little toe, two points on both feet. 〈Indications〉dystocia, headache, dizziness, and diabetes. 〈Method〉Puncture 0.1~0.2 cun with a filiform, needle. Moxibustion is applicable.

●小指头[xiǎo zhǐ tóu] 经外穴别名。即小指尖。见该条。

Xiaozhitou Another name for the extra point Xiaozhijian(EX-UE). →小指尖(p.504)

●小指爪纹[xiǎo zhǐ zhǎo wén] 经外穴名。出《千金要方》。在手小指背侧,爪甲根部,左右计二穴。〈主治〉喉痹。点刺出血。

Xiaozhizhaowen (EX-UE) An extra point,

from *Qianjin Yaofang* (*Essential Prescriptions Worth a Thousand Gold*). 〈Location〉on the dorsal aspect of the little finger, at the root of the nail, two points on both hands. 〈Indication〉inflammation of the throat. 〈Method〉Prick to cause bleeding.

●小竹[xiǎo zhú] 经穴别名。出《太平圣惠方》。即眉冲。见该条。

Xiaozhu Another name for Meichong (BL 3), a meridian point from *Taiping Shenghui Fang* (*Imperial Benevolent Prescriptions*). → 眉冲(p. 265)

●小炷灸[xiǎo zhù jiǔ] 灸法术语。又称小壮灸,指用较小艾炷灸治的方法。

Small Moxa Cone Moxibustion A moxibustion term, also known as cone moxibustion, referring to moxibustion treatment with small moxa cones.

●小壮灸[xiǎo zhuàng jiǔ] 灸法术语,即小炷灸,见该条。

Cone Moxibustion A moxibustion term, synonymous with small moxa cone moxibustion. → 小炷灸(p. 505)

●小肘尖[xiǎo zhǒu jiān] 经外穴别名。斗肘穴别名。见该条。

Xiaozhoujian Another name for the extra point Douzhou(EX-UE). → 斗肘(p. 85)

●歇[xiē] 经闭的别名。见该条。

Pause Another name for amenorrhea. → 经闭(p. 208)

●歇经[xiē jīng] 经闭的别名。见该条。

Menopause Another name for amenorrhea. → 经闭(p. 208)

●胁[xié] 部位名,腋下到肋骨尽处统称为胁。

Hypochondrium A body part, i.e. the region from the armpit to the termination of the ribs.

●胁窌[xié jiào] 经穴别名。出《针灸甲乙经》。即章门,见该条。

Xiejiao Another name for Zhangmen (LR 13), a meridian point from *Zhenjiu Jia-Yi Jing* (*A-B Classic of Acupuncture and Moxibustion*). → 章门(p. 585)

●胁堂[xié táng] 经外穴名。见《外台秘要》。在侧胸部,当腋窝下二寸凹陷中。灸治心内膜炎、胸胁支满、喘逆、肝病、胸膜炎等。

Xietang (EX-CA) An extra point, seen in *Waitai Miyao* (*Clandestine Essentials from the Imperial Library*). 〈Location〉on the side of chest, in the depression 2.0 cun below the armpit. 〈Indications〉endocarditis, fullness in the chest and hypochondrium, dyspnea, liver diseases and pleuritis, etc. 〈Method〉Moxibustion.

●胁痛[xié tòng] 病证名。出《灵枢·缪刺论》等篇。泛指一侧或双侧胁肋部疼痛而言,胁肋为足厥阴、足少阳两经循行所过,故发病多与肝胆疾患有关。根据受邪的性质不同,胁肋痛可分为肝郁胁痛、湿热胁痛、瘀血胁痛、阴虚胁痛。详见各条。

Hypochondriac Pain A syndrome from *Lingshu: Miuci Lun* (*Miraculous Pivot: Treatise on Contralateral Insertion*), generally referring to hypochondriac pain in one or both sides. The Meridians of Foot-Jueyin and Foot-Shaoyang run through the hypochondriac region, so hypochondriac pain is mostly related to disorders of the liver and gallbladder. According to the different nature of pathogenic factors, hypochondriac pain can be divided into hypochondriac pain due to the stagnation of liver-qi; hypochondriac pain due to damp-heat; hypochondriac pain due to blood stasis and hypochondriac pain due to yin-deficiency. → 肝郁胁痛(p. 129)、湿热胁痛(p. 372)、瘀血胁痛(p. 570)、阴虚胁痛(p. 562)

●斜刺[xié cì] 刺法术语,指针体与穴位表面呈30°～60°角刺入。对肌肉较薄和邻近重要脏器的胸胁、上背等处的穴位,均可采用,斜刺可防止刺伤脏器。此外,为了使气至病所,也可采用斜刺法。参见"迎随补泻"条。

Oblique Insertion A needling method, referring to inserting the acupuncture needle at an angle of 30°～60° formed by the needle and the acupoint surface. It is applicable to acupoints on thin muscles or on the chest, hypochondrium and upper back with important internal organs near by. Oblique insertion can avoid damaging internal organs. In addition, it can also make the needling sensation go to the diseased area. → 迎随补泻(p. 567)

● 斜视 [xié shì] 病证名。见《世医得效方》。又称风牵偏视。多因脾胃之气不足，络脉空虚，风邪乘虚侵袭，目系拘急；或肝肾素亏，精血不足，目系失养，目珠维系失调所致，症见一眼或双眼黑睛偏向内眦或外眦，转动受限，严重者视一为二，若起病突然，发热、头痛、恶心、呕吐，苔白脉浮者为外感风邪；若起病缓慢，头晕目眩，视物昏朦，耳鸣，舌淡脉沉细者为肝肾亏损，治宜祛风通络，补益肝肾，取四白、合谷、风池、足三里、肝俞、肾俞、内斜视加太阳、瞳子髎；外斜视加睛明、攒竹，外感加风府、太阳，肝肾阴虚加太溪，照海。

Strabismus A syndrome, seen in *Shiyi De Xiaofang* (*Effective Prescriptions Handed Down to Generations*), also known as paralytic strabismus, mostly due to insufficiency of the qi of the spleen and stomach and deficiency of the collaterals leading to the invasion of the wind-evil and contracture by the eye system; or to deficiency of the liver and kidney and insufficiency of the essence and blood which leads to the failure to nourish the eye system and an inability to hold the eye and eyeball. ⟨Manifestations⟩ one eye or both eyes slanting to the inner or outer canthus, limitation of eye movement, or even diplopia. Sometimes, it occurs suddenly and manifests fever, headache, nausea, vomiting, whitish tongue coating and floating pulse. These manifestations are caused by the attack of exogenous wind evil. On the other hand, slow onset, dizziness with blurred vision, tinnitus, pale tongue, deep and thready pulse, are caused by deficiency of the liver and kidney. ⟨Treatment principle⟩ Dispel wind and dredge the meridians, tonifying the liver and kidney. ⟨Point selection⟩ Sibai (ST 2), Hegu (LI 4), Fengchi (GB 20), Zusanli (ST 36), Ganshu (BL 18), and Shenshu (BL 23). Add Taiyang (EX-HN 5) and Tongziliao (GB 1) for inner strabismus; add Jingming (BL 1) and Cuanzhu (BL 2) for outer strabismus; add Fengfu (DU 16) and Taiyang (EX-HN 5) for attack of exopathogen; and add Taixi (KI 3) and Zhaohai (KI 6) for deficiency of the yin of the liver and kidney.

● 泻方补圆 [xiè fāng bǔ yuán] 刺法用语。出《素问·八正神明论》。与泻圆补方不同。此是指针刺必须等待气血盛衰之时而施补泻。

Reducing Square and Reinforcing Round A needling method, from *Suwen*: *Ba Zheng Shenming Lun* (*Plain Questions*: *On Eight Natural Qi and Divinity*), different from reducing round and reinforcing square. This method means that the reinforcing or reducing method is applied when qi and blood are in an excessive or exhaustive state.

● 泻南补北 [xiè nán bǔ běi] 配穴法之一。见《难经·七十五难》。此法根据五行生克关系，提出对肝实肺虚而脾土无恙的病症，要用泻心火、补肾水的方法来治疗，东方（肝）实，西方（肺）虚，泻南方（心），补北方（肾）。因为火是木之子，泻火能抑木，又能减去克金的作用；水是木之母，金之子，补水能加强克火，又能济金抑木。所谓"子能令母实，母能令子虚"这种治法是对"虚者补其母，实者泻其子"的补充，说明五脏之间互相影响，治疗方法不能局限于补母泻子，并可据此推演，如心实肾虚，要泻脾补肝；脾实肝虚，要泻肺补心；肺实心虚，要泻肾补脾；肾实脾虚，要泻肝补肺。

Reducing South and Reinforcing North One of the methods of point selection, seen in *Nanjing*: *Qishiwu Nan* (*The Classic of Questions*: *Question 75*). This method, based on the restrictions of the five elements, indicates that the therapy of reducing heart-fire and reinforcing kidney-water should be applied to syndromes due to liver-excess and lung-deficiency but without symptoms of the spleen. The east direction (the liver) means excess while the west direction (the lung) deficiency, reducing south (the heart), reinforcing north (the kidney). Fire is the "son" of wood, so reducing fire can restrain wood and also decrease the function of counteracting metal; water is the "mother" of wood and the "son" of metal, so reinforcing water can strengthen the function of counteracting fire and also help metal restrain wood. This is the theory of "son can cause mother to become excessive, mother can cause son to become deficient". This therapy is the supplement to "reinforcing the mother organs when treating cases of deficiency and reducing the son when treating cases of excess". It shows the interacting relationship

of the five viscera. The therapy can not be limited to reinforcing the mother and reducing the son. It can also be further inferred according to the above mentioned therapy that one can reduce the spleen and reinforce the liver when treating cases of heart-excess and kidney-deficiency; reduce the lung and reinforce the heart when treating cases of spleen-excess and liver-deficiency; reduce the kidney and reinforce the spleen when treating cases of lung-excess and heart-deficiency; and reduce the liver and reinforce the lung when treating cases of kidney-excess and spleen-deficiency.

●泻圆补方[xiè yuán bǔ fāng] 刺法用语。见《灵枢·官针》。为补泻法的要领。意指泻法有如圆规,多用旋转,有利于祛邪,补法有如角尺,端端正正。不多转动,有利于扶正。

Reducing Round and Reinforcing Square A term for needling method, seen in *Lingshu: Guanzhen (Miraculous Pivot: Official Needles)*. This is the essential point of the reinforcing and reducing method. The reducing method uses the twirling and rotating manipulation most of the time, like a pair of compasses, which is beneficial to reducing pathogenic factors; the reinforcing method uses upright manipulation without more turning and rotating like a square angle, which is beneficial to strengthening the body resistance.

●泻子随母[xiè zǐ suí mǔ] 针刺补泻方法。出《流注指微赋》。又名子母补泻法。参见该条。

Reducing Son According to Mother A kind of reinforcing-reducing needle manipulation from *Liuzhu Zhiwei Fu (Ode to Subtleties of Flow)*, also named mother-child reinforcing-reducing method. →子母补泻法(p. 625)

●泄[xiè] ①宣泄。一般指宣泄肺气。②同"泻",多种腹泻的总称。③指泻法或用泻剂。④指筋缓缩不能收持之症。

1. **Dispersing** Generally referring to dispersing the flow of lung-qi.
2. The same as "泻"(xiè), a general name for various types of diarrhea.
3. **Purgative Prescription** Referring to the reducing method or a purgative prescription.
4. **A morbid condition** Referring to the slow contraction of the tendons.

●泄泻[xiè xiè] 病名。见《三因极一病证方论》。简称泻或泄。指大便稀薄,如水样,次数增多。本病分急性和慢性两类,前者因感受外邪或饮食所伤,实证居多。后者因脾胃虚弱,肝木侮土,或肾阳衰微所致,虚证居多。临床又可分为寒湿泻、湿热泻、伤食泻、肝郁泻、脾虚泻、肾虚泻。详见各条。

Diarrhea A syndrome, from *San Yin Ji Yi Bingzhengfang Lun (Treatise on the Three Categories of Pathogenic Factors of Diseases and the Prescriptions)*, a short form for an evacuation or excretion, referring to frequent watery stools. It is clinically divided into acute and chronic types. The former is due to the attack of exogenous pathogens or improper diet, mostly excess syndromes; the latter is due to deficiency of the spleen and stomach, the liver affecting the spleen or exhaustion of the kidney-yang, mostly deficiency syndromes. In the clinic, it is also divided into diarrhea due to cold-dampness; diarrhea due to damp-heat; diarrhea due to improper diet; diarrhea due to stagnation of the liver-qi; diarrhea due to spleen deficiency and diarrhea due to kidney deficiency. →寒湿泻(p. 157)、湿热泻(p. 372)、伤食泻(p. 349)、肝郁泻(p. 129)、脾虚泻(p. 296)、肾虚泻(p. 367)

●解脉[xiè mài] 出《素问·刺腰痛篇》。指足太阳散在腘窝部的血络。解,是分散或关节的意思。腰痛可刺委中、委阳部的血络。

Separative Vessel Originally from *Suwen: Ci Yaotong Pian (Plain Questions: On Treatment of Lumbago with Acupuncture)*, referring to the superficial venules of the Meridian of Foot-Taiyang scattered in the popliteal fossa. Here, "解"(xiè) means scatter or joint. The superficial venules in Weizhong(BL 40) and Weiyang(BL 39) regions can be punctured for treating lumbago.

●心[xīn] 耳穴名。①位于甲腔中心凹陷处。用于治疗失眠、心悸、癔病、盗汗、心绞痛、心动过速、心律不齐、无脉症、神经衰弱、口舌生疮。②位于耳背上部。〈主治〉疖肿、失眠、多梦、高血压、头痛。

Heart (MA) An auricular point. 〈Location ①〉in the depression of the middle cavity of concha. 〈Indications〉 insomnia, palpitation,

hysteria, night sweating, angina pectors, tachycardia, arrythmia, pulseless disease, neurosism and ulcer in the mouth and tongue. ⟨Location②⟩on the upper part of the back of ear. ⟨Indications⟩swelling furuncle, insomnia, dreamy sleep, hypertension and headache.

●心包经[xīn bāo jīng]　手厥阴心包经之简称。见

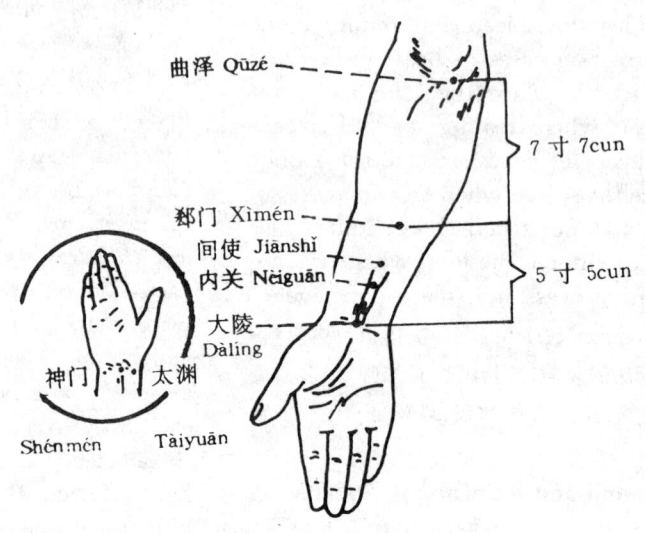

图66　心包经穴（前臂部）

Fig 66　Points of Pericardium Meridian

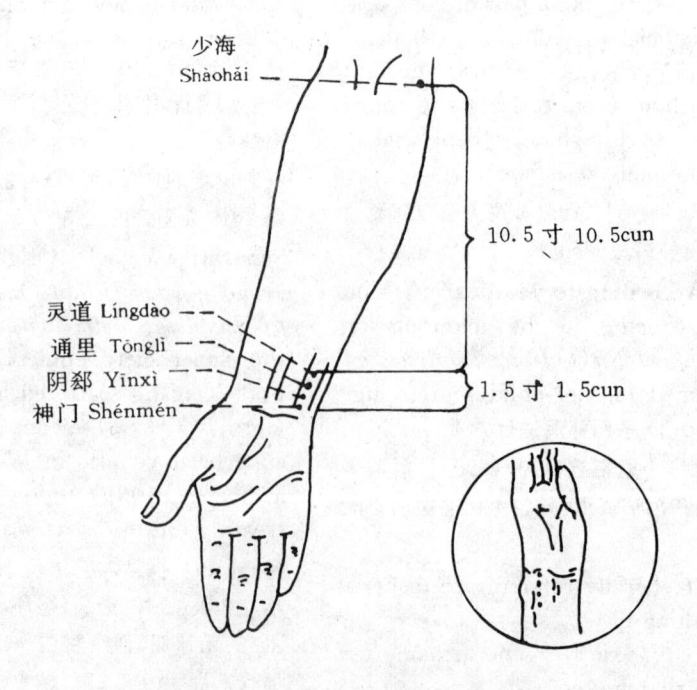

图67　心经穴（前臂部）

Fig 67　Points of Heart Meridian

该条。

Pericardium Meridian The short form for the Pericardium Meridian of Hand-Jueyin. → 手厥阴心包经(p. 390)

●心火亢盛尿血[xīn huǒ kàng shèng niào xuè] 尿血证型之一。多因心火亢盛，下移小肠所致。证见尿血鲜红，小便热赤，心烦口渴，口舌生疮，舌尖红，脉数。治宜清营血，泻心火。取关元、劳宫、然谷、少府。

Hematuria due to Flaring Heart-Fire A type of hematuria, mostly due to exuberant heart-fire moving downward to the small intestine. 〈Manifestations〉hematuria in bright-red color, dark and hot urine, irritability and thirst, ulcers in the mouth and tongue, red tongue tip, and rapid pulse. 〈Treatment principle〉Clear heat evil in the blood, purge pathogenic fire of the heart. 〈Point selection〉Guanyuan (RN 4), Laogong (PC 8), Rangu (KI 2) and Shaofu(HT 8).

●心悸[xīn jì] 病证名。见《千金要方·心脏》又名惊悸、怔忡。指以心中悸动，胸闷，心慌，善惊易怒为主症。多由气虚、血虚、痰火、瘀血所致。临床可分为气虚、血虚、痰火、瘀血心悸，详见各条。

Palpitation A disease, seen in *Qianjin Yaofang: Xinzang (Essential Prescriptions Worth a Thousand Gold: The Heart)*, also called palpitation due to fright or severe palpitation, referring to the syndrome characterized by rapid beating of the heart, suffocation of the chest, nervousness, susceptibility to fright and anger. Mostly caused by deficiency of qi and blood, phlegm-fire and blood stasis. Clinically, it is divided into palpitation due to qi deficiency; palpiration due to blood deficency; palpitation due to phlegm-fire and palpitation due to blood stasis. →气虚心悸(p. 310)、血虚心悸(p. 529)、痰火心悸(p. 423)、瘀血心悸(p. 570)

●心经[xīn jīng] 手少阴心经之简称。见该条。

Heart Meridian Short form for the Heart Meridian of Hand-Shaoyin. →手少阴心经(p. 395)

●心脾两虚不寐[xīn pí liǎng xū bù mèi] 不寐证型之一。由思虑忧愁，耗伤心脾，气血虚弱，心神失养所致。证见夜来不易入寐，寐则多梦易醒，心悸，健忘，容易出汗，面色少华，精神疲乏，脘痞，便溏，舌质淡，苔薄白，脉细弱，治宜补气养血。取脾俞、心俞、神门、三阴交、百会、四神聪。

Insomnia due to Deficiency of the Heart and Spleen A type of insomnia, caused by excessive worries consuming the heart and spleen deficiency of qi and blood and loss of nourishment of the heart. 〈Manifestations〉difficulty in falling asleep, dream-disturbed sleep or liability to waking, palpitations, forgetfulness, frequent sweating, pale complexion, lassitude, mass in the stomach, watery stools, pale tongue with thin and whitish coating, thready and weak pulse. 〈Treatment principle〉Invigorate qi and nourish blood. 〈Point selection〉Pishu(BL 20), Xinshu(BL 15), Shenmen(HT 7), Sanyinjiao (SP 6), Baihui (DU 20) and Sishencong(EX-HN 1).

●心手少阴之脉[xīn shǒu shào yīn zhī mài] 手少阴心经的原名。见该条。

Heart Vessel of Hand-Shaoyin The original name for the Heart Meridian of Hand-Shaoyin. →手少阴心经(p. 395)

●心俞[xīn shū] 经穴名。出《灵枢·背俞》。属足太阳膀胱经，为心的背俞穴。〈定位〉在背部，当第五胸椎棘突下，旁开1.5寸(图7)。〈层次解剖〉皮肤→皮下组织→斜方肌→菱形肌下缘→竖脊肌。浅层布有第五、六胸神经后支的内侧皮支及伴行的动、静脉。深层有第五、六胸神经后支的肌支和相应肋间后动、静脉背侧支的分支或属支。〈主治〉癫狂、痫证、惊悸、失眠、心悸、健忘、心烦、咳嗽、吐血、梦遗、心痛、胸引背痛，斜刺0.5～0.8寸；可灸。

Xinshu (BL 15) A meridian point, from *Lingshu: Beishu (Miraculous Pivot: Back-Shu Points)*, a point on the Bladder Meridian of Foot-Taiyang, and the Back-Shu point of the heart. 〈Location〉on the back, below the spinous process of the 5th thoracic vertebra, 1.5 cun lateral to the posterior midline (Fig. 7). 〈Regional anatomy〉skin→subcutaneous tissue→trapezius muscle→inferior border of rhomboid muscle→erector spinal muscle. In the superficial layer, there are the medial cutaneous branches of the posterior branches of the 5th and 6th thoracic nerve and the accompanying arteries and veins. In the deep layer, there are the muscular branches of the posteri-

or branches of the 5th and 6th thoracic nerves and the branches or tributaries of the dorsal branches of the related posterior intercostal arteries and veins. 〈Indications〉 manic-depressive psychosis, epilepsy, palpitations due to fright, insomnia, palpitations, forgetfulness, irritability, cough, hemoptysis, nocturnal emission, cardiac pain, back pain caused by the chest. 〈Method〉 Puncture obliquely 0.5~0.8 cun. Moxibustion is applicable.

● 心痛 [xīn tòng] 病证名。出《内经》。为胃脘部和心前区疼痛的总称。

Cardialgia A syndrome, from *Neijing* (*The Canon of Internal Medicine*), the general term for epigastric pain and precordial pain.

● 心系 [xīn xì] 指心脏周围的脉管组织。出《灵枢·经脉》。

Heart System The vasalium (meridians and collaterals) around the heart, originally from *Lingshu: Jingmai* (*Miraculous Pivot: Meridians*).

● 心下痛 [xīn xià tòng] 病证名。因胃脘作痛多在心窝处(剑突下，故名)。详见"胃痛"条。

Epigastric Pain A syndrome, so named because epigastric pain usually occurs in the scrobiculus cordis (below the xiphoid process). →胃痛(p.467)

● 心主 [xīn zhǔ] ①经脉名。出《灵枢·经脉》，指手厥阴心包经。②因各经以其原穴为代表，故心主又指手厥阴心包经的原穴大陵。

Heart Dominator ① The Pericardium Meridian of Hand-*Jueyin*. A meridian, originally from *Lingshu: Jingmai* (*Miraculous Pivot: Meridians*). ② Refers to Daling (PC 7), Each Yuan (Primary) point represents its own meridian, so it refers to Daling (PC 7), the Yuan (Primary) point of the Pericardium Meridian of Hand-Jueyin.

● 心主手厥阴心包络之脉 [xīn zhǔ shǒu jué yīn xīn bāo luò zhī mài] 手厥阴心包经原名，见该条。

Percardium Vessel of Hand-Jueyin The original name for the Pericardium Meridian of Hand-Jueyin. →手厥阴心包经(p.390)

● 辛頞鼻渊 [xīn è bí yuān] 即鼻渊。见该条。

Xin E Rhinorrhea →鼻渊(p.19)

● 新集明堂灸法 [xīn jí míng táng jiǔ fǎ] 书名。撰人不详，三卷。见宋《崇文总目》。书佚。

Xin Ji Mingtang Jiufa (New Collection of Mingtang Moxibustion) A book with an unknown author, 3 volumes, seen in *Chongwen Zongmu* (*Chong Wen Complete Catalogue*) of the Song Dynasty. The book is no longer extant.

● 新建 [xīn jiàn] 经外穴名。出《新针灸学》。位与居■同。见该条。

Xinjian (EX) An extra point, from *Xin Zhenjiuxue* (*New Science of Acupuncture and Moxibustion*). Its location is the same as that of Juliao (GB 29). →居髎(p.225)

● 新设 [xīn shè] 经外穴名。出《新针灸学》。在项部，当斜方肌外缘，后发际下1.5寸处。〈主治〉后头痛、项强、落枕、肩胛疼痛等。直刺0.5~1.0寸；可灸。

Xinshe (EX-HN) A meridian point, from *Xin Zhenjiuxue* (*New Science of Acupuncture and Moxibustion*). 〈Location〉 on the nape, on the lateral border of the trapezius muscle, 1.5 cun below the posterior hairline. 〈Indications〉 back headache, stiffness of the nape, stiffneck, pain in the scapular area. 〈Method〉 Puncture perpendicularly 0.5~1.0 cun. Moxibustion is applicable.

● 囟会 [xìn huì] 经穴名。出《灵枢·热病》。属督脉，又名顶门。〈定位〉在头部，当前发际正中直上2寸(百会前3寸)(图28)。〈层次解剖〉皮肤→皮下组织→帽状腱膜→腱膜下疏松组织。布有额神经及左、右颞浅动、静脉和额动、静脉的吻合网。〈主治〉头痛、目眩、面赤暴肿、鼻渊、鼻衄、鼻痔、鼻痛、癫疾、嗜睡、小儿惊风。平刺0.3~0.5寸，小儿禁刺；可灸。

Xinhui (DU 22) A meridian point, from *Lingshu: Rebing* (*Miraculous Pivot: Febrile Diseases*). A point on the Du Meridian, also named Dingmen. 〈Location〉 on the head, 2 cun directly above the midpoint of the anterior hairline and 3 cun anterior to Baihui (DU 20) (Fig. 28). 〈Regional anatomy〉 skin→subcutaneous tissue→epicranial aponeurosis→subaponeurotic loose tissue. There are the frontal nerve and the anastomotic network of the left and right superficial temporal arteries and veins with the left and right frontal arteries

and veins in this area. 〈Indications〉headache, blurring of vision, flushed face with sudden swelling, rhinorrhea, epistaxis, nasal polyp, nasal carbuncle, disorder of the brain, drowsiness, infantile convulsion. 〈Method〉Puncture perpendicularly 0.3~0.5 cun, needling forbidden for children. Moxibustion is applicable.

●囟中[xìn zhōng] 经外穴名。见《千金要方》。约与囟会穴同位。〈主治〉小儿暴痫，目反上视，眸子动。用灸法。

Xinzhong(EX-HN) An extra point, seen in *Qianjin Yaofang* (*Essential Prescriptions Worth a Thousand Gold*). 〈Location〉about the same location as Xinhui(DU 22). 〈Indications〉sudden epilepsy in children, abnormal vision of the eye with looking superiorly, abnormal moving of the pupil. 〈Method〉moxibustion.

●兴隆[xīng lóng] 经外穴名。见《凌氏汉章针灸全书》。在上腹部，当脐上一寸，旁开一寸处。〈主治〉心中冷急，气上攻结成痞块。直刺0.5~1寸；可灸。

Xinglong (EX-CA) An extra point, seen in *Lingshi Hanzhang Zhenjiu Quanshu* (*Ling Hanzhang's Complete Book of Acupuncture and Moxibustion*). 〈Location〉on the upper abdomen, 1 cun above the umbilicus and 1 cun lateral to the anterior midline. 〈Indications〉cold feeling in the heart, mass accumulated due to uprising attack of qi. 〈Method〉Puncture perpendicularly 0.5~1.0 cun. Moxibustion is applicable.

●惺惺[xīng xīng] ①经穴别名。出《肘后备急方》。即风府。见该条。②经外穴别名。见《医学入门》。即夺命。见该条。

Xingxing Another name for ①Fengfu(DU 16), a meridian point from *Zhouhou Beiji Fang*(*A Handbook of Prescription for Emergencies*). →风府(p. 111); ②an extra point seen in *Yixue Rumen* (*An Introduction to Medicine*). →夺命(p. 91)

●行痹[xíng bì] 痹证证型之一。出《素问·痹论》。由风寒湿邪闭阻经络，风邪偏盛所致。症见肢体关节酸痛，游走不定，关节屈伸不利；或见恶风发热，苔薄白，脉浮弦。治宜疏通经络，祛邪止痛，取膈俞、血海、大椎、风池、风府。肩部痛取肩髎、肩髃、臑俞。肘臂痛取曲池、合谷、天井、外关、尺泽。腕部痛取阳池、外关、阳溪、腕骨。背脊痛取身柱、腰阳关。臀部痛取环跳、居髎、悬钟。股部痛取秩边、承扶、阴陵泉。膝部痛取犊鼻、梁丘、阳陵泉、膝阳关。踝部痛取申脉、照海、昆仑、丘墟。

Migratory Arthralgia A type of arthralgia syndrome from *Suwen: Bi Lun* (*Plain Questions: On Bi-Syndromes*), mostly caused by attack of wind, cold, and damp evils, which block the meridians and collaterals with predominantly wind-evil. 〈Manifestations〉aching of the limbs and joins with migratory pain, limitation of the joints; or aversion to wind and fever, thin and whitish tongue coating, floating and wiry pulse. 〈Treatment principle〉Remove the obstruction of the meridians and collaterals, expel pathogenic factors to relieve pain. 〈Point selection〉Geshu(BL 17), Xuehai (SP 10), Dazhui(DU 14), Fengchi(GB 20), and Fengfu(DU 16). For pain in the shoulder region, select Jianliao(SJ 14), Jianyu(LI 15) and Naoshu(SI 10). For pain on the arm, select Quchi(LI 11), Hegu(LI 4), Tianjing(SJ 10), Waiguan(SJ 5) and Chize(LU 5). For pain on the wrist, select Yangchi(SJ 4), Waiguan(SJ 5), Yangxi(LI 5) and Wangu(SI 4). For pain on the back, select Shenzhu(DU 12), Yaoyangguan(DU 3). For pain in the thigh, select Huantiao(GB 30), Juliao(GB 29) and Xuanzhong(GB 39). For pain in the femur region, select Zhibian(BL 54), Chengfu (BL 36) and Yinlingquan(SP 9). For pain in the knee select Dubi(ST 35), Liangqiu(ST 34), Yanglingquan(GB 34) and Xiyangguan (GB 33). For pain at the ankle, select Shenmai(BL 62), Zhaohai(KI 6), Kunlun(BL 60) and Qiuxu(GB 40).

●行间[xíng jiān] 经穴名。出《灵枢·本输》。属足厥阴肝经，为本经荥穴。〈定位〉在足背侧，当第一、二趾间，趾蹼缘的后方赤白肉际处(图17.2)。〈层次解剖〉皮肤→皮下组织→拇趾近节趾骨基底部与第二跖骨头之间，布有腓深神经的趾背神经和趾背动、静脉。〈主治〉月经过多、闭经、痛经、白带、阴中痛、遗尿、淋症、疝气、胸胁满痛、呃逆、咳嗽、洞泻、头痛、眩晕、目赤痛、青盲、中风、癫痫、瘈疭、失眠、口㖞、膝肿、下肢内侧痛、足跗肿痛。直刺0.5~0.8寸；可灸。

Xingjian (LR 2)   A meridian point, from

Lingshu: Benshu (*Miraculous Pivot: Meridian Points*), the *Ying* (Spring) point of the Liver Meridian of Foot-Jueyin. ⟨Location⟩ on the instep of the foot, between the 1st and 2nd toes, at the junction of the red and white skin proximal to the margin of the web (Fig. 17.2). ⟨Regional anatomy⟩ skin → subcutaneous tissue → between base of proximal phalangeal bone of great toe and head of 2nd metatarsal bone. There are the dorsal digital nerve of the deep peroneal nerve and the dorsal digital artery and vein in this area. ⟨Indications⟩ profuse menstruation, amenorrhea, dysmenorrhea, leukorrhea, urethralgia, enuresis, stranguria, hernia, pain and fullness in the chest and hypochondrium, hiccup, cough, diarrhea, headache, dizziness, redness and pain in the eye, optic atrophy, apoplexy, epilepsy, clonic convulsion, insomnia, deviation of mouth, swelling knee, pain in the medial side of the lower extremities, swelling and pain on the back of foot. ⟨Method⟩ Puncture perpendicularly 0.5～0.8 cun. Moxibustion is applicable.

●行气法 [xíng qì fǎ] 针灸术语，指能促使针感扩散和传导的手法。行气法，又可统称调气法。参见该条。

Qi-Promoting Method A needling manipulation, referring to manipulations employed in acupuncture to spread and direct the transmission of the needling response. The qi-promoting method can also be named the qi-regulating method. →调气法 (p. 438)

●行针 [xíng zhēn] 针刺术语。又称运针。①指进针后，为了使之得气，调节针感以及进行补泻而施行的各种针刺手法。②指施行和运用针刺疗法。

Needle Transmission A term for needling manipulation, also named needle conveying, referring to ①various manipulations applied to regulate needle sensation and conduct reinforcing and reducing activities in order to achieve qi after needle insertion; ②manipulating and applying acupuncture therapy.

●行针指要赋 [xíng zhēn zhǐ yào fù] 针灸歌诀名。见《针灸聚英》。歌中列举一些常见证候的用穴。《针灸大成》载此，略有修改。全文如下：或针风，先向风府、百会中；或针水，水分侠脐上边取；或针结，针着大肠泻水穴；或针劳，须向膏肓及百劳；或针虚，气海、丹田、委中奇；或针嗽，肺俞、风门须用灸；或针痰，先针中脘、三里间；或针吐，中脘、气海、膻中补；翻胃，吐食一般医。针中有妙少人知。

Xingzhen Zhiyao Fu (Ode to the Essentials of Acupuncture) A verse on acupuncture and moxibustion, seen in *Zhenjiu Juying* (*Essentials of Acupuncture and Moxibustion*). Points used for some commonly seen syndromes are listed in the verse, and recorded in *Zhenjiu Dacheng* (*A Great Compendium of Acupuncture and Moxibustion*) with little revision. The full text of the verse is as follows: Fengfu (DU 16) and Baihui (DU 20) for treating diseases due to wind, Shuifen (RN 9) above the umbilicus for treating diseases due to water, points on the large intestine to reduce water for needling mass. Gaohuang (BL 43) and Bailao (EX) for needling pulmonary tuberculosis, Qihai (RN 6), Dantian (elixir field) and Weizhong (BL 40) for needling deficiency, Feishu (BL 13) and Fengmen (BL 12) by moxibustion for cough, Zhongwan (RN 12) and Sanjian (LI 3) for needling phlegm, Zhongwan (RN 12), Qihai (RN 6) and reinforcing Danzhong (RN 17) for needling vomiting, general treatment of regurgitation and vomiting. Few people know the wonders of this type of needling mentioned in the verse.

●行针总要歌 [xíng zhēn zǒng yào gē] 针灸歌赋名。见《针灸大成》卷三。内容是概括针法的要点，通俗易懂，易于上口。不足为仅举头面及颈部正中各穴，未及其它穴位。

Xingzhen Zongyao Ge (A Verse on Generals of Acupuncture) A verse on acupuncture and moxibustion, seen in Vol. 3 of *Zhenjiu Dacheng* (*A Great Compendium of Acupuncture and moxibustion*). A generalization of the primary needling methods of some important points in popular words and easy to read and understand. Yet, only the points on the face and the middle of the neck were listed without touching upon the others.

●胸 [xiōng] ①部位名。指缺盆下，腹之上。②耳穴名。位于胸椎穴内侧近耳腔缘。⟨主治⟩胸闷、胸痛、乳

腺炎、泌乳不足。

1. Chest A body part, referring to the region below the supracla vicular fossa and above the abdomen.

2. Chest(MA) An auricular point. ⟨Location⟩ on the border of the cavity of the ear and on the medial side of Thoracic Vertabra(MA). ⟨Indications⟩ oppressive feeling in the chest, chest pain, mastitis, and insufficient lactation.

●**胸痹**[xiōng bì] 病证名。出《灵枢·本藏》，是以胸痛彻背，上气喘息，咳唾为主的一种病证。多因心气虚衰，心阳不振，七情郁结，劳累受寒，饱食肥甘而致痰湿内蕴，气血运行不畅，心脉瘀阻而发，临床分虚寒型、痰浊型、瘀血型胸痹等，详见各条。

Obstruction of Qi in the Chest A syndrome from *Lingshu: Benzang* (*Miraculous Pivot: Zang Organs Proper*), characterized by chest pain rediating to the back, shortness of breath, and coughing. Mostly due to deficiency or exhaustion of heart-qi, hypofunction of heart-yang, stagnation of the seven emotions, overworking and invasion of cold, overeating of greasy and fleshy food leading to accumulation of phlegm-dampness, obstruction of qi and blood circulation and blockage of the heart meridian. It is clinically divided into obstrction of qi in the chest due to cold-deficiency, obstruction of qi in the chest due to phlegm turbidity and obstruction of qi in the chest due to blood stasis. →**虚寒胸痹**(p. 515)、**痰浊胸痹**(p. 426)、**瘀血胸痹**(p. 571)

●**胸薜**[xiōng bì] 薜息别名。见《经外奇穴汇编》。见该条。

Xiongbi Another name for Bixi(EX), also seen in *Jingwai Qixue Huibian* (*An Expository Manual of Extra Acupoints*). →**薜息**(p. 20)

●**胸腔区**[xiōng qiāng qū] 头针刺激区。在胃区与前后正中线之间，发际上下各引二厘米长直线。⟨主治⟩支气管哮喘，胸部不适等症。

Thoracic Cavity Area The region for stimulation of scalp acupuncture, located between the gastric region and anterior-posterior midline. Draw a straight line 2cm in length respectively above and below the hairline. ⟨Indications⟩ bronchial asthma and discomfort in the chest region.

●**胸堂**[xiōng táng] ①经穴别名。见《备急千金要方》即膻中。见该条。②经外穴名。出《针灸孔穴及其疗法便览》。在胸部，当两乳之间，胸骨之两缘。⟨主治⟩咳嗽、喘息、噎膈、咯血、心悸、怔忡、乳少、乳房痛等。用灸法。

1. Xiongtang Another name for Danzhong (RN 17), a meridian point seen in *Beiji Qianjin Yaofang* (*Essential Prescriptions Worth a Thousand Gold for Emergencies*). →**膻中**(p. 75)

2. Xiongtang(EX-CA) An extra point, originally from *Zhenjiu Kongxue Jiqi Liaofa Bianlan* (*Guide to Acupoints and Acupuncture Therapeutics*) ⟨Location⟩ on the chest, between the two breasts and two borders of the thoracic bones. ⟨Indications⟩ cough, dyspnea, hiccup, hemoptysis, palpitation, severe palpitation, insuffcient lactation, pain in the breasts, etc. ⟨Method⟩ moxibustion.

●**胸通谷**[xiōng tōng gǔ] 经外穴名。见《千金要方》，在胸部，当乳头下二寸处。⟨主治⟩心痛、胁痛、乳腺炎等。用灸法。

Xiongtonggu(EX-CA) An extra point, from *Qianjin Yaofang* (*Essential Prescriptions Worth a Thousand Gold*). ⟨Location⟩ on the chest, 2 cun below the nipples. ⟨Indications⟩ cardiac pain, hypochondriac and mastitis, etc. ⟨Method⟩ moxibustion.

●**胸乡**[xiōng xiāng] 经穴名。出《针灸甲乙经》。属足太阴脾经。⟨定位⟩在胸外侧部，当第三肋间隙，距前正中线6寸(图39.3和图40)。⟨层次解剖⟩皮肤→皮下组织→胸大肌→胸小肌。浅层布有第三肋间神经外侧皮支和胸腹壁静脉的属支。深层有胸内、外侧神经的分支，胸肩峰动、静脉的胸肌支和胸外侧动、静脉的分支或属支。⟨主治⟩胸胁胀痛、胸引背痛不得卧，斜刺或向外平刺0.5～0.8寸；可灸。

Xiongxiang(SP 19) A meridian point, originally from *Zhenjiu Jia-Yi Jing* (*A-B Classic of Acupuncture and Moxibustion*), a point of the spleen Meridian of Foot-Taiyin. ⟨Location⟩ on the lateral side of the chest, in the 3rd intercostal space, 6 cun lateral to the anterior midline (Figs. 39. 3 &40). ⟨Regional anatomy⟩ skin→subcutaneous tissue→greater

pectoral muscle → smaller pectoral muscle. In the superficial layer, there are the lateral cutaneous branches of the 3rd intercostal nerve and the tributaries of the thoracoepigastric vein. In the deep layer, there are the branches of the medial pectoral nerve and the lateral pectoral nerve, the pectoral branches of the thoracoacromial artery vein and the branches of tirbutaries of the lateral thoracic artery and vein. ⟨Indications⟩ sensation of fullness and pain in the chest and hypochondriac region, chest pain rediating to the back and inability to lie flat. ⟨Method⟩ Puncture obliquely or subcutaneously 0.5～0.8 cun toward the lateral side. Moxibustion is applicable.

●胸之阴俞[xiōng zhī yīn shū] 经穴别名。见《西方子明堂灸经》。即长强。见该条。

Xiongzhiyinshu Another name for Changqiang(DU 1), a meridian point seen in *Xi Fang Zi Mingtang Jiujing*(*Xi Fang Zi Classic of Moxibustion*). → 长强(p. 39)

●胸椎[xiōng zhuī] 耳穴名。位于轮屏切迹至对耳轮上、下脚分叉处分为五等分, 中五分之二为胸椎。具有强脊益髓的作用, 主治胸胁疼痛、乳腺炎、泌乳不足、经前乳房胀痛。

Thoracic Vertebrae（MA） An auricular point. ⟨Location⟩ There are five equal shares from the incisure of helix to the branching point of the upper and lower crus of helix, the middle two fifths is the point. ⟨Functions⟩ Strengthen the spine and benefit marrow. ⟨Indications⟩ pain in the chest and hypochondriac region, mastitis, insufficient lactation, and distension and pain in the breast before the menses.

●休息痢[xiū xī lì] 痢疾证型之一。见《诸病源候论·痢疾诸候》。多因治疗失宜, 或气血虚弱, 脾肾不足, 以致正虚邪恋, 湿热伏于肠胃而成。证见下痢时发时止, 日久难愈, 倦怠怯冷, 嗜卧, 临厕里急腹痛, 大便夹有粘液或见赤色, 舌质淡、苔腻, 脉濡软或虚数。治宜温中祛邪, 疏调肠胃。针合谷、天枢、上巨虚、脾俞、胃俞、肾俞、关元。可加灸。

Chronic Dysentery with Frequent Relapse A type of dysentery, seen in *Zhubing Yuanhou Lun: Liji Zhuhou*(*General Treatise on the Etiology and Symptomatology of Diseases: Causes and Symptoms of Dysentery*), mostly caused by improper treatment, deficiency of qi and blood, and insufficiency of the spleen and kidney leading to the struggle of the weak body-resistance and pathogenic factors and the retention of dampheat in the intestines and stomach. ⟨Manifestations⟩ intermittent dysentery with chronic course and a tendency to relapse, listlessness and aversion to cold, drowsiness, contraction of genital organ and abdominal pain, sticky fluid and blood in the stools, pale tongue with greasy coatting, soft or weak and rapid pulse. ⟨Treatment principle⟩ Warm the middle-*jiao* to remove evils; regulate the intestines and stomach. ⟨Point selection⟩ Hegu (LI 4), Tianshu (ST 25), Shangjuxu (ST 37), Pishu (BL 20), Weishu (BL 21), Shenshu (BL 23) and Guanyuan(RN 4). Moxibustion is applicable.

●绣球风[xiù qiú fēng] 即肾囊风。见该条。

Scrotal Eczema → 肾囊风(p. 365)

●虚秘[xū bì] 便秘证型之一。见《卫生宝鉴》。多因病后、产后气血未复, 气虚转运无力, 血虚肠失润下所致。证见小腹不适, 有便意而努责乏力, 多汗, 短气, 疲惫, 面色少华, 心悸, 目眩, 无力排出大便, 粪质松散如糟粕, 舌淡白, 脉细弱无力。治宜补气养血。取脾俞、胃俞、大肠俞、三阴交、足三里、关元。

Constipation of Insufficiency Type A type of constipation seen in *Weisheng Baojian*(*A Treasured Mirror of Health Protection*), mostly caused by deficiency of qi and blood after illness or delivery, general debility due to qi deficiency and loss of intestine nourishment due to blood deficiency. ⟨Manifestations⟩ discomfort of the lower abdomen, inability to discharge stools in spite of efforts, profuse sweating, shortness of breath, fatigue, pale complexion, palpitation, blurring of vision, unable to discharge stools, loose stools like dross, pale tongue and thready and weak pulse. ⟨Treatment principle⟩ Invigorate qi and nourish blood. ⟨Point selection⟩ Pishu(BL 20), Weishu (BL 21), Dachangshu(BL 25), Sanyinjiao(SP 6), Zusanli(ST 36) and Guanyuan(RN 4).

●虚寒呕吐[xū hán ǒu tù] 呕吐证型之一。由于脾胃虚弱, 中阳不振, 胃失和降所致。证见饮食稍有不

慎。即易呕吐,时作时止,面色㿠白,倦怠无力,口干而不欲饮,四肢不温,大便溏稀,舌质淡,脉濡弱。治宜健脾益胃。针脾俞、胃俞、足三里、阴陵泉、中脘、章门、内关。加灸。

Vomiting due to Cold of Insufficiency Type A type of vomiting, due to deficiency of the spleen and stomach, dysfunction of the middle-yang and failure of the stomach-qi to descend. 〈Manifestations〉 vomiting after improper diet with intermittent condition, pale complexion, lassitude, dry mouth without wanting a drink, cold limbs, loose stools, pale tongue, and soft and weak pulse. 〈Treatment principle〉 Invigorate the spleen and stomach. 〈Point selection〉 Pishu(BL 20), Weishu(BL 21), Zusanli(ST 36), Yinlingquan(SP 9), Zhongwan(RN 12), Zhangmen(LR 13) and Neiguan(PC 6). 〈Method〉 Moxibustion is applicable in addition to acupuncture.

●**虚寒胸痹**[xū hán xiōng bì] 胸痹证型之一。多因素体阳衰,胸阳不足,阴寒之邪乘虚侵袭,寒凝气滞,痹阻胸阳所致。证见胸痛彻背,心悸,胸闷短气,恶寒,肢冷,受寒则甚,苔白滑,脉沉迟。治宜助阳散寒。针心俞、厥阴俞、内关、通里、气海、关元。可加灸。

Obstruction of Qi in the Chest due to Cold of Insufficiency Type A type of obstruction of qi in the chest. Mostly due to yang-exhaustion of the body, insufficiency of chest-yang, or invasion of yin-cold evil when the body is deficient leading to the stasis of cold and qi which blocks the chest-yang. 〈Manifestations〉 chest pain radiating to the back, palpitation, full feeling in the chest and shortness of breath, aversion to cold, cold limbs, even more serious when attacked by cold-evil, whitish and smooth tongue coating deep and slow pulse. 〈Treatment principle〉 Strengthen yang to dispel cold. 〈Point selection〉 Xinshu(BL 15), Jueyinshu(BL 14), Neiguan(PC 6), Tongli(HT 5), Qihai(RN 6) and Guanyuan(RN 4). Moxibustion is applicable in addition to acupuncture.

●**虚寒胃痛**[xū hán wèi tòng] 胃痛证型之一。由脾胃虚寒,脏腑脉络失于温养所致。证见胃痛隐隐、泛吐清水。喜暖喜按,纳食减少,神疲乏力,甚则手足欠温,大便溏薄,舌质淡,脉软弱。治宜温中补虚止痛。针脾俞、胃俞、章门、中脘、足三里、内关、关元、公孙。可加灸。

Stomachache due to Cold of Insufficiency Type A type of gastric pain, due to deficiency cold of the spleen and stomach and failure to warm and nourish the zang-fu organs and meridians. 〈Manifestations〉 sensation of dull pain in the stomach, vomiting clear water from mouth, relieved by warmness and pressing, poor appetite, lassitude, cold hands and feet and watery stools, pale tongue and soft and weak pulse. 〈Treatment principle〉 Warm the middle-jiao and reinforce the deficiency to stop pain. 〈Point selection〉 Pishu(BL 20), Weishu(BL 21), Zhangmen(LR 13), Zhongwan(RN 12), Zusanli(ST 36), Neiguan(PC 6), Guanyuan(RN 4) and Gongsun(SP 4). Moxibustion is applicable in addition to acupuncture.

●**虚火牙痛**[xū huǒ yá tòng] 牙痛证型之一。因肾阴不足,虚火上炎所致。证见牙痛隐隐。时作时止,牙齿浮动,口不臭,舌尖红,脉细,治宜滋阴降火。取太溪、行间、合谷、下关、颊车。

Toothache due to Deficiency Fire A type of toothache, caused by insufficiency of the kidney-yin and flaring-up of deficiency-fire. 〈Manifestations〉 intermittent dull toothache, loose tooth, without foul smell in the mouth, red tip of the tongue and thready pulse. 〈Treatment principle〉 Nourish yin to reduce the deficiency-fire. 〈Point selection〉 Taixi(KI 3), Xingjian(LR 2), Hegu(LI 4), Xiaguan(ST 7) and Jiache(ST 6).

●**虚里**[xū lǐ] 胃之大络名。出《素问·平人气象论》。其脉从腰贯膈,上络于肺,而出于左乳之下,当心尖搏动处。

Xuli(Collateral) The Main Collateral of the Stomach, originally from *Suwen: Pingren Qixiang Lun* (*Plain Questions: On Normal People's Physiology*). The meridian, begins at the waist, ascends upward through the diaphragm to connect the lung and emerges below the left breast, at the beating point of the cardiac apex.

●**虚热咽喉肿痛**[xū rè yān hóu zhǒng tòng] 咽喉肿痛证型之一,因肾阴亏耗,阴液不能上润咽喉,虚火

上炎,灼于咽喉所致。证见咽喉稍见红肿、疼痛较轻、口干舌燥、颊赤唇红、手足心热、舌质红、脉细数。治宜滋阴降火。取太溪、照海、鱼际。

Swelling and Pain of the Throat due to Heat of Deficiency Type One type of swelling and pain of the throat, due to consumption of kidney-yin, failure of the yin-fluid to ascend to nourish the throat, causing flaring-up of deficiency-fire which burns the throat. 〈Manifestations〉 slight redness and swelling of the throat with slight pain, dry mouth and tongue, flushed face and red lip, fever in the palm and sole, red tongue and thready and rapid pulse. 〈Treatment principle〉 Nourish yin to reduce pathogenic fire. 〈Point selection〉 Taixi(KI 3), Zhaohai(KI 6) and Yuji(LU 10).

●虚热经行先期[xū rè jīng xíng xiān qī] 经行先期的证型之一。多因久病之后损气伤阴,阴血不足,虚热内生,冲任不固所致。证见经期提前,经量较少,色红质稠,潮热盗汗,手足心热,腰膝酸软,舌红苔少,脉细数。治宜养阴清热。取关元、血海、三阴交、复溜、然谷。

Preceded Menstrual Cycle due to Heat of Deficiency Type A type of advanced menstruation, generally caused by the impairment of qi and yin after a prolonged illness, insufficiency of yin-blood, deficiency-heat in the interior leading to debility of the Chong and Ren Meridians. 〈Manifestations〉 advanced menstrual period, small amount of menses, red and thick menses, hectic fever and night sweat, fever in the palm and sole, aching and weakness of the waist and knee, red tongue with thin coating, thready and rapid pulse. 〈Treatment principle〉 Nourish yin and clear heat. 〈Point selection〉 Guanyuan(RN 4), Xuehai(SP 10), Sanyinjiao(SP 6), Fuliu(KI 7) and Rangu(KI 2).

●虚则补之[xū zé bǔ zhī] 针灸治疗原则之一。出《灵枢·经脉》。与"盛则泻之"相对,又称虚则实之。意指对虚证宜用补法以实其正气,如虚寒证则可用温灸法。

Illness of Deficiency Type should be Treated by Tonifying Method One of the principles of acupuncture treatment, from *Lingshu: Jingmai*(*Miraculous Pivot: Meridians*), the opposite of the principle of "Illness of excess type should be treated by reducing method", also known as the principle of deficiency disorders should be strengthened", referring to the application of the reinforcing method in deficiency syndromes aimed at strengthening the body resistance, e. g. warming moxibustion can be apllied to deficiency cold syndrome.

●徐春甫[xú chūn fǔ] 人名。明代医学家,字汝元,祁门(今属安徽)人。其博览医书,兼通针灸,曾任太医院医官。编辑《古今医统》百卷,刊于1556年。书内有其自撰的《经穴发明》和《针灸直指》两卷,主张良医治病应针灸、药物并用。

Xu Chunfu A famous physician in the Ming Dynasty, who styled himself Ruyuan, from Qimen County(of Anhui Province today). He read a great variety of medical books and was also good at acupuncture and moxibustion. He was once appointed a medical officer in an imperial hospital. He compiled *Gu Jin Yitong* (*The General Medicine of the Past and Present*) in 100 volumes, which was published in 1556. In the book, he himself wrote two volumes: *Jingxue Faming*(*Invention On Meridian Points*) and *Zhenjiu Zhizhi*(*Straightforward Exposition of Acupuncture and Moxibustion*), in which he maintained that a good physician should apply acupuncture, moxibustion and drugs at the same time in clinic.

●徐而疾则实[xú ér jí zé shí] 针刺补法的要领,与泻法"疾而徐则虚"对举,出《灵枢·九针十二原》。指缓慢地进针,迅速地出针,能使正气实,即为补。后世补法用三进一退,或二进一退即出于此。参见"徐疾补泻"条。又指补法要缓慢地出针,并迅速按住穴位。参见"开阖补泻"条。

Reinforcement Can Be Achieved by Slow-yet-Rapid Needling The principle of using the reinforcing method in acupuncture, contrary to "reduction can be achieved by rapid-yet-slow needling", from *Lingshu: Jiu Zhen Shier Yuan*(*Miraculous Pivot: On Nine Needles and Twelve Sources*). It means that slow insertion and rapid withdrawal can cause the body resistance to become strong, which is regarded as reinforcing. In later generations, three in-

sertions with one withdrawal, or two insertions with one withdrawal of reinforcing method developed from the above mentioned principle. See "slow-rapid reinforcing-reducing method". It also means in using the reinforcing method, withdrawal of the needle should be slow and the selected acupoint should be pressed rapidly. →开阖补泻(p. 230)

●徐凤[xú fēng] 人名。明代针灸家,字廷瑞,弋阳石塘(今属江西)人。学针于倪孟仲、彭九思。晚年著《针灸大全》。又自撰《金针赋》、《子午流注逐日按时定穴歌》等。

Xu Feng An acupuncture-moxibustion expert in the Ming Dynasty, who styled himself Ting Rui, a native of Shitang, Yiyang (in Jiangxi province today). He learned acupuncture from Ni Mengzhong and Peng Jiusi, and wrote *Zhenjiu Daquan* (*A Complete Collection of Acupuncture and Moxibustion*) in his later years, and composed *Jin Zhen Fu* (*Ode to Gloden Needle*) and *Ziwu Liuzhu Zhuri Anshi Dingxue Ge* (*Verses on Midnight-Noon Ebb-Flow to Match the Hour in Point Selection*), etc.

●徐疾补泻[xú jí bǔ xiè] 针刺补泻法之一。见《灵枢·九针十二原》。以进针和退针的快(疾)阳(徐)来区分补泻。即徐进针疾出针为补,疾进针徐出针为泻。

Slow-Rapid Reinforcing-Reducing Method One of the reinforcing-reducing methods in acupuncture therapy from *Lingshu: Jiu Zhen Shier Yuan* (*Miraculous Pivot: On Nine Needles and Twelve Sources*). Reinforcing and reducing are distinguished according to the speed with which the needle is inserted and withdrawn. Slow insertion and rapid withdrawal is reinforcement; rapid insertion and slow withdrawal is reduction.

●徐廷璋[xú tíng zhāng] 人名。明代针灸家,里籍不详。精针术,撰《活人妙法针经》二卷,已佚。见《中国医籍考》。

Xu Tingzhang An acupuncture-moxibustion expert in the Ming Dynasty, his native place unknown, skillful in acupuncture and compiler of *Huoren Miaofa Zhenjing* (*Acupuncture Canon of Magical Methods for Saving Life*) in 2 volumes, which is no longer extant. See *Zhongguo Yiji Kao* (*Study on Chinese Ancient Books on Medicine*).

●徐文中[xú wén zhōng] 人名。元代针灸家,字用和,安微宣城人,善针灸。事见《宣城县志》。

Xu Wenzhong An acupuncture-moxibustion expert in the Ming Dynasty, who styled himself Yonghe, from Xuancheng of Anhui Province, good at acupuncture and moxibustion. See *Xuanchengxian Zhi* (*Annals of Xuancheng County*).

●徐悦[xú yuè] 人名,隋代针灸家。撰《体疗杂病疾源》三卷,又与龙衔素合著《针经并孔穴蝦蟇图》三卷,均佚。

Xu Yue An acupuncture-moxibustion expert in the Sui Dynasty, who wrote *Tiliao Zabing Jiyuan* (*Physical Practice, Miscellaneous Diseases and Etiology*) in 3 volumes, and composed *Zhenjing Bing Kongxue Hama Tu* (*Frog Charts of Acupuncture Meridians and Points*) in 3 volumes in collaboration with Long Xiansu. These two books are no longer extant.

●许希[xǔ xī] 人名。宋代医家,开封人。以医为业,擅长针灸,翰林医学。1034年(景祐元年)仁宗病,侍医数进药不效,希得荐而施针刺心下包络之法治愈。命为翰林医官,后为殿中省尚药奉御,撰有《神应针经要诀》一卷。

Xu Xi A medical expert in the Song Dynasty, a native of Kaifeng. He specialized in medicine and was skillful in acupuncture and moxibustion and medicine of the Imperial Academy. Renzong (an emperor of the Song Dynasty) fell ill in 1034 (the first year of Jingyou's reign). The attendant physician failed to cure him of the disease after continuous administration. Xu Xi was recommended and cured the emperor by puncturing the pericardium collateral below the heart. He was appointed an official of the Medical Bureau and later he became the imperial chief pharmacologist. He wrote one volume of *Shen-ying Zhengjing Yaojue* (*Essentials of Acupuncture Canon of Divine Resonance*).

●许裕卿[xǔ yù qīng] 人名。清代针灸家,徽州(今属安徽)人。常往来于歙县、休宁之间,善以手指代

针,治疗多奇效,撰有《遯气符医纪》。

Xu Yuqing An acupuncture-moxibustion expert in the Qing Dynasty, from Huizhou (in Anhui Province today). Frequently coming and going in Shexian and Xiuning counties, he was good at acupuncture treatment with fingers instead of needles and achieved noticeable effect. He wrote *Dunqi Fuyi Ji* (*Records of Mediceal Treament with a Tally for Preventing Qi Disorder*).

●絮针[xù zhēn] 古代生活用针具。絮,指棉絮,盖以此针粗大,用于缝制被服,故名。《灵枢·九针论》中的圆针、锋针,均取法于絮针。

Xu-Needle A needle used in ancient times. Here "絮"(xù) means cotton. It was so named because of its thick and big body and its use for sewing clothes and quilt. Round-sharp and lance needles mentioned in *Lingshu: Jiuzhen Lun* (*Miraculous Pivot: On Nine Needles*) were derived from xu-needle.

●蓄血成胀[xù xuè chéng zhàng] 即血鼓,详该条。

Abdominal Distension due to Accumulated Blood. →血鼓(p. 524)

●玄悟会要针经[xuán wù huì yào zhēn jīng] 书名。宋代王处明撰,五卷。现已佚。见《宋史·艺文志》。

Xuanwu Huiyao Zhenjing (*Canon for Understanding the Essentials of Acupuncture*) A book, written by Wang Chuming in the Song Dynasty, 5 volumes in all, no longer extant. Cf *Songshi: Yi Wen Zhi* (*The History of the Song Dynasty: Records of Art and Literature*).

●玄悟四神针法[xuán wù sì shén zhēn fǎ] 书名。撰人不详,一卷,现已佚。见《崇文总目》。

Xuanwu Sishen Zhenfa (*Comprehension of Four-Spirit Methods of Acupuncture*) A book, its author unknown, 1 volume and no longer extant. Cf. *Chongwen Zongmu* (*Chong Wen Complete Catalogue*).

●旋耳疮[xuán ěr chuāng] 病名。见《医宗金鉴》。即耳部湿疹,好发于耳廓周围。症见皮肤潮红,奇痒,搔之糜烂,渗水,结痂。若发于耳后,可见耳后褶缝如刀割之状。见"湿疹"条。

Eczema of the Ear A disease, seen in *Yizong Jinjian* (*Gold Mirror of Orthodox Medical Lineage*), namely, eczema which occurs on the ear region, usually seen around the auricle. 〈Manifestations〉hectic redness on the skin, severe itch, rot induced by scratching, oozing water, and scab. If it occurs behind the ear, it is manifested as the crease behind the ear like a cut by a knife. →湿疹(p. 373)

●旋机[xuán jī] 经穴别名。出《备急千金要方》。即璇玑。见该条。

Xuanji(旋机) Another name for Xuanji (RN 21), a meridian point from *Beiji Qianjin Yao Fang* (*Essential Prescriptions Worth a Thousand Gold for Emergencies*). →璇玑(p. 520)

●旋玑[xuán jī] 经穴别名。出《太平圣惠方》。即璇玑。见该条。

Xuanji(旋玑) Another name for Xuanji (RN 21), a meridian point from *Taiping Shenghui Fang* (*Imperial Benevolent Prescriptions*). →璇玑(p. 520)

●悬浆[xuán jiāng] 经穴别名。出《铜人腧穴针灸图经》。即承浆。见该条。

Xuanjiang Another name for Chengjiang (RN 24), a meridian point from *Tongren Shuxue Zhenjiu Tujing* (*Illustrated Manual of Points for Acupuncture and Moxibustion on a Bronze Stature with Acupoints*). →承浆(p. 43)

●悬厘[xuán lí] 经穴名。出《针灸甲乙经》。属足少阳胆经,为手足少阳、阳明之会。〈定位〉在头部鬓发上,当头维与曲鬓弧形连线的上3/4与下1/4交点处(图28)。〈层次解剖〉同颔厌穴。〈主治〉偏头痛、面肿、目外眦痛、耳鸣、上齿痛。向后平刺0.5～0.8寸;可灸。

Xuanli(GB 6) A meridian point from *Zhenjiu Jia-Yi Jing* (*A-B Classic of Acupuncture and Moxibustion*), a point on the Gallbladder Meridian Foot-Shaoyang, the Crossing point of Shaoyang Meridians of Hand and Foot and Yangming Meridians. 〈Location〉on the head, in the hair above the temples, at the junction of the upper three fourths and lower one-fourth of the curved line connecting Touwei (ST 8) and Qubin (GB 7) (Fig. 28). 〈Regional anatomy〉Same as Hanyan (GB 4). 〈Indications〉migraine, swelling of the face, pain in the outer canthus, tinnitus, pain in the upper teeth. 〈Method〉Puncture subcutaneously 0.5～0.8 cun towards the posterior aspect. Moxibustion is applicable.

●**悬颅**[xuán lú] 经穴名。出《灵枢·寒热病》。属足少阳胆经,为手足少阳、阳明之会。〈定位〉在头部鬓发上,当头维与曲鬓弧形连线的中点处(图28)。〈层次解剖〉同颔厌穴。〈主治〉偏头痛、面肿、目外眦痛,向后平刺0.5～0.8寸;可灸。

Xuanlu(GB 5) A meridian point, from *Ling Shu: Han Re Bing* (*Miraculous Pivot: Cold and Heat Diseases*), a point on the Gallbladder meridians of Foot-Shaoyang, the crossing point of Shaoyang Meridian of Hand and Foot and Yangming Meridians. 〈Location〉on the head, in the hair above the temples, at the midpoint of the curved line connecting Touwei (ST 8) and Qubin (GB 7) (Fig. 28). 〈Regional anatomy〉Same as Hanyan (GB 4). 〈Indications〉migraine, swelling of the face, pain in the outer canthus. 〈Method〉Puncture subcutaneously 0.5～0.8 cun towards the posterior aspect. Moxibustion is applicable.

●**悬命**[xuán mìng] 经外穴名。出《千金要方》。又名鬼禄。在口腔内,当上唇系带之中点处。〈主治〉癫狂、昏迷诂语、小儿惊痫等。直刺0.1～0.2寸。

Xuanming (EX-HN) An extra point, from *Qianjin Yaofang* (*Essential Prescriptions Worth a Thousand Gold*), also known as Guilu. 〈Location〉in the mouth, at the midpoint of the frenum of the upper lip. 〈Indications〉epilepsy, coma and delirium, and infantile convulsion, etc. 〈Method〉Puncture perpendicularly 0.1～0.2 cun.

●**悬起灸**[xuán qǐ jiǔ] 艾条的一种。与实按灸相对。将艾条空悬于穴位上方施灸,不致灼伤皮肤。操作时可集中熏灸一处,或作较大范围的回旋灸,也可作一起一落的雀啄灸,参见"回旋灸"及"雀啄灸"条。

Suspended Moxibustion A form of moxa-cone moxibustion, the opposite of pressing moxibustion. Suspend a moxa roll and ignite it. The moxibustion is done a certain distance over the selected acupoint so as not to burn the skin. The moxa roll can be concentrated on one point during the treatment, or revolved over a large area or used in bird-pecking moxibustion. →回旋灸(p.177)、雀啄灸(p.328)

●**悬泉**[xuán quán] 经穴别名。出《备急千金要方》。即中封。见该条。

Xuanquan Another name for Zhongfeng (LR 4), a meridian point from Beiji *Qianjin Yaofang* (*Essential Prescriptions Worth a Thousand Gold for Emergencies*). →中封(p.609)

●**悬枢**[xuán shū] 经穴名。出《针灸甲乙经》,属督脉,又名悬柱。〈定位〉在腰部。当后正中线上,第一腰椎棘突下凹陷中(图12.2和图7)。〈层次解剖〉皮肤→皮下组织→棘上韧带→棘间韧带。浅层主要布有第一腰神经后支的内侧支和伴行的动、静脉。深层有棘突间的椎外(后)静脉丛,第一腰神经后支的分支和第一腰动、静脉脊侧支的分支或属支。〈主治〉腰脊强痛、腹胀、腹痛、完谷不化、泄泻、痢疾。直刺0.5～1.0寸;可灸。

Xuanshu (DU 5) A meridian point, from *Zhenjiu Jia-Ji Jing* (*A-B Classic of Acupuncture and Moxibustion*), a point on the *Du* Meridian, also known as Xuanzhu. 〈Location〉on the low back, on the posterior midline, in the depression below the spinous process of the lst lumbar vertebra (Figs. 12.2 &7). 〈Regional anatomy〉skin→subcutaneous tissue→supraspinal ligament→interspinal ligament. In the superficial layer, there are the medial branches of the posterior branches of the lst lumbar nerve and the accompanying artery and vien. In the deep layer, there are the external (posterior) vertebral venous plexus between the adjacent spinous processes, the branches of the posterior branches of the lst lumbar nerve and the branches or tributaries of the dorsal branches of the lst lumbar artery and vien. 〈Indications〉pain and stiffness of the lower back, abdominal distention, abdominal pain, diarrhea with undigested food, dysentery. 〈Method〉Puncture perpendicularly 0.5～1.0 cun. Moxibustion is applicable.

●**悬钟**[xuán zhōng] 经穴名。出《针灸甲乙经》。属足少阳胆经,八会穴的髓会。又名绝骨。〈定位〉在小腿外侧,当外踝尖上3寸,腓骨前缘(图8.1)。〈层次解剖〉皮肤→皮下组织→趾长伸肌→小腿骨间膜。浅层布有腓肠外侧皮神经。深层有腓深神经的分支,如穿透小腿骨间膜可刺中腓动、静脉。〈主治〉半身不遂、颈项强痛、胸腹胀满、胁肋疼痛、膝腿痛、脚气、腋下肿,直刺0.5～0.8寸;可灸。

Xuanzhong (GB 39) A meridian point, from *Zhenjiu Jia-Yi Jing* (*A-B Classic of Acupunc-

ture and Moxibustion) a point on the Gallbladder Meridian of Foot-Shaoyang, the influential point of the marrow of the Eight Influential Points. also known as Juegu. 〈Location〉on the lateral side of the leg, 3 cun above the tip of the external malleolus, on the anterior border of the fibula (Fig. 8.1). 〈Regional anatomy〉 skin→subcutaneous tissue→long extensor muscle of toes→interosseous membrane of leg. In the superficial layer, there is the lateral sural cutaneous nerve. In the deep layer, there are the branches of the peroneal nerve. If the needle penetrates through the interosseous membrane of the leg, the peroneal artery and vein may be injured. 〈Indications〉 hemiplegia, neck rigidity, fullness of the chest, abdominal distention, pain in the hypochondriac region, pain in the knee and leg, beriberi, and swelling in armpit. 〈Method〉 Puncture perpendicularly 0.5～0.8 cun. Moxibustion is applicable.

●悬柱[xuán zhù]经穴别名。出《医学入门》。即悬枢。见该条。

Xuanzhu Another name for Xuanshu (DU 5), a meridian point from *Yixue Rumen* (*An Introduction to Medicine*).→悬枢(p.519)

●璇玑[xuán jī] 经穴名。出《针灸甲乙经》。属任脉，又名旋机、旋玑。〈定位〉在胸部，当前正中线上，天突下1寸(图40)。〈层次解剖〉皮肤→皮下组织→胸大肌起始腱→胸骨柄。主要布有锁骨上内侧神经和胸廓内动、静脉的穿支。〈主治〉咳嗽、气喘、胸满痛、喉痹咽肿、胃中有积。平刺0.3～0.5寸；可灸。

Xuanji (RN 21) A meridian point, originally from *Zhenjiu Jia-Yi Jing* (*A-B Classic of Acupuncture and Moxibustion*), a point on the Ren Meridian, also called Xuanji(旋机)and (旋玑) (different in Chinese character). 〈Location〉on the chest and on the anterior midline, 1 cun below Tiantu(RN 22)(Fig. 40). 〈Regional anatomy〉 skin→subcutaneous tissue → origin of greater pectoral muscle → manubrium of sternum. There are the medial supraclavicular nerve and the perforating branches of the internal thoracic artery and vein in this area. 〈Indications〉 cough, asthma, fullness and pain in the chest, inflammation of the throat, swelling of the throat, retention of food in the stomach. 〈Method〉 Puncture subcutaneously 0.3～0.5 cun. Moxibustion is applicable.

●选饭[xuǎn fàn] 即恶阻。见该条。

Choosing Food →恶阻(p.93)

●选穴法[xuǎn xué fǎ] 临症选取穴位的方法。又称取穴法。参见该条。

Method of Choosing Acupoints The method choosing effective acupoints according to the differential diagnosis of TCM, also known as method of the point selection in acu-moxibustion.→取穴法(p.326)

●眩晕[xuàn yùn] 病证名。见《素问·至真要大论》等篇。又称头眩。眩，眼花。晕，头旋。指病人自觉头昏眼花，视物旋转翻覆，不能坐立，常伴有恶心、呕吐，出汗等症。本病多因痰湿内壅，肾水不足，肝风内动，命门火衰，虚阳上浮等所致。临床可分为眩晕实证和眩晕虚证。详见各条。

Dizziness A syndrome, seen in *Suwen*: *Zhizhen Yaoda Lun* (*Plain Questions*: *Great Treatise on Extremely True Gist*), also known as vertigo, referring to a subjective feeling of unsteady movement within the head, revolving and overturning of vision, inability to sit or stand, accompanied by nausea, vomiting and heat. Mostly due to the accumulation of the phlegm-dampness, insufficiency of kidney water, up-stirring of liver-wind, decline of the fire of life-gate and floating of deficiency-yang. In clinic, it is divided into excess syndrome of dizziness and deficiency syndrome of dizziness. →眩晕实证(p.520)、眩晕虚证(p.521)

●眩晕实证[xuàn yùn shí zhèng] 眩晕证型之一。多因肝阳偏亢，风阳内动，或风阳挟痰浊上扰清空所致。证见眩晕呈阵发性，视物旋转翻覆，头胀痛或昏重如裹，多烦易怒，胸胁胀闷，恶心，呕吐痰涎，不思饮食，舌质偏红苔黄腻，脉弦或滑数。治宜平肝潜阳，和胃化痰。取翳风、颔厌、印堂、会宗、阴陵泉、行间、水泉。

Excess Syndrome of Dizziness A type of dizziness, usually caused by slight hyperactivity of liver-yang, upstirring of the wind-yang, or by disturbing of the orifices resulting from wind-yang and phlegm-turbidity. 〈Manifesta-

tions⟩ paroxysmal dizziness, revolving and overturning of vision, distending pain of the head as if it were bound up by cloth, irritability and liability to anger, distention and fullness in the chest and hypochondriac qi region, nausea, vomiting with phlegm fluid, loss of appetite, red tongue with yellowish and greasy coating, wiry or slippery, rapid pulse. ⟨Treatment principle⟩ Calm the liver and supress yang hyperactivity of the liver, regulate the function of the stomach to remove phlegm. ⟨Point selection⟩ Yifeng(SJ 1), Hanyan(GB 4), Yintang(EX-HN 3), Huizong(SJ 7), Yinlinquan(SP 9), Xingjian(LR 2) and Shuiquan(KI 5).

●眩晕虚证[xuàn yùn xū zhèng] 眩晕证型之一。多因心脾两虚,气血化源不足,不能上荣头目;或肾阴亏虚,不能生精补髓,髓海空虚所致。证见头晕目眩,但视物无旋转翻覆之感,劳累易于复发或症状加重,面色少华,神情疲倦,心悸,少寐,腰酸,时有耳鸣,舌质淡,脉细。治宜补益气血。取百会、完骨、脾俞、胃俞、三焦俞、肾俞、足三里。可灸。

Deficiency Syndrome of Dizziness A type of dizziness, usually caused by deficiency of both the heart and spleen, insufficiency of both qi and blood, leading to failure to nourish the head and eye; or by deficiency of kidney-yin leading to failure to produce essence to nourish the marrow and insufficiency of the marrow-sea. ⟨Manifestations⟩ dizziness and blurring of vision, without the feeling of revolving and overturning, liability to a relapse or a serious case induced by overworking, pale comlpexion, lassitude, palpitation, insomnia, aching of the lower back, intermittent tinnitus, pale tongue with thready pulse. ⟨Treatment principle⟩Invigorate qi and nourish blood. ⟨Point selection⟩ Baihui(DU 20), Wangu(GB 12), Pishu(BL 20), Weishu(BL 21), Sanjiaoshu(BL 22), Shenshu(BL 23) and Zusanli(ST 36). Moxibustion is applicable in addition to acupuncture.

●薛己[xuē jǐ] 人名,明代医学家,字新甫,号立斋,吴县(今属江苏)人。世业医,先后任御医及太医院使。通各科,尤精于疡科和针灸。自著及注释医书多种,如《内科摘要》等。后人将薛己的经验、医案整理成《薛氏医案》。

Xue Ji A medical expert of the Ming Dynasty, who styled himself Xinfu and assumed the name of Lizhai, a native of Wuxian County (of Jiangsu Province today). He came from a long line of doctors and was once an imperial physician and later an official of the Institute of the Imperial physicians. He specialized in various medical subjects and was especially proficient at the specialty of ulcers and acupuncture. He compiled and annotated many kinds of medical books such as *Neike Zhaiyao* (*Summary of Internal Medicine*), etc. His experience and records in medicine were sorted out into *Xueshi Yian*(*Xue's Medical Records*) for posterity.

●薛立斋[xuē lì zhāi] 人名。即明代薛己。见"薛己"条。

Xue Lizhai The assumed name of Xue Ji of the Ming Dynasty. →薛己(p. 521)

●穴[xué] 腧穴的简称。见该条。

Points The short form for acupoints. →腧穴(p. 407)

●穴道[xué dào] 腧穴的别称。见《太平圣惠方》。见"腧穴"条。

Point Channel Another name for an acupoint, seen in *Taiping Shenghui Fang*(*Imperial Benevolent Prescriptions*). →腧穴(p. 407)

●穴位[xué wèi] 即腧穴。又指腧穴的所在部位。详见"腧穴"条。

Locus An acupoint and also the location of an acupoint. →腧穴(p. 407)

●穴位超声刺激法[xué wèi chāo shēng cì jī fǎ] 针刺治疗法之一,借助于发射声能的音头,将一定强度的高频声能透入穴位的治疗方法。其剂量可根据音头与穴位的间距,以及调节强度和作用时间来控制。

Point-Ultrasonic Stimulation Therapy A form of acupuncture therapy, referring to the therapy of radiating, with the help of a sound-emitting head, a high-frequency sound of a certain strength which can penetrate into the selected point. The amount of stimulation can be controlled in accordance with the distance between the sound-emitting head and the point, and the regulation of the sound strength and the time it takes to work on the point.

●穴位磁疗法[xué wèi cí liáo fǎ] 治病方法之一。利用磁性物体作用于穴位以治病的方法。金代刘完素《素问玄机原病式》有：含浸针砂酒，以磁石附耳治疗耳聋；宋代严用和《济生方》有用鸣聋散（磁石、穿山甲）塞耳，口含生铁，治疗暴聋和耳鸣记载。现代临床主要有静磁法、动磁法、电磁法等。静磁法的磁场恒定，以贴敷为主。动磁法的磁场强度和方向随时变化，须旋动。电磁法，主要应用电磁治疗机所产生的低频交变磁场进行治疗。所用磁体材料有铈钴铜合金、钐钴合金、钡铁氧体、锶体氧体、铝镍钴磁钢等。一般所用磁场强度为100～4000高斯。贴敷法，即将磁体贴敷或固定于穴位上。多用于高血压、扭伤、腱鞘囊肿等。旋转法，即将旋转机对准穴位进行治疗；或将磁体置于穴位表面摩擦转动。多用于头痛、带状疱疹等。电磁法即选择合适的磁头置于穴位上，多用于支气管炎、肺炎、腰肌劳损、关节炎等。对磁治过敏或头晕，恶心乏力，嗜睡，失眠等副作用严重者停用，孕妇下腹部、婴幼儿及严重心脏病患者的心前区，均禁用。

Acupoint Magnetotherapy A therapeutic method, referring to the treatment of diseases by means of magnetic objects acting on acupoints. It was recorded in *Suwen*: *Xuanji Yuanbingshi* (*Exploration to Mysterious Etiology in Plain Questions*), by Liu Wansu of the Jin Dynasty that a magnet was attached to the ear, while kept in the patient's mouth was some wine, in which some needles had been dipped, to treat deafness; in *Jisheng Fang* (*Recipes for Saving Lives*) by Yan Yonghe of the Song Dynasty, it is written that Ming Long powder (magnetite and Chuanshanjia) was used to fill up the ear while some pig iron was kept in the patient's mouth to treat sudden deafness and tinnitus. In modern clinics it is classified as static magnetotherapy, motive magnetotherapy and electromagnetic therapy, etc. Since the magnetic field is constant, static magnetotherapy is mainly applied with mounting method; the intensity and direction of the magnetic field in motive magnetotherapy changes all the time, so revolving it is necessary. Electromagnetic-therapy is applied to treat diseases with the use of a kind of electromagnetic therapeutic machine/meter, which produces a low-frequency magnetic field. The magnetic materials can be alloy of cerium, cobalt and copper, alloy of samarium and cobalt, oxide of barium and iron, oxide of strontium, and magnetic steel of aluminium, nickel and cobalt, etc. The common intensity used is 100-4000 gauss. The mounting method fixes the magnet on the selected point for the treatment of hypertension, sprain and thecal cyst, etc. The revolving method is to aim the megnet at the selected point or to place the magnet at the selected point and rub and revolve it to treat headache and herpes zoster. The electromagnetic method is to choose a suitable magnetic head and place it on the point for the treatment of bronchitis, pneumonia, lumbar muscle strain and arthritis, etc. Application of magnetotherapy for patient allergic to it or having severe side-effects such as dizziness, nausea, fatigue, sleepiness and insomnia, etc. Should be stopped. Its application on the abdomen of a pregnant woman, or on the precardium of a body of a child or a patient with severe heart disease is forbidden.

●穴位封闭疗法[xué wèi fēng bì liáo fǎ] 治病方法之一。指穴位注射疗法中，采用麻醉性药物者，参见"穴位注射法"条。

Acupoint Block Therapy A therapeutic method, referring to point-injection therapy with narcotic drugs. →穴位注射法(p.523)

●穴位激光疗法[xué wèi jī guāng liáo fǎ] 治疗方法之一。又称激光针、光针。是在针灸疗法基础上，利用激光束照射穴位以治疗疾病的方法。最常使用为氦——氖激光疗法。应用小功率氦——氖激光照射穴位治疗(功率一般为1～30mA)，也可用光导纤维对准穴位照射治疗，穿透组织深度为10～15mm。照射距离，一般为20～30mm，特殊为100mm，可根据患者具体情况选择。每日照射一次，每次取2～4穴，每穴照射2～5分钟，照射10次为一疗程。病情较顽固者，可照射3个疗程，或3个疗程以上，每个疗程间隔7～10天，此法具有通经活络，消炎止痛等作用，可用于治疗头痛、偏头痛、鼻旁窦炎、支气管炎、哮喘、胃和十二指肠溃疡、高血压、慢性结肠炎、神经炎和各种神经痛、神经衰弱、关节炎、小儿遗尿及妇科病等各种病症。采用激光照射中，医者要戴激光防护镜，不

可对视光束,以免损伤眼睛。

Laser Therapy on the Acupoint A therapeutic method also known as laser needle or light needle. The therapy, on the basis of acupuncture therapy, can be used to treat diseases by irradiating points with a laser beam. The most frequently used therapy is the Helium Neon Laser therapy. A Helium—Neon laser with small power (usu. 1-30 Ma) is employed to irradiate the points for treatment. Optical fibers can also be used to irradiate the selected points, to a depth of 10-15 *mm*. The irradiating distance is usually 20-30 *mm*, in special cases, 100 *mm* can be used according to the patient's concrete conditions. The irradiation is done once a day on 2-4 acupoints, 2-5 minutes for each point, 10 times as one course of treatment. Three or more courses for severe cases with an interval of 7-10 days between two courses. This therapy has such functions as removing inflammation to stop pain. 〈Indications〉 headache, migraine, nasosinusitis, bronchitis, asthma, stomach and duodenal ulcer, hypertension, chronic colitis, neuritis and various neuralgia, neurosism, arthritis, infantile enuresis and various common diseases in gynecology. The doctors should wear laser-protecting glasses in the course of laser irradiation and avoid the laser beam in case it damages the eye.

●穴位冷敷法[xué wèi lěng fū fǎ] 治病方法。见《本草纲目》。在穴位上给予寒冷刺激以治疗疾病的方法。例如用白矾填满脐中,以水滴之,以治疗二便不通。现代有用氯乙烷或二氧化碳等冷凝剂,在穴位上进行适量喷射者。

Cold-Application at Acupoints A therapeutic method, from *Bencao Gangmu (Compendium of Materia Medica)*, referring to the therapy by which the acupoints are given cold stimulation for the treatment of diseases. For instance, fill the umbilicus with alum and drop some water on it to treat difficult urination and defecation. In modern times, an appropriate amount of some cryogens such as ethylene chloride and carbondioxide, etc. can be sprayed upon the points.

●穴位埋线法[xué wèi mái xiàn fǎ] 针刺法之一。将铬制羊肠线埋入穴位皮下或肌肉深层,用其持续刺激作用来治疗。一般采用特制埋线针,选取腹、背及四肢肌肉丰满处的穴位,每次埋线1～2穴。可用于消化性溃疡、慢性胃肠炎、慢性支气管炎、哮喘、神经官能症、小儿麻痹后遗症等。

Catgut Embedding at Acupoints A needling method. Implant a piece of chromium-made catgut in the acupoint subcutaneously in the muscles or in the deep layer to maintain a continuous stimulation to treat diseases. Generally, a specially-made needle is used for catgut implantation on the acupoints selected on the abdomen, the back and four limbs with chubby muscles, 1-2 points each time. 〈Indications〉 digestive ulcer, chronic gastroenteritis, chronic bronchitis, asthma, psychoneurosis and sequela of infantile paralysis, etc.

●穴位吸引器[xué wèi xī yǐn qì] 一种抽气拔罐用具。由带有阀门的橡皮球和底有管口的特制玻璃罐组成,两者用橡皮管接通。手捏橡皮球抽吸罐内空气,造成负压(可高达240毫米汞柱左右),将玻璃罐吸附在穴位局部皮肤上。

Point Aspirator An instrument for aspirating and cupping, composed of a rubber ball with a valve and a specially made glass cup with a pipe-mouth at the bottom, connected by a rubber pipe. Hold the rubber ball between fingers to aspirate the air in the glass cup until a negative pressure forms, thus attacking the glass cup to the local skin around the selected acupoint.

●穴位照射法[xué wèi zhào shè fǎ] 针刺治疗方法。利用光辐射在穴位上的作用来治病的方法。现代有以红外线、紫外线、激光等照射穴位的治法。

Point-Rediation Therapy A needling therapy, referring to the method by which light is used to irradiate acupoints. There are point-radiation therapies with infrared ray, ultraviolet ray or laser in modern times.

●穴位注射法[xué wèi zhù shè fǎ] 针刺法之一。为水针之别称。见该条。

Point-Injection Therapy One form of needling methods, another name of hydro-acupuncture therapy. →水针(p.411)

523

● 血闭 [xuè bì]　即经闭,详见该条。
Blood Stoppage　→经闭(p.208)

● 血鼓 [xuè gǔ]　鼓胀证型之一。见《石室秘录·内伤门》。又称蓄血成胀。因气血瘀滞,水湿不能运行所致。证见脘腹胀大坚硬,脐周青筋暴露,胁下癥结,腿见血缕,皮肤甲错,头颈胸臂可现血痣,大便色黑,舌质紫黯或有瘀斑,脉细弦或涩,治宜疏通肝脾,活血化瘀。针期门、血海、石门、三阴交。

Tympanitis due to Blood Stasis　A type of tympanitis, originally seen in *Shishi Milu: Neishang Men (Secret Records in the Stone House: Discussion on Internal Injuries)*, also known as abdominal distention induced by accumulated blood, caused by the stagnation of qi and blood, and the accumulation of fluid in the body. 〈Manifestations〉 hard distention of the abdomen, engorged veins around the umbilicus, mass in the hypochondriac region, congestions of the leg, cyanosis of skin, vascular nevus seen on the head, the neck, the chest and the arm, melena; purplish dark tongue with stasis, thready and wiry or choppy pulse. 〈Treatment principle〉 Dredge the liver and spleen, promote blood circulation to resolve blood stasis. 〈Point selection〉 Qimen (LR 14), Xuehai (SP 10), Shimen (RN 5) and Sanyinjiao (SP 6).

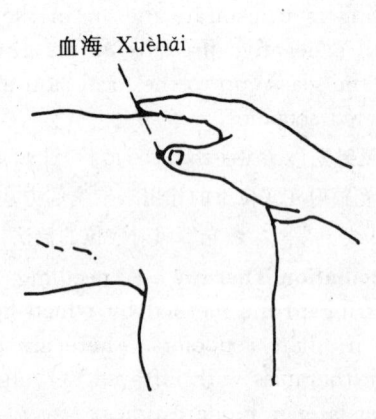

图68　血海穴
Fig 68　Xuehai point

● 血海 [xuè hǎi]　①四海之一,指冲脉。出《灵枢·海论》。又称十二经之海。冲脉上循脊里,与十二经脉会聚而贯通全身,故称。②经穴名。出《针灸甲乙经》。又名血郄、百虫窠。属足太阴脾经。〈定位〉屈膝,在大腿内侧,髌底内侧端上2寸,当股四头肌内侧头的隆起处(图68)。〈层次解剖〉皮肤→皮下组织→股内侧肌。浅层布有股神经前皮支,大隐静脉的属支。深层有股动、静脉的肌支和股神经的肌支。〈主治〉月经不调、崩漏、经闭、瘾疹、湿疹等。直刺1.0～1.5寸;可灸。③指肝脏。肝有贮藏和调节血液的功能,故称。

1. Sea of Blood, the　One of the four seas, referring to the Chong Meridian, from *Lingshu: Hai Lun (Miraculous Pivot: On Seas)*, also known as the Sea of the Twelve Meridians. The Chong Meridian ascends and runs inside the vertebral column, converges with the Twelve Meridians and passes through the whole body, thus the name.

2. Xuehai (SP 10)　A meridian point, originally from *Zhenjiu Jia-Yi Jing (A-B Classic of Acupuncture and Moxibustion)*, also known as Xuexi and Baichongke, a point on the Spleen Meridian of Foot-Taiyin. 〈Location〉 with the knee flexed, on the medial side of the thigh, 2 cun above the superior medial corner of the patella, on the prominence of the medial head of the quadriceps muscle of the thigh (Fig. 68). 〈Regional anatomy〉 skin→subcutaneous tissue→medial vastus muscle of thigh. In the superficial layer, there are the anterior cutaneous branches of the femoral nerve and the tributaries of the great saphenous vein. In the deep layer, there are the muscular branches of the femoral artery and vein and the muscular branches of the fermoral nerve. 〈Indications〉 irregular menstruation, metrorrhagia and metrostaxis, amenorrhea, urticaria and eczema, etc. 〈Method〉 Puncture perpendicularly 1.0～1.5 cun. Moxibustion is applicable.

3. Referring to the liver. It is so referred to because liver has the function of restoring and regulating the blood.

● 血寒经迟 [xuè hán jīng chí]　即血寒经行后期的别名。详见该条。

Delayed Menses due to Blood-Cold　Retarded menstruation due to blood-cold. →血寒经行后期(p.525)

●**血寒经行后期**[xuè hán jīng xíng hòu qī] 是经行后期的证型之一。又称血寒经迟。多因经产之时,感受寒凉,寒邪乘虚侵入胞宫,血为寒滞,运行失常所致。症见经期错后,量少色黯有块,小腹绞痛,得热痛减,面色青白,形寒畏冷。治宜温经行滞。取气海、气穴、三阴交、归来、天枢。可加灸。若见经血量少,色淡质稀,小腹隐痛,喜热喜按,面色㿠白,头晕气短,腰痠乏力等,则为冲任虚寒,血行无力所致。治宜温经养血。取气海、气穴、三阴交、命门、太溪,可加灸。

Delayed Menstruation due to Blood-Cold
One type of delayed menstruation, also known as delayed menses due to blood-cold, mostly caused by the attack of cold during delivery, and the invasion of cold upon the uterus which leads to the stagnation of blood and disorder of the blood circulation.〈Manifestations〉delayed menstrual period, oligomenorrhea with dark color and blood clots, colicky pain in the lower abdomen which can be relieved by hot compress, pale complexion, cold body and intolerance to cold.〈Treatment principle〉Warm the meridians to relieve stagnation.〈Point selection〉Qihai (RN 6), Qixue (KI 13), Sanyinjiao(SP 6), Guilai(ST 29)and Tianshu(ST 25). Moxibustion can be applied in addition to acupuncture. If the disease is manifested with oligomenorrhea in pink color with thin discharge, dull pain in the lower abdomen, relieved by hot compress and pressing, pale complexion, dizziness and shortness of breath, aching of the lower back and fatigue, it is caused by deficiency-cold of the Chong and Ren Meridians, leading to weakness in blood circulation. 〈Treatment principle〉Warm the meridians and nourish the blood.〈Point selection〉 Qihai(RN 6), Qixue (KI 13), Sanyinjiao(SP 6), Mingmen(DU 4) and Taixi(KI 3). Moxibustion can be applied in addition to acupuncture.

●**血寒月经过少**[xuè hán yuè jīng guò shǎo] 是月经过少的证型之一。多因素体阳虚,阴寒内生,化气生血功能不足,冲任血少所致。症见经期血量过少,色淡或黯,质稀,形寒畏冷,小腹冷痛,喜得温热。治宜温经养血。取关元、气海、肾俞、命门、足三里。多灸。

Scanty Menstruation due to Blood-Cold
One type of hypomenorrhea, usually caused by yang-deficiency with formation of yin-cold in the body, deficiency in the function of transmitting qi and generating blood leading to the lack of blood in the Chong and Ren Meridians.〈Manifestations〉scanty menstruation with dark pale or dark menses, thin discharge accompanied by intolerance to cold, cold pain over the lower abdomen with a desire for warmth.〈Theatment principle〉Warm the meridians and nourish the blood.〈Point selection〉Guanyuan(RN 4), Qihai(RN 6) Shenshu(BL 23), Mingmen(DU 4) and Zusanli(ST 36). More moxibustion is applicable.

●**血厥**[xuè jué] 厥证证型之一,指因失血过多或暴怒气逆,而引起的昏厥重证。血厥有虚实之分。失血过多,突然昏厥,面色苍白,口唇无华,四肢震颤,目陷口张,自汗肤冷,呼吸微弱,舌质淡,脉细数无力者为虚证,治宜救逆固脱。取百会、气海、关元。用灸法。病起暴怒之后,突然昏仆,不省人事,牙关紧闭,面赤唇紫,舌红,脉沉弦者为实证,治宜苏厥开窍。取水沟、内关、行间、涌泉。

Syncope due to Excessive Loss of Blood One type of syncope, referring to a sudden loss of consciousness resulting from excessive bleeding or adverse rising of qi after a rage. There are two types of syncope due to excessive bleeding: excess and deficiency.〈Manifestations of the deficiency type〉excessive bleeding, sudden syncope, pale complexion, lusterless lip, vibration of the four limbs, depression of the eye with the mouth open, spontaneous perspiration with cold skin, faint breath, pale tongue with thready, rapid and weak pulse.〈Treatment principle〉Recuperate depleted yang and rescue the patient from collapse.〈Point selection〉Baihui(DU 20), Qihai(RN 6), and Guanyuan(RN 4).〈Method〉Moxibustion.〈Manifestations of the excess type〉sudden syncope after a rage, loss of consciousness, lockjaw, flushed face with purplish lip, red tongue with deep and wiry pulse.〈Treatment principle〉Restore consciousness and induce resuscitation.〈Point selection〉Shuigou (DU 26), Neiguan(PC 6), Xingjian(LR 2) and Yongquan(KI 1).

●**血亏经闭**[xuè kuī jīng bì] 经闭的证型之一。多

因久病失血,或早婚房事过度,生育过多等耗伤精血,以致阴虚血亏,先见经期错后,量少,逐渐无血下达,冲任胞宫空虚,终成经闭。症见面色㿠白,皮肤干燥,形体消瘦,不思饮食,舌淡脉细,治宜滋阴补血。取胃俞、脾俞、膈俞、足三里、三阴交。

Amenorrhea due to Deficiency of Blood A type of amenorrhea, mostly due to chronic illness and loss of blood or early marriage and excessive sexual intercourse and excessive child birth leading to consumption of essence and blood, yin-deficiency and lack of blood. First seen as delayed menstrual period with scanty menstrual discharge, then the gradual stopping of menstruation and emptiness of the Chong and Ren Meridians, eventually leading to amenorrhea. 〈Manifestations〉 pale complexion, dry skin, emaciation, loss of appetite, pale tongue with thready pulse. 〈Treatment principle〉 Nourish yin and enrich blood. 〈Point selection〉 Weishu(BL 21), Pishu(BL 20), Geshu(BL 17), Zusanli(ST 36) and Sanyinjiao(SP 6).

●**血淋**[xuè lìn] 淋证证型之一。出《诸病源候论·淋病诸候》。多因湿热下注膀胱,热盛伤络,迫血妄行所致。证见小便频急,热涩刺痛,尿中带血,夹有血丝血块,小腹微有胀痛,苔黄腻,或舌红少苔,脉细数。治宜清利湿热,通淋止痛。取膀胱俞、中极、阴陵泉、少海、太溪、行间、血海、三阴交。

Stranguria Complicated by Hematuria One type of stranguria, from *Zhubing Yuanhou Lun: Linbing Zhuhou* (*General Treatise on the Etiology and Symptomatology of Diseases Causes and Symtoms of Stranguria*), mostly caused by damp-heat flowing downward to attack the urinary bladder and accumulation of heat attacking the collaterals which leads to bleeding. 〈Manifestations〉 frequent urination with difficulty and pain, blood in urine with congestion and blood clots, slight distention and pain in the lower abdomen, yellowish and greasy tongue coating, or red tongue with thin coating, thready and rapid pulse. 〈Treatment principle〉 Clear heat and promote diuresis, promote stranguria and arrest pain. 〈Point selection〉 Pangguangshu(BL 28), Zhongji(RN 3), Yinlingquan(SP 9), Shaohai(HT 3), Taixi (KI 3), Xingjian(LR 2), Xuehai(SP 10) and Sanyinjiao(SP 6).

●**血络**[xuè luò] 指位于机体浅表的细小络脉。出《灵枢·血络论》。又称络脉,亦称血脉。临床上常用作诊断和刺血治病。

Superficial Venules The thin and minute collaterals located subcutaneously in the body's shallow surface, from *Lingshu: Xueluo Lun* (*Miraculous Pivot: On Superficial Venules*). Also known as collateral branches of large meridians or blood vessels. Clinically, it is often used for diagnosis and for treating diseases by pricking to bleed.

●**血脉**[xuè mài] ①经脉。出《灵枢·九针论》。简称脉,是气血运行的通道。②血络的别名。详见该条。

1. **Meridian** Originally from *Lingshu: Jiu Zhen Lun* (*Miraculous Pivot: On Nine Needles*), called vessel for short, the passage in which qi and blood circulate.
2. Another name for superficial venules. →**血络**(p.526)

●**血门**[xuè mén] 经外穴名。出《医经小学》。〈定位〉在小腹部,当脐上4寸,旁开腹正中线3寸处,〈主治〉妇人腹中血块、胃痛、消化不良、急性胃炎等。直刺0.5~1.0寸;可灸。

Xuemen(EX-CA) An extra point, originally from *Yijing Xiaoxue* (*Elementary Collections of Medical Classics*). 〈Location〉 on the upper abdomen, 4 cun above the umbilicus, 3 cun lateral to the anterior midline. 〈Indications〉 blood clots in the abdomen, gastric pain, indigestion and acute gastritis, etc. 〈Method〉 Puncture perpendicularly 0.5-1.0 cun. Moxibustion is applicable.

●**血纳包络**[xuè nà bāo luò] 子午流注针法用语。与气纳三焦相对。《针灸大全》论子午流注之法:"三焦乃阳气之父,包络乃阴血之母。""阴干注脏,乙、丁、己、辛、癸而重见者,血纳包络。"意指当阴干的重现时,分别按生他的关系取心包经的五输穴。如乙日乙酉时,开肝经井穴;丁亥时,取心经荥穴;乙丑时,取脾经输穴;辛卯时,取肺经经穴;癸巳时,取肾经合穴;至乙未时重见乙,取心包经荥(火)穴。乙属木,为木生火关系。

Blood-Reflowing to Pericardium Meridian A term in midnight-noon ebb-flow needling,

as opposed to qi-reflowing to Sanjiao Meridian. As is stated on the theory of mid-night noon ebb-flow in *Zhenjiu Daquan*(*A Complete Work of Acupuncture and Moxibustion*), Sanjiao is the father of yang-qi, while the Pericardium Meridian is the mother of yin-blood. Yin stems pour into the zang organs, Yi (2nd), Ding(4th), Ji(6th), Xin(8th) and Gui (the 10th of the ten Heavenly Stems) are seen in serious cases, blood should reflow to the Pericardium Meridian, meaning when Yin stem is seen once again, select respectively the Five-Shu Points of the Pericardium Meridian in accordance with their interpromoting relation. For instance, select the Jing(Well) point of the Liver Meridian in the Yi-You period (5p. m. -7p. m.) on the day of Yi(the 2nd of the ten Heavenly Stems); Ying(Spring)Point of the Heart Meridian in the period of Ding-Hai (9 p. m. -11p. m.); the Shu (Stream) point of the Spleen Meridian in the period of Yi-Chou(1 a. m. -3 a. m.); the Jing (River) Point of the Lung Meridian in the period of Xin-Mou(5a. m. -7a. m.); the He(Sea) point in the period of Gui-Si(9a. m. -11a. m.); in the period of Yi-Wei(1p. m. -3p. m.), when Yi is seen again, select the Ying (Fire) Point of the Pericardium Meridian. Yi belongs to wood, which can promote fire.

● 血热崩漏[xuè rè bēng lòu] 是崩漏的证型之一。多因外感邪热，或食辛辣助阳之品，热伤冲任，迫血妄行所致。症见血崩色深红，气味臭秽，血质浓稠，口干喜饮，心烦易怒，舌红苔黄，脉滑数。治宜清热凉血。取气海、三阴交、隐白、血海、水泉。

Metrorrhagia and Metrostaxis due to Blood-Heat One type of metrorrhagia and metrostaxis, mostly caused by the attack of exogenous heat evil, or the intake of pungent food leading to heat attacking the Chong and Ren Meridians and irregular uterine bleeding. 〈Manifestations〉bleeding in dark-red color with foul smell, thick bleeding discharge, dry mouth with preference for drink, irritability and liability to rage, red tongue with yellowish coating, smooth and rapid pulse. 〈Treatment principle〉Eliminate pathogenic heat from the blood. 〈Point selection〉Qihai(RN 6), Sanyinjiao(SP 6), Yinbai(SP 1), Xuebai(SP 10) and Shuiquan(KI 5).

● 血热经行先期[xuè rè jīng xíng xiān qī] 经行先期的证型之一。又称血热经早。多因素体内热，过嗜辛辣食物，或感受热邪，以致热扰冲任，迫血妄行。证见经期提前七、八天以上，血量较多，色紫红，质稠粘，心烦口渴，面赤，小便黄，大便干，舌红苔黄，脉滑数。治宜清热凉血。取曲池、少海、血海、阴陵泉、太冲。

Preceded Menstrual Cycle due to Blood-Heat One type of preceded menstruation, also known as early menstruation due to blood heat. Mostly caused by interior heat of body, overeating of pungent food, or the attack of Heat-evil leading to heat attacking the Chong and Ren Meridians and abnormal bleeding. 〈Manifestations〉bleeding 7 or 8 days or more before the menstrual cycle, profuse menstrual discharge in purplish-red color, thick and sticky, irritability and thirst, flushed face, yellowish urine, dry stools, red tongue with yellowish coating, slippery and rapid pulse. 〈Treatment principle〉Remove pathogenic heat from the blood. 〈Point selection〉Quchi (LI 11), Shaohai(HT 3), Xuehai(SP 10), Yinlingquan(SP 9) and Taichong(LR 3).

● 血热经早[xuè rè jīng zǎo] 即血热经行先期。见该条。

Earlier-than-Usual Menstruation due to Blood Heat →血热经行先期(p. 527)

● 血热月经过多[xuè rè yuè jīng guò duō] 月经过多的证型之一。多因素体阳盛内热，或过嗜辛辣，热伏冲任，迫血妄行所致。证见经血量多，或经行持续时间延长，血色深红，或紫，稠粘或有臭秽气味。面红身热，口干作渴，时作烦躁，治宜清热凉血。取曲池、气海、曲骨、血海、三阴交、水泉、太冲。

Menorrhagia due to Blood-Heat One type of menorrhagia, mostly caused by excessive Yang and interior heat of the body, or overeating of purgent food leading to heat accumulation in the Chong and Ren Meridians and bleeding. 〈Manifestations〉profuse menstrual discharge, or prolonged menstrual cycle, dark red or purplish color, sticky and thick menses with foul smell, flushed face and fever, dry mouth and thirst, intermittent irritability.

⟨Treatment principle⟩ Remove pathogenic heat from the blood. ⟨Point selection⟩ Quchi(LI 11), Qihai(RN 6), Qugu(RN 2), Xuehai(SP 10), Sanyinjiao(SP 6), Shuiquan(KI 5) and Taichong(LR 3).

●血少不孕[xuè shǎo bù yùn]　血虚不孕的别名。见该条。

Sterility due to Insufficiency of Blood →血虚不孕(p.528)

●血丝疔[xuè sī dīng]　即红丝疔。见该条。

Blood-Streaked Infection →红丝疔(p.164)

●血郄[xuè xì]　①经穴别名。出《铜人腧穴针灸图经》。即委中。见该条。②经外穴别名。即百虫窝。见该条。

Xuexi　Another name for ① Weizhong(BL 40), a meridian point, originally from *Tongren Shuxue Zhenjiu Tujing* (*Illustrated Manual of Points for Acupuncture and Moxibustion on a Bronze Statute with Acupoints*).→委中(p.461) ② the extra point Baichongwo(EX-LE 3). →百虫窝(p.11)

●血虚不孕[xuè xū bù yùn]　是不孕的证型之一。又称血少不孕。多由素体脾胃虚弱，或久病失血伤阴，阴血不足，冲任空虚，胞脉失养所致。证见月经量少色淡，周期错后，身体瘦弱，面色萎黄，疲倦乏力，头晕心悸，舌质淡，脉沉细。治宜补益精血，调理冲任。取关元、气户、子宫、三阴交、足三里。

Sterility due to Blood Deficiency　One type of Sterility, also known as sterility due to insufficiency of blood, mostly due to deficiency of the spleen and stomach, or prolonged illness with bleeding and Yin damage leading to insufficiency of Yin-blood and emptiness of the Chong and Ren Meridians with failure to nourish the uterine collaterals. ⟨Manifestations⟩ scanty menstruation with pink color, delayed menstrual cycle, emaciation, sallow complexion, fatigue, dizziness and palpitation, pale tongue, deep and thready pulse. ⟨Treatment principle⟩ Replenish and invigorate the essence and blood, regulate the Chong and Ren Meridians. ⟨Point selection⟩ Guanyuan(RN 4), Qihu(ST 13), Zigong(EX-CA 1), Sanyinjiao(SP 6) and Zusanli(ST 36).

●血虚产后头痛[xuè xū chǎn hòu tóu tòng]　产后头痛证型之一，多因产后失血过多，血虚不能上荣于脑，髓海空虚所致。临床可见头痛较缓，头目昏重，神疲乏力，小腹隐痛，面色苍白，舌淡，脉细弱。治宜补血益气。取百会、气海、肝俞、脾俞、肾俞、足三里。

Postpartum Headache due to Blood Deficiency　One type of postpartum headache, mostly caused by excessive bleeding after delivery, deficiency of blood with failure to nourish the head leading to emptiness of the reservoir of marrow. ⟨Manifestations⟩ mild headache, dizziness and heaviness of the head and eye, lassitude and fatigue, dull pain in the lower abdomen, pale compelxion, pale tongue, thready and weak pulse. ⟨Treatment principle⟩ Enrich blood and replenish qi. ⟨Point selection⟩ Baihui(DU 20), Qihai(RN 6), Ganshu(BL 18), Pishu(BL 20), Shenshu(BL 23) and Zusanli(ST 36).

●血虚风燥牛皮癣[xuè xū fēng zào niú pí xuǎn]　牛皮癣证型之一。由于日久不愈，营血不足，血虚化燥生风，皮肤经络失于濡养，以致患处皮肤粗糙脱落白屑。其证除见牛皮癣的一般症状外，病程较长，局部干燥，肥厚，脱屑，状如牛领之皮，苔薄，脉细。治宜养血润燥。取曲池、足三里、血海、三阴交、膈俞、阿是穴。详见"牛皮癣"条。

Neurodermatitis due to Blood Deficiency and Wind-Dryness　One type of neurodermatitis due to prolonged illness without being cured, insufficiency of Yin-Blood, blood deficiency transforming into dryness and producing wind in the skin, meridians and collaterals, loss of nourishment of blood, leading to dry and rough skin with white-bits coming off. ⟨Manifestations⟩ prolonged course of disease, dryness and thickness of local skin with white-bits coming off, looking like the skin of a cattle collar, thin tongue coating and thready pulse, in addition to the general symptoms. ⟨Treatment principle⟩ Enrich the blood and moisten the dryness. ⟨Point selection⟩ Quchi(LI 11), Zusanli(ST 36), Xuehai(SP 10), Sanyinjiao(SP 6), Geshu(BL 17) and Ashi points. →牛皮癣(p.285)

●血虚经行后期[xuè xū jīng xíng hòu qī]　经行后期证型之一。多因素患失血，或大病、久病，或产育过多，耗伤阴血，以致血海空虚，冲任不足，胞宫不得按

时满溢,导致月经过期而来,症见经期错后在七、八天以上,血量少色淡,经质清稀,面色苍白,头晕目眩,心悸少寐,舌淡苔少,脉细无力。治宜补血益气。取气海、气穴、三阴交、足三里、心俞、脾俞、膈俞。

Delayed Menstruation due to Blood Deficiency One type of delayed menstruation, mostly caused by habitual bleeding, severe or chronic illness, or excessive childbirths, the comsumption and damage of Yin-blood leading to the emptiness of the blood reservoir, insufficiency of the Chong and Ren Meridians with failure to fill the uterine collaterals on time which causes delayed menstrual cycle. 〈Manifestations〉menstruation occurring 7 or 8 days later than usual, scanty menstruation in pink color, thin mentrual blood, pale complexion, dizziness and blurring of vision, palpitation and insomnia, pale tongue with thin coating, thready and weak pulse. 〈Treatment principle〉Enrich the blood and replenish qi. 〈Point selection〉Qihai (RN 6), Qixue (KI 13), Sanyinjiao (SP 6), Zusanli (ST 36), Xinshu (BL 15), Pishu (BL 20) and Geshu (BL 17).

●**血虚湿疹**[xuè xū shī zhěn] 湿疹证型之一。多由湿疹久延失治,血虚生风化燥,肌肤失于濡养所致。证见病情反复,病程较长,皮肤损害处颜色黯褐,粗糙肥厚,瘙痒,并有脱屑等,舌质淡,苔薄白,脉细弦。治宜养血润燥。取足三里、三阴交、大都、郄门、列缺、照海。

Eczema due to Blood Deficiency One type of eczema, mostly caused by prolonged eczema and postponed treatment, blood deficiency bringing about wind and dryness, leading to the failure to nourish the skin. 〈Manifestations〉a relapsed case with prolonged course of the disease, dark-brown color of the impaired skin, rough and thick skin with itching sensation and white-bits coming off, pale tongue with thin and whitish coating, thready and wiry pulse. 〈Treatment principle〉Enrich the blood and moisten dryness. 〈Point selection〉Zusanli (ST 36), Sanyinjiao (SP 6), Dadu (SP 2), Ximen (PC 4), Lieque (LU 7) and Zhaohai (KI 6).

●**血虚头痛**[xuè xū tóu tòng] 头痛证型之一。见《兰室秘藏》卷中。由血虚不能上荣所致,证见头昏而痛,痛势绵绵,休息痛减,神疲,心悸,面色少华,有久病及失血史。舌质淡,脉细。治宜益气养血,和络止痛。取上星、百会、头维、血海、足三里、三阴交。

Headache due to Blood Deficiency A type of headache, originally seen in Vol. 2 of the 3-volume book *Lanshi Micang* (*Secret Records of the Chamber of Orchids*), caused by blood-deficiency with failure to nourish the head. 〈Manifestations〉dizziness and pain in the head, continuous pain relieved by rest, lassitude, palpitation, lusterless complexion with a history of prolonged illness and bleeding; pale tongue and thready pulse. 〈Treatment principle〉Replenish qi and enrich blood, regulate the collaterals and relieve pain. 〈Point selection〉Shangxing (DU 23), Baihui (DU 20), Touwei (ST 8), Xuehai (SP 10), Zusanli (ST 36) and Sanyinjiao (SP 6).

●**血虚心悸**[xuè xū xīn jì] 心悸证型之一。见《医学入门》。多由心血不足,心失所养所致。证见心悸不宁,思虑劳累尤甚,面色少华,头晕目眩,短气,舌质淡红,脉细数。若心中烦热,少寐多梦,口干,耳鸣,面赤,舌质淡红,脉细数,则为阴虚火旺。治宜养血定惊。取膈俞、肝俞、脾俞、通里、神堂、足三里。阴虚火旺加太溪、肾俞、神门。

Palpitation due to Blood Deficiency One type of palpitation, seen in *Yixue Rumen* (*An Introduction to Medicine*), mostly caused by insufficiency of heart-blood with failure to nourish the heart. 〈Manifestations〉palpitation and restlessness which are aggravated by overstrain and worries, lusterless complexion, dizziness and blurring of vision, shortness of breath, pale red tongue, thready and rapid pulse. If seen as irritability and fever in the heart, insomnia and dreamy sleep, dry mouth, tinnitus, flushed face, pale red tip of tongue, thready and rapid pulse, it is caused by hyperactivity of fire due to yin-deficiency. 〈Treatment principle〉Enrich the blood and arrest convulsion. 〈Point selection〉Geshu (BL 17), Ganshu (BL 18), Pishu (BL 20), Tongli (HT 5) Shentang (BL 44), Zusanli (ST 36), plus Taixi (KI 3), Shenshu (BL 23), and Shenmen (HT 7) for palpitation due to hyperactivity of fire due to yin-deficiency.

●血虚月经过少[xuè xū yuè jīng guò shǎo] 月经过少证型之一。多因素体虚弱,久病失血伤阴,或脾胃损伤,生化之源不足,冲任血虚所致。症见月经量少,或点滴一、二天便净,色淡红,质稀,面色萎黄,头晕心悸,小腹空痛,治宜补血益气健脾。取脾俞、胃俞、肾俞、膈俞、气海、足三里、三阴交。

Scanty Menstruation due to Blood Deficiency

One type of scanty menstruation, mostly caused by general weakness of the body, prolonged illness and bleeding leading to yin damage, or impairment of the spleen and stomach, insufficiency of the source for production and transformation leading to blood deficiency of the Chong and Ren Meridians. 〈Manifestations〉scanty menstruation, or little discharge for only one or two days, pink and thin menses, sallow complexion, dizziness, palpitation, hollow pain in the lower abdomen. 〈Treatment principle〉Enrich the blood, replenish qi and invigorate the spleen. 〈Point selection〉 Pishu (BL 20), Weishu (BL 21), Shenshu (BL 23), Geshu (BL 17), Qihai (RN 6) Zusanli (ST 36), and Sanyinjiao (SP 6).

●血瘀崩漏[xuè yū bēng lòu] 崩漏证型之一。多因瘀血停滞于内,冲任失调,血不归经所致,症见崩漏血中挟有瘀块,腹痛拒按,瘀块排出后痛减,舌质黯红,脉沉涩。治宜调血祛瘀止崩。取气海、三阴交、隐白、地机、气冲、冲门。

Metrorrhagia and Metrotaxis due to Blood Stasis One type of metrorrhagia and metrotaxis, mostly caused by accumulation of blood stasis, dysfunction of the Chong and Ren Meridians with failure to hold blood in the meridians. 〈Manifestations〉stasis clots in uterine bleeding, abdominal pain and tenderness which is relieved by the discharge of blood clots, dark red tongue, deep and choppy pulse. 〈Treatment principle〉Regulate blood to remove blood stasis and arrest uterine bleeding. 〈Point selection〉Qihai (RN 6), Sanyinjiao (SP 6), Yinbai (SP 1), Diji (SP 8), Qichong (ST 30) and Chongmen (SP 12).

●血瘀不孕[xuè yū bù yùn] 不孕证型之一。多因情志内伤气血运行不畅,瘀血停滞,内阻冲任胞脉所致。症见经期错后,经行涩滞不畅,血块较多,腹痛拒按,烦躁易怒,乳房胀痛,舌质黯或有瘀斑,脉涩。治宜活血化瘀,理气行滞。取中极、气冲、四满、地机、内关、太冲。

Sterility due to Blood Stasis One type of sterility, mostly caused by difficult circulation of qi and blood, accumulation of blood stasis in the Chong and Ren Meridians and the uterus resulting from emotional internal damage. 〈Manifestations〉difficult menstruation with profuse blood clots, abdominal pain and tenderness, irritability and liability to a rage, distending pain in the breast, dark tongue or with ecchymosis, and choppy pulse. 〈Treatment principle〉Promote blood circulation by removing blood stasis, regulate the flow of qi and remove retention. 〈Point selection〉 Zhongji (RN 3), Qichong (ST 30), Siman (KI 14), Diji (SP 8), Neiguan (PC 6) and Taichong (LR 3).

●血瘀产后头痛[xuè yū chǎn hòu tóu tòng] 产后头痛证型之一。多因恶露停留胞宫,循经上冲于脑所致。临床可见头痛较剧,小腹刺痛,拒按,舌紫黯,脉涩。治宜活血化瘀。取上星、头维、血海、太冲、中都。

Postpartum Headache due to Blood Stasis One type of postpartum headache, mostly caused by the retention of lochia in the uterus attacking the head along the meridians. 〈Manifestations〉severe headache, pricking pain in the lower abdomen and tenderness, purplish dark tongue, and choppy pulse. 〈Treatment Principle〉Promote blood circulation by removing blood stasis. 〈Point selection〉Shangxing (DU 23), Touwei (ST 8), Xuehai (SP 10), Taichong (LR 3) and Zhongdu (LR 6).

●血瘀经行后期[xuè yū jīng xíng hòu qī] 经行后期证型之一。多因气滞,寒凝,以致瘀血内阻冲任,经血不能按时下达胞宫所致。气滞血瘀者,症见经期错后,经量涩少,血色紫黯,血块较多,小腹胀痛。治宜行气活血化瘀。取气海、气穴、三阴交、中极、四满、太冲、大敦。寒凝血瘀者,症见小腹冷痛,拒按,血块祛后则舒,四肢不温,治宜温经活血化瘀。取气海、气穴、三阴交、关元、中极、血海、膈俞。

Delayed Menstruation due to Blood Stasis One type of delayed menstruation mostly caused by stagnation of qi and accumulation of cold evil leading to the obstruction of blood stasis in the Chong and Ren Meridians with

the failure of menstrual blood to flow down to the uterus on time. 〈Manifestations of blood stasis due to stagnation of qi〉 delayed menstrual cycle, scanty menstruation with difficult discharge, purplish dark menses with profuse blood clots, distention and pain in the lower abdomen. 〈Treatment principle〉 Regulate the flow of qi and promote blood circulation to remove blood stasis. 〈Point selection〉 Qihai(RN 6), Qixue(KI 13), Sanyinjiao(SP 6), Zhongji(RN 3), Siman(KI 14), Taichong(LR 3) and Dadun(LR 1). 〈Manifestations of blood stasis due to accumulation of cold-evil〉 cold pain in the lower abdomen and tenderness, which is relieved by the discharge of blood clots, cold limbs. 〈Treatment principle〉 Warm the meridians and promote blood circulation to remove blood stasis. 〈Point selection〉Qihai(RN 6), Qixue (KI 13), Sanyinjiao (SP 6), Guanyuan(RN 4)Zhongji(RN 3), Xuehai(SP 10)and Geshu(BL 17).

●**血瘀痛经**[xuè yū tòng jīng] 痛经证型之一。多因经期产后，余血未尽，继受寒凉，或因情志内伤等，致使宿血停滞，凝结成瘀，内阻冲任胞脉，碍血下行所致。症见经前或经行之时，小腹刺痛拒按，经血量少，有块，血块下后痛减，舌紫黯，有瘀斑，脉弦涩。治宜活血化瘀，通络止痛。取膈俞、地机、气海、归来、次髎、血海。

Dysmenorrhea due to Blood Stasis One type of dysmenorrhea, mostly caused by the accumulation of blood stasis blocking the Chong and Ren Meridians and the uterus preventing the blood from flowing downward, resulting from unfinished diacharge of lochia or menses after delivery or menstrual cycle followed by the attack of cold or from internal impairment in emotion. 〈Manifestations〉pricking pain in the lower abdomen and tenderness before or during the menstrual cycle, scanty menstruation with blood clots, which is relieved by the discharge of blood clots, purplish dark tongue with ecchymosis, wiry and choopy pulse. 〈Treatment principle〉Promote blood circulation to remove blood stasis and dredge the collaterals to arrest pain. 〈Point selection〉Geshu (BL 17), Diji(SP 8), Qihai(RN 6), Guilai(ST 29), Ciliao(BL 32) and Xuehai(SP 10).

●**血瘀月经过少**[xuè yū yuè jīng guò shǎo] 月经过少证型之一。多见寒凝气滞，瘀血内停，冲任血行不畅所致。症见经行量少，色黯有块，小腹刺痛拒按，血块排出后痛减，舌边瘀斑，脉涩。治宜活血化瘀。取膈俞、血海、气海、中极、地机。

Scanty Menstruation due to Blood Stasis One type of hypomenorrhea, mostly caused by the accumulation of cold and the stagnation of qi, the retention of blood stasis, leading to the blockage of blood circulation into the Chong and Ren Meridians. 〈Manifestations〉scanty dark menstruation with blood clots, pricking pain in the lower abdomen and tenderness, which is relieved by the discharge of blood clots, ecchymosis at the edge of the tongue, choppy pulse. 〈Treatment principle〉Promote blood circulation to remove blood stasis. 〈Point selection〉Geshu(BL 17), Xuehai(SP 10), Qihai(RN 6), Zhongji(RN 3) and Diji (SP 8).

●**熏灸**[xūn jiǔ] 灸法的一种。见《五十二病方》。水煮艾或其他药物以其热气熏患处，或用火燃点后，以其烟熏患处。

Fumigating Moxibustion One form of moxibustion, originally seen in *Wushier Bingfang* (*Prescriptions for Fifty-Two Diseases*), referring to fumigating the affected part with steam produced by boiling the moxa or other herbs or with smoke of burning them.

●**熏脐法**[xūn qí fǎ] 间接灸一种。为蒸脐治病法之别称。见该条。

Fumigating the Umbilicus A type of indirect moxibustion, another name for treating a disease by steaming the umbilicus. →**蒸脐治病法** (p.599)

●**循法**[xún fǎ] 针刺辅助手法名。十四法之一。见《素问·离合真邪论》。指用手指沿经络部位，在腧穴的上下部位轻柔地循按。可激发经气的运行，使针刺容易得气。此法在《针经指南》、《针灸大成》中均有论述。

Massage along the Meridian An auxiliary manipulation in acupuncture, one of the fourteen methods, seen in *Su wen: Lihe Zhenxie Lun* (*Plain Questions: On the Expelling and*

Parting of Evil-Qi from Vital Qi), referring to a procedure for promoting the needling effect by pressing with the fingers gently on the upper or lower parts of the related acupoints along the meridians and collaterals. It can promote the flow of meridian-qi and make the needling response appear more easily. It is expounded in *Zhenjing Zhinan* (*A Guide to the Classics of Acupuncture*) and *Zhenjiu Dacheng* (*A Great Compendium of Acupuncture and Moxibustion*) as well.

●循脊[xún jǐ] ①经穴别名。见《针灸集成》。即天枢。见该条。②经外穴别名。出《针灸集成》。即长谷。见该条。

Xunji Another name for ① Tianshu (ST 25), a meridian point, seen in *Zhenjiu Jicheng* (*A Collection of Acupuncture and Moxibustion*). →天枢(p. 434) ② Changgu (EX-CA), an extra point, originally from *Zhenjiu Jicheng* (*A Collection of Acupuncture and Moxibustion*). →长谷(p. 39)

●循际[xún jì] ①经穴别名。出《备急千金要方》。即天枢。见该条。②经外穴别名。出《千金要方》。即长谷。见该条。

Xunji Another name for ① Tianshu (ST 25), a meridian point originally from *Beiji Qianjin Yaofang* (*Essential Prescriptions Worth a Thousand Gold for Emergencies*). →天枢(p. 434) ② the extra point, Changgu (EX-CA), originally from *Qianjin Yaofang* (*Essential Prescriptions Worth a Thousand Gold*). →长谷(p. 39)

●循经考穴编[xún jīng kǎo xué biān] 书名。撰人不详，两卷，约成书于十七世纪初（明末）。本书按十四经顺序，对经脉经穴做了详细考证，并附奇经内容及脏腑图。

Xunjing Kaoxue Bian (*Studies on Acupoints along Meridians*) A two-volume book with its author unknown, completed in the early years of the 17th century (end of the Ming Dynasty). In the book, detailed research was done on the Fourteen Meridians, and on the acupoints of the meridians, attached to it were an illustration of extra meridians and a diagram of zang-fu organs.

●循经感传现象[xún jīng gǎn chuán xiàn xiàng] 指沿经络路线出现的一些特殊感觉传导现象。参见"经络现象"条。

Sensation Transmission along the Meridians Transmission of some special sensations, occurring along the course of the meridians and collaterals. →经络现象(p. 211)

●循元[xún yuán] ①经穴别名。出《医学纲目》。即天枢。见该条。②经外穴别名。出《针灸集成》。即长谷。见该条。

Xunyuan Another name for ① Tianshu (ST 25), a meridian point originally from *Yixue Gangmu* (*An Outline of Medicine*). →天枢(p. 434) ② Changgu (EX-CA), an extra point, originally from *Zhenjiu Jicheng* (*A Collection of Acupuncture and Moxibustion*). →长谷(p. 39)

Y

●丫叉毒[yā chā dú] 即虎口疔。见该条。

Nail-Like Boil around Tiger's Mouth →虎口疔(p. 168)

●丫指[yā zhǐ] 即虎口疔，见该条。

Y-Shaped Finger →虎口疔(p. 168)

●压痛点[yā tòng diǎn] 指通过按压或撮捏体表时所发现的疼痛处或敏感处，腧穴的初级阶段，即以压痛反应作为定穴的依据。参见"压诊"、"阿是穴"条。

Pressing Pain Points The painful and sensitive sites found when the body surface is pressed or pinched. In the beginning, acupuncture points are located on the basis of the reaction of the pressing pain points. →压诊(p. 532)、阿是穴(p. 1)

●压诊[yā zhěn] 又称按诊。是指用按压循摄等手

法,寻找经络穴位上的异常变化,以协助诊断的方法。临床一般用拇指指腹循摄或用拇、食指撮捏,以探索皮下浅层异常反应,用拇指按压揉动以探查较深层异常反应,用力要均匀,左右进行对比,检查背腰部时,可以两手拇指紧贴脊椎棘突两侧,自下而上分段按压,并注意棘突间距离及有无偏斜,再推压两侧髂嵴和肩胛骨内侧缘。穴位压诊法的重点是夹脊穴及背俞、募、郄、合等穴。可见有皮下结节条索状物、压痛点、麻木区及肌胀隆起、硬结凹陷、松弛、变色、温度异常等反应。检查所得结果,须结合四诊和全身情况进行综合分析,以辨证选穴。

Diagnosis by Pressing Also known as pressing for diagnosis, referring to the pressing or molding manipulation, by which abnormal changes can be found on the acupoints, so as to help make a diagnosis. In clinic, usually the thumb is used to give pressure or to mold the skin around the acupoint in order to search for an abnormal reaction in the subcutaneous parts. Use the thumb to press and knead the deeper layer so as to probe the abnormal reaction there. The manipulation should be applied in an even movement with a balance of left and right. When checking the back and lumbar area, use the two thumbs to attach closely to the two sides of the vertebral process, and give pressure in parts from inferior to superior, paying attention to the distance between the processes and seeing that it is done slantwise before pressing forwards along the medial border of the iliac muscle and scapula on both sides. The emphasis in diagnosis by pressure is on the following points: Back-Shu points, Front-Mu points, Xi (Cleft) points, He (Sea) points, as well as Huatuojiaji points. The abnormal reaction may be: subcutaneous node or streaks, pressure pain point, numb region and eminence of muscular distention, depression, flabby, change of color of the masses and the body temperature, etc. To check the results obtained, make a comprehensive analysis in combination with the four diagnostic methods and the general condition of the whole body before selecting points by differentiating syndromes and signs.

●**押手法**[yā shǒu fǎ] 针刺术语。毫针进针时一般以左手按押穴位,协助进针,故左手通常称为押手。根据按押方式不同,又分别称为指切押手(爪切进针)、舒张押手(撑开进针)、夹持押手(捏起进针)、骈指押手(夹持进针)法等。

Hand-Pressing Method An acupuncture term. Press the acupoint generally with the left hand so as to help insert it, when the filiform needle is inserted. According to the different ways of pressing, it can be divided into hand pressing with fingers, hand pressing with fingers stretching, hand pressing by means of holding the skin, and hand pressing by means of holding the needle between fingers.

●**牙**[yá] 耳穴名。位于耳垂分区的1区。耳垂分区的方法是:从屏间切迹软骨下缘至耳垂下缘划三条等距水平线,再在第二水平线上引两条垂直等分线,由内向外、由上而下把耳垂分成1、2、3、4、5、6、7、8、9九个区。

Tooth (MA) An auricular point. 〈Location〉 on the lst of the ear lobe sections. The way of dividing the ear lobe is: from the lower border of the cartilage of the intertragic notch to the lower border of the ear lobe, draw three horizontal lines with equal distance between each two, and then, crossing the 2nd horrizontal line, draw two vertical lines by which the area is vertically and equally divided. From inferior to exterior, superior to inferior, the auricularlobe is divided into sections numbered with 1-9.

●**牙痛**[yá tòng] 症状名。为口腔疾病患中常见的症状。本症有虚实之分,实痛多因胃火、风火引起。虚痛多由肾阴不足所致。临床分为风火牙痛、实热牙痛和虚火牙痛。详见各条。

Toothache A symptom, commonly seen in oral diseases. It is divided into two types: excess and deficiency, mostly caused by stomach-fire and wind-fire. The deficiency-toothache is mostly due to insufficiency of kidney-yin. In clinic, it is divided into: toothache due to wind-fire, toothache due to excess-heat and toothache due to deficiency-fire. →风火牙痛(p. 112)、实热牙痛(p. 386)、虚火牙痛(p. 515)

●**哑门**[yǎ mén] 经穴名。《素问·气穴论》名瘖门,

近作哑门。属督脉,为督脉、阳维之会。又名舌横、横舌、舌厌。〈定位〉在项部,当后发际正中直上0.5寸,第一颈椎下(图28和图7)。〈层次解剖〉皮肤→皮下组织→左、右斜方肌之间→项韧带(左、右头夹肌之间→左、右头半棘肌之间)。浅层布有第三枕神经和皮下静脉。深层有第二、第三颈神经后支的分支,椎外(后)静脉丛和枕动、静脉的分支或属支。〈主治〉舌缓不语、音哑、头重、头痛、颈项强急、脊强反折、中风尸厥、癫狂、痫证、癔病、鼻衄、重舌、呕吐。伏案正坐位,使头微向前倾,项肌放松,向下颌方向缓慢刺入0.5~1寸;禁灸。

Yamen（DU 15） A meridian point, whose original name was Yinmen presented in *Suwen: Qixue Lun (Plain Questions: On Loci of Qi)*. It is a point on the Du Meridian, the crossing point of the Du and the Yangwei Meridians, also named Sheheng, Hengshe and Sheyan.〈Location〉on the nape, 0.5 cun directly above the midpoint of the posterior hairline, below the lst cervical vertebra (Figs. 28&7).〈Regional anatomy〉 skin→subcutaneous tissue→between left and right trapezius muscles→ nuchal ligament (between left and right splenius muscles of head)→between left and right semispinal muscles of head. In the superficial layer, there are the 3rd occipital nerve and the subcutaneous vein. In the deep layer, there are the branches of the posterior branches of the 2nd and 3rd cervical nerves, the external (posterior) vertebral venous plexus and the branches or tributaries of the occipital artery and vein.〈Indications〉 stiffness of tongue with aphasia, hoarseness of voice, heaviness of the head, headache, stiffness of the neck and nape, back rigidity, apoplexy with corpse-like syncope, mental disorder, epilepsy, hysteria, nose-bleeding, double tongue, vomiting.〈Method〉Have the patient sit straight at a table with the head sloping forward slightly and with the muscles of the nape relaxed, puncture 0.5~1.0 cun slowly toward the mandible. Moxibustion is forbidden.

●**咽喉**[yān hóu] 耳穴名。位于耳屏内侧面的上二分之一处。具有清咽利喉作用。〈主治〉声音嘶哑,急、慢性咽炎,扁桃体炎等。

Pharynx-Larynx（MA-T 3） An auricular point.〈Location〉at the upper half of the medial aspect of the tragus.〈Function〉Remove intense heat from the pharynx and larynx, relieve sorethroat.〈Indications〉hoarseness, acute and chronic pharyngitis and tonsillitis, etc.

●**咽喉肿痛**[yān hóu zhǒng tòng] 病证名。属于喉痹、乳蛾范畴。是咽喉病患中常见的病证之一。临床分风热咽喉肿痛、实热咽喉肿痛二种。参见各条。

Swelling and Pain of the Throat A disease, belonging to the category of sore-throat tonsillitis, one of the common diseases related to the throat. It is clinically divided into two types—swelling and pain of the throat due to wind-heatpathogen and swelling and pain of the throat due to excessive heat. →风热咽喉肿痛(p.114)、实热咽喉肿痛(p.386)

●**言语二区**[yán yǔ èr qū] 头针刺激区。〈定位〉从顶骨结节后下方2厘米处引一平行于前后正中线的直线,向下取3厘米长直线(图59.4)。〈主治〉命名失语(又称健忘性失语,病人称呼"名称"能力障碍,如病人不会叫"椅",只说是"坐的";其他人叫椅时,他能听懂。)

The Second Speech Area Stimulation area of scalp acupuncture.〈Location〉This area is a 3 cm straight line, starting from a point 2 cm posterior and inferior to the parietal tubercle, parallel to the anterior-posterior midline (Fig. 59.4).〈Indications〉nominal aphasia, also called amnestic aphasia, e.g. the patient is unable to say "chair", but knows a chair is something that can be sat on and understands what it is when someone else mentions "chair".

●**言语三区**[yán yǔ sān qū] 头针刺激区。晕听区中点向后引4厘米长的水平线。主治感觉性失语。(病人理解言语能力障碍,常答非所问。)

The Third Speech Area Stimulation area of scalp acupuncture.〈Location〉4 cm horizontal line backward from the midpoint of the vertigo-auditory area.〈Indication〉sensory aphasia (disturbance of language comprehension with frequent irrelevant answers).

●**严振**[yán zhèn] 人名。明针灸学家,号漫翁。疑著《循经考穴编》。参见该条。

Yan Zhen An acupuncture-moxibustion ex-

pert in the Ming Dynasty, who assumed the name Manwong and is supposed to have written *Xunjing Kaoxue Bian* (*Studies on Acupoints Along Meridians*). →循经考穴编(p. 532)

●沿皮刺[yán pí cì]　又称横刺、平刺。指针体与穴位皮肤表面呈10～20度角沿皮下刺入。适用于头面、胸部等肌肉浅薄处或正当骨面上的穴位。

Subcutaneous Needling　Also called horizontal needling or flat puncture, referring to inserting the needle subcutaneously to form an angle of 10°—20° with the skin. It is applied to points on the superficial and thin muscles such as the face, head, chest, etc. and the points just on the surface of the bones.

●研子[yán zǐ]　经外穴名。见《千金要方》。又名两手研子骨。在腕部背侧，当尺骨茎突之高点处。灸治热病后发豌豆疮。

Yanzi（EX-UE）　An extra point, seen in *Qianjin Yaofang* (*Essential Prescriptions Worth a Thousand Gold*), also named Liangshouyanzigu. 〈Location〉on the dorsum of the wrist, the highest spot on the styloid process of the ulna. 〈Indication〉sore of the pisiform after febrile disease. 〈Method〉moxibustion.

●盐哮[yán xiāo]　经外穴别名。即小指尖。详见该条。

Yanxiao　Another name for the extra point Xiaozhijian. →小指尖(p. 504)

●颜[yán]　部位名。额之中部，又称天庭、庭。一说指眉目之间；一说指面部前中央。

Central Forehead　A body part on the center of the forehead, which is also named "heaven court" or "court". One opinion about this is that the area is between the eyebrows and another is that it is the anterior centre of the face.

●眼[yǎn]　耳穴名。位于5区，参见"牙"条。用于治疗急性结膜炎、电光性眼炎、假性近视、麦粒肿。

Eye（MA-L 11）　An auricular point on the fifth area. 〈Indications〉acute conjunctivitis, electric ophthalmitis, pseudomyopia, hordeolum eye. →牙(p. 533)

●眼睑下垂[yǎn jiǎn xià chuí]　病证名。又称上胞下垂、睑废、雎目。多因先天禀赋不足，肾气虚弱，以致眼睑松弛，复多因脾虚气弱，肌肉弛纵，风邪外袭，脉络失和为病，亦可由外伤所致。证见上眼睑下垂，遮掩瞳孔，无力睁眼，双侧下垂者影响瞻视，重者眼球转动不灵，视一为二。中气不足者，兼有精神疲乏，食欲不振、眩晕、面色少华，眼睑麻木不仁，脉虚力无。治宜健脾益气。取攒竹、丝竹空、阳白、足三里、三阴交。风邪伤络者，多突然发病，并兼有其他肌肉麻痹症状。治宜疏风通络。取攒竹、丝竹空、阳白、风池、合谷。

Blepharoptosis　A disease, also named ptosis of the upper eyelid, dysfunction of the eyelid, or eyes of the vulture. Frequently due to congenital defect, deficiency of kidney-qi leading to blepharochalasis, accompanied by insufficiency of the spleen, muscular relaxation, affection by exopathogenic wind, resulting in lack of coordination between the meridians and collaterals. Or, it is due to trauma. 〈Manifestations〉blepharoptosis covering the pupil, weakness in opening eyes, difficulty in looking up due to blepharoptosis on both sides, poor movement of the eyeball and double vision in serious cases. Cases of qi-deficiency of the middle-jiao are accompanied by fatigue, lack of appetite, dizziness, dim complexion, numbness of the eyelid, feeble and weak pulse. 〈Treatment principle〉Strengthen the spleen and replenish qi. 〈Point selection〉Cuanzhu (BL 2), Sizhukong (SJ 23), Yangbai (GB 14), Zusanli (ST 36) and Sanyinjiao (SP 6). 〈Manifestations〉those with impairment of collaterals by pathogenic wind: sudden onset of the illness accompanied by numbness of other muscles. 〈Treatment principle〉Dispel wind and remove obstruction in the meridians. 〈Point selection〉Cuanzhu (BL 2), Sizhukong (SJ 23), Yangbai (GB 14), Fengchi (GB 20) and Hegu (LI 4).

●眼系[yǎn xì]　目系的别名。见该条。

Eye System　→目系(p. 273)

●燕口[yàn kǒu]　经外穴名。出《千金要方》。在口吻两旁赤白肉际。主治癫狂、面瘫、三叉神经痛等。沿皮刺0.3～0.5寸。

Yankou（EX-HN）　An extra point, originally from *Qianjin Yaofang* (*Essential Prescriptions Worth a Thousand Gold*). 〈Location〉on the junction of the red and white skin lateral

to both angles of the mouth. 〈Indications〉 manic-depressive psychosis, facial paralysis and trigeminal neuralgia, etc. 〈Method〉 Puncture subcutaneously 0.3-0.5 cun.

●阳白[yáng bái] 经穴名。出《针灸甲乙经》。属足少阳胆经,为足少阳、阳维之会。〈定位〉在前额部,当瞳孔直上,眉上1寸(图28和图5)。〈层次解剖〉皮肤→皮肤下组织→枕额肌额腹。布有眶上神经外侧支和眶上动、静脉外侧。〈主治〉头痛、目眩、目痛、外眦疼痛、眼睑瞤动、雀目。平刺0.5~0.8寸;可灸。

Yangbai(GB 14) A meridian point, originally from *Zhenjiu Jia-yi Jing* (*A-B Classic of Acupuncture and Moxibustion*), a point on the Gallbladder Meridian of Foot-Shaoyang, the crossing point of the Meridian of Foot-Shaoyang and the Yangwei Meridian. 〈Location〉 on the forehead, directly above the pupil, 1 cun above the eyebrow (Figs. 28 & 5). 〈Regional anatomy〉 skin → subcutaneous tissue → frontal belly of occipitofrontal muscle. There are the lateral branches of the supraorbital artery and vein in this area. 〈Indications〉 headache, dizziness, pain in the eye, pain in the outer canthus, flickering eyelid, nyctalopia. 〈Method〉 Puncture horizontally 0.5~0.8 cun. Moxibustion is applicable.

●阳池[yáng chí] 经穴名。出《灵枢·本输》。属手少阳三焦经,本经原穴。又名别阳。〈定位〉在腕背横纹中,当指伸肌腱的尺侧缘凹陷处(图44.4)。〈层次解剖〉皮肤→皮下组织→腕背侧韧带→指伸肌腱(桡侧)与小指伸肌腱之间→桡腕关节。浅层布有尺神经手背支、腕背静脉网、前臂后皮神经的末支。深层有尺动脉腕背支的分支。〈主治〉腕痛、肩臂痛、耳聋、疟疾、消渴、口干、喉痹。直刺0.3~0.5;可灸。

Yangchi (SJ 4) A meridian point, originally from *Lingshu: Benshu* (*Miraculous Pivot: Meridian Points*), the Yuan(Primary) point of the Sanjiao Meridian of Hand-Shaoyang, also named Bieyang. 〈Location〉 at the midpoint of the dorsal crease of the wrist, in the depression on the ulnar side or the tendon of the extensor muscle of the fingers (Fig. 44.4). 〈Regional anatomy〉 skin → subcutaneous tissue → ligament of dorsum of wrist-between tendons of extensor muscle of fingers and extensor muscle of little finger → radiocarpal joint. In the superficial layer, there are the dorsal branches of the ulnar nerve, the dorsal venous network of the wrist and the terminal branches of postericx cutaneous nerve of the forearm. In the deep layer, there are the branches of the dorsal carpal branch of the ulnar artery. 〈Indications〉 pain in the wrist, pain of the shoulder and arm, deafness, malarial disease. diabetes, dry mouth, inflammation of the throat. 〈Method〉 Puncture perpendicularly 0.3-0.5 cun. Moxibustion is applicable.

●阳刺[yáng cì] 刺法名。出《黄帝内经太素》卷二十二。今本《灵枢·官针》作扬刺。参见该条。

Yang Needing An ancient acupuncture technique, originally from Vol. 22 of *Huangdi Neijing Tai Su* (*Comprehensive Notes to the Yellow Emperor's Inner Canon*). It is called centre-square needling in the present edition of *Lingshu: Guan Zhen* (*Miraculous Pivot: Official Needle*). → 扬刺 (p.542)

●阳辅[yáng fǔ] 经穴名。出《灵枢·本输》。属足少阳胆经,为本经经穴。又名分肉、绝骨。〈定位〉在小腿外侧,当外踝尖上4寸,腓骨前缘稍前方(图8.2)。〈层次解剖〉皮肤→皮下组织→趾长伸肌→拇长伸肌→小腿骨间膜→胫骨后肌。浅层布有腓肠外侧皮神经和腓浅神经。深层有腓动、静脉。〈主治〉偏头痛、目外眦痛、缺盆中痛、腋下痛、瘰疬、胸、胁、下肢外侧痛、疟疾、半身不遂。直刺0.5~0.8寸;可灸。

Yangfu(GB 38) A meridian point, originally from *Ling Shu: Benshu* (*Miraculous Pivot: Meridian Points*), the Jing(River) point of the Gallbladder Meridian of Foot-Shaoyang, also named Fenrou or Juegu. 〈Location〉on the lateral side of the leg, 4 cun above the tip of the external malleous, slightly anterior to the anterior border of the fibula (Fig. 8.2). 〈Regional anatomy〉skin → subcutaneous tissue → long extensor muscle of toes → long extensor muscle of the great toe → interosseous membrane of leg → posterior tibial muscle. In the superficial layer, there are the lateral sural cutaneous nerve and the superficial peroneal nerve. In the deep layer, there are the peroneal artery and vein. 〈Indications〉 migraine, pain in the outer canthus, pain in the supraclavicular fossa

and in the armpit, scrofula, pain in the chest, the hypochondriac region and the lateral surface of the lower limbs, malarial disease, hemiplegia. 〈Method〉Puncture perpendicularly 0. 5-0. 8 cun. Moxibustion is applicable.

●阳刚[yáng gāng] ①经穴别名。见《太平圣惠方》。即阳纲。参见该条。②经外穴名。见《古今医统》。位于命门穴旁开1寸。〈主治〉消渴、黄疸、肠风下血、痔疮、腰痛、遗尿、遗精等。直刺0.5～1寸;可灸。

1. **Yanggang** Another name for Yanggang (阳纲)(BL 48), a meridian point, seen in *Taiping Shenghuifang* (*Imperial Benevolent Prescriptions*).→阳纲(p. 537)

2. **Yanggang** (EX-B) An extra point, seen in *Gujin Yitong* (*The General Medicine of the Past and Present*).〈Location〉1 cun lateral to Mingmen(DU 4).〈Indications〉diabetes, jaundice, hematochezia, hemorrhoid, lumbago, enuresis, emission.〈Method〉Puncture perpendicularly 0. 5-1. 0 cun. Moxibustion is applicable.

●阳纲[yáng gāng] 经穴名。出《针灸甲乙经》。属足太阳膀胱经,又名阳刚。〈定位〉在背部,当第十胸椎棘突下,旁开3寸(图7)。〈层次解剖〉皮肤→皮下组织→背阔肌→下后锯肌→竖脊肌。浅层布有第十、十一胸神经后支的外侧皮支和伴行的动、静脉。深层有第十、十一胸神经后支的肌支和相应的肋间后动、静脉背侧支的分支或属支。〈主治〉肠鸣、腹痛、泄泻、黄疸、消渴。斜刺0.5～0.8寸;可灸。

Yanggang (BL 48) A meridian point, originally from *Zhenjiu Jia-Yi Jing* (*A-B Classic of Acupuncture and Moxibustion*), a point on the Bladder Meridian of Foot-Taiyang, also named Yanggang(阳·刚).〈Location〉on the back, below the spinous process of the 10th thoracic vertebra, 3 cun lateral to the posterior midline (Fig. 7).〈Regional anatomy〉skin→subcutaneous tissue → latissimus muscle of back → inferior posterior serratus muscle → erector spinal muscle. In the superficial layer, there are the lateral cutaneous branches of the posterior branches of the 10th and 11th thoracic nerves and the accompanying arteries and veins. In the deep layer, there are the muscular branches of the posterior branches of the 10th and 11th thoracic nerves and the branches or tributaries of the dorsal branches of the related posterior intercostal arteries and veins.〈Indications〉borborygmus, abdominal pain, diarrhea, jaundice, diabetes.〈Method〉Puncture obliquely 0. 5-0. 8 cun. Moxibustion is applicable.

●阳谷[yáng gǔ] 经穴名.出《灵枢·本输》。属手太阳小肠经,为本经经穴。〈定位〉在手腕尺侧,当尺骨茎突与三角骨之间的凹陷处(图65.2)。〈层次解剖〉皮肤→皮下组织→尺侧腕伸肌腱的前方。浅层有尺神经手背支,贵要静脉等分布。深层有尺动脉的腕背支等结构。〈主治〉颈颔肿、臂外侧痛、手腕痛、热病无汗、头眩、目赤肿痛、癫狂妄言、胁痛项肿、疥疮生疣、痔漏、耳聋、耳鸣、齿痛。直刺0.3～0.4寸;可灸。

Yanggu (SI 5) A meridian point, originally from *Lingshu*: *Ben Shu* (*Miraculous Pivot*: *Meridian Points*), the Jing (River) Point of the Small Intestine Meridian of Hand-Taiyang.〈Location〉on the ulnar border of the wrist, in the depression between the styloid process of the ulna and trianguar bone (Fig. 65. 2).〈Regional anatomy〉 skin→subcutaneous tissue→anterior side of tendon of ulnar extensor muscle of wrist. In the superficial layer, there are the dorsal branches of the ulnar nerve and the basilic vein. In the deep layer, there are the dorsal branches of the ulnar artery.〈Indications〉 swelling of the neck and jaw, pain in the lateral surface of the arm, pain in the wrist, febrile disease without sweat, dizziness, redness, swelling and pain of the eyes, ravings due to epilepsy, hypochondriac pain, swelling of the nose, verruca from scabies, hemorrhoid complicated by anal fistula, deafness, tinnitus, toothache.〈Method〉Puncture perpendicularly 0. 3-0. 4 cun. Moxibustion is applicable.

●阳关[yáng guān] 经穴别名。一属督脉,在腰;一属胆经,在膝。《针灸大全》称前者为背阳关,后者为足阳关;近代多称前者为腰阳关,后者为膝阳关。见各条。

Yangguan Another name for two meridian points. One is on the loin, and belongs to the Du Meridian; the other is on the knee and belongs to the Gallbladder Meridian. In *Zhenjiu*

Daquan(*A Complete Work of Acupuncture and Moxibustion*), the former was named Beiyangguan, the latter, Zuyangguan. In modern times, the former one is named Yaoyangguan(DU 3), the latter one Xiyangguan(GB 33).→背阳关(p.17)、足阳关(p.645)、腰阳关(p.546)、膝阳关(p.484)

●阳黄[yáng huáng] 黄疸证型之一。见《景岳全书·黄疸》。多因感受湿热外邪,内蕴肝胆,湿郁热蒸,以致疏泄功能阻滞,胆液横溢所致。证见目肤色黄,鲜明如橘,身热口渴,腹部胀满,胸中懊憹,小便短黄,大便秘结,苔黄腻,脉弦数。治宜清热化湿,疏利肝胆。取至阳、腕骨、阳陵泉、太冲。

Yang Jaundice A type of jaundice from *Jingyue Quanshu: Huangdan (Jingyue's Complete Works: Jaundice)*, mostly caused by affection of exogenous pathogenic damp-heat, in the liver and the gallbladder, heat due to blockage of dampness, leads to a disorder in the dispelling and purging functions and overflow of bile. ⟨Manifestations⟩ yellowish eyes and skin like colour of a fresh orange, fever, thirst, abdominal distension, vexation, scanty dark urine, constipation, yellowish and greasy tongue coating, wiry and rapid pulse. ⟨Treatment principle⟩ Clear heat, eliminate dampness and smooth the liver and gallbladder. ⟨Point selection⟩ Zhiyang (DU 9), Wangu (SI 4), Yanglingquan (GB 34) and Taichong (LR 3).

●阳交[yáng jiāo] 经穴名。出《针灸甲乙经》。属足少阳胆经,为阳维脉的郄穴。又名别阳、足髎。⟨定位⟩在小腿外侧,当外踝尖上7寸,腓骨后缘(图8.1)。⟨层次解剖⟩皮肤→皮下组织→小腿三头肌→腓骨长肌→后肌间隔→拇长屈肌。浅层布有腓肠外侧皮神经。深层有腓动、静脉,胫后动、静脉和胫神经。⟨主治⟩胸胁胀满疼痛、面肿、惊狂、癫疾、瘈疭、膝股痛、下肢痿痹。直刺0.5～0.8寸;可灸。

Yangjiao (GB 35) A meridian point, originally from *Zhenjiu Jia-Yi Jing (A-B Classic of Acupuncture and Moxibustion)*, a point on the Gallbladder Meridian of Foot-Shaoyang, the Xi (Cleft) point of the Yanwei Meridian, also named Bieyang or Zuliao. ⟨Location⟩ on the lateral side of the leg, 7 cun above the tip of the external malleolus, on the posterior border of the fibula (Fig. 8.1). ⟨Regional anatomy⟩ skin→subcutaneous tissue→tricpes muscle of calf→long peroneal muscle→posterior intermusclar septum→long flexor muscle of great toe. In the superficial layer, there is the lateral sural cutaneous nerve. In the deep layer, there are the peroneal artery and vein, the posterior tibial artery and vein, and the tibial nerve. ⟨Indications⟩ fullness and pain in the chest and hypochondrium, edema of the face, mania due to fright, disorder of the head, clonic convulsion, pain in the knee and thigh, flaccidity and numbness of the lower limbs. ⟨Method⟩ Puncture perpendicularly 0.5～0.8 cun. Moxibustion is applicable.

●阳窟[yáng kū] 肠窟之误。见《针灸聚英》。即腹结。参见该条。

Yangku A slip of pen of *Changku*, seen in *Zhenjiu Juying (Essentials of Acupuncture and Moxibustion)*, referring to Fujie (SP 14). →腹结(p.121)

●阳陵[yáng líng] ①经穴别名。见《标幽赋》。即阳陵泉。详见该条。②经穴别名。见《针灸大全》。即阳关。详见该条。

Yangling Another name for ① Yanglingquan (GB 34), a meridian point seen in *Biaoyou Fu (Lyrics of Recondite Principles)*→阳陵泉(p.538) ② Yangguan, a pair of meridian points, seen in *Zhenjiu Daquan (A Compete Work of Acupuncture and Moxibustion)*. →阳关(p.537)

●阳陵泉[yáng líng quán] 经穴名。出《灵枢·邪气藏府病形》。属足少阳胆经。为本经合穴,八会穴之筋会。又名阳之陵泉、阳陵。⟨定位⟩在小腿外侧,当腓骨头前下方凹陷处(图8.2)。⟨层次解剖⟩皮肤→皮下组织→腓骨长肌→趾长伸肌。浅层布有腓肠外侧皮神经。深层有胫前返动、静脉,膝下外侧动、静脉的分支或属支和腓总神经分支。⟨主治⟩半身不遂、下肢痿痹、麻木、膝肿痛、脚气、胁肋痛、口苦、呕吐、黄疸、小儿惊风、破伤风。直刺或斜向下刺1～1.5寸;可灸。

Yanglingquan (GB 34) A meridian point originally from *Ling Shu: Xieqi Zangfu Bingxing (Miraculous Pivot: Pathogenic Evils, Zang-Fu Organs and Manifestations)*, on the Gallbladder Meridian of Foot-Shaoyang, the influential point of the tendons of the 8 Influential

Points, also named Yangzhilingquan or Yangling. ⟨Location⟩ on the lateral side of the leg, in the depression anterior and inferior to the head of the fibula(Fig. 8.2). ⟨Regional anatomy⟩ skin → subcutaneous tissue → long peroneal muscle → long extensor muscle of toes. In the superficial layer, there is the lateral sural cutaneous nerve. In the deep layer, there are the anterior recurrent tibial artery and vein, the branches or tributaries of the lateral inferior genicular artery and vein, and the branches of common peroneal nerve. ⟨Indications⟩ hemiplegia, flaccidity and numbness of the lower limbs, swelling and pain of the knee, beriberi, pain in the hypochondriac region, bitter taste, vomiting, jaundice, infantie convulsion, tetanus. ⟨Method⟩ Puncture perpendicularly or obliquely downwards 1.0～1.5 cun. Moxibustion is applicable.

●阳络[yáng luò]　①经络名。出《灵枢·百病始生》。与阴络相对,指位于浅表的络脉。②指自手、足三阴经分出的络脉。③专指足阳明胃的络脉,与足阳明胃的经脉相对之称。

Yang Collaterals　①A catelogue of collaterals, originally from *Ling Shu*: *Baibing Shisheng* (*Miraculous Pivot*: *Occurrence of Diseases*), as opposed to yin collaterals, referring to those distributed superficially. ②Referring to the collaterals diverging from the three yang meridians of hand and foot. ③Referring especially to the Stomach Collaterals of Foot-yangming as opposed to the Stomach Meridian of Foot-yangming.

●阳明脉[yáng míng mài]　早期经脉名。出《帛书》。与足阳明胃经类似。参见该条。

Yangming Vessel　Early name of a meridian, originally from *Bo Shu* (*Silk Book*), similar to Foot-Yangming Meridian. →足阳明胃经(p. 647)

●阳跷[yáng qiāo]　①经脉名。指阳跷脉。见该条。②经穴别名。见《针灸大全》。即申脉。见该条。

1. Yangqiao　A meridian, referring to the Yangqiao Meridian. →阳跷脉(p. 539)

2. Yangqiao　Another name for Shenmai(BL 62), a meridian point seen in *Zhenjiu Daquan* (*A Complete Work of Acupuncture and Moxibustion*). →申脉(p. 359)

●阳跷病[yáng qiāo bìng]　奇经八脉病候之一。出《难经·二十九难》。可见下肢活动不利、不寐、目痛等。

Diseases of Yangqiao　One of the pathological manifestations of the Eight Extra Meridians, originally from *Nanjing*: *Ershijiu Nan* (*The Classic of Questions*: *Question* 29). ⟨Manifestations⟩ difficulty in movement of the lower limbs, insomnia, pain in the eye, etc.

●阳跷脉[yáng qiāo mài]　奇经八脉之一。其循行起于足跟外侧,经行踝上行腓骨后缘,沿股部外侧和胁后上肩,过颈部上挟口角,进入目内眦,与阴跷脉会合,再沿足太阳经上额,与足少阳经合于风池。

Yangqiao Meridian　One of the Eight Extra Meridians, which starts from the lateral surface of the heel, goes along the lateral malledus to the posterior border of the fibula, ascends along the lateral surface of the thigh, crosses the other meridians to the shoulder, passes through the neck to reach the angle of the mouth, then enters the inner canthus, joins the Yinqiao Meridian, goes along the Meridian of Foot-Taiyang to the forehead, and at last meets the Meridian of Foot-Shaoyang at Fengchi(GB 20).

●阳水[yáng shuǐ]　水肿证型之一。出《丹溪心法·水肿》。由肺气失宣,三焦壅滞,不能通调水道下输膀胱所致。证见头面先肿,渐及全身,腰部以上肿甚,按之凹陷,恢复较快,皮肤光泽,小便短少,恶寒发热,肢体酸痛,咳嗽气粗,舌苔薄黄,脉浮数。治宜清热散寒,疏风利水。取肺俞、三焦俞、偏历、阴陵泉、合谷。

Yang Type of Edema　A type of edema, originally from *Danxi Xinfa*: *Shuizhong* (*Danxi's Experience*: *Edema*), due to obstruction of the lung-qi, blockage of Sanjiao causing failure to clear and regulate the water passages to make the body fluid metabolize to the urinary bladder. ⟨Manifestations⟩ first, swelling of the face and head, then of the whole body, severe swelling of the area above the loin, hollow with pressure, quick recovery, lustrous skin, oliguria, aversion to cold, fever, aching of the body, cough, short breath, thin and yellowish tongue coating, superficial and rapid pulse.

⟨Treatment principle⟩Clear heat, dispel cold and wind and induce diuresis. ⟨Point selection⟩Feishu(BL 13), Sanjiaoshu(BL 22), Pianli (LI 6), Yinlingquan(LI 9), and Hegu(LI 4).

●阳燧锭灸[yáng suì dìng jiǔ]　灸法的一种。出《针灸逢源》。阳燧锭是由硫磺加上其他药物混合制成，放在穴位上燃点施灸。本法可用于风湿痹痛、关节扭伤、手足挛急等症。

Sulfur-Made Lozenge Moxibustion　A kind of moxibustion, originally from *Zhenjiu Fengyuan* (*The Origin of Acupuncture and Moxibustion*), which is made of sulfur and other herbal medicines, and ignited on the points for moxibustion. ⟨Indications⟩ rheumatalgia, sprain of joints, contracture and tight sensation of hands and feet.

●阳维病[yáng wéi bìng]　奇经八脉病候之一。出《难经·二十九难》。证见恶寒、发热、腰痛等。

Diseases of Yangwei Meridian　One of the pathological manifestations of the Eight Extra Meridians, originally from *Nan Jing: Ershijiu Nan* (*The Classic of Quetions: Question 29*). ⟨Manifestations⟩aversion to cold, fever, lumbago, etc.

●阳维脉[yáng wéi mài]　奇经八脉之一。出《素问·刺腰痛篇》。其循行，起于足跟外侧，向上经过外踝，沿足少阳经上行髋关节部，经胁肋后侧，从腋后上肩，至前额，再到项后，合于督脉。

Yangwei Meridian　One of the Eight Extra Meridians, originally from *Su Wen: Ci Yaotong Pian* (*Plain Questions: On Treatment of Lumbago with Acupuncture*). It begins on the lateral surface of the heel, goes upward across the lateral malleolus, ascends along the Meridian of Foot-Shaoyang to the hip joint, then along the posterior surface of the hypochondrium, goes from the posterior surface of the armpit to the shoulder and the forehead, then to the posterior surface of the nape and finally meets the Du Meridian.

●阳维穴[yáng wéi xué]　①阳维脉交会穴。下肢部交会足太阳经的金门、足少阳经的阳交，肩部交会手太阳经的臑俞、手少阳经的天髎、足少阳经的肩井；头部交会足少阳经的风池、脑空、承灵、正营、目窗、头临泣、阳白、本神，督脉的哑门、风府。②经穴别名。见《针经指南》。即外关。见该条。③经外穴名。出《千金翼方》。在耳廓后，当手拉耳向前时，于眼部所出现的弦筋上，与耳门穴相平处。⟨主治⟩耳鸣、耳聋、中耳炎等。直刺0.1～0.2寸；可灸。

1. Yangwei Xue　The confluence points of the Yangwei Meridian. Those on the lower limbs are Jinmen(BL 63) of the Meridian of Foot-Taiyang and Yangjiao(GB 35) of the Meridian of Foot-Shaoyang; on the shoulder are Naoshu (SI 10) of the Meridian of Hand-Taiyang, Tianliao(SJ 15) of the Meridian of Hand-Shaoyang and Jianjing (GB 21) of the Meridian of Foot-Shaoyang; on the head are Fengchi (GB 20), Naokong (GB 19), Chengling (GB 18), Zhengying (GB 17), Muchuang (GB 16), Toulingqi (GB 15), Yangbai(GB 14), and Benshen(GB 13) of the Meridian of Foot-Shaoyin; Yamen (DU 15) and Fengfu(DU 16) of the Du Meridian.

2. Yangwei　Another name for Waiguan(SJ 5), a meridian point, seen in *Zhenjing Zhinan* (*Guide to the Classics of Acupuncture*). →外关(p. 453)

3. Yangwei(EX-HN)　An extra point, originally from *Qianjin Yifang* (*Supplement to the Essential Prescriptions Worth a Thousand Gold*). ⟨Location⟩on the area posterior to the ear, at the tight tendons appearing in the back of the ear while pulling the ear foreward, at the same level on *Ermen*(SJ 21). Indications: tinnitus, deafness, otits media, etc. ⟨Method⟩ Puncture perpendicularly 0.1～0.2 cun. Moxibustion is applicable.

●阳萎[yáng wěi]　病证名。见《景岳全书·杂证谟》。又称阴痿。指男子未到性功能衰退时期，出现阴茎不举，或举而不坚，或时间短暂以致影响正常性生活的病证。多因房劳过度，命门火衰所致。亦有因肝肾虚火，心脾受损，惊恐不释，抑郁伤肝所致者。临床分为阳萎实证、阳萎虚证。参见各条。

Impotence　A disease, seen in *Jingyue Quanshu: Zazhenmo* (*Jingyue's Complete Works: Strategies on Miscellaneous Diseases*), also named weakness of the penis, referring to the disease characterized by poor erection or erection that lasts only for a few seconds. A dysfunction which affects normal sexual life,

mostly caused by intemperance in sexual life, decline of fire from the gate of life. or fire due to deficiency of the liver and kidney, impairment of the heart and the spleen, long term fright and terror, impairment of the liver due to melancholia in some cases. It is clinically divided into excess syndrome of impotence and deficiency syndrome of impotence. →阳萎实证(p.541)、阳萎虚证(p.541)

●阳萎实证[yáng wěi shí zhèng] 阳萎证型之一。多由湿热下注,宗筋弛纵所致。证见阴茎虽能勃起,但时间短暂,每多早泄,阴囊潮湿,臊臭,下肢酸重,小便黄赤,舌苔黄腻,脉濡数。治宜清利湿热。取肾俞、气海、阴陵泉、三阴交、足三里、蠡沟、八髎。

Excess Syndrome of Impotence A type of impotence, mostly due to the downward flow of damp-heat and relaxation of the assembled tendons. 〈Manifestations〉erection but only for a short time, frequent prospermia, wet scrotum with foul smell, aching and heavy sensation of the lower limbs, dark urine, yellowish and greasy tongue coating, soft and rapid pulse. 〈Treatment principle〉Eliminate dampness and heat. 〈Point selection〉Shenshu(BL 23), Qihai(RN 6), Yinlingquan(SP 9), Sanyinjiao(SP 6), Zusanli(ST 36), Ligou(LR 5) and Baliao(BL 31,32,33,34).

●阳萎虚证[yáng wěi xū zhèng] 阳萎证型之一。多因纵欲过度,宗筋弛纵所致。证见阴茎勃起困难,时时滑精,精薄清冷,头晕,耳鸣,心悸短气,面色㿠白,精神不振,腰膝酸软,畏寒肢冷,舌淡白,脉沉细。治宜温补肾阳。取肾俞、命门、腰阳关、关元、复溜、大赫。

Deficiency Syndrome of Impotence A type of impotence, mostly due to intemperance in sexual life and relaxation of assembled tendons. 〈Manifestations〉difficulty in erection, frequent spermatorrhoea, thin and cold sperm, dizziness, tinnitus, palpitation, short breath, pale complexion, lassitude, lassitude in the loin and knees, aversion to cold, cold limbs, pale tongue, deep and thready pulse. 〈Treatment principle〉Warm and supplement the kidney-yang. 〈Point selection〉Shenshu (BL 23), Mingmen (DU 4), Yaoyangguan (DU 3), Guanyuan (RN 4), Fuliu (KI 7) and Dahe (KI 12).

●阳溪[yáng xī] 经穴名。出《灵枢·本输》。属手阳明大肠经,为本经经穴。又名中魁。〈定位〉在腕背横纹桡侧,手指向上翘起时,当拇短伸肌腱与拇长伸肌腱之间的凹陷中(图6.3)。〈层次解剖〉皮肤→皮下组织→拇短伸肌腱与拇长伸肌腱之间→桡侧腕长伸肌腱前方。浅层布有头静脉和桡神经浅支等。深层有桡动、静脉的分支或属支。〈主治〉头痛、耳聋、耳鸣、咽喉肿痛、龋齿痛、目赤、目翳、热病心烦、臂腕痛、癫、狂、直刺0.3—0.5寸;可灸。

Yangxi(LI 5) A meridian point, originally from *Lingshu: Ben Shu* (*Miraculous Pivot: Meridian Points*), the Jing (River) point of the Large Intestine Meridian of Hand-Yangming, also named Zhongkui. 〈Location〉at the radial end of the crease of the wrist, in the depression between the tendons of the short extensor and long extensor muscles of the thumb when the thumb is tilted upward (Fig. 6.3). 〈Regional anatomy〉skin→subcutaneous tissue→between short extensor muscle tendon of thumb and long extensor muscle tendon of thumb → front part of long radial extensor muscle of wrist. In the superficial layer, there are the branches of the cephalic vein and the superficial branches of the radial nerve. In the deep layer, there are the branches or tributaries of the radial artery and vein. 〈Indications〉 headache, deafness, tinnitus, sweelling and pain of the throat, pain of the dental caries, conjunctivel congestion, nebula in the eye, vexation due to rebrile disease, pain in the arm and the wrist, vertex, mania and epilepsy. 〈Method〉Puncture perpendicularly 0.3~0.5 cun. Moxibustion is applicable.

●阳虚崩漏[yáng xū bēng lòu] 崩漏证型之一。多因肾阳虚惫,失于封藏,冲任失于固摄所致。证见血崩下血,或淋漓不绝,血色淡红,小腹冷痛,四肢不湿,喜热畏寒,大便溏薄,舌淡苔白,脉沉细。治宜湿补肾阳,收摄经血。取关元、三阴交、肾俞、交信、气海、命门、复溜。

Metrorrhagia and Metrostaxia due to Yang Insufficiency A type of metrorrhagia and methrastaxis, mostly due to insufficiency of kindney-yang, dysfunction in storing essence, debility of the Chong and Ren Meridians.

⟨Manifestations⟩ bleeding due to metrorrhagia, or pale, dripping blood, cold-pain in the lower abdomen, cold limbs, preference for warm, aversion to cold, loose stools, pale tongue with whitish coating, deep and thready pulse. ⟨Treatment principle⟩ Warm and recuperate the kidney yang, astringe to arrest menstruation. ⟨Point selection⟩ Guanyuan(RN 4), Sanyinjiao(SP 6), Shenshu(BL 23), Jiaoxin(KI 8), Qihai(RN 6), Mingmen(DU 4) and Fuliu(KI 7).

●阳虚呃逆[yáng xū è nì] 呃逆证型之一。多因脾胃虚弱,虚气上逆所致。证见呃逆声低弱无力,气不得续,面色苍白,手足不温,食少困倦,舌淡苔白,脉沉细弱。治宜温补脾胃,和中降逆。针天突、膈俞、足三里、内关、气海、中脘、脾俞、胃俞。

Hiccup due to Yang Insufficiency A type of hiccup, mostly due to deficiency of the spleen and stomach, adverse up-moving of qi of deficiency type. ⟨Manifestations⟩ hiccup with low voice, short breath, pale tongue with whitish coating, deep, thready and weak pulse. ⟨Treatment principle⟩ Warm and invigorate the spleen and stomach; regulate the middle-jiao and keep the adverse qi downward. ⟨Point selection⟩ Tiantu(RN 22), Geshu(BL 17), Zusanli(ST 36), Neiguan(PC 6), Qihai(RN 6), Zhongwan(RN 12), Pishu(BL 20) and Weishu(BL 21).

●阳虚腹痛[yáng xū fù tòng] 腹痛证型之一。多因中阳不足,内失温养所致。证见腹痛隐隐,时作时止,痛时腹部喜按,大便溏泄,面色少华,舌质淡胖,边有齿痕,舌苔白,脉沉细而迟。治宜补脾温肾。针脾俞、肾俞、章门、关元。

Abdominal Pain due to Yang Insufficency A type of abdominal pain, mostly due to weakened yang of the middle-jiao, internal lack of warmth and nourishment. ⟨Manifestations⟩ occasional dull abdominal pain from time to time, relieved when pressed, loose stools, dim complexion, pale and enlarged tongue with marks of the teeth on the edge of the tongue, whitish coating, deep, thready and slow pulse. ⟨Treatment principle⟩ Reinforce the spleen and warm the kidney. ⟨Point selection⟩ Pishu(BL 20), Shenshu(BL 23), Zhangmen(LR 13) and Guanyuan(RN 4).

●阳泽[yáng zé] 经穴别名。出《千金翼方》。即曲池。详见该条。

Yangze Another name for Quchi(LI 11), a meridian point from *Qianjin Yifang* (*A Supplement to Essential Prescriptions Worth a Thousand Gold*). →曲池(p. 323)

●阳之陵泉[yáng zhī líng quán] 经穴别名。出《灵枢·九针十二原》。即阳陵泉。详见该条。

Yangzhilingquan Another name for Yanglingquan(GB 34), a meridian point from *Lingshu: Jiu Zhen Shier Yuan* (*Miraculous Pivot: Nine Needles and Twelve Yuan (Primary) Points*). →阳陵泉(p. 538)

●阳中隐阴[yáng zhōng yǐn yīn] 针刺手法名。出《金针赋》。与阴中隐阳相对,为先补后泻法。其法当先浅部运针,行紧按慢提九数,觉微热,再进到深部运针,行紧提慢按六数,觉微凉,稍停片刻,出针。用于先寒后热的病证。

Yin Occluded in Yang A needling method, originally from *Jinzhen Fu* (*Ode to Gold Needle*), as compared with yang occluded in yin, a method of reinforcing followed by reducing. Apply the needle superficially. First thrust it rapidly and lift it slowly 9 times. When the patient feels slightly warm, apply the needle in the deep part. Lift it rapidly and thrust it slowly 6 times, retain the needle for a while when the patient feels slightly cold and then withdraw the needle. ⟨Indications⟩ diseases with cold symptoms before fever.

●扬刺[yáng cì] 《内经》刺法名。出《灵枢·官针》。为十二刺之一。又名阳刺。扬是分散的意思,其法正中刺一针,周围刺四针,刺得较浅,以治疗范围较大的寒痹等,与齐刺相对,同属多针类刺法。

Central-Square Needlling One of the 12 needing methods from *Lingshu: Guan Zhen* (*Miraculous Pivot: Official Puncture*), also named Yang Ci (阳刺). Yang (扬) means "to spread". ⟨Method⟩ Insert superficially one needle at the centre of the affected area and another four around it. ⟨Indications⟩ cases of relatively widespread and superficial cold arthralgia. It is compared to triple puncture, and they both belong to the method of multineedle

puncture.

●杨继洲[yáng jì zhōu] 人名。明代著名针灸学家,名济时,三衢(今浙江衢县)人,家世医,曾任太医院医官,他博览群书,临证经验丰富,尤精于针灸。在家传《卫生针灸玄机秘要》的基础上,结合个人经验,编成《针灸大成》一书。此书内容丰富,取材广泛,可称集明以前针灸学之精华,对针灸学的发展作出了重要贡献。

Yang Jizhou A famous acupuncture moxibustion expert in the Ming Dynasty, whose given name was Jishi, a native of Sanqu (today's Quxian County, Zhejiang Province). He came from a long line of doctors and was once a medicinal official in the Institute of Imperial Physicians. Reading extensively, he was rich in clinical experience and especially proficient in acupuncture and moxibustion. On the basis of *Weisheng Zhenjiu Xuanji Miyao* (*Mysterious Clandestine Essentials of Acupuncture and Moxibustion for Health Protection*), handed down in the family, and combined with his own experience, he compiled *Zhenjiu Dacheng* (*A Great Compendium of Acupuncture and Moxibustion*). The book has substantial content, draws extensive materials, collects the acumoxibustion cream prior to the Ming Dynasty, and is a significant contribution to the development of acupuncture and moxibustion.

●杨介[yáng jiè] 人名。北宋医家,字吉老,泗洲(今江苏盱眙)人。对政和三年(1113年)绘制的解剖图加以校正,作《存真图》一卷,在解剖学和针灸学方面做出贡献。原书已佚。其图曾为《针灸聚英》和《针灸大成》所引用。

Yang Jie A famous physician in the Northern Song Dynasty, who styled himself Jilao, a native of Sizhou(today's Yuyi County, Jiangsu Province). He made corrections on the anatomic charts drawn in the third year of Zhenghe (1113), and compiled *Cunzhen Tu* (*Pictures of Reserving the True*), a book of a single volume, which was a contribution to anatomy, acupuncture and moxibustion. Although the book is no longer extant, the charts have been adopted by *Zhenjiu Juying* (*Essentials of Acupuncture and Moxibustion*) and *Zhenjiu Dacheng* (*A Great Compendium of Acupuncture and Moxibustion*).

●杨敬斋针灸全书[yáng jìng zhāi zhēn jiǔ quán shū] 书名。又名《秘传常山敬斋杨先生针灸全书》。原题陈言撰(实系托名),刊于1591年,分上、下两卷。其特点为增入各种病证的针穴图达104幅,为他书所未见。杨敬斋,常山人,事迹不详。

Yang Jingzhai Zhenjiu Quanshu (Yang Jingzhai's Complete Book of Acupuncture and Moxibustion) A two-volume book, also named *Michuan Changshan Jingzhai Yangxianshen Zhenjiu Quanshu* (*A Secretly Bequeathed and Complete Book of Acupuncture and Moxibustion of Mr. Yang Jingzhai from Changshan*) with Chen Yan inscribed on the book as the author. Published in 1591, the book was characterized by the addition of as many as 140 charts of acupoints for various diseases never seen in other medical works. Yang Jingzhai, was a native of Changshan, whose deeds are unknown.

●杨上善[yáng shàng shàn] 人名。隋唐时期医学家,籍贯不详。大业中(605～616年)曾任太医侍御,很有名望。撰有《黄帝内经太素》三十卷,是注解《内经》最早的医家之一,对后世研究《内经》作出了较大贡献。又著《黄帝内经明堂类成》。

Yang Shangshan A famous medical expert in the Sui and Tang Dynasties, whose native place is unknown. He was a famous court physician in the reign of Da Ye (605-616) and the compiler of *Huangdi Neijing Taisu* (*Comprehensive Notes to the Yellow Emperor's Canon of Internal Medicine*) in 30 volumes. He was one of the earliest physicians who annotated *Neijing* (*The Canon of Internal Medicine*), and contributed a great deal to its studies by later generations. He also compiled *Huangdi Neijing Mingtang Leicheng* (*Classification of Acupoints of the Yellow Emperor's Canon of Internal Medicine*).

●杨珣[yáng xún] 人名。明代医家,陕西人。曾在太医院供职,广览医书,擅长针灸。撰《针灸集书》、《针灸详说》、《伤寒撮要》(已佚)等。

Yang Xun A famous physician of the Ming Dynasty, a native of Shanxi Province. He worked in the Institute of Imperial Physi-

cians, read medical books extensively, and was proficient in acupuncture and moxibustion. He was the compiler of *Zhenjiu Jishu*(*A Book Collection of Acupuncture and Moxibustion.*), and *Shanghan Cuoyao*(*Essentials of Exogenous Cold-Induced Diseases*)(nonextant), etc.

●杨颜齐[yáng yán qí] 人名。宋代针灸家,里籍不详。《宋史·艺文志》载有颜齐《灸经》十卷。佚。

Yang Yanqi An acupuncture-moxibustion expert in the Song Dynasty, whose native place is unknown. His 10-volume *Jiu Jing*(*Classic of Moxibustion*)(nonextant) was recorded in *Songshi:Yi Wen Zhi*(*The History of the Song Dynasty:Records of Art and Literature*).

●仰靠坐位[yǎng kào zuò wèi] 针灸体位名。患者身体正坐,背靠于椅,头往后仰,面部朝上的体位,适用于取前头、面、颈和胸上部的腧穴。

Facing-Upward Sitting Posture Posture for acupuncture and moxibustion. The patient sits straight in a chair, against its back, with his head backwards and his face upwards. It is used for the selection of acupoints on the front head, face, neck and chest.

●仰卧位[yǎng wò wèi] 针灸体位名。患者身体平卧于床,头面、胸腹朝上的体位。适用于取头、面、颈、胸、腹及上、下肢的部分腧穴。

Dorsal Position Posture for acupuncture and moxibustion, with the patient lying on a bed, his face, chest and abdomen facing upwards for the convenience of selecting acupoints on the head, face, neck, chest, abdomen, upper and lower limbs.

●养老[yǎng lǎo] 经穴名。出《针灸甲乙经》。属手太阳小肠经,为本经郄穴。〈定位〉在前臂背面尺侧,当尺骨小头近端桡侧凹陷中(图65.2)。〈层次解剖〉皮肤→皮下组织→尺侧腕伸肌腱。浅层布有前臂内侧皮神经,前臂后皮神经,尺神经手背支和贵要静脉属支等。深层有腕背动、静脉网等。〈主治〉目视不明、肩背肘臂痛、急性腰痛。掌心向胸时直刺0.3~0.5寸,或斜刺0.5~0.8寸;可灸。

Yanglao(SI 6) A meridian point, from *Zhenjiu Jia-Yi Jing*(*A-B Classic of Acupuncture and Moxibustion*), the Xi(Cleft) point of the Small Intestine Meridian of Hand-Taiyang.〈Location〉on the ulnar side of the posterior surface of the forearm, in the depression proximal to and on the radial side of the head of the ulna(Fig. 65.2).〈Regional anatomy〉skin→subcutaneous tissue→tendon of ulnar extensor muscle of wrist. In the superficial layer, there are the medial cutaneous nerve of the forearm, the posterior cutaneous nerve of the forearm, the dorsal branches of the ulnar nerve and the tributaries of the basilic vein. In the deep layer, there is the network of the dorsal carpal arteries and veins.〈Indications〉blurring of vision, pain in the shoulder, back, elbow and arm, acute lumbago.〈Method〉Puncture perpendicularly 0.3~0.5 cun or obliquely 0.5~0.8 cun with the palm facing the chest. Moxibustion is applicable.

●腰骶椎[yāo dǐ zhuī] 耳穴名。位于轮屏切迹至对耳轮上、下脚分叉分为五等分,上五分之二为腰骶椎。具有强脊益髓的作用。〈主治〉腰骶部疼痛、腹痛、腰腿痛、腹膜炎等。

Lumbosacral Vertebrae(MA) An otopoint.〈Location〉Divide the area from the muscle of incisure of helix to the branching spot of the upper and lower cruse of the anthelicis into five equal parts, the 2nd from the top of which is the point.〈Function〉Strengthen the vertebra and replenish the spinal cord.〈Indications〉pain in the lower back, abdominal pain, pain in the waist and lower extremities and peritonitis, etc.

●腰户[yāo hù] 经穴别名。出《针灸甲乙经》。即腰俞,详见该条。

Yaohu Another name for *Yaoshu*(DU 21), a meridian point from *Zhenjiu Jia-Yi Jing*(*A-B Classic of Acupuncture and Moxibustion*).→腰俞(p.545)

●腰脊痛[yāo jǐ tòng] 症状名。出《素问·标本病传论》。指腰椎及其周围疼痛。即腰痛。详见该条。

Pain Along the Spinal Column A symptom from *Suwen:Biao Ben Bing Chuan Lun*(*Plain Questions:On the Primary and Sencondary Aspects and the Progress of Diseases*), referring to a pathologic state of pain along and around the spinal column. i.e. lumbago.→腰痛(p.545)

●腰目[yāo mù] 经外穴名。出《千金要方》。在腰部,当肾俞穴直下3寸处。灸治消渴、小便频数等。

Yaomu(EX-B) An extra point, from *Qianjin Yaofang* (*Essential Prescriptions Worth a Thousand Gold*). 〈Location〉on the low back, 3 cun straight down from Shenshu(BL 23). 〈Indications〉 diabetes, frequent urination. 〈Method〉moxibustion.

●腰目骱[yāo mù jiào] 经外穴别名。即腰眼。详见该条。

Yaomujiao. →腰眼(p. 546)

●腰奇[yāo qí] 经外穴名。见《中医杂志》。〈定位〉在骶部,当尾骨端直上2寸,骶角之间凹陷中(图61)。〈层次解剖〉皮肤→皮下组织→棘上韧带。布有第二、第三骶神经后支的支及伴行的动、静脉。〈主治〉癫狂。向上沿皮刺2~3寸。

Yaoqi(EX-B 9) An extra point from *Zhongyi Zazhi*(*Journal of Traditional Chinese Medicine*). 〈Location〉on the low back, 2 cun directly above the tip of the coccyx, in the depression between the sacral horrns(Fig. 61). 〈Regional anatomy〉skin→subcutaneous tissue→supraspinal ligament. There are the branches of the posterior branches of the 2nd and 3rd sacral nerves and the accompanying artery and vein in this area. 〈Indication〉epilepsy. 〈Method〉Puncture subcutaneously 2~3 cun upward.

●腰俞[yāo shū] 经穴名。出《素问·缪刺论》。属督脉。又名背解、髓空、腰户、腰注、腰柱、髓俞。〈定位〉在骶部,当后正中线上,适对骶管裂孔(图12.2和图7)。〈层次解剖〉皮肤→皮下组织→骶尾背侧韧带→骶管。浅层主要布有第五骶神经的后支。深层有尾丛。〈主治〉腰脊强痛、腹泻、便秘、痔疾、脱肛、便血、癫痫、淋浊、月经不调、下肢痿痹。向上斜刺0.5~1.0寸;可灸。

Yaoshu(DU 2) A meridian point from *Suwen*:*Miuci Lun*(*Plain Questions*:*On Contralateral Collateral Needling*),a point on the Du Meridian,also named Beijie, Suikong, Yaohu, Yaozhu(*注,*柱)and Suishu. 〈Location〉on the sacrum, on the posterior midline, just at the sacral hiatus (Figs. 12. 2&7). 〈Regional anatomy〉skin→subcutaneous tissue→dorsal sacrococcgyeal ligament→sacral canal. In the superficial layer, there are the posterior branches of the 5th sacral nerve. In the deep layer, there is the coccygeal plexus. 〈Indications〉sharp pain along the spinal column, diarrhea, constipation, hemorrhoid, proctoptosis, hemafecia, epilepsy, stranguria with turbid urine, irregular menstruation, numbness of the lower limbs. 〈Method〉Puncture obliquely 0.5~1.0 cun. Moxibustion is applicable.

●腰痛[yāo tòng] 病证名。出《素问·刺腰痛论》等。又称腰脊痛。指腰部一侧或两侧疼痛,或痛连脊椎的病证。多因肾虚或感受寒湿之邪,以及血瘀挫闪而成。可分为寒湿、劳损和肾虚腰痛三种。详见各条。

Lumbar Pain(Lumbago) A disease from *Suwen*:*Ci Yaotong Lun*(*Plain Questions*:*On Treatment of Lumbago with Acupuncture*), also named pain along the spinal column, referring to pathologic pain in one or both sides of the waist, or along the spinal column, mostly caused by deficiency of the kidney, or affection of pathogenic cold-dampness, blood stasis, sprain and contusion. It can be divided into three types—lumbar pain due to cold dampness, lumbar pain due to overstrain *and* lumbar due to deficiency of the kidney. →寒湿腰痛(p. 157)、劳损腰痛(p. 238)、肾虚腰痛(p. 367)

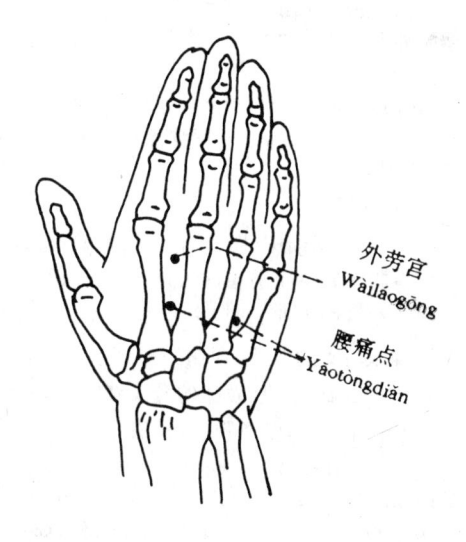

图69 腰痛点和外劳宫穴

Fig 69 Yaotongdian and Wailaogong points

●腰痛点[yāo tòng diǎn] 又名腰痛穴。在手背侧，当第2、3掌骨及第4、5掌骨之间，当腕横纹与掌指关节中点处一侧二穴(图69)。〈层次解剖〉一穴：皮肤→皮下组织→指伸肌腱和桡侧腕短伸肌腱。另一穴：皮肤→皮下组织→小指伸肌腱与第四指伸肌腱之间。该二穴处布有手背静脉网和掌背动脉，有桡神经的浅支和布有尺神经的手背支。〈主治〉急性腰扭伤。向掌心斜刺0.5～1.0寸。

Yaotongdian (EX-UE 7) A set of extra points, also named Yaotongxue. 〈Location〉on the dorsum of the hand, between the 2nd, 3rd, 4th and 5th metacarpal bones lateral to the midpoint of the cross striation and the metacarpophalangeal articulation, two points on each side (Fig. 69). 〈Regional anatomy〉First point: skin→subcutaneous tissue→tendons of digital extensor muscle and short radial extensor muscle of wrist. Another point: skin→subcutaneous tissue→between tendons of extensor muscle of little finger and extensor muscle of the 4th finger. There are the dorsal venous netwoek of the hand, the dorsal palmar artery, the superficial branches of the radial nerve and the dorsal branches of the hand from the unlnar nerve in the area of these two poinst. 〈Indication〉 acute lumbar sprain. 〈Method〉 Puncture 0.5～1.0 cun obliquely toward the palm.

●腰痛穴[yāo tòng xué] 经外穴别名。即腰痛点。详见该条。

Yaotongxue Another name for the extra point Yaotongdian.→腰痛点(p.546)

●腰眼[yāo yǎn] 经外穴名。见《肘后备急方》。又名鬼眼、腰目窌。〈定位〉在腰部，当第四腰椎棘突下，旁开约3.5寸凹陷中(图61)。〈层次解剖〉皮肤→皮下组织→胸腰筋膜浅层和背阔肌腱膜→髂肋肌→胸腰筋膜深层→腰方肌。浅层主要布有臀上皮神经和第四腰神经后支的皮支。深层主要有第四腰神经后支的肌支和第四腰动、静脉的分支或属支。〈主治〉瘰疬、腰痛、小腹痛，以及肾下垂、睾丸炎、腰肌劳损、腰部软组织扭挫伤等。直刺1.0～1.5寸；可灸。

Yaoyan (EX-B 7) An extra point originally from *Zhouhou Beiji Fang* (*A Handbook of Prescriptions for Emergencies*), also named Guiyan or Yaomujiao. 〈Location〉on the low back, below the spinous process of the 4th lumbar vertebra, in the depression 3.5 cun lateral to the posterior midline (Fig. 61). 〈Regional anatomy〉 skin→subcutaneous tissue→superficial layer of thoracolumbar fascia and aponeurosis of latissimus muscle of back→iliocostal muscle → deep layer of thoracolumbar fasicia→quadrate muscle of loins. In the superficial layer, there are the superior clunial nerve and the cutaneous branches of the posterior branch of the 4th lumbar nerve. In the deep layer, there are the muscular branches of the posterior branch of the 4th lumbar nerve and the branches or tributaries of the 4th lumbar artery and vein. 〈Indications〉 tuberculosis, lumbar pain, pain in the lower abdomen, nephroptosia, orchitis, lumbar muscle strain, contusion of soft tissue in the lumbar region. 〈Method〉 Puncture 1.0～1.5 cun perpendicularly. Moxibustion is applicable.

●腰阳关[yāo yáng guān] 经穴名。出《素问·骨空论》王冰注。属督脉，原名阳关，后加腰字。又名背阳关。〈定位〉在腰部，当后正中线上，第四腰椎棘突下凹陷中(图12.2和图7)。〈层次解剖〉皮肤→皮下组织→棘上韧带→棘间韧带→弓间韧带。浅层主要布有第四腰神经后支的内侧支和伴行的动、静脉。深层有棘突间的椎外(后)静脉丛，第四腰神经后支的分支和第四腰动、静脉的背侧支的分支或属支。〈主治〉腰骶疼痛、下肢痿痹、月经不调、赤白带下、遗精、阳萎、便血。直刺0.5～1.0寸；可灸。

Yaoyangguan (DU 3) A meridian point, originally from Wang Bing's annotation for *Su Wen*: *Gukong Lun* (*Plain Questions*: *On the Apertures of Bones*), a point on the Du Meridian, originally named Yangguan (with Yao(腰)added later), also called Beiyangguan. 〈Location〉on the low back and on the posterior midline, in the depression below the spinous process of the 4th lumbar vertebra (Figs. 12.2&7). 〈Regional anatomy〉 skin→subcutaneous tissue→supraspinal ligament→interspinal ligament→interarcuate ligament. In the superficial layer, there are the medial branches of the posterior branches of the 4th lumbar nerve and the accompanying artery and vein. In the deep layer, there are the external (posterior) vertebral venous plexus between the adjacent spinous processes, the branches of the posterior branches of the 4th

lumbar nerve and the branches or tributaries of the dorsal branches of the 4th lumbar artery and vein. ⟨Indications⟩ pain in the lumbosacral portion, paraparesis, irregular menstruation, leukorrhea with reddish discharge, emission, impotence, hemafecia. ⟨Method⟩ Puncture 0.5-1.0 cun perpendicularly. Moxibustion is applicable.

●腰宜[yāo yí] 经外穴名。见《针灸孔穴及其疗法便览》。⟨定位⟩在腰部，当第四腰椎棘突下，旁开3寸（图61）。⟨层次解剖⟩皮肤→皮下组织→胸腰筋膜浅层→竖脊肌（或臀大肌内上缘）。浅层主要布有臀上皮神经。深层主要有第四腰神经后支的肌支，第四腰动、静脉背侧支的分支或属支。⟨主治⟩妇人血崩、腰痛、脊柱肌痉挛等。直刺0.5～1寸；可灸。

Yaoyi (EX-B 6) An extra point, seen in *Zhenjiu Kongxue Jiqi Liaofa Bianlan*(*Guide to Acupoints and Acupuncture Therapeutics*). ⟨Location⟩ on the loin, 3 cun below the spinous process of the 4th lumbar vertebra (Fig. 61). ⟨Regional anatomy⟩skin→subcutaneous tissue→superficial layer of the thoracolumbar fascia→erector spinal muscle(or medial margin of the greatest gluteal muscle). In the superficial layer, there are the cutaneous nerves of arm. In the deep layer, there are the muscular branches of the posterior branch of the 4th lumbar nerves and the branches or tributaries of the dorsal branch of the 4th lumbar artery and vein. ⟨Indications⟩metrorrhagia in women, lumbago, myospasm muscular spasm along the spinal column. ⟨Method⟩ Puncture perpendicularly 0.5～1.0 cun. Moxibustion is applicable.

●腰注[yāo zhù] 经穴别名。见《太平圣惠方》。即腰俞。详见该条。
Yaozhu Another name for Yaoshu (DU 21), a meridian point originally seen in *Taiping Shenghui Fang*(*Imperial Benevolent prescrptions*).→腰俞(p.545)

●腰柱[yāo zhù] 经穴别名。见《外台秘要》。即腰俞。详见该条。
Yaozhu Another name for Yaoshu (DU 21), a meridian point seen in *Waitai Miyao* (*Clandestine Essentials from the Imperial Library*).→腰俞(p.545)

●摇柄法[yáo bǐng fǎ] 为摇法之别称。详见该条。
Handle-Rotating Manipulation Another name for rotating manipulation.→摇法(p.547)

●摇法[yáo fǎ] 针刺手法名，十四法之一。见《针经指南》。又称摇柄法、针摇。指入针后，以右手持针柄作左右摆动的一种辅助方法。与其他手法配合应用，有加强得气的作用。
Rotating One of the 14 needling methods, seen in *Zhenjing Zhinan*(*Guide to the Classics of Acupuncture*), also called handle-rotating manipulation or needle rotating, referring to rotating the needle left and right with the needle handle held in the right hand after the insertion of the needle——an auxiliary method used in association with other manipulations, functioning to strengthen the obtaining of qi.

●药饼灸[yào bǐng jiǔ] 间接灸的一种。系用辛温芳香的药物制成药饼放在穴位上，再加放艾炷施灸。有温中散寒，行气活血作用。临床应用有椒饼灸和豉饼灸等多种。参见各条。
Tablet Moxibustion A type of indirect moxibustion. Apply to the point a tablet made of drugs pungent in flavor, warm and fragrant in property, with a moxa-stick placed on a point for moxibustion. ⟨Function⟩ Warm the middle-jiao to dispel cold and promote flow of qi and blood circulation. Applied in clinic are various methods of moxibustion such as pepper-paste moxibustion and fermented soybean-cake moxibustion, etc.→椒饼灸(p.199)、豉饼灸(p.47)

●药锭灸[yào dìng jiǔ] 灸法之一。将多种药物研末，和硫黄熔化在一起，制成药锭，置于穴位上施灸。
Ingot-Shaped Tablet Moxibustion A type of moxibustion. Grind various herbal medicines into a fine powder, mix it with sulphur and melt it to make an ingot-shaped tablet. Apply it to the selected point for moxibustion.

●药捻灸[yào niǎn jiǔ] 灸法之一。用棉纸紧裹药末捻成细条，剪成小段，贴于穴位上施灸。如蓬莱火即为药捻灸的一种。参见"蓬莱火"条。
Medicated-Stick Moxibustion A type of moxibustion. Roll medicinal powder into a piece of cotton paper to form a stick, cut it into pieces and stick them on the selected points for moxibustion. Penglai Fire Moxibustion, for instance, is an example of medicated-stick moxibustion.→蓬莱火(p.291)

●药筒法[yào tǒng fǎ] 即煮药拔罐法。详见该条。

Medicinal Cupping →煮药拔罐法(p.621)

●**药物艾卷**[yào wù ài juǎn] 指含有药末的艾卷。如太乙神针、雷火神针、念盈药条等。详见各条。

Moxa Rolls with Medicinal Powder Moxa rolls containing medicinal powder, such as great monad herbal moxa stick, thunder-fire herbal moxa stick, and moxa roll with more medicinal powder. →太乙神针(p.421)、雷火神针(p.239)、念盈药条(p.284)

●**药物发泡灸**[yào wù fā pào jiǔ] 刺灸法之一。又名药物发泡疗法,即天灸。详见各条。

Medicinal Blister-Causing Moxibustion One of the methods of needling and moxibustion, also called medicinal blister-causing therapy. i.e. vesiculation. →药物发泡疗法(p.548)、天灸(p.432)

●**药物发泡疗法**[yào wù fā pào liáo fǎ] 即药物发泡灸。详见该条。

Medicinal Blister-Causing Therapy →药物发泡灸(p.548)

●**药薰蒸气灸**[yào xūn zhēng qì jiǔ] 灸法之一。见《五十二病方》。是利用药液蒸气熏灸经络穴位,而达到治疗目的一种灸法。临床上因药物处方及熏灸部位不同,适应证也有所区别。

Moxibustion by Steaming with Herbal Medicine A kind of moxibustion seen in *Wushier Bing Fang* (*Prescriptions for Fifty-Two Diseases*), referring to a moxibustion method of steaming the acupoints with herbal medicinal fluid to achieve the purpose of treatment. Its indications are clinically different because of the different prescriptions of herbal medicine and different body parts to be steamed.

●**噎膈**[yē gé] 病证名。见《济生方》卷二。又名噎塞、膈噎。噎,指进食吞咽困难。膈,指饮食梗阻胸膈。噎证既可单独发生,又可为膈证的前兆,因此并称为噎膈。多因忧愁思虑过度,而致气痰凝血瘀,或因暴食饮酒,损伤津液,精血干枯所致。初起时,先有不同程度的吞咽困难和胸闷,胸痛,进固体食物则梗阻难下,即食即吐。带有痰涎,呃逆,嗳气,病人渐消瘦,精神疲惫,舌苔薄白或腻,脉弦滑。随着梗阻日渐加重,流食亦难咽下,饮食极少。津液亏乏,致大便少而秘结,状如羊矢,小便黄赤,舌色光绛,无苔,脉细数。治宜调理脾胃,滋阴降逆。取天突、膻中、足三里、内关、上脘、胃俞、脾俞、膈俞。便秘加照海,短气加气海,肢冷、脉微加命门、肾俞。

Dysphagia A disease, seen in Vol. 2 of *Ji Sheng Fang* (*Recipes for Saving Lives*) also named choke or diaphragm obstruction. *Ye*(噎), refers to the difficulty in swallowing food while eating. *Ge*(膈), refers to the retention of food in the chest and diaphragm. Since the former may either occur along in the clinic, or be the warning sign of the latter, these two are jointly known as Yege(噎膈)(dysphagia). It is mostly due to severe melancholy and anxiety, resulting in stagnation of qi, phlegm-coagulation and blood stasis, or due to over eating and drinking, leading to the impairment of body fluid, exhaustion of essence and blood. It is initially manifested as difficulty swallowing to different degrees, oppressive feeling in the chest, chest pain, obstruction while eating solid food, instant vomiting after food intake, accompanied by sputum and saliva, hiccup, belching, progressive marasmus of the patient, lassitude, thin and white or greasy tongue coating, wiry and slippery pulse. It is gradually manifested as severe obstruction, even difficulty in swallowing liquid diet, severe decrease of food intake, over consumption of the body fluids, resulting in constipation or little stools, like sheep dung, scanty darkish urine, deep-red tongue with little coating, thready and rapid pulse. 〈Treatment principle〉 Regulate the spleen and stomach, nourish yin and lower the adverse flow of qi. 〈Point selection〉 Tiantu(RN 22), Danzhong (RN 17) Zusanli(ST 36), Neiguan(PC 6), Shangwan(RN 13), Weishu(BL 21), Pishu (BL 20), Geshu(BL 17). For constipation, add Zhaohai(KI 6); for short breath, add Qihai(RN 6); for cold limbs and weak pulse, add Mingmen(DU 4) and Shenshu(BL 23).

●**噎塞**[yē sè] 病证名。见《千金要方》卷十六。即噎膈。详见该条。

Choke A disease, seen in Vol. 16. of *Qianjin Yaofang* (*Essential Prescriptions Worth a Thousand Gold*), synonymous with dysphagia. →噎膈(p.548)

●**叶茶山**[yè chá shān] 人名。清针灸家。参见"叶

广祚"条。

Ye Chashan An acupuncture-moxibustion expert in the Qing Dynasty. →叶广祚(p.549)

●叶广祚[yè guǎng zuò] 人名。清针灸家,字明传,岭南(今广东番禺)人。其祖父叶澄泉,得人传授灸法,传至三代,治疗多验。于康熙七年(1668年),由广祚编成《采艾编》四卷,署名"茶山草木隐"。其后有署名"叶茶山"者,续编《采艾编翼》。

Ye Guangzuo An acupuncture expert in the Qing Dynasty, who styled himself Mingchuan, a native of Lingnan (today's Fanyu in Guangdong Province). His grandfather, Ye Chengquan, learned moxibustion therapy and the therapy was passed on for 3 generations and proved miraculously effective in treatment. In the 7th year of Kangxi (1668), Guangzuo compiled *Cai Ai Bian* (*Collecting Mugwort Floss*) in 4 volumes, the signature on which was "Chashan Caomuyin". Later someone, with the undersigned as "Ye Chashan", supplementarily compiled *Cai Ai Bian Yi* (*A Supplement to Collecting Mugwort Floss*).

●夜光[yè guāng] 经穴别名。出《针灸甲乙经》。即攒竹。详见该条。

Yeguang Another name for *Canzhu* (BL 2), a meridian point originally from *Zhenjiu Jia-Yi Jing* (*A-B Classic of Acupuncture and Moxibustion*). →攒竹(p.58)

●液门[yè mén] 经穴名。出《灵枢·本输》。属手少阳三焦经,为本经荥穴。又名腋门、掖门。〈定位〉在手背部,当第四、五指间,指蹼缘后方赤白肉际处(图48和44.4)。〈层次解剖〉皮肤→皮下组织→第四与第五指近节指骨基底部之间→第四骨间背侧肌和第四蚓状肌。浅层布有尺神经的指背神经,手背静脉网。深层有指动、静脉结构。〈主治〉头痛、目赤、耳痛、耳鸣、耳聋、喉痹、疟疾、手臂痛。直刺0.3～0.5寸;可灸。

Yemen (SJ 2) A meridian point, originally from *Lingshu*: *Benshu* (*Miraculous Pivot*: *Meridian Points*), the Ying (Spring) point of the Sanjiao Meridian of Hand-Shaoyang, also named Yemen (腋门), Yemen (掖门). 〈Location〉on the dorsum of the hand, between the 4th and 5th fingers, at the junction of the red and white skin, proximal to the margin of the web (Figs. 48&44.4). 〈Regional anatomy〉skin→subcutaneous tissue→between bases of 4th and 5th proximal phalangeal bones→4th dorsal interosseous muscle and 4th lumbrical muscle. In the superficial layer, there are the dorsal digital nerve of the ulnar nerve and the dorsal venous network of the hand. In the deep layer, there are the dorsal digital artery and vein. 〈Indications〉headache, conjunctival congestion, pain of the ear, tinnitus, deafness, inflammation of the throat, malarial disease, pain in the hand and arm. 〈Method〉Puncture perpendicularly 0.3～0.5 cun. Moxibustion is applicable.

●掖间[yè jiān] 经穴别名。即液门。详见该条。

Yejian Another name for the meridia point Yemen (ST 2). →液门(p.549)

●掖门[yè mén] ①经外穴名。见《千金要方》。又名腋门、掖间。在侧胸部,腋正中线上,当腋窝下1寸处。灸治诸风惊妄、呃逆、狐臭、瘰疬等。②经穴别名。即液门。详见该条。

1. **Yemen** (掖门) (EX-CA) An extra point, seen in *Qianjin Yaofang* (*Essential Prescriptions Worth a Thousand Gold*), also named Yemen (腋门). 〈Location〉on the lateral part of the chest, at the middle axillary line, 1 cun below the armpit. 〈Indications〉mania due to fright and pathogenic wind, hiccup, bromhidrosis, scrofula, etc. 〈Method〉moxibustion.

2. **Yemen** (掖门) Another name for the meridian point Yemen (SJ 2) (液门). →液门(p.549)

●腋[yè] 部位名。在肩下胁上之窝陷。

Armpit A body part, referring to the lacuna above the hypochondrium and under the shoulder.

●腋门[yè mén] ①经穴别名。见《针灸甲乙经》。即液门。详见该条。②经穴别名。出《针灸甲乙经》。即大巨。详见该条。③经外穴别名。即掖门,详见该条。

Yemen (腋门) Another name for ①Yemen (液门)(SJ 2), a meridian point seen in *Zhenjiu Jia-Yi Jing* (*A-B Classic of Acupuncture and Moxibustion*). →液门(p.549) ②Daju (ST 27),

a meridian point originally from *Zhenjiu Jia-YiJing* (*A-B Classic of Acupuncture and Moxibustion*). →大巨(p. 64)③the extra point Yemen(掖门)(EX-CA)→掖门(p. 549)

●腋气[yè qì] 经外穴名。见《医经小学·漏经穴法》。位于腋下毛中,先用快刀剃净腋毛,以搽粉后出现黑点为是。灸治狐臭。

Yeqi(EX-CA) An extra point, seen in *Yijing Xiaoxue*: *Loujing Xuefa* (*Collection of Elementary Medical Classics*: *Selection of Points for Uterine Bleeding*). 〈Location〉on the centre of the axillary hair, the black spot seen after having the axillary hair cut and the axillary region powdered. 〈Indication〉bromhidrosis.〈Method〉moxibustion.

●腋下穴[yè xià xué] 经外穴名。见《千金要方》。在胸侧部当腋中线上,腋窝直下1.5寸处。主治噫嗳、胸膈满闷、狐臭,以及肋间神经痛等。斜刺0.3～0.5寸;可灸。

Yexiaxue(EX-CA) An extra point, seen in *Qianjin Yaofang* (*Essential Prescriptions Worth a Thousand Gold*).〈Location〉on the middle axillary line of the lateral part of the chest, 1.5 cun directly below the armpit.〈Indications〉eructation, hiccup, fullness and oppressive feeling in the chest and diaphragm, bromhidrosis, intercostal neuralgia.〈Method〉Puncture obliquely 0.3～0.5 cun. Moxibustion is applicable.

●哕[yè] 见《类证活人书》。即干呕。详见该条。

Noisy Nausea without Food Retching, seen in *Leizheng Huoren Shu*(*A Book of Differential Diagnosis and Treatment for Saving Lives*).→干呕(p. 123)

●一夫法[yī fū fǎ] 横指同身寸的别称。详见该条。

Finger Breadth Measurement Another name for finger breadth cun. →横指同身寸(p. 164)

●一进三退[yī jìn sān tuì] 刺法用语。又称三退一进。透天凉等泻法中用此。其法与三进一退的补法相对。针一直进到深层,分三层退针,即逐步由深层、中层退到浅层。可反复施行。一次进,三次退,体现了疾入徐出,从荣置气的泻法原则。

One Insertion and Three Liftings A term for a needling technique, also named three liftings and one insertion, used in reducing methods such as thorough heaven cool, the opposite of the reinforcing method of three insertions and one lifting.〈Method〉Thrust the needle directly to the deep layer, then lift it separately from the deep to the middle and superficial layers. This can be repeated several times. This technique, one insertion and three liftings, embodies the reducing principle of quick insertion and slow liftings and getting qi from the Ying system.

●一阳[yī yáng] 经络名。出《素问·阴阳别论》。指少阳。详见"三阳三阴"条。

One Yang A meridian, originally from *Suwen*: *Yin Yang Bie Lun* (*Plain Questions*: *Supplementary Exposition of Yin and Yang*), referring to Shaoyang. →三阳三阴(p. 345)

●一月经再行[yī yuè jīng zài xíng] 即经行先期。详见该条。

Menstruation Twice a Month Another name for preceded menstrual cycle. →经行先期(p. 214)

●医工针[yī gōng zhēn] 针具。见《针灸聚英》卷三。指医疗用针具,用以与其他针相区分。

Medical Needle A kind of needle, seen in Vol. 3 of *Zhenjiu Juying* (*Essentials of Acupuncture and Moxibustion*), referring to needles for medical treatment, which are different from other kinds of needles.

●医缓[yī huǎn] 人名。春秋时秦国名医。据《左传》记载:晋候病,求医于秦,医缓前往诊治,谓其疾不可治,在肓之上,膏之下,攻(灸)之不可,达(针)之不及,药不能及。这是史书中关于使用针灸治病的早期记载。

Yi Huan A famous physician in the Qin State of the Spring and Autumn period. It was recorded in *Zuo Zhuan* (*Commentary on the Spring and Autumn Annals*) that the Marquis of the Jin was ill and asked the Qin State to send a doctor. Yi Huan went to make a diagnosis and give treatment. He said the disease was incurable because the affected part was just above the diaphragm and below the heart. Moxibustion was inappilcable there, acupuncture could not reach it, and herbal medicine could not get there either. This is an

early record on treatment by applying acupuncture and moxibustion in historical literature.

● 医经小学[yī jīng xiǎo xué] 书名。综合性医书，六卷，明代刘纯撰，刊于1388年。作者集诸家之说，以韵语等形式编纂而成。刘纯为朱震亨再传弟子，故书中多反映朱氏之经验。卷三为经络专篇，把十二经脉、八脉交会八穴、经脉流注、周身经穴等，编成歌诀十一首，便于诵记。

Yijing Xiaoxue（Collection of Elementary Medical Classics） A synthetical book of medicine in 6 volumes, written by Liu Chun in the Ming Dynasty, published in 1388. The author collected the theories of many medical families and applied the form of verse to compile and write the book. Liu Chun was an apprentice in the second generation of Zhu Zhenheng, therefore, much of Zhu's experience was recorded in the book. In Vol. 3, a specific chapter on meridians and collaterals, the twelve meridians, eight confluence points, ebb-flow of the meridians and acupoints of the whole body, etc. were compiled into eleven verses for easy memory.

● 医学纲目[yī xué gāng mù] 书名。明代楼英编著，全书共分十部，《刺灸》载于第一部。内容以阴阳脏腑为纲，分门别类，便于研究。对营气、卫气、宗气的运行，以及络脉传注等，提出新的见解，对针灸理论有所发挥。

Yixue Gangmu（An Outline of Medicine） A book in 10 volumes, compiled by Lou Ying in the Ming Dynasty. Acupuncture and moxibustion was recorded in the first volume which took yin-yang and zang-fu as the key to put different categories in order for studying conveniently. The author advanced many new views on the circulation of ying-qi, defensive-qi and pectoral qi as well as the ebb-flow of the collaterals, which somehow developed the theories of acupuncture and moxibustion.

● 医学入门[yī xué rù mén] 书名。综合性医书。明代李挺编撰，刊于1575年。本书以《医经小学》为蓝本，参考诸家学说，并附以己见，分类编纂而成，共七卷。卷一为针灸篇，首载子午八法及杂病穴法、针法、灸法、炼脐法及各种禁忌。正文为歌赋，加注文以补充说明，是一部较有影响的医学经书。

Yixue Rumen（An Introduction to Medicine） A comprehensive medical book in 7 volumes, compiled by Li Chan in the Ming Dynasty and published in 1575. Taking *Yijing Xiaoxue*（*Elementary Collections of Medical Classics*）as its chief resource, consulting the theories of various schools and adding his own viewpoints, he classified and compiled the book. Vol 1 is on acupuncture and moxibustion, in which the eight methods of midnight-noon, point selection, acupuncture and moxibustion therapy for miscellaneous diseases, method of training and various kinds of contraindications were recorded. It is an influential medical classic with the text in verse and notes for explanation.

● 医宗金鉴[yī zōng jīn jiàn] 书名。丛书，九十卷，十五种。是清政府组织编写的大型医学丛书，由吴谦等主编。全书内容丰富完备，叙述系统扼要，包括基础理论及临床各科内容，成书于1742年。其中《刺灸心法要诀》为针灸方面的专书。参见该条。

Yizong Jinjian（Gold Mirror of Orthodox Medical Lineage） A series of books in 90 volumes with 15 classifications, a full-length medical series which were organized and compiled by the government of the Qing Dynasty with Wu Qian and some others as chief editors. It had substantial contents with systematic but brief relations, including basic theory and clinical knowledge, which was finished in 1742. Among them, *Cijiu Xinfa Yaojue*（*Essentials of Acupuncture and Moxibustion in Verse*）is a monograph on acupuncture and moxibustion. →刺灸心法要诀（p. 55）

● 胰胆[yí dǎn] 耳穴名。位于肝肾两穴之间。用于治疗胆囊炎、胆石症、胆道蛔虫症、带状疱疹、中耳炎、耳鸣、听力减退、胰腺炎、偏头痛。

Pancreas-Gallbladder（MA-SC 6） An auricular point.〈Location〉between the two points of Liver（MA-SC 5）and Kidney（MA）.〈Indications〉cholecystitis, cholelithiasis, ascariasis of biliary tract, herpes zoster, otitis media, tinnitus, hypoacusis, pancreatitis and migraine.

● 胰俞[yí shū] 经外穴别名。即胃脘下俞。详见该

Yishu Another name for the extra point Weiwanxiashu(EX-CA). →**胃脘下俞**(p. 468)

●**遗道**[yí dào] 经外穴名。见《千金要方》。在下腹部,当脐下4寸旁开2.5寸处。治遗尿。

Yidao (EX-CA) An extra point, seen in *Qianjin Yaofang*(*Essential Prescriptions Worth a Thousand Gold*). 〈Location〉on the abdomen, 2.5 cun lateral to the part 4 cun inferior to the navel. 〈Indication〉enuresis.

●**遗精**[yí jīng] 病证名,见《丹溪心法·梦遗》。又名失精、遗泄。指男子不经性交而精液遗泄的病证。多由肾气不固引起。其中有梦而遗精的,名为梦遗。无梦而遗精的,甚或清醒时精液流出的,名为滑精。详见"梦遗"、"滑精"条。

Emission A disease, seen in *Danxi Xinfa*: *Mengyi*(*Danxi's Experience*: *Nocturnal Emission*), also named loss of sperm and leaking of the seminal fluid, referring to the male disease marked by leaking of the seminal fluid without sexual intercourse, mostly caused by unconsolidation of the kidney-qi. The case occurring during dreams is called nocturnal emission and the case without dream or even in waking state is called spermatorrhea. →**梦遗**(p. 266)、**滑精**(p. 168)

●**遗泄**[yí xiè] 见《杂病源流犀烛·遗泄源流》。即遗精。详见该条。

Leaking of the Seminal Fliud Emission seen in *Zabing Yuanliu Xizhu*: *Yixie Yuanliu*(*Bright Candle to Pathology of Miscellaneous Diseases*: *Pathology of Emission*). →**遗精**(p. 552)

●**颐**[yí] 部位名。指下颌正中部,又可解释为口角后、腮之前。

Central Jaw A part of the body, referring to the centre of the jaw, indicating also the part posterior to the angle of the mouth and anterior to the parotid.

●**以痛为输**[yǐ tòng wéi shū] 针灸治疗原则之一。出《灵枢·经筋》。意指对于某些病证,可以在病痛局部或找压痛点作为穴位进行治疗。因为这种穴位既无定名,也无定位,故后世有阿是穴、不定穴、天应穴之称。详见各条。

Painful Locality Taken as Acupoint A principle of acupuncture and moxibustion treatment originally from *Lingshu*: *Jingjin*(*Miraculous Pivot*: *Muscle Regions Along Meridians*), referring to selecting the local affected region or pressure pain point as the acupoint to treat some diseases. Since these points do not have fixed names or locations, they are called Ashi points, un-fixed points and natural reactive points. →**阿是穴**(p. 1)、**不定穴**(p. 28)、**天应穴**(p. 436)

●**异经取穴**[yì jīng qǔ xué] 取穴法之一。与本经取穴相对,又称他经取穴。指在与病变经脉相关的其他经脉上选取穴位,包括表里经、同名经等。如胃痛取足太阴脾经公孙,痔痛取手太阴肺经的孔最等。

Point Selection on Disparate Meridians A kind of point selection, as opposed to point selection on the affecetd meridian, also called point selection on other meridians, referring to selecting points on other meridians which are related to the affected meridian including interior-exterior related meridians and same-name meridians, e.g. selecting Gongsun(SP 4) on the Spleen Meridian of Foot-Taiyin for stomachache; Kongzui(LU 6) on the Lung Meridian of Hand-Taiyin for pain due to hemorrhoids, etc.

●**疫毒痢**[yì dú lì] 痢疾证型之一。因疫毒之邪侵犯肠腑,熏蒸三焦,气血阻滞,传导失常所致。其发病急重,证见便次频繁,痢下脓血多而粪便少,腐臭异常,腹痛剧烈,里急后重,高热口渴,烦躁不安。甚则神昏痉厥,舌红绛,苔黄燥,脉大而滑数。治宜清热解毒,疏调肠胃。取合谷、天枢、上巨虚、大椎、十宣。

Fulminant Dysentery A type of dysentery due to invasion of epidemic pathogenic factors steaming the intestines and Sanjiao by the dominant heat, resulting in the stagnation of qi and blood and disorder in transportation. This acute and severe disease is manifested as frequent defecation with more pus blood and less stool and an extremely foul smell, sharp pain in the abdomen, tenesmus, thirst due to severe pyrexia, dysphoria, even coma and convulsions or falling down, deep red tongue with yellowish and dry coating, large, slippery and rapid pulse. 〈Treatment principle〉Clear heat and detoxify, regulate the intestines and stom-

●疫咳[yì ké] 顿咳的别名。详见该条。

Pertussis Another name for cough at a draught. →顿咳(p. 90)

●意舍[yì shě] 经穴名。出《针灸甲乙经》。属足太阳膀胱经。〈定位〉在背部,当第十一胸椎棘突下,旁开3寸(图7)。〈层次解剖〉皮肤→皮下组织→背阔肌→下后锯肌→竖脊肌。浅层布有第十一、十二胸神经后支的外侧皮支和伴行的动、静脉。深层有第十一、十二胸神经后支的肌支和相应肋间后动、静脉背侧支的分支或属支。〈主治〉腹胀、肠鸣、泄泻、呕吐、饮食不下。斜刺0.5~0.8寸;可灸。

Yishe (BL 49) A meridian point, originally from *Zhenjiu Jia-Yi Jing (A-B Classic of Acupuncture and Moxibustion)*, a point on the Bladder Meridian of Foot-Taiyang. 〈Location〉 on the back, below the spinous process of the 11th thoracic vertebra, 3 cun lateral to the posterior midline (Fig. 7). 〈Regional anatomy〉 skin→subcutaneous tissue→latissimus muscle of back→inferior posterior serratus muscle→erector spinal muscle. In the superficial layer, there are the lateral cutaneous branches of the posterior branches of the 11th and 12th thoracic nerves and the accompanying arteries and veins. In the deep layer, there are the muscular branches of the posterior branches of the 11th and 12th thoracic nerves and the branches or tributaries of the dorsal branches of the related posterior intercostal arteries and veins. 〈Indications〉 abdominal distension, borborygmus, diarrhea, vomiting, lack of appetite. 〈Method〉 Puncture obliquely 0.5~0.8 cun. Moxibustion is applicable.

●嗌乳[yì rǔ] 即伤乳吐的别名。详见该条。

Milk Vomiting Another name for milk vomiting due to improper feeding. →伤乳吐(p. 349)

●譩譆[yì xǐ] 经穴名。出《素问·骨空论》。属足太阳膀胱经。〈定位〉在背部,当第六胸椎棘突下,旁开3寸(图7)。〈层次解剖〉皮肤→皮下组织→斜方肌→菱形肌→竖脊肌。浅层布有第六、七胸神经后支的皮支和伴行的动、静脉。深层有肩胛背神经,肩胛背动、静脉,第六胸神经后支的肌支和相应的肋间后动、静脉的背侧支的分支和属支。〈主治〉咳嗽、气喘、肩背痛、季肋引少腹痛、目眩、鼻衄、疟疾、热病汗不出。斜刺0.5~0.8寸;可灸。

Yixi (BL 45) A meridian point, originally from *Suwen: Gu Kong Lun (Plain Questions: On the Apertures of Bones)*, a point on the Bladder Meridian of Foot-Taiyang. 〈Location〉 on the back, below the spinous process of the 6th thoracic vertebra, 3 cun lateral to the posterior midline (Fig. 7). 〈Regional anatomy〉 skin→subcutaneous tissue→trapezius muscle→rhomboid muscle→erector spinal muscle. In the superficial layer, there are the cutaneous branches of the posterior branches of the 6th and 7th thoracic nerves and the accompanying arteries and veins. In the deep layer, there are the dorsal scapular nerve, the dorsal scapular artery and vein, the muscular branches of the posterior branches of the 6th thoracic nerve and the branches or tributaries of the dorsal branches of the related posterior intercostal arteries and veins. 〈Indications〉 cough, dyspnea, pain of the shoulder and back, hypochondriac pain radiating to the lower abdomen, blurred vision, epistaxis, malarial disease, febrile disease with no sweat. 〈Method〉 Puncture obliquely 0.5~0.8 cun. Moxibustion is applicable.

●翳风[yì fēng] 经穴名。出《针灸甲乙经》。属手少阳三焦经,为手、足少阳之会。〈定位〉在耳垂后方,当乳突与下颌角之间的凹陷处(图28和图50)。〈层次解剖〉皮肤→皮下组织→腮腺。浅层布有耳大神经和颈外静脉的属支,深层有颈外动脉的分支耳后动脉,面神经等。〈主治〉耳鸣、耳聋、口眼㖞斜、牙关紧闭、颊肿、瘰疬。直刺0.8~1.2寸;可灸。

Yifeng (SJ 17) A meridian point, originally from *Zhenjiu Jia-yi Jing (A-B Classic of Acupuncture and Moxibustion)*, a point on the Sanjiao Meridian of Hand-Shaoyang, the Crossing Point of the Meridians of Hand- and Foot-Shaoyanng. 〈Location〉 posterior to the ear lobe, in the depression between the mastoid process and mandibular angle (Fig. 28&50). 〈Regional anatomy〉 skin→subcutaneous tissue→parotid gland. In the superficial

layer, there are the great auricular nerve and the tributaries of the external jugular vein. In the deep layer, there are the posterior auricular artery of the extranal carotid artery and the facial nerve. ⟨Indications⟩ tinnitus, deafness, deviation of the eye and mouth, lockjaw, swelling of the cheek, scrofula. ⟨Method⟩ Puncture perpendicularly 0.8~1.2 cun. Moxibustion is applicable.

●**翳明**[yì míng] 经外穴名。出《中华医学杂志》。⟨定位⟩在项部,当翳风后1寸(图56)。⟨层次解剖⟩皮肤→皮下组织→胸锁乳突肌→头夹肌→头最长肌。浅层布有耳大神经的分支,深层有静深动、静脉。⟨主治⟩近视、远视、夜盲、头痛、耳鸣、眩晕、失眠、白内障、青光眼、视神经萎缩、腮腺炎、精神病等。直刺1.0~1.5寸。

Yiming (EX-HN 14) An extra point, originally from *Zhonghua Yixue Zazhi* (*Journal of Chinese Medicine*). ⟨Location⟩ on the nape. 1 cun posterior to Yifeng (SJ 17) (Fig. 56). ⟨Regional anatomy⟩ skin→subcutaneous tissue → sternocledomastoid muscle → splenius muscle of head→muscle of head. In the subperficial layer, there are the branches of the great auricular nerve. In the deep layer, there are the deep cervical artery and vein. ⟨Indications⟩ myopia, hyperopia, night blindness, headache, tinnitus, dizziness, insomnia, cataract, glaucoma, optic atrophy, parotitis, psychosis, etc. ⟨Method⟩ Puncture perpendicularly 1.0~1.5 cun.

●**阴包**[yīn bāo] 经穴名。出《针灸甲乙经》。属足厥阴肝经。又名阴胞。⟨定位⟩在大腿内侧,当股骨内上髁上4寸,股内肌与缝匠肌之间(图41和图49)。⟨层次解剖⟩皮肤→皮下组织→缝匠肌与股薄肌之间→大收肌。浅层布有闭孔神经的皮支,大隐静脉的属支。深层有股神经的肌支,隐神经,股动、静脉等结构。⟨主治⟩月经不调、遗尿、小便不利、腰骶痛引小腹。直刺0.8~1寸;可灸。

Yinbao (LR 9) A meridian point, originally from *Zhenjiu Jia-Yi Jing* (*A-B Classic of Acupuncture and Moxibustion*), a point on the Liver Meridian of Foot-Jueyin, also named Yinbao(阴胞). ⟨Location⟩ on the medial side of the thigh, 4 cun above the medial epicondyle of the femur, between the medial vastus muscle and sartorius muscle (Figs. 41&49). ⟨Regional anatomy⟩ skin→subcutaneous tissue → between sartorius muscle and graclilis muscle→great adductor muscle. In the superficial layer, there are the cutaneous branches of the obturator nerve and the tributaries of the great saphenous vein. In the deep layer, there are the muscular branches of the femoral nerve, the saphenous nerve and the femoral artery and vein. ⟨Indications⟩ irregular menstruation, enuresis, difficulty in urination, and pain in the lumbosacral region extending to the lower abdomen. ⟨Method⟩ Puncure perpendicularly 0.8~1.0 cun. Moxibustion is applicable.

●**阴胞**[yīn bāo] 经穴别名。见《太平圣惠方》。即阴包,详见该条。

Yinbao(阴胞) Another name for Yinbao(LR 9)(阴包), a meridian point originally from *Taiping Shenghui Fang* (*Imperial Benevolent Prescriptions*). →阴包(p. 554)

●**阴部瘙痒**[yīn bù sāo yǎng] 即阴痒。详见该条。

Pruritus in Female Pudendum Another name for pruritus vulva. →阴痒(p. 562)

●**阴刺**[yīn cì] 《内经》刺法名。出《灵枢·官针》。是十二刺之一。阴刺是左右两侧穴位同用的刺法。如下肢寒厥,可同刺左右两侧的足少阴肾经的原穴太溪,以治阴寒。

Yin Puncture An acupuncture term in *Neijing* (*The Inner Canon of Huangdi*), originally from *Lingshu: Guanzhen* (*Miraculous Pivot: Official Needles*), one of the Twelve Methods of Needling, referring to bilateral points being selecied at the same time in acupuncture treatment. e. g. puncturing bilaterally Taixi(KI 3), the Yuan(Primary) point of the Kidney Meridian of Foot-Shaoyin to treat cold lower limbs.

●**阴鼎**[yīn dǐng] 经穴别名。出《针灸甲乙经》。即阴市。详见该条。

Yinding Another name for Yinshi(ST 33), a meridian point originally from *Zhenjiu Jia-Yi Jing* (*A-B Classic of Acupuncture and Moxibustion*). →阴市(p. 558)

●**阴都**[yīn dū] ①经穴名。出《针灸甲乙经》属足少阴肾经,为冲脉、足少阴之会。又名食宫、石宫、通关。⟨定位⟩在上腹部,当脐中上4寸,前正中线旁开0.5寸(图40)。⟨层次解剖⟩皮肤→皮下组织→腹直肌鞘前

壁→腹直肌。浅层布有腹壁浅静脉，第七、八、九胸神经前支的前皮支及伴行的动、静脉。深层有腹壁上动、静脉的分支或属支，第七、八、九胸神经前支的肌支和相应的肋间动、静脉。〈主治〉腹胀、肠鸣、腹痛、便秘、不孕、胸胁痛、疟疾。直刺0.5～0.8寸；可灸。② 经外穴别名。出《针灸集成》。即经中。详见该条。

1. **Yindu** (KI 19)　A meridian point, originally from *Zhenjiu Jia-Yi Jing* (*A-B Classic of Acupuncture and Moxibustion*), a point on the Kidney Meridian of Foot-Shaoyin, the crossing point of the Chong and the Foot-Shaoyin Meridians, also named Shigong, tongguan. 〈Location〉on the upper abdomen, 4 cun above the centre of the umbilicus and 0.5 cun lateral to the anterior midline (Fig. 40). 〈Regional anatomy〉skin→subcutaneous tissue→anterior sheath of rectus muscle of abdomen→rectus muscle of abdomen. In the superficial layer, there are the superficial epigastric vein, the anterior cutaneous branches of the anterior branches of the 7th to 9th thoracic nerves and the accompanying arteries and veins. In the deep layer, there are the branches or tributaries of the superior epigastric artery and vein, the musclar branches of the anterior branches of the 7th to 9th thoracic nerves and the related intercostal arteries and veins. 〈Indications〉 abdominal distension, borborygmus, abdominal pain, constipation, sterility, pain in the chest and hypochondrium, and malarial disease. 〈Method〉Puncture perpendicularly 0.5～0.8 cun. Moxibustion is applicable. 2. **Yindu**　Another name for Jingzhong (EX-HN), an extra point originally from *Zhenjiu Jicheng* (*A Collection of Acupuncture and Moxibustion*). →经中(p.217)

●阴独八穴[yīn dú bā xué]　经外穴别名。出《针灸集成》。即八风。详见该条。

Yindubaxue　Another name for Bafeng(EX-LE 10), a set of extra points, originally from *Zhenjiu Jicheng* (*A Collection of Acupuncture and Moxibustion*). →八风(p.4)

●阴谷[yīn gǔ]　经穴名。出《灵枢·本输》。属足少阴肾经，为本经合穴。〈定位〉在腘窝内侧，屈膝时，当半腱肌肌腱与半膜肌肌腱之间(图46)。〈层次解剖〉皮肤→皮下组织→半膜肌肌腱与半膜肌肌腱之间→腓肠肌内侧头。浅层布有股后皮神经和下皮静脉。深层有膝上内侧动、静脉的分支或属支。〈主治〉阳萎、疝痛、月经不调、崩漏、小便难、阴中痛、癫狂、膝股内侧痛。直刺0.8～1.2寸；可灸。

Yingu (KI 10)　A meridian points, originally from *Lingshu: Benshu* (*Miraculous Pivot: Meridian Point*), the He (Sea) point on the Kidney Meridian of Foot-Shaoyin. 〈Location〉 on the medial side of the popliteal fossa, between the tendons of the semitendinous and semimembranous muscles when the knee is fixed (Fig. 46). 〈Regional anatomy〉 skin → subcutaneous tissue → between tendons of semimembranous muscle and semitendinous muscle → medial head of gastrocnemius muscle. In the superficial layer, there are the posterior cutaneous nerve of the thigh and the subcutaneous vein. In the deep layer, there are the branches or tributaries of the superior medial genicular artery and vein. 〈Indications〉 impotence, hernia, irregular menstruation, metrorrhagia and metrostaxis, difficulty in urination, pain in pudendum, manic depressive disorder, pain along the medial side of both the knee and thigh. 〈Method〉Puncture perpendicularly 0.8～1.2 cun. Moxibustion is applicable.

●阴关[yīn guān]　①经穴别名。出《针灸甲乙经》。即承扶。详见该条。②经穴别名。出《针灸甲乙经》。即大赫。详见该条。

Yinguan　Another name for ① Chengfu(BL 36), a meridian point originally from *Zhenjiu Jia-Yi Jing* (*A-B Classic of Acupuncture and Moxibustion*). →承扶(p.42)② Dahe(KI 12), a meridian point originally from *Zhenjiu Jia-Yi Jing* (*A-B Classic of Acupuncture and Moxibustion*). →大赫(p.62)

●阴狐疝[yīn hú shàn]　即狐疝。详见该条。

Scrotal Inguinal Hernia　→狐疝(p.167)

●阴黄[yīn huáng]　黄疸证型之一。见《景岳全书·黄疸》。多因酒食不节，饥饱失宜，或劳倦过度，损伤脾胃，健运失常，湿郁气滞，以致肝胆瘀积，胆汁排泄不畅，外溢肌肤而致。证见目肤俱黄，其色晦暗，或如烟熏，畏寒，神疲，纳少，脘痞，口淡不渴，大便不实，舌淡苔白而润或腻，脉濡缓或沉迟。治宜温化寒湿，健脾利胆，取脾俞、足三里、胆俞、阳陵泉、三阴交、气海。

Yin Jaundice　A type of jaundice, seen in

555

Jingyue Quanshu: Huangdan (Complete Works of Zhang Jingyue: Jaundice), generally due to immoderate drinking, improper diet, or overtiredness, leading to impairment of the spleen and stomach, dysfunction of the spleen in transportation, damp stagnancy and qi stagnation, resulting in stagnation of the liver and gallbadder with cholestasis and bile overflowing to the muscle and skin. ⟨Manifestations⟩ yellow tinged sclera and skin with dim and lusterless appearance, intolerance of cold, lassitude, poor appetite, fullness in the stomach, lack of taste, lack of thirst, loose stools, pale tongue with whitish and moist or greasy coating, soft and leisurely pulse or deep and slow pulse. ⟨Treatment principle⟩ Warm and resolve cold-dampness, invigorate the spleen and normalize the function of the gallbladder. ⟨Point selection⟩ Pishu (BL 20), Zusanli (ST 36), Danshu (BL 19), Yanglingquan (GB 34), Sanyinjiao (SP 6) and Qihai (RN 6).

●阴交[yīn jiāo] 经穴名。出《针灸甲乙经》。属任脉，为任脉、冲脉、足少阴之会。又名少关、横户。⟨定位⟩在下腹部，前正中线上，当脐中下1寸（图40）。⟨层次解剖⟩皮肤→皮下组织→腹白线→腹横筋膜→腹膜外脂肪→壁腹膜。浅层主要布有第十一胸神经前支的前皮支，脐周静脉网。深层有第十一胸神经前支的分支。⟨主治⟩绕脐冷痛、腹满水肿、泄泻、疝气、阴痒、小便不利、奔豚、血崩、带下、产后恶露不止、小儿陷囟、腰膝拘挛。直刺0.5～1寸；可灸。孕妇慎用。

Yinjiao (RN 7) A meridian point, originally from *Zhenjiu Jia-Yi Jing* (*A-B Classic of Acupuncture and Moxibustion*), a point on the Ren Meridian, the Crossing Point of the Ren, Chong and Foot-Shaoyin Meridians, also named Shaoguan and Henghu. ⟨Location⟩ on the lower abdomen and on the anterior midline, 1 cun below the center of the umbilicus (Fig. 40). ⟨Regional anatomy⟩ skin→subcutaneous tissue→linea alba→transverse fascia→extraperitoneal fat tissue→parietal peritoneum. In the superficial layer, there are the anterior cutaneous branches of the anterior branch of the 11th thoracic nerve and the periumbilical venous network. In the deep layer, there are the branches of the anterior branch of the 11th thoracic nerve. ⟨Indications⟩ cold pain around the navel, fullness of the abdomen and edema, diarrhea, hernia, pruritus vulvae, difficulty in urination, sensation of rushing gas, metrorrhagia, morbid leukorrhea, lochiorrhea, sunken fontanel in infants, muscular spasm of the loin and knees. ⟨Method⟩ Puncture perpendicularly 0.5～1.0 cun. Moxibustion is applicable. This kind of needling must be carefully applied to pregnant women.

●阴结[yīn jié] 1.病证名。①见《素问·兰室秘藏》。即冷秘。详见该条。②指虚秘，凡阳虚阴凝，传送失常，或精血亏耗，大肠干燥者均称阴结。参见"虚秘"条。2.脉象名，指脉沉迟弦硬，连连强直，如摸索竹竿子一样。是阴气偏盛所致。

1. Yin-Accumulation A type of constipation, referring to ① yin-constipation, seen in *Su Wen: Lanshi Micang* (*Plain Questions: Secret Records of the Chamber of Orchids*), synonymous with constipation of cold type. →冷秘 (p. 241) ② constipation of deficiency type due to insufficiency of yang and stagnation of yin, resulting in abnormal transportation, or due to exhaustion of essence and blood, leading to dryness in the large intestine. →虚秘 (p. 514)

2. Yin Knotted Pulse A type of pulse condition, marked by deep, slow, taut, hard and constant stiff pulse, which is just like feeling a bamboo pole, caused by excess of yin-qi.

●阴茎穴[yīn jīng xué] 经外穴名。见《肘后备急方》。又名势头。在男性尿道口上方宛宛中，灸治癫痫、阴缩。

Yinjingxue (EX-CA) An extra point, seen in *Zhouhou Beiji Fang* (*A Handbook of Prescriptions for Emergencies*), also named Shitou. ⟨Location⟩ in the depression above meatus urinarius in male. ⟨Indications⟩ epilepsy and flaccid constriction of penis.

●阴廉[yīn lián] 经穴名。出《针灸甲乙经》。属足厥阴肝经。⟨定位⟩在大腿内侧，当气冲直下2寸，大腿根部，耻骨结节的下方，长收肌的外缘（图17.1）。⟨层次解剖⟩皮肤→皮下组织→长收肌→短收肌→小收肌。浅层布有股神经前皮支，大隐静脉和腹股沟浅淋巴结。深层有闭孔神经的前、后支，旋股内侧动、静脉的肌支。⟨主治⟩月经不调、赤白带下、少腹疼痛、股内侧痛、下肢痉挛。直刺0.8～1寸；可灸。

Yinlian (LR 11) A meridian point on the

Liver Meridian of Foot-Jueyin, originally from *Zhenjiu Jia-Yi Jing* (*A-B Classic of Acupuncture and Moxibustion*). ⟨Location⟩ on the medial side of the thigh, 2 cun directly below Qichong(ST 3), at the proximal end of the thigh, below the pubic tubercle and on the lateral border of the long abductor muscle of the thigh(Fig. 17. 1). ⟨Reginal anatomy⟩ skin →subcutaneous tissue→long adductor muscle → short adductor muscle → small adductor muscle. In the superficial layer, there are the anterior cutaneous branches of the femoral nerve, the great saphenous vein and the superficial inguinal lymph nodes. In the deep layer, there are the anterior and posterior branches of the obturator nerve and the muscular branches of the medial femoral circumflex artery and vein. ⟨Indications⟩ irregular menstruation, leukorrhea with reddish discharge, pain in the lower abdomen, pain in the medial side of thigh, spasm of the lower limbs. ⟨Method⟩ Puncture perpendicularly 0.8~1.0 cun. Moxibustion is applicable.

●阴陵[yīn líng]　经穴别名。出《标幽赋》。即阴陵泉。详见该条。

Yinling　Another name for Yinlingquan(SP 9), a meridian point originally from *Biao You Fu*(*Lyrics of Recondite Principles*). →阴陵泉(p.557)

●阴陵泉[yīn líng quán]　经穴名。出《灵枢·本输》。属足太阴脾经,为本经合穴。又名阴之陵泉、阴陵。⟨定位⟩在小腿内侧,当胫骨内侧髁后下方凹陷处(图39.4)。⟨层次解剖⟩皮肤→皮下组织→半腱肌腱→腓肠肌内侧头。浅层布有隐神经的小腿内侧皮支,大隐静脉和膝降动脉分支。深层有膝下内侧动、静脉。⟨主治⟩腹胀、喘逆、水肿、黄疸、暴泄、小便不利或失禁、阴茎痛、妇人阴痛、遗精、膝痛。直刺0.5~1寸;可灸。

Yinlingquan (SP 9)　A meridian point, originally from *Ling Shu*: *Benshu*(*Miraculous Pivot*: *Meridian Points*), the He(Sea) point of the Spleen Meridian of Foot-Taiyin, also named Lingquan or Yinling. ⟨Location⟩ on the medial side of the leg, in the depression posterior and inferior to the medial condyle of the tibia (Fig. 39.4). ⟨Regional anatomy⟩ skin→subcutaneous tissue → tendon of semitendinous muscle→medial head of gastrocnemius muscle. In the superficial layer, there are the medial cutaneous branches of the leg from the saphenous nerve, the great saphenous vein and the branches of the descending genicular artery. In the deep layer, there are the medial inferior genicular artery and vein. ⟨Indications⟩ abdominal distension, asthma, edema, jaundice, sudden diarrhea, difficulty in urination or incontinence of urine, pain in the penis, pain in the pudendum of women, emission, pain in the knee. ⟨Method⟩Puncture perpendicularly 0.5~1.0 cun. Moxibustion is applicable.

●阴络[yīn luò]　①络脉名。出《灵枢·百病始生》。与阳络相对,指位置较深的络脉。②泛指从手、足三阴经的络脉。

Yin Collaterals　① A category of collaterals, originally from *Lingshu*: *Baibing Shisheng* (*Miraculous Pivot*: *Beginning of Various Diseases*), opposite to the yang collaterals, referring to the collaterals distributed deeply. ② Referring generally to the collaterals branching out from the three yin meridians of hand and foot.

●阴门瘙痒[yīn mén sāo yǎng]　即阴痒。详见该条。
Pruritus of Vaginal Orifice　→阴痒(p.562)
●阴门痒[yīn mén yǎng]　即阴痒。详见该条。
Itching of Vaginal Orifice　→阴痒(p.562)

●阴囊缝[yīn náng fèng]　经外穴名。见《千金要方》。又名囊下缝。在阴囊下部正中线上。灸治卒癫、狂风骂詈挝斫人,名为热阳风证。

Yinnangfeng(EX-CA)　An extra point, seen in *Qianjin Yaofang* (*Essential Prescriptions Worth a Thousand Gold*), also named Nangxiafeng. ⟨Location⟩ at the midline of the lower part of the scrotum. ⟨Indications⟩ depressive psychosis, and madness, etc. ⟨Method⟩ Moxibustion.

●阴囊下横纹[yīn náng xià héng wén]　经外穴名。见《类经图翼》。在阴囊下第一横纹中点处。灸治卒中急风、闷乱欲死、眼反、口噤、腹中切痛。

Yinnangxiahengwen（EX-CA)　An extra point, seen in *Leijing Tuyi*(*Illustrated Supplements to Classified Canon of Internal*

Medicine of the Yellow Emperor). ⟨Location⟩ at the midpoint of the first transverse crease in the lower part of the scrotum. ⟨Indications⟩ acute apoplexy, severe case of oppressive feeling in the chest and dysphoria, superduction, lockjaw, and severe pain in the abdomen.

●阴跷病[yīn qiāo bìng] 奇经八脉病候之一。见《难经·二十九难》。可见多眠、癃闭、下肢活动不利。

Diseases of Meridian One of the Yinqiao pathological maninfestations of Eight Extra Meridians, originally from *Nanjing: Ershijiu Nan* (*The Classic of Questions: Question 29*). ⟨Manifestations⟩ Drowsiness, uroschesis, difficulty in the movement of the lower limbs.

●阴跷脉[yīn qiāo mài] 奇经八脉之一。见《灵枢·脉度》,其循行,以足少阴肾分出,起于然谷之后,上行内踝的上方,向上沿大腿内侧,进入前阴部,然后沿着腹部上入胸内,入于缺盆,向上出人迎的前面,皮达鼻旁,连属目内眦,与足太阳经、阳跷脉会合。

Yinqiao Meridian One of Eight Extra Meridian, originally from *Lingshu: Mai Du* (*Miraculous Pivot: Courses and Lengths of Meridians*). ⟨Course⟩ Branching from the Kidney Meridian of Foot-Shaoyin, it begins behind the navicular bone and goes upward to the superior part of the medial malleolus. Running along the medial side of the thigh, it enters the interior pudendum, goes upward along the abdomen, and enters the chest and supraclavicular fossa, then runs anteriorly to Renying (ST 9) and reaches the lateral part of the nose, links the inner canthus, and finally converges with the Meridians of Foot-Taiyang and Yangqiao.

●阴跷穴[yīn qiāo xué] 经穴别名。见《针经指南》。即照海。详见该条。

Yinqiaoxue Another name for Zhaohai (KI 6), a meridian point seen in *Zhenjing Zhinan* (*A Guide to the Classics of Acupuncture*). → 照海(p.586)

●阴茄[yīn qié] 即阴挺。详见该条。

Prolapse of Uterus Another name for prolapse of uterus and vagina. → 阴挺(p.559)

●阴市[yīn shì] 经穴名。出《针灸甲乙经》。属足阳明胃经。又名阴鼎。⟨定位⟩在大腿前面,当髂前上棘与髌底外侧端线的连线上,髌底上3寸(图60.2)。⟨层次解剖⟩皮肤→皮下组织→股直肌腱与股外侧肌之间→股中间肌,浅层布有股神经前皮支和股外侧皮神经,深层有旋肌外侧动、静脉的降支和股神经肌支。⟨主治⟩膝腿麻痹、酸痛、屈伸不利、下肢不遂、腰痛、寒疝、腹胀腹痛。直刺0.5～1寸;可灸。

Yinshi (ST 33) A meridian point, originally from *Zhenjiu Jia-Yi Jing* (*A-B Classic of Acupuncture and Moxibustion*), a point on the Stomach Meridian of Foot-Yangming, also named Yinding. ⟨Location⟩ on the anterior side of the thigh and on the line connecting the anterior superior iliac spine and the superiolateral corner of the patella, 3 cun above this corner (Fig. 60.2). ⟨Regional anatomy⟩ skin → subcutaneous tissue → between tendons of rectus muscle and lateral vastus muscle of thigh → intermediate vastus muscle of thigh. In the superficial layer, there are the anterior cutaneous branches of the femoral nerve and the lateral cutaneous nerve of the thigh. In the deep layer, there are the descending branches of the lateral cricumflex femoral artery and vein and the muscular branches of the femoral nerve. ⟨Indications⟩ numbness and aching of the knee and leg, difficulty in flexion and extension, paralysis of the lower limbs, lumbago, periumbilical colic due to invasion of cold, distension and pain in the abdomen. ⟨Method⟩ Puncture perpendicularly 0.5～1.0 cun. Moxibustion is applicable.

●阴水[yīn shuǐ] 水肿证型之一。出《丹溪心法·水肿》。由脾阳不振,肾阳虚衰,不能运化水湿所致。证见足跗先肿,渐及周身,腰以下肿甚,按之凹陷,皮色晦暗,便溏,四肢倦怠,面色苍白,舌淡苔白,脉多沉迟。治宜健脾温肾,助阳利水。取脾俞、肾俞、水分、气海、太溪、足三里。

Yin Edema A type of edema, originally from *Danxi Xinfa* (*Danxi's Experience: Edema*) generally due to insufficiency of the spleen yang and the kindey-yang, leading to inability to transport and transform water and dampness. ⟨Manifestations⟩ first, pitted edema of the back of feet, gradually extending to the whole body, with the part below the waist more serious, dim skin, loose stools, lassitude

of limbs, pale complexion, pale tongue with white coating, frequent, deep and slow pulse. 〈Treatment principle〉Strengthen the spleen and warm the kidney, restore yang and remove dampness by diursis. 〈Point selection〉Pishu(BL 20), Shenshu(BL 23), Shuifen(RN 28), Qihai(RN 6), Taixi(KI 3) and Zusanli(ST 36).

●阴挺[yīn tǐng] 病证名,见《诸病源候论》。又称阴㿗、阴茄、阴挺下脱、茄病、下瘤、鸡冠疮等,包括子宫脱垂、阴道壁膨出、阴痔、阴脱等,详见"子宫脱垂"条。

Prolapse of Uterus and Vagina A disease, originally from *Zhubing Yuanhou Lun* (*General Treatise on the Etiology and Symptomatology of Diseases*), also named prolapse of vagina, fall-off uterus and vagina, prolapse of uterus, eggplant-like prolapse, appearing of the uterus or cockscomb sore, invoving hysteroptosis, protrusion of vaginal wall, prolapse of uterus, and fall-off of uterus. →子宫脱垂(p. 625)

●阴挺下脱[yīn tǐng xià tuō] 即阴挺。详见该条。参见"子宫脱垂"条。

Fall-Off of Uterus and Vagina Another name for prolapse of uterus and vagina. →子宫脱垂(p. 625)

●阴突[yīn tū] 即阴挺。详见该条,参见"子宫脱垂条"。

Prolapse of Vagina →子宫脱垂(p. 625)

●阴脱[yīn tuō] 即子宫脱垂。详见该条。

Falling of Uterus →子宫脱垂(p. 625)

●阴维病[yīn wéi bìng] 奇经八脉病候之一。出《难经·二十九难》。可见心痛、呕吐、胁肋痛等。

Diseases of the Yinwei Meridian One of the pathological manifestations of the Eight Extra Meridians, originally from *Nanjing: Ershijiu Nan* (*The Classics of Questions: Question* 29) 〈Manifestations〉cardiac pain, vomiting, and pain in the hypochondriac region, etc.

●阴维脉[yīn wéi mài] 奇经八脉之一。出《素问·刺腰痛篇》。其循行起于小腿内侧,沿大腿内侧上行到腹部,与足太阴经相合过胸部,与任脉会于颈部。

Yinwei Meridian One of the Eight Extra Meridians, originally from *Suwen: Ci Yaotong Pian* (*Plain Questions: On the Treatment of Lumbago with Acupuncture*). It begins at the medial side of the shank, goes upward along the medial side of the thigh to the abdomen, joins the Foot-Taiyin Meridian on the chest and the Ren Meridian on the neck.

●阴维穴[yīn wéi xué] 1.阴维脉交会穴。下肢部交会足少阴经的筑宾;腹部交会足太阴经的冲门、府舍、大横、腹哀及足厥阴经的期门;颈部交会任脉的天突、廉泉。2.经穴别名。①见《针经指南》。即内关。详见该条。②出《针灸甲乙经》。即大赫。详见该条。

1. Yinwei points The crossing points on the Yinwei Meridian. The crossing point on the lower limbs is Zhubin(KI 9) of the Meridian of Foot-Shaoyin; the Crossing Points on the abdomen are: Chongmen(SP 12), Fushe(SP 13), Daheng(SP 15) and Fu'ai(SP 16) of the Meridian of Foot-Taiyin, and Qimen(LR 14) of the Meridian of Foot-Jueyin; the Crossing Points on the neck are: Tiantu(RN 22) and Lianquan(RN 23) of the Ren Meridian.

2. Yinwei Another name for ① Neiguan(PC 6), a meridian point seen in *Zhenjing Zhinan* (*Guide to the Classics of Acupuncture*). →内关(p. 278)② Dahe(KI 12), a meridian point, originally from *Zhenjiu Jia-Yi Jing* (*A-B Classic Acupuncture and Moxibustion*). →大赫(p. 62)

●阴痿[yīn wěi] 出《灵枢·邪气藏府病形篇》等。即阳痿。详见该条。

Flaccidness of Penis Impotence originally from *Lingshu: Xieqi Zangfu Bingxing Pian* (*Miraculous Pivot: Pathogenic Evils, Zang-Fu Organs and Manifestations*). →阳痿(p. 540)

●阴郄[yīn xì] 经穴名。《针灸甲乙经》名手少阴郄,《备急千金要方》名阴郄。属手少阴心经,为本经郄穴。〈定位〉在前臂掌侧,当尺侧腕屈肌腱的桡侧缘,腕横纹上0.5寸(图49和图51)。〈层次解剖〉皮肤→皮下组织→尺侧腕屈肌腱桡侧缘→尺神经。浅层有前臂内侧皮神经,贵要静脉属支等分布。深层有尺动、静脉。〈主治〉心痛、惊恐、心悸、骨蒸、盗汗、吐血、衄血、失语。直刺0.2～0.5寸;可灸。

Yinxi (HT 6) A meridian point, named Shoushaoyinxi in *Zhenjiu Jia-Yi Jing* (*A-B Classic of Acupuncture and Moxibustion*), and Yinxi in *Beiji Qianjin Yaofang* (*Essential Pre-*

scriptions for Emergencies Worth a Thousand Gold), the Xi (Cleft) point on the Heart Meridian of Hand-Shaoyin. 〈Location〉 on the palmer side of the forearm and on the radial side of the tendon of the ulnar flexor muscle of the wrist, 0.5 cun proximal to the crease of the wrist (Figs. 49&51). 〈Regional anatomy〉 skin→subcutaneous tissue→radial border of tendon of ulnar flexor muscle of wrist→ulnar nerve. In the superficial layer, there are the medial cutaneous nerve of the forearm and the tributaries of the basilic vein. In the deep layer, there are the ulnar artery and vein. 〈Indications〉 cardiac, pain, fright and terror, palpitation, hectic fever due to yin deficiency, night sweat, hematemesis, epistaxis, and aphasia. 〈Method〉 Puncture perpendicuary 0.2～0.5 cun. Moxibustion is applicable.

●**阴虚崩漏**[yīn xū bēng lòu] 崩漏证型之一。多因肾阴不足,虚火妄动,精血失守所致,证见血崩下血,或淋漓不绝,出血量少,血色鲜红,头晕耳鸣,五心烦热,失眠盗汗,腰膝痠软,舌红苔少,脉细数。治宜调补肾阴,取关元、三阴交、肾俞、交信、然谷、阴谷。

Metrorrhagia and Metrostaxis due to Yin Deficiency A type of metrorrhagia and metrostaxis, mostly due to insufficiency of the kidney-yin, resulting in hyperactivity of fire of deficiency type leading to failure to control blood. 〈Manifestations〉 profuse menses or incessant menses with small amount and scarlet color, dizziness, tinnitus, dysphozia with feverish sensation in chest, palm and soles, insomnia, night sweat, soreness and debility of waist and knees, red tongue with little coating, thready and rapid pulse. 〈Treatment principle〉 Regulate and tonify the kidney-yin. 〈Point selection〉 Guanyuan (RN 4), Sanyinjiao (SP 6), Shenshu (BL 23), Jiaoxin (KI 8), Rangu (KI 2) and Yingu (KI 10).

●**阴虚呃逆**[yīn xū è nì] 呃逆证型之一。因胃阴不足,失于濡润,气失顺降所致。证见呃逆声音急促而不连续,口干舌燥,烦躁不安,舌质红而干或有裂纹,脉细数。治宜生津养胃,止呃平逆。取天突、膈俞、内关、足三里、胃俞、中脘、太溪。

Hiccup due to Yin Deficiency A type of hiccups due to deficiency of stomach-yin, resulting in a failure to moisten and the descending of the stomach-qi. 〈Manifestations〉 rapid but intermittent hiccups, dry mouth and tongue, dysphoria, red and dry tongue or tongue with cracks, thready and rapid pulse. 〈Treatment principle〉 Promote the production of the body fluid to nourish the stomach and relieve the hiccups. 〈Point selection〉 Tiantu (RN 22), Geshu (BL 17), Neiguan (PC 6), Zusanli (ST 36), Weishu (BL 21), Zhongwan (RN 12) and Taixi (KI 3).

●**阴虚火旺不寐**[yīn xū huǒ wàng bù mèi] 不寐证型之一。由肾阴不足,不能上济于心,心火独亢,热扰神明,神志不宁所致。证见虚烦不寐,或寐则易醒,手足心热,惊悸,出汗,口干咽燥,头晕耳鸣,健忘,遗精,腰痠,舌红,脉细数。治宜滋阴降火。取大陵、通里、复溜,太冲。

Insomnia due to Yin Deficiency and Hyperactivity of Fire A type of insomnia due to deficiency of Kidney-yin, and failure to nourish the heart, this leads to the flaring of heart-fire, which results in mental disorder due to heat, and mental restlessness. 〈Manifestations〉 insomnia due to vexation, or aptness to wake during sleep, feverish sensation in the palms and soles, palpitation, dry mouth and throat, dizziness tinnitus, amnesia, emission, soreness of waist, red tongue, thready and rapid pulse. 〈Treatment principle〉 Nourish yin to reduce pathogenic fire. 〈Point selection〉 Daling (PC 7), Tongli (HT 5), Fuliu (KI 7) and Taichong (LR 3).

●**阴虚火旺咳血**[yīn xū huǒ wàng ké xuè] 咳血证型之一。多由阴虚火旺,肺络损伤所致。证见咳嗽少痰,痰中带血,血色鲜红,潮热盗汗,口干咽燥,颧部红艳,形体消瘦,舌红苔少,脉细数。治宜益阴养肺,清热止血,取尺泽、鱼际、孔最、百劳、然谷。

Hemoptysis due to Yin Deficiency and Hyperactivity of Fire A type of hemoptysis resulting from impairment of pulmonary vessels, mostly caused by hyperactivity of fire due to yin deficiency. 〈Manifestations〉 cough with a little phlegm mixed with scarlet blood, tidal fever and night sweat, dry mouth and throat, flush of zygomatic region, emaciation, red tongue with little coating, thready and rapid

pulse. ⟨Treatment principle⟩ Supplement yin and nourish the lung, clear heat to stop bleeding. ⟨Point selection⟩ Chize(LU 5), Yuji(LU 10), Kongzui(LU 6), Bailao(EX-B) and Rangu(KI 2).

●阴虚火旺尿血 [yīn xū huǒ wàng niào xuè] 尿血证型之一。多因肾阴不足，阴虚火旺，下移小肠所致。证见尿血，小便短赤，头晕耳鸣，潮热盗汗，腰腿酸软，舌红少苔，脉细数。治宜养阴清热，降火止血。取关元、阴谷、太溪、大敦。

Hematuria due to Yin Deficiency and Hyperactivity of Fire A type of hematuria, mostly due to deficiency of kindey-yin, and hyperactivity of fire due to yin deficiency, which moves down to the small intestine. ⟨Manifestations⟩ hematuria, scanty dark urine, dizziness, tinnitus, tidal fever, night sweat, lassitude in loin and legs, red tongue with little coating, thready and rapid pulse. ⟨Treatment principle⟩ Nourish yin, remove heat and reduce pathogenic fire to stop bleeding. ⟨Point selection⟩ Guanyuan(RN 4), Yingu(KI 10), Taixi(KI 3) and Dadun(LR 1).

●阴虚咳嗽 [yīn xū ké sòu] 咳嗽证型之一。多因肺阴不足，肺失滋润，肺燥气逆所致。证见干咳无痰，或痰少而粘，咽燥喉痛，午后发热，手足心热，或痰中带血，舌红少津，脉细数。治宜润肺止咳，滋阴清热。取肺俞、太渊、太溪、廉泉。

Cough due to Yin Deficiency A type of cough, generally due to deficiency of lung-yin, leading to failure to nourish the lung and resulting in dryness of the lung and reversed flow of qi. ⟨Manifestations⟩ dry cough without phlegm, or with a little thick phlegm mixed with blood, dry and sore throat, fever in the afternoon, feverish sensation in the palms and soles, red and dry tongue, thready and rapid pulse. ⟨Treatment principle⟩ Nourish the lung to arrest cough and nourish yin to clear heat. ⟨Point selection⟩ Feishu(BL 13), Taiyuan(LU 9), Taixi(KI 3) and Lianquan(RN 23).

●阴虚瘰疬 [yīn xū luǒ lì] 瘰疬证型之一，多由肺肾阴虚，虚火内灼所致，其证除见瘰疬的一般症状外，兼见骨蒸潮热、盗汗、咳嗽、虚烦不寐，头晕神疲，舌红少苔，脉细数。治宜滋阴降火。取天井、少海、百劳、肾俞、脾俞。参见"瘰疬"条。

Scrofula due to Yin Deficiency A type of scrofula, mostly due to Yin deficiency of the lung and the kidney, interior scorching fire of deficiency type. ⟨Manifestations⟩ in addition to the general symptoms of scrofula, hectic fever due to yin deficiency, night sweat, cough, insomnia due to vexation, dizziness, mental fatigue, red tongue with a little coating, thready and rapid pulse are also seen. ⟨Treatment principle⟩ Nourish yin to reduce pathogenic fire. ⟨Point selection⟩ Tianjing(SJ 10), Shaohai(HT 3), Bailao(EX-B), Shenshu(BL 23), Pishu(BL 20). →瘰疬(p. 258)

●阴虚呕吐 [yīn xū ǒu tù] 呕吐证型之一。由胃阴不足，胃失濡养，气失和降所致。证见呕吐反复发作，时作干呕，口燥咽干，似饥而不欲食，舌红津少，脉多细数，治宜养阴益胃。取脾俞、胃俞、血海、三阴交、足三里、内关。

Vomiting due to Yin Deficiency A type of vomiting due to deficiency of stomach-yin, leading to failure to nourish the stomach and abnormal descending of qi. ⟨Manifestations⟩ frequent vomiting, dry mouth and throat, anorexia, red tongue with a little fluid, thready and rapid pulse. ⟨Treatment principle⟩ Nourish the stomach-yin to reinforce the stomach. ⟨Point selection⟩ Pishu(BL 20), Weishu(BL 21), Xuehai(SP 10), Sanyinjiao(SP 6), Zusanli(ST 36) and Neiguan(PC 6).

●阴虚乳癖 [yīn xū rǔ pǐ] 乳癖证型之一。多因肝肾阴虚，经络失养而成痼疾。其证除见乳癖的一般症状外，兼见午后潮热，颧红，头晕耳鸣，腰背酸痛，疲倦，月经量少色淡，舌红，脉细数。治宜补益肝肾。取太溪、太冲、外关、中渚、乳根、肾俞。参见"乳癖"条。

Breast Nodules due to Yin Deficiency A type of breast nodules mostly due to yin deficiency of the liver and kidney, resulting in failure to nourish the meridians. ⟨Manifestations⟩ besides the general symptoms, it is accompanied by tidal fever in the afternoons, flush of zygomatic region, dizziness, tinnitus, pain in the back and loin, tiredness, scanty and light-colored menstruation, red tongue, thready and rapid pulse. ⟨Treatment principle⟩ Tonify the liver and kidney. ⟨Point selection⟩ Taixi(KI

3), Taichong (LR 3), Waiguan (SJ 5), Zhongzhu(SJ 3), Rugen(ST 18) and Shenshu (BL 338). →乳癖(p. 338)

●阴虚胃痛[yīn xū wèi tòng] 胃痛证型之一。多因胃痛日久,或郁热伤阴,胃失濡养所致。证见胃痛隐隐,口燥咽干,大便干结,舌红少津,脉细数。治宜养阴益胃止痛,取脾俞、胃俞、章门、中脘、足三里、内关、血海、三阴交。

Stomachache due to Yin Deficiency A type of stomachache, generally due to lingering stomachache, or impairment of yin due to stagnated heat, leading to failure to nourish the stomach. 〈Manifestations〉 dull pain in the stomach, dry mouth and throat, constipation, red tongue with a little fluid, thready and rapid pulse. 〈Treatment principle〉 Nourish yin and reinforce the stomach to alleviate pain. 〈Point selection〉 Pishu(BL 20), Weishu (BL 21), Zhangmen(LR 13), Zhongwan(RN 12), Zusanli(ST 36), Neiguan(PC 6), Xuehai (SP 10) and Sanyinjiao(SP 6).

●阴虚胁痛[yīn xū xié tòng] 胁痛证型之一。由湿热久羁,郁火伤阴,肝络失养所致。证见胁痛隐隐,痛无定处,无膜胀重着感,劳累或体位变动时,疼痛明显,颧红,低热,自汗,头晕目眩,心悸,舌质偏红,少苔,脉细数。治宜滋阴养血,和络定痛。取阴郄、心俞、血海、三阴交、太溪。

Hypochondriac Pain due to Yin Deficiency A type of hypochondriac pain due to lingering retention of damp-heat and impairment of yin by stagnated fire, leading to failure to nourish the liver collaterals. 〈Manifestations〉 dull and moveable pain in the hypochondriac region without sensation of distension or pressure, which is worsened by tiredness or change of posture, flush of zygomatic region, low fever, spotaneous perspiration, dizziness, palpitation, reddish tongue with thin coating, thready and rapid pulse. 〈Treatment principle〉 Nourish yin and blood, regulate collaterals and alleviate pain. 〈Point selection〉 Yinxi(HT 6), Xinshu (BL 15), Xuehai(SP 10) Sanyinjiao(SP 6) and Taixi(KI 3).

●阴阳配穴法[yīn yáng pèi xué fǎ] 配穴法之一。指阴经穴与阳经穴配伍应用,如内关配足三里治疗胃病。三阴交配足三里治疗消化不良。列缺配合谷治疗感冒等。其互为表里的阴、阳两经的穴位配合使用。则称表里配穴法。详见该条。

The Combination of Points on Yin Meridians with Those on Yang Meridians One form of point prescriptions, referring to the mixed application of points on yin and yang meridians. For instance, select Neiguan(PC 6) coordinated with Zusanli(ST 36) to treat gastropathy; Sanyinjiao(SP 6) with Zusanli(ST 36) to treat dyspeptic; Lieque(LU 7) with Hequ(LI 4) to treat common cold. The coordinating application based on the exterior-interior relationship of yin and yang meridians is named the combination of the exterior-interior points. →表里配穴法(p. 24)

●阴阳穴[yīn yáng xué] ①经外穴名。出《千金要方》。在拇趾趾节横纹内侧端。灸治卒中恶风、赤白带下、泻泄、肠疝。②经外穴别名。出《千金要方》。即营池。详见该条。

1. Yinyangxue (EX-LE) An extra point, originally from *Qianjin Yaofang*(*Essential Prescriptions Worth a Thousand Gold*). 〈Location〉 at the medial end of the transverse crease of the hallucis joint. 〈Indications〉 acute apoplexy, leukorrhea with reddish discharge, diarrhea, hernia. 〈Method〉 moxibustion.

2. Yinyangxue Another name for Yingchi (EX-LE), an extra point originally from *Qianjin Yaofang* (*Essential Prescriptions Worth a Thousand Gold*). →营池(p. 568)

●阴痒[yīn yǎng] 病证名。出《肘后备急方》。又称阴门痒、阴门瘙痒、阴部瘙痒。是以妇女阴道内或外阴部瘙痒,甚则痒痛难忍,坐卧不宁为特征的一种病证,多由于脾虚湿盛,肝郁化热,湿热蕴结,流注于下,或因外阴不洁,久坐湿地,病虫侵袭阴部所致。证见外阴部或阴道内瘙痒,甚则疼痛,奇痒难忍,心烦少寐,坐立不安,胃脘满闷,口苦而粘,小便黄赤,带下量多,黄稠腥臭,舌苔黄腻,脉弦数或滑数,治宜清热利湿,佐以疏肝。取中极、下髎、血海、三阴交、蠡沟、曲骨、大敦、间使。

Pruritus Vulvae A disease, originally from *Zhouhou Beiji Fang* (*A Handbook of Prescriptions for Emergencies*), also named itching of vaginal orifice, pruritus of vaginal orifice and pruritus in femals pudendum, character-

ized by pruritus in the vulva or vagina, even with intolerable pruritus leading to restlessness. Generally caused by excess of dampness due to insufficiency of the spleen, transformation of the depressive liver-qi into heat downward flow of accumulated damp-heat, or dirty vulva, long-time sitting on damp earth, and invasion of germs to the vulva. 〈Manifestations〉 pruritus, and pain in severe cases, intolerable pruritus in vulva or vagina, vexation, insomnia, restlessness, fullness in the stomach, sticky mouth with bitter taste, dark urine, leukorrhea with yellowish, thick and foul discharge, yellowish and greasy coating, taut and rapid or slippery and rapid pulse. 〈Treatment principle〉Clear heat and promote diuresis in combination with relieving the depressed liver. 〈Point selection〉Zhongji(RN 3), Xialiao (BL 34), Xuehai(SP 10), Sanyinjiao(SP 6), Ligou(LR 5), Qugu(RN 2), Dadun(LR 1) and Jianshi(PC 5).

●阴之陵泉[yīn zhī líng quán] 经穴别名。出《灵枢·九针十二原》。即阴陵泉。详见该条。

Yinzhilingquan Another name for Yinlingquan(SP 9), a meridian point originally from *Lingshu: Jiu Zhen Shier Yuan*[*Miraculous Pivot: Nine Needles and Twelve Yuan (Primary) Points*]. →阴陵泉(p.557)

●阴中隐阳[yīn zhōng yǐn yáng] 针刺手法名。出《金针赋》。与阳中隐阴对称，为先泻后补法，其法当先深部运针，行紧提慢按六数，觉微凉，再退到浅部运针，行紧按慢提九数，觉微热，稍停片刻，出针。用于先热后寒的病证。

Yang Occluded in Yin An acupuncture manipulation term, originally from *Jinzhen Fu (Ode to Gold Needle)*, opposite to yin occluded in Yang, the method of reducing before reinforcing. 〈Method〉Manipulate the needle in the deep region first with a quick lifting and slow thrusting movement six times, lift the needle to the shallow layer when slight coolness is felt and manipulate the needle with quick thrusting and slow lifting nine times. Retain the needle for a while when slight warmth is felt, then withdraw the needle. 〈Indications〉diseases with fever prior to cold.

●殷榘[yīn jǔ] 人名。明针灸家，字度卿，号方山，仪真(今江苏仪征)人，世医出身，治病有良效，且不计报酬。曾开棺针刺暴死产妇，得活。事见《仪真县志》。

Yin Ju An acupuncture and moxibustion expert in the Ming Dynasty, who styled himself Duqing and assumed the name of Fangshan, a native of Yizhen(now Yizheng in Jiangsu Province). Born in a family of doctors for generations, he treated diseases with excellent effects and never cared about the pay. He once opened a coffin and rescued a parturient by needling her who had suddenly died. The story can be seen in *Yizhenxian Zhi*(*Records of Yizhen County*).

●殷门[yīn mén] 经穴名。出《针灸甲乙经》。属足太阳膀胱经。〈定位〉在大腿后面，当承扶与委中的连线上，承扶下6寸(图35.3)。〈层次解剖〉皮肤→皮下组织→股二头肌长头及半腱肌。浅层布有股后皮神经。深层有坐骨神经及并行动、静脉，股深动脉穿支等结构。〈主治〉腰脊强痛、不可俯仰、大腿疼痛。直刺1.5~2.5寸；可灸。

Yinmen(BL 37) A meridian point on the Bladder Meridian of Foot-Taiyang, originally from *Zhenjiu Jia-Yi Jing* (*A-B Classic of Acupuncture and Moxibustion*).〈Location〉on the posterior side of the thigh and on the line connecting Chengfu(BL 36) and Weizhong (BL 40), 6 cun below Chengfu(BL 36)(Fig. 35.3).〈Regional anatomy〉 skin→subcutaneous tissue→long head of biceps muscle of thigh and semitendinous muscle. In the superficial layer, there is the posterior femoral cutaneous nerve. In the deep layer, there are the sciatic nerve and the accmpanying artery and vein and the perforating branches of the deep femoral artery.〈Indications〉rigidity and pain along the spinal column, inability to bend forward and backward, and pain in the thigh. 〈Method〉Puncture perpendicularly 1.5~2.5 cun. Moxibustion is applicable.

●瘖门[yīn mén] 经穴别名。见《素问·气穴论》。即哑门。详见该条。

Yinmen(瘖门) Another name for Yamen (DU 15), a meridian point originally from *Suwen: Qixue Lun*(*Plain Questions: On Loci of*

● 寅门[yín mén] 经外穴名。见《千金要方》。在头部，当前正中线入发际1.8寸。〈主治〉黄疸病。沿皮刺0.3～0.5寸。

Yinmen (EX-HN) An extra point, originally from *Qianjin Yaofang* (*Essential Prescriptions Worth a Thousand Gold*). 〈Location〉 on the head, 1.8 cun directly above the midpoint of the anterior hairline. 〈Indication〉 jaundice. 〈Method〉 Puncture subcutaneously 0.3～0.5 cun.

● 银针[yín zhēn] 针具名。以银质为主制成的医用针具。其传热和导电性能较好，多用于温针。

Silver Needle A kind of needle instrument made of silver, frequently used as the warm needle for its good conductivity of heat and electricity.

● 龂交[yín jiāo] 经穴别名。出《针灸甲乙经》。即龈交。详见该条。

Yinjiao(断交) Another name for Yinjiao(DU 28), a meridian point originally from *Zhenjiu Jia-Yi Jing* (*A-B Classic of Acupuncture and Moxibustion*). →龈交(p.564)

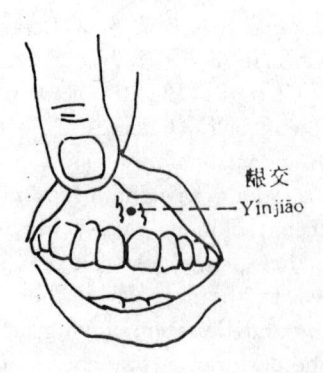

图70 龈交穴
Fig 70 Yinjiao point

● 龈交[yín jiāo] 经穴名。出《素问·气府论》。属督脉。又名断交。〈定位〉在上唇内，唇系带与上齿龈的相接处(图70)。〈层次解剖〉上唇系带与牙龈之移行处→口轮匝肌深面与上颌骨牙槽弓之间，布有上颌神经的上唇支以及眶下神经与面神经分支交叉形成的眶下丛和上唇动、静脉。〈主治〉齿龈肿痛、口㖞口噤、口臭、齿衄、鼻渊、面赤颊肿、唇吻强急、面部疮癣、两腮生疮、癫狂、项强。向上斜刺0.2～0.3寸；禁灸。

Yinjiao (DU 28) A meridian point, originally from *Suwen*: *Qi Fu Lun* (*Plain Questions*: *On House of Qi*), a point on the Du Meridian, also named Yinjiao(断交). 〈Location〉 inside the upper lip, at the junction of the labial frenum and upper gum (Fig. 70). 〈Regional anatomy〉 transitional border of superior labial frenulum and upper gum→between deep surface of orbicular muscle of mouth and alveolar arch of maxillary bone. There are the superior labial branches of the maxillary nerve, the infraorbital plexus formed by the branches of the infraorbital and facial nerves, and the superior labial artery and vein in this area. 〈Indications〉 gingivitis, wiry mouth, lockjaw, foul breath, bleeding from the gum, rhinorrhea with turbid discharge, flushed face and swollen cheek, spasm of lips, sore and tinea on the face, sore on the cheeks, manic-depressive disorder, and stiff-neck. 〈Method〉 Puncture upward obliquely 0.2～0.3 cun. Moxibustion is forbidden.

● 引火法[yǐn huǒ fǎ] 天灸的一种。见《串雅外编》。为药物贴敷的一种，用吴茱萸60克。研为细末，掺和面粉30克，用水调整和成糊状，涂在布上，贴涌泉穴。或用附子1个研为细末，用醋调为膏状，贴于涌泉穴。治疗手足不温、四肢厥冷等。

Inducing Fire Method A form of medicinal vesiculation, originally from *Chuan Ya Waibian* (*External Treatise on Folk Medicine*). 〈Method〉 Grind *Wu Zhu Yu* (*Fructus Eaodiae*) (60g) into powder and mix it with flour (30g), and then stir it into paste with water. Put it on a piece of cloth and apply it to Yongquan(KI 1). Or grind one piece of *Fu Zi* (*Radix Aconiti Praeparata*) into powder and mix it with vinegar into a paste, then apply the paste to Yongquan(KI 1). 〈Indications〉 lack of warmth in hands and feet, cold limbs, etc.

● 引针[yǐn zhēn] 为出针法之别称。详见该条。

Pulling Away the Needle Another name for withdrawing the needle. →出针法(p.51)

●**饮郄**[yǐn xì] 经外穴名。见《外台秘要》。在胸部，当第6肋间隙中，距前正中线6寸处。〈主治〉腹痛、肠鸣、胸胁痛，以及肺炎、胸膜炎、肝区痛等，斜刺0.3～0.5寸；可灸。

Yinxi（EX-CA） An extra point, seen in *Waitai Miyao*(*Clandestine Essentials from the Imperial Library*).〈Location〉on the chest, in the 6th intercostal space, 6 cun lateral to the anterior midline.〈Indications〉abdominal pain, borborygmus, pain in hypochodriac region, pneumonia, pleurisxy and hepatalgia, etc.〈Method〉Puncture obliquely 0.3～0.5 cun. Moxibustion is applicable.

●**隐白**[yǐn bái] 经穴名。出《灵枢·本输》。属足太阴脾经，为本经井穴。又名鬼垒。〈定位〉在足大趾末节内侧，距趾甲角0.1寸(指寸)(图39.1)。〈层次解剖〉皮肤→皮下组织→甲根，布有足背内侧皮神经的分支，趾背神经和趾背动、静脉。〈主治〉腹胀、暴泄、善呕、烦心善悲、胸痛、心痛、胸满、咳嗽、喘息、慢惊风、昏厥、月经过期不止、崩漏、吐血、衄血、尿血、便血、癫狂、多梦、尸厥。斜刺0.1寸，或点刺出血；可灸。

Yinbai（SP 1） A meridian point, originally from *Lingshu*: *Ben Shu*（*Miraculous Pivot*: *Meridian Points*）, the Jing(Well)point on the Spleen Meridian of Foot-Taiyin, also named Guilei.〈Location〉on the medial side of the distal segment of the great toe, 0.1 cun from the corner of the toenail(Fig. 39.1).〈Regional anatomy〉skin→subcutaneous tissue→root of nail. There are the branches of the medial dorsal cutaneous nerve of the foot, the dorsal digital nerve and the dorsal digital artery and vein in this area.〈Indications〉abdominal distension, spouting diarrhea, frequent vomiting, vexation, susceptiblility to sorrow, pain in the chest, cardiac pain, full sensation in the chest, cough, syndrome characterized by dyspnea, chronic infantile convulsion, fainting spell, menostaxis, metrorrhagia and metrostaxis, hematemesis, nose bleeding, hematuria, hemafecia, manic-depressive disorder, dreaminess, corpselike syncope.〈Method〉Puncture obliquely 0.1 cun, or prick to cause bleeding. Moxibustion is applicable.

●**瘾疹**[yǐn zhěn] 即风疹。详见该条。

Urticaria →风疹(p.116)

●**印堂**[yìn táng] ①经外穴名。见《扁鹊神应针灸玉龙经》。〈定位〉在额部，当两眉头中间(图10)。〈层次解剖〉皮肤→皮下组织→降眉间肌。布有额神经的分支滑车上神经，眼动脉的分支额动脉及伴行的静脉。〈主治〉头痛、眩晕、呕吐、失眠、鼻渊、鼻衄、目痛、眼昏、眉棱骨痛、颜面疔疮、小儿急、慢惊风、产后血晕、子痫、以及感冒、鼻炎、高血压、三叉神经痛等。沿皮刺0.5～1.0寸；可灸。②部位名，指两眉之间和眉上方。又名阙、眉心。

1. Yintang（EX-HN 3） An extra point, seen in *Bian Que Shenying Zhenjiu Yulong Jing* (*Bian Que's Jade Dragon Classics of Acupuncture and Moxibustion*).〈Location〉on the forehead, at the midpoint between the eyebrows(Fig. 10).〈Regional anatomy〉skin → subcutaneous tissue → procerus muscle. There are the supratrochlear branch of the frontal nerve and the frontal artery from the ophthalmic artery and the accompanying vein in this area.〈Indications〉headache, vertigo, vomiting, insomnia, rhinorrhea, with turbid discharge, epistaxis, pain in the eye, blurring of vision, pain in the supra-orbital bone, facial furuncle, acute or chronic infantile convulsion, puerperal faintness, eclampsia gravidarum, common cold, rhinitis, hypertension and prosopalgia.〈Method〉Puncture subcutaneously 0.5～1.0 cun. Moxibustion is applicable.

2. Glabella A part of the body, referring to the part between and above the eyebrows, also named que or the centre between eyebrows.

●**应突**[yìng tū] 经外穴名。出《外台秘要》。在胸部，当乳头外开2寸直下，第6肋间隙下1寸处。〈主治〉饮食不下、腹满肠鸣泄泻，以及肋间神经痛。沿皮刺0.3～0.5寸；可灸。

Yingtu（EX-CA） An extra point, originally from *Waitai Miyao* (*Clandestine Essentials from the Imperial Library*).〈Location〉on the chest, 2 cun lateral to the nipple and directly downward, 1 cun below the 6th intercostal space.〈Indications〉lack of appetite, fullness of abdomen, borborygmus, diarrhea,

intercostal neuralgia. ⟨Method⟩ Puncture subcutaneously 0.3~0.5 cun. Moxibustion is applicable.

●缨脉[yīng mài] 经脉名。出《素问·通评虚实论》。指颈旁足阳明胃经脉。

The Stomach Meridian in Neck A meridian, originally from *Suwen: Tongping Xushi Lun* (*Plain Question: A Thorough Discussion on Deficiency and Excess*), referring to the Meridian of Foot-Yangming in the lateral part of the neck.

●膺[yīng] 部位名。胸前两旁肌肉隆起之处，即胸大肌。

Pectoral Muscle A body part, referring to the prominence of the pectoral major muscle, i.e. great pectoral muscle.

●膺窗[yīng chuāng] 经穴名。出《针灸甲乙经》。属足阳明胃经。⟨定位⟩在胸部，当第三肋间隙，距前正中线4寸(图40)。⟨层次解剖⟩皮肤→皮下组织→浅筋膜→胸大肌→肋间肌。浅层布有肋间神经的外侧皮支、胸腹壁静脉的属支。深层有胸内、外侧神经、胸肩峰动、静脉的分支或属支，第三肋间神经和第三肋间后动、静脉。⟨主治⟩咳嗽、气喘、胸胁胀痛、乳痈。直刺0.2~0.4寸，或向内斜刺0.5~0.8寸；可灸。

Yingchuang (ST 16) A meridian point, originally from *Zhenjiu Jiayi Jing* (*A-B Classic of Acupuncture and Moxibustion*), a point on the stomach meridian of Foot-Yangming. ⟨Location⟩ on the chest, in the 3rd intercostal space, 4 cun lateral to the anterior midline (Fig. 40). ⟨Regional anatomy⟩ skin→subcutaneous tissue→greater pectoral muscle→intercostal muscle. In the superficial layer, there are the lateral cutaneous branches of the intercostal nerve and the tributaries of the thoracoepigastric vein. In the deep layer, there are the medial and lateral pectoral nerves, the branches or tributaries of the thoracoacromial artery and vein, the third intercostal nerve and the third posterior intercostal artery and vein. ⟨Indications⟩ cough, dyspnea, distending pain in hypochondrium, acute mastitis. ⟨Method⟩ Puncture perpendicularly 0.2~0.4 cun, or medially and obliquely 0.5~0.8 cun. Moxibustion is applicable.

●膺俞[yīng shū] 经穴别名。即中府。详见该条。

Yingshu Another name for the meridian point Zhongfu(LU 1). →中府(p. 609)

●膺中[yīng zhōng] ①部位名，指胸前两旁高处。②经穴别名。即中府。详见该条。

1. Prominence of Pectoral Muscle A body part, i.e. the protruding part lateral to the anterior chest.

2. Yingzhong Another name for the meridian point Zhongfu(LU 1). →中府(p. 609)

●膺中俞[yīng zhōng shū] 经穴别名，出《针灸甲乙经》。即中府。详见该条。

Yingzhongshu Another name for Zhongfu (LU 1), a meridian point originally from *Zhenjiu Jia-Yi Jing* (*A-B Classic of Acupuncture and Moxibustion*). →中府(p. 609)

●迎而夺之[yíng ér duó zhī] 刺法用语。见《灵枢·小针解》。与随而济之相对，为迎随泻法的原则。意指泻法要逆着经脉循行而刺，以损夺其有余。详见"随而济之"条。

Reducing by Puncturing against the Direction of Meridian-Qi An acupuncture technique, originally from *Lingshu: Xiaozhen Jie* (*Miraculous Pivot: Explanation of Delicate Needling*), the opposite of reinforcing by puncturing along the direction of meridian-qi the principle of reducing by puncturing against the direction of meridians. Referring to needling with the needle tip against the direction of the meridians to remove excessive pathogenic factors. →随而济之(p. 416)

●迎风冷泪[yíng fēng lěng lèi] 迎风流泪证型之一。多因肝肾两虚，精血亏耗，泪窍狭窄，风邪外引，泪液外溢所致。证见眼睛不红不痛，泪下无时，迎风更甚，泪水清稀，流泪时无热感。治宜补益肝肾。取睛明、攒竹、风池、肝俞、肾俞。

Epiphora with Cold Tears Induced by Wind A type of epiphora induced by wind, frequently due to deficiency of the liver and kidney, exhaustion of essence and blood, stricture of puncta lacrimalis, exterior inducement of pathogenic wind, leading to overflowing. ⟨Manifestations⟩ epiphora without soreness or pain of eyes, timeless epiphora which become worse when facing the wind, clear, thin and cold tears. ⟨Treatment principle⟩ Tonify the

liver and kidney.〈Point selection〉Jingming (BL 1), Cuanzhu (BL 2), Fengchi (GB 20), Ganshu (BL 18) and Shenshu (BL 23).

●迎风流泪[yíng fēng liú lèi] 病证名。见《眼科捷径》。多由肝肾不足、或肝经郁热所致。证见遇风流泪,甚者泪下如雨。有冷泪和热泪之分。详见"迎风冷泪"、"迎风热泪"条。

Epiphora Induced by Wind A disease, seen in *Yangke Jiejing* (*A Shortcut of Ophthalmology*), generally due to yin deficiency of the liver and kidney, or stagnated heat in the liver meridian.〈Manifestations〉epiphora with wind, even with plenty of tears in severe cases. It is divided into cold tears and warm tears.→迎风冷泪(p.566)、迎风热泪(p.567)

●迎风热泪[yíng fēng rè lèi] 是迎风流泪的证型之一。多因肝火炽盛,或风热外袭所致。证见眼睛红肿,焮痛,羞明,泪下粘浊,迎风加剧。流泪时有热感,治宜疏风清热,舒肝明目。取睛明、攒竹、合谷、阳白、太冲。

Epiphora with Warm Tears Induced by Wind
A type of epiphora induced by wind, generally due to excessive liver-fire, or invasion by exogenous pathogenic wind-heat.〈Manifestations〉red and swelling eyes with burning pain, photophobia, warm and thick tears, which becomes serious when against the wind.〈Treatment principle〉Dispel wind and remove heat, relieve the depressed liver to improve acuity of vision.〈Point selection〉Jingming (BL 1), Cuanzhu (BL 2), Hegu (LI 4), Yangbai (GB 14) and Taichong (LR 3).

●迎随[yíng suí] 刺法用语。迎,意为逆;随,意为顺。此指针刺补泻法的区分原则,又用以统称各式补泻法。参见"迎随补泻"条。

Puncturing along or against the Direction of Meridians An acupuncture technique. "Ying"(迎) means "against" and "Sui"(随) means "along". The classifying principle of reinforcing and reducing methods, also used as the general designation for various reinforcing and reducing methods.→迎随补泻(p.567)

●迎随补泻[yíng suí bǔ xiè] 针刺补泻方法。出《难经·七十二难》。又称针向补泻。系以顺经针刺或逆经针刺来区分补泻。针尖顺着经脉方向刺为补,针尖逆着经脉方向针刺为泻。

Reinforcing and Reducing by Puncturing along and agaist the Direction of the Meridians Respectively A method of reinforcing and reducing, originally from *Nanjing: Qishier Nan* (*The Classic of Questions: Question 72*), also named reinforcing or reducing depending on needling direction, referring to distinguishing reinforcing and reducing by means of needling with or against the direction of the meridians. Needling along the direction of meridian is reinforcing while needling against it is reducing.

●迎香[yíng xiāng] 经穴名。属手阳明大肠经,为手、足阳明之会。又名冲阳。〈定位〉在鼻翼外缘中点旁,当鼻唇沟中(图5和图28)。〈层次解剖〉皮肤→皮下组织→提上唇肌。浅层布有上颌神经的眶下神经分支。深层布有面神经颊支,面动、静脉的分支或属支。〈主治〉鼻塞、不闻香臭、鼻衄、鼻渊、口眼歪斜、面痒、面浮肿、鼻瘜肉。直刺0.1～0.2寸,或向鼻方向斜刺0.3～0.5寸;不宜灸。

Yingxiang (LI 20) A meridian point of the Large Intestine Meridian of Hand-Yangming, the Crossing Point of the Meridians of Hand-Yangming and Foot-Yangming, also named Chongyang.〈Location〉in the nasolabial groove, beside the midpoint of the lateral border of the nasal ala (Figs. 5&28).〈Regional anatomy〉skin→subcutaneous tissue→levator muscle of the upper lip. In the superficial layer, there are the branches of the infraorbital nerve from the maxillary nerve. In the deep layer, there are the buccal branches of the facial nerve and the branches or tributaries of the facial artery and vein.〈Indications〉stuffy nose, anosmia, epistaxis, rhinorrhea with turbid discharge, deviation of the eye and mouth, itching of the face, edema of face, nasal polyp.〈Method〉Puncture perpendicularly 0.1～0.2 cun, or puncture obliguely towards the nose 0.3～0.5 cun. Moxibustion is not advisable.

●荥输治外经[yíng shū zhì wài jīng] 《内经》取穴法则之一,指各经的荥穴和输穴,主治从脏腑外行的经脉病候,参见"合治内腑"条。

Selecting Ying (Spring) and Shu (Stream) Points for Treating Meridian Disorder One

of the principles of point selection in *Neijing* (*The Canon of Internal Medicine*) referring to treating disorders which occur on the meridian running out from the zang-fu organs by needling Ying (Spring) points and Shu (Stream) points. →合治内腑(p.162)

●荥穴[yíng xué] 五腧穴之一。荥穴多位于掌指或跖趾关节之前,喻脉气稍大,象水成小流。用于治疗发热等疾患。

Ying (Spring) Points One of the Five Shu Points, generally located in front of the metacarpophalangeal joint and the mertatarsophalangeal joint with stronger meridian-qi like water converging into a stream, used for treating fever and other diseases.

●营池[yíng chí] 经外穴名。出《千金要方》。又名阴阳穴。在足内踝下缘前、后之凹陷中,每侧二穴,左右计四穴。〈主治〉月经过多、赤白带下。直刺0.2~0.3寸;可灸。

Yingchi (EX-LE) An extra point, originally from *Qianjin Yaofang* (*Essential Prescriptions Worth a Thousand Gold*), also named Yinyangxue. 〈Location〉in the depressions anterior and posterior to the lower border of medial malleolus, two points on each side and four points in all. 〈Indications〉menorrhagia, leukorrhea with reddish discharge. 〈Method〉Puncture perpendicularly 0.2~0.3 cun. Moxibustion is applicable.

●瘿气[yǐng qì] 病证名。出《尔雅》。又名大脖子。以颈部肿大为主证。古典医书将本病分为气瘿、血瘿、肉瘿、筋瘿和石瘿五类。以气瘿尤为多见。详见"气瘿"条。

Goiter A disease, originally from *Erya* (*Definition and Pronunciation of Characters*), also called big neck, manifested by deroncus. It is divided in classical medical works into five types: qi goiter, hemangioma of the neck, fleshy goiter with visible varicose veins and stony goiter, of which qi goiter is the most commonly seen. →气瘿(p.313)

●痈疽神秘灸经[yōng jū shén mì jiǔ jīng] 书名。又名《痈疽灸经》。元代胡元庆撰,明代薛已校补。是讨论灸法痈疽的专书,成书于1354年。《薛氏医案》中可见。

Yongju Shenmi Jiujing (**Mysterious Canon of Moxibustion for Carbuncle**) A book, also named *Yongju Jiujing* (*Moxibustion Canon for Carbuncles*), written by Hu Yuanqing in the Yuan Dynasty, proofread and supplemented by Xue Ji in the Ming Dynasty and published in 1354. It is a monograph dealing with the treatment of carbuncle and cellulitis by moxibustion. It can be seen in *Xueshi Yian* (*Xue's Medical Records*).

●痈疽神妙灸经[yōng jū shén miào jiǔ jīng] 书名。明代彭用光撰,成书于1561年。现辑入彭氏《简易普济良方》第五卷,为灸法治痈疽的专篇。

Yongju Shenmiao Jiujing (**Wonderful Canon of Moxibustion for Carbuncles**) A book written by Peng Yongguang in the Ming Dynasty, published in 1561. It was compiled in Vol. 5 of *Jianyi Puji Liangfang* (*Simple and Effective Prescriptions for Universal Relief*), a monograph for treating carbuncle and cellulitis by moxibustion.

●勇泉[yǒng quán] 经穴别名。见《素问》王冰注。即涌泉。见该条。

Yongquan(勇泉) Another name for Yongquan(涌泉)(KI 1), a meridian point originally from annotation of *Su Wen* (*Plain Questions*) by Wang Bing. →涌泉(p.568)

●涌泉[yǒng quán] 经穴名。出《灵枢·本输》。属足少阴肾经,为本经井穴。又名地冲、地卫、足心。〈定位〉在足底部,卷足时足前部凹陷处,约当足底二、三趾趾缝纹头端与足跟连线的前1/3与后2/3交点上(图71)。〈层次解剖〉皮肤→皮下组织→足底腱膜(跖腱膜)→第二趾足底总神经→第二蚓状肌。浅层布有足底内侧神经的分支,深层有第二趾底总神经和第二趾足底总动、静脉。〈主治〉头痛、头晕、眼花、咽喉痛、舌干、失音、小便不利、大便难、小儿惊风、足心热、癫疾、霍乱转筋、昏厥。直刺0.5~0.8寸;可灸。

Yongquan (KI 1) A meridian point, originally from *Lingshu: Benshu* (*Miraculous Pivot: Meridian Points*), the Jing (Well) Point of the Kidney Meridian of Foot-Shaoyin. also named Dichong, Diwei and Zuxin. 〈Location〉on the sole, in the depression appearing on the anterior part of the sole when the foot is in the planter flexion, approximately at the junction

of the anterior third and posterior two-thirds of the line connecting the base of the 2nd and 3rd toes and the heel (Fig. 71). 〈Regional anatomy〉 skin→subcutaneous tissue→plantar aponeurosis → 2nd common digital nerve of sole→2nd lumbrical muscle. In the superficial layer, there are the branches of the medial planter nerve. In the deep layer, there are the 2nd common digital nerve of the sole and the 2nd common digital artery and vein of the sole. 〈Indications〉 headache, dizziness, dim eyesight, sore throat, dry tongue, aphonia, diffculty in urination, defecation, infantile convulsion, feverish sensation in the soles, epilepsy, cramp in cholera morbus, syncope. 〈Method〉 Puncture perpendicularly 0.5～0.8 cun. Moxibustion is applicable.

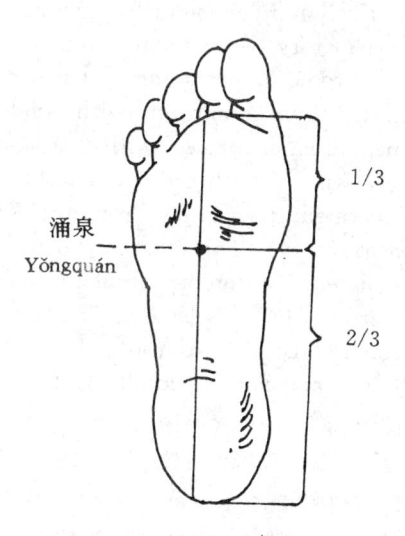

图71 涌泉穴
Fig 71 Yongquan point

●幽门 [yōu mén] ①指胃的下口，为七冲门之一。②经穴名，出《针灸甲乙经》。属足少阴肾经，为冲脉、足阴之会。又名上门。〈定位〉在上腹部，当脐中上6寸，前正中线旁开0.5寸（图40）。〈层次解剖〉皮肤→皮下组织→腹直肌鞘前壁→腹直肌。浅层布有第六、七、八胸神经前支的前皮支及伴行的动、静脉。深层有腹壁上动、静脉的分支或属支，第六、七、八胸神经前支的肌支和相应的肋间动、静脉。〈主治〉腹痛、呕吐、善哕、消化不良、泄泻、痢疾。直刺0.5～0.8寸；可灸。不可深刺，以免伤及内脏。③经穴别名。出《圣济总录》。即下脘，见该条。

1. **Pylorus** The lower orifice of the stomach, one of the Seven Important Portals.
2. **Youmen** (KI 21) A meridian point originally from *Zhenjiu Jiayi Jing* (*A-B Classic of Acupuncture and Moxibustion*), a point on the Kidney Meridian of Foot-Shaoyin, the crossing point of the Chong Meridian and the Foot-Shaoyin Meridian, also named Shangmen. 〈Location〉 on the upper abdomen, 6 cun above the centre of the umbilicus and 0.5 cun lateral to the anterior midline (Fig. 40). 〈Regional anatomy〉 skin→subcutaneous tissue→anterior sheath of rectus muscle of abdomen→rectus muscle of abdomen. In the superficial layer, there are the anterior cutaneous branches of the anterior branches of the 6th to 8th thoracic nerves and the accompanying arteries and veins. In the deep layer, there are the branches or tributaries of the superior epigasrtic artery and vein, the muscular branches of the anterior branches of the 6th to 8th thoracic nerves and the related intercostal arteries and veins. 〈Indications〉 abdominal pain, vomiting, susceptility to hiccup, dyspesia, diarrhea and dysentery. 〈Method〉 Puncture perpendicularly 0.5～0.8 cun. Moxibustion is applicable. 〈Cautions〉 deep insertion should be avoided in case it injures internal organs.
3. **Youmen** Another name for Xiawan (RN 10), a meridian point, originally from *Shengji Zonglu* (*Imperial Medical Encyclopaedia*). →下脘 (p. 490)

●油风 [yóu fēng] 病证名。出《外科正宗》。又名鬼舐头，即斑秃。详见该条。

Alopecia Areata due to Pathogenic Wind A disease originally from *Waike Zhengzong* (*Orthodox Manual of External Diseases*), also called haircut by ghost. →斑秃 (p. 12)

●油捻灸 [yóu niǎn jiǔ] 灸法的一种。以纸捻沾植物油点然后，在穴位处进行熏灸。多用于治皮肤病。

Oil Wick Moxibustion A kind of moxibustion. ⟨Method⟩ Dip a paper wick into vegetable oil and ignite it, then give moxibustion with it on the selected points. This method is mostly used for treatment of dermatoses.

●右关[yòu guān] 经穴别名。出《太平圣惠方》。即石关。详见该条。

Youguan Another name for Shiguan (KI 18), a meridian point originally from *Taiping Shenghui Fang* (*Imperial Benevolent Prescriptions*). →石关(p. 384)

●右玉液[yòu yù yè] 经外穴名。见"金津玉液"条。

Youyuye (EX-HN) An extra point. →金津玉液(p. 202)

●瘀血头痛[yū xuè tóu tòng] 头痛证型之一。因头部外伤或因久痛入络,瘀血阻滞脉络所致。证见头痛如刺,经久不愈,痛处固定不移,视物昏黑,记忆减退,舌微紫,脉细或涩。治宜活血化瘀,行气定痛。取百会、太阳、阿是穴、合谷、三阴交、血海。

Headache due to Blood Stasis A type of Headache, due to head trauma or chronic pain affecting the collaterals, resulting in blood stasis blocking the meridians and collaterals. ⟨Manifestations⟩ stabbing, fixed and obstinate pain in the head, poor vision, hypomnesis, light purple tongue, and thready or choppy pulse. ⟨Treatment principle⟩ Promote blood criculation by removing blood stasis, promote circulation of qi to relieve pain. ⟨Point selection⟩ Baihui (DU 20), Taiyang (EX-HN 5), Ahshi Point, Hegu (LI 4), Sanyinjiao (SP 6) and Xuehai (SP 10).

●瘀血胃痛[yū xuè wèi tòng] 胃痛证型之一。多因病延日久,或气病及血,瘀血内阻,络脉不通所致。证见胃脘疼痛,痛有定处而拒按,或痛有针刺感,食后痛甚,甚见吐血便黑,舌质紫黯,脉涩,治宜活血化瘀止痛,取中脘、足三里、内关、膈俞、期门、公孙、三阴交。

Stomachache due to Blood Stasis A type of stomachache, mostly caused by obstruction of the meridians and collaterals by blood stasis resulting from lingering stomach disorder or pathological change from qi to blood. ⟨Manifestations⟩ fixed or stabbing pain in the stomach with tenderness, which becomes even worse after eating. One can even see melena and hematemesis. Dark purplish tongue, choppy pulse. ⟨Treatment Principle⟩ Promote blood circulation by removing blood stasis to relieve pain. ⟨Point selection⟩ Zhongwan (RN 12), Zusanli (ST 36), Neiguan (PC 6), Geshu (BL 17), Qimen (LR 14), Gongsun (SP 4) and Sanyinjiao (SP 6).

●瘀血胁痛[yū xuè xié tòng] 胁痛证型之一,因跌仆闪挫,胁肋脉络损伤,经脉气血阻滞,血运不畅所致。证见胁痛固定不移,持续不断,有跌仆外伤史或慢性胁痛史,胁下胀痛拒按,或有痞块,舌质偶见瘀点、瘀斑、脉弦 或细涩。治宜活血通络,行气止痛,取大包、京门、行间、膈俞、三阴交。

Hypochondriac pain due to Blood Stasis A type of hypochondriac pain due to traumatic injury, resulting in the impairment of hypochondriac meridians and collaterals, leading to the stagnation of qi and blood. ⟨Manifestations⟩ fixed and persistent hypochondriac pain, with a history of traumatic injury, or a history of chronic hypochondriac pain, distending in the hypochondrium with tenderness or mass, tongue proper with occasional ecchymosis, wiry or thready and choppy pulse. ⟨Treatment principle⟩ Promote blood circulation to remove obstruction in the meridians and collaterals, promote circulation of qi to relieve pain. ⟨Point selection⟩ Dabao (SP 21), Jingmen (GB 25), Xingjian (LR 2), Geshu (BL 17) and Sanyinjiao (SP 6).

●瘀血心悸[yū xuè xīn jì] 心悸证型之一。多由气滞血瘀,心脉瘀阻,心失所养所致。证见心悸持续多年,日渐加重,动则气喘,或有阵发性胸痛,面色黄瘦,唇舌紫黯,脉细涩结代。甚则心阳不振,怔忡不已,形寒肢冷,咳喘不得卧,冷汗、浮肿,脉微欲绝。治宜活血强心。取曲泽、少海、气海、血海。脉微欲绝加百会、太渊。浮肿加灸水分。

Palpitation due to Blood Stasis A type of Palpitation. Generally due to stagnation of qi and blood stasis, resulting in obstruction of the cardiac meridians and failure to nourish the heart. ⟨Manifestations⟩ progressive palpitations for many years, shortness of breath during physical activity, or paroxysmal chest pain, sallow complexion, dark purple lips and

tongue, thready, choppy or knotted and intermittent pulse. In severe cases, insufficiency of the heart-yang, severe palpitation, cold body and extremities, inability to lie flat due to cough with dyspnea, cold sweat, edema, feeble pulse. 〈Treatment principle〉 Promote blood circulation to strengthen functions of the heart. 〈Point selection〉 Quze(PC 3), Shaohai (HT 3), Qihai (RN 6), Xuehai (SP 10); for cases with feeble pulse, add Baihui (DU 20) and Taiyuan (LU 9); for cases with edema, use moxibustion on Shuifen (RN 9).

●瘀血胸痹 [yū xuè xiōng bì] 胸痹证型之一。由气郁日久，瘀血内停，络脉不通，痹阻胸阳所致。证见胸痛如刺，或绞痛阵发，痛彻肩背，唇舌紫暗，脉细涩或结代。治宜活血化瘀，通络止痛，取膻中、巨阙、膈俞、阴郄、心俞。

Obstruction of Qi in the Chest due to Blood Stasis A type of obstruction of qi in the chest, caused by long-term depressed qi, resulting in stagnation of blood blockage of the collaterals leading to obstruction of yang-qi in the chest. 〈Manifestations〉 stabbing or paroxysmal colic pain in the chest radiating to shoulder and back, purple lips and tongue, thready, choppy or knotted pulse. 〈Treatment principle〉 Promote blood circulation by removing blood stasis, relieve pain by removing obstruction in the meridians and collaterals. 〈Point selection〉 Danzhong (RN 17), Juque (RN 14), Geshu (BL 17), Yinxi (HT 6) and Xinshu (BL 15).

●于法开 [yú fǎ kāi] 人名。晋代僧人、针灸家。本姓吴，字道林。从释支遁，研习医典，明晓医术。撰有《议论备豫方》一卷，已佚。

Yu Fakai A monk and an acupuncture-moxibustion expert of the Jin Dynasty, originally surnamed Wu, who styled himself Daolin. He followed Zhi Dun, studied medical classics, was well versed in medical skills and compiled *Yilun Beiyu Fang* (*A Discussion on Reserved Formulas*), which is no longer extant.

●鱼 [yú] 部位名。大拇指后掌侧隆起之肉。

Thenar Eminence A body part, referring to the projected muscle on the palm to the rear of connecting with the thumb.

●鱼肠 [yú cháng] 经穴别名。见《循经考穴编》。即承山。见该条。

Yuchang Another name for Chengshan (BL 57), a meridian point originally from *Xunjing Kaoxue Bian* (*Studies on Acupoints Along Meridians*) →承山 (p. 45)

●鱼腹 [yú fù] 经穴别名。出《针灸甲乙经》。即承山。详见该条。

Yufu Another name for Chengshan (BL 57), a meridian point originally from *Zhenjiu Jia-Yi Jing* (*A-B Classic of Acupuncture and Moxibustion*). →承山 (p. 45)

●鱼际 [yú jì] 经穴名。出《灵枢·本输》。属手太阴肺经，为本经荥穴。〈定位〉在手拇指本节（第1掌指关节）后凹陷处，约当第1掌骨中点桡侧，赤白肉际处（图16和图49）。〈层次解剖〉皮肤→皮下组织→拇短展肌→拇对掌肌→拇短屈肌。浅层有正中神经掌皮支及桡神经浅支等分布。深层有正中神经肌支和尺神经肌支等结构。〈主治〉咳嗽、咳血、失音、喉痹、咽干、身热、乳痈、肘挛、掌心热。直刺0.5～0.8寸；可灸。

Yuji (LU 10) A meridian point, originally from *Ling Shu*: *Benhu* (*Miraculous Pivot*: *Meridian Points*), the Ying (Spring) point of the Lung Meridian of Hand-Taiyin. 〈Location〉 in the depression proximal to the 1st metacarpophalangeal joint, on the radial side of the midpoint of the 1st metacarpal bone, and on the junction of the red and white skin (Figs. 16&49). 〈Regional anatomy〉 skin→subcutaneous tissue→short abductor muscle of thumb→opponens muscle of thumb→short flexor muscle of thumb. In the superficial layer, there are the cutaneous branches of the median nerve and the superficial branches of the radial nerve. In the deep layer, there are the muscular branches of the median and ulnar nerves. 〈Indications〉 cough, hemoptysis, aphonia, inflammation of the throat, dry throat, fever, acute mastitis, elbow spasm, feverish sensation in the palm. 〈Method〉 Puncture perpendicularly 0.5～0.8 cun. Moxibustion is applicable.

●鱼络 [yú luò] 指大拇指本节后内侧（大鱼际）的络脉。出《灵枢·邪气藏府病形》。临床上可从鱼际部

络脉的色泽变化以诊察肠胃病。如该处色青,主胃中寒;色赤主肠胃有热等。

Collaterals Located at the Thenar Eminence
The collaterals at the internal posterior aspect of thenar eminence, originally from *Lingshu: Xie Qi Zang Fu Bing Xing* (*Miraculous Pivot: Pathogenic Evils, Zang-Fu Organs and Manifestations*). In clinic, some enterogastric diseases can be discovered and diagnosed according to changes of color and lustre of collaterals located at the thenar eminence, for instance, blue color represents cold syndrome of the stomach, red indicates heat syndrome of the stomach and intestine, etc.

●鱼尾[yú wěi] ①经外穴名。出《银海精微》。在眼外眦横纹尽处。〈主治〉头痛、头晕,目疾,以及面神经麻痹等。沿皮刺0.3~0.5寸。②经穴别名。出《扁鹊神应针灸玉龙经》。即瞳子髎。详见该条。

1. **Yuwei**(EX-HN) An extra point, originally from *Yinhai Jingwei* (*Essentials of Ophthalmology*).〈Location〉at the end of the cross striation of the outer canthus.〈Indications〉headache, dizziness, ophthalmopathy and facial paralysis, etc.〈Method〉puncture subcutaneously 0.3~0.5 cun.

2. **Yuwei** Another name for Tongziliao(GB 1), a meridian point, originally from *Bianque Shenying Zhenjiu Yulong Jing* (*Bian Que's Jade Dragon Classics of Acupuncture and Moxibustion*). →瞳子髎(p. 443)

●鱼腰[yú yāo] ①经外穴名。出《扁鹊神应针灸玉龙经》。〈定位〉在额部,瞳孔直上,眉毛中(图10)。〈层次解剖〉皮肤→皮下组织→眼轮匝肌→枕额肌额腹。布有眶上神经外侧支,面神经的分支和眶上动、静脉的外侧支。〈主治〉偏正头痛、目赤肿痛、目翳、近视,以及角膜炎、结膜炎、眼肌麻痹、眶上神经痛、面神经麻痹等。沿皮刺0.3~0.5寸。②经穴别名。见《针方六集·神照集》。即承山。详见该条。③《东医宝鉴》误作印堂别名。④《银海精微》所载的光明穴,与本穴同位。参见"光明"条。

1. **Yuyao**(EX-HN 4) An extra point, originally from *Bian Que Shenying Zhenjiu Yulong Jing* (*Bian Que's Jade Dragon Classics of Acupuncture and Moxibustion*).〈Location〉at the frontal part, directly above the pupil, at the midpoint of the eyebrows(Fig. 10).〈Regional anatomy〉skin→subctaneous tissue→orbiclar muscle of eye→frontal belly of occipitofrontal muscle. There are the lateral branches of the supraorbital nerve, the branches of the facial nerve and the lateral branches of the supraorbital artery and vein in this area.〈Indications〉migraine, headache, redness swelling and pain in the eye, conjunctivitis, myopia, keratitis ocular paralysis, ophthalmoplegia, supraorbital neuralgia, facial paralysis, etc.〈Method〉Puncture subcutaneously 0.3~0.5 cun.

2. **Yuyao** Another name for Chengshan(BL 57), a meridian point seen in *Zhenfang Liuji: Shenzhao Ji* (*Six Collections of Acupuncture Prescriptions: Collection under God's Brightness*). →承山(p. 45)

3. **Yuyao** mistaken for another name for Yintang(EX-HN 3)in *Dongyi Baojian* (*Treasured Mirror of Oriental Medicine*).

4. **Guangming** A point, recorded in *Yinhai Jingwei* (*Essentials of Ophthalmology*), located in the same position as Yuyao→光明(p. 149)

●髃骨[yú gǔ] 部位名。又称肩端骨。为肩胛上部(肩胛岗)与巨骨结合处。即肩胛岗之肩峰突。

Acromion Scapulae A body part, also called acromion bone, referring to the joint of supra scapular region(spine of scapula) and clavicle, namely, the acromion protrusion of the spine of scapula.

●玉房俞[yù fáng shù] 经穴别名。见《中国针灸学》。即白环俞。详见该条。

Yufangshu Another name for Baihuanshu (BL 30), a meridian point, seen in *Zhongguo Zhenjiuxue* (*Chinese Acupuncture and Moxibustion*). →白环俞(p. 10)

●玉匮针经[yù guì zhēn jīng] 书名。吴时吕广撰,已佚。见《隋书·经籍志》。

Yugui Zhenjing(**Canon of Acupuncture of the Jade Chamber**) A book written by Lü Guang in the Wu Kingdom, which is no longer extant. See *Suishu: Jingji Zhi* (*The History of the Sui Dynasty: Records of Classics and Books*).

●玉户[yù hù] 经穴别名。出《针灸甲乙经》。即天

突。详见该条。

Yuhu Another name for Tiantu (RN 22), a meridian point originally from *Zhenjiu Jia-Yi Jing* (*A-B Classic of Acupuncture and Moxibustion*). →天突(p. 434)

●玉环俞[yù huán shū] 经穴别名。见《中国针灸学》。即白环俞。详见该条。

Yuhuanshu Another name for Baihuanshu (BL 30), a meridian point seen in *Zhongguo Zhenjiuxue* (*Chinese Acupuncture and Moxibustion*). →白环俞(p. 10)

●玉龙赋[yù lóng fù] 针灸歌赋名。撰人不详。内容依据《玉龙歌》,文字简括,便于诵习。见《针灸聚英》。

Yulong Fu (**Jade Dragon Ode**) Verse of acupuncture and moxibustion, whose author is unknown. It was written on the basis of *Yu Long Ge* (*Jade Dragon Verses*), which is concisely written and easy to recite. See *Zhenjiu Juying* (*Essentials of Acupuncture and Moxibustion*).

●玉门头[yù mén tóu] 经外穴名。又名女阴缝、鬼藏。在女性外生殖器部,阴蒂头是穴。主治妇人阴疮、癫狂。针0.3寸;可灸。

Yumantou (EX-CA) An extra point, also called Nüyinfeng and Guicang. 〈Location〉 on the external genital organs in female, at the gland of clitoris. 〈Indications〉 pundendal sores of women, manic-depressive psychosis. 〈Method〉 Puncture 0.3 cun. Moxibustion is applicable.

●玉泉[yù quán] ①经穴别名。出《针灸甲乙经》。即中极。详见该条。②经外穴名。见《千金要方》。在脐下6.5寸,当男子阴茎根上正中央,耻骨联合下缘处。主治癫疝、睾丸炎等。直刺0.3～0.5寸;可灸。③经外穴名。见《幼幼新书》。在后头部,当枕外隆凸上缘,旁开正中线1.5寸,再直下1寸。灸治瘖钩不语。

1. **Yuquan** Another name for Zhongji (RN 3), a meridian point originally from *Zhenjiu Jia-Yi Jing* (*A-B Classic of Acupuncture and Moxibustion*). →中极(p. 611)

2. **Yuquan** (EX-CA) An extra point, seen in *Qianjin Yaofang* (*Essential Prescriptions Worth a Thousand Gold*). 〈Location〉 6.5 cun below the umbilicus, right in the middle of the penis root, at the lower border of the pubic symphysis. 〈Indications〉 swelling of the scrotum, orchitis, etc. 〈Method〉 Puncture perpendicularly 0.3～0.5 cun. Moxibustion is applicable.

3. **Yuquan** (EX-HN) An extra point, seen in *Youyou Xinshu* (*A New Book of Pediatrics*). 〈Location〉 at the upper border of the external occipital protuberance on the back of the head, 1.5 cun lateral to the medial line, and 1 cun below it. 〈Indications〉 aphonia and aphasia. 〈Method〉 moxibustion.

●玉堂[yù táng] 经穴名。出《难经·三十一难》。属任脉。又名玉英。〈定位〉在胸部,当前正中线上,平第三肋间(图40)。〈层次解剖〉皮肤→皮下组织→胸骨体。主要布有第三肋间神经前皮支和胸廓内动、静脉的穿支。〈主治〉膺胸疼痛、咳嗽、气短、喘息、喉痹咽肿、呕吐寒痰、两乳肿痛。平刺0.3～0.5寸;可灸。

Yutang (RN 18) A meridian point, originally from *Nanjing*: *Sanshiyi Nan* (*The Classic of Question*: *Question 31*), a point on the Ren Meridian, also called Yuying. 〈Location〉 on the chest, at the anterior midline, on the level of the 3rd intercostal space (Fig. 40). 〈Regional anatomy〉 skin→subcutaneous tissue→sternal body. There are the anterior cutaneous branches of the 3rd intercostal nerve and the perforating branches of the internal thoracic artery and vein in this area. 〈Indications〉 chest pain, cough, shortness of breath, asthma, inflammation of the throat, vomiting of cold-phlegm and swelling and pain in breasts. 〈Method〉 Puncture subcutaneously 0.3～0.5 cun. Moxibustion is applicable.

●玉田[yù tián] 经外穴名。见《针灸孔穴及其疗法便览》。在骶部,当第四骶骨嵴下凹陷处。〈主治〉难产、腰骶痛,以及腓肠肌痉挛等。沿皮刺0.5-1寸;可灸。

Yutian (EX-B) An extra point, originally from *Zhenjiu Kongxue Jiqi Liaofa Bianlan* (*Guide to Acupoints and Acupuncture Therapeutics*). 〈Location〉 on the sacrum, in the depression below the 4th articular sacral crest. 〈Indications〉 difficult labour, pain in the waist and sacrum, systremma, etc. 〈Method〉 Puncture subcutaneously 0.5～1.0 cun. Moxibustion is applicable.

●玉液[yù yè] ①经外穴名。见"金津玉液"条。②道家养生术语。指人工炼造的可以服食的丹药。③指唾液。

1. Yuye(EX—HN 13)　An extra point. →金津玉液(p. 202)

2. **Dao Medicine for Health Preservation**　A term for health preservation from the Taoist school, referring to man-made dan medicine for edible use.

3. Yuye　Saliva.

●玉英[yù yīng]　经穴别名。出《针灸甲乙经》。即玉堂。详见该条。

Yuying　Another name for Yutang(RN 18), a meridian point originally from *Zhenjiu Jia-Yi Jing* (*A-B Classic of Acupuncture and Moxibustion*). →玉堂(p. 573)

●玉枕[yù zhěn]　经穴名。出《针灸甲乙经》。属足太阳膀胱经。〈定位〉在后头部，当后发际正中直上2.5寸，旁开1.3寸，平枕外隆凸上缘的凹陷处(图28和图31)。〈层次解剖〉皮肤→皮下组织→枕额骨枕腹。浅层布有枕大神经，枕动、静脉。深层为腱膜下疏松结缔组织和颅骨外膜。〈主治〉头痛、恶风寒、呕吐、不能远视、目痛、鼻塞。平刺0.3～0.5寸；可灸。

Yuzhen(BL 9)　A meridian point, originally from *Zhenjiu Jia-Yi Jing* (*A-B Classic of Acupuncture and Moxibustion*), a point on the Bladder Meridian of Foot-Taiyang. 〈Location〉on the occiput, 2.5 cun directly above the midpoint of the posterior hairline and 1.3 cun lateral to the midline, in the depression on the level of the upper border of the external occipital protuberance (Figs. 28 &31). 〈Regional anatomy〉 skin→subcutaneous tissue→epicranial aponeurosis. In the superficial layer, there are the greater occipital nerve and the occipital artery and vein. In the deep layer, there are the subaponeurotic loose connective tissue and the pericranium. 〈Indications〉 headache, aversion to wind and cold, vomiting, myopia, pain in the eye, stuffy nose. 〈Method〉Puncture subcutaneously 0.3～0.5 cun. Moxibustion is applicable.

●玉枕骨[yù zhěn gǔ]　部位名。即枕骨两旁高起之骨，现称枕骨之上项线。

Projecting Bones Bilateral to the Occipital Bone　A body part, referring to the convex bones on both sides of the occipital bone. Now called the upper line of the nape of the occipital bone.

●玉柱[yù zhù]　经穴别名。见《太平圣惠方》。即承山。详见该条。

Yuzhu　Another name for Chengshan(BL 57), a meridian point, seen in *Taiping Shenghui Fang*(*Imperial Benevolent Prescriptions*). →承山(p. 45)

●宛陈则除之[yù chén zé chú zhī]　《内经》针灸治则之一。见《灵枢·九针十二原》。宛通"郁"。宛陈，是郁积陈久的意思，指对气血瘀滞，邪在血分的一些病证。宜用刺络出血的方法。

Removing the Stagnation of Blood, Qi and Other Pathogenic Factors in the Xue Stage　One of treatment principles of acupuncture and moxibustion in *Neijing*(*The Canon of Internal Medicine*), seen in *Lingshu: Jiu Zhen Shier Yuan* (*Miraculous Pivot: Nine Needles and Twelve Yuan-*(*Primary*)*Points*). "Yu(宛)" indicates stagnation, "yuchen(宛陈)" means long-time stagnation. This principle refers to the treatment of some diseases caused by stagnation of qi and blood, and pathogens in the xue stage. It is advisable to apply bloodletting needling.

●郁冒[yù mào]　产后血晕的别名。详见该条。

Oppressive Feeling and Dizziness　Another name for postpartum faint. →产后血晕(p. 37)

●郁证[yù zhèng]　病证名。①泛指郁而不发的病证。如《素问·六元正纪大论》所载之木、火、土、金、水，五气之郁，又称五郁；《丹溪心法》所载之气、血、湿、热、痰、食，六郁；《景岳全书》所载之怒、思、悲、恐、忧、惊，情志之郁；《赤水玄珠》所载之心、肝、脾、肺、肾，五脏本气之郁等。②见《张氏医通·郁》。是指由情志忧郁，气滞不畅引起的病证。郁证包括的病证很多，临床以"梅核气"、"脏躁"最为多见。详见"梅核气"、"脏躁"。

Melancholia　A disease, ① generally referring to all oppressive and stuffed syndromes, e. g. melancholia of wood, fire, earth, metal and water, also called melancholia of the five-qi, originally from *Su Wen: Liu Yuan Zhengji Da Lun*(*Plain Questions: On the Laws of the Six Climatic Changes*); melancholia due to the

stagnation of qi, blood, dampness, heat, phlegm and food, i. e. six melancholia originally from *Danxi Xinfa* (*Danxi's Experience*); melancholia due to anger, anxiety, grief, fear, melancholy and terror, i. e. melancholia due to emotions, originally from *Jingyue Quanshu*(*Complete Works of Zhang Jingyue*); melancholia of the heart, liver, spleen, lung and kidney, ie. the melancholia of five zang-organs qi, etc. ② referring to syndromes due to melancholic emotions leading to impeded circulation of qi, originally from *Zhangshi Yi Tong*: *Yu* (*Zhang's Treatise on General Medicine*: *Depression*). There is a variety of syndromes reflected in melancholia, but globus hystericus and hysteria are commonly seen in clinic. →梅核气(p. 265)、脏躁(p. 582)

● 郁中[yù zhōng] 耳穴别名。即上耳根,详见该条。

Middle Stasis(MA) Another name for the auricular point Upper Root of Auricle(MA). →上耳根(p. 351)

● 彧中[yù zhōng] 经穴名。出《针灸甲乙经》。属足少阴肾经。又名或中、域中。〈定位〉在胸部,当第一肋间隙,前正中线旁开2寸(图40)。〈层次解剖〉皮肤→皮下组织→胸大肌。浅层布有第一肋间神经的前皮支、锁骨上内侧神经和胸廓内动、静脉的穿支。深层有胸内、外侧神经的分支。〈主治〉咳嗽、气喘、痰壅、胸胁胀满、不嗜食。斜刺或平刺0.5～0.8寸;可灸。

Yuzhong(KI 26) A meridian point, originally from *Zhenjiu Jia-Yi Jing* (*A-B Classic of Acupuncture and Moxibustion*), a point on the Kidney Meridian of Foot-Shaoyin, also named Huozhong and Yuzhong. 〈Location〉on the chest, in the lst intercostal space, 2 cun lateral to the anterior midline (Fig. 40). 〈Regional anatomy〉skin → subcutaneous tissue → great pectoral muscle. In the superficial layer, there are the anterior cutaneous branches of the lst intercostal nerve, the medial supraclavicular nerve and the perforating branches of the internal thorcic artery and vein. In the deep layer, there are the branches of the medial and lateral pectoral nerves. 〈Indications〉cough, dyspnea, abundant expectoration, fullness in the chest and hypochondrium, anorexia. 〈Method〉 Puncture obliquely or subcutaneously 0.5～0.8 cun. Moxibustion is applicable.

● 域中[yù zhōng] 经穴别名。出《医学入门》。即彧中。详见该条。

Yuzhong Another name for Yuzhong (KI 26), a meridian point originally from *Yixue Rumen* (*An Introduction to Medicine*). →彧中(p. 575)

● 渊液[yuān yè] 经穴别名。见《针灸聚英》。即渊腋。详见该条。

Yuanye(渊液) Another name for Yuanye(渊腋)(GB 22), a meridian point, seen in *Zhen Jiu Ju Ying* (*Essentials of Acupuncture and Moxibustion*). →渊腋(p. 575)

● 渊腋[yuān yè] 经穴名。出《灵枢·痈疽》。属足少阳胆经。又名渊液、泉液。〈定位〉在侧胸部,举臂,当腋中线上,腋下3寸,第四肋间隙中(图72)。〈层次解剖〉皮肤→皮下组织→前锯肌→肋间外肌。浅层布有第三、四、五肋间神经外侧皮支,胸长神经和胸外侧动、静脉。深层有第四肋间神经和第四肋间后动、静脉。〈主治〉胸满、胁痛、腋下肿、臂痛不举。斜刺0.5～0.8寸;可灸。

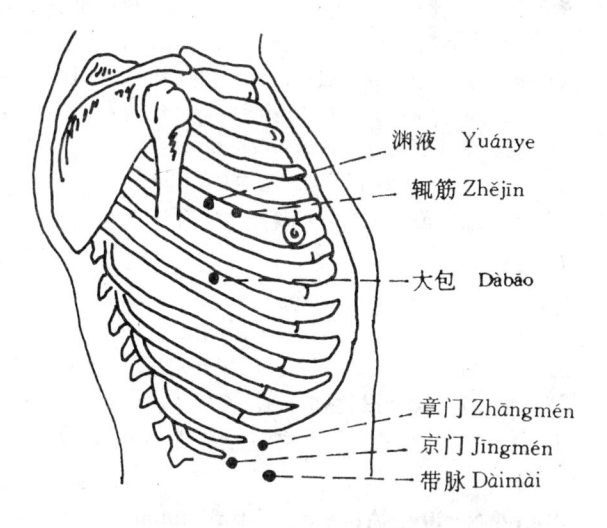

图72 渊腋、辄筋和带脉穴
Fig 72 Yuanye, Zhejin and Daimai points

Yuanye(GB 22) A meridian point, originally from *Lingshu*: *Yong Ju* (*Miraculous Pivot*: *Carbuncle and Other Suppurative Inflammations*), a point on the Gallbladder Meridian of

Foot-Shaoyang, also named Yuanye (渊液) and Quanye. 〈Location〉 on the lateral side of the chest, on the midaxillary line when the arm is raised, 3 cun below the axilla, in the 4th intercostal space (Fig. 72). 〈Regional anatomy〉 skin → subcutaneous tissue → anterior serratus muscle → external intercostal muscle. In the superficial layer, there are the lateral cutaneous branches of the 3rd to 5th intercostal nerves, the long thoracic nerve and the lateral thoracic artery and vein. In the deep layer, there are the 4th intercostal nerve and the 4th posterior intercostal artery and vein. 〈Indications〉 fullness of the chest, pain in the hypochondrium, subaxillary swelling, pain in the arm and inability to raise the arm. 〈Method〉 Puncture obliquely 0.5～0.8 cun. Moxibustion is applicable.

●元儿[yuán ér] 经穴别名。出《针灸甲乙经》。即膻中。详见该条。

Yuaner Another name for Danzhong (RN 17), a meridian point originally from *Zhenjiu Jia-Yi Jing* (*A-B Classic of Acupuncture and Moxibustion*). →膻中(p. 75)

●元见[yuán jiàn] 经穴别名。见《针灸大成》。即膻中。详见该条。

Yuanjian Another name for Danzhong (RN 17), a meridian point originally from *Zhenjiu Dacheng* (*A Great Compendium of Acupuncture and Moxibustion*). →膻中(p. 75)

●员在[yuán zài] 经穴别名。出《针灸甲乙经》。即攒竹。详见该条。

Yuanzai Another name for Cuanzhu (BL 2), a meridian point originally form *Zhenjiu Jia-Yi Jing* (*A-B Classic of Acupuncture and Moxibustion*). →攒竹(p. 58)

●员针[yuán zhēn] 针具名。员，古通"圆"。见"圆针"条。

Round Needle An acupuncture apparatus. In ancient China, the word "yuan" (员) was synonymous with the word "yuan" (圆). →圆针 (p. 576)

●员柱[yuán zhù] 经穴别名。见《外台秘要》。即攒竹。详见该条。

Yuanzhu Another name for Cuanzhu (BL 2), a meridian point originally from *Waitai Miyao* (*Clandestine Essentials from the Imperial Library*). →攒竹(p. 58)

●圆利针[yuán lì zhēn] 针具名。见《灵枢·九针十二原》。古代九针之一。其针针尖稍大且尖，圆而且锐，针身略粗，长1.6寸。〈主治〉痈肿、痹证。可深刺之。

Round-Sharp Needle A needling apparatus, seen in *Lingshu:Jiu Zhen Shier Yuan* (*Miraculous Pivot: Nine Needles and Twelve Yuan (Primary) Points*), one of the nine needles of ancient China, with a slightly large, round and sharp tip and slightly thick body, 1.6 cun in length. 〈Indications〉 carbuncle and swelling on the body surface, arthralgia-syndrome. 〈Method〉 deep puncturing.

●圆针[yuán zhēn] 针具名。见《灵枢·九针十二原》。古代九针之一。后人称圆头针。其针头卵圆，身如圆柱，长1.6寸。用以按摩体表，治疗筋肉方面的病痛。

Round Needle A needling apparatus, seen in *Ling Shu:Jiu Zhen Shier Yuan* (*Miraculous Pivot:Nine Needles and Twelve Yuan (Primary) Points*), one of the nine needles of ancient China, also called round-head needle, with an ovoid tip and cylinder-like body, 1.6 cun in length, used to massage the body surface for treating diseases of tendons and muscles.

●圆柱[yuán zhù] 经穴别名。见《古今医统》。即攒竹。详见该条。

Yuanzhu Another name for Cuanzhu (BL 2), a meridian point seen in *Gu Jin Yitong* (*The General Medicine of the Past and Present*). →攒竹(p. 58)

●原络配穴法[yuán luò pèi xué fǎ] 配穴法之一。指以本经原穴与其表里经的络穴配合使用，治疗表里经同病或本经疾病的方法。参见表里配穴法、主客原络配穴法。

Combined Selection of the Yuan (Primary) Point and the Luo (Connecting) Point One of the point selecting methods, referring to the method of puncturing the Yuan (Primary) point and the Luo (Connecting) point of its exterior-interior meridian to treat diseases of

表20　　　　　　　　　十 二 经 原 穴
Table 20　　　　The Yuan(Primary)points of the 12 Meridians

手三阴经 Three Yin Meridians of Hand	肺经 Lung Meridian 太渊 Taiyuan (LU 9)	心经 Heart Meridian 神门 Shenmen (HT 7)	心包经 Pericardium Meridian 大陵 Daling(PC 7)
手三阳经 Three Yang Meridians of Hand	大肠经 Large Intestine Meridian 合谷 Hegu(LI 4)	小肠经 Small Intestine Meridian 腕骨 Wangu(SI 4)	三焦经 Sanjiao Meridian 阳池 Yangchi (SJ 4)
足三阴经 Three Yin Meridians of Foot	脾经 Spleen Meridian 太白 Taibai(SP 3)	肾经 Kidney Meridian 太溪 Taixi(KI 3)	肝经 Liver Meridian 太冲 Taichong(LR 3)
足三阳经 Three Yang Meridians of Foot	胃经 Stomach Meridian 冲阳 Chongyang (ST 42)	膀胱经 Bladder Meridian 京骨 Jinggu(BL 64)	胆经 Gallbladder Meridian 丘墟 Qiuxu (GB 40)

the exterior-interior meridians or of the meridian corresponding to the Yuan(Primary) point. →表里配穴法(p. 24)、主客原络配穴法(p. 621)

●原穴[yuán xué]　经穴分类名。出《灵枢·九针十二原》和《灵枢·本输》。是脏腑原气经过留止的腧穴。十二经各有一原穴，阴经的原穴与五腧穴中的输穴相同。原穴关系到原气，原气通过三焦散布到各原穴。因而原穴能主治五脏六腑的疾病。各经原穴见表20。

Yuan(Primary) Points　A category of acupoints, originally from *Lingshu: Jiu Zhen Shier Yuan (Miraculous Pivot: Nine Needles and Twelve Yuan (Primary) Points)* and *Ling Shu: Ben Shu (Miraculous Pivot: Meridian Points)*, referring to the place where the primordial qi of zang-fu organs passes and stays. There is one Yuan(Primary)point for each of the Twelve Meridians. The Yuan(Primary) points of yin meridians are also their Shu (Stream)points. The primordial qi spreads via the sanjiao to every Yuan (Primary) point. Therefore, puncturing the Yuan (Primary) point can cure diseases of the five-zang and six-fu organs. See Table 20.

●缘中[yuán zhōng]　耳穴名。又称脑点。位于对屏尖与轮屏切迹之间。具有益脑安神作用。〈主治〉智能发育不全，遗尿、内耳眩晕症。

Central Rim(MA)　An auricular point, also called Brain point(MA).〈Location〉between the tip of antitragus and helix notch.〈Function〉Tonify the brain to achieve tranquilization.〈Indications〉intellectual maldevelopment, enuresis, and oticodinia.

●远道取穴[yuǎn dào qǔ xué]　取穴法之一。又称远隔取穴，简称远取，指远离病痛部位选穴。其具体应用可分本经取穴、异经取穴等。详见各条。

Distant Point Selection　One of the point selection methods, also called distal selection, or distant selection, referring to selecting points distal to the region with disease. Its clinical application can be divided into selecting points of the same meridian and selecting points of other meridians. →本经取穴(p. 18)、异经取穴(p. 552)

●远隔取穴[yuǎn gé qǔ xué]　即远道取穴。详见该条。

Distal Point Selection　→远道取穴(p. 577)

●远节段取穴[yuǎn jié duàn qǔ xué]　现代取穴法的一种。指在临床治疗或针麻时所选用的穴位，与病痛或手术部位不属于同一或邻近的脊髓节段所支配。例如头部疾患或颅脑手术，取用下肢部穴位；腰腿部疾患，取用上肢穴。参见"近节段取穴"条。

Distal Segment Point Selection　One of the modern point selection methods, referring to

points selected for treating diseases or for acupuncture anesthesia distant from the disease or near the spinal segment which the diseased or operative region belongs to, e. g. selecting points on lower limbs for diseases on the head or operations on the cranium, or points on the upper limbs for lumbo-crural problems. →近节段取穴(p. 207)

●远近配穴法[yuǎn jìn pèi xué fǎ] 配穴法之一。指远离病痛部位的穴与邻近的穴配合应用,即远道取穴与近道取穴相结合。例如胃病远取内关、足三里,近取中脘等。

Distal-Proximal Point Association A form of point association, referring to points distal to and near the affected region being associated for treatment, namely, the combination of distal point selection and proximal point selection, e. g. selecting distal Neiguan (PC 6) and Zusanli (ST 36) and proximal Zhongwan (RN 12) for gastric disease, etc.

●远取[yuǎn qǔ] 远道取穴的简称。见该条。

Distant Selection The short form of distant point selection. →远道取穴(p. 577)

●约纹[yuē wén] 又作约文,即横纹,特指关节部的皱纹。

The Wrinkle Aslo written as Yuewen (约文), a synonym of transverse crease, especially referring to creases near the joints.

●哕[yuě] 病证名。①呃逆。参见"呃逆"条。②干呕。见《丹溪心法·呕吐》。参见"干呕"条。

Hiccough A syndrome, referring to ① hiccup. →呃逆(p. 92) ② retching, seen in *Danxi Xinfa: Outu (Danxi's Experience: Vomiting)*. →干呕(p. 123)

●月闭[yuè bì] 即经闭。详见该条。

Closing of Menstruation Another name for amenia. →经闭(p. 208)

●月不通[yuè bù tōng] 即经闭。详见该条。

Obstruction of Menstruation Another name for amenia. →经闭(p. 208)

●月候不调[yuè hòu bù tiáo] 即月经不调。详见该条。

Irregular Monthly Coming Another name for irregular menstruation. →月经不调(p. 578)

●月候过多[yuè hòu guò duō] 即月经过多。详见该条。

Hypermenorrhea Another name for menorrhagia. →月经过多(p. 579)

●月忌[yuè jì] 古代针灸宜忌说之一。出《千金翼方》卷二十八。将十二月配属十二地支,按其变化推算血忌日、血支日、月厌日、四激日、月杀日、月刑日、六(月)害日等。据以避忌针灸。

Monthly Forbidding One of the ancient theories on the compatibility and incompatibility of acupuncture and moxibustion, originally from Vol. 28 of *Qianjin Yifang (Supplement to the Essential Prescriptions Worth a Thousand Gold)*. The theory, in which the twelve months in a year match with the Twelve Earthly Branches, was used for calculating blood-forbidden days, blood-divided days, monthly-tired days, four-irritability days, monthly-killing days, monthly-penalized days and six(monthly)-harming days, etc, and then deciding the compatibility and incompatibility of acupuncture and moxibustion according to the changes of the months matching with the Twelve Earthly Branches.

●月经不调[yuè jīng bù tiáo] 病证名。见《千金要方》。又称月水不调、月使不调、月经不匀、月候不调、失信、经水无常、经水不定、经水不调、经不调、经气不调、经血不定、经脉不调、经候不匀、经候不调等。泛指月经的周期、血量、血色和经质的异常。常见的有经行先期,经行后期,经行先后无定期及月经过多,月经过少等。参见各条。

Irregular Menstruation A disease, originally from *Qianjin Yaofang (Essential Prescriptions Worth a Thousand Gold)*, also called irregular monthly flow, irregular monthly envoy, irregular menses, irregular monthly coming, failing to keep the monthly coming, disorder of menstrual flow, irregularity of menstrual flow, irregular menstrual flow, menoxenia, irregular menstrual qi, disorder of menstrual blood, irregular menstrual vessel, disorder of menstrual coming, irregular menstrual time, etc. It generally refers to abnormality of the menstrual cycle, blood quantity, blood color and quality. The most commonly seen irregular menses are preceded menstrual cycle, delayed menstrual

cycle, disorder of menstrual cycle, menorrhagia, scanty menstruation, etc. →经行先期(p. 214)、经行后期(p. 214)、经行先后无定期(p. 214)、月经过多(p. 579)、月经过少(p. 579)

●月经不通[yuè jīng bù tōng]　即经闭。详见该条。

Blockage of Menstruation　Another name for amenia. →经闭(p. 208)

●月经不行[yuè jīng bù xíng]　即经闭。详见该条。

No menstruation　Another name for amenia. →经闭(p. 208)

●月经不匀[yuè jīng bù yún]　即月经不调。详见该条。

Irregular Menses　Another name for irregular menstruation. →月经不调(p. 578)

●月经过多[yuè jīng guò duō]　病证名。见《圣济总录》。又称月候过多、经来乍多。指月经周期虽准，但血量超过正常，或经行时间延长，超过七、八天以上，量亦增多。临床分气虚月经过多，血热月经过多，劳伤月经过多。详见各条。

Menorrhagia　A disease, seen in *Shengji Zonglu* (*Imperial Medical Encyclopaedia*) also called hypermenorrhea and profuse menstruation, referring to timely menstrual cycle with excessive blood discharge, or menstrual period delayed more than 7-8 days, and with more than normal blood. It is clinically divided into menorrhagia due to deficiency of qi, menorrhagia due to blood-heat and menorrhagia due to overstrain. →气虚月经过多(p. 310)、血热月经过多(p. 527)、劳伤月经过多(p. 238)

●月经过少[yuè jīng guò shǎo]　病症名。又称月经涩少、月经滞涩、经水否涩、经水涩少、经乍来少等。指月经周期虽准，但血量少于正常，或经行时间过短，量亦过少，甚至点滴，一、二日即净。临床多见血虚月经过少，血寒月经过少，血瘀月经过少，肾虚月经过少，痰湿月经过少。详见各条。

Scanty Menstruation　A disease, also called oligomenorrhea, infrequent menstruation, hard-coming of the menstrual flow, oligohypomenorrhea, hypomenorrhea, etc, referring to a timely menstrual cycle with little blood, or a short menstrual period with little blood, even only several drops for 1-2 days. It is clinically divided into scanty menstruation due to deficiency of blood, scanty menstruation due to blood-cold, scanty menstruation due to blood stasis, scanty menstruation due to deficiency of the kidney and scanty menstruation due to phlegm-dampness. →血虚月经过少(p. 530)、血寒月经过少(p. 525)、血瘀月经过少(p. 531)、肾虚月经过少(p. 367)、痰湿月经过少(p. 424)

●月经落后[yuè jīng luò hòu]　即经行后期。详见该条。

Backward Menstruation　Another name for delayed menstrual cycle. →经行后期(p. 214)

●月经涩少[juè jīng sè shǎo]　即月经过少。详见该条。

Oligomenorrhea　Another name for scanty menstruation. →月经过少(p. 579)

●月经先期[yuè jīng xiān qī]　即经行先期。详见该条。

Forward Menstruation　Another name for preceded menstrual cycle. →经行先期(p. 214)

●月经滞涩[yuè jīng zhì sè]　即月经过少。详见该条。

Infrequent Menstruation　Another name for scanty menstruation. →月经过少(p. 579)

●月使不调[yuè shǐ bù tiáo]　即月经不调。详见该条。

Irregular Monthly Envoy　Another name for irregular menstruation. →月经不调(p. 578)

●月使不来[yuè shǐ bù lái]　即经闭。详见该条。

No-Coming of Monthly Envoy　Another name for amenia. →经闭(p. 208)

●月事不来[yuè shì bù lái]　即经闭。详见该条。

Disappearance of Menses　Another name for amenorrhea. →经闭(p. 208)

●月事不通[yuè shì bù tōng]　即经闭。详见该条。

Obstruction of Menstruation　Another name for amenorrhea. →经闭(p. 208)

●月水来腹痛[yuè shuǐ lái fù tòng]　即痛经。详见该条。

Abdominal Pain in Menstrual Period　Another name for dysmenorrhea. →痛经(p. 444)

●月水不来[yuè shuǐ bù lái]　即经闭。详见该条。

No-Arrival of Menstrual Flow　Another name for amenorrhea. →经闭(p. 208)

●月水不调[yuè shuǐ bù tiáo]　即月经不调。详见该

条。

Irregular Menstrual Flow Another name for irregular menstruation. →月经不调(p. 578)

●**月水不通**[yuè shuǐ bù tōng] 即经闭。详见该条。

Obstruction of Menstrual Flow Another name for amenorrhea. →经闭(p. 208)

●**云门**[yún mén] 经穴名。出《素问·水热穴论》。属手太阴肺经。〈定位〉在胸前壁的外上方,肩胛骨喙突上方,锁骨下窝凹陷处,距前正中线6寸。(图49和图75)。〈层次解剖〉皮肤→皮下组织→三角肌→锁胸筋膜→喙锁韧带。浅层有头静脉,锁骨上中间神经。深层有胸肩峰动、静脉支,胸内、外侧神经的分支。〈主治〉咳嗽、气喘、胸痛、肩背痛、胸中烦热。向外斜刺0.5～0.8寸;可灸。

Yunmen (LU 2) A meridian point, from *Suwen: Shui Re Xue Lun* (*Plain Questions: On Acupoints for Edema and Febrile Diseases*), a point on the Lung Meridian of Hand-Taiyin. 〈Location〉in the superior lateral part of the anterior thoracic wall, superior to the coracoid process of the scapula, in the depression of the infraclavicular fossa, 6 cun lateral to the anterior midline (Figs. 49&75). 〈Regional anatomy〉skin→subcutaneous tissue→deltoid muscle→clavipectoral fascia→coracoclavicular ligament. In the superficial layer, there are the cephalic vein and the intermediate supraclavicular nerve. In the deep layer, there are the branches of the thoracoacromial artery and vein, the branches of the medial and lateral pectoral nerves. 〈Indications〉cough, dyspnea, pain in the chest, pain of the shoulder and back, dysphoria with a smothering sensation in the chest. 〈Method〉Puncture obliquely outward 0.5～0.8 cun. Moxibustion is applicable.

●**云岐子**[yún qí zǐ] 人名。金代医家张璧的别名,为张元素之子,易州(今河北易水)人,继承父业,医名闻于当时。所著针灸专著《云岐子论经络迎随补泻法》,即《洁古·云岐针法》。收入《济生拔萃》中。

Yun Qizi Another name for Zhang Bi, a medical expert of the Jin Dynasty, Zhang Yuansu's son, a native of Yizhou County (today's Yishui County, Hebei Province). He carried on his father's medical profession and was well-known at the time. His acupuncture monograph, *Yun Qizi Lun Jingluo Yingsui Buxie Fa* (*Yun Qizi's Treatise on Reinforcing and Reducing Techniques of Opposing and Following the Meridians*), namely, *Jie Gu: Yun Qi Zhenfa* (*Acupuncture Techniques of Jie Gu and Yun Qi*), was compiled in *Jisheng Bacui* (*Selected Materials Beneficial to Life*).

●**运动区**[yùn dòng qū] 头针刺激区。上点在前后正中线中点往后0.5厘米处;下点在眉枕线和鬓角发际前缘相交处。如果鬓角不明显,可以从颧弓中点向上引垂直线,此线与眉枕线交叉处向前移0.5厘米为运动区下点。上下两点连线即为运动区。运动区又可分为上、中、下三部。①上部:是运动区的上1/5,为下肢、躯干运动区。②中部:是运动区的中2/5,为上肢运动区。③下部:是运动区的下2/5,为面运动区,亦称言语一区。主治:①上部:对侧下肢、躯干部瘫痪。②中部:对侧上肢瘫痪。③下部:对侧中枢性面神经瘫痪,运动性失语(部分或完全丧失语言能力,但基本上保留理解语言的能力),流涎,发音障碍。

The Motor Area A stimulation area of scalp acupuncture. 〈Location〉Take the point 0.5 cun posterior to the mid-point of anteroposterior midline as the upper point, and the point of intersection of the eyebrow-occiput line and the anterior border of the hairline of the temple as the lower point. If the hairline of the temple is not clear, take the point 0.5 cun anterior to the point of intersection of the eyebrow-occiput line and the line perpendicularly upward from the midpoint of the zygomatic arch as the lower point. The connecting line between the upper and lower point is the motor area. This area can be divided into three parts:①The upper part:the upper 1/5 is the motor area for the lower limbs and trunk. ②The middle part:the middle 2/5, are the motor area for the upper limbs. ③The lower part:the lower 2/5 are the motor area for the face, also called the first speech area. 〈Indications〉①the upper part can be used to treat paralysis of the opposite side upper limbs. ②The middle part can be used to treat paralysis of the opposite side upper limbs. ③The lower part can be used to treat opposite side central

facial paralysis, motor aphasia (partial or completeloss of linguistic ability, but still able to comprehend language), salivation and dysphonia.

●运气法 [yùn qì fǎ] 针刺手法名,其法在施术之时,先行六阴之数(慢按紧提),若觉针不气满,便向病所倒卧针身,令患者吸气五口,使气至病所,然后引针退出。可治疼痛之疾。

Directing-Qi Method A needling technique. While manipulating the needle, first slowly thrust and quickly lift the needle for six times (in Yin number), and the doctor feels the needling sensation under the needle, then ledge the needle with the tip toward the affected area, ask the patient to inhale for five times and make qi get to the affected area, and then withdraw the needle. It can be applied to pain diseases.

●运用区 [yùn yòng qū] 头针刺激区。从顶骨结节起分别引一垂直线和与该线夹角40度的前后两线,长度均为3厘米。〈主治〉失用症。

The Usage Area A stimulation area of scalp acupuncture. 〈Location〉 Take the parietal tubercle as a starting point, draw a vertical line from the point, at the some time draw two other lines from the point separately forwards and backwards, at 40° angles with the vertical line, each of the three lines is 3 cun long. 〈Indication〉 apraxia.

●运针 [yùn zhēn] 为行针之别称。详见该条。

Needling Manipulation Another name for needling transmission. →行针(p. 512)

●晕灸 [yùn jiǔ] 灸法术语。指病人在灸治过程中发生晕厥现象。多因体质虚弱,情绪紧张,或艾炷过大,火力过猛所引起。临床表现及处理方法,参见"晕针"条。

Fainting During Moxibustion A moxibustion term, referring to a patient becoming faint during moxibustion, commonly due to delicate constitution, nervous tension, or excess fire of too big a moxa cone. For its clinical manifestations and treatment, see fainting during acupuncture. →晕针(p. 581)

●晕听区 [yùn tīng qū] 头针刺激区。从耳尖直上1.5厘米处,向前及向后各引2厘米的水平线。〈主治〉眩晕、耳鸣、听力降低。

The Vertigo-Auditory Area A stimulation area of scalp acupuncture. 〈Location〉 4 cun horizontal straight line on the site 1.5 cun directly above the auricular apex. 〈Indications〉 vertigo, tinnitus and hypoacusis.

●晕针 [yùn zhēn] 针法术语。指由于针刺而产生晕厥现象。当针刺时,患者感觉头晕、恶心、目眩、心悸,继而面色苍白,冷汗出,四肢厥逆,血压降低,脉象微弱,甚至突然意识丧失者,即为晕针。多因患者体质虚弱,精神紧张,饥饿疲劳,或针刺体位不当,针体较粗,刺激过重,针感太强而发生。一旦晕针,应及时处理,免致不良后果。首先应立即停止针刺,将已刺之针迅速拔出,然后将患者平卧,头部稍低,松开衣带,喂予温水或糖水,休息十至十五分钟,一般可以恢复。重者在行上述处理后,可指压或针刺水沟、素髎、中冲、内关、合谷、太冲、涌泉、足三里等,亦可灸百会、气海、关元等。

Fainting During Acupuncture An acupuncture term, referring to fainting resulting from needling. 〈Manifestation〉 During a needling course, the patient is suddenly troubled with dizziness, nausea, vertigo, palpitation, pale complexion, cold sweating, cold extremities, drop of blood pressure, feeble pulse, and even a loss of consciousness. 〈Pathogenesis〉 commonly due to delicate constitution, nervous tension, hunger and fatigue or due to improper posture for needling, excessive thickness of the needle, excessive needling stimulation and sensation. 〈Treatment〉 Treatment should be given quickly in order to avoid serious consequence. First, stop needling immediately and withdraw all needles. Then, help the patient to lie down flat with his head in a lower position, loosen his clothes, give him warm water or water with sugar. The patient will usually recover after a rest of 10-15 minutes. In severe cases, on the basis of the above-mentioned treatments, press hard with the finger-nails or needles Shuigou(DU 26), Suliao(DU 25), Zhongchong(PC 9), Neiguan(PC 6), Hegu(LI 4), Taichong(LR 3), Yongquan(KI 1), Zusanli(ST 36), etc., or apply moxibustion to Baihui(DU 20), Qihai(RN 6), Guanyuan(RN 4), etc.

Z

●匝风[zā fēng] 经穴别名。出《针灸甲乙经》。即脑户。见该条。

Zafeng Another name for Naohu(DU 17), a meridian point from *Zhenjiu Jia-Yi Jing*(*A-B Classic of Acupuncture and Moxibustion*). → 脑户(p.276)

●杂病十一证歌[zá bìng shí yī zhèng gē] 针灸歌赋名。为七言韵诗,共十一首。见《针灸大全》。

Zabing Shiyi Zheng Ge(**Eleven Verses For Miscellaneous Diseases**) Verses on acupuncture and moxibustion, seven characters in each line, eleven verses in all, seen in *Zhenjiu Daquan*(*A Complete Work of Acupuncture and Moxibustion*).

●赞刺[zàn cì] 《内经》刺法名。见《灵枢·官针》。为十二刺之一。其法:直入直出,多针而浅刺出血。用于治疗痈肿,丹毒等证。具有赞助其消散之功,故称赞刺。本法与九刺中的络刺,五刺中的豹文刺,同是放血刺法,只是归类不同。

Repeated Shallow Puncture A needling method in *Neijing* (*The Inner Canon of Huangdi*), from *Lingshu: Guanzhen*(*Miraculous Pivot: Official Needles*), one of the Twelve Needling Methods. Manipulation: Insert and withdraw the needle perpendicularly, repeatedly, and shallowly for blood-letting. ⟨Indications⟩carbuncle and erysipelas, etc. It is so named for the effect of promoting the subsidence of the disease with the function of letting blood. It is the same as the collateral needling of the Nine Needling Methods and the leopard-spot puncturing of the Five Needling Techniques. They only vary in classification.

●脏病取原[zàng bìng qǔ yuán] 见《内经》。治疗原则之一。出《灵枢·九针十二原》。指五脏有病,取其原穴治疗。如肺病取太渊,心病取神门,脾病取太白,肾病取太溪,肝病取太冲等。

Selecting Yuan(Primary) Points for Diseases of Zang Organs One of the treatment principles in *Neijing* (*The Canon of Internal Medicine*), from *Lingshu: Jiu Zhen Shier Yuan* [*Miraculous Pivot: Nine Needles and Twelve Yuan (Primary) Points*], referring to the selection of Yuan(Primary) points for diseases of the five zang organs, eg., use Taiyuan(LU 9) for lung diseases, Shenmen(HT 7) for heart diseases, Taibai(SP 3) for spleen diseases, Taixi(KI 3)for kidney diseases and Taichong (LR 3)for liver diseases.

●脏燥[zàng zào] 病证名。多由忧郁不解,伤及心脾,阴血暗耗,心失所养而致。证见精神恍惚,情感失常,时时悲泣,喜怒无常,每因精神激惹而发作,舌苔薄白,脉弦细。如兼脘痞食少,心悸,不寐,神倦,面色少华,舌淡,脉虚缓为心脾两虚;如兼眩晕,耳鸣,面色泛红,手足心热多汗,腰痠,健忘,虚烦不寐,舌红少苔,脉细数,为心肾两虚。治宜滋阴益气,养心调神。取膈俞、肾俞、心俞、内关、神门、三阴交。心脾两虚加脾俞、足三里、通里;心肾两虚加照海、太溪。

Hysteria A disease, commonly due to prolonged melancholy, damage of the heart and spleen and consumed blood which lead to failure to nourish the heart. ⟨Manifestations⟩ trance, abnormal emotion, regular grief and weeping, joy and anger without reason, often caused by mental stimulation, thin white coating, stringy, taut and thready pulse. If it is accompanied by fullness in the stomach and little food intake, palpitations, insomnia, mental fatigue, dim complexion, pale tongue, slightly slow, deficient pulse, it is a syndrome of deficiency of qi and blood of the heart and spleen; if accompanied by vertigo, tinnitus, red complexion, feverish sensation in palms and soles, hyper-hidrosis, soreness of waist, amnesia, insomnia due to vexation, red tongue with little coating, thready and rapid pulse, the syndrome

is caused by deficiency of yin of the heart and kidney. 〈Treatment principle〉 Nourish yin and supplement qi, nourish the heart to regulate the mind. 〈Point selection〉 Geshu (BL 17), Shenshu (BL 23), Xinshu (BL 15), Neiguan (PC 6), Shenmen (HT 7), Sanyinjiao (SP 6). Supplementary points: for deficiency of qi and blood in the heart and spleen, Pishu (BL 20), Zusanli (ST 36) and Tongli (HT 5) are added; for deficiency of yin in the heart and kidney, Zhaohai (KI 6) and Taixi (KI 3).

● 藏俞 [zàng shū] ①经穴别名。见《备急千金要方》。即神道。详见该条。②指五脏诸阴经的井、荥、输、经、合各穴。

1. **Zangshu** Another name for Shendao (DU 11), a meridian point from *Beiji Qianjin Yaofang* (*Essential Prescriptions Worth a Thousand Gold for Emergencies*). →神道 (p.)

2. **Zang Organ Points** The Jing (Well) point, Ying (Spring) point, Shu (Stream) point, Jing (River) point and He (Sea) point of the yin-meridians corresponding to the five zang organs.

● 藏输 [zàng shū] 经外穴名。出《千金要方》。在背部,当第五胸椎棘突高点处。主治卒病恶风、失欠、内痹等。用灸法。

Zangshu (EX-B) An extra point, from *Qianjin Yaofang* (*Essential Prescriptions Worth a Thousand Gold*). 〈Location〉 on the back, at the tip of the spinous process of the fifth thoracic vertebra. 〈Indications〉 sudden onset of disease with aversion to wind, inability to raise oneself slightly, numbness, etc. 〈Method〉 moxibustion.

● 燥热咳嗽 [zào rè ké sòu] 咳嗽证型之一。因外感风热燥邪,耗伤肺津所致。证见干咳少痰,或痰不易咳,鼻燥咽干,咳甚则胸痛,或有形寒身热,舌尖红,苔薄黄,脉细而数。治宜滋阴润肺,清热止咳。取太溪、肺俞、列缺、照海。

Cough due to Dry-Heat Pathogen One of the syndromes of cough, due to pathogenic wind, heat and dryness factors leading to impairment of fluid in the lung. 〈Manifestations〉 dry cough with little sputum, or difficult to expectorated sputum, dryness of nose and throat, severe cough leading to pain in the chest, or chills with fever, red tip of tongue, thin and yellow tongue coating, thready and rapid pulse. 〈Treatment principle〉 Nourish yin and moisten the lung, clear heat to relieve cough. 〈Point selection〉 Taixi (KI 3), Feishu (BL 13), Lieque (LU 7) and Zhaohai (KI 6).

● 炸腮 [zhà sāi] 即痄腮的别名。详见该条。

Epidemic Parotiditis Another name for mumps. →痄腮 (p. 583)

● 痄腮 [zhà sāi] 病证名。见《幼科金针》。又称炸腮、含腮疮、蛤蟆瘟。是小儿常见的急性传染病。以冬春两季为多见。主要是由风温病毒从口鼻而入,壅阻少阳经络,郁而不散,结于腮颊所致。临床以发病急,耳下腮部肿胀、疼痛为其特征。轻者,耳下腮部酸痛肿胀,咀嚼不便,伴有恶寒发热,全身轻度不适等证,舌苔微黄,脉浮数。治宜疏风解表,清热解毒。取颊车、翳风、外关、合谷。重者,腮部焮热肿痛,咀嚼困难,高热头痛,烦躁口渴,大便干结,小便短赤,或伴有呕吐,睾丸肿痛,甚则神昏惊厥,舌苔黄,脉滑数。治宜清热解毒,通络消肿。取耳和髎、外关、关冲、合谷、曲池、少商、丰隆。睾丸肿痛加太冲、曲泉。

Mumps A disease, originally from *Youke Jin Zhen* (*Gold Needle of Pediatrics*), also called epidemic parotiditis, an acute viral infectious disease causing suppurative lesions in the cheek and pyogenic inflammation of cheeks. It occurs more commonly in children during the winter and spring. 〈Pathogenesis〉 due to invasion by a wind-warm virus into the mouth and nose which blocks the meridians of Shaoyang and stagnates in the cheek. 〈Manifestations〉 sudden onset, swelling and pain in the parotid region under the ear. The mild type is characterized by swelling of the parotid region under the ear, difficulty in chewing, accompanied by aversion to cold, fever, a bit of malaise all over the body, etc., slightly yellow tongue coating, superficial and rapid pulse. 〈Treatment principle〉 Dispel wind to relieve exterior syndrome and clear heat and toxins. 〈Point selection〉 Jiache (ST 6), Yifeng (SJ 17), Waiguan (ST 5), Hegu (LI 4). Severe cases show redness, swelling and pain of the parotid region, difficulty in chewing, high fever and headache, irritability, thirst, constipation, scanty dark urine, sometimes accompa-

nied by vomiting, swelling and pain of the testis, even coma and convulsion, yellow tongue coating, slippery and rapid pulse. ⟨Treatment principle⟩ Clear heat and toxins and remove obstruction in meridians and collaterals to reduce edema. ⟨Point selection⟩ Erheliao(SJ 22), Waiguan(SJ 5), Guanchong(SJ 1), Hegu(LI 4), Quchi(LI 11), Shaoshang (LU 11), Fenglong(ST 40), for the swelling and pain of the testis, add Taichong(LR 3) and Ququan(LR 8).

●张介宾[zhāng jiè bīn] 人名。明代著名医学家。字景岳,号会卿,会稽(今浙江绍兴)人。他对《素问》、《灵枢》很有研究,历三十年,著《类经》、《类经图翼》、《类经附翼》,其中对针灸理论与临床论述很多。晚年结合过去临床经验,撰《景岳全书》。

Zhang Jiebin A famous medical expert in the Ming Dynasty, who styled himself Jingyue and assumed Huiqing, a native of Huiji(today's Shaoxing, Zhejiang Province). He made a profound study on *Su Wen* (*Plain Questions*) and *Lingshu* (*Miraculous Pivot*), and spent 30 years completing *Leijing* (*Classified Canon of Internal Medicine of the Yellow Emperor*), *Leijing Tuyi* (*Illustrated Supplements to Classified Canon of Internal Medicine of the Yellow Emperor*), and *Leijing Fuyi* (*Supplements to Classified Canon of Internal Medicine of the Yellow Emperor*), in which there is much exposition on the theory and clinical practice of acupuncture and moxibustion. In his later years, he summed up his clinical experience and compiled *Jingyue Quanshu* (*Complete Works of Zhang Jingyue*).

●张权[zhāng quán] 人名。明针灸家。里籍不详。辑《十四经发挥合纂》十六卷。

Zhang Quan An acupuncture-moxibustion expert in the Ming Dynasty, the author of *Shisi Jing Fahui Hezuan* (*Joint Edition of an Elaboration of the Fourteen Meridians*), 16 volumes in all. His native place is unknown.

●张元素[zhāng yuán sù] 人名。金代著名医学家。字洁古,易州(今河北易水)人。其治病不泥于古方,且善于针灸。曾撰《洁古刺诸痛法》。其子张璧,承父业,亦擅针。

Zhang Yuansu A well-known medical expert in the Jin Dynasty, who styled himself Jiegu. A native of Yi County(today's Yishui County, Hebei Province). He was good at acupuncture and moxibustion, never formalistic in classical prescriptions and the compiler of *Jiegu Ci Zhutong Fa* (*Jiegu's Methods of Acupuncture for Treating Pains*). Zhang Bi, his son, carried on his cause and was also good at acupuncture.

●张志聪[zhāng zhì cōng] 人名。清代医学家。字隐庵,浙江钱塘(今杭州)人。精于医,通针灸,其主持集注《灵枢》,开集体注释之先河。所撰《针灸秘传》,佚,见《清史稿》。

Zhang Zhicong A medical expert in the Qing Dynasty who styled himself Yin'an, a native of Qiantang(today's Hangzhou). He was conversant in Chinese medicine, good at acupuncture and moxibustion and a pioneer of collective annotation. He took charge of annotating *Lingshu* (*Miraculous Pivot*). His work *Zhenjiu Michuan* (*Secretly Bequeathed Methods of Acupuncture and Moxibustion*) is no longer extant. See *Qingshi Gao* (*A Historical Text of the Qing Dynasty*).

●张仲景[zhāng zhòng jǐng] 人名。东汉末年杰出的医学家。名机,南阳(今河南南阳)人。其"勤求古训,博采众方",著成《伤寒杂病论》。经后人整理成《伤寒论》与《金匮要略》两书。前书中运用六经辨证,是对经络理论的发展。两书虽以药物治疗为主,但兼以针灸,包括温针、熏、熨各法的宜忌。

Zhang Zhongjing An outstanding medical expert in the last years of the Eastern Han Dynasty, also named Ji, a native of Nanyang (Today's Nanyang, Henan Province). He wrote *Shanghan Zabing Lun* (*Treatise on Cold-Induced and Miscellaneous Diseases*) by "diligently searching into ancient classics and widely collecting various prescriptions". The book was rearranged into two books, *Shanghan Lun* (*Treatise on Cold-Induced Diseases*) and *Jingui Yaolue* (*Synopsis of the Golden Chamber*). The former was a development of the theory of meridians and collaterals because of its application of the dialectics of the Six Meridians. Both of the books deal with treatments using herbal medicine, but also devote

quite a few pages to acupuncture and moxibustion, including the compatibility and incompatibility of acupuncture with needles warmed by burning moxa, treatment with smoke and the topical application of heated drugs.

●章迪[zhāng dí]　人名。宋针灸家。字吉老，无为（今属安徽）人。善针，疗效好。事见《无为县志》。

Zhang Di An acupuncturist of the Song Dynasty who styled himself Jilao, a native of Wuwei (of Anhui Province today). He was good at acupuncture and treated diseases with good effects. His deeds were recorded in *Wuweixian Zhi* (*Annals of Wuwei County*).

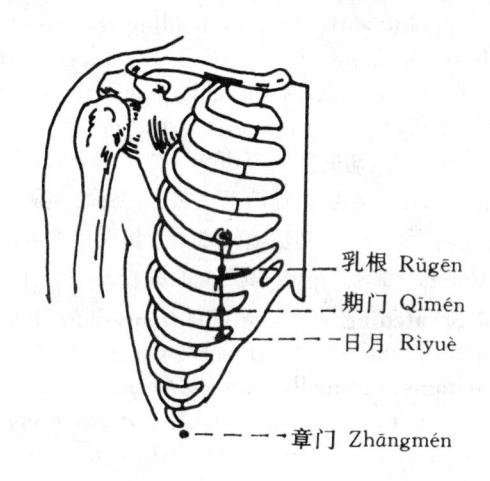

图73　章门和期门穴
Fig 73　Zhangmen and Qimen points

●章门[zhāng mén]　经穴名。出《针灸甲乙经》。属足厥阴肝经，为脾之募穴，八会穴之脏会，足厥阴、少阳之会。又名长平、肋髎、季肋。〈定位〉在侧腹部，当第十一肋游离端的下方（图72和图73）。〈层次解剖〉皮肤→皮下组织→腹外斜肌→腹内斜肌→腹横肌。浅层布有第十及第十一胸神经前支的外侧皮支，胸腹壁浅静脉的属支。深层有第十及第十一胸神经和肋间后动、静脉的分支或属支。〈主治〉腹痛，腹胀，肠鸣，泄泻，呕吐，神疲肢倦，身瞤动，胸胁肋痛，黄疸，痞块，小儿疳疾，脊背痛。斜刺0.5至0.8寸；可灸。

Zhangmen (LR 13) A meridian point, originally from *Zhenjiu Jia-Yi Jing* (*A-B Classic of Acupuncture and Moxibustion*), also named Changping, Leijiao or Jilei. A point on the Liver Meridian of Foot-Jueyin, the Front (Mu) point of the spleen, the influential point of the zang organs and the crossing point of the Foot-Jueyin and Shaoyang Meridian. 〈Location〉on the lateral side of the abdomen, below the free end of the 11th rib (Figs. 72 & 73). 〈Regional anatomy〉 skin→subcutaneous tissue→external oblique muscle of abdomen→internal oblique muscle of abdomen→transverse muscle of abdomen. In the superficial layer, there are the lateral cutaneous branches of the anterior branches of the 10th and 11th thoracic nerves and the tributaries of the superficial thoracoepigastric vein. In the deep layer, there are the 10th and 11th thoracic nerves and the branches or tributaries of the 10th and 11th posterior intercostal arteries and veins. 〈Indications〉 abdominal pain, abdominal distention, borborygmus, diarrhea, vomiting, mental fatigue and lassitude, muscular twitching, pain in the chest and hypochondrium, jaundice, mass in the abdomen, infantile malnutrition and pain in the back and loin. 〈Method〉Puncture obliquely 0.5～0.8 cun. Moxibustion is applicable.

●掌中[zhǎng zhōng]　经穴别名。见《针灸资生经》。即劳宫。见该条。

Zhangzhong Another name for Laogong (PC 8), a meridian point originally from *Zhenjiu Zisheng Jing* (*Acupuncture-Moxibustion Classic for Saving Life*). →劳宫 (p. 237)

●胀[zhàng]　①病症名。出《素问·胀论》。又名胀病，鼓胀，单腹胀。以腹部膨大胀满为主证，故名。详见臌胀条。②指膨胀不适的自觉症状，如头胀，胁胀，腹胀等。

1. Distention A disease, originally from *Suwen: Zhang Lun* (*Plain Questions: On Distention*), also called disease of distention, tympanites or abdominal distention alone, referring to a disease, the main symptom of which is abdominal intumescence with distention and fullness, hence the name. →臌胀 (p. 146)

2. Fullness The uncomfortable symptom of inflation, such as fullness of the head, fullness of the hypochondrium, and fullness of the abdomen, etc.

●胀病[zhàng bìng] 病证名。见《医门法律》卷六。即鼓胀。见该条。

Disease of Distention A disease, originally from Vol. 6 of *Yimen Falü* (*Principles and Prohibition for Medical Profession*). → 鼓胀 (p. 146)

●瘴疟[zhàng nüè] 疟疾证型之一。出《肘后方》。指因感受山岚瘴毒而发的一种危重疟疾。临证可分为热瘴、冷瘴两类。详见各条。

Malignant Malaria A type of malaria, originally from *Zhouhou Fang* (*A Handbook of Prescriptions*), referring to critical malaria caused by suffering from mountainous evil air. The disease is clinically divided into malignant malaria due to heat mountainous evil air and malignant malaria due to cold mountainous evil air. → 热瘴 (p. 332)、冷瘴 (p. 241)

●爪法[zhǎo fǎ] 针刺手法名。十四法之一。指针刺时用指甲掐切穴位以帮助进针。在《难经·七十八难》、《针经指南》、《针灸大成》、《针灸问对》中均有论述。

Nail-Pressing A needling manipulation, one of the Fourteen Methods, referring to pressing the point with nail to aid insertion while needling, expounded in *Nanjing: Qishiba Nan* (*The Classic of Questions: Question 78*), *Zhenjing Zhinan* (*Guide to the Classics of Acupuncture*), *Zhenjiu Dacheng* (*A Great Compendium of Acupuncture and Moxibustion*), and *Zhenjiu Wendui* (*Catechism of Acupuncture and Moxibustion*).

●爪切[zhǎo qiē] 针刺手法名。指进针前用左手大指甲端压切穴位,以便进针。

Nail-Pressing A needling manipulation, referring to pressing the acupoint with the left thumb nail to make insertion of the needle easier.

●爪切进针[zhǎo qiē jìn zhēn] 进针方法之一。又称指切进针法。其法两手配合,用左手拇指或食指的指甲压切穴位,右手持针沿着指甲旁迅速刺入,适用于短针的进针。爪切能固定穴位,帮助进针,减轻疼痛并可增强针感。参见"爪切"条。

Nail-Pressing Insertion One of the methods of needle insertion, also called finger-pressing insertion, that is, using both hands, press the acupoint with the nail of the thumb or the index finger, hold the needle with the right hand and keep the needle tip closely against the border of the nail of the left hand. Then quickly insert the needle into the skin. The method is suitable for puncturing with short needles. The nail pressing can fix the acupuncture point, aid insertion, reduce pain while inserting and strengthen the needling sensation. → 爪切 (p. 586)

●爪切押手[zhǎo qiē yā shǒu] 押手方式之一。用手指按切穴位,另一手(刺手)持针使针尖部紧贴指甲缘刺入穴内。参见"爪切进针"条。

Nail-Pressing Technique One of the techniques of hand pressing, referring to pressing the acupoint with the nail, holding the needle with other hand (the puncturing hand) and keeping the needle tip closely against the edge of the nail, and then inserting the needle into the skin. → 爪切进针 (p. 586)

●爪摄[zhǎo shè] 针刺辅助手法名。出《针灸大成》。为十二字手法之一。其法随经络上下用大指爪甲切之,针下邪气滞涩不行者,其气可自通行。

Nail-Scratching An auxiliary needling manipulation, one of the Twelve-Character Manipulations, originally from *Zhenjiu Dacheng* (*A Great Compendium of Acupuncture and Moxibustion*), referring to scratching along the meridian with the nail of the thumb to promote the movement of stagnated pathogens while the needle is inserted.

●照海[zhào hǎi] 经穴名。出《针灸甲乙经》。属足少阴肾经,八脉交会穴之一,通于阴跷脉。又名太阴跷、阴跷穴。〈定位〉在足内侧,内踝尖下方凹陷处(图46和图81)。〈层次解剖〉皮肤→皮下组织→胫骨后肌腱。浅层布有隐神经的小腿内侧皮支,大隐静脉的属支。深层有胟内侧动、静脉的分支或属支。〈主治〉咽干,痫证,失眠,嗜卧,惊恐不宁,目赤肿痛,月经不调,痛经,赤白带下,阴挺,阴痒,疝气,小便频数,脚气。直刺0.5至0.8寸;可灸。

Zhaohai (KI 6) A meridian point, originally from *Zhenjiu Jia-Yi Jing* (*A-B Classic of Acupuncture and Moxibustion*), a point on the Kidney Meridian of Foot-Shaoyin, one of the eight confluent points which connects with

the Yinqiao Meridian, also named Taiyinqiao and Yinqiaoxue.〈Location〉on the medial side of the foot, in the depression below the tip of the medial malleolus(Figs. 46&81).〈Regional anatomy〉 skin→subcutaneous tissue→tendon of posterior tibial muscle. In the superficial layer, there are the medial cutaneous branches of the saphenous nerve to the leg and the tributaries of the great saphenous vein. In the deep layer, there are the branches or tributaries of the medial tarsal artery and vein. 〈Indications〉dry throat, epilepsy, insomnia, drowsiness, restlessness with terror and fear, redness and swelling, pain of the eye, irregular menstruation, dysmenorrhea, morbid leukorrhea, prolapse of the uterus, pruritus vulvae, hernia, frequency of micturition, beriberi. 〈Method〉Puncture perpendicularly 0.5～0.8 cun. Moxibustion is applicable.

●折针[zhé zhēn] 针刺术语。见《千金方》卷二十五。又称断针。指针刺时,针身误断在体内而言。多因针身有损伤,针刺时用力过猛或病员突然变动体位所造成。故针刺前应注意检查针具,避免过猛、过强运针,应嘱患者不要随便更换体位,预防其折针。残端显露体外时,可用手指或镊子起出;情况严重者应手术切开取出。

Breaking of the Inserted Needle An acupuncture term, originally from Vol. 25 of *Qianjin Fang*(*Prescriptions Worth a Thousand Gold*), also called snapping of the inserted needle, referring to accidental breaking of a needle in the body during acupuncture, commonly due to an impaired body of the needle, excessively heavy manipulation while needling, or a sudden change of the patient's posture.〈Caution〉Before needling, examine the needles carefully; while needling, avoid sudden and heavy manipulation; after inserting, advise the patient not to change posture. 〈Treatment〉If the broken part sticks out of the skin, remove it with fingers or forceps; if the broken part is completely under the skin, a surgical operation is necessary.

●辄筋[zhé jīn] 经穴名。出《针灸甲乙经》。属足少阳胆经。〈定位〉在侧胸部,渊腋前1寸,平乳头,第四肋间隙中(图23和图72)。〈层次解剖〉皮肤→皮下组织→前锯肌→肋间外肌。浅层布有第三、四、五肋间神经外侧皮支和胸外侧动、静脉的分支或属支。深层有第四肋间神经和第四肋间后动、静脉。〈主治〉胸胁痛,喘息,呕吐,吞酸,腋肿,肩臂痛。斜刺0.5至0.8寸;可灸。

Zhejin(GB 23) An meridian point, originally from *Zhenjiu Jia-Yi Jing*(*A-B Classic of Acupuncture and Moxibustion*), a point on the Gallbladder Meridian of Foot-Shaoyang.〈Location〉on the lateral side of the chest, 1 cun anterior to Yuanye(GB 22), on the level of the nipple, and in the 4th intercostal space (Figs. 23&72).〈Regional anatomy〉 skin→subcutaneous tissue→anterior serratus muscle →external intercostal muscle. In the superficial layer, there are the lateral cutaneous branches of the 3rd to 5th intercostal nerves and the branches or tributaries of the lateral thoracic artery and vein. In the deep layer, there are the 4th intercostal nerve and 4th posterior intercostal artery and vein.〈Indications〉pain in the chest and hypochondrium, dyspnea, vomiting, acid regurgitation, axillary swelling, pain in the shoulder and back. 〈Method〉Puncture obliquely 0.5～0.8 cun. Moxibustion is applicable.

●针[zhēn] 原作鍼、箴。原意均指缝衣用具,后来以之作为医疗用具。从古代的砭石、竹针,发展到现代的金属针。《黄帝内经》所载医用针具分九种,总称九针。详见九针条。近代的针刺工具种类很多,如毫针、皮肤针、三棱针等,详见各条。

Acupuncture Needle Originally written as zhen(鍼) or zhen(箴), initially referring to sewing utensils, and later, used as medical apparatus. The needle underwent a long development process from ancient Bian stone and bamboo needles to modern metal ones. In *Huangdi Neijing* (*The Yellow Emperor's Inner Canon*), the medical needling apparatus was divided into nine types, generally called Nine Needles. →九针(p. 221) In modern times, there are various needling apparatus, such as filiform needles, cutaneous needles, three-edged needles and embedding needles, etc. →毫针(p. 159)、皮肤针(p. 292)、三棱针(p. 344)

●**针艾** [zhēn ài] 针灸术语。见《灵枢·官能》。针用于刺，艾用于灸、针艾是从用具而言，刺灸是从应用而言。

Needle-Moxa An acupuncture and moxibustion term, seen in *Lingshu: Guan Neng* (*Miraculous Pivot: Functions and Abilities*). A needle is used for acupuncture while moxa is used for moxibustion. Needle-moxa is named in terms of its appliance, and acupuncture-moxibustion in terms of its application.

●**针柄灸** [zhēn bǐng jiǔ] 灸法的一种。为温针灸之别称。见该条。

Needle-Handle Moxibustion A kind of moxibustion, another name for needle warming through moxibustion. →温针灸(p. 471)

●**针博士** [zhēn bó shì] 古代太医署人员职位名。负责掌管针灸专业的教授和考核。官阶约八品。

Professor of Acupuncture A post of the stuff in the office of Imperial Physicians in ancient times. The official on the post was to take charge of teaching and testing on acupuncture and moxibustion. It was roughly analogous to the official of the 8th rank.

●**针刺补泻法** [zhēn cì bǔ xiè fǎ] 针刺手法名。出《黄帝内经》。临床上为了起到补虚泻实的作用，将针刺方法分为补法和泻法。补法在于顺其气，或将气向内推进，使正气有所补益；泻法则是逆其气，折其病势，将气向外引伸，使邪气有所散逸。补泻手法贯穿于从进针到出针的整个过程中，其效应还受到病人体质和功能状态的影响。临床上应根据具体情况选用适当的补泻手法。参见"徐疾补泻"、"提插补泻"、"捻转补泻"、"迎随补泻"、"呼吸补泻"、"开阖补泻"等条。

Reinforcing and Reducing Manipulations in Acupuncture Therapy A needling manipulation, originally from *Huangdi Neijing* (*The Yellow Emperor's Inner Canon*). For tonifying deficiency and purging excess, the needling methods are clinically divided into reinforcing method and reducing method. Reinforcement refers to being obedient to the qi flow or carrying the qi inward to tonify the vital-qi. Reduction refers to being against the qi flow to purge the excessive qi or carrying the qi outward to dispel pathogens. The reinforcing and reducing methods run through the whole process from insertion to withdrawal of the needle and its effect is influenced by the constitution and functional state of patient. In clinic, the proper reinforcing and reducing manipulation should be selected according to the concrete conditions. →徐疾补泻(p. 517)、提插补泻(p. 427)、捻转补泻(p. 283)、迎随补泻(p. 567)、呼吸补泻(p. 167)、开阖补泻(p. 230)

●**针刺感应** [zhēn cì gǎn yīng] 针刺术语。为针感之别称。详见该条。

Needling Response Another name for needling sensation. →针感(p. 590)

●**针刺角度** [zhēn cì jiǎo dù] 针刺术语。指针刺时针体与穴位皮肤表面所呈的夹角。临床上根据针刺部位的解剖特点和刺法的要求，分别采用不同的角度进针。一般分为直刺、斜刺和横刺（平刺）三种。参见各条。

Angle of Needle Insertion An acupuncture term, referring to the angle between the body of needle and the surface of the acupoint. Clinically, according to the anatomic characteristic of the acupoint and the demand of the needling method, different insertion angles are adopted. The insertion angles are commonly divided into three types: perpendicular insertion, oblique insertion and transverse (horizontal) insertion. →直刺(p. 602)、斜刺(p. 505)、横刺(平刺)(p. 163)

●**针刺麻醉** [zhēn cì má zuì] 又称针麻。系指针刺穴位以起镇痛和调节等作用，而使病人能在神志清醒状态下接受手术的一种方法。这是我国医务人员在针刺治病的基础上，发展起来的一项研究成果。本法不需要复杂的器械设备，操作简便安全。在术中不用或少用麻醉药，病人不会发生麻醉意外和出现麻醉药的副作用。在手术中保持清醒状态，除痛觉变迟钝外，其他感觉和运动机能保持正常。术后疼痛较轻，一般不会出现恶心、呕吐等反应，而且可以早期进食和早期活动，更由于针刺具有调动和加强体内抗病因素的作用，还能加速术后康复过程。临床上适用于甲状腺、上颌窦、青光眼、颅脑、颈椎前路、全喉截除、肺叶切除、胃大部切除、脾切除、剖腹产、腹式输卵管结扎、前列腺切除、膝外侧半月板摘除等手术。一般认为应用于头、颈、胸部手术的效果较好。针

麻所应用的刺激方法有手法运针、电针、穴位注射等,有时也适当采用少量辅助药物。但针麻目前存在镇痛不全,手术部肌肉松弛不够,未能完全控制内脏牵拉反应等问题,有待进一步提高。

Acupuncture Anesthesia Also called needling anesthesia, referring to the method by which a patient can be operated on in a conscious state by needling acupoints to achieve the effect of analgesia and regulation, etc. The method, as an achievement in scientific research, has been developed on the basis of acupuncture treatment by medical staff in China. The method needs no complex instruments or devices, and is convenient and safe. During the operation no or little drugs are needed, so there are no anesthetic accidents or side effects of the drugs. The patient is in a concious state and the feeling and motor functions are normal except hypoalgesia. After the operation, the patient has only slight pain, without nausea, vomiting, etc. and can eat and act at an early time. Acupuncture can arouse and strengthen the internal disease-resistant factors, so the recovery process can be accelerated. 〈Indications〉operation on thyroid, maxillary sinus, glaucoma, cranium and cervical vertebrae, and total laryngectomy, pulmonary lobectomy, gastrectomy, splenectomy, cesarean section, gastrotubotomy, prostatectomy, lateral knee meniscectomy, etc. It is commonly thought that the method is better for operations on the head, neck and chest. 〈Method〉manual needling manipulation, electrotherapy, point-injection therapy, etc., sometimes with a few supplementary drugs. This method still has some problems, such as incomplete analgesia, incomplete muscular relaxation in the part operated on, and incomplete control of the stretching reaction of the organs, etc., which needs further improvement.

●针刺手法[zhēn cì shǒu fǎ] 针刺术语。概指针刺治疗时采用的各种操作手法。包括毫针,三棱针,皮肤针,皮内针等。各种不同针具的施术方法,参见"毫针刺法"及有关条。

Acupuncture Manipulations An acupuncture term, generally referring to the various manipulations used in a needling course which include the needling methods of the filiform needle, the three-edged needle, the cutaneous needle, the intradermal needle, etc. →毫针刺法(p. 160)

●针法[zhēn fǎ] 针刺术语。①又称刺法,指针刺治疗疾病的方法。②各种针具的针刺操作方法的总称,如毫针的各种针刺手法,三棱针的点刺法,皮肤针的叩刺法等。参见"针刺手法""毫针刺法"等有关条。

Needling Method A term of acupuncture. ①Also called puncturing techniques, referring to the methods used to treat patients with acupuncture. ② The general term for the puncturing and manipulating methods of various needling instruments, such as the various needling methods of filiform needles, the spot pricking method of the three-edged needle, the tapping method of the cutaneous needle, etc. →针刺手法(p. 589)、毫针刺法(p. 160)

●针方[zhēn fāng] 书名。唐·甄权撰。见于《新唐书·艺文志》一卷。书佚。

Zhenfang (Acupuncture Prescriptions) A book, written by Zhen Quan in the Tang Dynasty, seen in Vol 1. of *Xin Tangshu: Yi Wen Zhi*(*The New History Book of the Tang Dynasty: Records of Art and Literature*). The book was lost.

●针方六集[zhēn fāng liù jí] 书名。针灸丛书。明·吴昆撰。成书于1618年。全书分六集。即神照集:介绍经络、腧穴、骨度法等,并附有图解;开蒙集:注释《标幽赋》,并论五门八法六十六穴;尊经集:引用《内经》原文,讲术针刺手法;旁通集:论述针与药的效用比较,附评《金针赋》;纷署集:叙述腧穴的主治和操作;兼罗集:辑录各家歌赋和灸法,兼有作者的评议和见解。

Zhenfang Liu Ji(Six Collections of Acupuncture Prescriptions) A series of books on acupuncture and moxibustion, compiled by Wu Kun in the Ming Dynasty, completed in 1618, divided into 6 volumes, i. e. *Shen Zhao Ji*(*Collection under Illumination of the Deity*), which introduces meridians and collaterals, acupoints, bone-length measurement, and related diagrams; *Kai Meng Ji*(*Collection of Enlightenment*), which annotates *Biao You Fu*(*Lyrics of Recondite Principles*) and dis-

cussed the five classes, eight therapeutic methods and the sixty-six points; *Zun Jing Ji* (*Collection of Respecting the Classics*) which quoted the original text of *Nei Jing* (*The Inner Canon of Huangdi*) and explained the manipulations of acupuncture; *Pang Tong Ji* (*Collection of Gaining a Comprehension by Analogy*), which discussed the effect of acupuncture and drugs, and commented on *Jin Zhen Fu* (*Ode to Gold Needle*); *Fen Shu Ji* (*Collection of Diversified Opinions*) which discussed the indications of acupoints and their manipulations; *Jian Luo Ji* (*Collection of Miscellanea*) which quoted the various acupuncture verses and moxibustion with the author's comments and opinions.

●针感[zhēn gǎn] 针刺术语。又称针刺感应。指病人对针刺所产生的局部或较大范围的痠、胀、重、麻等感觉,以及医生手指所感觉到的针下沉紧等反应。针感的出现,因不同部位的解剖特点而有所不同。如肌肉肥厚的部位,多出现痠胀感和针下沉紧感;神经干分布的部位,多出现痠麻感;感觉迟钝的部位,多出现痠感,四肢末端和敏感部位,多出现疼痛感。参见"得气"条。

Needling Sensation An acupuncture term, also called needling response, referring to the patient's local or wider feelings of soreness, distention, heaviness and numbness, etc., and the operator's sensation of tenseness and dragging around the needle. Needling sensations vary with different anatomical characteristics of different regions. The feeling of soreness and distention and the tenseness and dragging sensation commonly appear in the part with rich muscles; the feeling of soreness and numbness generally appears in the part where nerve trunks distribute ; the soreness feeling commonly appears insensitive areas; the pain feeling in the distal part of limbs and sensitive regions. →得气(p. 77)

●针工[zhēn gōng] 古代太医署人员职位名。见《旧唐书·职官志》。

Acupuncture Operator A post in the office of Imperial Physicians in ancient times, seen in *Jiu Tangshu: Zhi Guan Zhi* (*The Old History Book of the Tang Dynasty: Records of Officials*).

●针盒[zhēn hé] 盒式藏针用具。多用金属制成,内部分成几格,安放不同规格的针具。便于消毒和应用。

Needle Box A box-shaped appliance for storing needles, commonly made of metal, divided into several shelves inside for the various types of needles and for the convenience of sterilization and application.

●针解法[zhēn jiě fǎ] 针刺手法名。见《奇效良方·针灸门》。〈方法〉欲使针下之气上行,以手指按压针刺部位下方;欲使针下之气下行,以手指按压针刺部位上方。

Method of Leading the Needling Sensation An acupuncture manipulation, originally from *Qixiao Liangfang: Zhenjiu Men* (*Prescriptions of Wonderful Efficacy: Field of Acupuncture and Moxibustion*). 〈Method〉Press the region inferior to the acupoint with the fingers to move the needling reaction upward; press the region superior to the acupoint with the fingers to make the needling reaction downward.

●针经[zhēn jīng] 书名。①《灵枢》的古称。②东汉涪翁撰《针经》,见《后汉书·郭玉传》。书佚。

Zhenjing (**Canon of Acupuncture**) A book, ① the archaic name of *Lingshu* (*Miraculous Pivot*). ② the one compiled by Fu Weng in the Eastern Han Dynasty, seen in *Hou Han Shu: Guo Yu Zhuan* (*The History of Late Han Dynasty: Biography of Guo Yu*). The book was lost.

●针经节要[zhēn jīng jié yào] 书名。撰人不详。初刊于1315年。由元·杜思敬辑入《济生拔萃》。内容为节录《针经》原文。其中有论十二经腧穴、十二经病证、十二经穴治证及六十六穴主治等。

Zhenjing Jieyao (**Essentials of Acupuncture Classics**) A book, whose author is unknown, initially published in 1315, compiled in *Ji Sheng Bacui* (*Selected Materials Beneficial to Life*) by Du Sijing in the Yuan Dynasty, contains excerpts from *Zhenjing* (*Canon of Acupuncture*), such as discussions on the acupoints of the Twelve Meridians, the diseases and syndromes of the Twelve Meridians, the

indications of the acupoints of the Twelve meridians and the indications of the sixty-six points, etc.

● 针经摘英集 [zhēn jīng zhāi yīng jí] 书名。元·杜思敬辑。本书摘录前人书籍中有关九针、腧穴折量、治疗手法等,切合临床,刊于1315年。载于《济生拔萃》中。

Zhenjing Zhaiying Ji (A Collection of Gems from Acupuncture Classics) A book, compiled by Du Sijing in the Yuan Dynasty, includes excerpts from the ancient books on the nine needles, location of acupoints, treating manipulations, suitable to the clinic, published in 1315, in *Jisheng Bacui (Selected Materials Beneficial to Life)*.

● 针经指南 [zhēn jīng zhǐ nán] 书名。一卷。金·窦杰撰。刊于1295年。内含《标幽赋》、《通玄指要赋》、《流注八穴》、《手指补泻法》等,为针灸学的参考书。为《针灸四书》之一。

Zhenjing Zhinan (Guide to the Classics of Acupuncture) A book with one volume, written by Dou Jie in the Jin Dynasty, published in 1295, including *Biao You Fu (Lyrics of Recondite Principles)*, *Tongxuan Zhiyao Fu (Ode to the Understanding of Abstruse Essentials of Acupuncture)*, *Liuzhu Ba Xue (Eight Points of Flow)*, *Shouzhi Bu Xie Fa (Finger Reinforcing and Reducing)*, etc., a reference book for acupuncture and moxibustion, and one of the *Zhenjiu Si Shu (Four Books on Acupuncture and Moxibustion)*.

● 针灸 [zhēn jiǔ] 针法、灸法的合称。针法是应用多种针具,通过经络穴位以治疗疾病的方法;灸法是以艾为主要材料,熏灼经络穴位以治疗疾病的方法。通称为针灸疗法。

Acupuncture and Moxibustion Combined term for the methods of acupuncture and moxibustion. Acupuncture is the therapy which treats diseases by puncturing acupoints and meridians with various needling instruments, while moxibustion is the therapy which treats diseases by smoking and burning points and meridians mainly with moxa. They are generally called acupuncture and moxibustion therapy.

● 针灸大成 [zhēn jiǔ dà chéng] 书名。为针灸学名著。十卷,明·杨继洲撰,靳贤校。刊于1601年。为杨氏在早年撰写的《卫生针灸玄机秘要》基础上扩充而成。卷一,辑录《内经》、《难经》等有关理论,并予以注释。卷二、三为针灸歌赋。卷四为针法。卷五为子午流注及灵龟八法。卷六、七为经络、俞穴。卷八为诸症针灸治疗。卷九为名医刺灸法和杨氏医案。卷十录陈氏《小儿按摩经》。本书总结了明以前针灸学的成就,具有较高参考价值。

Zhenjiu Dacheng (A Great Compendium of Acupuncture and Moxibustion) A book containing well-known works on acupuncture and moxibustion, 10 volumes in all, collected by Yang Jizhou of the Ming Dynasty, proofread by Jin Xian, published in 1601, an expansion on the basis of *Weisheng Zhenjiu Xuanji Miyao (Mysterious Clandestine Essentials of Acupuncture and Moxibustion for Health Protection)* written by Mr. Yang in his early years. In Vol. 1, some theories are extracted from *Neijing (The Canon of Internal Medicine)*, *Nanjing (The Classic of Questions)*, etc. Vols. 2-3 are valued for the verses on acupuncture and moxibustion. Vol. 4 deals with needling methods. Vol. 5 records midnight-noon ebb-flow and the eight methods of intelligent turtle. Vols. 6-7 refers to the meridians and collaterals and acupoints. Vol. 8 talks about the treatments of various syndromes with acupuncture and moxibustion. Vol. 9 introduces famous doctors' methods of acupuncture and moxibustion, and Mr. Yang's medical records and Vol. 10 is an excerpt from *Chen's Xiaoer Anmojing (Classic of Massage of Children's Diseases)*. The book is a summary of the achievements in acupuncture and moxibustion before the Ming Dynasty and therefore is a valuable reference.

● 针灸大全 [zhēn jiǔ dà quán] 书名。又名《针灸捷法大全》,六卷。明·徐凤撰。是综合性的针灸书籍。卷一,载针灸歌赋。卷二,为《标幽赋》加注。卷三,为周身经穴歌。卷四,载窦氏八法。卷五,载《金针赋》及《论子午流注之法》。卷六,为灸法。该书的另一特点是附有插图。

Zhenjiu Daquan (A Complete Work of Acupuncture and Moxibustion) A book, also named *Zhenjiu Jiefa Daquan (Complete*

Collection of Swiftly Effective Methods of Acupuncture and Moxibustion), 6 Volumes in all, written by Xu Feng of the Ming Dynasty, a comprehensive book on acupuncture and moxibustion. Vol. 1, records the verses on acupuncture and moxibustion. Vol. 2 annotates Biao You Fu(Lyrics of Recondite Principles). Vol. 3 contains the verses of meridians points all over the body. Vol. 4 introduces Dou's Eight Methods. Vol. 5 contains Jin Zhen Fu(Ode to Gold Needle)and Lun Zi Wu Liu Zhu Zhi Fa(Treatise on Midnight-Noon Ebb-Flow) and Vol. 6 deals with moxibustion therapy. It is a book with illustrations.

●针灸疗法[zhēn jiǔ liáo fǎ] 针灸术语。指用针刺与艾灸治疗疾病方法的总称。参见"针法""灸法"条。

Acupuncture and Moxibustion Therapy An acupuncture and moxibustion term, a general term for the treating methods by needling and moxa-burning. →针法(p. 589)、灸法(p. 223)

●针灸感应现象[zhēn jiǔ gǎn yīng xiàn xiàng] 又称经络感传现象,详见该条。

Phenomenon of Acupuncture-Moxibustion Response Another name for meridian transmission. →经络感传现象(p. 209)

●针灸歌赋[zhēn jiǔ gē fù] 针灸诗歌韵文的总称。歌,又称诀、歌括;赋,是辞句对称的韵文。元明期间针灸歌赋的编写最多。

Verse-Fu on Acupuncture and Moxibustion A general term for the verses and prose in rhyme on acupuncture and moxibustion. The verse is also called rhymed formula and rhymed direction. The Fu is rhymed prose interspersed with verses. The verse-Fu on acupuncture and moxibustion were mostly compiled in the Yuan and Ming Dynasties.

●针灸集成[zhēn jiǔ jí chéng] 书名。又名《勉学堂针灸集成》。清·廖润鸿撰。四卷。刊于1874年。卷一论针灸法,针灸禁忌,别穴,奇穴等;卷二论骨度法及诸病针治法;卷三、四为十四经经穴及经外奇穴。故有前两卷称《针灸集成》,后两卷称《经穴详集》的说法。其内容多录自张介宾的《类经图翼》。

Zhen Jiu Ji Cheng(A Collection of Acupuncture and Moxibustion) A book, also named Mian Xue Tang Zhenjiu Jicheng(Mian Xue Tang Compendium of Acupuncture and Moxibustion) written by Liao Runhong of the Qing Dynasty, 4 volumes in all, published in 1874. Vol. 1 is on the techniques and contraindications of acupuncture and moxibustion, special points and fantastic points, Vol. 2 is on bone-length measurement and treating methods of acupuncture for various diseases and Vols. 3-4 are on the points of the fourteen meridians and extraordinary points. The first 2 volumes are called Zhenjiu Jicheng(A Collection of Acupuncture and Moxibustion)and the latter 2 are called Jingxue Xiangji(Detailed Work on Meridian Points). The contents of the book were mostly quoted from Leijing Tuyi(Illustrated Supplements to Classified Canon of Internal Medicine of the Yellow Emperor)written by Zhang Jiebin.

●针灸甲乙经[zhēn jiǔ jiǎ yǐ jīng] 书名。原名《黄帝三部针灸甲乙经》,又名《黄帝甲乙经》、《黄帝三部针经》,简称《甲乙经》。原书以十天干分卷,故简称"甲乙"。晋·皇甫谧著。该书以《素问》、《针经》、《明堂孔穴针灸治要》三书为依据编写而成。今传本为十二卷本。书中系统阐述了中医理论,并详载全身六百四十九个经穴的部位与主治,刺灸方法等。是我国现存最早,内容较系统的一部针灸学名著。

Zhenjiu Jia-Yi Jing(A-B Classic of Acupuncture and Moxibustion) A book, initially entitled Huangdi San Bu Zhenjiu Jia-Yi Jing (Three Collections of the Yellow Emperor's A-B Classic of Acupuncture and Moxibustion), Huangdi San Bu Zhenjing(Three Collections of the Yellow Emperor's Classic of Acupuncture), and Jia-Yi Jing(A-B Classic) for short, divided into volumes according to the ten heavenly stems and so called Jia-Yi (A-B) for short, written by Huangpu Mi of the Jin Dynasty, on the basis Suwen (Plain Questions), Zhenjing (Needling Classic) and Mingtang Kongxue Zhenjiu Zhiyao(An Outline of Points for Acupuncture and Moxibustion). The present edition of the book has twelve volumes in all, systematically expounds the Chinese medical therapy, and records in detail the locations, indications and needling methods of the 649 meridian points all over the body. It is the earliest and most

systematic work on acupuncture and moxibustion ever kept in China.

●针灸经穴图考[zhēn jiǔ jīng xué tú kǎo] 书名。黄竹斋编著,人民卫生出版社1957年出版。八卷。全书以十四经为纲,365穴及奇穴拾遗为目,对每个穴位进行了考证。卷一为针法、灸法辑要;卷二至六为十二经穴考证;卷七为任脉、督脉经穴考证;卷八为冲、带、维、跷脉经穴及奇穴考证。后附引用书目,有一定参考价值。

Zhenjiu Jingxue Tukao (Study on Acupoints Illustrations of Acupuncture and moxibustion) A book of 8 volumes written by Huang Zhuzhai, published by the People's Medical Publishing House in 1957. Taking the Fourteen Meridians as the key link, and 365 points and the omissions of extraordinary points as the objective, the book tested every point. Vol. 1 is a summary of acupuncture and moxibustion methods; Vols. 2-6, textual research into the points of the twelve meridians; Vol. 7, textual research into the points of the Ren and Du Meridians; Vol. 8, textual research into the points of Chong, Dai, Wei and Qiao Meridians and extraordinary points. Attached to the book is a biliography which is valuable for reference.

●针灸节要[zhēn jiǔ jié yào] 书名。为《针灸素难要旨》之别称。见该条。

Zhenjiu Jieyao (Essentials of Acupuncture and Moxibustion) Another name for *Zhenjiu Su Nan Yaozhi (The Essentials of Acupuncture and Moxibustion in "Plain Questions" and "The Classic of Questions")*. →针灸素难要旨 (p. 593)

●针灸聚英[zhēn jiǔ jù yīng] 书名。又名《针灸聚英发挥》。明·高武撰、四卷。刊于1529年。载针灸学基本理论、诸病治法及多种歌赋。多以按语的形式陈述作者个人见解。

Zhenjiu Juying (Essentials of Acupuncture and Moxibustion) A book in 4 volumes, also named *Zhenjiu Juying Fahui (An Elaboration of Essentials of Acupuncture and Moxibustion)*, written by Gao Wu of the Ming Dynasty, published in 1529. The book records the essential theories on acupuncture and moxibustion, treating methods for various diseases, and various verse-Fu. The author's personal opinions are mostly stated in the notes.

●针灸聚英发挥[zhēn jiǔ jù yīng fā huī] 书名。为《针灸聚英》之别称。见该条。

Zhenjiu Juying Fahui (An Elaboration of Essentials of Acupuncture and moxibustion) Another title for *Zhenjiu Juying (Essentials of Acupuncture and Moxibustion)* →针灸聚英 (p. 593)

●针灸全生[zhēn jiǔ quán shēng] 书名。又名《铜人明堂针灸》。清·肖福庵撰。两卷。刊于1831年。首为十四经经穴及周身经穴图解、歌诀,次为各种病证的针灸取穴。内容简要。

Zhenjiu Quansheng (A Book on Acupuncture and Moxibustion for Saving Life) A book in 2 volumes, also entitled *Tongren Mingtang Zhenjiu (Acupuncture and Moxibustion on a Bronze Statue with Acupoints)*, written by Xiao Fuan of the Qing Dynasty, published in 1831. The book briefly illustrates the points of the Fourteen Meridians and verses for the meridian points all over the body, and then discusses point selection for various diseases.

●针灸四书[zhēn jiǔ sì shū] 书名。为丛书。元·窦桂芳辑。1311年刊行。为《子午流注针经》、《针经指南》、《灸膏肓腧穴法》、《黄帝明堂灸经》四书的合称。附窦氏的《针灸杂说》。该书的内容亦可见于《普济方》针灸门中。

Zhenjiu Si Shu (Four Books on Acupuncture and Moxibustion) A series of books, compiled by Dou Guifang of the Yuan Dynasty, published in 1311, a combined term for the 4 books of *Ziwu Liuzhu Zhenjing (Acupuncture Classics on Midnight-Noon Ebb-Flow)*, *Zhenjing Zhinan (Guide to the Classics of Acupuncture)*, *Jiu Gaohuang Shuxue Fa (Methods of Moxibustion on Gaohuang Point)* and *Huangdi Mingtang Jiujing (The Yellow Emperor's Classic of Acupoints and Moxibustion)*, with the attachment of *Zhenjiu Zashuo (Miscellaneous Remarks on Acupuncture and Moxibustion)* written by Mr. Dou. The contents of this book can also be seen in the chapter on acupuncture and moxibustion of *Puji Fang (Prescriptions for Universal Relief)*.

●针灸素难要旨[zhēn jiǔ sù nàn yào zhī] 书名。又

名《针灸节要》、《针灸要旨》。明•高武撰。刊于1531年。三卷。本书为《内经》、《难经》有关针灸的论述分类汇编而成,以针灸理论及经脉流注为主,解释与发挥不多。

Zhenjiu Su Nan Yaozhi (The Essentials of Acupuncture and Moxibustion in "Plain Questions" and "The Classic of Questions") A book in 3 volumes, also named *Zhenjiu Jieyao* (*Essentials of Acupuncture Classics*) and *Zhenjiu Yaozhi* (*Essential Exposition of Acupuncture and Moxibustion*), written by Gao Wu of the Ming Dynasty, published in 1531. The book is a classified collection of the exposition on acupuncture and moxibustion from *Neijing* (*The Inner Canon of Huangdi*) and *Nanjing* (*The Classic of Questions*), mainly with theories on acupuncture and moxibustion and the ebb-flow of meridians, but with few explanations and elaborations.

●**针灸体位**[zhēn jiǔ tǐ wèi] 针灸术语。简称体位。指针灸取穴和施术时患者身体应处的位置。体位分坐位、卧位和立位三种,其中以坐位、卧位常用,立位容易引起晕针。详见坐位、卧位。

Postures for Acupuncture and Moxibustion An acupuncture and moxibustion term, called posture for short, referring to the postures adopted by patients for point selection and manipulation of acupuncture and moxibustion. Postures are of three types, sitting, lying and standing. The former two postures are commonly used clinically, while the standing posture can easily cause fainting during acupuncture treatment. →坐位(p.649)、卧位(p.471)

●**针灸图经**[zhēn jiǔ tú jīng] 书名。撰人不详。见《隋书•经籍考》,书佚。

Zhenjiu Tujing (Illustrated Canon of Acupuncture and Moxibustion) A book, with its author unknown, no longer extant, originally from *Suishu: Jing Ji Kao* (*The History of the Sui Dynasty: Records of Classics and Books*).

●**针灸图要诀**[zhēn jiǔ tú yào jué] 书名。撰人不详。见《隋书•经籍志》,书佚。

Zhenjiu Tu Yaojue (Essentials of the Diagrams of Acupuncture and Moxibustion) A book, whose author is unknown, no longer extant, originally from *Suishu: Jing Ji Zhi* (*The History of the Sui Dynasty: Annals of Classics and Books*).

●**针灸问答**[zhēn jiǔ wèn dá] 书名。《针灸问对》的别称。见该条。

Zhenjiu Wen Da (Questions and Answers on Acupuncture and Moxibustion) Another title of *Zhenjiu Wen Dui* (*Catechism of Acupuncture and Moxibustion*). →针灸问对(p.594)

●**针灸问对**[zhēn jiǔ wèn duì] 书名。又名《针灸问答》。明•汪机撰。刊于1530年。三卷。全书采用问答体裁。上卷介绍针灸经络的基本理论,中卷介绍针法,下卷介绍灸法并附经络穴位的歌诀。内容均取自《素问》、《灵枢》等,对元明流行的针灸学说持不同意见。

Zhenjiu Wen Dui (Catechism of Acupuncture and Moxibustion) Title of a book, also named *Zhenjiu Wen Da* (*Question and Answers on Acupuncture and Moxibustion*), written by Wang Ji of the Qing Dynasty and published in 1530 in 3 volumes. The book was written with the style of questions and answers. The lst volume was an introduction to the basic theories of the meridians and collaterals in acupuncture and moxibustion; the 2nd discussed needling methods and the 3rd showed moxibustion with the meridians and acupoints in verse attached. The contents of the book were all taken from *Suwen* (*Plain Questions*) and *Lingshu* (*Miraculous Pivot*), etc., also, the author held different points of view to the theories prevalent in the Yuan and Ming Dynasties.

●**针灸学**[zhēn jiǔ xué] ①中医学的学科之一。包括基础和临床两部分。基础以经络、腧穴等为主;临床有刺法、灸法、治疗等。②书名。江苏省中医学校针灸学教研组编。于1957年江苏人民出版社出版。分经络、腧穴、刺法、灸法、治疗、参考六篇。既是教学讲义,又是对古针灸学理论的系统整理。③书名。全国高等医药院校试用教材,南京中医学院主编。1961年人民卫生出版社出版,1964、1975、1979、1985年分别修订,由上海科学技术出版社出版。内容为上、中、下三部分,分别论述针灸学源流、经络与腧穴、刺灸方法和治疗等。末附原著、歌赋、子午流注等。④书名。

上海中医学院编。1974年人民卫生出版社出版。分经络、穴位、刺灸法、治疗四篇。近年经络穴位，针灸作用的研究等资料丰富。
Science of Acupuncture and Moxibustion
①One branch of traditional Chinese medicine, composed of basic and clinical parts, with the former mainly dealing with the meridians, collaterals and acupoints, etc., and the latter acupuncture techniques, moxibustion techniques and treatments, etc. ②Title of a book, compiled by the Teaching and Research Group of Acupuncture and Moxibustion of the Traditional Chinese Medical School of Jiangsu Province, and published by the Jiangsu Publishing House in 1957. The book consists of six chapters: meridians, collaterals, needling methods, moxibustion methods, treatment of diseases and references. It is not only a teaching material but also a systematization of ancient theories on acupuncture and moxibustion. ③Title of a book, a trial teaching material for medical colleges and universities of the whole country, compiled by Nanjing Traditional Chinese Medical College, published by the People's Hygiene Publishing House in 1961, and revised in 1964, 1975, 1979 and 1985. The revised editions were published by Shanghai Science and Technology Publishing House, including three sections dealing respectively with the origin and development of acupuncturology, meridians and collaterals, acupoints, methods of acupuncture and moxibustion, and treatment, etc., and with the appendix of the original verse on acupuncture and moxibustion and midnight-noon ebb-flow. ④Title of a book, compiled by Shanghai Traditional Medical College and published by the People's Hygiene Publishing House in 1974, including four sections on meridians and collaterals, methods of acupuncture and moxibustion and treatment with a great number of materials about research on meridians and collaterals, acupoints and the actions of acupuncture and moxibustion in recent years.

●针灸要旨[zhēn jiǔ yào zhǐ] 书名。为《针灸素难要旨》的别称。
Zhenjiu Yaozhi (Essentials of Acupuncture and Moxibustion) Title of a book, another name for *Zhenjiu Sunan Yaozhi* (*The Essentials of Acupuncture and Moxibustion in "Plain Questions" and the "Classic of Questions"*).

●针灸易学[zhēn jiǔ yì xué] 书名。清·李守先撰。刊于1798年。两卷。卷上为针灸源流、手法和认证三部分，介绍针灸方法及要穴的应用。卷下记述十四经穴及奇穴。
Zhenjiu Yi Xue (Acupuncture and Moxibustion Are Easy to Learn) A book in 2 volumes, written by Li Shouxian in the Qing Dynasty, and published in 1798. The 1st volume dealt with the origin and development of acupuncture and moxibustion, manipulations and differentiation of syndromes, it introduced methods of acupuncture and moxibustion and the application of some important points. The 2nd volume listed the acupoints of the fourteen meridians and the extra points.

●针灸杂说[zhēn jiǔ zá shuō] 书名。见《针灸四书》条。见该条。
Zhenjiu Zashuo (Miscellaneous Remarks on Acupuncture and Moxibustion) Title of a book. →针灸四书(p.593)

●针灸择日编集[zhēn jiǔ zé rì biān jí] 书名。明·全循义、全义孙合编。刊于1447年。书中主要辑录明以前文献中有关针灸选择日时的资料，加以比较，依干支日时定针灸的可否。
Zhenjiu Zeri Bianji (A Collection of Acupuncture and Moxibustion on Selected Days) Title of a book, written by Quan Xunyi and Quan Yisun in the Ming Dynasty, published in 1447. The book recorded material concerning the selection of the day and the hour for acupuncture and moxibustion from documents prior to the Ming Dynasty, compared them and determined the time for acupuncture and moxibustion in accordance with the Heavenly Stems and Earthly Branches matching the day and hour.

●针灸治疗刺激点[zhēn jiǔ zhì liáo cì jī diǎn] 刺激点的别称。见该条。
Stimulation Point for Acupuncture and Moxibustion Another name for stimulation point. →刺激点(p.53)

●针灸资生经[zhēn jiǔ zī shēng jīng] 书名。宋·王执中著。七卷。刊于1220年。卷一论人体各部腧穴，并附图；卷二论针灸方法，卷三至七论多种病的取穴治

疗。该书对灸法也较重视，并纠正了古书中的一些错误。

Zhenjiu Zisheng Jing (Acupuncture-Moxibustion Classic for Saving Life) A book in 7 volumes, written by Wang Zhizhong in the Song Dynasty and published in 1220. The lst volume presented the points of the human body with illustrations, the 2nd discussed the methods of acupuncture and moxibustion, the 3rd to the 7th dealt with treatments for many kinds of diseases. Greater importance was attached to moxibustion method and some errors in the ancient works were corrected in this book.

●针灸纂要[zhēn jiǔ zuàn yào]　书名。①撰人不详。见于明《医藏目录》，一卷。书佚。②吴炳耀撰，吴韵桐绘图。成于1933年。两册。上册说内景、阴阳、五行、诊法、经络、针刺法及治疗；下册载多种歌赋及经脉经穴图。③邱茂良编著。1958年江苏人民出版社出版。其对针灸史、学习方法、针灸学基本理论及治疗等均有论述。

Zhenjiu Zuanyao (A Compilation of Essentials of Acupuncture and Moxibustion) ①A book in a single volume with its author unknown, and no longer extant, originally from *Yi Cang Mulu* (*Catalogue of Books in Medical Treasury*) in the Ming Dynasty. ②A book in 2 volumes, written by Wu Bingyao, illustrated by Wu Yuntong and published in 1933. The lst volume introduced the inner distribution of yin-yang and five elements, diagnostic methods, meridians and collaterals, acupuncture methods and treatments, the 2nd volume contained many verses about acupuncture and moxibustion. ③A book compiled by Qiu Maoliang and published by Jiangsu People's Hygiene Publishing House in 1958, in which the history of acupuncture and moxibustion, studying method, basic theories and therapeutics of acupuncturology were expounded.

●针麻[zhēn má]　为针刺麻醉之简称。见该条。

A. A.　abbreviation for Acupuncture Anesthesia→针刺麻醉(p.588)

●针麻定量[zhēn má dìng liàng]　针麻术语。指在针刺麻醉过程中对针麻刺激参数所进行的显示和测定。

Quantification of Acupuncture Anesthesia A term of acupuncture anesthesia, referring to the display and determination of the stimulation parameters in the course of acupuncture anesthesia.

●针麻诱导期[zhēn má yòu dǎo qī]　针麻术语。指针刺麻醉过程中，从针刺入穴位，获得针感，并施以一定的刺激方式开始，直至达到镇痛效果而可以进行手术的这一段时间。其持续时间的长短与所用穴位的特点和刺激方法有关，一般以15至30分钟为宜。若针刺穴位在神经干或支上，诱导期持续时间可稍短，如针刺穴位远离手术区，诱导期持续时间可稍长。手法运针刺激的诱导期持续时间一般比电针刺激要略长。

Induced Period of Acupuncture Anesthesia A term of acupuncture anesthesia, referring to the period from insertion of the needle with the occurrence of the needling response and the application of certain proper stimulation forms until the analgesic effect is produced so that the surgical operation can be performed. The duration of the period mainly depends on the characteristics of the selected acupoints and stimulation forms, usually 15-30 minutes. If the acupoints is located on the nerve trunk or branch, the induced period may take less time, while if the acupoint is far from the area of operation, the induced period may last a little longer. In general, the duration of the induced period with the needle manipulated by hand is a bit longer than that with electrical acupuncture.

●针师[zhēn shī]　指掌握针法的医师。古代太医署设有针师职位。见《旧唐书·职官志》。

Acupuncturist Referring to the doctor who masters the needling methods. In ancient times, there was an acupuncturist post in the Office of Imperial Physicians, originally from *Jiu Tangshu: Zhiguan Zhi* (*The Old History Book of the Tang Dynasty: Records of Official Posts and Ranks*)

●针石[zhēn shí]　古针具名。又作*箴石、砭石的一种，即筒形类似针状的细棒。参见"砭石"条。

Needling Stone An acupuncture instrument used in ancient times, also called zhen-stone, a kind of stone used for needling, i.e. a needle-

shaped thin stone stick. →砭石(p. 22)

●**针头补泻**[zhēn tóu bǔ xiè] 针刺术语。见《针灸大成》，为手指补泻之别称，详见该条。

Reinforcing and Reducing by Needle Tip An acupuncture term, originally from *Zhenjiu Dacheng* (*A Great Compendium of Acupuncture and Moxibustion*), another name for finger reinforcing and reducing. →手指补泻法(p. 404)

●**针退**[zhēn tuì] 针刺手法名。十二字手法之一。见《针灸大成》。指在用泻法时，退针、出针的方法。

Needle Lifting A form of needling manipulation, one of the 12-character manipulations, referring to the method of lifting or withdrawing the needle while the reducing method is applied, originally from *Zhenjiu Dacheng* (*A Great Compendium of Acupuncture and Moxibustion*).

●**针向补泻**[zhēn xiàng bǔ xiè] 针刺补泻法。见《图注八十一难经》。指以针芒顺逆分补泻。参见"迎随补泻"条。

Reinforcing and Reducing According to Needling Direction A needling method for reinforcing and reducing in acupuncture treatment, seen in *Tu Zhu Bashiyi Nanjing* (*Illustrated Annotation on the Classic of Eighty-One Questions*), referring to differentiating reinforcing and reducing according to the direction of the needle tip, along or against the meridians. →迎随补泻(p. 567)

●**针眼**[zhēn yǎn] 病证名。出《诸病源候论》。又称偷针，土疳，麦粒肿。多因外感风热客于眼睑；或过食辛辣炙煿等物，脾胃湿热上攻于目，以致营卫失调，气血凝滞，热毒壅阻于眼睑皮肤经络之间所致。初起眼睑痒痛并作，患部睫毛根部毛囊皮肤红肿、硬结、形如麦粒，推之不移。继则红肿热痛加剧，垂头时疼痛加剧。轻者数日内可未成脓肿而自行消散。较重者要经3至4天后，于睫毛根部附近或相应的睑结膜上出现黄色脓点，不久可自行溃破，排出脓液而愈。本症有惯发性，多生于一目，但也有两目同时而发，或一目肿后，他目又起。因脾胃湿热者，兼有口臭、心烦、口渴、苔黄腻、脉濡数。治宜清脾胃湿热。取合谷、承泣、四白、上巨虚、阴陵泉。因外感风热者，则有恶寒、发热、头痛、咳嗽、苔薄、脉浮数。治宜疏风清热。取睛明、攒竹、行间、太阳。

Stye A disease, originally from *Zhubing Yuanhou Lun* (*General Treatise on the Etiology and Symptomatology of Diseases*), also called stealing needle or , hordeolum, mostly due to retention of exogenous pathogenic wind-heat in the eyelid, or over-eating acrid and fried food resulting in the upward invasion of damp-heat in the spleen and stomach to the eyes, leading to disharmony between ying and wei, stagnation of qi and blood, and obstruction of noxious heat in the collaterals of eyelid. 〈Manifestations〉in the initial period, itching and pain of the eyelid, redness and swelling of the eyelid skin with grain-like unmovable scleroma. Followed by severe redness, swelling, heat and pain of the eyelid, which is intensified when lowering the head. In mild cases, the scleroma may resolve by itself without pyogenesis in a few days; In severe cases, after 3 or 4 days, a yellowish pustule occurs around the root of the eyelash or relevant palpebral conjunctiva which can be ulcerated by itself and ends in discharge of pus. Styes are of a habitual nature, they mostly occur in one eye but sometimes in both eyes at the same time, or the swelling of one eye may be followed by that of the other. For cases due to damp-heat in the spleen and stomach, accompanied by foul breath, vexation, thirstiness, yellowish and greasy tongue coating, soft and rapid pulse. 〈Treatment principle〉Remove damp-heat from the spleen and stomach.〈Point selection〉Hegu (LI 4), Chengqi (ST 1), Sibai (ST 2), Shangjuxu (ST 37) and Yinlingquan (SP 9). For cases due to exogenous wind-heat, accompanied by aversion to cold, fever, headache, cough, thin tongue coating, superficial and rapid pulse. 〈Treatment principle〉Dispel wind and remove heat.〈Point selection〉Jingming (BL 1), Cuanzhu (BL 2), Xingjian (LR 2) and Taiyang (EX-HN 5).

●**针摇**[zhēn yáo] 针刺手法名。出《针灸大成》。为十二手法之一。为摇法之别称。见该条。

Needle Shaking A needling manipulation, originally from *Zhenjiu Dacheng* (*A Great Com-

pendium of Acupuncture and Moxibustion), one of the Twelve Manipulations, another name for shaking method. →摇法(p. 547)

●真肠[zhēn cháng] 经穴别名。出《太平圣惠方》。即承筋,见该条。

Zhenchang Another name for Chengjin (BL 56), a meridian point, originally from *Taiping Shenghui Fang* (*Imperial Benevolent Prescriptions*). →承筋(p. 43)

●甄权[zhēn quán] 人名。隋唐时针灸学家。许州扶沟(今河南扶沟)人。颇有医名。针术有奇效。事见《旧唐书》撰《明堂人形图》,一卷,《针经钞》一卷,《针方》一卷。三书均佚。

Zhen Quan An expert in acupuncture and moxibustion in the Sui and Tang Dynasties, a native of Fugou of Xuzhou (now Fugou in Henan Province), famous for his miraculous effects of acupuncture, which were recorded in *Jiu Tangshu* (*The Old History Book of the Tang Dynasty*). He wrote *Mingtang Renxing Tu* (*Chart of Acupoints as Shown on Human Figure*) in 1 volume, *Zhenjing Chao* (*Transcribed Passages from the Canon of Acupuncture*) in 1 volume and *Zhenfang* (*Acupuncture Prescriptions*) in 1 volume, but none is extant.

●箴石[zhēn shí] ①指砭石。②分指针与石。

1. Knife-Shaped Stone
2. Needle and Stone

●枕[zhěn] 耳穴名。位于对耳屏外侧的后上方。具有镇静止痛、安神熄风作用。〈主治〉头昏、头晕、头痛、失眠、支气管哮喘、癫痫、神经衰弱。

Occiput (MA) An auricular point. 〈Location〉at the posterior superior corner of the lateral aspect of the antitragus. 〈Functions〉tranquilizing the mind, alleviating pain and calming the wind. 〈Indications〉dizziness, headache, insomnia, bronchial asthma, epilepsy and neurosism.

●枕骨[zhěn gǔ] ①经穴别名。出《针灸聚英》。即头窍阴,见该条。②部位名。指后头中央隆起之骨,俗称后山骨,现称枕骨结骨。

1. **Zhengu** Another name for Touqiaoyin (GB 11), a meridian point, originally from *Zhenjiu Juying* (*Essentials of Acupuncture and Moxibustion*). →头窍阴(p. 444)

2. **Occipital Node** A body part, referring to the protruding bone in the center of occiput, popularly called the hind mountain bone.

●振埃[zhèn āi] 《内经》刺法名。出《灵枢·刺节真邪》。为刺法五节之一。指气逆于上,充满于胸中,而致胸部胀满,呼吸摇肩,或气喘,坐伏不能平卧,害怕尘埃烟薰,呼吸不畅一类病证。取天容、廉泉等穴以降逆,疏通血络,其效验有如振落尘埃。

Shaking off Dust A needling method mentioned in *Neijing* (*The Canon of Internal Medicine*), originally from *Lingshu: Ci Jie Zhen Xie* (*Miraculous Pivot: Acupuncture Principles and Diseases*), one of the Five Needling Techniques, used for diseases caused by adverse rising of qi resulting in fullness of the chest and leading to distension and fullness in the chest, shaking shoulders when breathing, or dyspnea, inability to lie flat and fear of dust and smoke. In the treatment, select Tianrong (SI 17), Lianquan (RN 23) and other points to lower the adverse flow of qi and dredge the meridians and collaterals, which can achieve remarkable and quick effect like shaking off dust.

●震颤法[zhèn chàn fǎ] 针刺手法名。见《神应经》。持住针柄作小幅度快频率的颤动动作,以增强针感。临床上多用于针准确地刺入到应刺部位的深度时,虽已得气,但很微弱之时。参见捣法。

Trembling Method A form of needling manipulation, originally from *Shen Ying Jing* (*Classic of God Merit*), referring to manipulation by vibrating the needle handle with small amplitude and high frequency to strengthen the needling response. In clinic, it is commonly used when the needle is inserted to the depth of the certain point to be needled and the needling sensation is obtained but very weak though. →捣法(p. 77)

●怔忡[zhēng chōng] 病证名。指心跳剧烈的一种病证。属心悸。详见"心悸"条。

Severe Palpitation A disease, characterized by violent heart-beat, one type of palpitation. →心悸(p. 509)

●蒸脐法[zhēng qí fǎ] 为蒸脐治病法之别称。详见该条。

Steaming the Navel Another name for navel-steaming therapy. →蒸脐治病法(p. 599)

●蒸脐治病法 [zhēng qí zhì bìng fǎ] 间接灸一种。又称蒸脐法、熏脐法、炼脐法。是将药末填满脐中,上置艾炷施灸的一种方法。所用的药物处方,因病而异,其操作方法亦有所别。如《针灸大成·卷九》蒸脐治病法用于预防疾病。药用五灵脂(生用)24克,青盐(生用)24克,乳香3克,没药3克,夜明沙6克,地鼠粪9克,葱头3克,木通9克,麝香少许,研为细末。用莜面团作圆圈围脐周围,将药末6克放于脐,用槐树皮剪成五分硬币大的圆放在药上,上置艾炷施灸。而《医学入门》载炼脐法治疗劳疾。药用麝香15克,丁香9克,青盐12克,夜明砂15克,乳香、没药各19克,小茴香12克,木香、虎骨、蛇骨、龙骨、朱砂各15克,雄黄9克,白附子15克,人参、附子、胡椒各21克,五灵脂15克,共为细末。另用白面作条,搁于脐上,将前药一料,分为三份,取一份。先填麝香五分入脐内,又将前药一份入面圈内,按药令紧,中插数孔,外用槐叶一片盖于药上,艾火灸之。灸至遍身大汗为度。适用于劳伤、失血、气虚体倦、阳萎、遗精、阴虚、痰火、妇人赤白带下、虚寒积滞等症,并可用健身防病。

The Navel-Steaming Therapy One form of indirect moxibustion, also called steaming the navel, umbilicus moxibustion method, or fumigating umbilicus method, etc. The umbilicus is filled up with the drug powder and with an ignited moxa cone on it for moxibustion. The prescribed drugs vary according to diseases and so do the moxibustion methods. For example, this therapy was used for prevention of disease in Vol. 9 of *Zhenjiu Dacheng*(*A Great Compendium of Acupuncture and Moxibustion*). Take *Wu Ling Zhi*(*Faeces Trogopterorum*)(24g)(raw use), salt(24g)(raw use), *Ru Xiang*(*Resina Olibani*)(3g), *Mo Yao*(*Resina Commiphorae Myrrhae*)(3g), *Ye Ming Sha*(*Faeces Vespertilionis*)(6g), feces of vole(9g), onion(3g), *Mu Tong*(*Caulis Akebiae*)(9g) and a little bit of *She Xiang*(*Moschus*). Grind these drugs into a fine powder, put a circle made of naked oat flour around the umbilicus, cover the powder with a piece of sophora japonica bark the size of a five-fen coin, and then put a moxa cone on it for moxibustion. Another example of this therapy, in *Yixue Rumen*(*An Introduction to Medicine*), is used for the treatment of consumptive disease. Use *She Xiang*(*Moschus*) 15g, *Ding Xiang*(*Flos Syzygii Aromatici*)9g, salt 12g, *Ye Ming Sha*(*Faeces Vespertilionis*) 15g, *Ru Xiang*(*Resina Olibani*)19g, *Mo Yao*(*Resina Commiphorae Myrrhae*)19g, *Xiao Hui Xiang*(*Fructus Foenicuii*)12g, *Mu Xiang*(*Radix Acuklandiae*)15g, *Hu Gu*(*Os Tigris*) 15g, Snake Bone 15g, *Long Gu*(Ss Draconis) 15g, *Zhu Sha*(Cinnabaris)15g, *Xionghuang*(*Realgar*)9g, *Bai Fu Zi*(*Rhizoma Typhonii*)15g, *Ren Shen*(*Radix Ginseng*)21g, *Fu Zi*(*Radix Aconiti Praeparata*)21g, pepper 21g, *Wu Ling Zhi*(*Faeces Trogopterorum*)15g. Grind them into a powder, put a circle made of flour around the umbilicus, then take the powder and divide it into three equal portions. First fill 1.5g of *She Xiang*(*Moschus*)into the umbilicus, then put one portion of the powder in the flour circle, press the powder to make it more close, punch several holes in the centre, then cover the powder with a piece of sophora leaf. Ignite a moxa cone on it for moxibustion until the patient is bathed in sweat. 〈Indications〉 internal injury caused by over-strain, loss of blood, lassitude due to qi deficiency, impotence, emission, yin deficiency, phlegm-fire, leukorrhea with reddish discharge, cold of insufficiency type and retention of food, etc. It is also used for keeping health and prevention of disease.

●正经 [zhèng jīng] ①指十二经脉,与奇经八脉相对而言。出《黄帝内经太素》卷十九。②指本经的意思。出《难经·四十九难》。如因经脉本身功能失常而发病的,称为正经自病。

1. Regular Meridians The Twelve Meridians, corresponding with the Eight Extra Meridians, originally from *Huangdi Neijing Taisu*(*Comprehensive Notes to the Yellow Emperor's Inner Canon*).

2. The Meridian Proper The meridian itself, originally from *Nanjing: Sishijiu Nan*(*The Classic of Questions: Question* 49). For instance, a disease caused by the irregularity of the function of the meridian is called the illness of the meridian proper.

● 正疟 [zhèng nüè] 疟疾证型之一。由疟邪侵入，伏于半表半里，与营卫相搏，正邪交争所致。证见寒战壮热，休作有时，先有呵欠乏力，继则寒栗鼓颔，寒罢则内外皆热头痛面赤，口渴饮引，终则遍身汗出，热退身凉，舌红苔薄白，脉弦。治宜祛邪截疟，和解表里。取丘墟、陶道、液门、曲池、间使。一般在发作前1至2小时针刺为宜。

Typical Malaria One type of malarial disease, caused by invasion of malarial pathogen hiding in half exterior and half interior part of the body and struggling with ying and wei. ⟨Manifestations⟩ intermittent rigor and high fever. At the initial stage, yawning and weariness followed by chill, high fever after chill, headache, flushed face, thirst and ending in sweating all over the body, disappearance of fever and cold body, red tongue with thin and white coating, wiry pulse. ⟨Treatment principle⟩ Eliminate malarial pathogen to prevent reoccurrence of malaria, regulate the interior and exterior. ⟨Point selection⟩ Qiuxu (GB 40), Taodao (DU 13), Yemen (SJ 2), Quchi (LI 11) and Jianshi (PC 5). It is advisable to give acupuncture 1-2 hours before onset.

● 正营 [zhèng yíng] 经穴名。出《针灸甲乙经》。属足少阳胆经，为足少阳、阳维之会。⟨定位⟩在头部，当前发际上2.5寸，头正中线旁开2.25寸（图28）。⟨层次解剖⟩皮肤→皮下组织→帽状腱膜→腱膜下疏松结缔组织。布有眶上神经和枕大神经的吻合支，颞浅动、静脉的顶支。⟨主治⟩头痛，头晕，目眩，唇吻强急，齿痛。平刺0.5～0.8寸；可灸。

Zhengying (GB 17) A meridian point, originally from *Zhenjiu Jia-Yi Jing* (*A-B Classic of Acupuncture and Moxibustion*), a point on the Gallbladder Meridian of Foot-Shaoyang, the crossing point of the Foot-Shaoyang Meridian and the Yangwei Meridian. ⟨Location⟩ on the head, 2.5 cun above the anterior hairline and 2.25 cun lateral to the midline of the head (Fig. 28). ⟨Regional anatomy⟩ skin→subcutaneous tissue→epicranial aponeurosis→loose connective tissue below aponeurosis. There are the anatomotic branches of the supraorbital and greater occipital nerves and the parietal branches of the superficial temporal artery and vein in this area. ⟨Indications⟩ headache, dizziness, spasm of the lips, toothache. ⟨Method⟩ Puncture subcutaneously 0.5～0.8 cun. Moxibustion is applicable.

● 政和圣济总录 [zhèng hé shèng jì zǒng lù] 方书名。即《圣济总录》，见该条。

Zhenghe Shengji Zonglu (*Zhenghe Imperial Medical Encyclopaedia*) A medical formulary. →圣济总录 (p.369)

● 支沟 [zhī gōu] 经穴名。出《灵枢·本输》。属手少阳三焦经，为本经经穴。又名飞虎、飞处。⟨定位⟩在前臂背侧，当阳池与肘尖的连线上，腕背横纹上3寸，尺骨与桡骨之间（图48和图44.3）。⟨层次解剖⟩皮肤→皮下组织→小指伸肌→拇长伸肌→前臂骨间膜。浅层布有前臂后皮神经，头静脉和贵要静脉的属支。深层有骨间后动、静脉和骨间后神经。⟨主治⟩暴暗，耳聋，耳鸣，肩背酸痛，呕吐，胁肋痛，便秘，热病。直刺0.5～1寸；可灸。

Zhigou (SJ 6) A meridian point, originally from *Ling Shu: Benshu* (*Miraculous Pivot: Meridian Points*), the Jing (River) point of the Sanjiao Meridian of Hand-Shaoyang, also named Feihu and Feichu. ⟨Location⟩ on the dorsal side of the forearm and on the line connecting Yangchi (SJ 4) and the tip of the olecranon, 3 cun proximal to the dorsal crease of the wrist, between the radius and ulna (Figs. 48&44.3). ⟨Regional anatomy⟩ skin→subcutaneous tissue→extensor muscle of little finger → long extensor muscle of thumb → interosseous membrane of forearm. In the superficial layer, there are the posterior cutaneous nerve of the forearm and the tributaries of the cephalic and basilic vein. In the deep layer, there are posterior interosseous artery and vein and the posterior interosseous nerve. ⟨Indications⟩ sudden loss of voice, deafness, tinnitus, soreness and pain in the shoulder and back, vomiting, hypochondriac pain constipation and febrile diseases. ⟨Method⟩ Puncture perpendicularly 0.5～1 cun. Moxibustion is applicable.

● 支节 [zhī jié] 支，指四肢；节，指骨节，又泛指穴位。

Limbs and Joints Limbs refer to the four extremities and joints the junctures of bones. The term also refers to the points in general.

●支正[zhī zhèng] 经穴名。出《灵枢·经脉》。属手太阳小肠经,为本经络穴。〈定位〉在前臂背面尺侧,当阳谷与小海的连线上,腕背横纹上5寸(图48和图44.3)。〈层次解剖〉皮肤→皮下组织→尺侧腕屈肌→指深屈肌→前臂骨间膜。浅层有前臂内侧皮神经,贵要静脉属支。深层有尺动、静脉和尺神经。〈主治〉项强,肘挛,手指痛,热病,头痛,目眩,癫狂,易惊,好笑喜忘,惊恐悲愁,消渴,疥疮生疣。直刺0.3~0.5寸;可灸。

Zhizheng(SI 7) A meridian point, originally from *Lingshu*: *Jingmai* (*Miraculous Pivot*: *Meridians*), the Luo(Connecting) point of the Small Intestine Meridian of Hand-Taiyang. 〈Location〉on the ulnar side of the posterior surface of the fore arm and on the line connecting Yanggu (SI 5) and Xiaohai (SI 8), 5 cun proximal to the dorsal crease of the wrist (Figs. 48 & 44.3). 〈Regional anatomy〉skin→subcutaneous tissue→ulnar. Flexor muscle of wrist → deep flexor muscle of fingers → interosseous membrane of forearm. In the superficial layer, there are the medial cutaneous nerve of the forearm and the tributaries of the basilic vein. In the deep layer, there are the ulnar artery and vein and the ulnar nerve. 〈Indications〉rigidity of the nape, spasm of the elbow, pain in the fingers, febrile diseases, headache, dizziness, manic-depressive disorder, susceptibility to fright, abnormal and frequent laughter, amnesia, emotional disorders such as terror, fear, grief and anxiety, diabetes, scabies and wart. 〈Method〉Puncture perpendicularly 0.3~0.5 cun. Moxibustion is applicable.

●知热感度测定法[zhī rè gǎn dù cè dìng fǎ] 指测定十二经脉的井穴或背俞穴对温热感觉的灵敏度,并比较其左右两侧的差异数值,从而分析各经虚实或不平衡现象。一般采用线香或知热感度测定仪来进行。如以线香为热源,则对准井穴作来回运动,每次约隔半秒,至病人觉烫时即停止,记录其次数作为该经的知热感度。或将热源对准穴位置于固定距离,测定病人感到烫热所需的时间。测定结束后,从所测十二个井穴或背俞穴知热数值的高低或左右两侧的差数来分析各经的虚实、不平衡等情况。所测井穴中,有些穴位的位置因测定的需要而有所更动,如足少阴经涌泉穴改为小趾甲角内侧,称内至阴穴等。

Determination of Heat Sensitivity A method of determining the sensitivity to heat of the Jing (Well) points of the Twelve Meridians and the Back-Shu points and comparing the numerical values of the difference at the left and right sides to analyse the deficiency-excess or imbalance of each meridian. Usually it is done by means of incense thread or a heat sensitivity determination instrument. If incense thread is used as the heat source, move it back and forth over the point, with an interval of 1/2 second after each movement until the patient feels a scorching feeling. The number of movements recorded the heat sensitivity of each meridian. Or, hold the heat source directly over the point at a fixed distance and determine how long it takes the patient before he/she has a scorching feeling. After the determination, analyse the condition of deficiency-excess or imbalance of each meridian according to the different determined values of heat sensitivity of the twelve Jing (Well) or Back-Shu points or the difference between the values of the left and the right sides. Among the Jing (Well) points, the locations of some points should be changed for the demand for determination, e.g., the point medial to the inner corner of the toenail, called Neizhiyin (EX-LE) point, is determined instead of Yongquan (KI 1) of the Foot-Shaoyin Meridian.

●蜘蛛鼓[zhī zhū gǔ] 见《医学入门·鼓胀》。详见鼓胀条。

Spider-Like Distention Seen in *Yixue Rumen*: *Gu Zhang* (*An Introduction to Medicine*: *Distention of Abdomen*). →鼓胀(p.146)

●直肠[zhí cháng] ①耳穴名。又称直肠下段、位于耳轮起始部,近屏上切迹处。治疗便秘、腹泻、脱肛、内外痔、里急后重。②经穴别名。见《针灸甲乙经》。即承筋。详见该条。

1. Rectum(MA-H2) An auricular point, also named Lower Portion of Rectum (MA). 〈Location〉on the end of the helix approximate to the superior tragic notch. 〈Indications〉constipation, diarrhea, prolapse of the rectum, inter-

nal and external hemorrhoids and tenesmus.
2. **Zhichang** Another name for Chengjin(BL 56), a meridian point seen in *Zhenjiu Jia-Yi Jing* (*A-B Classic of Acupuncture and Moxibustion*). →承筋(p. 43)

●直肠下段[zhí cháng xià duàn] 为直肠之别称。见该条1。

Lower Portion of Rectum(MA) Another name for Rectum(MA-H 2). →直肠1(p. 601)

●直刺[zhí cì] 刺法术语。指针体与穴位皮肤表面呈90度角左右刺入。适用于肌肉丰厚的腰、臀、腹及四肢部的穴位。对肌肉较薄和接近重要脏器的穴位，采用直刺时不可深入，宜采用斜刺或沿皮刺。

Perpendicular Insertion An acupuncture technique, referring to inserting the needle perpendicularly, forming an angle of 90° with the skin surface. This method is usually applied to points on regions with thick muscles such as the lumbar buttock regions, abdomen and extremities. For points on regions with thin muscles or close to important zang-organs, do not insert the needle deeply when applying perpendicular insertion; it is usually appropriate to adopt oblique or subcutaneous insertion on these occasions.

●直耳[zhí ěr] 经穴别名。出《针灸甲乙经》。即本神，见该条。

Zhier Another name for Benshen(GB 13), a meridian point originally from *Zhenjiu Jia-Yi Jing* (*A-B Classic of Acupuncture and Moxibustion*). →本神(p. 18)

●直骨[zhí gǔ] 经外穴名。见《针灸集成》。在胸部，当乳头直下一横指处。主治小儿温疟，咳嗽，气逆等。用灸法。

Zhigu(EX-CA) An extra point, originally from *Zhenjiu Jicheng* (*A Collection of Acupuncture and Moxibustion*). ⟨Location⟩ in the chest, one finger-width directly below nipples. ⟨Indications⟩ pyrexial malaria in children, cough and dyspnea. ⟨Method⟩ moxibustion.

●直接灸[zhé jiē jiǔ] 艾炷灸的一种。又称着肤灸、着肉灸、明灸。是将艾炷直接放在穴位上施灸的一种方法。根据施灸的程度不同，可分为化脓灸、非化脓灸两种。详见各条。

Direct Moxibustion A form of moxa-cone moxibustion, also called moxibustion on skin, moxibustion on muscle or open moxibustion. Referring to placing a moxa cone directly on a point for moxibustion. According to the different degrees of moxibustion, it is divided into suppurative moxibustion and non-suppurative moxibustion. →化脓灸(p. 169)、非化脓灸(p. 106)

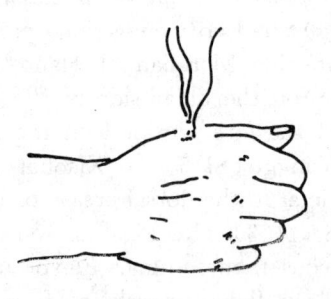

图74 直 接 灸

Fig 74 Direct moxibustion

●直鲁古[zhí lǔ gǔ] 人名。辽代针灸家。其在战争中为辽太祖所俘。后曾任太医，擅针灸，著《脉诀》、《针灸书》，已佚。见《辽史》及道光十年《承德府志》。

Zhi Lugu An expert in acupuncture and moxibustion in the Liao Dynasty, once captured by the crown ancestor of the Liao Dynasty in war and appointed imperial physician. Later, he became proficient in acupuncture and moxibustion and wrote *Maijue* (*Sphygmology in Verse*) and *Zhenjiu Shu* (*A Book of Acupuncture and Moxibustion*), already lost. cf. *Liaoshi* (*The History of the Liao Dynasty*) and *Chengdefu Zhi* (*Annals of Chengde*) of the 10th year of Daoguang.

●直针刺[zhí zhēn cì] 《内经》刺法名。见《灵枢·官针》。现多称沿皮刺、横刺、平刺。是十二刺之一。指捏起皮肤沿皮下针刺，以治疗寒气侵犯较浅的痹证。多用于肌肉浅薄部位。

Straight Puncture An acupuncture tech-

nique in *Neijing* (*The Inner Canon of Huangdi*), originally from *Ling shu: Guanzhen* (*Miraculous Pivot: Official Needles*), usually called subcutaneous insertion, transverse insertion or horizontal insertion, one of the Twelve Needling Methods, referring to pinching up the skin around the point and then inserting the needle subcutaneously in order to treat aching and numbness due to shallow invasion by pathogenic cold. It is commonly applied to portions with thin muscles in the shallow layer.

●指[zhǐ] 耳穴名。位于将耳舟部分为六等份，自上而下，第一等份为指。治疗指部疾患如甲沟炎、手指疼痛、麻木。

Finger (MA-SF 1) An auricular point. 〈Location〉Divide scaphoid fossa into six equal parts, from superior to inferior, the 1st equal part is the Finger (MA-SF 1). 〈Indications〉disorders of the fingers such as paronychia, pain and numbness.

●指拔[zhǐ bá] 针刺手法名。见《针灸大成》。十二字手法之一。指出针之时，将针提至皮下，待针气缓不觉沉紧时再拔针的方法。

Finger Pulling An acupuncture manipulation, originally from *Zhenjiu Dacheng* (*A Great Compendium of Acupuncture and Moxibustion*), one of the Twelve-Character Manipulations, referring to lifting the needle to the subcutaneous level, then waiting until feeling of the needling qi subsides and there is no tight or heavy feeling in the hand, and then pulling the needle out.

●指拨法[zhǐ bō fǎ] 针刺时用手指拨动针柄以增强针感的方法。其法用拇、食指捏持针柄，以中指轻轻拨动针体，以增强针感。

Finger Plucking A manipulation of plucking the handle of the needle with a finger to strengthen the needling response, while performing acupuncture. 〈Method〉Hold the handle of the needle with the thumb and index finger and pluck the body of the needle gently with the middle finger so as to strengthen the needling response.

●指持[zhǐ chí] 针刺手法名。见《针灸大成》。十二字手法之。指针刺以前以右手持住针柄，用心专著，使针在穴上着力一旋一插，直透腠理的操作方法。

Finger Holding An acupuncture manipulation, seen in *Zhenjiu Dacheng* (*A Great Compendium of Acupuncture and Moxibustion*). One of the Twelve-Character Manipulations. 〈Method〉Before acupuncture, hold the handle of the needle with the right hand, then, slowly and forcefully rotate and thrust the needle on the point very attentively and get the needle tip directly through the skin and superficial muscles.

●指搓[zhǐ cuō] 针刺手法名。见《针灸大成》。十二字手法之一。指针刺后的捻转方法。如搓线状。参见"搓法"条。

Finger Rotating An acupuncture manipulation, seen in *Zhenjiu Dacheng* (*A Great Compendium of Acupuncture and Moxibustion*), one of the Twelve-Character Manipulations, referring to twirling or rotating manipulation after insertion as if twisting thread. →搓法(p. 59)

●指寸定位法[zhǐ cùn dìng wèi fǎ] 经穴定位方法之一。指依据患者本人手指所规定的分寸以量取腧穴的方法。参见"同身寸"条。

Locating Point by Finger-Cun Measurement One of the methods for locating acupoints, referring to locating an acupoint according to the stipulated length and breadth of the patient's fingers as a unit. →同身寸(p. 442)

●指疔[zhǐ dīng] 病证名。生于手指部疔疮的总称。外伤感染或脏腑火毒郁发所致。患指赤肿剧痛，易溃脓者顺。若肿势上延，甚而损及掌指筋骨，或并发疔疮走黄者逆。治同疔疮。见该条。

Felon A disease, a general term for furuncles and sores in fingers, commonly due to traumatic infection or stirring up of fire-toxin smoldering in zang-fu organs. 〈Manifestations〉redness, swelling and severe pain of the affected finger. The quick appearance of diabrosis indicates a favorable prognosis. If the swelling develops in the upper part, causes the impairment of the metacarpal tendon and bone, or is accompanied by septicemia, this indicates an unfavorable prognosis. The treatment of felon is the same as that of furuncle. →疔疮(p. 82)

● 指根[zhǐ gēn] 经外穴名，又名下四缝。〈定位〉位于第二、三、四、五指指掌横纹之中点处，左右计八穴。〈主治〉手部疔疮，五指尽痛，腹痛呕吐，发热。三棱针点刺出血。

Zhigen（EX-UE） An extra point, also named Xiasifeng.〈Location〉at the midpoint of palmar digital cross striation of the 2nd to the 5th fingers, 8 points in all on both sides.〈Indications〉hand furuncle, pain in the five fingers, abdominal pain, Vomiting and fever.〈Methed〉Prick with a three-edged needle to cause bleeding.

● 指留[zhǐ liú] 针刺手法名。见《针灸大成》。十二字手法之一。指在出针时不立即将针拔出，而将针提至天部在皮下停留一段时间，使荣卫之气疏散，不致随针外逸的一种方法。

Finger Retaining An acupuncture manipulation, seen in *Zhenjiu Da Cheng*(*A Great Compendium of Acupuncture and Moxibustion*), one of the Twelve-Character Manipulations, referring to the manipulation of not pulling the needle out immediately when withdrawing the needle, but lifting the needle to the Heaven Portion and retaining the needle tip beneath the skin for a while so as to make nutrient and defensive qi spread and not escape with the withdrawal of the needle.

● 指迷赋[zhǐ mí fù] 针灸歌赋名。元·窦默撰。见《广平府志·艺文略》。赋未见。

Zhi Mi Fu (Ode for Dispelling Confusions) A verse on acupuncture and moxibustion, written by Dou Mo in the Yuan Dynasty, seen in *Guangpingfu Zhi*: *Yi Wen Lue* (*Annals of the Prefecture of Guangping*: *Summary of Art and Literature*), but the verse is not in it.

● 指捻[zhǐ niǎn] 针刺手法名。见《针灸大成》。十二字手法之一。指以捻转为基础，目的在于行气的一种方法。可在通关过节时配合应用。参见"捻法"条。

Finger Twirling An acupuncture manipulation, seen in *Zhenjiu Dacheng*(*A Great Compendium of Acupuncture and Moxibustion*), one of the Twelve-Character Manipulations, referring to taking the twirling method as the basic manipulation for the purpose of promoting the circulation of qi. It may be used when the meridian qi passes through joints. →捻法(p.283)

● 指切进针[zhǐ qiē jìn zhēn] 进针方法之一。为爪切进针之别称，见该条。

Finger-Pressing Insertion One of the methods of needle inserting, another name for Nail-Pressing Insertion. →爪切进针(p.586)

● 指循[zhǐ xún] 针刺手法名。见《针灸大成》。十二字手法之一。指针刺而气不至，可用指循导气法来催动经气的方法。参见"循法"条。

Finger Pressing An acupuncture manipulation, seen in *Zhenjiu Dacheng*(*A Great Compendium of Acupuncture and Moxibustion*), one of the Twelve-Character Manipulations, referring to the method used to promote meridian qi by pressing the skin with the fingers along the meridian course when the meridian qi does not arrive after insertion. →循法(p.531)

● 指压进针法[zhǐ yā jìn zhēn fǎ] 进针法之一。其法：右手持针，拇、食指捏住针根部，以中指或无名指直抵穴位，针身紧靠指旁，然后运用拇、食指的压力，将针迅速刺入穴位。本法适用于短针的进针，可单手操作，不须左手按压。

Inserting the Needle Under Pressure of Finger One of the methods for inserting the needle.〈Method〉Hold the root of the needle with the thumb and index fingers of the right hand, press straight on the acupoint with the middle or the ring finger, keep the body of the needle closely against the finger, then insert the needle into the point quickly, using the pressure of the thumb and index fingers. This method is suitable for the insertion of the short needle and can be manipulated only with one hand without the help of pressing of the other hand.

● 指针[zhǐ zhēn] 意指以手代针，如按压、掐切或揉动等法均是。

Needle-Like Finger Pressing Methods to use fingers rather than needles, such as pressing, finger-nail pressing or poking, etc.

● 趾[zhǐ] 耳穴名。位于对耳轮上脚的外上角。用于治疗趾部疼痛、甲沟炎。

Toe(MA) An auricular point.〈Location〉on the external superior angle of the superior

crus of anthelix. 〈Indications〉pain of the toe and paronychia.

●至宫[zhì gōng] 经穴别名。见《普济方》。即目窗,见该条。
Zhigong Another name for *Muchuang* (GB 16), a meridian point seen in *Puji Fang* (*Prescriptions for Universal Relief*). →目窗(p. 272)

●至荣[zhì róng] 经穴别名。即目窗,见该条。
Zhirong Another name for the meridian point *Muchuang* (GB 16). →目窗(p. 272)

●至阳[zhì yáng] 经穴名。出《针灸甲乙经》。属督脉。〈定位〉在背部,当后正中线上,第七胸椎棘突下凹陷中(图12.2和图7)。〈层次解剖〉针刺经过的层次结构同脊中穴。浅层主要布有第七胸神经后支的内侧皮支和伴行的动、静脉。深层有棘突间的椎外后静脉丛,第七胸神经后支的分支和第七肋间后动、静脉背侧支的分支或属支。〈主治〉胸肋胀痛,腹痛黄疸,咳嗽气喘,腰背疼痛,脊强,身热。斜刺0.5~1.0寸;可灸。
Zhiyang (DU 9) A meridian point, originally from *Zhenjiu Jia-Yi Jing* (*A-B Classic of Acupuncture and Moxibustion*), a point on the Du Meridian. 〈Location〉 on the back and on the posterior midline, in the depression below the spinous process of the 7th thoracic vertebra (Figs. 12.2&7). 〈Regional anatomy〉The layer structures of the needle insertion are the same as those in Jizhong (Du 6). In the superficiald layer, there are the medial cutaneous branches of the posterior branches on the 7th thoracic nerve and the accompanying artery and vein. In the deep layer there are the external (posterior) vertebral venous plexus between the adjacent spinous processes, the branches of the posterior branches of the 7th thoracic nerve and the branches or tributaries of the dorsal branches of the 7th posterior intercostal artery and vein. 〈Indications〉distending pain in the chest and hypochondrium, abdominal pain, jaundice, cough, dyspnea, pain in the loin and back, back rigidity and fever. 〈Method〉 Puncture obliquely 0.5~1.0 cun. Moxibustion is applicable.

●至阴[zhì yīn] 经穴名。出《灵枢·本输》。属足太阳膀胱经,为本经井穴。〈定位〉在足小趾末节外侧,距趾甲角0.1寸(指寸)(图35.2)。〈层次解剖〉皮肤→皮下组织→甲根。布有足背外侧皮神经的趾背神经和趾背动、静脉网。〈主治〉头痛,鼻塞,鼻衄,目痛,足下热,胞衣不下,胎位不正,难产。斜刺0.2寸,或点刺出血;可灸。
Zhiyin (BL 67) A meridian point, orginally from *Lingshu*: *Benshu* (*Miraculous Pivot*: *Meridians Points*), the Jing (Well) point of the Bladder Meridian of Foot-Taiyang. 〈Location〉on the lateral side of the distal segment of the little toe, 0.1 cun from the corner of the toenail (Fig. 35.2). 〈Regional anatomy〉 skin → subcutaneous tissue → root of nail. There are the dorsal digital nerve of the lateral dorsal cutaneous nerve of the foot and the arteriovenous network of the dorsal digital arteries and veins in this area. 〈 Indications 〉 headache, stuffy nose, epistaxis, pain of the eye, feverish sensation in the sole, retention of placenta, malposition of fetus and difficult labour. 〈Method〉Puncture obliquely 0.2 cun, or prick to cause bleeding. Moxibustion is applicable.

●至营[zhì yíng] 经穴别名。出《针灸甲乙经》。即目窗,见该条。
Zhiying Another name for *Muchuang* (GB 16), a meridian point originally from *Zhenjiu Jia-Yi Jing* (*A-B Classic of Acupuncture and Moxibustion*). →目窗(p. 272)

●志室[zhì shì] 经穴名。出《针灸甲乙经》。属足太阳膀胱经。又名精宫。〈定位〉在腰部,当第二腰椎棘突下,旁开3寸(图7)。〈层次解剖〉皮肤→皮下组织→背阔肌腱膜→竖脊肌→腰方肌。浅层布有第一、二腰神经后支的外侧皮支和伴行的动、静脉。深层有第一、二腰神经的肌支和相应的腰动、静脉背侧支的分支或属支。〈主治〉遗精,阳萎,阴部肿痛,小便淋沥,水肿,腰脊强痛。直刺0.8~1.0寸;可灸。
Zhishi (BL 52) A meridian point, originally from *Zhenjiu Jia-Yi Jing* (*A-B Classic of Acupuncture and Moxibustion*), a point on the Bladder Meridian of Foot-Taiyang, also named Jinggong. 〈Location〉 on the low back, below the spinous process of the 2nd lumbar vertebra, 3 cun lateral to the posterior midline (Fig. 7). 〈Regional anatomy〉 skin → subcutaneous tissue → aponeurosis of latissimus muscle of

back→erector spinal muscle→lumbar quadrate muscle. In the superficial layer, there are the lateral cutaneous branches of the posterior branches of the lst and 2nd lumbar nerves and the accompanying arteries and veins. In the deep layer, there are the muscular branches of the posterior branches of the lst and 2nd lumbar nerves and the branches or tributaries of the related lumbar arteries and veins. 〈Indications〉 seminal emission, impotence, swelling and pain in the pudendum, dribbling urination, edema, stiffness and pain along the spinal column. 〈Method〉 Puncture perpendicularly 0.8～1.0 cun. Moxibustion is applicable.

●治喘[zhì chuǎn] 经外穴别名。即定喘。见该条。
Zhichuan Another name for the extra point Dingchuan(EX-B 1).→定喘(p. 84)

●治腑者治其合[zhì fǔ zhě zhì qí hé] 《内经》取穴法则之一。语见《素问·咳论》。指治疗六腑病应取其位在足三阳经上的合穴。
Selecting Related He (Sea) Points to Treat Diseases of Fu Organs One of the principles of point selection in *Neijing* (*Canon of Internal Medicine*), seen in *Suwen: Ke Lun* (*Plain Questions: Treatise on Cough*), referring to selecting the respective He(Sea) points on the Three Yang Meridians of the Foot to treat diseases of the six fu organs.

●治痿独取阳明[zhì wěi dú qǔ yáng míng] 《内经》治痿选穴原则。语出《素问·痿论》。指治疗痿证取阳明经腧穴的重要性。
Selecting Points on Only the Yangming Meridians for the Treatment of Flaccidity Syndromes The principle of point selection for the treatment of flaccidity syndromes in *Neijing* (*The Canon of Internal Medicine*), originally from *Suwen: Wei Lun* (*Plain Questions: On Flaccidity Syndromes*), referring to the importance of selecting points on the Yangming Meridians in the treatment of flaccidity syndromes.

●治脏者治其俞[zhì zàng zhě zhì qí shù] 《内经》取穴法则之一。语出《素问·咳论》指治五脏病症应取该经五腧穴中的输穴。
Selecting Related Shu (Stream) Points to Treat Diseases of Zang Organs One of the principles of point selection in *Neijing*: (*Canon of Internal Medicine*). Originally from *Su Wen: Ke Lun* (*Plain Questions: Treatise on Cough*). It means that the Shu(Stream) points of the Five Shu points should be selected in the treatment of diseases of the five zang organs.

●秩边[zhì biān] 经穴名。出《针灸甲乙经》。属足太阳膀胱经。〈定位〉在臀部,平第四骶后孔,骶正中嵴旁开3寸(图7)。〈层次解剖〉皮肤→皮下组织→臀大肌→臀中肌→臀小肌。浅层布有臀中皮神经和臀下皮神经。深层有臀上、下动、静脉和臀上、下神经。〈主治〉腰骶痛,下肢痿痹,大小便不利,阴痛,痔疾。直刺1.5～2.0寸;可灸。
Zhibian(BL 54) A meridian point, originally from *Zhenjiu Jia-Yi Jing* (*A-B Classic of Acupuncture and Moxibustion*), a point on the Bladder Meridian of Foot-Taiyang. 〈Location〉 on the buttock and on the level of the 4th posterior sacral foramen, 3 cun lateral to the median sacral crest (Fig. 7). 〈Regional anatomy〉 skin→subcutaneous tissue→greatest gluteal muscle→middle gluteal muscle→least gluteal muscle. In the superficial layer, there are the middle and inferior clunial nerves. In the deep layer, there are the superior and inferior gluteal arteries and veins, and the superior and inferior gluteal. 〈Indications〉 lumbosacral pain, flaccidity and numbness of the lower limbs, difficulty in urination and defecation, pain in the pudendum and hemorrhoids. 〈Method〉 Puncture perpendicularly 1.5～2.0 cun. Moxibustion is applicable.

●痔疮[zhì chuāng] 病证名。见《素问·生气通论》。是发生于肛肠部的一种慢性疾病。临床按痔核发生的位置,分为内痔,外痔,和混合痔,统称为痔疮。本病多因久坐久立,饮食失调,泻痢日久,长期便秘;或劳倦、胎产等引起肛肠气血不调,经脉阻滞,蕴生湿热所致。临床分湿热痔疮,气虚痔疮两类。详见各条。
Hemorrhoid A disease, seen in *Suwen: Shengqi Tong Tian Lun* (*Plain Questions: Treatise on the Communication of the Force of Life with Heaven*) referring to a chronic disease occurring in the anal and rectal region. Clinically, it is divided into internal hemorrhoid, external hemorrhoid and mixed hemor-

rhoid according to the location. It is commonly due to long-term sitting or standing, improper diet, protracted dysentery, diarrhea, and constipation, or overtiredness, pregnancy and labor, etc. which result in the derangement of qi and blood in the anal and rectal region, stagnation and stasis in the meridians and retention of damp-heat. It is clinically divided into hemorrhoid due to damp-heat pathogen, and hemorrhoid due to qi-deficiency. →湿热痔疮(p. 373)、气虚痔疮(p. 311)

●痔核点[zhì hé diǎn] 为肛门之别称见该条。

Hemorrhoid Nucleus(MA) Another name for Anus(MA-H 5). →肛门(p. 131)

●滞产[zhì chǎn] 病证名。见《千金要方》。又称难产,产难。是指产妇临产后总产程超过24小时者。临床可分气血虚弱、气滞血瘀二种。气血虚弱者,多因体质虚弱,正气不足;或产时用力过早,耗血伤气;或临床胞水早破,浆血干枯,以致气血虚弱,产力不足所致。证见产时腹部疼痛微弱,坠胀不甚,或下血量多,色淡,久产不下,面色苍白,神疲倦怠,心悸气短,脉大而虚或沉细而弱。治宜补养气血,益气催产。取足三里、三阴交、复溜、至阴。气滞血瘀者,多因妊娠期间过度安逸,导致气滞不行,血流不畅,或临产感受寒邪,寒凝气滞,气机不利所致。证见腰腹剧痛,下血量少,色黯红,久产不下,面色青黯,精神紧张,胸脘胀闷,时欲呕恶,舌质黯红,脉沉实而至数不匀。治宜理气行血,调气催产。取合谷、三阴交、独阴。

Protracted Labor A disease, seen in *Qianjin Yaofang* (*Prescriptions Worth a Thousand Gold*), also called difficult labor or delivery with difficulty, referring to delivery with parturition of more than 24 hours. In clinic, it may be divided into two types: ①Deficiency of qi and blood. This is mostly due to a weak constitution with poor vital-qi due to exhaustion of blood, and the impairment of qi because of earlier exertion of force during childbearing, or consumption of blood and fluid resulting from premature rupture of the amniotic membrane, leading to insufficiency of qi and blood and inadequate force of labour. ⟨Manifestations⟩ some dull paroxysnal pain with slightly heavy and distending sensations, or profuse and light-colored bleeding, prolonged course of delivery, pale complexion, fatigue and listlessness, palpitation and shortness of breath, large but empty, or deep, weak and thready pulse. ⟨Treatment principle⟩ Invigorate qi and nourish blood, tonify qi to promote labor. ⟨Point Selection⟩Zusanli(ST 36), Sanyinjiao(SP 6), Fuliu(KI 7), and Zhiyin(BL 67). ②Stagnation of qi and stasis of blood. This is mostly due to lack of antepartum exercises resulting in the stagnation of qi and stasis of blood, or due to the invasion of pathogenic cold during parturient, leading to stagnation of blood and disorder of qi. ⟨Manifestations⟩ sharp pain in the lower back and abdomen, scanty bleeding dark blood, protracted labor, bluish complexion, nervousness, distention and fullness in the chest and epigastrium, feeling nauseous and vomiting now and then, dark red tongue, deep, rapid but uneven pulse. ⟨Treatment principle⟩Regulate the flow of qi and activate blood circulation to promote labor. ⟨Point selection⟩Hegu(LI 4), Sanyinjiao(SP 6)and Duyin(EX-LE 11).

●滞下[zhì xià] 痢疾的古称。见《千金要方·脾病》。因排便有脓血粘腻,滞涩难下,故名。详见"痢疾"条。

Prolonged Defecation with Difficulty An archaic term for dysentery, seen in *Qianjin Yaofang* (*Essential Prescriptions Worth a Thousand Gold*), it is so named because of the prolonged and difficult defecation with purulent and bloody stools. →痢疾(p. 244)

●滞针[zhì zhēn] 针刺异常现象之一。在行针或留针后,医者感觉针下涩滞,捻转、提插、出针均感困难,而病人则感觉痛剧,称滞针。多因病人精神过度紧张致肌肉收缩或因捻转过度,留针过久,体位变动等情况引起。可在穴位旁轻轻按摩或在附近再刺一针,使滞针部肌肉放松,然后轻轻转动退出。

Stuck Needle An abnormal condition of acupuncture in which the doctor twirls, lifts or thrusts and withdraws the needle with difficulty and there is a stagnant feeling after inserting or retaining the needle. Meanwhile, the patient feels a sharp pain. The condition is mostly caused by local muscle spasm due to nervousness, or over-twirling, prolonged retaining of the needle or a change in the

patient's posture. In this condition the doctor can massage slightly around the point or insert another needle nearby to relax the state of the muscle spasm, and then gently twirl and withdraw the needle.

●置针[zhì zhēn] 为留针之别称。详见该条。

Retention of the Needle Another name for retaining the needle. →留针(p. 251)

●中病旁取[zhōng bìng páng qǔ] 《内经》取穴法则之一。指中部的病症取用其周围穴。参见"气反"条。

Selecting Side Points to Treat Diseases in the Middle One of the principles of point selection in *Neijing* (*The Canon of Internal Medicine*), referring to selecting points in the lateral areas to treat diseases in the middle. →气反(p. 304)

●中冲[zhōng chōng] 经穴名。出《灵枢·本输》。属手厥阴心包经,为本经井穴。〈定位〉在手指末节尖端中央(图49和图45)。〈层次解剖〉皮肤→皮下组织。布有正中神经的指掌侧固有神经末梢,指掌侧固动、静脉的动、静脉网。皮下组织内富含纤维束。纤维束外连皮肤,内连远节指骨骨膜。〈主治〉中风昏迷,舌强不语,中暑,昏厥,小儿惊风,热病,舌下肿痛。浅刺0.1寸;或点刺出血;可灸。

Zhongchong(PC 9) A meridian point, originally from *Lingshu:Benshu*(*Miraculous Pivot: Meridian Points*), the *Jing*(Well) point of the Pericardium Meridian of Hand-Jueyin. 〈Location〉 at the centre of the tip of the middle finger (Figs. 49&45). 〈Regional anatomy〉 skin →subcutaneous tissue. There are the terminal branches of the proper palmar digital nerve of the median nerve, and the arteriovenous network of the proper palmar digital arteries and veins in this area. Inside the subcutaneous tissue are the rich fiber bundles between the skin and the periosteum of the distal phalanx. 〈Indications〉apoplexy, coma, stiff tongue, aphasia, heatstroke, syncope, infantile convulsion, febrile diseases and sublingual swelling and pain. 〈Method〉Puncture shallowly 0.1 cun, or prick to cause bleeding. Moxibustion is applicable.

●中刺激[zhōng cì jī] 针灸术语。刺激强度介于强、弱刺激之间的针灸强度。〈操作〉以中等强度均匀的捻转、提插,病人反应明显但不强烈,有时针感也可向近处扩散;艾灸则予中等量的艾炷灸或艾条熏灸。

Moderate Stimulation An acupuncture-moxibustion term, referring to the stimulating intensity of acupuncture and moxibustion, between strong and weak stimulations. 〈Manipulation〉 The practitioner evenly twirls, lifts and thrusts the needle with a moderate stimulation intensity, the needling sensation of the patient is obvious but not too strong and sometimes spreads nearby. For moxibustion, a moderate amount of cones or sticks made of moxa should be used in fumigation.

●中都[zhōng dū] ①经穴名。出《针灸甲乙经》。属足厥阴肝经,为本经郄穴。又名中郄。〈定位〉在小腿内侧,当足内踝尖上7寸,胫骨内侧面的中央(图17.2和图81)。〈层次解剖〉皮肤→皮下组织→胫骨骨面。布有隐神经的小腿内侧皮支,大隐静脉。〈主治〉胁痛,腹胀,泄泻,疝气,小腹痛,崩漏,恶露不尽。平刺0.5~0.8寸;可灸。②经穴别名。出《针灸甲乙经》。即神门,见该条。③经外穴名。八邪之一。在手中指、无名指本节岐骨间。又名液门。〈主治〉手臂红肿,直刺0.1寸;可灸。

1. Zhongdu(LR 6) A meridian point, originally from *Zhenjiu Jia-Yi Jing* (*A-B Classic of Acupuncture and Moxibustion*), the Xi (Cleft) point of the Liver Meridian of Foot-Jueyin, also named Zhongxi. 〈Location〉on the medial side of the leg, 7 cun above the tip of the medial malleolus, on the midline of the medial surface of the tibia (Figs. 17.2&81). 〈Regional anatomy〉 skin→subcutaneous tissue→medial surface of tibia. There are the medial cutaneous branches of the leg from the saphenous nerve and the great saphenous vein in this area. 〈Indications〉 hypochondriac pain, abdominal distention, diarrhea, hernia, pain in the lower abdomen, metrorrhagia and metrostaxis, and lochiorrhea. 〈Method〉 Puncture subcutaneously 0.5~0.8 cun. Moxibustion is applicable.

2. Zhongdu Another name for Shenmen(HT 7), a meridian point originally from *Zhenjiu Jia-Yi Jing*(*A-B Classic of Acupuncture and Moxibustion*).→神门(p. 362)

3. **Zhongdu**(EX-UE)　　An extra point, one of the eight points of Baxie(EX-UE 9).〈Location〉between the bone junctures of the 3rd and 4th metacarpophalangeal joints.〈Indication〉redness and swelling of the hand and arm.〈Method〉Puncture perpendicularly 0.1 cun. Moxibustion is applicable.

●中渎[zhōng dú]　经穴名。出《针灸甲乙经》。属足少阳胆经。又名中犊、下犊。〈定位〉在大腿外侧,当风市下2寸,或在横纹上5寸,股外侧肌与股二头肌之间(图8.1和图8.3)。〈层次解剖〉皮肤→皮下组织→髂胫束→股外侧肌→股中间肌。浅层布有股外侧皮神经。深层有旋股外侧动、静脉降支的肌支和股神经的肌支。〈主治〉下肢痿痹,麻木,半身不遂。直刺1.0~1.5寸;可灸。

Zhongdu(GB 32)　　A meridian point, originally from *Zhenjiu Jia-Yi Jing*(*A-B Classic of Acupuncture and Moxibustion*), a point on the Gallbladder Meridian of Foot-Shaoyang, also named Zhongdu(中犊) and Xiadu.〈Location〉on the lateral side of the thigh, 2 cun. below Fengshi(GB 31) or 5 cun above the poplifeal crease, between the lateral vastus muscle and biceps muscle of the thigh(Figs. 8.1&8.3).〈Regional anatomy〉skin→subcutanous tissue→iliotibial tract→lateral vastus muscle of thigh→intermediate vastus muscle of thigh. In the superficial layer, there is the lateral cutaneous nerve of the thigh. In the deep layer, there are the muscular branches of the descending branches of the lateral circumflex femoral artery and vein and the muscular branches of the femoral nerve.〈Indications〉flaccidity, numbness and pain of the lower limbs and hemiplegia.〈Method〉Puncture perpendicularly 1.0~1.5 cun. Moxibustion is applicable.

●中犊[zhōng dú]　经穴别名。出《针灸甲乙经》。即中渎,见该条。

Zhongdu　　Another name for Zhongdu(GB 32), a meridian point originally from *Zhenjiu Jia-Yi Jing*(*A-B Classic of Acupuncture and Moxibustion*).→中渎(p.609)

●中封[zhōng fēng]　经穴名。出《灵枢·本输》。属足厥阴肝经,为本经经穴。又名悬泉。〈定位〉在足背侧,当足内踝前,商丘与解溪连线之间,胫骨前肌腱的内侧凹陷处(图17.2和图81)。〈层次解剖〉皮肤→皮下组织→胫骨前肌腱内侧→距骨和胫骨内踝之间。布有足背内侧皮神经的分支,内踝前动脉,足背浅静脉。〈主治〉疝气,阴茎痛,遗精,小便不利,黄疸,胸胁胀满,腰痛,足冷,内踝肿痛。直刺0.5~0.8寸;可灸。

Zhongfeng(LR 4)　　A meridian point, originally from *Lingshu*: *Ben Shu*(*Miraculous Pivot*: *Meridian Points*), the Jing(River)Point of the Liver Meridian of Foot-Jueyin, also named Xuanquan.〈Location〉on the instep of the foot, anterior to the medial malleolus, on the line connecting Shangqiu（SP 5）and Jiexi（ST 41）, in the depression medial to the tendon of the anterior tibial muscle(Figs. 17.2&81).〈Regional anatomy〉skin→subcutaneous tissue→medial side of tendon of anterior tibial muscle→between talus and medial malleolus of tibia. There are the branches of the medial dorsal cutaneous nerve of the foot, the medial anterior malleolar artery and the superficial dorsal vein of the foot in this area.〈Indications〉hernia, penis pain, seminal emission, difficulty in micturition, jaundice, fullness and distention in the chest and hypochondrium, lumbago, cold feet, swelling and pain of the medial malleolus.〈Method〉Puncture perpendicularly 0.5~0.8 cun. Moxibustion is applicable.

●中府[zhōng fǔ]　经穴名。出《针灸甲乙经》。属手太阴肺经,为本经募穴,手、足太阴交会穴。又名膺俞,膺中俞,膺中,府中俞,龙颔。〈定位〉在胸前壁的外上方,云门下1寸,平第1肋间隙,距前正中线6寸(图49和图23)。〈层次解剖〉皮肤→皮下组织→胸大肌→胸小肌→胸腔。浅层布有锁骨上中间神经、第一肋间神经外侧皮支,头静脉等。深层有胸肩峰动、静脉和胸内、外侧神经。〈主治〉咳嗽,气喘,胸中烦满,胸痛,肩背痛,腹胀,呕逆,喉痹,浮肿。向外斜刺0.5~0.8寸;可灸。不可向内侧深刺,免伤肺脏。

Zhongfu(LU 1)　　A meridian point, originally from *Zhenjiu Jia-Yi Jing*(*A-B Classic of Acupuncture and Moxibustion*), the front(mu) point of the Lung Merdian of Hand-Taiyin, the crossing point of the Meridians of Hand-Taiyin and Foot-Taiyin, also named Yingshu, Yingzhongshu, Yingzhong, Fuzhongshu or

Longhe. ⟨Location⟩ in the superior lateral part of the anterior thoracic wall, 1 cun below Yunmen(LU 2), on the level of the 1st intercostal space, 6 cun lateral to the anterior midline (Figs. 49&23). ⟨Regional anatomy⟩ skin→subcutaneous tissue→greater pectoral muscle→smaller pectoral muscle→axillary cavity. In the superficial layer, there are the intermediate supraclavicular nerve, the lateral cutaneous branches of the first intercostal nerve and the cephalic vein and so on. In the deep layer, there are the thoracoacromial artery and vein, the medial and lateral pectoral nerves. ⟨Indications⟩ cough, dyspnea, irritability and fullness in the chest, chest pain, pain in the shoulder and back, abdominal distention, vomiting, inflammation of the throat and edema. ⟨Method⟩ Puncture obliquely 0.5~0.8 cun towards the lateral. Moxibustion is applicable. ⟨Caution⟩ Do not puncture too deeply towards the medial side in case the lung is hurt.

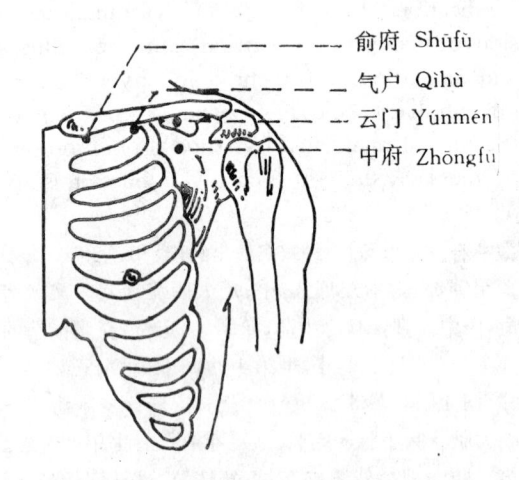

图75 中府和云门穴

Fig. 75 Zhongfu and Yunmen points

●中诰孔穴图经[zhōng gào kǒng xué tú jīng] 书名。撰人不详。见《素问·气府论》等篇，王冰注。

Zhonggao Kongxue Tujing (Zhong Gao Canon of Acupoints with Illustrations) A book, no details are known about its author, seen in Wang Bing's Annotation on *Suwen: Qifu Lun (Plain Questions: On Houses of Qi)*, etc.

●中管[zhōng guǎn] 经穴别名。出《脉经》。即中脘，见该条。

Zhongguan Another name for Zhongwan (RN 12), a meridian point originally from *Maijing (The Classic of Sphygmology)*. →中脘(p.614)

●中国针灸学[zhōng guó zhēn jiǔ xué] 书名。承淡庵著。1955年人民卫生出版社出版。全书分针科学、灸科学、经穴学及治疗学四篇。以经穴和治疗为主，且吸收近代研究成果。书中病名采用中西对照方式。

Zhongguo Zhenjiuxue (Chinese Acupuncture and Moxibustion) A book compiled by Cheng Dan'an and published by the People's Hygiene Press in 1955, composed of four chapters: Acupuncture, Moxibustion, Meridians and Points, and Therapeutics. Information on meridians, acupoints, treatment and also recent research achievements are collected. The names of diseases both in TCM and western medicine are given in contrast in the book.

●中国针灸治疗学[zhōng guó zhēn jiǔ zhì liáo xué] 书名。承淡庵编著。于1931年出版。全书全总论、经穴、手法、治疗四编。并辅以简要的汤剂丸散。后附内、外景两篇，作为分类选穴的参考。

Zhongguo Zhenjiu Zhiliao Xue (Therapeutics of Chinese Acupuncture and Moxibustion) A book compiled by Cheng Dan'an and published in 1931, which contains four chapters: General Treatise, Meridians and Acupoints, Manipulations, and Treatment, with brief prescriptions of decoction, pills and powders, and two chapters respectively on internal conditions and external conditions are appendixed at the end of the book, which serves as a reference to point classification and selection.

●中华针灸学[zhōng huá zhēn jiǔ xué] 书名。原名《针灸秘籍纲要》，赵尔康编著，1953年出版。全书分针科学、灸科学、经穴学、治疗学四编。经穴部分除有插图外，对每穴的主治作了较详的文献考证；治疗部分对每病的治法阐述了治理，并选录古代灸验方。

Zhonghua Zhenjiuxue (Acupuncture and Moxibustion of China) A book, originally entitled *Zhenjiu Mi Ji Gangyao (An Outline of Secret Books of Acupuncture and Moxibustion)*, written by Zhao Erkang, published in

1953, composed of four chapters: Acupuncture, Moxibustion, Meridians and Acupoints, and Therapeutics. In the chapters on meridians and acupoints, apart from illustrations, the author did detailed texual research on the indications of each point. In the chapter on therapeutics, the author expounded the therapeutic mechanisms on the treatment of various diseases, and selected some proven prescriptions of acupuncture and moxibustion of ancient times.

●中极[zhōng jí] 经穴名。出《素问·骨空论》。属任脉,为膀胱之募穴,足三阴、任脉之会。又名玉泉、气泉。〈定位〉在下腹部,前正中线上,当脐中下4寸(图40)。〈层次解剖〉皮肤→皮下组织→腹白线→腹横筋膜→腹膜外脂肪→壁腹膜。浅层主要布有髂腹下神经的前皮支和腹壁浅动、静脉的分支或属支。深层主要有髂腹下神经的分支。〈主治〉小便不利,遗溺不禁,阳萎,早泄,遗精,白浊,疝气偏坠,积聚疼痛,月经不调,阴痛,阴痒,痛经,带下,崩漏,阴挺,产后恶露不止,胞衣不下,水肿。直刺0.5～1.0寸,可灸。

Zhongji (RN 3) A meridian point, originally from *Suwen*: *Gu Kong Lun* (*Plain Questions*: *On the Apertures of Bones*), a point on the Ren Meridian, the Front (Mu) point of the bladder and the crossing point of the Three Yin Meridians of Foot and the Ren Meridian, also named Yuquan and Qiquan. 〈Location〉 on the lower abdomen and on the anterior midline, 4 cun below the centre of the umbilicus (Fig. 40). 〈Regional anatomy〉 skin→subcutaneous tissue→linea alba→transverse fascia→extraperitoneal fat tissue→parietal peritoneum. In the superficial layer, there are the anterior cutaneous branches of the iliohypogastric nerve and the branches or tributaries of the superficial epigastric artery and vein. In the deep layer, there are the branches of the iliohypogastric nerve. 〈Indications〉 difficulty in urination, enuresis, impotence, premature ejaculation, seminal emission, cloudy urine, hernia, abdominal mass with pain, irregular menstruation, pain or itching in the pudendum, dysmenorrhea, morbid leukorrhea, metrorrhagia and metrostaxis, prolapse of uterus, persistent lochia, retention of placenta and edema. 〈Method〉 Puncture perpendicularly 0.5～1.0 cun. Moxibustion is applicable.

●中肩井(zhōng jiān jǐng) 经穴别名。见《针灸甲乙经》。即肩髎。见该条。

Zhongjianjing Another name for Jianliao (SJ 14), a meridian point seen in *Zhenjiu Jia-Yi Jing* (*A-B Classic of Acupuncture and Moxibustion*).→肩髎(p. 189)

●中矩[zhōng jǔ] 经外穴名。见《医心方》。又名垂矩。在口腔下颌骨内侧,口底与齿龈粘膜移行部之中线处。主治中风,舌强不语,舌干燥等。直刺0.2～0.3寸。禁灸。

Zhongju (EX-HN) An extra point, seen in *Yi Xin Fang* (*The Heart of Medical Prescriptions*), also named Chuiju. 〈Location〉 in the mouth and inner side of the marrdible, at the intersection of the midline of the mouth base and gingival mucosa. 〈Indications〉 apoplexy, stiff tongue, aphasia and dry tongue, etc. 〈Method〉 Puncture perpendicularly 0.2～0.3 cun. Moxibustion is forbidden.

●中空[zhōng kōng] 经穴别名。出《针灸大成》。即中髎,见该条。

Zhongkong Another name for Zhongliao (BL 33), a meridian point originally from *Zhenjiu Dacheng* (*A Great Compendium of Acupuncture and Moxibustion*).→中髎(p. 612)

●中魁[zhōng kuí] ①经穴别名。出《针灸甲乙经》。即阳溪,见该条。②经外穴名。见《玉龙经》。〈定位〉在中指背侧近侧指间关节的中点处(图76)。〈层次解剖〉皮肤→皮下组织→指背腱膜。该处布有指背神经,其桡侧支来自桡神经,其尺侧支来自尺神经。血管有来自掌背动脉的指背动脉和掌背静脉网的属支指背静脉。〈主治〉呕吐、噎膈、鼻衄、牙痛、白癜风等。可灸。

1. **Zhongkui** Another name for Yangxi (LI 5), a meridian point originally from *Zhenjiu Jia-Yi Jing* (*A-B Classic of Acupuncture and Moxibustion*).→阳溪(p. 541)
2. **Zhongkui** (EX-UE 4) An extra point, seen in *Yulong Jing* (*Jade Dragon Classic*). 〈Location〉 on the dorsal side of the middle finger, at the centre of the proximal interphalangeal joint (Fig. 76). 〈Regional anatomy〉

skin → subcutaneous tissue → dorsal digital aponeurosis. There is the dorsal digital nerve in this area. Its radial branch originates from the radial nerve, and its ulnar branch originates from the ulnar nerve. There are the dorsal digital artery from the dorsal palmar artery and the dorsal digital vein to the dorsal venous network of the palm. 〈Indications〉vomiting, dysphagia, epistaxis, toothache and vitiligo, etc. 〈Method〉moxibustion.

●中髎[zhōng liáo] 经穴名。出《针灸甲乙经》。属足太阳膀胱经。又名中空。〈定位〉在骶部,当次髎下内方,适对第三骶后孔处(图7)。〈层次解剖〉皮肤→皮下组织→臀大肌→竖脊肌。浅层布有臀中皮神经。深层有第三骶神经和骶外侧动、静脉的后支。〈主治〉月经不调,赤白带下,腰痛,小便不利,便秘。直刺0.8～1.0寸;可灸。

Zhongliao(BL 33) A meridian point, originally from *Zhenjiu Jia-Yi Jing*(*A-B Classic of Acupuncture and Moxibustion*), a point on the Bladder Meridian of Foot-Taiyang, also named Zhongkong. 〈Location〉on the sacrum, medial and inferior to Ciliao(BL 32), just at the 3rd posterior sacral foramen (Fig. 7). 〈Regional anatomy〉skin → subcutaneous tissue→greatest gluteal muscle→erector spinal muscle. In the superficial layer, there is the middle clunial nerve. In the deep layer, there are the posterior branches of the 3rd sacral nerve and the lateral sacral artery and vein. 〈Indication〉irregular menstruation, leukorrhea with reddish discharge, lumbago, difficulty in urination and constipation. 〈Method〉Puncture perpendiculously 0.8～1.0 cun. Moxibustion is applicable.

●中膂[zhōng lǚ] 经穴别名。出《灵枢·刺节真邪》。即中膂俞,见该条。

Zhonglü Another name for Zhonglüshu(BL 29), a meridian point originally from *Lingshu*: *Ci Jie Zhen Xie*(*Miraculous Pivot*: *Acupuncture Principles and Diseases*). →中膂俞(p. 612)

●中膂内俞[zhōng lǚ nèi shū] 经穴别名。见《铜人腧穴针灸图经》。即中膂俞,见该条。

Zhonglüneishu Another name for Zhonglüshu(BL 29), a meridian point, seen in *Tongren Shuxue Zhenjiu Tujing*(*Illustrated Manual of Acupoints for Acupuncture and Moxibustion on a Bronze Statue with Acupoints*). →中膂俞(p. 612)

●中胂输[zhōng lǚ shū] 经穴别名。出《备急千金要方》。即中膂俞。见该条。

Zhonglüshu Another name for Zhonglüshu (中膂俞)(BL 29), a meridian point originally from *Beiji Qianjin Yaofang*(*Prescriptions Worth a Thousand Gold for Emergencies*). →中膂俞(p. 612)

●中膂俞[zhōng lǚ shū] 经穴名。出《针灸甲乙经》。属足太阳膀胱经。又名中膂内俞、中膂、中胂输、脊内俞。〈定位〉在骶部,当骶正中嵴旁1.5寸,平第三骶后孔(图7)。〈层次解剖〉皮肤→皮下组织→臀大肌→骶结节韧带。浅层布有臀中皮神经。深层有臀上、下动、静脉的分支或属支及臀下神经的属支。〈主治〉痢疾,疝气,腰脊强痛,消渴。直刺0.8～1.0寸;可灸。

Zhonglüshu(BL 29) A meridian point, originally from *Zhenjiu Jia-Yi Jing*(*A-B Classic of Acupuncture and Moxibustion*), a point on the Bladder Meridian of Foot-Taiyang, also named Zhonglüneishu, Zhonglü, Zhonglüshu, and Jineishu. 〈Location〉on the sacrum and on the level of the 3rd posterior sacral foramen, 1.5 cun lateral to the median sacral crest (Fig. 7). 〈Regional anatomy〉skin → subcutaneous tissue→greatest gluteal muscle→sacrotuberous ligament. In the superficial layer, there are the middle clunial nerves. In the deep layer, there are the branches or tributaries of the superior and inferior gluteal arteries and veins and the branches of the inferior gluteal nerve. 〈Indications〉dysentery, hernia, stiffness and pain along the spinal column and diabetes. 〈Method〉Puncture perpendicularly 0.8～1.0 cun. Moxibustion is applicable.

●中平[zhōng píng] 经外穴名。见《经外奇穴治疗诀》。在中指指掌横纹中央。〈主治〉口腔炎。直刺0.2～0.3寸;可灸。

Zhongping(EX-UE) An extra point, seen in *Jingwai Qixue Zhiliao Jue*(*Pithy Formulas for Treatment with Extra Acupoints*). 〈Location〉at the midpoint of palmar transverse crease of the middle finger. 〈Indication〉stom-

atitis. 〈Method〉Puncture perpendicularly 0.2~0.3 cun. Moxibustion is applicable.

●中气法[zhōng qì fǎ] 针刺手法名。出《针灸大成》。为纳气法之别称。见该条。

Qi-Intaking Method Another name for Qi-receiving method, an acupuncture manipulation originally from *Zhenjiu Dacheng*(*A Great Compendium of Acupuncture and Moxibustion*). →纳气法(p. 275)

●中泉[zhōng quán] 经外穴名。出《奇效良方》。〈定位〉在腕背侧横纹中,当指总伸肌腱桡侧的凹陷处。〈层次解剖〉皮肤→皮下组织→指伸肌腱与桡侧腕短伸肌腱之间。该处布有前臂后皮神经和桡神经浅支的分支,手背静脉网,桡动脉腕背支的分支。〈主治〉心痛,胸中气满不得卧,肺胀满膨膨然,目中白翳,掌中热,胃气上逆,唾血及腹中诸气痛等。直刺0.3~0.5寸;可灸。

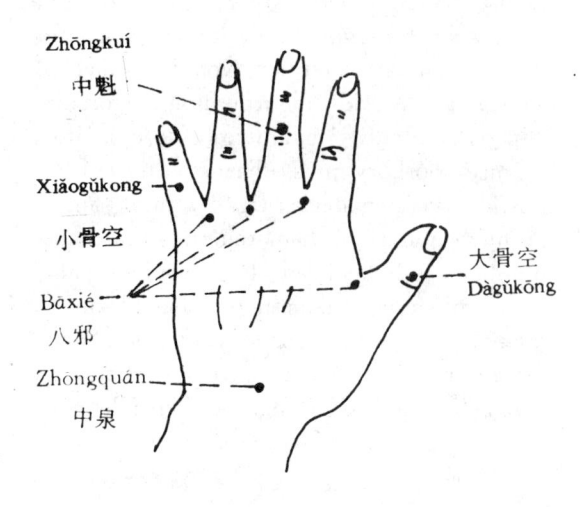

图76 中泉等经外穴(手背部)
Fig. 76 Zhongquan and other extra points (Dorsum of hand)

Zhongquan(EX-UE 3) An extra point originally from *Qixiao Liangfang* (*Prescriptions with Wonderful Efficacy*). 〈Location〉on the dorsal crease of the wrist, in the depression on the radial side of the tendon of the common extensor muscle of the fingers. 〈Regional anatomy〉 skin → subcutaneous tissue → between tendons of extensor muscle and short radial extensor muscle of wrist. There are posterior cutaneous nerve of the forearm, the branches of the superficial branch of the radial nerve, the dorsal venous network of the hand and the branches of the dorsal carpal branch of the artery in this area. 〈Indications〉precordial pain, fullness of qi in the chest and failure of the body to lie down, severe distention and fullness of the lung, nebula, adverse rising of stomach qi, feverish sensation in the palms, spitting blood and pain due to disorder of qi in the abdomen. 〈Method〉Puncture perpendicularly 0.3~0.5 cun. Moxibustion is applicable.

●中守[zhōng shǒu] 经穴别名。出《备急千金要方》。即水分,见该条。

Zhongshou Another name for Shuifen(RN 9), a meridian point originally from *Beiji Qianjin Yaofang*(*Prescriptions Worth a Thousand Gold for Emergencies*). →水分(p. 409)

●中枢[zhōng shū] 经穴名。出《素问·气府论》。王冰注。属督脉。又名中柱。〈定位〉在背部,当后正中线上,第十胸椎棘突下凹陷中(图12.2和图7)。〈层次解剖〉针刺经过的层次结构同脊中穴。浅层主要布有第十胸神经后支的内侧皮支和伴行的动、静脉。深层有棘突间的椎外(后)静脉丛,第十胸神经后支的分支和第十肋间后动、静脉背侧支的分支或属支。〈主治〉黄疸,呕吐,腹满,胃痛,食欲不振,腰背痛。斜刺0.5~1寸;可灸。

Zhongshu(DU 7) A meridian point, originally from *Su Wen*: *Qi Fu Lun*(*Plain Questions*: *On House of Qi*), annotated by Wang Bing, a point on the Du Meridian, also named Zhongzhu. 〈Location〉on the back and on the posterior midline, in the depression below the spinous process of the 10th thoracic vertebra (Figs. 12.2&7). 〈Regional anatomy〉 the layer structures of the needle insertion are the same as those in Jizhong(DU 6). In the superficial layer, there are the medial cutaneous branches of the posterior branches of the 10th thoracic nerve and the accompanying artery and vein. In the deep layer, there are the external(posterior) vertebral venous plexus between the adjacent spinous processes, the branches of the posterior branches of the 10th thoracic nerve and the branches or tributaries

of the dorsal branches of the 10th posterior intercostal artery and vein. 〈Indications〉jaundice, vomiting, fullness of the abdomen, stomachache, poor appetite and pain in the loin and back. 〈Method〉Puncture obliquely 0.5～1.0 cun. Moxibustion is applicable.

●**中庭**[zhōng tíng] 经穴名。出《针灸甲乙经》。属任脉。又名龙颔。〈定位〉在胸部,当前正中线上,平第5肋间,即胸剑结合部(图43.2和图40)。〈层次解剖〉皮肤→皮下组织→胸肋辐状韧带和肋剑突韧带→胸剑结合部。布有第六肋间神经的前皮支和胸廓内动、静脉的穿支。〈主治〉胸腹胀满,噎膈,呕吐,心痛,梅核气。平刺0.3～0.5寸;可灸。

Zhongting(RN 16) A meridian point, originally from *Zhenjiu Jia-Yi Jing*(*A-B Classic of Acupuncture and Moxibustion*), a point on the Ren Meridian, also named Longhe. 〈Location〉on the chest and on the anterior midline, on the level of the 5th intercostal space, on the xiphosternal synchondrosis (Figs. 43. 2&40). 〈Regional anatomy〉 skin→subcutaneous tissue → radiate sternocostal ligament and costoxiphoid ligament→xiphosternal synchondrosis. There are the anterior cutaneous branches of the 6th intercostal nerve and the perforating branches of the internal thoracic artery and vein in this area. 〈Indications〉distention and fullness in the chest and abdomen, dysphagia, vomiting, precordial pain and globus hystericus. 〈Method〉Puncture subcutaneously 0.3～0.5 cun. Moxibustion is applicable.

●**中脘**[zhōng wǎn] 经穴名。出《针灸甲乙经》。属任脉,为胃之募穴,又为手太阳、少阳,足阳明、任脉之会。为八会穴之腑会。又名太仓、大仓、胃脘、胃管、中管、上纪。〈定位〉在上腹部,前正中线上,当脐中上4寸(图43.2和图40)。〈层次解剖〉皮肤→皮下组织→腹白线→腹横筋膜→腹膜外脂肪→壁腹膜。浅层主要布有第八胸神经前支的前皮支和腹壁浅静脉的属支。深层主要布有第八胸神经的前支分支。〈主治〉胃脘痛,腹胀,呕吐,呃逆,翻胃,吞酸,纳呆,食谷不化,疳积,膨胀,黄疸,肠鸣,泄利,便秘,便血,胁下坚痛,虚劳吐血,哮喘,头痛,失眠,惊悸,怔忡,脏躁,癫狂,痫证,尸厥,惊风,产后血晕。直刺0.5～1.0寸;可灸。

Zhongwan(RN 12) A meridian point, originally from *Zhenjiu Jia-Yi Jing*(*A-B Classic of Acupuncture and Moxibustion*), a point on the Ren Meridian, the Front(Mu) point of the stomach, the crossing point of the Meridians of Hand-Taiyang, Hand-Shaoyang, Foot-Yangming, and the Ren meridian, the influential point of fu organs, also named Taicang, Dacang, Weiwan, Weiguan, Zhongguan and Shangji. 〈Location〉 on the upper abdomen and on the anterior midline, 4 cun above the centre of the umbilicus(Figs. 43. 2&40). 〈Regional anatomy〉 skin→subcutaneous tissue→ linea alba→transverse fascia→extraperitoneal fat tissue→parietal peritoneurn. In the superficial layer, there are the anterior cutaneous branches of the anterior branch of the 8th thoracic nerve and the tributaries of the superficial epigastric vein. In the deep layer, there are the branches of the anterior branch of the 8th thoracic nerve. 〈Indications〉 epigastric pain, abdominal distention, vomiting, hiccup, regurgitation, acid regurgitation, anorexia, dyspepsia, infantile malnutrition, tympanites, jaundice, borborygmus, diarrhea, dysentery, constipation, hemafecia, rigidity and pain in the hypochondrium, hematemesis due to consumption, asthma, headache, insomnia, palpitation, hysteria, manic-depressive disorder, epilepsy, corpse-like syncope, infantile convulsion and postpartum syncope due to deficiency of blood. 〈Method〉Puncture perpendicularly 0.5～1.0 cun. Moxibustion is applicable.

●**中恶**[zhōng wù] 经外穴名。见《医宗金鉴》。在胸侧部,乳头外侧3寸许,约当第四肋间隙。〈主治〉疰忤,腹痛,胸胁痛,肋间神经痛等。用灸法。

Zhongwu(EX-CA) An extra point, seen *in Yizong Jinjian*(*The Gold Mirror of Orthodox Medical Lineage*). 〈Location〉on the lateral side of the chest, about 3 cun lateral to nipples, in the 4th intercostal space. 〈Indications〉 latent disease, abdominal pain, pain in the chest and hypochondrium and intercostal neuralgia, etc. 〈Method〉 moxibustion.

●**中郄**[zhōng xì] ①经穴别名。出《针灸甲乙经》。即中都,见该条。②经穴别名。见《中国针灸学》。即委中,见该条。

Zhongxi Another name for ①Zhongdu（LR 6）, a meridian point originally from *Zhenjiu Jia-Yi Jing*（*A-B Classic of Acupuncture and Moxibustion*）.→中都（p.608）②Weizhong（BL 54）, a meridian point originally from *Zhongguo Zhenjiuxue*（*Chinese Acupuncture and Moxibustion*）.→委中（p.461）

●中消[zhōng xiāo] 消渴证型之一。出《丹溪心法·消渴》。由脾胃积热，化燥伤津所致。证见食量倍增，消谷善饥，嘈杂，烦热，多汗，形体消瘦，或见大便干结。兼见多饮多尿，舌苔黄燥，脉滑数。治宜清胃泻火，调中养阴。针脾俞，胃俞，三阴交，内庭，足三里，胰俞。

Diabetes Involving the Middle-Jiao A type of diabetes, originally from *Danxi Xinfa：Xiao Ke*（*Danxi's Experience：Diabetes*）, due to accumulation of heat in the spleen and the stomach. The heat transforms into dryness, resulting in impairment of the body fluid.〈Manifestations〉polyphagia, polyorexia, gastric discomfort with acid regurgitation, restlessness with feverish sensation, hyperhidrosis, emaciation, or constipation with dry stools, accompanied by polydipsia, polyuria, dry and yellowish tongue coating, slippery and rapid pulse.〈Treatment principle〉Clear heat and fire in the stomach; regulate the functions of the middle jiao and nourish yin.〈Point selection〉Pishu（BL 20）, Weishu（BL 21）, Sanjinjiao（SP 6）, Neiting（ST 44）, Zusanli（ST 36）and Yishu（EX-B）.

●中指节[zhōng zhǐ jié] 经外穴名。见《千金翼方》。又名中指之节，手中指第一节穴。在手中指背侧，远端指节横纹中点稍前方凹陷中。灸治牙齿痛。

Zhongzhijie（EX-UE） An extra point, seen in *Qianjin Yifang*（*A Supplement to the Essential Prescriptions Worth a Thousand Gold*）, also named Zhongzhizhijie or Shouzhongzhi diyijiexue.〈Location〉on the dorsal side of the middle finger, in the depression slightly distal to the midpoint of the oreast the distal interphalangeal joint.〈Indication〉toothache.〈Method〉moxibustion.

●中指同身寸[zhōng zhǐ tóng shēn cùn] 同身寸的一种。即以患者的中指中节桡侧两端纹头（拇中指屈曲成环形）之间的距离作为一寸。

Middle Finger Cun A proportional unit of the body. When the middle finger and the thumb are bent to form a circle, the distance between the two radial ends of the creases of the interphalangeal joints is taken as one cun.

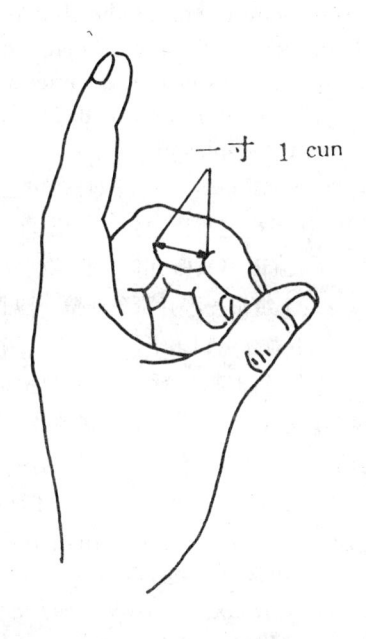

图77 中指寸
Fig. 77 Middle finger cun

●中渚[zhōng zhǔ] 经穴名。出《灵枢·本输》。属手少阳三焦经，为本经输穴。又名下都。〈定位〉在手背部，当环指本节（掌指关节）的后方，第四、五掌骨间凹陷处（图48和图44.4）。〈层次解剖〉皮肤→皮下组织→第四骨肌背侧肌。浅层布有尺神经的指背神经，手背静脉网的尺侧部。深层有第四掌背动脉等结构。〈主治〉头痛，目眩，目赤，目痛，耳聋，耳鸣，喉痹，肩背肘臂酸痛，手指不能屈伸，脊膂痛，热病，直刺0.3～0.5寸；可灸。

Zhongzhu（SJ 3） A meridian point, originally from *Lingshu：Benshu*（*Miraculous Pivot：Meridian Points*）, a point on the Sanjiao Meridian of Hand-Shaoyang, also named Xiadu.〈Location〉on the dorsum of the hand, proximal to the 4th metacarpophalangeal joint, in the depression between the 4th and 5th metacarpal bones（Figs. 48&44.4）.〈Regional anatomy〉skin→subcutaneous tissue→4th dorsal interosseous muscle. In the superfi-

cial layer, there are the dorsal digital nerve of the ulnar nerve and the ulnar part of the dorsal venous network of the hand. In the deep layer, there is the 4th dorsal metacarpal artery. 〈Indications〉headache, dizziness, redness and pain of the eye, deafness, tinnitus, sore throat, aching pain of the shoulder, back, elbow and arm, motor impairment of fingers, pain of the muscles near the spine and febrile diseases. 〈Method〉Puncture 0.3～0.5 cun. Moxibustion is applicable.

●中注[zhōng zhù] 经穴名。出《针灸甲乙经》。属足少阴肾经,为冲脉、足少阴之会。〈定位〉在中腹部,当脐中下一寸,前正中线旁开0.5寸(图40)。〈层次解剖〉皮肤→皮下组织→腹直肌鞘前壁→腹直肌。浅层布有脐周皮下静脉网和第十、十一、十二胸神经前支的前皮支及伴行的动、静脉。深层有腹壁下动、静脉的分支或属支,第十、十一、十二胸神经前支的肌支及相应的肋间动、静脉。〈主治〉月经不调,腰腹疼痛,大便燥结,泄泻,痢疾。直刺0.8～1.2寸;可灸。

Zhongzhu (KI 15) A meridian point, originally from *Zhenjiu Jia-Yi Jing* (*A-B Classic of Acupuncture and Moxibustion*), a point on the Kidney Meridian of Foot-Shaoyin. 〈Location〉on the lower abdomen, 1 cun below the centre of the umbilicus and 0.5 cun lateral to the anterior midline (Fig. 40). 〈Regional anatomy〉skin→subcutaneous tissue→anterior sheath of rectus muscle of abdomen→rectus muscle of abdomen. In the superficial layer, there are the periumbilical subcutaneous venous network, the anterior cutaneous branches of the anterior branches of the 10th to 12th thoracic nerves and the accompanying arteries and veins. In the deep layer, there are the branches or tributaries of the inferior epigastric artery and vein, the muscular branches of the anterior branches of the 10th to 12th thoracic nerves and the related intercostal arteries and veins. 〈Indications〉irregular menstruation, pain of the loin and abdomen, constipation, diarrhea and dysentery. 〈Method〉Puncture 0.8～1.2 cun. Moxibustion is applicable.

●中柱[zhōng zhù] 经穴别名。出《医学入门》。即中枢,见该条。

Zhongzhu Another name for Zhongshu (DU 7), a meridian point originally from *Yixue Rumen* (*An Introduction to Medicine*). →中枢(p. 613)

●踵[zhǒng] 部位名。指足跟部。

Heel A part of the body, referring to the hindmost part of the foot.

●中风[zhòng fēng] 病证名。见《灵枢·邪气藏府病形》等篇。亦称卒中。指猝然昏仆,不省人事,或突然口眼喎斜,半身不遂,言语不利的病证。多由年高气衰,劳累太过,肾阴不足,肝阳偏亢,阴阳相失,气血逆乱所致。忧思,恼怒,嗜酒等常可诱发本病。临床分为中脏腑,中经络两种证型。详见各条。

Apoplexy A disease, from *Lingshu: Xieqi Zangfu BingXing* (*Miraculous Pivot: Pathogenic Evils, ZangFu Organs and Manifestations*), also named apoplectic stroke. 〈Manifestations〉sudden syncope, distortion of face, hemiplegia and dysphasia. Mostly due to qi-deficiency with agedness, overstrain and the rising of liver yang caused by insufficiency of kidney yin, leading to imbalance of yin and yang and derangement of qi and blood. Melancholy, anger and addiction to drink are common predisposing causes of the disease. It is divided into apoplexy involving zang and fu and apoplexy involving the meridians and collaterals. →中脏腑(p. 618)、中经络(p. 617)

●中风不语穴[zhòng fēng bù yǔ xué] 经外穴名。见《经穴治疗学》。在背部,当第2及第5胸椎棘突高点处。〈主治〉中风不语。用灸法。

Zhongfengbuyuxue (EX-B) An extra point, originally from *Jing Xue Zhiliao Xue* (*Therapeutics of Acupuncture Points*). 〈Location〉on the back, at the high point of the spinous processes of the 2nd and 5th thoracic vertebra. 〈Indications〉aphasia from apoplexy. 〈Method〉Moxibustion.

●中风七穴[zhòng fēng qī xué] 指治疗中风的七个经验穴。见《太平圣惠方》。一、百会;二、耳前发际;三、肩井;四、风市;五、足三里;六、绝骨;七、曲池。〈主治〉中风,言语蹇涩,半身不遂。同时灸此七穴。

Seven Points for Apoplexy The seven experienced points used to treat apoplexy, originally from *Tai Ping Shenghui Fang* (*Imperial Benevolent Prescriptions*). They are Baihui

(DU 20), Erqianfaji(耳前发际), Jianjing(GB 21), Fengshi(GB 31), Zusanli(ST 36), Juegu(GB 39) and Quchi(LI 11).〈Indications〉apoplexy, aphasia, hemiplegia.〈Method〉moxibustion on the 7 points at the same time.

●中经络[zhòng jīng luò] 中风证型之一。多因肝风内动,痰浊瘀血阻滞经络所致。病位较浅,病情较轻。证见半身不遂,麻木不仁,口眼歪斜,舌强语涩,神志尚清,多愁善怒,舌苔黄腻,脉弦劲或缓滑。证宜醒脑开窍,通经活络。取内关、水沟、极泉、少海、委中、三阴交。口角㖞斜取地仓、颊车、合谷。舌强语涩取哑门、廉泉、通里。初病宜泻,久病宜补。

Apoplexy Involving the Meridians and Collaterals A type of apoplexy, mostly caused by the stirring of liver wind in the interior, and the block of the meridians and collaterals due to phlegm and blood stagnation. The position of the disease is shallower and the condition milder.〈Manifestations〉hemiplegia, numbness, distortion of the face, dysphasia, consciousness, emotional ability, yellow and greasy coating of the tongue, spring-taut pulse or leisurely and slippery pulse.〈Treatment principle〉Activiate the brain and regain consciousness; clear and activate the meridians and collaterals.〈Point selection〉Neiguan(PC 6), Shuigou(DU 26), Jiquan(HT 1), Shaohai(HT 3), Weizhong(BL 40), Sanyinjiao(SP 6).〈Supplementary points〉For deviation of the mouth, add Dicang(ST 4), Jiache(ST 6), and Hegu(LI 4); for stiff tongue and dysphasia, add Yamen(DU 15), Lianquan(RN 23) and Tongli(HT 5).〈Method〉Reducing is appropriate for patients in the early stage of the disease and reinforcing for patients affected for a long time.

●中暑[zhòng shǔ] 病名。见《三因极一病证方论·叙中暑论》。亦称中暍。指夏季气候炎热,感受暑邪而发生的一种急性病证。由于病情程度的轻重和证候表现各异,可分为中暑轻证和重证。详见各条。

Heatstroke A disease originally from *Sanyin Ji Yi Bing Zheng Fang Lun: Xu Zhong Shu Lun* (*Treatise on the Three Categories of Pathogenic Factors of Diseases and the Prescriptions: Introduction to Heatstroke*), also named sunstroke, referring to the acute disease which is caused by the attack of pathogenic summer-heat in hot summer, divided into mild heatstroke and serious heatstroke according to the seriousness and manifestations of the disease. →中暑轻证(p. 617)、中暑重证(p. 617)

●中暑轻证[zhòng shǔ qīng zhèng] 中暑证型之一。由于暑热夹湿,郁于肌表所致。证见头晕,头痛,身热,少汗,懊憹,呕吐,烦渴,倦怠思睡,舌苔白腻,脉濡数。治宜解表清暑,和中化湿。取大椎、合谷、陷谷、内关、足三里。

Mild Heatstroke A type of heatstroke, due to stagnant summer-heat and dampness in the exterior part of the body.〈Manifestations〉dizziness, headache, fever, lack of perspiration, heartburn, vomiting, restlessness, thirst, lassitude, and drowsiness, white and greasy coating of the tongue, soft and rapid pulse.〈Treatment principle〉Eliminate summer-heat from the body by diaphoresis, and regulate the function of the middle-Jiao to dispel dampness.〈Point selection〉Dazhui(DU 14), Hegu(LI 4), Xiangu(ST 43), Neiguan(PC 6) and Zusanli(ST 36).

●中暑重证[zhòng shǔ zhòng zhèng] 中暑证型之一。由暑热燔灼,蒙蔽心包所致。证见壮热无汗,肌肤灼热,面红目赤,口唇干燥,烦渴多饮,神志昏迷,烦燥不安,抽搐,瘈疭,舌红少津,苔黄,脉洪数。甚则热盛而气阴两伤,汗出如珠,面色苍白,呼吸浅促,四肢逆冷,昏迷深沉,舌绛少苔,脉细数无力。治宜清泄暑热,醒神。取水沟、十宣、曲泽、委中、曲池。意在急救。

Serious Heatstroke A type of heatstroke, due to the burning of summer-heat which leads to mental confusion.〈Manifestations〉high fever, lack of perspiration, red face and eyes, dry lips, morbid thirst, coma, restlessness, convulsion, clonic convulsion, red tongue with little body fluid, yellow coating, surging and rapid pulse. Severe cases are manifested by the deficiency of both qi and yin due to the domination of heat, profuse perspiration, pale face, short breath, cold limbs, deep coma, deep red tongue with little coating, thin, rapid and weak pulse.〈Treatment principle〉Clear summer-heat and regain consciousness.〈Point selection〉Shuigou(DU 26), Shixuan(EX-UE

11), Quze (PC 3), Weizhong (BL 40) and Quchi (LI 11). These points are punctured for first-aid.

●中暍[zhòng yè] 古病名。出《金匮要略·痉湿暍病脉证并治》。即中暑。详见该条。

Sunstroke An archaic name of a disease, originally from *Jingui Yaolüe: Jing Shi Ye Bing Mai Zheng Bing Zhi* (*Synopsis of the Gold Chamber: Pulse Conditions, Symptoms and Treatments of Convulsions, Dampness and Summer-Heat Syndromes*). →中暑(p. 617)

●中脏腑[zhòng zàng fǔ] 中风证型之一。多因风阳暴升,与痰火相搏,迫使血气并走于上,蒙蔽心窍所致。病位较深,病情较重,证见肢体瘫痪,神昏,失语等脏腑失调证候。根据病因病机不同,又可分为中脏腑闭证和中脏腑脱证。详见各条。

Apoplexy Involving Zang and Fu A type of apoplexy, mostly due to the sudden upward movement wind-yang and phlegm-fire stirring each other up, leading to upward qi and blood and mental confusion. The position of the disease is relatively deep, and the condition relatively serious. 〈Manifestations〉 paralysis of limbs, coma and aphasia, etc., as caused by the imbalance of zang and fu. According to the different aetiology and pathogenesis, it is further classified into excess-syndrome of the apoplexy involving zang and fu and collapse-syndrome of the apoplexy involving zang and fu. →中脏腑闭证(p. 618)、中脏腑脱证(p. 618)

●中脏腑闭证[zhòng zàng fǔ bì zhèng] 中风中脏腑证型之一。多因气火冲逆,血菀于上,肝火鸱张,痰浊壅盛所致。证见神志不清,牙关紧闭,两手握固,面赤,气粗,喉中痰鸣,大小便閉塞,苔黄腻,脉弦滑而数。治宜熄风开窍,清心豁痰。取水沟、十二井、太冲、丰隆、劳宫。可刺络。

Excess-Syndrome of Apoplexy Involving Zang and Fu One type of apoplexy involving zang and fu, mostly due to the reversed flow of qi and fire, blood stasis in the upper part, hyperactivity of liver-fire and abundant expectoration. 〈Manifestations〉 unconsciousness, trismus, clenched fist, red face, short breath, rale in the throat, constipation, anuresis, yellow and greasy coating of the tongue, spring-taut, slippery and rapid pulse. 〈Treatment principle〉 Calm the endopathic wind and regain consciousness; remove heat from the heart and eliminate phlegm. 〈Point selection〉 Shuigou (DU 26), the Twelve Jing (Well) points, Taichong (LR 3), Fenglong (ST 40), Laogong (PC 8). 〈Method〉 Collateral puncture is applicable.

●中脏腑脱证[zhòng zàng fǔ tuō zhèng] 中风中脏腑证型之一。由于真气衰微,元阳暴脱所致。证见昏沉不醒,目合,口张,手撒,遗尿,鼻鼾息微,四肢逆冷,舌痿,脉细弱或沉微。治宜益气,回阳,固脱。取百会、关元、神阙、足三里。重灸。

Collapse-Syndrome of Apoplexy Involving Zang and Fu A type of apoplexy involving zang and fu, due to the deficiency of genuine qi and the sudden collapse of the primary-yang. 〈Manifestations〉 deep coma, closing of eyes, opening of mouth, relaxed hand, incontinence of urine, nasal snore, respiratory failure, cold limbs, flaccid tongue, thin and weak pulse, or deep and feeble pulse. 〈Treatment principle〉 Supplement qi, restore yang and arrest collapse. 〈Point selection〉 Baihui (DU 20), Guanyuan (RN 4), Shenque (RN 8), Zusanli (ST 36). 〈Method〉 moxibustion with more or bigger moxa cones.

●周谷[zhōu gǔ] 经穴别名。即二间,见该条。

Zhougu Another name for the meridian point Erjian (LI 2). →二间(p. 101)

●周汉卿[zhōu hàn qīng] 人名。元明间针灸家。松阳(今属浙江)人。通医兼外科,尤善针灸,治疗有神效。事见《明史》、《宋濂集》。

Zhou Hanqing An acupuncture-moxibustion expert of the Yuan and Ming Dynasties, a native of Songyang (in Zhejiang Province today). Conversant with medical science and external diseases, he was especially good at acupuncture and moxibustion with miraculous therapeutic effect. His deeds are seen in *Mingshi* (*History of the Ming Dynasty*) and *Song Lian Ji* (*A Collection of Song Lian*).

●周荣[zhōu róng] 经穴名。《针灸甲乙经》名周营,《备急千金方》后诸书名周荣。属足太阴脾经。〈定位〉在胸外侧部,当第二肋间隙,距前正中线6寸(图39.3和图23)。〈层次解剖〉皮肤→皮下组织→胸大肌→胸

小肌。浅层布有第二肋间神经的外侧皮支和浅静脉。深层有胸内、外侧神经和胸肩峰动、静脉的胸肌支。〈主治〉胸胁胀满,咳嗽,气喘,胁肋痛,食不下。平刺或斜刺0.5～0.8寸;可灸。

Zhourong (SP 20)　A meridian point, named Zhouying in *Zhenjiu Jia-Yi Jing* (*A-B Classic of Acupuncture and Moxibustion*). Zhourong is named in books after *Beiji Qianjin Fang* (*Essential Prescriptions Worth a Thousand Gold for Emergencies*), a point on the Spleen Meridian of Foot-Taiyin. 〈Location〉 on the lateral side of the chest and in the 2nd intercostal space, 6 cun lateral to the anterior midline (Figs. 39.3 & 23). 〈Regional anatomy〉 skin → subcutaneous tissue → great pectoral muscle → smaller pectoral muscle. In the superficial layer, there are the lateral cutaneous branches of the 2nd intercostal nerve and the superficial vein. In the deep layer, there are the medial pectoral nerve, the lateral pectoral nerve and the pectoral branches of the thoracoacromial artery and vein. 〈Indications〉 distention and fullness in the chest and hypochondrium, cough, dyspnea, pain of hypochondrium, loss of appetite. 〈Method〉 Puncture horizontally or obliquely 0.5～0.8 cun. Moxibustion is applicable.

●**周营**[zhōu yíng]　经穴别名。出《针灸甲乙经》。即周荣,见该条。

Zhouying　Another name for Zhourong (SP 20), a meridian point, originally from *Zhenjiu Jia-Yi Jing* (*A-B Classic of Acupuncture and Moxibustion*). →周荣(p.618)

●**肘**[zhōu]　耳穴名。位于将耳舟部分为六等份,自上而下,第三等份为肘。用于治疗肘部疾患、肱骨外上髁炎、甲状腺疾患。

Elbow (MA-SF 3)　An ear point. 〈Location〉 Divide the scapha area into six equal parts, the third from superior is the point. 〈Indications〉 diseases in the elbow area, external humeral epicondylitis and diseases of the thyroid gland.

●**肘后备急方**[zhǒu hòu bèi jí fāng]　书名。初名为《肘后救卒方》。简称《肘后方》。八卷。晋·葛洪撰。本书是作者将其所撰《玉函方》中摘录可供急救医疗,实用有验的单验方及简要灸法汇编而成。书中介绍了一百多个针灸医方,其中大多是灸法,而且对危重病症灸法记载较多。

Zhouhou Beiji Fang (*A Handbook of Prescriptions for Emergencies*)　A book, originally entitled *Zhouhou Jiu Cu Fang* (*A Handbook of Prescriptions for emergencies*) and *Zhouhou Fang* (*A Handbook of Prescriptions*) for short, in 8 volumes, written by Ge Hong in the Jin Dynasty. The present book is an extraction of some practical and effective prescriptions for emergency and simple moxibustion methods from *Yu Han Fang* (*Prescriptions Kept in Jade Case*) by the same author. Introduced in the book are more than 100 prescriptions of acupuncture and moxibustion, most of which are for moxibustion. It deals more with moxibustion methods for critical diseases.

●**肘后歌**[zhǒu hòu gē]　针灸歌赋名。见《针灸聚英》。作者不详。为七言韵语,列举一些常见病证的远近配穴法,对临床有参考价值。其名称仿《肘后方》,意在取用方便。

Zhouhou Ge (*A Verse for Convenience of Acupuncture and Moxibustion*)　A verse on acupuncture and moxibustion, originally from *Juying* (*Essentials of Acupuncture and Moxibustion*), no details are known about the author. It is a verse with seven characters to a line, enumerating some methods of distant-local selection of points for common diseases, which are usable in clinical practice. The title is an imitation of *Zhouhou Fang* (*A Handbook of Prescriptions*), easy to use.

●**肘尖**[zhǒu jiān]　①经外穴名。见《千金要方》。〈定位〉在肘后部,屈肘,当尺骨鹰嘴的尖端。〈层次解剖〉皮肤→皮下组织→鹰嘴皮下囊→肱三头肌腱。该处布有前臂后皮神经和肘关节周围动、静脉网。〈主治〉瘰疬。用灸法。②部位名。指尺骨鹰嘴突起之尖端。③经穴别名。见《外科枢要》,即肘髎。见该条。

1. Zhoujian (EX-UE 1)　An extra point originally from *Qianjin Yaofang* (*Essential Prescriptions Worth a Thousand Gold*). 〈Location〉 on the posterior side of the elbow, at the tip of the olecranon when the elbow is flexed. 〈Regional anatomy〉 skin → subcutaneous tissue → subcutaneous bursa of olecranon

→ tendon of brachial triceps muscle. There are the posterior cutaneous nerve of the forearm and the arteriovenous network around the elbow joint in this area. 〈Indication〉 scrofula. 〈Method〉 moxibustion.

2. A part of the body, referring to the tip of the olecranon.

3. **Zhoujian** Another name for Zhouliao(LI 12), a meridian point originally from *Waike Shuyao*(*Essentials of External Diseases*) →肘髎(p. 620)

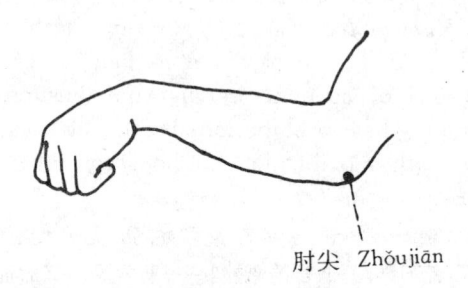

图78 肘尖穴
Fig. 78 Zhoujian point

●肘聊[zhǒu liáo] 经穴别名。见《太平圣惠方》。即肘髎,见该条。

Zhouliao Another name for Zhouliao(肘髎)(LI 12), a meridian point originally from *Taiping Shenghui Fang*(*Imperial Benevolent Prescriptions*). →肘髎(p. 620)

●肘髎[zhǒu liáo] 经穴名。出《针灸甲乙经》。属手阳明大肠经。又名肘尖、肘聊。〈定位〉在臂外侧,屈肘,曲池上方1寸,当肱骨边缘处(图48和图53)。〈层次解剖〉皮肤→皮下组织→肱桡肌→肱骨。浅层布有前臂后皮神经等结构。深层有桡侧副动、静脉的分支或属支。〈主治〉肘臂痛,拘挛,麻木,嗜卧。直刺0.5～0.8寸;可灸。

Zhouliao(LI 12) A meridian point, originally from *Zhenjiu Jia-Yi Jing*(*A-B Classic of Acupuncture and Moxibustion*), a point on the Large Intestine Meridian of Hand-Yangming, also named Zhoujian or Zhouliao(肘聊). 〈Location〉 with the elbow flexed, on the lateral side of the upper arm, 1 cun above Quchi(LI 11), on the border of the humerus (Figs. 48&53). 〈Regional anatomy〉 skin→subcutaneous tissue→brachioradial muscle→brachial muscle. In the superficial layer, there is the posterior cutaneous nerve of the forearm. In the deep layer, there are the branches or tributaries of the radial collateral artery and vein. 〈Indications〉 pain of the elbow and arm, contracture, numbness and drowsiness. 〈Method〉 Puncture perpendicularly 0.5～0.8 cun. Moxibustion is applicable.

●肘俞[zhǒu shū] 经外穴名。见《针灸孔穴及其疗法便览》。在肘关节后面,当鹰嘴突起与桡骨小头之间的凹陷处。〈主治〉肘关节及其周围软组织疾患等。直刺0.3寸;可灸。

Zhoushu(EX-UE) An extra point from *Zhenjiu Kongxue Ji Qi Liaofa Bianlan*(*Guide to Acupoints and Acupuncture Therapeutics*). 〈Location〉on the posterior aspect of the elbow joint, in the depression between the projection of the olecranon and the small head of radius. 〈Indications〉 diseases of the elbow joint and the soft tissue around it. 〈Method〉Puncture perpendicularly 0.3～0.5 cun. Moxibustion is applicable.

●肘椎[zhǒu zhuī] 经外穴名。出《肘后备急方》。在腰部。取穴时,患者俯卧,垂肘贴身,以两肘尖连线与后正中线交点及旁开左右各1寸处,共三穴。〈主治〉霍乱转筋,吐泻、心腹胀痛等。用灸法。

Zhouzhui(EX-B) An extra point, originally from *Zhouhou Beiji Fang*(*A Handbook of Prescriptions for Emergencies*). 〈Location〉on the low back, at the junction of the line connecting the two tips of the elbows and the posterior midline, and also one cun bilateral to the junction, three points in all. 〈Indications〉 cramp in cholera morbus, vomiting, diarrhea, distending pain of the heart and abdomen. 〈Method〉 moxibustion.

●珠顶[zhū dǐng] 为屏尖之别称,详见该条。

Zhuding(MA) Another name for Tragic Apex(MA-T 2)→屏尖(p. 298)

●珠形隆起[zhū xíng lóng qǐ] 耳廓解剖名称。耳轮脚后沟近头皮处的珠形软骨隆起。

Pearl-like Projection An anatomical name of the auricle surface, referring to the pearl-like projection of cartilage at the posterior sulcus to the crus of helix close to the scalp.

●主客 [zhǔ kè] 配穴用语。针灸配穴中称主要穴为"主",相配伍穴为"客"。一主一客相配伍,称"主客相应"。如八脉交会穴中将内关与公孙,后溪与申脉,外关与临泣,列缺与照海相配合应用。又原穴与络穴配用,称主客原络配穴法。详见该条。

Host and Guest A term in point combination. In the point combination of acupuncture, the main point is called a "host" and the adjunct point a "guest". The combination of a host and a guest is called the host-guest correspondence. Among the Eight Confluence Points, for example, Neiguan (PC 6) and Gongsun (SP 4), Houxi (SI 3) and Shenmai (BL 62), Waiguan (SJ 5) and Linqi (GB 41), Lieque (LU 7) and Zhaohai (KI 6) are used in combination. The use of the Yuan (Primary) and Luo (Connecting) points in combination is called the host-guest combination of Yuan (Primary) and Luo (Connecting) points. →主客原络配穴法 (p. 621)

●主客配穴法 [zhǔ kè pèi xué fǎ] 为主客原络配穴法之别称。见该条。

The Host-Guest Combination of Acupoints Another name for The Host-Guest Combination of Yuan (Primary) and Luo (Connecting) points. →主客原络配穴法 (p. 621)

●主客原络配穴法 [zhǔ kè yuán luò pèi xué fǎ] 配穴法之一。见《针灸大成》。又称原络配穴、主客配穴法。这是根据各经所属病证,取其本经的原穴为"主",再配用与其相为表里经脉的络穴为"客"。一主一客,配合应用。

The Host-Guest Combination of Yuan (Primary) and Luo (Connecting) Points One of the combination methods of points, originally from *Zhenjiu Dacheng* (*A Great Compendium of Acupuncture and Moxibustion*), also called the combination of Yuan (Primary) and Lou (Connecting) points and the host-guest combination of acupoints. According to the pathological manifestations of each meridian, the Yuan (Primary) point of the meridian is selected as the "host", with the Luo (Connecting) points of the internally- and externally-related meridian selected as the "guest". One host and one guest are applied in combination.

●煮拔筒 [zhǔ bá tǒng] 水罐法的一种。见《外台秘要》卷十三。其操作参见水罐法、煮药拔罐条。

Decocting the Cupping Tube A form of cupping with decocted cup, originally from Vol. 13 of *Waitai Miyao* (*Clandestine Essentials from the Imperial Library*). For manipulation, see cupping with boiled cup and post-decoction cupping →水罐法 (p. 410)、煮药拔罐法 (p. 621)

●煮药拔罐法 [zhǔ yào bá guàn fǎ] 水罐法的一种。又称药筒、煮拔筒。以竹罐与中药液同煮后,即行拔罐的方法。参见"水罐法"条。

Post-Decoction Cupping A form of cupping with decocted cup, also named medical tube or decocting the bamboo tube. ⟨Method⟩ Decoct a bamboo tube together with medical herbs and immediately cup with it. →水罐法 (p. 410)

●煮针法 [zhǔ zhēn fǎ] 针具消毒方法。此为古代针具炼煮方法。在元·危亦林《世医得效方》、《针灸大成》、《针灸聚英》中均有论述,但现已不用此法。

Boiling the Needle The sterilization of the acupuncture instrument, a method of boiling the acupuncture instrument in ancient times. It is stated in *Shiyi De Xiaofang* (*Effective Prescriptions Handed down for Generations*) written by Wei Yilin of the Yuan Dynasty, *Zhenjiu Dacheng* (*A Great Compendium of Acupuncture and Moxibustion*) and *Zhenjiu Juying* (*Essentials of Acupuncture and Moxibustion*), but no longer in use nowadays.

●注射式进针 [zhù shè shì jìn zhēn] 进针法之一。又称快插进针。其法:以拇、食指夹住针身下段,露出针尖2分左右,对准穴位,快速刺入,适用于直刺。

Inserting the Needle as if Injecting One of the needle insertion methods, also named rapid needle insertion. ⟨Method⟩ Hold the lower part of the needle body with the thumb and index finger, with a length of 0.2 cun above the tip of the needle exposed, insert the needle into the point rapidly. It is suitable for perpendicular puncture.

●注市 [zhù shì] ①经外穴名。见《千金要方》。又名㾴布。在胸侧部,腋中线上,当第7肋间隙处。⟨主治⟩㾴,胸胁痛,腹痛等。斜刺0.3~0.5寸。可灸。②旁廷穴的俗名,见该条。

1. Zhushi(EX-CA) An extra point, originally from *Qianjin Yaofang* (*Essential Prescriptions Worth a Thousand Gold*), also named Zhubu. ⟨Location⟩ in the lateral position of the chest, on the middle axillary line, in the 7th intercostal space. ⟨Indications⟩ chronic infectious disease, pain of the chest and hypochondrium, abdominal pain, etc. ⟨Method⟩ Puncture obliquely 0.3～0.5 cun. Moxibustion is applicable.

2. Zhushi A popular name of the point Pangting(EX-CA). →旁廷 (p. 288)

●注夏[zhù xià] 经外穴名。见《类经图翼》。在手掌侧,当第2掌骨桡侧缘之中点,与合谷相对处。⟨主治⟩夏令食欲不振,消化不良,呕吐,腹泻等。直刺0.3～0.5寸;可灸。

Zhuxia(EX-UE) An extra point, originally from *Leijing Tuyi* (*Supplements to Illustrated Classified Canon of Internal Medicine of the Yellow Emperor*). ⟨Location⟩ on the palm, at side of the hand, at the midpoint of the radial border of the 2nd metacarpal bone, opposite to Hegu(LI 4). ⟨Indications⟩ poor appetite, dyspepsia, vomiting and diarrhea in summer. ⟨Method⟩ Puncture perpendicularly 0.3～0.5 cun. Moxibustion is applicable.

●柱骨[zhù gǔ] 部位名。大椎上接脑下之椎骨,即颈椎。

Column Bone Cervical vertebral bone, a body part, referring to the vertebrae from Dazhui(DU 14) to the lower part of the brain.

●祝定[zhù dìng] 人名。明针灸家。字伯静,丽水(今属浙江)人。曾任医学提举。注《窦太师标幽赋》,已佚。见《处州府志》。

Zhu Ding An acupuncturist in the Ming Dynasty, who styled himself Bo Jing, a native of Lishui (in Zhejiang Province today), once in charge of medical promotion, annotater of *Dou Taishi Biao You Fu* (*Master Dou's Lyrics of Recondite Principles*), which is no longer extant, seen in *Chuzhoufu Zhi* (*Annals of Chuzhoufu*).

●疰布[zhù bù] 经外穴名。出《针灸集成》。即注市。见该条。

Zhubu Another name for Zhushi(EX-CA), an extra point originally from *Zhenjiu Jicheng* (*A Collection of Acupuncture and Moxibustion*). →注市①. (p. 621)

●筑宾[zhù bīn] 经穴名。出《针灸甲乙经》。又称筑滨。属足少阴肾经,为阴维之郄穴。⟨定位⟩在小腿内侧,当太溪与阴谷的连线上,太溪上5寸,腓肠肌肌腹的内下方(图49和图82)。⟨层次解剖⟩皮肤→皮下组织→小腿三头肌。浅层布有隐神经的小腿内侧皮支和浅静脉。深层有胫神经和胫后动、静脉。⟨主治⟩癫狂,痫证,呕吐涎沫,疝痛,小儿脐疝,小腿内侧痛。直刺0.5～0.8寸;可灸。

Zhubin(KI 9) A meridian point, originally from *Zhenjiu Jia-Yi Jing* (*A-B Classic of Acupuncture and Moxibustion*), a point on the Kidney Meridian of Foot-Shaoyin, also called Zhubin(筑滨), the Xi(Cleft) point of the Yinwei Meridian. ⟨Location⟩ on the medial side of the leg, on the line connecting Taixi(KI 3) and Yingu(KI 10), 5 cun above Taixi(KI 3), medial and inferior to the gastrocnemius muscle belly (Figs. 49&82). ⟨Regional anatomy⟩ skin→subcutaneous tissue→triceps muscle of calf. In the superficial layer, there are the medial cutaneous branches of the saphenous nerve to the leg and the superficial veins. In the deep layer, there are the tibial nerve and the posterior tibial artery and vein. ⟨Indications⟩ manic-depressive disorder, epilepsy, sialemesis, hernia pain, umbilical hernia in children and pain in the medial aspect of the leg. ⟨Method⟩ Puncture perpendicularly 0.5～0.8 cun. Moxibustion is applicable.

●筑滨[zhù bīn] 经穴别名。出《医学入门》。即筑宾。见该条。

Zhubin Another name for Zhubin(筑宾)(KI 9), a meridian point, originally from *Yixue Rumen* (*An Introduction to Medicine*). →筑宾 (p. 622)

●箸针[zhù zhēn] 针具名。见《外科正宗》卷四。指以竹筷扎针,作刺血或火针用。近人则有以竹筷头横扎缝衣针七枚,用以扣击皮肤,作皮肤针用,也属此类。

Bamboo Needle A kind of acupuncture instrument, originally from Vol. 4 of *Waike Zhengzong* (*Orthodox Manual of External*

Diseases), referring to puncturing with a bamboo chopstick to cause bleeding, or used as a fire needle. In recent years, some people fix 7 sewing needles horizontally at the end of a bamboo chopstick to percuss the skin as a cutaneous needle.

●转谷[zhuǎn gǔ] 经外穴名。出《外台秘要》。在侧胸部,当腋前皱襞直下,第3肋间隙处。〈主治〉胸胁支满,食欲不振,呕吐,以及肋间神经痛等。斜刺0.3~0.5寸;可灸。

Zhuangu(EX-CA) An extra point, originally from *Waitai Miyao* (*Clandestine Essentials from the Imperial Library*). 〈Location〉 in the lateral side of the chest, directly below the anterior axillary fold, in the 3rd intercostal space. 〈Indications〉 fullness in the chest and hypochondrium, poor appetite, vomiting and intercostal neuralgia. 〈Method〉 Puncture obliquely 0.3~0.5 cun. Moxibustion is applicable.

●腨[zhuàn] 部位名。又写作踹。指腓肠肌部。

Zhuan(腨) A body part, also written as "踹(zhuàn)", referring to the gastrocnemius.

●腨肠[zhuàn cháng] ①经穴别名。出《针灸甲乙经》。即承筋。详见该条。②部位名。见《灵枢·本输》。指腓肠肌部。

1. Zhuanchang Another name for Chengjin (BL 56), a meridian point, originally from *Zhenjiu Jia-Yi Jing* (*A-B Classic of Acupuncture and Moxibustion*). →承筋(p. 43)

2. Calf A part of the body, originally from *Lingshu*: *Benshu* (*Miraculous Pivot*: *Meridian Points*), referring to the gastrocnemius muscle.

●庄俞[zhuāng shū] 经穴别名。出《针灸集成》。即神道,见该条。

Zhuangshu Another name for Shendao(DU 11), a meridian point originally from *Zhenjiu Jicheng* (*A Collection of Acupuncture and Moxibustion*). →神道(p. 360)

●壮[zhuàng] 灸法术语。出《灵枢·经水》。①艾炷的计量单位,每灸一个艾炷称为一壮。②指艾炷。如大壮灸是指用较大的艾炷施灸,小壮灸是指用较小的艾炷施灸。

Zhuang A term for moxibustion treatment, originally from *Lingshu*: *Jingshui* (*Miraculous Pivot*: *Qi and Blood of Meridians*). ① a measurement unit of moxa cones, one moxa cone is called one zhuang. ② Moxa cone, e.g. big zhuang moxibustion refers to moxibustion with bigger moxa cones, while small zhuang moxibustion indicates moxibustion with smaller moxa cones.

●椎顶[zhuī dǐng] 经外穴别名。即崇骨。见该条。

Zhuiding Another name for the extra point Chonggu(EX). →崇骨(p. 80)

●頄[zhuō] 1.①部位名。见《灵枢·经脉》、《黄帝内经太素》指眼下、颧骨部。②部位名。见《医宗金鉴·刺灸心法要诀》。指属上颌骨部分。2.经穴别名。出《外台秘要》。即禾髎,见该条。

1. Zhuo A body part, ① originally from *Lingshu*: *Jingmai* (*Miraculous Pivot*: *Meridians*) and *Huangdi Neijing Taisu*(*Comprehensive Notes to the Yellow Emperor's Canon of Internal Medicine*), referring to the part below the eyes and the zygomatic bone. ② A body part, originally from *Yizong Jinjian*: *Cijiu Xinfa Yaojue* (*Gold Mirror of Orthodox Medical Lineage*: *Essentials of Acupuncture and Moxibustion in Verse*), referring to the upper jaw bone.

2. Zhuo Another name for Heliao(LI 19), a meridian point originally from *Waitai Miyao* (*Clandestine Essentials from the Imperial Library*). →禾髎(p. 160)

●着痹[zhuó bì] 痹证证型之一。出《素问·痹论》。由风寒湿邪痹阻经络,以湿邪偏盛所致。证见肢体关节酸痛沉重,肌肤微肿,不红,痛有定处,阴雨风冷天气每易发作,舌苔白腻,脉濡。治宜散寒除湿,通络止痛。取足三里、商丘、阴陵泉。近部与循经取穴详见行痹条。针灸并施。

Fixed Bi A type of arthralgia syndrome, originally from *Su Wen*: *Bi Lun* (*Plain Questions*: *On Bi-Syndromes*), caused by pathogenic wind cold and dampness blocking the meridians, especially caused by excess of pathogenic dampness. 〈Manifestations〉 aching and heaviness of the limbs and joints, slight swelling without redness of the skin, fixed pain, mostly occurring on cloudy, rainy, windy and cold days, white and greasy tongue coat-

ing, soft pulse. 〈Treatment principle〉 Dispel cold and remove dampness, remove obstructions in the meridians to relieve pain. 〈Point selection〉 Zusanli(ST 36), Shangqiu(SP 5), Yinlingquan(SP 9). For the selection of points in the local region and along the meridians, Cf. Wandering Bi (p.). 〈Method〉 Apply acupuncture and moxibustion at the same time. →行痹(p. 511)

●着肤灸[zhuó fū jiǔ] 直接灸之别称。见该条。
Moxibustion on Skin Another name for direct moxibustion. →直接灸(p. 602)

●着肉灸[zhuó ròu jiǔ] 直接灸之别称。见该条。
Moxibustion on Muscle Another name for direct moxibustion. →直接灸(p. 602)

●资脉[zī mài] 经穴别名。出《针灸甲乙经》。即瘛脉,见该条。
Zimai Another name for Chimai(SJ 18), a meridian point originally from *Zhenjiu Jia-Yi Jing* (*A-B Classic of Acupuncture and Moxibustion*). →瘛脉(p. 48)

●子豹[zǐ bào] 人名。战国时医家,为扁鹊的弟子。
Zi Bao A physician in the Warring States period, a disciple of Bian Que.

●子病[zě bìng] 即恶阻。详见该条。
Disease due to Fetus Another name for morning sickness. →恶阻(p. 93)

●子宫[zǐ gōng] ①内脏名,系指奇恒之腑之女子胞。②经外穴名。〈定位〉在下腹部,当脐中下4寸,中极旁开3寸。〈层次解剖〉皮肤→皮下组织→腹外斜肌腱膜→腹内斜肌→腹横肌→腹横筋膜。浅层主要布有髂腹下神经的外侧皮支和腹壁浅静脉。深层主要有髂腹下神经的分支和腹壁下动静脉的分支或属支。〈主治〉子宫脱垂,月经不调,痛经、不孕症等。直刺0.5～1.0寸,可灸。③耳穴名,即内生殖器穴,见该条。

1. **Zigong** A viscera name, i. e. the uterus, one of the extraordinary organs.
2. **Zigong(EX-CA 1)** An extra point. 〈Location〉at the lower abdomen, 4 cun below the centre of the umbilicus and 3 cun lateral to Zhongji(RN 3). 〈Regional anatomy〉 skin→subcutaneous tissue→aponeurosis of external oblique muscle of abdomen→internal oblique muscle of abdomen→transverse fascia of abdomen. In the superficial layer, there are the lateral cutaneous branches of the iliohypogastric nerve and the superficial epigastric vein. In the deep layer, there are the branches of the iliohpogastic nerve and the branches or tributaries of the inferior epigastric artery and vein. 〈Indications〉 prolapse of uterus, irregular menstruation, dysmenorrhea, infertility, etc. 〈Method〉Puncture perpendicularly 0.5～1.0 cun. Moxibustion is applicable.
3. **Zigong(MA)** An auricular point, another name for Neishengzhiqi(MA). →内生殖器(p. 280)

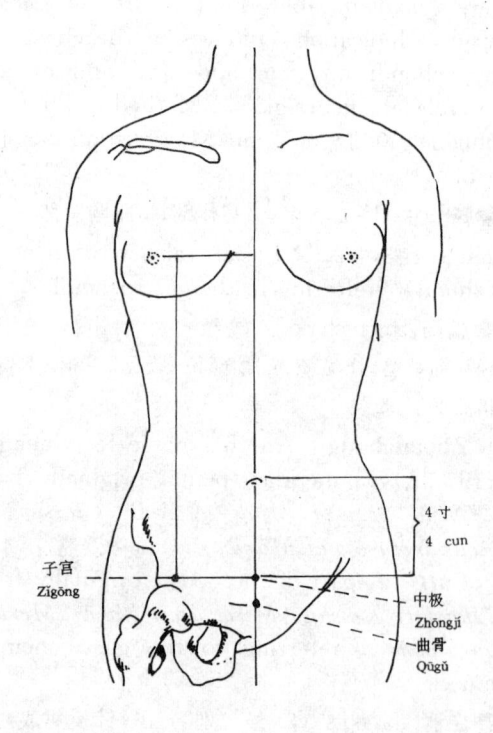

图79 子宫穴
Fig. 79 Zigong point

●子宫不收[zǐ gōng bù shōu] 即子宫脱垂。详见该条。
Contraction Failure of Uterus Another name for hysteroptosis. →子宫脱垂(p. 625)

●子宫脱出[zǐ gōng tuō chū] 即子宫脱垂。详见该

条。

Prolapse of Uterus Another name for hysteroptosis. →子宫脱垂(p. 625)

●**子宫脱垂**[zǐ gōng tuō chuí] 病证名。又称子宫脱出，阴脱，子宫不收。俗称吊茄子。与阴挺病相似。指妇女子宫下坠，甚至脱出阴道口外。多因气虚下陷，带脉失约，冲任虚损；或多产，难产，产时用力过度，产后过早参加重体力劳动等，损伤胞络及肾气，而使胞宫失于维系所致。证见子宫位置下垂，或脱出阴道口外，甚则连同阴道壁或膀胱直肠一并膨出。临床分气虚子宫脱垂，肾虚子宫脱垂。详见各条。

Hysteroptosis A disease, also called prolapse of uterus, pudendal prolapse and contraction failure of uterus, with the popular name "hanging eggplant". Similar to the disease of vaginal hernia, referring to the falling down of the uterus, or protrusion of the uterus through the vaginal orifice. Generally caused by the qi deficiency, dysfunction of the Dai Meridian, deficiency and injury of the Chong and Ren Meridians or by multigravida dystocia, overstrain while delivering, early participation of heavy labor after delivery, which leads to damage of the collateral of the uterus and kidney-qi, and thus makes the uterus unable to hold itself in the place. 〈Manifestations〉 metroptosis, or protrusion of the uterus through the vaginal orifice, sometimes with the prolapse of the vaginal orifice, sometimes with the prolapse of the vaginal wall, bladder and rectum. Clinically, it is divided into hysteroptosis due to qi deficiency and hysteroptosis due to deficiency of the kidney. →气虚子宫脱垂(p. 311)、肾虚子宫脱垂(p. 368)

●**子户**[zǐ hù] ①经穴别名。出《针灸甲乙经》。即气穴，见该条。②经外穴名。见胞门、子户条。

1. **Zihu** Another name for Qixue(KI 13), a meridian point originally from *Zhenjiu Jia-Yi Jing* (*A-B Classic of Acupuncture and Moxibustion*). →气穴(p. 311)

2. **Zihu** An extra point. →胞门、子户(p. 14)

●**子冒**[zǐ mào] 即子痫。详见该条。

Eclampsia Another name for eclampsia gravidarum. →子痫(p. 627)

●**子母补泻法**[zǐ mǔ bǔ xiè fǎ] 针刺补泻法之一。出《难经》。又称补母泻子法。补法选用五输穴中的母穴，泻法选用子穴。脏腑经脉分属五行，其五输穴也各配五行，阴经为井木、荥火、输土、经金、合水；阳经为井金、荥水、输木、经火、合土。据五行相生关系，每经各有一"母穴"和"子穴"。如肺经属金，金之母为土，即输穴太渊；金之子为水，即合穴尺泽。临床可根据"实则泻其子，虚则补其母"的原则来选用。如肺经虚证，可补本经(金)母穴太渊(土)，或母经(脾经)的穴位，称为虚则补其母(土生金)；又如肺经实证，可泻本经(金)子穴尺泽(水)，或子经(肾)的穴位，称实则泻其子(金生水)。

Mother-Child Reinforcing-Reducing Method One of the reinforcing-reducing methods of acupuncture, originally from *Nanjing* (*The Classic of Questions*), also called reinforcing-mother and reducing-child method. Select the mother-point of the Five-Shu Points for the reinforcing method and child-point for the reducing method, zang and fu and the meridians pertain to the five elements respectively, and the Five-Shu Points are also correlated respectively to the five elements. Yin meridians are Jing (Well)-wood, Ying (Spring)-fire, Shu (Stream)-earth, Jing (River)-metal and He (Sea)-water; Yang meridians include Jing (Well)-metal, Ying (Spring)-water, Shu (Stream)-wood, Jing (River)-fire and He (Sea)-earth. According to the interpromoting relationship of the five elements, each meridian has one "mother-point", and one "child-point", for example, the Lung Meridian belongs to metal, and metal's mother is earth, i.e. the Shu (Stream) point Taiyuan (LU 9); metal's child is water, i.e. the He(Sea) point Chize (LU 5). In clinic, the principle "reducing the child-point in the syndrome of excess type and reinforcing the mother-point in the syndrome of deficiency type" is usually adhered to. For example, to treat deficiency of the Lung Meridian, we can reinforce the mother-point Taiyuan (LU 9) of the meridian (metal) or the point of the mother meridian (Spleen Meridian), which is called reinforcing the mother-point in the syndrome of deficiency type (earth produces metal) to treat the excess syndrome of the Lung Meridian; we can reduce the child-point Chize (LU 5) of the meridian (metal) or the points of the child

meridian (Kidney), which is called reducing the child-point in the syndrome of excess type (metal produces water).

● 子痛[zǐ tòng] 即妊娠腹痛。详见该条。

Pain due to Fetus →妊娠腹痛(p. 335)

● 子午八法[zǐ wǔ bā fǎ] 子午流注针法和灵龟八法的合称。《医学入门》"言子午八法者,子午流注兼奇经八法也"。

Zi-Wu (Midnight-Noon) Eight Methods A general term for the acupuncture techniques of midnight-noon ebb-flow and the Eight Methods of Intelligent Turtle. In *Yixue Rumen (An Introduction to Medicine)*, it is recorded that "The Zi-Wu (Midnight-Noon) Eight Methods mean midnight-noon ebb-flow and also the Eight Methods of Extra Meridians".

● 子午补泻[zǐ wǔ bǔ xiè] 针刺补泻手法名。出《针灸大成》。即左右捻转补泻。左转为顺转,从子位转向午位;右转为逆转,从午位退向子位。参见"捻转补泻"条。

Reinforcing and Reducing Method at Zi-Wu Portions An acupuncture manipulation of reinforcing and reducing, originally from *Zhenjiu Dacheng (A Great Compendium of Acupuncture and Moxibustion)*, referring to reinforcing and reducing by twirling and rotating the acupuncture needle right and left. Twirling left is the normal direction, i. e. from zi portion to wu, twirling right is the adverse direction, i. e. from wu portion to zi. →捻转补泻(p. 283)

● 子午捣臼[zǐ wǔ dǎo jiù] 针刺手法名。出《金针赋》。子午捣臼是一种捻转提插相结合的针刺手法。子午,指左右捻转;捣臼,指上下提插。〈其法〉进针得气后,先紧按慢提九数,再紧提慢按六数,同时结合左右捻转,反复施行。本法导引阴阳之气,补泻兼施,又有消肿利水的作用。可用于水肿,气证等证。

Zi-Wu Dao Jiu Needling A kind of acupuncture manipulation, originally from *Jinzhen Fu (Ode to Gold Needle)*, a kind of needling technique using the combination of twirling, lifting and thrusting. Zi-wu refers to twirling left and right, while dao jiu refers to lifting and thrusting. 〈Method〉On arrival of qi after insertion, first thrust quickly and lift gently nine times, then, lift swiftly and thrust gently six times with the coordination of left and right twirling at the same time and apply the method repeatedly. This method has the function of inducing the qi of yin and yang, reinforcing and reducing simultaneously and inducing diuresis to alleviate edema. 〈Indications〉edema and diseases of qi.

● 子午法[zǐ wǔ fǎ] 针刺补泻方法。见《席弘赋》。为捻转补泻之别称。见该条。

Zi-Wu Method A kind of reinforcing and reducing method of acupuncture originally from *Xi Hong Fu (Ode of Xi Hong)*, another name for reinforcing and reducing by twirling and rotating the needle. →捻转补泻(p. 283)

● 子午经[zǐ wǔ jīng] 书名。旧题秦越人撰。一卷。内载针灸歌诀。现残存针灸避忌部分,收于《说郛》第一百零九卷。

Zi-Wu Jing (Classic on Midnight-Noon) A one volume book originally written by Qin Yueren, recording verses on acupuncture and moxibustion. Part of the book on contraindications of acupuncture and moxibustion was included in Vol. 109 of *Shuo Fu (Explanation of Outer City)*.

● 子午流注[zǐ wǔ liú zhù] ①子午流注针法所依据的理论。②书名。旧题窦汉卿撰,一卷。书佚。见《中国医籍考》。

1. Midnight-Noon Ebb-flow The theory of the needling method of midnight-noon ebb-flow was based upon.

2. Zi-Wu Liu Zhu (Midnight-Moon Ebb-Flow) A one-volume book, originally written by Dou Hanqing, the book has been lost. cf. *Zhongguo Yiji Kao (A Study on Chinese Medical Books)*.

● 子午流注针法[zǐ wǔ liú zhù zhēn fǎ] ①按时配穴法的一种。系以日时干支推算人体气血流注盛衰的时间,据此选配各经五输穴进行针刺治疗。子午,表示昼夜时间的变化;流注,表示气血的运行。气血循经运行随着时间变化而有盛衰,气血盛时穴"开";气血衰时穴"阖"。具体见气纳三焦,血纳包络,五门十变,纳甲、纳子等法。②书名。由承淡庵、陈璧疏、徐惜年合著。江苏人民出版社1957年出版。本书全面介绍了子午流注及八脉八法的应用。

1. **Needling Methods of Midnight-Noon Ebb-Flow**　A type of adjunct acupuncture point selection according to time, i. e. calculating the excessive and deficient time of the flowing and ebbing of qi and blood by the designated days and hours in terms of the Heavenly Stems and the Earthly Branches, prediction of which can be used for the selection of the Five Shu points of each meridian in acupuncture therapy. Zi-wu (midnight-noon) means the circulation of qi and blood. The flow of qi and blood changes with the time. The points open with the excess of qi and blood and close with deficiency. →气纳三焦(p. 309)、血纳包络(p. 526)、五门十变(p. 477)、纳甲法(p. 275)、纳子法(p. 275)

2. **Zi-Wu Liu Zhu Zhenfa (Needling Methods of Midnight-Noon Ebb-Flow)**　A book written by Cheng Danan, Chen Biliu and Xu Xinian, published in 1957 by the People's Publishing House of Jiangsu, an all-round introduction to midnight-noon ebb-flow and Eight Methods of the Eight Extra Meridians.

●子午流注针经[zǐ wǔ liú zhù zhēng jīng]　书名。金·何若愚撰，阎明广注。三卷。卷上为《流注指微赋》、《平人气象论经隧周环图》，及十二经脉循行、主病图形，卷中论子午流注；卷下为《井荥歌诀》及图。为子午流注学说的专书。现存《针灸四书》中。

Zi-Wu Liu Zhu Zhenjing (Acupuncture Classic on Midnight-Noon Ebb-Flow)　A book in 3 volumes, written by He Ruoyu in the Jin Dynasty, and annotated by Yan Mingguang. The 1st volume included *Liu Zhu Zhiwei Fu (Ode of the Subtleties of Flow), Pingren Qixiang Lun Jing sui Zhou Huan Tu (Normal People's Physiology and Circulatory Diagram of the Course of Meridians)* and the course and the indications of the twelve meridians. The 2nd volume dealt with midnight-noon ebb-flow and the 3rd was *Jing Ying Gejue [Verse on Jing (Well) and Ying (Spring) points]* and pictures. It is a monograph on the theory of midnight-noon ebb-flow, which is now recorded in *Zhenjiu Si Shu (Four Books on Acupuncture and Moxibustion)*.

●子午流注逐日按时定穴歌[zǐ wǔ liú zhù zhú rì àn shí dìng xué gē]　针灸歌诀名。明·徐凤作。载《针灸大全》。为十首七言韵语，内容按十天干分述各日时子午流注用穴，是子午流注配穴法的主要歌诀。

Zi-Wu Liu Zhu Zhu Ri An Shi Ding Xue Ge (Rhymes for Selecting Points in Terms of Heavenly Stems and Time of Each Day of Midnight-Noon Ebb-Flow)　A verse on acupuncture and moxibustion, written by Xu Feng in the Ming Dynasty, included in *Zhen Jiu Da Quan (A Complete Work of Acupuncture and Moxibustion)*. Ten verses with seven words in each rhyme, dealing respectively with the points for each day and hour of midnight-noon ebb-flow according to the Ten Heavenly Stems, the main verses of adjunct acupuncture points according to midnight-noon ebb-flow.

●子痫[zǐ xián]　病证名、出《诸病源候论》。又名妊娠痓，妊娠风痓，风痓，妊娠痫证，儿晕，儿风，儿痉，子冒，胎风。多因平素肝肾阴虚，孕后阴血聚而养胎，血不养肝，肝木失养，肝风内动所致。症见妊娠后期，头目眩晕，面色潮红，口苦咽干，下肢浮肿。病发时卒然昏倒，不省人事，四肢抽搐，牙关紧闭，目睛直视，口吐白沫，少时自醒，间歇发作，舌红或绛，脉弦数或弦滑。治宜育阴潜阳，平肝熄风。取百会、风池、内关、太冲、三阴交、太溪。

Eclampsia Gravidarum　A disease, originally from *Zhubing Yuanhou Lun (General Treatise on the Etiology and Symptomatology of Diseases)*, also called convulsion during pregnancy, wind-convulsion during pregnancy, wind-convulsion, epilepsy during pregnancy, dizziness due to fetus, wind-syndrome due to fetus, convulsion due to fetus, eclampsia, wind-syndrome due to pregnancy. Mostly caused by the constitutional yin deficiency of the liver and kidney, lack of blood in the liver due to the accumulation of blood in the fetus during pregnancy, malnutrition of the liver (wood) and stirring of the liver wind in the interior. 〈Manifestations〉in the later period of pregnancy, dizziness, flushed face, bitter taste and dry throat, edema of the lower limbs, sudden coma, unconsciousness, convulsion of the limbs with the jaw closed, eye fixed, frothy salivation, and consciousness after a while, intermittent attack, red or deep-red tongue, wiry and

rapid or wiry and slippery pulse. ⟨Treatment principle⟩ Nourish yin and suppress excessive yang, calm the liver to stop wind. ⟨Point selection⟩ Baihui (DU 20), Fengchi (GB 20), Neiguan (PC 6), Taichong (LR 3), Sanyinjiao (SP 6) and Taixi (KI 3).

●子脏冷无子[zǐ zàng lěng wú zǐ] 胞寒不孕的别名。详见该条。

Infertility due to Cold Uterus. →胞寒不孕 (p. 13)

●紫宫[zǐ gōng] 经穴名。出《针灸甲乙经》。属任脉。⟨定位⟩在胸部,当前正中线上,平第二肋间(图40)。⟨层次解剖⟩皮肤→皮下组织→胸大肌起始腱→胸骨体。主要布有第二肋间神经前皮支和胸廓内动、静脉的穿支。⟨主治⟩咳嗽,气喘,胸胁支满,胸痛,喉痹,吐血,呕吐,饮食不下。平刺0.3~0.5寸;可灸。

Zigong (RN 19) A meridian point, originally from *Zhenjiu Jia-Yi Jing* (*A-B Classic of Acupuncture and Moxibustion*), a point on the Ren Meridian. ⟨Location⟩ on the chest, on the anterior mid-line, at the level of the 2nd intercostal space (Fig. 40). ⟨Regional anatomy⟩ skin→subcutaneous tissue→origin of greater pectoral muscle→sternal body. There are the anterior cutaneous branches of the 2nd intercostal nerve and the perforating branches of the internal thoracic artery and vein in this area. ⟨Indications⟩ cough, dyspnea, fullness in the chest and hypochondriun, chest pain, sore throat, hematemesis, vomiting, poor appetite. ⟨Method⟩ Puncture subcutaneously 0.3~0.5 cun. Moxibustion is applicable.

●自灸[zì jiǔ] ①灸法术语。出《庄子·盗跖》。指自行施灸。②灸法的一种,"天灸"之别称。见该条。

1. A moxibustion term, originally from *Zhuang Zi : Dao Zhi* (*The Book of Zhuangcius : Bandit Zhi*), referring to self-moxibustion.
2. A kind of moxibustion, another name for medicinal vesication. →天灸 (p. 432)

●宗筋[zōng jīn] ①前阴部。出《素问·痿论》。前阴部是宗筋会聚的场所。②指阴茎、睾丸。出《灵枢·五音五味》。③专指阴茎。出《素问·痿论》。宗筋弛纵,就会产生筋痿。

1. **Urogenital Region** Orginally from *Suwen : Wei Lun* (*Plain Question : On Flaccidity Syndromes*), the confluence of tendons.
2. **Penis and Testis** Originally from *Lingshu : Wu Yin Wu Wei* (*Miraculous Pivot : On Five Sounds and Five Tastes*).
3. **Penis** Originally from *Suwen : Wei Lun* (*Plain Questions : On Flaccidity Syndromes*). The laxation of Zong Jin may cause mysthenia.

●宗脉[zōng mài] 经脉名。出《灵枢·口问》。指汇聚于眼和耳部的经脉。

Assembled Meridians A category of meridians, originally from *Lingshu : Kou Wen* (*Miraculous Pivot : Query*), referring to the meridians assembled in the eye and ear areas.

●综合手法[zōng hé shǒu fǎ] 针刺手法分类名。与基本手法及辅助手法相对而言。指针刺手法中由一些单一的手法互相结合起来的较复杂的手法。如《金针赋》所载的烧山火、透天凉、阳中隐阴、阴中隐阳等法均是。其中有的属补法,有的属泻法,有的属补泻结合法,有的属行气方法。

Comprehensive Manipulations A category of acupuncture manipulation, as compared to the basic techniques and auxiliary ones. Referring to the relatively complicated needling methods composed of some single manipulations, e.g. methods of setting the mountain on fire, making penetrating-heaven coolness, yin occluded in yang, and yang occluded in yin, etc. Some of them belong to the reinforcing method, some to the reducing method, some to a combination of both, and some to the method of promoting the flow of qi.

●走罐法[zǒu guàn fǎ] 为推罐之别称。见该条。

Moving Cupping Another name for cupping by pushing the cup. →推罐法 (p. 449)

●足大趾丛毛[zú dà zhǐ cóng máo] 穴位名。又称足大趾聚毛。指大敦穴。

Zudazhicongmao Dadun (LR 1), a meridian point also known as *Zudazhijumao*.

●足第二指上[zú dì èr zhǐ shàng] 经外穴名。见《类经图翼》。在足背部,当第2、3趾夹缝上1寸。⟨主治⟩水病;可灸。

Zudierzhishang (EX-LE) An extra point, seen in *Leijing Tuyi* (*Supplement to Illustrat-*

ed *Classified Canon of Internal Medicine of the Yellow Emperor*). ⟨Location⟩on the instep of the foot, 1 cun proximal to the margin of the web between the 2nd and 3rd toes. ⟨Indication⟩edema. ⟨Method⟩moxibustion.

●足窌[zú jiào] 经穴别名。出《针灸甲乙经》。即阳交,见该条。

Zujiao Another name for Yangjiao (GB 35), a meridian point originally from *Zhenjiu Jia-Yi Jing* (*A-B Classic of Acupuncture and Moxibustion*). →阳交(p.538)

●足巨(钜)阳脉[zú jù yáng mà] 早期经脉名。出《帛书》。与足太阳经类似。

Vessel of Foot-Juyang An earlier name of a meridian, originally in *Bo Shu* (*The Silk Book*), similiar to the Meridian of Foot-Taiyang.

●足卷阴脉[zú juǎn yīn mài] 早期经脉名。出《帛书》。与足厥阴经类似。

Vessel of Foot-Juanyin An earlier name of a meridian, seen in *Boshu* (*The Silk Book*), similiar to the Meridian of Foot-Jueyin.

●足厥阴标本[zú jué yīn biāo běn] 十二经脉标本之一。出《灵枢·卫气》。足厥阴之本,在行间上五寸,约当中封穴处;标在背部,约当肝俞穴处。

Superficiality and Origin of Foot-Jueyin One of the superficialities and origins of the Twelve Regular Meridians, originally from *Lingshu: Wei Qi* (*Miraculous pivot: Defensive Qi*). The origin of Foot-Jueyin is approximately at Zhongfeng (LR 4), 5 cun above Xingjian (LR 2). The superficiality is at Ganshu (BL 18) on the back.

●足厥阴肝经[zú jué yīn gān jīng] 十二经脉之一。原称肝足厥阴之脉。出《灵枢·经脉》。其循行从大趾背毫毛部开始,向上沿着足背内侧,离内踝一寸,上行小腿内侧,离内踝八寸处交出足太阴脾经之后,上膝腘内侧,沿着大腿内侧,进入阴毛中,环绕阴部,至小腹,夹胃旁边,属于肝,络于胆,向上通过膈肌,分布胁肋,沿喉咙之后,向上进入颃颡,连接目系,上行出于额部,与督脉交会于头顶。它的支脉,从目系下向颊里,环绕唇内。另一支脉,从肝分出,通过膈肌,向上流注于肺,接手太阴肺经。

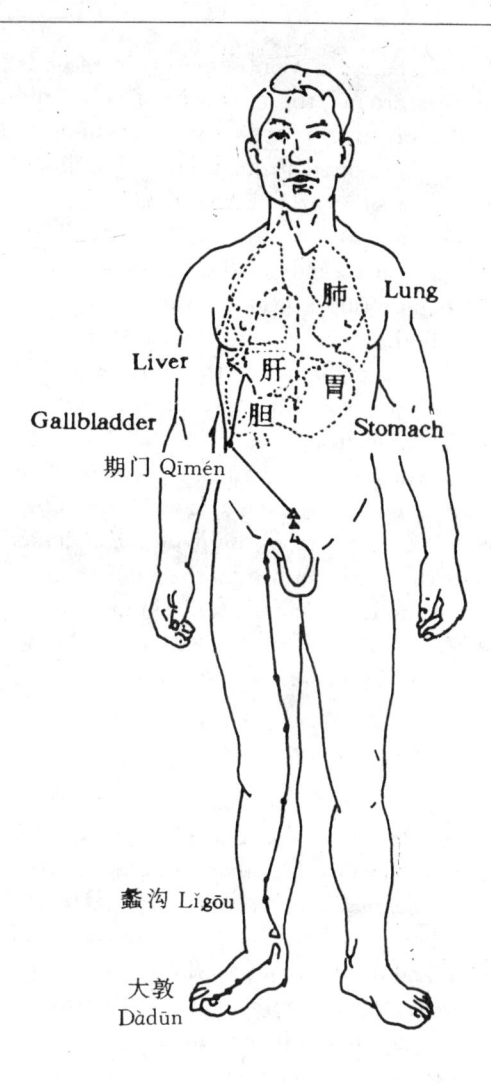

图80 足厥阴肝经
Fig. 80 Liver Meridian of Foot-Jueyin

The Liver Meridian of Foot-Jueyin One of the Twelve Regular Meridians, originally known as the Liver Vessel of Foot-Jueyin, originally from *Lingshu: Jingmai* (*Miraculous Pivot: Meridians*). The meridian starts from the dorsal hair of the great toe, runs upward along the dorsum of the foot, and passes through a point, 1 cun in front of the medial malleolus; it ascends to the area 8 cun above the medial malleolus, where it runs across and behind the Spleen Meridian of Foot-Taiyang. Then it runs upward to the medial aspect of the knee, and along the medial aspect of thigh into the pubic hair region, where it curves around the external genitalia and goes up to

the lower abdomen. Continuously, it ascends and curves around the stomach to enter the liver—the organ it pertains to, and connects with the gallbladder. From there it continues to ascend, passing through the diaphragm and branching out in the costal and hypochondriac region. Then it ascends to the nasopharynx along the posterior aspect of the throat and links with the "eye system". Runing further upward, it emerges from the forehead and meets with the Du Meridian at the vertex. One of its branches arises from the "eye system" and runs downward into the cheek, then curves around the inner surface of the lips. Another one arises from the liver and ascends through the diaphragm into the lung to connect with the Lung Meridian of Hand-Taiyin.

●足厥阴肝经病[zú jué yīn gān jīng bìng] 十二经脉病候之一。出《灵枢·经脉》。本经主要病候为：腰痛，疝气，小腹部肿胀，咽喉干，面垢如尘，神色晦暗等。

Diseases of the Liver Meridian of Foot-Jueyin One of the pathological manifestations of the Twelve Meridians, originally from *Lingshu: Jingmai (Miraculous Pivot: Meridians)*. 〈Main manifestations〉 lumbago, hernia, swelling and distention of the lower abdomen, dry throat, dirty complexion, as if covered with dust, and dark, gloomy look, etc.

●足厥阴经别[zú jué yīn jīng bié] 十二经别之一。原称足厥阴之正。出《灵枢·经别》。足厥阴经别，从足背上足厥阴经分出，向上到达外阴部，和足少阳经别会合并行。

Divergent Meridian of Foot-Jueyin One of the Twelve Divergent Meridians, originally known as the Divergence of Foot-Jueyin, originally from *Lingshu: Jingbie (Miraculous Pivot: Divergent Meridians)*. The Divergent Meridian of Foot-Jueyin emerges from the part of the Meridian of Foot-Jueyin on the dorsum of foot, and runs upward to the region of external genitals to converge into and run alongside the divergent meridian of Foot-Shaoyang.

●足厥阴经筋[zú jué yīn jīng jīn] 十二经筋之一。出《灵枢·经筋》。足厥阴经筋，起始于足大趾的上边，向上结于内踝前方，向上沿胫骨内侧，结于胫骨内髁之下，再向上沿大腿内侧，结于阴器部位而与诸筋相联络。

Muscle Region of the Foot-Jueyin One of the Twelve Muscle Regions, originally from *Lingshu: Jingjin (Miraculous Pivot: Muscle Along Meridians)*. The muscle region starts from the upper part of the great toe and goes upwards to concentrate at the front of the medial malleolus. Then it runs along the medial side of the tibia and masses under the internal-condyle of the tibia. Continuously, it ascends along the medial aspect of the thigh to concentrate at the region of the external genitalia and links with all other muscle regions.

●足厥阴经筋病[zú jué yīn jīng jīn bìng] 十二经筋病候之一。出《灵枢·经筋》。足厥阴经筋发病，可见足大趾支撑不适，内踝前部疼痛，内辅骨处亦痛，大腿内侧疼痛转筋，前阴不能运用，若房劳过度，耗伤阴精则阳萎不举，伤于寒则阴器缩入，伤于热则阴器挺长不收等。

Diseases of the Muscle Region of Foot-Jueyin One of the pathological manifestations of the Twelve Muscle Regions, originally from *Lingshu: Jingjin (Miraculous Pivot: Muscle Regions Along Meridians)*. 〈Manifestations〉 sustaining disturbance of the great toe, aching at the front of the medial malleolus, pain at medial aspect of the knee joint, spasm and pain of the medial aspect of the thigh, dysfunction of external genitalia, impotence due to consumption of yin-essence resulting from excessive sexual intercourse, flaccid constriction of penis due to pathogenic cold, prolonged erection of the penis due to pathogenic heat, etc.

●足厥阴络脉[zú jué yīn luò mài] 十五络脉之一。原称足厥阴之别。出《灵枢·经脉》。足厥阴络脉名为蠡沟。其脉循行在离内踝上五寸处蠡沟穴分出，走向足少阳经脉，其分支经过胫骨部，上行到睾丸部，结在阴茎处。

Collateral of Foot-Jueyin One of the Fifteen Main Collaterals, originally known as the branch of Foot-Jueyin, originally from *Lingshu: Jingmai (Miraculous Pivot: Meridians)*. Its name is Ligou (LR 5). The collateral de-

rives from Ligou(LR 5), 5 cun above the medial malleolus and runs to the Foot-Shaoyang Meridian. Its branch passes along the tibia and ascends to the testes to concentrate at the penis.

●足厥阴络脉病[zú jué yīn luò mài bìng] 十五络脉病候之一。出《灵枢·经脉》。其病气厥逆则睾丸肿胀，突发疝气。实证可见阳强不倒；虚证可见阴部暴痒。取足厥阴络穴治疗。

Diseases of Collateral of Foot-Jueyin One of the pathological manifestations of the Fifteen Main Collaterals, originally from *Lingshu: Jingmai* (*Miraculous Pivot: Meridians*). 〈Manifestations〉 swelling and distention of the testes resulting from reversed flow pathogenic qi, sudden onset of hernia. The excess type is manifested as prolonged erection; the deficiency type is manifested as sudden itching at the external genitalia. The Luo (Connecting) point of Foot-Jueyin should be selected for the treatment of these diseases.

●足厥阴脉[zú jué yīn mài] 早期经脉名。出《帛书》。与足厥阴经类似。

The Foot-Jueyin Vessel An earlier name of a meridian, originally from *Bo Shu* (*Silk Book*), similiar to the Foot-Jueyin Meridian.

●足厥阴之别[zú jué yīn zhī bié] 足厥阴络脉的原名。见该条。

The Branch of Foot-Jueyin The original name of the Collateral of the Foot-Jueyin. → 足厥阴络脉(p. 630)

●足厥阴之正[zú jué yīn zhī zhèng] 足厥阴经别的原名。见该条。

The Divergence of Foot-Jueyin The original name of the Divergent Meridian of Foot-Jueyin. → 足厥阴经别(p. 630)

●足临泣[zú lín qì] 经穴名。《灵枢·本输》名临泣。属足少阳胆经，为本经输穴。八脉会穴之一，通于带脉。〈定位〉在足背外侧，当足四趾本节(第四跖趾关节)的后方，小趾伸肌腱的外侧凹陷处(图8.1和图8.2)。〈层次解剖〉皮肤→皮下组织→第四骨间背侧肌和第三骨间足底肌(第四与第五跖骨之间)。布有足背静脉网，足背中间皮神经，第四跖背动、静脉和足底外侧神经的分支等。〈主治〉头痛，目外眦痛，目眩，乳痈，瘰疬，胁肋痛，疟疾，中风偏瘫，痹痛不仁，足跗肿痛。直刺0.5～0.8寸；可灸。

Zulinqi(GB 41) A meridian point, originally known as Linqi in *Lingshu: Benshu* (*Miraculous Pivot: Meridian Points*), the Shu(Stream) point of the Gallbladder Meridian of Foot-Shaoyang and one of the Eight Confluence Points which links with the Dai Meridian. 〈Location〉 on the lateral side of the instep of the foot, posterior to the 4th metatarsophalangeal joint, in the depression lateral to the tendon of the extensor muscle of the little toe (Figs. 8.1&8.2). 〈Regional anatomy〉 skin→subcutaneous tissue→4th dorsal interosseous muscle and 3rd plantar interosseous muscle. There are the venous network of the dorsum of the foot, the intermediate dorsal cutaneous nerve of the foot, the 4th dorsal metatarsal artery and vein, and the branches of the lateral plantar nerve in this area. 〈Indications〉 headache, aching of the outer canthus, vertigo, breast abscess, scrofula, pain flaccidity and numbness, swelling and aching of the dorsum of the foot. 〈Method〉 Puncture perpendicularly 0.5～0.8 cun. Moxibustion is applicable.

●足窍阴[zú qiào yīn] 经穴名。《灵枢·本输》名窍阴，《针灸资生经》称足窍阴。属足少阳胆经，为本经井穴。〈定位〉在足第四趾末节外侧，距趾甲角0.1寸(指寸)(图8.1和图8.2)。〈层次解剖〉皮肤→皮下组织→甲根。布有足背中间皮神经的趾背神经，趾背动、静脉和趾底固有动、静脉构成的动、静脉网。〈主治〉偏头痛，目眩，目赤肿痛，耳聋，耳鸣，喉痹，胸胁痛，足跗肿痛，多梦，热病。直刺0.1～0.2寸；可灸。

Zuqiaoyin(GB 44) A meridian point, known as Qiaoyin in *Lingshu: Benshu* (*Miraculous Pivot: Meridian Points*), but named Zuqiaoyin in *Zhenjiu Zisheng Jing* (*Acupuncture-Moxibustion Classic for Saving Life*). The Jing (Well) point of the Gallbladder Meridian of Foot-Shaoyang. 〈Location〉 on the lateral side of the distal segment of the 4th toe, 0.1 cun from the corner of the toenail(Figs. 8.1&8.2). 〈Regional anatomy〉 skin→subcutaneous tissue→root of nail. There are the dorsal digital nerve of the intermediate dorsal cutaneous nerve of the foot, and the arteriovenous network formed by the dorsal digital arteries and

veins of the foot with the proper plantar arteries and veins in this area. 〈Indications〉 migraine, vertigo, redness, swelling and pain of the eye, deafness, tinnitus, sore throat, pain in the chest and hypochondriac region, aching and swelling of the dorsum of the foot, dream-disturbed sleep, febrile disease. 〈Method〉 Puncture perpendicularly 0.1~0.2 cun. Moxibustion is applicable.

●足三里[zú sān lǐ] 经穴名。《内经》原名三里;《圣济总录》称足三里。属足阳明胃经,为本经合穴。又名下陵、下陵三里、鬼邪、下三里。〈定位〉在小腿前外侧,当犊鼻下3寸,距胫骨前缘一横指(中指)(图60.5和图6.1)。〈层次解剖〉皮肤→皮下组织→胫骨前肌→小腿骨间膜→胫骨后肌。浅层布有腓肠外侧皮神经等结构。深层有胫前动、静脉的分支或属支等。〈主治〉胃痛,呕吐,腹胀,肠鸣,消化不良,泄泻,便秘,痢疾,疳疾,喘嗽痰多,乳痈,头晕,耳鸣,心悸,气短,癫狂,中风,脚气,水肿,膝胫酸痛,鼻疾,产后血晕。直刺0.5~1.5寸;可灸。

Zusanli(ST 36) A meridian point originally known as Sanli in *Neijing*(*The Canon of Internal Medicine*), named Zusanli in *Shengji Zonglu*(*Imperial Medical Encyclopaedia*), the He(Sea) point of the Stomach Meridian of Foot-Yangming, also called Xialing, Xialingsanli, Guixie and Xiasanli, etc. 〈Location〉 on the anteriolateral side of the leg, 3 cun below Dubi(ST 35), one finger breadth (middle finger) from the anterior crest of the tibia (Figs. 60.5&6.1). 〈Regional anatomy〉 skin →subcutaneous tissue→anterior tibial muscle → interosseous membrane of leg → posterior tibial muscle. In the superficial layer, there is the lateral cutaneous nerve of the calf. In the deep layer, there are the branches or tributaries of the anterior tibial artery and vein. 〈Indications〉gastric pain, vomiting, abdominal distention, borborygum, indigestion, diarrhea, constipation, dysentery and infantile malnutrition, cough and asthma with profuse sputum, breast abscess, dizziness, tinnitus, palpitation, shortness of breath, manic-depressive psychosis, apoplexy, beriberi, edema, soreness and pain of the knee and ankle, nasal disorders and postpartum faintness, etc. 〈Method〉 Puncture perpendicularly 0.5~1.0 cun. Moxibustion is applicable.

●足三阳经[zú sān yáng jīng] 经脉名。出《灵枢·逆顺肥瘦》。足阳明胃经、足太阳膀胱经,足少阳胆经的总称。足三阳经从头走足,分布于人体前、侧、后面。见各条。

Three Yang Meridians of Foot The name of meridians, originally from *Lingshu*:*Nishun Fei Shou* (*Miraculous Pivot*: *Circulatory Direction of Meridians and Body Constitution*), the general term for the Stomach Meridian of Foot-Yangming, Bladder Meridian of Foot-Taiyang and Gallbladder Meridian of Foot-Shaoyang. The three yang meridians run downwards from the head to the foot, and are distributed separately on the anterior, lateral and posterior aspects of the body. →足阳明胃经(p.647)、足太阳膀胱经(p.640)、足少阳胆经(p.633)

●足三阴经[zú sān yīn jīng] 经络名。出《灵枢·逆顺肥瘦》。足太阴经,足少阴经,足厥阴经的总称。足三阴经从足走腹,分布于下肢内侧,上达腹部及胸部。

Three Yin Meridians of Foot The name of meridians, originally from *Lingshu*: *Ni Shun Fei Shou*(*Miraculous Pivot*:*Circulatory Direction of Meridians and Body Constitution*), general term for the Meridians of Foot-Taiyin, Foot-Shaoyin and Foot-Jueyin. The three yin meridians run upwards from the foot to the abdomen, and are distributed separately on the medial side of the lower limbs, then reach the abdominal and chest regions.

●足上廉[zú shàng lián] 经穴别名。见《圣济总录》。即上巨虚,见该条。

Zushanglian Another name for Shangjuxu (ST 37), a meridian point seen in *Shengji Zonglu*(*Imperial Medical Encyclopaedia*). → 上巨虚(p.352)

●足少阳标本[zú shào yáng biāo běn] 十二经标本之一。出《灵枢·卫气》。足少阳之本,在足上,约当足窍阴穴;标在耳前,约当听会穴。

The Superficiality and Origin of Foot-Shaoyang One of the superficialities and origins of the Twelve Meridians, originally from *Lingshu*:*Wei Qi*(*Miraculous Pivot*:*Defensive*

Qi). The origin of foot-Shaoyang is at Zuqiaoyin (GB 44) on the foot, and the superficiality is approximately at Tinghui (GB 2) in front of the ear.

●**足少阳胆经**[zú shào yáng dǎn jīng] 十二经脉之一。原称胆足少阳之脉。出《灵枢·经脉》。其循行从外眼角开始，上行到额角，下耳后，沿颈旁，**行手少阳三焦经之前**，至肩上退后，交出手少阳三焦经之后，进入缺盆。它的支脉，从耳后进入耳中，走耳前，至外眼角后。另一支脉，从外眼角分出，下向大迎，会合于手少阳三焦经至眼下，下边盖过颊车，下行颈部，会合于缺盆，由此下向胸中，通过膈肌，络于肝，属于胆，沿胁里，出于气街，绕阴部毛际，横向进入髋关节部。它的主干，从缺盆下向腋下，胸侧过季胁，向下会合于髋关节部。由此向下，沿大腿外侧，出膝外侧，下向腓骨头前，直下到腓骨下段，下出外踝之前，沿足背进入第四趾外侧。它的支脉，从足背分出，进入大趾趾缝间，沿第一、二趾骨间，出趾端，回转来通过爪甲，出于趾背毫毛部，接足厥阴肝经。

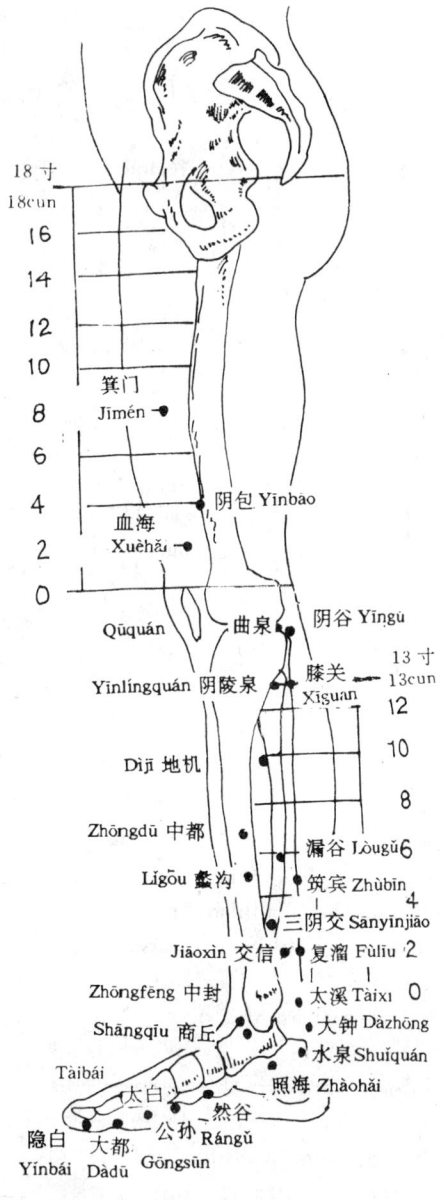

图81 足三阴经

Fig. 81 Three Yin Meridians of Foot

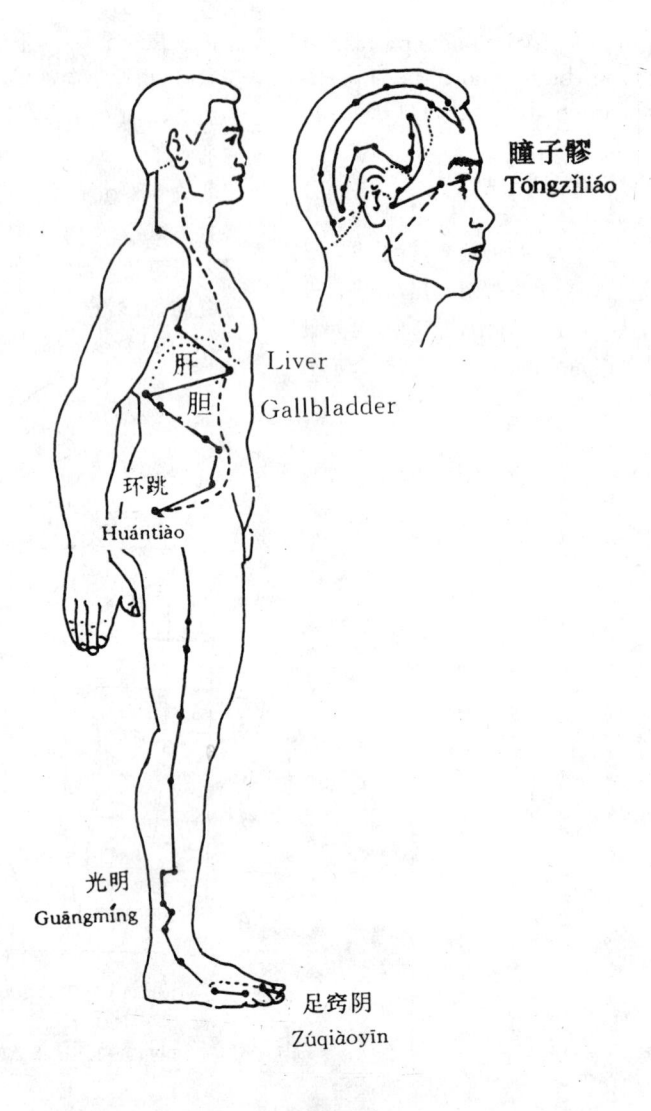

Fig. 82 Gallbladder Meridian of Foot-Shaoyang

The Gallbladder Meridian of Foot-Shaoyang

One of the Twelve Regular Meridians, originally known as the Gallbladder Vessel of Foot-Shaoyang, originally from *Lingshu: Jingmai* (*Miraculous Pivot: Meridians*). This meridian originates from the outer canthus, and ascends to the corner of the forehead, then curves downwards to the retroauricular region and runs along the side of the neck in front of the Sanjiao Meridian of Hand-Shaoyang to the shoulder. Turning back, it traverses and passes behind the Sanjiao Meridian of Hand Shaoyang down to the supraclavicular fossa. The retroauricular branch arises from the retroauricular region and enters into the ear, then comes out and passes the preauricular region to the posterior aspect of the outer canthus. The branch arising from the outer canthus runs downwards to Daying (ST 5) and meets with the Sanjiao meridian of Hand-Shaoyang in the infraorbital region. Then, passing through Jiache (ST 6), it descends to the neck and enters the supraclavicular fossa where it meets the other branch which has already reached the place. From there, it descends into the chest, passes

through the diaphragm to connect with the liver and enters into the gallbladder, the organ it pertains to. Then it runs inside the hypochondriac region, and emerges from the qi street. From there it runs superficially along the margin of the pubic hair and goes traversely into the hip region. The straight portion of this meridian runs downwards from the supraclavicular fossa, passes in front of the axilla along the lateral aspect of the chest and through the floating ribs to the hip region, where it meets with the previous meridian. From there it descends along the lateral aspect of the thigh to the lateral side of the knee. Going further downwards along the anterior aspect of the fibula all the way to its lower end, it reaches the anterior aspect of the external malleolus. Along the dorsum of the foot, it enters the lateral side of the tip of the 4th toe. The branch of the dorsum of the foot springs from Zulinqi (GB 41), runs between the 1st and 2nd metatarsal bones to the distal portion of the great toe and passes through the nail, and terminates at its hairy region, where it links with the Liver Meridian of Foot-Jueyin.

● 足少阳胆经病 [zú shào yáng dǎn jīng bìng] 十二经脉病候之一。出《灵枢·经脉》。本经主要病候：口苦，嗳气，胸胁痛，面色灰暗，头侧痛，目外眦痛，耳聋，颈部肿痛，瘰疬，寒热，疟疾，自汗，经脉所过处疼痛。

Diseases of the Gallbladder Meridian of Foot-Shaoyang One of the pathological manifestations of the Twelve Meridians, originally from *Lingshu: Jingmai (Miraculous Pivot: Meridians)*. 〈Main manifestations〉 bitter taste, eructation, aching in the hypochondriac, region, grey complexion, migraine, aching of the outer canthus, deafness, swelling and pain of the neck, scrofula, chills and fever, malaria, spontaneous perspiration, pain in the region along this meridian.

● 足少阳经别 [zú shào yáng jīng bié] 十二经别之一，原称足少阳之正。出《灵枢·经别》。足少阳经别，从足少阳胆经分出，绕过大腿前侧进入外阴部，同足厥阴经别会合，分支从外阴部进入浮肋之间，沿着腹腔里，归属于胆，散布到肝脏，上贯心中，挟着食道，浅出于下颌之间，散布在面部，联系眼球后面通入颅腔。当外眦部与足少阳经脉会合。

Divergent Meridian of Foot-Shaoyang One of the Twelve Divergent Meridians, originally known as the Divergence of Foot-Shaoyang, seen in *Lingshu: Jingbie (Miraculous Pivot: Divergent Meridians)*. The divergent meridian derives from the Gallbladder Meridian of Foot-Shaoyang, and curves around the anterior aspect of the thigh. Then it enters the external genitalia region to meet the Divergent Meridian of Foot-Jueyin. Arising from the external genitalia region, its branch enters the intercostal space, and runs inside the abdominal cavity to the gallbladder and the organ it pertains to and spreads in the liver. Then, the branch passes through the heart and goes upwards along the esophagus, and emerges superficially from the middle of the mandible. Continuously, it spreads over the face and links with the posteriority of the eye, then runs into the cranial cavity. This divergent meridian meets the Meridian of Foot-Shaoyang at the outer canthus.

● 足少阳经筋 [zú shào yáng jīng jīn] 十二经筋之一。出《灵枢·经筋》。足少阳经筋，起于第四趾，上结于外踝，再向上沿胫外侧结于膝外侧。其分支另起于腓骨部，上走大腿外侧，前边结于伏兔，后边结于骶部。直行的经侧腹季胁，上走腋前方，联系于胸侧和乳部，结于缺盆。直行的上出腋部，通过缺盆，走向太阳经的前方，沿耳后上绕到额角，交会于头顶，向下走向颔，上方结于鼻旁，分支结于外眦成"外维"。

Muscle Region of Foot-Shaoyang One of the Twelve Muscle Regions, originally from *Lingshu: Jingjin (Miraculous Pivot: Muscle Regions Along Meridians)*. The muscle region starts from the tip of the 4th toe, and concentrates at the lateral malleolus. Then it goes upwards along the lateral side of the tibia to mass at the lateral side of the knee. Its branch starts from the fibula and ascends along the lateral aspect of the thigh, then masses anteriorly at the muscular retus femoris and posteriorly at the sacrum. One straight portion of the muscle region ascends to the anteriority of the armpit along the lateral abdomen and hypochondri-

um, and links with the lateral aspect of the chest and the breast region, then concentrates in the supraclavicular fossa. After deriving from the armpit and passing through the supraclavicular fossa, another straight portion of the muscle region goes forward to the anteriority of the Foot-Taiyang Meridian and curves along the retroauricular region to the corner of the forehead. Then, it assembles at the vertex, and descends to the jaw to concentrate superiorily at the nasal sides. Its branch masses at the outer canthus to construct the "external dimension".

●足少阳经筋病[zú shào yáng jīng jīn bìng] 十二经筋病候之一。出《灵枢·经筋》。足少阳经筋发病,可见第四趾支撑不适,掣引转筋,并牵连膝外侧转筋,膝不能随意屈伸;腘部的经筋拘急,前面牵连髀部,后面牵引尻部,向上牵及胁下空软处及胁部咋痛,向上牵引缺盆;胸侧、颈部所维系的筋发生拘急。如果从左侧向右侧维络的筋拘急时,则右眼不能张开。因此筋上过的额角与跻脉并行,阴阳跻脉在此互相交叉,左右之筋也是交叉的,左侧的维络右侧,所以左侧的额角筋伤,会引起右足不能活动,这叫维筋相交。

Diseases of the Muscle Region of Foot-Shaoyang One of the pathological manifestations of the Twelve Muscle Regions, originally from *Lingshu: Jingjin(Miraculous Pivot: Muscle Along Meridians)*. 〈Manifestations〉 sustaining disturbance of the 4th toe, spasm of the toe connecting to the lateral side of the knee, failure of the knee to flex and stretch, contracture of the muscles in the popliteal fossa and connecting anteriorly to the upper half of the thigh, posteriorly to the sacral region, and superiorly to the hypochondriac region and the supraclavicular fossa, contracture of the muscles of the chest and the neck. If contracture occurs in the muscles which bind from the left to the right, the right eye is unable to open. This is because the muscle region reaches and passes through the right corner of the forehead and runs together with the Qiao Meridian. The Yinqiao Meridian crosses the Yangqiao Meridian here, and the left muscle region also crosses the right muscle region, so the left muscle region controls the right. Therefore, the injury of the muscle in the left corner of the forehead should lead to the failure of the right eye to move, which is known as the crossing of binding muscles.

●足少阳络脉[zú shào yáng luò mài] 十五络脉之一。原称足少阳之别。出《灵枢·经脉》。足少阳络脉名曰光明。在距离外踝上五寸光明穴处分出,走向足厥阴经脉,向下联络足背。

Collateral of Foot-Shaoyang One of the Fifteen Main Collaterals, originally known as the Branch of Foot-Shaoyang, from *Lingshu: Jingmai (Miraculous Pivot: Meridians)*, the collateral of Foot-Shaoyang is named Guangming. The collateral derives from Guangming (GB 3), 5 cun above the external malleolus, and goes to the Foot-Jueyin Meridian to run downwards and connect the dorsum of the foot.

●足少阳络脉病[zú shào yáng luò mài bìng] 十五络脉病候之一。出《灵枢·经脉》。其实证可见足部厥冷;虚证可见下肢瘫痪,不能起立。可取足少阳络穴治疗。

Diseases of the Collateral of Foot-Shaoyang One of the pathological manifestations of the Fifteen Main Collaterals, originally from *Lingshu: Jingmai (Miraculous Pivot: Meridians)*. Excess type is manifested as numb and cold feet; deficiency type is manifested as paralysis of the lower limbs and failure to stand up. The Luo (Connecting) point of Foot-Shaoyang Should be selected for the treatment of the disease.

●足少阳脉[zú shào yáng mài] 早期经脉名。出《帛书》。与足少阳经类似。

The Foot-Shaoyang Vessel An early name of a meridian, originally from *Bo Shu (Silk Book)*, similiar to the Foot-Shaoyang Meridian.

●足少阳穴[zú shào yáng xué] 经外穴名。见《千金要方》。在足背部当第2趾正中线第2跖趾关节之后方1寸处。〈主治〉胆石,腹中不安。直刺0.2寸。

Zushaoyangxue(EX-LE) An extra point, seen in *Qianjin Yaofang (Essential Prescriptions Worth a Thousand Gold)*. 〈Location〉on

the instep of the foot and on the midline of the 2nd toe, 1 cun posterior to the 2nd metatarsophalangeal joint. 〈Indications〉 excess syndrome of the gallbladder, abdominal distention and mass. 〈Method〉 Puncture 0.2 cun perpendicularly.

●足少阳之别[zú shào yáng zhī bié] 足少阳络脉的原名。见该条。

The Branch of Foot-Shaoyang The original name of the Collateral of Foot-Shaoyang. →足少阳络脉(p. 636)

●足少阳之正[zú shào yáng zhī zhèng] 足少阳经别的原名。见该条。

The Divergence of Foot-Shaoyang The original name of the Divergent Meridian of Foot-Shaoyang. →足少阳经别(p. 635)

●足少阳、足厥阴经别[zú shào yáng zú jué yīn jīng bié] 十二经别中的一合。出《灵枢·经别》。足少阳经别经过离、入、出的循行后，最后合于本经。足厥阴经别经过离、入、出的循行后，合于与其相表里的足少阳经。参见足少阳经别、足厥阴经别条。

Divergent Meridians of Foot-Shaoyang and Foot-Jueyin One confluence of the Twelve Divergent Meridians, originally from *Lingshu: Jingbie* (*Miraculous Pivot: Divergent Meridians*). The Divergent Meridian of Foot-Shaoyang finally joins its own regular meridian in the processes of deriving, entering and emerging. The Divergent Meridian of Foot-Jueyin finally joins into its externally-internally related meridian, the Foot-Shaoyang Meridian, in the processes of deriving, entering and emerging. →足少阳经别(p. 635)、足厥阴经别(p. 630)

●足少阴标本[zú shào yīn biāo běn] 十二经脉标本之一。出《灵枢·卫气》。足少阴之本，在内踝下三寸处，约当然谷穴处；标在背俞与舌下两脉，约当肾俞穴与廉泉之处。

The Superficiality and Origin of Foot-Shaoyin One of the superficialities and origins of the Twelve Regular Meridians. Originally from *Lingshu: Wei Qi* (*Miraculous Pivot: Defensive Qi*). The origin of Foot-Shaoyang is at Rangu(KI 2), 3 cun inferior to the internal malleolus, while the superficiality is at the Back-Shu point and the two vessels beneath the tongue, approximately at Shenshu(BL 23) and Lianquan(RN 23).

●足少阴经别[zú shào yīn jīng bié] 十二经别之一。原称足少阴之正。出《灵枢·经别》。足少阴经别，从本经脉在腘窝部分出后，与足太阳经别相合并行，上至肾脏，在十四椎处分出来，归属于带脉，其直行的继续上行，联系于舌根，再出来到项部，仍归入足太阳经别。

The Divergent Meridian of Foot-Shaoyin One of the Twelve Divergent Meridians, originally known as the Divergence of Foot-Shaoyang, originally from *Lingshu: Jingbie* (*Miraculou Pivot: Divergent Meridians*). The divergent meridian derives from its own regular meridian at the popliteal fossa, then runs together with the Divergent meridian of Foot-Taiyang, ascends to the kidney and emerges from the 14th vertebra to the Dai Meridian, the meridian it pertains to. The straight portion of the divergent meridian ascends continously to link with the base of the tongue, and emerges again from here to reach the nape and join the Divergent Meridian of Foot-Taiyang.

●足少阴经筋[zú shào yīn jīng jīn] 十二经筋之一。出《灵枢·经筋》。足少阴经筋，起于足小趾下边，入足心部同足太阴经筋斜至内踝下方，结于足跟，与足太阳经筋会合，向上结于胫骨内髁下，同足太阴经筋一起向上行，沿大腿内侧，结于阴部，沿脊旁肌肉内夹脊，上后项结于枕骨，与足太阳经筋会合。

Muscle Region of Foot-Shaoyin One of the Twelve Muscle Regions, originally from *Lingshu: Jingjin* (*Miraculous Pivot: Muscles along Meridians*), starting from the inferior aspect of the small toe and entering the sole, running obliquely to the region below the medial malleolus with the muscle region of Foot-Taiyin, connecting with the heel, and joining the muscle region of Foot-Taiyang. It runs from there upwards to connect the lower part of the medial condyle of the tibia and continuously upwards along the medial aspect of the thigh to connect with the pudendum and runs upwards in the muscles alongside the spine to the posterior top to connect with the occipital bone, and join the muscle region of Foot-

Taiyang.

●足少阴经筋病 [zú shào yīn jīng jīn bìng] 十二经筋病候之一。出《灵枢·经筋》。足少阴经筋发病，可见足下转筋，所经过和所结聚的总部位，都有疼痛和转筋的证候，病在足少阴经筋，主要有痫证，抽搐和项背反张等证，病在背侧的不能前俯，在胸腹侧的不能后仰，背为阳，腹为阴，阳筋病，项背部筋急，而腰向后反折，身体不能前俯，阴筋病，腹部筋急，而身不能后仰。

Diseases of the Muscle Region of Foot-Shaoyin One of the pathological manifestations of the Twelve Muscle Regions, originally from *Lingshu: Jingjin* (*Miraculous Pivot: Muscles Regions Along Meridians*). ⟨Manifestations⟩ spasm of the sole, pain and spasm along the root of the meridian, pain and spasm of the connected region, epilepsy, convulsion, opisthotonos, antexed dyscinesia when the symptoms are felt in the back, and retroflexion dyscinesia when the symptoms are seen in the chest and abdomen. Because the back belongs to yang, and the abdomen to yin, when the yang-muscle regions are found with such disease, the muscles on the neck and back contract, and the loin is retroflexed, and can not bend forward; when the yin-muscle regions are diseased, the muscles on the abdomen contract, and the body cannot bend backward.

●足少阴络脉 [zú shào yīn luò mài] 十五络脉之一。原称足少阴之别。出《灵枢·经脉》。足少阴络脉名曰大钟。其脉在内踝后足跟部大钟穴分出，走向足太阳经。其支脉与本经相并上行，走到心包下，外行通过腰脊部。

Collateral of Foot-Shaoyin One of the Fifteen Main Collaterals named the Branch of Foot-Shaoyin, originally from *Lingshu: Jingmai* (*Miraculous Pivot: Meridians*). The collateral of Foot-Shaoyin is Dazhong, deriving from Dazhong (KI 4) at the heel posterior to the medial malleolus (Dazhong KI 4), and running to join the meridian of Foot-Taiyang. The branch goes upwards parallel to its own meridian to the region below the pericardium, and runs outwards through the part of the loin and spine.

●足少阴络脉病 [zú shào yīn luò mài bìng] 十五络脉病候之一。出《灵枢·经脉》。其病症脉气厥逆，可见心胸烦闷。实证可见二便不通；虚证可见腰痛。可取足少阴络穴治疗。

Diseases of the Collateral of Foot-Shaoyin One of the pathological manifestations of the Fifteen Main Collaterals, originally from *Lingshu: Jingmai* (*Miraculous Pivot: Meridians*). ⟨Manifestations⟩ vexation and oppressive feeling in the chest due to reversed flow of the meridian qi, difficulty in urination and defecation in the syndrome of excess type and lumbago in the syndrome of deficiency type. The Luo (Connecting) point can be selected to treat the diseases.

●足少阴脉 [zú shào yīn mài] 早期经脉名。出《帛书》。与足少阴经类似。

Vessel of Foot-Shaoyin An early name of a meridian, originally from *Boshu* (*Silk Book*), similar to the Meridian of Foot-Shaoyin.

●足少阴肾经 [zú shào yīn shèn jīng] 十二经脉之一。原称肾足少阴之脉。出《灵枢·经脉》。其循行从足小趾下边开始，斜向足底心，出于舟骨粗隆下，沿内踝之后，分支进入足跟中，上向小腿内，出腘窝内侧，上大腿内后侧，通过脊柱，属于肾，络于膀胱。它直行的脉，从肾向上，通过肝、膈，进入肺中，沿着喉咙，夹舌根旁。它的支脉从肺出来，络于心，流注于胸中，接手厥阴心包经。

The Kidney Meridian of Foot-Shaoyin One of the Twelve Meridians, originally named the Kidney Vessel of Foot-Shaoyin, from *Lingshu: Jingmai* (*Miraculous Pivot: Meridians*). It starts from the inferior aspect of the small toe, runs obliquely towards the sole and emerges from the lower aspect of the tuberosity of the navicular bone, along the region posterior to the medial malleolus, one branch entering the heel, then it ascends along the medial side of the leg to the medial side of the popliteal fossa, and goes further upward along the posteriomedial aspect of the thigh towards the vertebral column, where it enters the kidney, its pertaining organ, and connects with the bladder. The straight portion of the meridian goes upwards from the kidney, passes through the liver and diaphragm, enters the lung, runs along the throat and terminates at

the root of the tongue. Another branch springs from the lung, joins the heart and runs into the chest to link with the Pericardium Meridian of Hand-Jueyin.

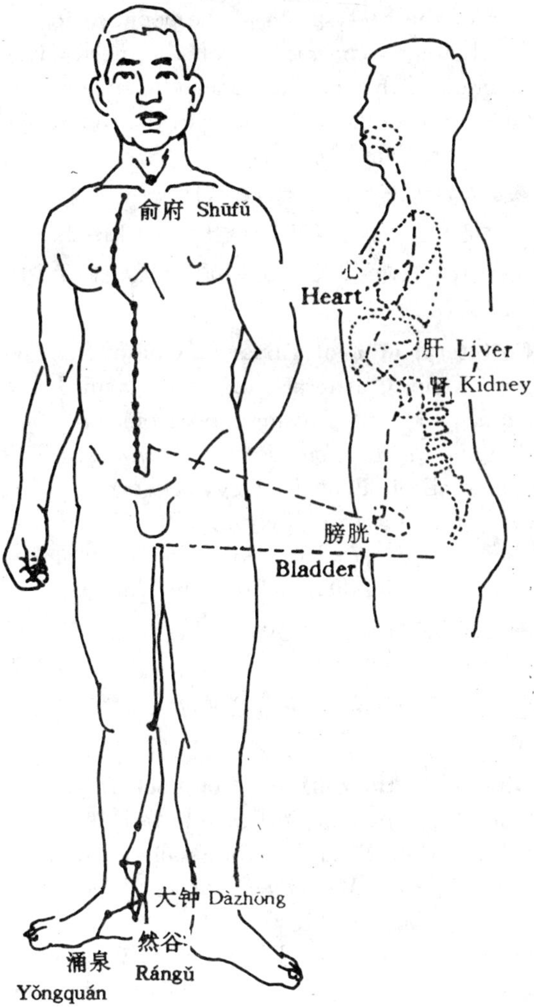

图83 足少阴肾经

Fig. 83 Kidney Meridian of Foot-Shaoyin

●**足少阴肾经病**[zú shào yīn shèn jīng bìng] 十二经脉病候之一。出《灵枢·经脉》。足少阴肾经主要病候为饥饿不思饮食，面色黯黑无光泽，咳嗽，痰中带血，气喘，口热，舌干，咽肿，喉咙干痛，心悸，惊惕，黄疸，泄泻，腰脊及股内后侧痛，痿软，厥冷，喜卧，足心热。

Diseases of the Kidney Meridian of Foot-Shaoyin One of the pathological manifestations of the Twelve Meridians, originally from *Lingshu*: *Jingmai* (*Miraculous Pivot*: *Meridians*). 〈Manifestations〉 anorexia, darkish and dim complexion, cough, phlegm with blood, dyspnea, hot breath, dry tongue, swelling of the throat, dryness and pain of the throat, palpitation, terror, jaundice, diarrhea, pain of the waist, spine and posteriomedial aspect of the thigh, flaccidity, cold limbs, drowsiness and fever in the sole.

●**足少阴之别**[zú shào yīn zhī bié] 足少阴络脉的原名。见该条。

The Branch of Foot-Shaoyin The original name of collateral of Foot-Shaoyin. →**足少阴络脉**(p. 638)

●**足少阴之正**[zú shào yīn zhī zhèng] 足少阴经别的原名。见该条。

The Divergence of Foot-Shaoyin The original name of the Divergent Meridian of Foot-Shaoyin. →**足少阴经别**(p. 637)

●**足太阳标本**[zú tài yáng biāo běn] 十二经标本之一。出《灵枢·卫气》。足太阳之本，在足跟上五寸，约当附阳穴处；标在两络命门(目)，约当睛明穴处。

The Superficiality and Origin of Foot-Taiyang One of the superficialities and origins of the Twelve Meridians, originally from *Lingshu*: *Wei Qi* (*Miraculous Pivot*: *Defensive Qi*). The origin of Foot-Taiyang is located in the region 5 cun above the heel, near the point Fuyang (BL 59); while the superficialities in the two collaterals Mingmen (eyes), near the point Jingming (BL 1).

●**足太阳经别**[zú tài yáng jīng bié] 十二经别之一。原称足太阳之正。出《灵枢·经别》。足太阳经别，在腘窝部从足太阳经脉分出，其中一条在骶骨下五寸处别行进入肛门，向里属于膀胱，散布联络肾脏，沿着脊柱两旁的肌肉，到心脏部进入散布在心内。直行的一条，循脊部两旁的肌肉处继续上行，浅出项部，仍归入足太阳本经。

Divergent Meridian of Foot-Taiyang One of the Twelve Divergent Meridians, originally named the Divergence of Foot-Taiyang, originally from *Lingshu*: *Jingbie* (*Miraculous Pivot*: *Divergent Meridians*). It diverges from the Meridian of Foot-Taiyang in the popliteal fossa, one branch entering the anus from the re-

gion 5 cun below the sacral bone, running into the pertaining organ, the bladder, distributing in and connecting with the kidney, running upwards in the muscles alongside the spine to the heart, and distributing in it, the straight one going continuously upward along the muscle beside the spine, emerging from the neck and returning to the Meridian of Foot-Taiyang proper.

●足太阳经筋[zú tài yáng jīng jīn] 十二经筋之一。出《灵枢·经筋》。足太阳经筋，起始于足小趾，上结于外踝，斜上结于膝部，下方沿足外侧结于足跟，向上沿跟腱结于腘部。其分支结于臀部，向上夹脊旁，上后项。分支入结于舌根。直行者结于枕骨，上向头项，由头的前方下行到颜面，结于鼻部。分支形成"目上纲"，下边结于鼻旁。背部的分支从缺盆出来，斜上结于鼻旁部。

Muscle Region of Foot-Taiyang One of the Twelve Muscle Regions, originally from *Lingshu: Jingjin (Miraculous Pivot: Muscles Along Meridians)*, starting from the little toe and connecting upward with the external malleolus, running upward obliquely to amass at the knee and then run downwards along the external aspect of the foot to amass at the heel, running on upward along the tendo calcaneus to amass at the popliteal fossa. One branch amasses at the gluteal region, runs upward alongside the spine to the posterior top, and terminates at the root of the tongue. The straight portion of the muscle region amasses at the occipital bone, runs upward to the top of the head, downward along the anterior side of the head to the face, amassing at the nose. The branch forms the upper border of the eye, and runs downward to amassing the region beside the nose. The branch on the back starts from the supraclavicular fossa, and runs upwards obliquely to amassing the region beside the nose.

●足太阳经筋病[zú tài yáng jīng jīn bìng] 十二经筋病候之一。出《灵枢·经筋》。其病可见足小趾支撑不适和足跟部掣引疼痛，腘窝部挛急，脊背反张，项筋拘急，肩不能抬举，腋部支撑不适，缺盆中如扭掣样疼痛，不能左右活动。

Diseases of the Muscle Region of Foot-Taiyang One of the pathological manifestations of the Twelve Muscle Regions, originally from *Lingshu: Jingjin (Miraculous Pivot: Muscles along Meridians)*. 〈Manifestations〉 uncomfortable sensation in the little toe, pulling pain of the heel, spasm in the popliteal fossa, opisthotonos, contracture of the neck, dysfunction of the shoulder, uncomfortable sensation in the axilla, pulling pain in the supraclavicular fossa and dyscinesia.

●足太阳络脉[zú tài yáng luò mài] 十五络脉之一。原称足太阳之别。出《灵枢·经脉》。足太阳络脉名曰飞扬。其脉在外踝上七寸处飞扬穴分出，走向足少阴经。

Collateral of Foot-Taiyang One of the Fifteen Main Collaterals, originally named the Branch of Foot-Taiyang, and from *Lingshu: Jingmai (Miraculous Pivot: Meridians)*. The collateral of Foot-Taiyang is Feiyang (BL 58), deriving from Feiyang (BL 58), 7 cun above the external malleolus and running towards the Meridian of Foot-Shaoyin.

●足太阳络脉病[zú tài yáng luò mài bìng] 十五络脉病候之一。出《灵枢·经脉》。实证见鼻塞，鼻流清涕，头痛，背痛；虚证见鼻流清涕，鼻出血。可取足太阳经络穴治疗。

Diseases of the Collateral of Foot-Taiyang One of the pathological manifestations of the Fifteen Main Collaterals, originally from *Lingshu: Jingmai (Miraculous Pivot: Meridians)*. 〈Manifestations〉 Of the excess type, stuffy nose, watery nasal discharge, headache, and back pain. Of the deficiency type, watery nasal discharge and epistaxis. The Luo (Connecting) point of Foot-Taiyang can be selected to treat the diseases.

●足太阳膀胱经[zú tài yáng páng guāng jīng] 十二经脉之一。原称膀胱足太阳之脉。出《灵枢·经脉》。其循行从内眼角开始，上行额部，交会于头顶。它的支脉，从头顶分出到耳上角。它的直行主干，从头顶入内络于脑，复出项部开下行。一支沿肩胛内侧，夹脊旁，到达腰中，进入脊旁筋肉，络于肾，属于膀胱。一支从腰分出，夹脊旁，通过臀部，进入腘窝中。背部另一支脉，从肩胛内侧分别下行，通过肩胛，经过髋关节部，沿大腿外侧后边下行，会合于腘窝中，由此

向下通过腓肠肌部，出外踝后方，沿第五跖骨粗隆，到小趾的外侧，接足少阴肾经。

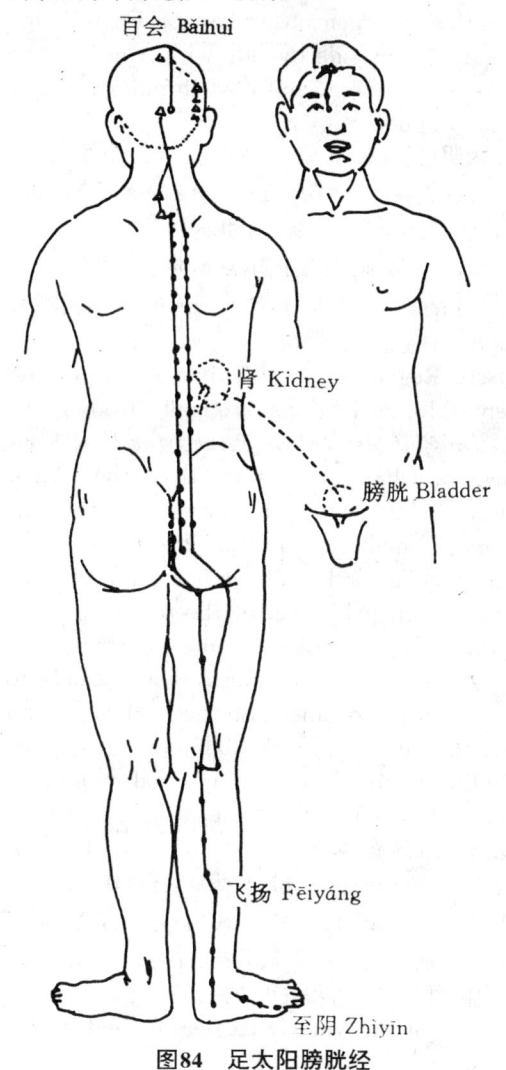

图84 足太阳膀胱经

Fig. 84　Bladder Meridian of Foot-Taiyang

The Bladder Meridian of Foot-Taiyang　One of the Twelve Meridians, originally named the Bladder Meridian of Foot-Taiyang, seen in *Lingshu: Jingmai* (*Miraculous Pivot: Meridians*), starting from the inner canthus and ascending to the forehead, joining the Du Meridian at the vertex. From here, a branch runs to the angle superior to the ear. The straight portion of the meridian enters the brain from the vertex and communicates with it. It then emerges and bigurcates to descend along the neck. A branch runs downward along the medial aspect of the scapula region and parallel to the vertebral column, reaches the lumbar region and enters the paravertebral muscle to connect the kidney and join its pertaining organ, the urinary bladder. The branch of the lumbar region descends alongside the spine, passing through the gluteal region and ending in the popliteal fossa. Another branch on the back descends along the medial aspect of the scapular region, passing through the scapula and hip joint. It converges in the popliteal fossa. From there, it descends through the gastrocnemius muscle to the posterior aspect of the external malleolus, then runs along the tuberosity of the 5th metatarsal bone, and reaches the lateral side of the little toe, where it links with the Kidney Meridian of Foot-Shaoyin.

●足太阳膀胱经病[zú tài yáng páng guāng jīng bìng] 十二经病候之一。出《灵枢·经脉》。本经主要病候可见头痛，目痛，鼻塞，衄血，项强，脊背痛，腰痛，痔，疟疾，癫狂，髋部不能屈，腘部掣痛，小腿肚及脚痛，小腹偏肿而痛，癃闭，遗溺。

Diseases of the Bladder Meridian of Foot-Taiyang　One of the pathological manifestations of the Twelve Meridians, originally from *Lingshu: Jingmai* (*Miraculous Pivot: Meridians*). 〈Manifestations〉headache, pain of eyes, stuffy nose, epistaxis, stiffness of the nape, back pain, lumbago, hemorrhoid, malaria, manic-depressive disorder, flexion dyscinesia of the hip, pulling pain of the popliteal fossa region, pain of the gastrocnemius muscle and foot, swelling and pain of the lower abdomen, uroschesis and enuresis.

●足太阳穴[zú tài yáng xué]　经外穴名。见《千金要方》。在外踝后一寸宛宛中。〈主治〉消渴，咽干，淋症，癫疝。用灸法。

Zutaiyangxue（EX-LE）　An extra point, originally from *Qianjin Yaofang* (*Essential Prescriptions Worth a Thousand Gold*). 〈Location〉in the depression 1 cun posterior to the external malleolus. 〈Indications〉diabetes, dry throat, stranguria and swelling of the scrotum. 〈Method〉moxibustion.

●足太阳之别[zú tài yáng zhī bié]　足太阳络脉的原名。见该条。

641

The Branch of Foot-Taiyang The original name of Collateral of Foot-Taiyang. →足太阳络脉(p. 640)

●足太阳之正[zú tài yáng zhī zhèng] 足太阳经别的原名。见该条。

The Divergence of Foot-Taiyang The original name of Divergent Meridian of Foot-Taiyang. →足太阳经别(p. 639)

●足太阳、足少阴经别[zú tài yáng zú shào yīn jīng bié] 十二经别中的一合。出《灵枢·经别》。足太阳经别经过离、入、出的循行后,最后合于本经。足少阴经别经过离、入、出的循行后,合于足太阳经。参见足太阳经别,足少阴经别条。

Divergent Meridians of Foot-Taiyang and Foot-Shaoyin One confluence of the Twelve Divergent Meridians, originally from *Lingshu：Jingbie*(*Miraculous Pivot：Divergent Meridians*). The Divergent Meridian of Foot-Taiyang finally joins the regular meridian after the circulation of derivation, entry and emergence, and the Kidney Divergent Meridian of Foot-Shaoyin joins the Meridian of Foot-Taiyang. →足太阳经别(p. 639)、足少阴经别(p. 637)

●足太阴标本[zú tài yīn biāo běn] 十二经脉标本之一。出《灵枢·卫气》。足太阴之本,在中封上四寸之中,约当三阴交穴处。标在背俞与舌本、约当脾俞与廉泉穴处。

The Superficiality and Origin of Foot-Taiyin

One of the superficialities and origins of the Twelve Meridians, originally from *Lingshu：Wei Qi*(*Miraculous Pivot：Defensive Qi*). The origin of Foot-Taiyin is located in the region 4 cun above Zhongfeng(LR 4), near the point Sanyinjiao(SP 6), and the superficiality in the Back-Shu point and the root of the tongue, near the point Pishu(BL 20) and the point Lianquan(RN 23).

●足太阴经别[zú tài yīn jīng bié] 十二经别之一。原称足太阴之正。出《灵枢·经脉》。足太阴经别,从足太阴经脉分出后到达大腿前面,和足阳明经的经别相合并行,向上结于咽喉,贯通到舌本。

Divergent Meridian of Foot-Taiyin One of the Twelve Divergent Meridians, originally named Zheng(main branch) of Foot-Taiyin, seen in *Lingshu：Jingmai*)(*Miraculous Pivot：Meridians*), deriving from the meridian of Foot-Taiyin, the Divergent Meridian of Foot-Taiyin reaches the anterior side of the thigh, joins the Divergent Meridian of Foot-Yangming, and runs side by side with it upward to amass at the throat and pass through the root of the tongue.

●足太阴经筋[zú tài yīn jīng jīn] 十二经筋之一。出《灵枢·经筋》。足太阴经筋,起始于足大趾内侧端,上行结于内踝,直行向上结于膝内辅骨,向上沿着大腿内侧,结于股前,会聚于阴器部,向上到腹部,结于脐,再沿着腹内结于肋骨,散布到胸中,在内的经筋则附着于脊旁。

Muscle Region of Foot-Taiyin One of the twelve Muscle Regions, originally from *Lingshu：Jingjin*(*Miraculous Pivot：Muscle Regions Along Meridians*). It starts from the medial aspect of the big toe, runs upward to amass at the medial malleolus, ascends directly to amass at the medial condyle of the tibia, runs upward along the medial aspect of the thigh to amass at the greater trochanter of the thigh, and converges in the pudendum, then ascends to the abdomen to amass at the umbilicus, and then the ribs along the abdomen cavity, distributing in the chest. The internal muscle region is attached to the spine.

●足太阴经筋病[zú tài yīn jīng jīn bìng] 十二经筋病候之一。出《灵枢·卫气》。其病症,可出现足大趾支撑不适,牵引内踝作痛,转筋,膝内辅骨痛,肌内侧牵引髀部作痛,阴器部有扭转疼痛,并可向上引脐及两胁作痛,且能牵引膺和脊内疼痛。

Diseases of the Muscle Region of Foot-Taiyin

One of the pathological manifestations of the Twelve Muscle Regions, originally from *Lingshu：Wei Qi*(*Miraculous Pivot：Defensive Qi*). 〈Manifestations〉 uncomfortable sensation of the big toe, pulling pain of the medial malleolus, spasm, pain of the knee and the medial condyle of the tibia, pain of the medial aspect of the thigh involving the greater trochanter, torsive pain of the external genitals, which may radiate to the umbilicus upward and hypochondrium, and pulling pain of the chest and spine.

●足太阴络[zú tài yīn luò] 经穴别名。见《针灸甲乙经》。即漏谷。见该条。

Zutaiyinluo Another name for Lougu(SP

7), a meridian point originally from *Zhenjiu Jia-Yi Jing* (*A-B Classic of Acupuncture and Moxi-bustion*). → 漏谷 (p. 256)

●足太阴络脉 [zú tài yīn luò mài] 十五络脉之一。原称足太阴之别。出《灵枢·经脉》。足太阴络脉名曰公孙。其脉在距离足大趾本节后方一寸处公孙穴分出，走向足阳明胃经，其支脉进入腹腔，与肠胃联络。

Collateral of Foot-Taiyin One of the Fifteen Main Collaterals, originally from *Lingshu: Jingmai* (*Miraculous Pivot: Meridians*). Its name is Gongsun (SP 4). The collateral of Foot-Taiyin derivs from Gongsun (SP 4) 1 cun posterior to the lst metatarsodigital joint, and runs towards the Stomach Meridian of Foot-Yangming. Its branch enters the abdominal cavity to connect with the intestines and stomach.

●足太阴络脉病 [zú tài yīn luò mài bìng] 十五络脉病候之一。出《灵枢·经脉》。其病可见气厥逆上，挥霍缭乱，上吐下泻。实证可见腹内绞痛。虚证可见腹部胀气。可取足太阴络穴治疗。

Diseases of the Collateral of Foot-Taiyin One of the pathological manifestations of the Fifteen Main Collaterals, originally from *Lingshu: Jingmai* (*Miraculous Pivot: Meridians*). ⟨Manifestations⟩ cholera morbus due to reversed flow of qi, vomiting and diarrhea, colicky pain of the abdomen in the syndrome of excess type, and flatulence of the abdomen in the syndrome of deficiency type. The Luo (Connecting) point of Foot-Taiyin can be selected to treat the diseases.

●足泰阴脉 [zú tài yīn mài] 早期经脉名。出《帛书》。与足太阴经类似。

Vessel of Foot-Taiyin (泰阴) An early name of a meridian, originally from *Boshu* (*Silk Book*), similar to the Meridian of Foot-Taiyin.

●足太阴脾经 [zú tài yīn pí jīng] 十二经脉之一。原称脾足太阴之脉。出《灵枢·经脉》。其循行从大趾末端开始，大趾足内侧赤白肉际，经核骨，上向内踝前边，上小腿内侧，沿胫骨后，交出足厥阴肝经之前，上膝股内侧前边，进入腹部，属于脾，络于胃，通过膈肌，夹食管旁，连舌根，散布舌下。它的支脉，从胃部分出，上过膈肌，流注心中，接手少阴心经。

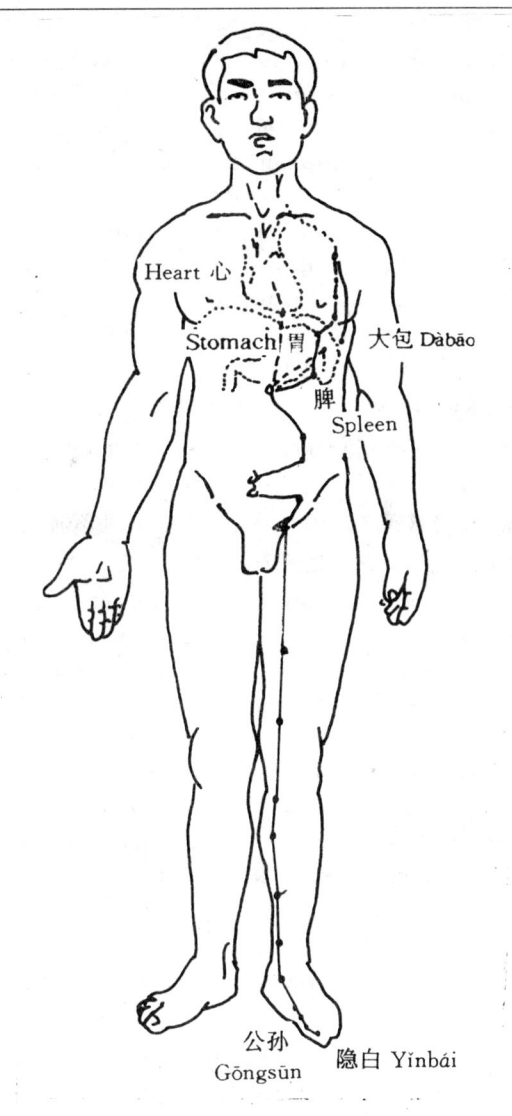

图85 足太阴脾经
Fig. 85 Spleen Meridian of Foot-Taiyin

The Spleen Meridian of Foot-Taiyin One of the Twelve Meridians, originally named Foot-Taiyin Meridian, and seen in *Lingshu: Jingmai* (*Miraculous Pivot: Meridians*). It starts from the tip of the big toe, runs along the medial aspect of the big toe at the junction of red and white skin, passes through the nodular process on the medial aspect of the lst metatarsophalangeal joint, ascends to the front of the medial malleolus and further up to the medial aspect of the leg, follows the posterior aspect of the tibia and passes through the front of the Liver Meridian of Foot-Jueyin. Going on along the anterior medial aspect of the knee and

then the thigh, it enters the abdomen, reaches the spleen, the organ it pertains to and connects with the stomach. From there it ascends, passing through the diaphragm and running along side the esophagus to connect with the root of the tongue and spread under the tongue. Its branch starts from the stomach, goes upwards through the diaphragm, and flows into the heart to link with the Heart Meridian of Hand-Shaoyin.

●足太阴脾经病[zú tài yīn pí jīng bìng] 十二经脉病候之一。出《灵枢·经脉》。本经的主要病证可见呕吐,胃脘痛,腹胀,嗳气,心烦,黄疸,腹中痞块,大便溏薄,全身感到沉重无力,心窝下急痛,小便不通,不能安睡,经脉所过之处痛厥。

Diseases of the Spleen Meridian of Foot-Taiyin One of the pathological manifestations of the Twelve Meridians, originally from *Lingshu : Jingmai* (*Miraculous Pivot : Meridians*). 〈Manifestations〉 vomiting, gastric pain, abdominal distension, eructation, vexation, jaundice, mass in the abdomen, diarrhea, heavy and weak feeling of the whole body, acute pain in the epigastrium, enuresis, insomnia, pain and cold in the region along the course of the meridian.

●足太阴之别[zú tài yīn zhī bié] 足太阴络脉的原名。见该条。

The Branch of Foot-Taiyin The original name of the Collateral of Foot-Taiyin. →足太阴络脉(p. 643)

●足太阴之正[zú tài yīn zhī zhèng] 足太阴经别的原名。见该条。

The Divergence of Foot-Taiyin The original name of the Divergent Meridian of Foot-Taiyin. →足太阴经别(p. 642)

●足泰阳脉[zú tài yáng mài] 早期经脉名。出《帛书》。与足太阳经类似。

Vessel of Foot-Taiyang (泰阳) An early name of a meridian, originally from *Bo Shu* (*Silk Book*), similar to the Meridian of Foot-Taiyang(太阳).

●足通谷[zú tōng gǔ] 经穴名。出《灵枢·本输》。原名通谷,属足太阳膀胱经,为本经荥穴。〈定位〉在足外侧,足小趾本节(第五跖趾关节)的前方,赤白肉际处(图35.2)。〈层次解剖〉皮肤→皮下组织→小趾近节趾骨底的跖侧面。布有足背外侧皮神经,足背静脉弓的属支,趾足底固有动、静脉。〈主治〉头痛,项痛,目眩,鼻衄,癫狂。直刺0.2～0.3寸;可灸。

Zutonggu (BL 66) A meridian point, originally from *Lingshu : Benshu* (*Miraculous Pivot : Meridian Points*), originally named Tonggu, a point on the Bladder Meridian of Foot-Taiyang, the Ying (Spring) point of the meridian. 〈Location〉 on the lateral side of the foot, anterior to the 5th metatarsophalangeal joint, at the junction of the red and white skin (Fig. 35.2). 〈Regional anatomy〉 skin → subcutaneous tissue → plantar surface of proximal end of little toe. There are the lateral dorsal cutaneous nerve of the foot, the tributaries of the arch of the dorsal veins of the foot, and the proper digital plantar arteries and veins in this area. 〈Indications〉 headache, pain of the neck, dizziness, epistaxis, manic depressive disorder. 〈Method〉 Puncture perpendicularly 0.2 ～ 0.3 cun. Moxibustion is applicable.

●足五里[zú wǔ lǐ] 经穴名。见《针灸资生经》。属足厥阴肝经。〈定位〉在大腿内侧,当气冲直下3寸,大腿根部,耻骨结节的下方,长收肌的外缘(图86)。〈层次解剖〉皮肤→皮下组织→长收肌→短收肌→大收肌。浅层布有股神经的前支,大隐静脉。深层有闭孔神经的前支和后支,股深动、静脉的肌支,旋股内侧动、静脉的肌支。〈主治〉小腹胀痛,小便不通,阴挺,睾丸肿痛,嗜卧,四肢倦怠,瘰疬。直刺0.5～0.8寸;可灸。

Zuwuli (LR 10) A meridian point, originally from *Zhenjiu Zisheng Jing* (*Acupuncture and Moxibustion Classic for Saving Life*), a point on the Liver Meridian of Foot-Jueyin. 〈Location〉 on the medial side of the thigh, 3 cun directly below Qichong (ST 30), at the proximal end of the thigh, below the pubic tubercle and on the lateral border of the long abductor muscle of the thigh (Fig. 86). 〈Regional anatomy〉 skin → subcutaneous tissue → long adductor muscle → short adductor muscle → great adductor muscle. In the superficial layer, there are the anterior cutaneous branches of the femoral nerve and the saphenous vein. In the deep layer, there are the anterior and posterior branches of the obturator nerve, the

muscular branches of the deep femoral artery and vein, and the muscular branches of the medial femoral circumflex arteries and veins. 〈Indications〉distending pain of the lower abdomen, retention of urine, prolapse of the uterus, swelling and pain of the testicle, drowsiness, weakness of the four limbs and scrofula. 〈Method〉Punctrue perpendicularly 0.5～0.8cun. Moxibustion is applicable.

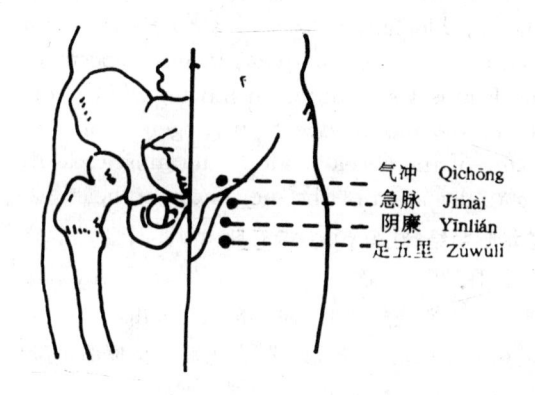

图86 足五里、阴廉和急脉穴
Fig. 86 Zuwuli, Yinlian and Jimai points

●足下廉[zú xià lián] 经穴别名。见《圣济总录》。即下巨虚,见该条。

Zuxialian Another name for Xiajuxu(ST 39), a meridian point originally from *Shengji Zonglu*(*Imperial Medical Encyclopaedia*). → 下巨虚(p.489)

●足心[zú xīn] ①经穴别名。即涌泉,见该条。②经外穴名。出《备急千金要方》。位于足底中线,第2趾尖端至足跟后缘连线的中点。〈主治〉崩漏、头痛、眩晕、癫疾、足底痛、休克等。直刺0.3～0.5寸;可灸。③部位名,约涌泉穴部位。

1. **Zuxin** Another name for the meridian point Yongquan(KI 1). →涌泉(p.568)
2. **Zuxin**(EX-LE) An extra point originally from *Beiji Qianjin Yaofang*(*Essential Prescriptions Worth a Thousand Gold for Emergencies*). 〈Location〉on the midline of the sole, at the midpoint of the line connecting the tip of the 2nd toe and the posterior border of the heel. 〈Indications〉metrorrhagia and metrostaxis, headache, dizziness, epilepsy, pain of the sole, and shock, etc. 〈Method〉Puncture perpendicularly 0.3～0.5 cun.
3. **Sole** A body part, near the point Yongquan(KI 1).

●足阳关[zú yáng guān] 经穴别名,即膝阳关,见该条。

Zuyangguan Another name for Xiyangguan (GB 33). →膝阳关(p.484)

●足阳明标本[zú yáng míng biāo běn] 十二经脉标本之一。出《灵枢·卫气》。足阳明之本,在厉兑。标在人迎、颊、挟颃颡。

The Superficiality and Origin of Foot-Yangming One of the superficialities and origins of the Twelve Meridians, originally from *Lingshu: Wei Qi*(*Miraculous Pivot: Defensive Qi*). The origin of Foot-Yangming is located in Lidui (ST 45), and the superficiality in Renying(ST 9), cheek and the part alongside the nasopharnx.

●足阳明经别[zú yáng míng jīng bié] 十二经别之一。原称足阳明之正。出《灵枢·经别》。足阳明经别,在大腿前面从足阳明分出,进入腹腔之内,属于胃腑,散布到脾脏,向上通连心脏,沿着食道浅出于口腔,上达于鼻根和眼眶下部,回过来联系到眼后与脑相连的组织,脉气仍会合于足阳明经。

Divergent Meridian of Foot-Yangming One of the Twelve Divergent Meridians, originally named the Divergence of Foot-Yangming, from *Lingshu: Jingbie*(*Miraculous Pivot: Divergent Meridians*). The Divergent Meridian of Foot-Yangming derives from the Meridian of Foot-Yangming anterior to the thigh, enters the abdominal cavity. It pertains to the stomach and distributes in the spleen, then it runs upward to connect with the heart, and emerges from the mouth cavity along the esophagus, reaches the root of the nose and the infraorbital region and winds back to communicate with the tissues posterior to eyes connecting with the brain. The meridian-qi also converges in the meridian of Foot-Yangming.

●足阳明经筋[zú yáng míng jīng jīn] 十二经筋之一。出《灵枢·经筋》。足阳明经筋,起始于足次趾,中趾及无名趾,结于足背,斜向外行加附于腓骨,上结于胫外侧,直上结于髀枢,又向上沿胁部属于脊。其直行的上沿胫骨,结于膝部。分支之筋结于外辅骨

部,合并足少阳经筋。直行的沿伏兔上行,结于大腿部而聚会于阴器。再向上分布到腹部,至缺盆处结聚。再向上至颈,夹口旁,合于鼻旁颧部,相继下结于鼻,从鼻旁合于足太阳经筋。太阳经筋为"目上纲",阳明经筋为"目下纲"。另一分支之筋,从面颊结于耳前部。

Muscle Region of Foot-Yangming One of the Twelve Muscle Regions originally from *Lingshu*: *Jingjin* (*Miraculous Pivot*: *Muscles Regions Along Meridians*). The Foot-Yangming Muscle Region starts from the 2nd, the middle and the 4th toes, gathers at the dorsum of the foot, runs obliquely outwards and attaches to the fibula, gathers at the lateral aspect of the tibia upwards and stretches directly to the greater trochanter, then ascends along the costal regions and pertains to the spine. The straight trunk ascends along the tibia, and enters the knee with branches assembling at the fibula, merging with the Foot-Shaoyang Muscle Region. The straight trunk continues going up along the muscles rectus femoris, reaches the thigh and gathers at the external genitals, then distributes to the abdomen and enters the supraclavicular fossa. It runs upwards to the neck, along the lateral side of the mouth, reaches the zygomatic portion, then descends to the nose, and merges with the Foot-Taiyang Muscle Region at the lateral side of the nose. The Taiyang Muscle Region forms the margin of the upper eyelid, the Yangming Muscle Region forms the margin of the lower eyelid. Another branch reaches and amasses at the proctic region from the the cheek.

●足阳明经筋病[zú yáng míng jīng jīn bìng] 十二经筋病候之一。出《灵枢·经筋》。其病可出现足中趾及胫部支撑不适,拘紧疼痛,足部活动感觉到僵硬不舒,股前拘紧疼痛,髀前部肿,疝气,腹部筋肉拘紧,向上牵制到缺盆和颊部,突然发生口角歪斜,如有寒邪则掣引眼睑不能闭合,如有热邪则筋松弛使眼睑不能睁开。颊筋有寒使筋脉紧急,牵引颊部致口角移动;有热时则筋肉松弛收缩无力,所以口歪。

Diseases of the Muscle Region of Foot-Yangming One of the pathological manifestations of the Twelve Muscle Regions, originally from *Lingshu*: *Jingjin* (*Miraculous Pivot*: *Muscle Regions Along Meridians*). ⟨Manifestations⟩ distension, constracture and pain of the middle toe and tibia, rigidity of foot, contracture, pain and swelling in the anterior portion of the thigh, hernia, contracture of abdominal muscles and tendons, which radiates to the supraclavicular fossa and the cheek, sudden occurrence of facial paralysis, sometimes accompanied by blepharospasm due to pathogenic cold, or blepharochalasis due to flaccidity of tendon caused by pathogenic heat, spasm of cheek muscles resulting in moving of the corner of the mouth due to pathogenic cold; relaxing of the cheek tendons and muscles leading to deviation of the mouth due to heat.

●足阳明络脉[zú yáng míng luò mài] 十五络脉之一。原称是阳明之别。出《灵枢·经脉》。足阳明络脉名曰丰隆,在距离外踝上八寸丰隆穴处分出,走向足太阴经。其支脉沿着胫骨外缘,向上联络头顶部,与各经的脉气相会合,向下联络喉咙和咽峡部。

The Collateral of Foot-Yangming One of the Fifteen Main Collaterals, formerly called the Branch of Foot-Yangming, originally from *Lingshu*: *Jingmai* (*Miraculous Pivot*: *Meridians*). It is named Fenglong (ST 40), a meridian point, from which the Foot-Yangming collateral originates, 8 cun above the lateral malleolus and runs towards the Foot-Taiyin Meridian with its branch going along the lateral border of tibia, reaching the top of the head, amassing there, converging with the qi of each meridian, and going downwards to connect with the laryngeal part of the pharynx and isthmus of fauces.

●足阳明络脉病[zú yáng míng luò mài bìng] 十五脉病候之一。出《灵枢·经脉》。其病见气逆,就会患喉部肿痛,突然音哑。实证可发生癫病,狂病;虚证可见足胫部弛缓无力,骨肉萎缩。可取足阳明络穴治疗。

Diseases of the Collateral of Foot-Yangming One of the pathological manifestations of the Fifteen Main Collaterals, originally from *Lingshu*: *Jingmai* (*Miraculous Pivot*: *Meridians*). Manifested as sore throat, sudden hoarseness due to reversed flow of qi; manic-depressive psychosis due to excessive pathogen

in the collateral; relaxation and myoatrophy of the leg due to deficiency of the collateral. Select the Luo(Connecting) point of Foot-Yangming Meridian for the treatment.

●足阳明脉 [zú yáng míng mài] 早期经脉名。出《帛书》。与足阳明经类似。

Foot-Yangming Vessel An early name of a meridian, originally from *Boshu*(*Silk Book*), similar to the Foot-Yangming Meridian.

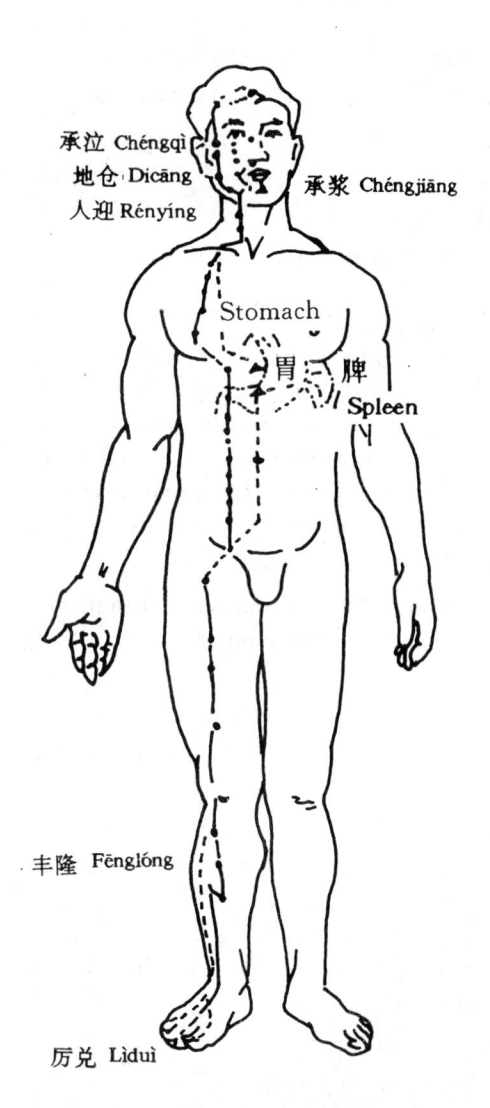

图87 足阳明胃经

Fig. 87 Stomach Meridian of Foot-Yangming

●足阳明胃经 [zú yáng míng wèi jīng] 十二经脉之一。原称足阳明之脉。出《灵枢·经脉》。其循行从鼻旁开始，交会鼻根中，旁边会足太阳经，向下沿鼻外侧，进入上齿槽中，回出来夹口旁环绕口唇，向下交会于颏唇沟，退回来沿下颌出面动脉部，再沿下颌角，上耳前，经颧弓上，沿发际，至额颅中部。它的支脉，从大迎前向下，经颈动脉部，沿喉咙，进入缺盆部，通过膈肌，属于胃，络于脾。外行的主干，从缺盆向下，经乳中，向下夹脐两旁，进入气街。它的支脉，从胃口向下，沿腹里，至腹股沟动脉部与前者会合。由此下行经髀关节前，到股四头肌隆起处，下向膝膑中，沿胫骨外侧，下行足背，进入中趾内侧趾缝，出次趾末端。它的支脉，从膝下三寸处分出，向下进入中趾外侧趾缝，出中趾末端。另一支脉，从足背部分出，进大趾趾缝，出大趾末端，接足太阴脾经。

The Stomach Meridian of Foot-Yangming One of the Twelve Regular Meridians, originally called the Foot-Yangming Vessel of the Stomach, from *Lingshu: Jingmai* (*Miraculous Pivot: Meridians*). ⟨Circulation⟩ The Stomach Meridian of Foot-Yangming starts from the lateral side of ala nasi and ascends to the bridge of the nose, where it meets the Bladder Meridian of Foot-Taiyang. Turning downwards along the lateral side of the nose, it enters the upper gum. Reemerging, it curves round the lips and descends to meet the Ren Meridian at the mentolabial groove. Then it runs posteriolaterally across the lower portion of the cheek at the facial artery. Winding along the angle of the mandible, it ascends in front of the ear and traverses the zygomatio arch. Then it follows the anterior hairline and reaches the forehead. The facial branch runs downwards in front of Daying (ST 5) to the carotid, from there goes along the throat and enters the supraclavicular fossa. Descending, it passes through the diaphragm, enters the stomach the organ it pertains to, and connects with the spleen. The straight portion of the meridian arises from the supraclavicular fossa and runs downward passing the nipple. It descends by the umbilicus and enters Qijie. The branch from the lower orifice of the stomach descends from inside the abdomen to the inguina artery to meet with the former. Running further downwards, through the anterior of the thigh joint, to the convex of quandriceps muscle of the thigh, it reaches the knee.

From there, it runs on downward and along the anterior border of the lateral aspect of the tibia, passes the dorsum of the foot, and reaches the lateral side of the tip of the 2nd toe. The tibial branch emerges from the point 3 cun below the knee, enters the lateral side of the middle toe, and terminates at the end of the middle toe. Another branch rises from the dorsum of the foot, enters the medial side of the tip of the big toe, and terminates at its end, where it links with the Spleen Meridian of Foot-Taiyin.

● 足阳明胃经病 [zú yáng míng wèi jīng bìng] 十二经脉病候之一。出《灵枢·经脉》。本经病可见寒热，疟疾，鼻塞，衄血，口喎，颈肿，喉痛，癫狂，温热病，自汗，腹胀满，大腹水肿，胃脘痛，恶心，呕吐，饮食不化或消谷善饥，经脉所过部肿痛。

Diseases of the Stomach Meridian of Foot-Yangming One of the pathological manifestations of the Twelve Regular Meridians, originally from *Lingshu: Jingmai (Miraculous Pivot: Meridians)*. ⟨Manifestations⟩ chills accompanied by fever, malaria, stuffy nose, nosebleeding, wry mouth, neck swelling, sore throat, manic-depressive psychosis, epidemic febrile disease, spontaneous perspiration, abdominal distension, ascites, epigastric pain, nausea vomiting, dyspepsia or polyorexia, swelling and pain along the course of the meridian.

● 足阳明之别 [zú yáng míng zhī bié] 足阳明络脉的原名。见该条。

The Branch of the Foot-Yangming Meridian The original name of the Foot-Yangming Collateral. →足阳明络脉 (p. 646)

● 足阳明之正 [zú yáng míng zhī zhèng] 足阳明经别的原称。见该条。

The Divergence of Foot-Yangming The original name of the divergent meridian of Foot-Yangming. →足阳明经别 (p. 645)

● 足阳明、足太阴经别 [zú yáng míng zú tài yīn jīng bié] 十二经别中的一合。出《灵枢·经别》。足阳明经别经过离、入、出的循行，最后合于本经。足太阴经别经过离、入、出的循行后，合于与其相表里的足阳明经。参见足阳明经别、足太阴经别条。

The Divergent Meridians of Foot-Yangming and Foot-Taiyin One convergence of the Twelve Divergent Meridians, originally from *Lingshu: Jingbie (Miraculous Pivot: Divergent Meridians)*. The Divergent Meridian of Foot-yangming finally converges into the Foot-Yangming Meridian through the course of departure, entrance and emergence; the Divergent Meridian of Foot-Taiyin Converges into the Foot-Yangming Meridian through the course of departure, entrance and emergence. →足阳明经别 (p. 645)、足太阴经别 (p. 642)

● 足运感区 [zú yùn gǎn qū] 头针刺激区。在前后正中线的中点旁开左右各1厘米，向后引3厘米长，平行于正中线。⟨主治⟩对侧下肢瘫痪，疼痛，麻木，急性腰扭伤，夜尿，皮质性多尿，子宫下垂等。

Foot Motor Sensory Area The specific stimulation area for scalp acupuncture. ⟨Location⟩ At the two points 1 cun bilateral to the midpoint of the anterior-posterior midline, draw two 3-centimetre long straight lines backwards, parallel to the midline. ⟨Indications⟩ contralateral lower extremity paralysis, pain and numbness, acute lumbar sprain, nocturia, cortical diuresis, hysteroptosis, etc.

● 阻病 [zǔ bìng] 恶阻的别名。详见该条。

Vomiting and Nausea during Pregnancy Another name for morning sickness. →恶阻 (p. 93)

● 组穴 [zǔ xué] 指由两个以上的穴位组合应用而重新命名者。如"四关"，由合谷、太冲组成。"六之灸"，由膈俞、肝俞、脾俞组成等。

The Grouped Points A set of more than two points which gains a new name when they are used in combination, e. g. Siguan is composed of Hegu (LI 4) and Taichong (LR 3); Liuzhijiu consists of Geshu (BL 17), Ganshu (BL 18) and Pishu (BL 20), etc.

● 纂 [zuǎn] 部位名。见篡条。

Zuan A body part. →篡 (p. 58)

● 左右配穴法 [zuǒ yòu pèi xué fǎ] 配穴法之一。指左右两侧同名穴位的配合应用。十二经脉左右同源，其穴位均两侧对称，临床上对于内脏疾病，左右两侧同取，以增强作用。例如胃病取两侧的胃俞或两侧的足三里等。

The Combination of the Left-Right Points
A kind of point selections in which bilateral points with same names are chosen for needling. The left and the right of the Twelve Regular Meridians have the same source, and the points are bilaterally symmetric. So the bilateral symmetric points are used for treating splanchnopathy in clinic, usually selected to strengthen curative effect, eg. bilateral Weishu (BL 21)and Zusanli(ST 36)can be selected to treat gastropathy,etc.

●左右转[zuǒ yòu zhuàn] 刺法用语。指针刺的捻转方向。一般用右手持针,当大指向前,食指退后,称为左转或外转;大指向后,食指向前,称为右转或内转。后世结合捻转提出补泻手法多种,参见"捻转补泻"条。

Left and Right Twirling An acupuncture technique, referring to the twirling and rotating direction of needling. Generally, hold the needle in the right hand. The manipulation in which the thumb goes forward and index finger backward, is called left rotation or outward rotation; the manipulation in which thumb goes backward and index finger forward is called right rotation or inward rotation. Chinese descendents have put forward many kinds of reinforcing and reducing methods on the basis of twirling or rotating method. →捻转补泻(p.283)

●坐骨神经[zuò gǔ shén jīng] 耳穴名。位于对耳轮下脚的中三分之一处。用于治疗坐骨神经痛。

Sciatic Nerve（MA-AH 6） An auricular point.〈Location〉at the middle 1/3 of the inferior antihelix crus.〈Indication〉sciatica.

●坐位[zuò wèi] 针灸体位名。又分仰靠坐位、俯伏坐位、侧伏坐位。详见各条。

Sitting Postures Postures for acupuncture and moxibustion treatment, also divided into sitting with back and head against a lazy back, sitting in flexion and sitting with one side of the face resting on a table. →仰靠坐位(p.544)、俯伏坐位(p.119)、侧伏坐位(p.31)

附录一
Appendix 1

中外针灸医家
Biographical Names

注：本附录辑录了国内外不同时期的针灸学家和对针灸医学具有重要贡献和影响的医学家，共258人。本附录以姓氏笔划为序。

Note: Compiled here in this appendix are the 258 biographical names of acu-moxibustion experts and of the famous physicians of different times who have had great contribution to and important effect on acu-moxbustion medicine both at home and abroad. They are arranged in the order of the number of strokes of the first Chinese character of their surnames.

二画(2 strokes)

1. 丁德用，里籍不详。宋代针灸家。
   Ding Deyong, his native place unknown, an acupuncturist of the Song Dynasty.

2. 丁毅，亦名德刚，江浦人(今江苏)，明代针灸家。
   Ding Yi, also named Ding Degang, Coming from Jiangpu(of today's Jiangsu Province), an acupuncturist of the Ming Dynasty.

三画(3 strokes)

3. 于法开，亦名吴道林，浙江人，晋代针灸家。
   Yu Fakai, also named Wn Daolin, a native of Zhejiang Province, an acupuncturist of the Jin Dynasty.

4. 万塚汶上，日本人，十九世纪针灸学者。
   Ayajami Manguka, a Japanese acupuncturist in the 19th Century.

5. 卫世杰，里籍不详，宋代针灸家。
   Wei Shijie, his native place unknown, an acupuncturist of the Song Dynasty.

6. 小阪元祐，日本人，亦名小板荣升，十九世纪针灸学者。
   Genyu Kosaka, also named Esho Kosaka, a Japanese acupuncturist in the 19th Century.

7. 马丹阳，亦名马从义、马宜甫、马钰，扶风(今属陕西)人，金代道家、针灸家。
   Ma Danyang, also named Ma Congyi, Ma Yifu, Ma Yü, a native of Fufeng (of today's Shanxi Province), a Taoist and acupuncturist of the Jin Dynasty.

8. 马嗣明，河内(今河南沁阳)人，北朝北齐针灸家。
   Ma Siming, A native of Henei (today's Qinyang, Henan Province), an acupuncturist of the Northern Qi of the Northern Dynasty.

9. 子杨，里籍不详，战国时针灸医家。
   Zi Yang, his birthplace not clear, an acupuncturist of the Warring States Period.

10. 子豹，里籍不详，战国时针灸医家。
    Zi Bao, his birthplace unknown, an acupuncturist of the Warring States Period.

四画 (4 strokes)

11. 王开，亦名启元、镜泽，兰溪(属浙江)人，元代针灸家。
    Wang Kai, also named Wang Qiyuan, Wang Jingze, a native of Lanxi (of today's Zhejiang Province), an acupuncturist of the Yuan Dynasty.

12. 王处明，里籍不详，宋代针灸家。
    Wang Chuming, his native place unknown, an acupuncturist of the Song Dynasty.

13. 王执中,亦名王叔权,瑞安(属浙江)人,南宋针灸家。
    Wang Zhizhong, also named Wang Shuquan, a native of Ruian (of today's Zhejiang Province), an acupuncturist of the Southern Song Dynasty.

14. 王冰,亦名启玄子,王太仆,唐代医学家。
    Wang Bing, also named Qi Xuanzi, Wang Taipu, a physician of the Tang Dynasty.

15. 王好古,亦名王海藏、王进之,赵州(属河北)人,元代医家。
    Wang Haogu, also called Wang Haicang, Wang Jinzhi, a native of Zhaozhou (of todday's Hebei Province), a physician of the Yuan Dynasty.

16. 王克明(1069—1135),亦名王彦昭,饶州乐平(属江西)人,南宋医家。
    Wang Keming (1069—1135), also called Wang Yanzhao, a native of Yueping, Raozhou, (of today's Jiangxi Province), a medical expert of the Southern Song Dynasty.

17. 王怀隐,睢阳(属河南)人,北宋医学家。
    Wang Huaiyin, a native of Suiyang (of today's Henan Province), a physician of the Northern Song Dynasty.

18. 王国瑞,兰溪(属浙江)人,元代针灸家。
    Wang Guorui, a native of Lanxi (of today's Zhejiang Province), a famous acupuncturist of the Yuan Dynasty.

19. 王禹,西晋针灸学者。里籍不详。
    Wang Yu, his native place unknown, an acupuncturist in the Western Jin Dynasty.

20. 王涌愚,江苏人,近代针灸家。
    Wang Yongyu, a native of Jiangsu Province, an acupuncturist of modern times.

21. 王焘 (约670—755),郿(陕西)人,唐代医家。
    Wang Tao (about A. D. 670~755), a native of Mei (of today's Shanxi Province), a physician of the Tang Dynasty.

22. 王惟一 (约987—1067)亦名惟德,北宋针灸家。
    Wang Weiyi (about 987~1067), also named Wang Weide, a well-known acupuncturist of the Northern Song Dynasty.

23. 王纂,海陵(属江苏)人,南朝刘宋针灸家。
    Wang Zuan, A native of Hailing, (of today's Jiangsu Province), an acupuncturist in the Liusong Period of the Southern Dynasties.

24. 王叔和,亦名王熙,高平(属江西)人,晋代著名医学家。
    Wang Shuhe, also named Wang Xi, a native of Gaoping (of today's Jiangxi Province), a famous physician of the Jin Dynasty.

26. 尤乘,亦名生洲,吴门(属江苏)人,明清间医家.
    You Cheng, also named Shengzhou, a native of Wumen (of today's Jiangsu Province), a physician of the Ming and Qing Dynasties.

27. 长桑君,古代医学家。
    Chang Sang Jun, an ancient physician.

28. 公孙克,里籍不详,宋代针灸家。
    Gongsun Ke, his hometown not clear, an acupuncturist in the Song Dynasty.

29. 丹波康赖,日本人,十九世纪针灸学家。
    Yasuyori Tanba, a Japanese acupuncturist in the 19th century.

30. 方慎庵(1893—1962),安徽人,近代针灸家。
    Fang Shenan (1893~1962), A native of Anhui Province, an acupuncturist of modern times.

31. 邓良仲,里籍不详,近代针灸家。
    Deng Liangzhong, his native place unknown, an acupuncturist of modern times.

32. 孔广培,亦名筱亭,萧山(属浙江)人,清代针灸家。

Kong Guangpei, also named Kong Xiaoting, a native of Xiaoshan (of Zhejiang Province), an acupuncturist of the Qing Dynasty.

五画 (5 strokes)

33. 石藏用,亦名石用之,北京人,宋代针灸家。

Shi Cangyong, also named Shi Yongzhi, a native of Beijing, an acupuncture expert of the Song Dynasty.

34. 龙衔素,里籍不详,隋朝针灸家。

Long Xiansu, his native place unknown, an acu-moxibustion expert of the Sui Dynasty.

35. 叶广祚,亦名叶明传,岭南(属广东)人,清代针灸家。

Ye Guangzuo, also named Ye Mingchuan, a native of Lingnan, Guangdong Province, an acu-moxibustion expert of the Qing Dynasty.

36. 叶茶山,里籍不详,清代针灸家。

Ye Chashan, his birthplace not clear, an acu-moxibustion expert of the Qing Dynasty.

37. 史谋,徽州(属安徽)人,清代针灸家。

Shi Mou, a native of Hui Zhou(of Anhui Province), an acu-moxibustion expert of the Qing Dynasty.

38. 丘珏,亦名延美,邵武(属福建)人,明代针灸家。

Qiu Jue, also called Qiu Tingmei, a native of Shaowu (of Fujian Province), an acu-moxibustion expert of the Ming Dynasty.

39. 丘经历,里籍不详,宋代针灸家。

Qiu Jingli, his native place unknown, an acu-moxibustion expert of the Song Dynasty.

40. 冯卓怀,里籍不详,清代针灸家。

Feng Zhouhuai, his native place unknown, an acupuncturist of the Qing Dynasty.

41. 冯衢,又名樽宜,丹徒(属江苏)人,清代女医家。

Feng Qu, also named Feng Zunyi, a native of Dantu (of Jiangsu Province), a woman medical expert of the Qing Dynasty.

42. 宁守道,扶沟(属河南)人,明代针灸家。

Ning Shoudao, A native of Fugou (of Henan Province), an acu-moxibustion expert of the Ming Dynasty.

六画 (6 strokes)

43. 过龙,亦名过云从,十足道人,吴县(属江苏)人,明代针灸家。

Guo Long, also named Guo Yuncong, Shizu Daoren, a native of Wuxian(of Jiansu Province), an acupuncturist of the Ming Dynasty.

44. 吕广,亦名吕博,三国时医家。

Lü Guang, also named Lü Bo, a medical expert in the Three Kingdoms Period.

45. 吕夔,亦名吕大章,明代针灸家。

Lü Kui, also named Lü Dazhang, an acu-moxibustion expert of the Ming Dynasty.

46. 朱之光,又名朱尔韬,鹤山里(属安徽)人,明代针灸家。

Zhu Zhiguang, also named Zhu Ertao, a native of He Shanli(of Anhui Province), an acu-moxibustion expert of the Ming Dynasty.

47. 朱权,凤阳(属安徽)人,明代针灸家。

Zhu Quan, a native of Fengyang (of Anhui Province), an acu-moxibustion expert of the Ming Dynasty.

48. 朱震亨 (1281—1358)亦名朱彦修,朱丹溪,义乌(属浙江)人,金元著名医家。

Zhu Zhenheng (1281—1358), also named Zhu Yanxiu, Zhu Danxi, a native of Yiwu (of today's Zhejiang Province), a well-known medical expert in the Jin and Yuan Periods.

49. 朱肱,又名朱翼中,朱奉议,北宋医学家。

Zhu Hong, also named Zhu Yizhong, Zhu Fenyi', a medical expert of the Northern Song Dynasty.

50. 朱琏,溧阳(江苏)人,现代针灸家。

    Zhu Lian, a native of Liyang (of Jiangsu Province), an acu-moxibustion expert of the modern times.

51. 朱棣,凤阳(字徽)人,明代医家。

    Zhu Di, a native of Fengyang (of Anhui Province), a medical expert in the Ming Dynasty.

52. 朱遂,又名米遂,唐代针灸家。

    Zhu Sui, also named Mi Sui, an acupuncturist of the Tang Dynasty.

53. 伏羲,传说中华民族的祖先,九针的创造者。

    Fu Xi, the legendary ancestry of the Chinese People, the Creator of the nine-needles.

54. 任作田,(1886—1950),辽宁人,近代针灸家。

    Ren Zuotian(1886—1950), a native of Liaoning Province, an acu-moxibustion expert of the modern times.

55. 华佗,(?—公元208年前),又名华元化,沛国谯(今安徽)人,东汉末年著名医家。

    Hua Tuo (?—208 B.C.), also named Hua Yuanhua, a native of Qiao County, Pei State (of today's Anhui Province), a famous physician of the late Eastern Han Dynasty.

56. 后腾仲介,日本人,十八世纪艾灸家。

    Chukai Goto, a Japanese moxibustion expert in the 18th Century.

57. 全循义,里籍不详,明代针灸家。

    Quan Xunyi, his native place unknown, an acupuncturist of the Ming Dynasty.

58. 刘元宾,又名通真子,安福(属江西)人,宋代针灸家。

    Liu Yuanbin, also named Tong Zhen Zi, a native of Anfu (of Jiangxi Province), an acu-moxibustion expert of the Song Dynasty.

59. 刘完素 (1110—1200),亦名守真。河间(属河北)人,金元著名医家。

    Liu Wansu(1110—1200), also named Liu Shouzhen, a native of Hejian (of today's Hebei Province), a famous medical expert of the Jin and Yuan Dynasties.

60. 刘纯,亦名宗厚,吴陵(属江苏)人,明代医家。

    Liu Chun, also named Liu Zonghou, a native of Wuling (of Jiangsu Province), a medical expert of the Ming Dynasty.

61. 刘党,亦名琼瑶真人,宋代针灸家。

    Liu Dang, also named Qiongyao Zhenren, an acu-moxibustion expert of the Song Dynasty.

62. 刘瑾,亦名刘永怀,刘恒庵,南昌(江西)人,明代针灸家。

    Liu Jin, also named Liu Yonghuai, Liu Heng'an, a native Nanchang (of Jiangxi Province), an acu-moxibustion expert of the Ming Dynasty.

63. 刘国光,清代灸学家。

    Liu Guoguang, an acu-moxibustion expert of the Qing Dynasty.

64. 刘润堂,沧县(属河北)人,清针灸家。

    Liu Runtang, A native of Cangxian (of Hebei Province), an acu-moxibustion expert of the Qing Dynasty.

65. 庄绰,亦名庄季裕,清源(属山西)人,南宋灸学家。

    Zhuang Chuo, also named Zhuang Jiyu, a native of Qingyuan (of Shanxi Province), an acu-moxibustion expert of the Southern Song Dynasty.

66. 安井之越,日本人,十八世纪针灸家。

    Yukikoshi Yasui, a Japanese acupuncturist in the 18th Century.

67. 许裕卿,徽州(属安徽),清代针灸家。

    Xu Yuqing, a native of Huizhou (of Anhui Province), an acupuncturist of the Qing Dynasty.

68. 许希,开封(河南)人,北宋针灸家。

Xu Xi, a native of Kaifeng (of Henan Province), an acu-moxibustion expert of the Northern Song Dynasty.

69. 许浚,朝鲜人,十七世纪医学家。
    Sui Jun, a Kerean medical expert in the 17th Century.

70. 许叔微（约 1079—1154）,亦名许知可,宋代医学家。
    Xu Shuwei (about 1079—1154), also named Xu Zhike, a physician of the Song Dynasty.

71. 许侄,朝鲜人,十八世纪针灸家。
    Sui Zhi, a Korean acu-moxibustion expert of the 18th century.

72. 孙卓三,浮梁北乡(江西)人,明代针灸家。
    Sun Zhuosan, a native of Beixiang, Fuliang (of Jiangxi Province), an acu-moxibustion expert of the Ming Dynasty.

73. 孙鼎宜,里籍不详,清代医学家。
    Sun Dingyi, his native place unknown, a medical expert of the Qing Dynasty.

74. 孙思邈,(公元 581—682),唐代著名医学家。
    Sun Simiao(581—682 A.D.), a famous medical expert of the Tang Dynasty.

七画(7 Etrokes)

75. 杜思敬,亦称宝善老人,铜鞮(属江西)人,元代医学家。
    Du Sijing, also called Baoshan Laoren, a native of Tongdi (of today's Jiangxi Province), a medical expert of Yuan Dynasty.

76. 杨上善,里籍不详,隋唐时代医学家。
    Yang Shangshan, his native place unknown, a medical expert of the Sui and Tang Dynasties.

77. 杨介,亦名吉老,泗州(江苏)人,北宋医学家。
    Yang Jie, also named Yang Jilao, a native of Sizhou (of Jiangsu Province), a physician of the Northern Song Dynasty.

78. 杨玄操,里籍不详,唐代医家。
    Yang Xuancao, his native place unknown, a medical expert of the Tang Dynasty.

79. 杨绚,陕西人,明代医家。
    Yang Xun, A native of Shanxi Province, a physician of the Ming Dynasty.

80. 杨继洲（约 1522—1620 年）,又名杨济时,衢州(属浙江)人,明代针灸学家。
    Yang Jizhou (about 1522—1620), also named Yang Jishi, a native of Qu Zhou (of Zhejiang Province), a famous acu-moxibustion expert of the Ming Dynasty.

81. 杨敬斋,常山人,明代针灸家。
    Yang Jingzhai, A native of Changshan, an acupuncturist of the Ming Dynasty.

83. 杨颜齐,里籍不详,宋代针灸家。
    Yang Yanqi, his native place unknown, an acupuncturist of the Song Dynasty.

83. 严振,亦名漫翁,明代针灸学家。
    Yan Zhen, also named Man Weng, an acu-moxibustion expert of the Ming Dynasty.

84. 李玉,亦名成章,六安(安徽)人,明代针灸家。
    Li Yu, also named Li Chengzhang, a native of Liuan (of Anhui Province), an acupuncturist of the Ming Dynasty.

85. 李庆嗣,洺州(河北)人,金代医家。
    Li Qingsi, A native of Ming Zhou(of Hebei Province), a medical expert of the Jing Dynasty.

86. 李守兴,字善述,长葛(河南)人,清代针灸家。
    Li Shouxing, also named Li Shanshu, a native of Changge (of today's Henan Province), an acupuncturist of the Qing Dynasty.

87. 李守道,亦名存吾,浦城(福建)人,明代针灸家。

Li Shoudao, also named Li Cunwu, a native of Pucheng (of Fujian Province), an acupuncturist of the Ming Dynasty.

88. 李时珍(1518—1655)亦名东璧,李濒湖,蕲州(湖北)人,明代杰出的医药学家。
Li Shizhen (1518—1655), also named Li Dongbi, Li Pinhu, a native of Qizhou (of Hubei Province), a distinguished medical and pharmaceutical expert of the Ming Dynasty.

89. 李学川,亦名李三源,吴县(属江苏)人,清代针灸学家。
Li Xunchuan, also named Li Sanyuan, a native of Wuxian (of Jiangsu Province), an acu-moxibustion expert of the Qing Dynasty.

90. 李杲(1180—1251),亦名李明之,真定(属河北)人,金元时医家。
Li Gao (1180—1251), also named Li Mingzhi, a native of Zhending (of today's Hebei Province), a famous medical expert in the Jin ang Yuan Period.

91. 李浩,蔡邑(属河南)人,金代针灸家。
Li Hao, a native of Caiyi (of today's Henan Province), an acu-moxibustion expert of the Jin Dynasty.

92. 李源,蔡邑(属河南)人,金代针灸家。
Li Yuan, A native of Caiyi (of today's Henan Province), an acu-moxibustion expert of the Jin Dynasty.

93. 李培卿(1865—1947),亦名李怀德,江苏嘉定人,近代针灸学家。
Li Peiqing (1865—1947), also named Li Huaide, a native of Jiading, Jiangsu Province, a contemporary acu-moxibustion expert.

94. 李梦周,鄞县(浙江)人,清代针灸家。
Li Mengzhou, a native of Yinxian (of Zhejiang Province), an acu-moxibustion expert of the Qing Dynasty.

95. 李梴,亦名健斋,南丰(属江西)人,明代医学家。
Li Chan, also named Li Jianzhai, a native of Nanfeng (of Jiangxi Province), a physician of the Ming Dynasty.

96. 李潭,清河(河北)人,北朝北魏针灸家。
Li Tan, a native of Qinghe (of Hebei Province), an acupuncturist of the Northern Wei Dynasty in the Bei Chao Period.

97. 医缓,春秋时秦国医家,针灸家。
Yi Huan, a physician and acupuncturist of the Qin Country in the Spring-Autumn Period.

98. 岐伯,传说中古代医学家,针灸学家。
Qi Bo, an ancient legendary expert of medicine and acu-moxibustion.

99. 吴之英,清末针灸医家。
Wu Zhiying, an acu-moxibustion expert in the late Qing Dynasty.

100. 吴文炳,明代针灸家。
Wu Wenbing, an acu-moxibustion expert in the Ming Dynasty.

101. 吴亦鼎,亦名砚丞,歙县(安微)人,清代针灸家。
Wu Yiding, also named Wu Yancheng, a native Shexian (of today's Anhui Province), an acu-moxibustion expert of the Qing Dynasty.

102. 吴延龄,亦名介石,浙江人,明代医家。
Wu Yanling, also named Wu Jieshi, a native of Zhejiang Province, a medical expert of the Ming Dynasty.

103. 吴复珪,明代针灸家。
Wu Fugui, an acu-moxibustion expert of the Ming Dynasty.

104. 吴崑(1552—1620),亦名山甫,歙县澄塘(属安微)人,明代针灸医家。
Wu Kun (1552—1620), also native Wu Shanfu, a native of Chengtang, Shexian (of today's Anhui Province), a medical expert of acu-moxibustion of the Ming Dynasty.

105. 吴谦亦名六吉,歙县(属安徽)人,清代医学家。

Wu Qian, also named Wu Liuji, a native of Shexian (today's Anhui province), a medical expert of the Qing Dynasty.

106. 吴嘉言,分水(浙江人),明代针灸家。
  Wu Jiayan, a native of Fenshui (of Zhejiang Province), an acupuncturist of the Ming Dynasty.

107. 吴櫂仙(1892—1976),亦名吴显宗,巴县(四川)人,现代针灸家。
  Wu Zhouxian(189—1976),also named Wu Xianzong, a native of Baxian (in Sichuan Province), an acu-moxibustion expert of the modern times.

108. 何若愚,金代著名针灸家。
  He Ruoyu, a famous acu-moxibustion expert of the Jin Dynasty.

109. 邱时敏,清代针灸家。
  Qiu Shimin, an acup-moxibustion expert of the Qing Dynasty.

110. 汪机,亦名汪省之、汪石山,祁门朴墅(属安徽)人,明代医学家。
  Wang Ji, also named Wang Xiangzhi, Wang Shishan, a native of Pushu, Qimen (of today's Anhui Province), a medical expert of the Ming Dynasty.

111. 汪昂(1615—?)亦名汪讱庵,休宁(属安徽)人,清代医学家。
  Wang Ang (1615—?), also named Wang Ren'an, a native of Xiuning (today Anhui Province), a medical expert of the Qing Dynasty.

112. 沈子禄,亦名沈承之,吴江(属江苏)人,明代医家。
  Shen Zilu, also named Shen Chengzhi, a native of Wu Jiang (of today's Jiangsu Province), a physician of the Ming Dynasty.

113. 沈好问,亦名裕生、沈启明,元代针灸家。
  Shen Haowen, also named Shen Yushen, Shen Qiming, an acu-moxibustion expert of the Ming Dynasty.

114. 沈彤,亦名沈冠元,吴江(属江苏)人,清代医家。
  Shen Tong, also named Shen Guanyuan, a native of Wujiang (of today's Jiangsu Province), a physician of the Qing Dynasty.

115. 沈绂,里籍不详,清代医家。
  Shen Fu, his native place unknown, a physician of the Qing Dynasty.

116. 宋子景,黄冈(属湖北)人,明代针灸家。
  Song Zijing, a native of Huanggang (of today's Hubei Province), an acu-moxibustion expert of the Ming Dynasty.

117. 张三锡,亦名张叔承,张嗣泉,明代医学家。
  Zhang Sanxi, also named Zhang Shuchen, Zhang Siquan, a medical expert of the Ming Dynasty.

118. 张山雷 (1872—1934),亦名张寿颐,嘉定(属上海市)人,近代医学家。
  Zhang Shanlei (1872—1934), also named Zhang Shouyi, a native of Jiading(of Shanghai City), a contemporary medical expert.

119. 张元素(约1130—?年),亦名张洁古,易州(今河北)人,金代针灸医家。
  Zhang Yuansu (1130—?), also, named Zhang Jiegu, a native of Yizhou(of today's Hebei Province), a medical expert of acu-moxibustion of the Jin Dynasty.

120. 张介宾(1563—1640),亦名张景岳、张惠卿,会稽(属浙江)人,明代著名医学家。
  Zhang Jiebin (1563—1640), also named Zhang Jingyue, Zhang Huiqing, a native of Huiji (of today's Zhejiang Province), a famous physician of the Ming Dynasty.

121. 张文仲,洛阳(属河南)人,唐代医家,善灸法。
  Zhang Wenzhong, a native of Luoyang (of Henan Province), a medical expert of the Tang Dynasty who was good at moxibustion.

122. 张权,里籍不详,明代针灸家,善经络学。

Zhang Quan, his native place unknown, an acu-moxibustion expert of the Ming Dynasty who was good at Jingluology.

123. 张仲景（公元150—219）亦名张机,南阳(属河南)人,东汉末杰出医学家。
Zhang Zhongjing (150—219 A.D.), also named Zhang Ji, a native of Nanyang (of Henan Province), a distinguished physician in the late Eastern Han Dynasty.

124. 张璧,易州(河北)人,元代针灸家。
Zhang Bi, a native of Yizhou (of Hebei Province), an acupuncturist of the Yuan Dynasty.

125. 张从正（约1156—1228）,亦名张子和,张戴人,考城(属河南)人,金元时医学家。
Zhang Congzheng (about 1156—1228), also named Zhang Zihe, Zhang Dairen, a native of Kaocheng (of today's Henan Province, a famous physician in the Jin and Yuan Dynasties.

126. 张志聪,(1610—1674),亦名张隐庵,钱塘(属浙江)人,清代医学家。
Zhang Zhicong (1610—1674), also named Zhang Yin'an, a native of Qinantang (of Zhejiang Province), a physician of the Qing Dynasty.

127. 张明,里籍不详,明代经络专家。
Zhang Ming, his native place unknown, a Jingluology expert of the Ming Dynasty.

128. 张祉,亦名张天与,铅山(江西)人,明代针灸家。
Zhang Zhi, also named Zhang Tianyu, a native of Qianshan(of Jiangxi Province), an acupuncturist of the Ming Dynasty.

129. 张济,无为军(属安徽)人,宋代医家,善针灸临床。
Zhang Ji, a native of Wuweijun (of today's Anhui Province), a physician of the Song Dynasty who was good at clinical acu-moxibustion.

130. 陆仲运,青阳(属安徽)人,元代医家,精于经络腧穴。
Lu Zhongyun, a native of Qingyang (of Anhui Province), a physician of the Yuan Dynasty who was good at meridians and acuponits.

131. 陆瘦燕,(1909—1969),亦名陆昌,昆山(属江西)人,现代针灸家。
Lu Shouyan (1909—1969), also named Lu Chang, a native of Kunshan(of today's Jiangxi Province), an acu-moxibustion expert of the modern times.

132. 陈会,亦名陈善同,张宏纲,丰城(属江西)人,明代针灸家。
Chen Hui, also named Chen Shantong, Zhang Honggang, a native of Fengcheng (of today's Jiangxi Province), an acu-moxibustion expert of the Ming Dynasty.

133. 陈廷铨,亦名陈隐荃,清泉(属河南)人,清代针灸家。
Chen Tingquan, also named Chen Yinyan, a native of Qingquan (of today's Henan Province), an acu-moxibustion expert of the Qing Dynasty.

134. 陈时荣,亦名陈颐春,华亭(属上海市)人,明代针灸家。
Chen Shirong, also named Chen Yichun, a native of Huating (of Shenghai City), an acupuncturist of the Ming Dynasty.

135. 陈言,福建建阳人,明代针灸家。
Chen Yan, a native of Jianyang, Fujian Province, an acu-moxibustion expert of the Ming Dynasty.

136. 陈景魁,亦名陈叔旦,陈斗岩,世居句岩(属江苏)人,明代针灸家。
Chen Jingkui, also named Chen Shudan, Chen Douyan, a native of Juyan, Shi ju (of today's Jiangsu Province), an acupuncturist of the Ming Dynasty.

137. 陈惠畴,亦名陈寿田,湘潭(湖南)人,清代针灸家。
Chen Huichou, also named Chen Shoutian, a native of Xiangtan (of Hunan Province), an acu-moxibustion expert of the Qing Dynasty.

八画 (8 strokes)

138. 直鲁左(公元915—1005),吐谷浑(属青海)人,五代(辽)针灸家。
 Zhi Luzuo (915—1005 A. D.), a native of Tuguhun (of today's Qinghai Province), an acu-moxibustion expert of the Liao Dynasty of the Five Dynasties.

139. 范九思,里籍不详,北宋针灸家。
 Fan Jiusi, his native place unknown, an acupuncturist of the Northern Song Dynasty.

140. 范培贤,亦名春坡,义乌(属浙江)人,清末针灸家。
 Fan Peixian, also named Fan Chunpo, a native of Yiwu (of today's Zhejiang Province), an acu-moxibustion expert in the late Qing Dynasty.

141. 范毓齮,亦名培兰,里籍不详,清针灸家。
 Fan Yuqi, also named Fan Peilan, his birthplace not clear, an acupuncturist of the Qing Dynasty.

142. 罗天益(1220—1290年),亦名罗谦甫,藁城(属河北)人,元代医学家。
 Luo Tianyi(1220—1290), also named Luo Qianfu, a native of Gaocheng (of Hebei Province), a physician of the Yuan Dynasty.

143. 罗兆琚(1888—1945),亦名佩琼,柳州(属广西)人,近代针灸家。
 Luo Zhaoju (1888—1945), also named Luo Peiqiong, a native of Liuzhou(of Guangxi Autonomous Region), an acu-moxibustion expert of the modern times.

144. 罗哲初(1878—1938),桂林(广西)人,近代针灸家。
 Luo Zhechu (1878—1938), A native of Guilin (of Guangxi Province), an acu-moxibustion expert of the modern times.

145. 知聪,南北朝僧人,中国针灸传播日本之先驱者。
 Zhi Cong, a Buddhist monk, the pioneer who propagated Chinese acu-moxibustion to Japan.

146. 金义孙,里籍不详,明代针灸家。
 Ji Yisun, his birthplace not clear, an acupuncturist of the Ming Dynasty.

147. 金孔贤,义乌(属浙江)人,明代经络学家。
 Ji Kongxian, a native of Yiwu (of today's Zhejiang Province), a Jingluological expert of the Ming Dynasty.

148. 金冶田,里籍不详,清代针灸学家。
 Ji Yetian, his native place unknown, an acu-moxibustion expert of the Qing Dynasty.

149. 忽泰必烈,亦名公泰,忽泰吉甫,元代针灸学家。
 Hu Taibilie, also named Gong Tai, Hutaijifu, an acu-moxibustion expert of the Yuan Dynasty.

150. 忽光济,里籍不详。元代针灸家。
 Hu Guangji, his native place unknown, an acupuncturist of the Yuan Dynasty.

151. 周孔田,里籍不详,清代经络医家。
 Zhou Kongtian, his birthplace not clear, an expert of the Jingluology of the Qing Dynasty.

152. 周汉卿,松阳(属浙江)人,元明间针灸家。
 ZHou Hangqing, a native of Songyang (of today's Zhejiang Province), an acupuncturist of the Yuan and Ming Dynasties.

153. 庞安时 (约1042—1099),亦名庞安常,蕲水(属湖北)人,北宋医家。
 Pang Anshi (about 1042—1099), also named Pang Anchang, a native of Qishui (of Hubei Province), a physician of the Northern Song Dynasty.

154. 承淡安 (约1899—1957年),亦名承澹庵,江阴(江苏)人,现代针灸家。
 Cheng Dan'an (1899—1957), also named Cheng Tan'an, a native of Jiangyin (of Jiangsu Province), an acupuncturist of the modern times.

155. 和气惟亨,日本人,十九世纪针灸家。

Iryo Waki, a Japanese acupuncturist in the 19th century.

156. 郑梅漳（约1727—1728年），亦名郑宏纲，郑纪元，歙县（属安徽）人，清名医。
Zheng Meijian (about 1727—1728), also named Zheng Honggang, Zheng Jiyuan, a native of Shexian (of today's Angui Province), a famous physician of the Qing Dynasty.

九画 (9 strokes)

157. 项世贤，亦名嗣宗，乐平（属江西）人，明代针灸家。
Xiang Shixian, also named Xiang Sizong, a native of Leping (of Jiangxi Province), an acupuncturist of the Ming Dynasty.

158. 胡元庆，里籍不详，元代针灸学家。
Hu Yuanqing. his birthplace not clear, an acupuncturist of the Yuan Dynasty.

159. 胡珏，亦名胡念庵，钱塘（属浙江）人，清代医家。
Hu Jue, also named Hu Nian'an, a native of Qiantang (of Zhejiang Province), a physician of the Qing Dynasty.

160. 胡最良（1853—1923年），无锡（江苏）人，近代针灸家。
Hu Zuiliang (1853—1923), a native of Wuxi (of Jiangsu Province), a contemporary acupuncturologist.

161. 赵献可，亦名赵养葵，鄞县（属浙江）人，明代经络学家。
Zhao Xianke, also named Zhao Yangkui, a native of Yinxian (of today's Zhejiang Province), an expert of Jing-luology of the Ming Dynasty.

162. 赵熙（1872—1938），亦名赵辑庵，赵遁山，代县（属山西）人，近代针灸家。
Zhao Xi (1877—1938), also named Zhao Ji'an, Zhao Dunshan, a native of Daixian (of today's Shanxi Province), a contemporary acupuncturologist.

163. 施沛，里籍不详，明代医家。
Shi Pei, his birthplace not clear, a physician of the Ming Dynasty.

164. 闻人耆年，檇李（属浙江）人，南宋针灸家。
Wen Renqinian, a native of Zuili (of Zhejiang Province), an acupuncturologist of the Southern Song Dynasty.

165. 祝定，亦名祝伯静，丽水（属浙江）人，明代针灸家。
Zhu Ding, also named Zhu Bojing, a native of Lishui (of today's Zhejiang Province), an acu-moxibustion expert of the Ming Dynasty.

166. 姚良，亦名姚亮，姚香卿，吴县（属江苏）人，明代针灸家。
Yao Liang, also named Yao Liang, Yao Xiangqing, a native of Wuxian (of today's Jiangsu Province), an acupuncturologist of the Ming Dynasty.

167. 皇甫谧（215—282年）亦名皇甫静，皇甫士安，安定朝定（属甘肃）人，魏晋针灸学家。
Huangfu Mi (215—282), also named Huangfu Jing, Huangfu Shi'an, coming from Chaoding, Anding (of today's Gansu Province), a acupuncturologist of the Wei and Jin Dynasties.

168. 秦鸣鹤，里籍不详，唐代针灸家。
Qin Minghe, his native place unknown. an acupuncturologist of the Tang Dynasty.

169. 秦承祖，里籍不详，南朝刘宋针灸家。
Qin Chengzu, his birthplace not clear, an acu-moxibustion expert in the Liusong Period of the Southern Dynasties.

170. 秦越人，亦名扁鹊，秦卢医，神应王，神应候，渤海郡鄚（属河北）人，战国时著名医学家。
Qin Yueren, also named Bian Que, Qin Luyi, Shenying Wang, Shenying Hou, a native of Moxian, Bohai Jun (of today's Hebei), an outstanding physician in the Warring States Periad.

171. 夏英，亦名时彦，杭州人，明代针灸家。
Xia Ying, also named Xia Shiyan, a native of Hangzhou City, an acupuncturologist of the Ming Dynasty.

172. 夏春农，邗上（属江苏）人，清末喉科针灸医家。
Xia Chunnong, a native of Honshang (of today's Jiangsu Province), a laryngologist and acupuncturist in the late

Qing Dynasty.

173. 徐凤（公元十四世纪），亦名徐廷瑞，弋阳石塘（属江西）人，明代针灸家。
    Xu Feng (14th century), also named Xu Tingrui, a native of Shitang, Yiyang (of today's Jiangxi Province), an acupuncturologist of the Ming Dynasty.

174. 徐梦符，里籍不详，宋代针灸学专家。
    Xu Mengfu, his native place unknown, an acu-moxibustion expert of the Song Dynasty.

175. 徐悦，里籍不详，隋代针灸家。
    Xu Yue, his native place unknown, an acu-moxibustion expert of the Sui Dynasty.

176. 徐文中，亦用徐用和，里籍不详，元代针灸家。
    Xu Wenzhong, also named Xu Yonghe, his birthplace not clear, an acupuncturologist of the Yuan Dynasty.

177. 徐文伯，亦名徐德秀，南朝刘宋医家。
    Xu Wenbo, also named Xu Dexiu, a physician of in the Liusong Period of the Southern Dynasties.

178. 徐师曾，亦名伯鲁，吴江（属江苏）人，明代经络专家。
    Xu Shizeng, also named Xu Bolu, a native of Wujiang (of today's Jiangsu Province), an expert of Jingluology of the Ming Dynasty.

179. 徐廷璋，里籍不详，明代针灸医家。
    Xu Tingzhang, his birthplace not clear, an acu-moxibustion expert of the Ming Dynasty.

180. 徐叔湘，浙江人，南朝刘宋针灸医家。
    Xu Shuxiang, a native of Zhejiang Province, an acu-moxibustion expert in the Liusong Period of the Southern Dynasties.

181. 徐春甫（1520—1590），亦名汝元，祁门（属安徽）人，明代医家。
    Xu Chunfu(1520—1596), also named Xu Ruyuan, a native of Qimen(of today's Anhui Province), a physician of the Ming Dynasty.

182. 徐秋夫，浙江人，南朝刘宋医家。
    Xu Qiufu, a native of Zhejiang Province, a physician in the Liusong Period of the Southern Dynasties.

183. 徐道度，浙江人，南朝刘宋针灸家。
    Xu Daodu, a native of Zhejiang Province, an acupuncturist in the Liusong Period of the Southern Dynasties.

184. 徐熙，亦名徐仲融，浙江人，晋代医学家。
    Xu Xi, also named Xu Zhongrong, a native of Zhejiang Province, a physician of the Jin Dynasty.

185. 倪孟仲，江西人，明代针灸家。
    Ni Mengzhong, a native of Jiangxi Province, an acupuncturist of the Ming Dynasty.

186. 殷榘，亦名殷度卿，殷方山，仪真（属江苏）人，明代针灸家。
    Yin Qu, also named Yin Duqing, Yin Fangshan, a native of Yizhen(of today's Jiangsu Province), an acupuncturologist of the Ming Dynasty.

187. 殷元，里籍不详，隋代针灸家。
    Yin Yuan, his birthplace not clear, an acupuncturologist of the Sui Dynasty.

188. 郭玉，亦名郭通直，汉雒（属四川）人，东汉针灸家。
    Guo Yu, also named Guo Tongzhi, a native of Luoxian(of today's Sichuan Province), an acupuncturologist of the Eastern Han Dynasty.

189. 郭忠，亦名恕甫，兴化（属江苏）人，北宋针灸家。
    Guo Zhong, also named Guo Shufu, a native of Xinghua (of today's Jiangsu Province), an acupuncturologist of the Northern Song Dynasty.

190. 高凤桐（1877—1962），北京人，近代针灸家。
    Gao Fengtong(1877—1962), a native of Beijing City, an acupuncturologist of the modern times.

191. 高武,别名梅孤子,四明(浙江)人,明代针灸医家。
    Gao Wu, also called Mei Gu Zi, a native of Siming (of today's Zhejiang Province), a famous acupuncturologist of the Ming Dynasty.
192. 高洞阳,里籍不详,元末针灸医家。
    Gao Dongyang, his birthplace not clear, an acu-moxibustion expert in the late stage of the Yuan Dynasty.
193. 席弘,亦名席弘远,江西人,宋代著名针灸学家。
    Xi Hong, also named Xi Hongyuan, a native of Jiangxi Province, a well-known, acupuncturologist of the Song Dynasty.
194. 席延赏,里籍不详,宋代针灸家。
    Xi Yanshang, his birthplace not clear, an acupuncturist of the Song Dynasty.
195. 凌千一,归安双林(属浙江)人,明代针灸家。
    Ling Qianyi, a native of Shuanglin, Gui'an (of today's Zhejiang Province), an acupuncturist of the Ming Dynasty.
196. 凌凤仪,亦名凌学川,虞山(属江苏)人,明代针灸家。
    Ling Fengyi, also named Ling Xuechuan, a native of Yushan (of today's Jiangsu Province), an acu-moxibustion expert of the Ming Dynasty.
197. 凌云,亦名凌汉章,凌卧岩,归安双林(属浙江)人,明代针灸学家。
    Ling Yun, also named Ling Hanzhang, Ling Woyan, a native of Shuanglin, Guian (of today's Zhejiang Province), an acupuncturologist of the Ming Dynasty.
198. 凌贞侯,归安双林(属浙江)人,明代针灸家。
    Ling Zhenhou, a native of Shuanglin, Guian (of today's Zhejing Province), an acupuncturologist of the Ming Dynasty.
199. 凌瑄,亦名凌双湖,浙江人,明代针灸家。
    Ling Xuan, also named Ling Shuanghu, a native of Zhejiang Province, an acupuncturologist of the Ming Dynasty.
200. 陶钦臣,彭泽(属江西)人,明代针灸家。
    Tao Qinchen, a native of Pengze (of today's Jiangxi Province), an acupuncturist of the Ming Dynasty.
201. 聂莹,里籍不详,明代针灸家。
    Nie Ying, his native place unknown, an acupuncturist of the Ming Dynasty.
202. 原昌克,原南阳,日本人,19世纪针灸学家。
    Masakapsu Hara a Japanese acupuncturologist in the 19th century.
203. 圆觉,里籍不详,清末针灸、气功家。
    Yuan Jue, his native place unknown, an expert of acupuncture and qigong in the late Qing Dynasty.
204. 钱镜湖,里籍不详,清代针灸家。
    Qian Jinghu, his birthplace not clear, an acu-moxibustion expert of the Qing Dynasty.
205. 钱雷,四明(属浙江)人,明代经络学家。
    Qian Lei, a native of Siming (of today's Zhejiang Province), a Jingluologist of the Ming Dynasty.
206. 翁藻,亦名翁稼江,武宁(属江西)人,清代医学家。
    Weng Zao, also named Weng Jiajiang, a native of Wuning (of today's Jiangxi Province), a physician of the Qing Dynasty.

十一画 (11 strokes)

207. 萧福安,里籍不详,清代针灸家。
    Xiao Fu'an, His birthplace not clear, an acu-moxibustion expert of the Qing Dynasty.
208. 巢元方,里籍不详,隋代医学家。
    Chao Yuanfang, his native place unknown, a physician of the Sui Dynasty.

209. 黄士真,里籍不详,元代针灸家。
Huang Shizhen, his hometown not clear, an acupuncturologist of the Yuan Dynasty.

210. 黄中子,里籍不详,元代艾师。
Huang Zhongzi, his native place unknown, an expert of moxibustion of the Yuan Dynasty.

211. 黄石屏,亦名黄灿,清江(属江西)人,清末针灸家。
Huang Shiping, also named Huang Can, a native of Qingjiang(of Jiangxi Province), an acupuncturologist in the late Qing Dynasty.

212. 黄竹斋(1886—1960),亦名黄维翰,长安(属陕西)人,现代针灸学家。
Huang Zhuzhai (1886—1960), also named Huang Weihan, a native of Chang'an (of Shanxi Province), an acupuncturologist of the modernitimes.

213. 黄学龙(1876—1958),东阳(属浙江)人,近代针灸家。
Huang Xuelong(1876—1958), a native of Dongyang(of today's Zhejiang Province), an acu-moxibustion expert of the modern times.

214. 黄帝,传说中中华民族的祖先。
Huang Di, One of the ancestors of the Chinese People in legend.

215. 黄宰,祁门(属安徽)人,明代针灸家。
Huang Zai, a native of Qimen (of today's Anhui Province), an acupuncturist of the Ming Dynasty.

216. 黄崇赞,安化(属甘肃)人,清末针灸医家。
Huang Chongzan, a native of Anhua (of Gansu Province), an acupuncturist in the late Qing Dynasty.

217. 黄鸿舫(1879—1944),亦名黄伊莘,江苏无锡人,近代针灸医家。
Huang Hongfang (1879—1944), also named Huang Yishen, a native of Wuxi, Jiangsu Province, an acupuncturologist of the modern times.

218. 黄渊,里籍不详,明代针灸家。
Huang Yuan, his birthplace not clear, an acupuncturist of the Ming Dynasty.

219. 黄岩,里籍不详,清代经穴图画家。
Huang Yan, his home town unknown, an artist of the Qing Dynasty specialized in the drawing of meridians and acupoints.

220. 崔知悌,鄢陵(属河南)人,唐代灸疗专家。
Cui Zhidi, a native of Yanling (of today's Henan Province), an expert of moxibustion in the Tang Dynasty.

221. 崔彧,亦名崔文若,东武城(属山东)人,北朝北魏针灸家。
Cui Yu, also named Cui Wenruo, a native of Dongwucheng (of today's Shandong Province), an acupuncturologist in the Northern Wei of the Northern Dynasties.

222. 章迪,亦名章吉老,无为(属安徽)人,北宋针灸家。
Zhang Di, also named Zhang Jilao, a native of Wuwei (of today's Anhui Province), an acupuncturist in the Northern Song Dynasty.

223. 涪翁,里籍不详,东汉初年针灸家。
Fu Weng, his native place unknown, an acupuncturist in the early Eastern Han Dynasty.

224. 淳于意,亦名淳仓公,齐临菑(属山东)人,西汉著名医家。
Chunyu Yi, also named Chun Canggong, a native of Linzi, Qi State (of Today's Shandoing Province), a famous physician of the Western Han Dynasty.

225. 商元,里籍不详,宋代针灸家。
Shang Yuan, his birthplace not clear, an acupuncturist of the Song Dynasty.

226. 曹翕,里籍不详,三国时期针灸家。
Cao Xi, his birthplace not clear, an acupuncturist in the Three Kingdoms Period.

227. 阎明广,里籍不详,金代针灸家。
　　　Yan Mingguang, his home town unknown, an acupuncturist of the Jin Dynasty.

十二画 12 strokes)

228. 葛可久(1305—1353),亦名葛乾孙,长洲(属江苏)人,元代医学家。
　　　Ge Kejiu (1305—1353), also named Ge Qiansun, a native of Changzhou (of today's Jiangsu Province), a physician of the Yuan Dynasty.

229. 葛洪(公元 261—341),亦名稚川,丹阳句岩(属江苏)人,东晋道家、医学家。
　　　Ge Hong (281—341), also named Ge Zhichuan, a native of Juyan, Danyang (of today's Jiangsu Province), a Taoist and physician of the Eastern Jin Dynasty.

230. 彭九思,里籍不详,明代针灸家。
　　　Peng Jiusi, his birthplace unknown, an acpuncturologist of the Ming Dynasty.

231. 彭用光,里籍不详,明代针灸学家。
　　　Peng Yongguang, his native place unknown, an acupuncturologist of the Ming Dynasty.

232. 韩贴丰,里籍不详,清代针灸家。
　　　Han Tiefeng, his birthplace not clear, an acupuncturist of the Qing Dynasty.

233. 程天祚,里籍不详,南北朝以前针灸家。
　　　Cheng Tianzuo, his hometown unknown, an acupuncturist before the Southern and Northern Dynasties.

234. 程兴阳,四川彭县人,近代针灸家。
　　　Cheng Xingyang, a native of Pengxian, Sichuan Province, a contemporary acupuncturologist.

235. 程约,亦名程孟搏,新安婺源(属江西)人,宋代针灸家。
　　　Cheng Yue, also named Cheng Mengbo, a native of Wuyuan, Xin'an (of today's Jiangxi Province), an acupuncturologist of the Song Dynasty.

236. 程玠,歙县(属安徽)人,明代医家。
　　　Cheng Jie, a native of Shexian (of Anhui Province), a physician of the Ming Dynasty.

237. 程高,里籍不详,东汉针灸家。
　　　Cheng Gao, his birthplace unknown, an acupuncturist of the Eastern Han Dynasty.

238. 焦蕴稳,海州(今江苏)人,明代针灸家。
　　　Jiao Yunwen, a native of Haizhou (of today's Jiangsu Province), an acupuncturist of the Ming Dynasty.

239. 释湛池,亦名还元,济宁(属山东)人,明代针灸家。
　　　Shi Zhanchi, also named Shi Huanyuan, a native of Jining (of today's Shandong Province), an acupuncturologist of the Ming Dynasty.

240. 释僧匡,亦名僧匡、僧康,里籍不详,隋针灸家。
　　　Shi Sengkuang, also named Seng Kuang, Seng Kang, his birthplace unknown, an acupuncturist in the Sui Dynasty.

241. 滑寿(1304—1386),亦名滑伯仁,元末明初著名医学家。
　　　Hua Shou (1304—1386), also named Hua Boren, a well-known physician of the Yuan and Ming Dynasties.

十三画(13 sfroke)

242. 楼英(1332—1402),亦名楼全善,萧山(属浙江)人,元明医学家。
　　　Lou Ying (1332—1401) also named Lou Quanshan, a native of Xiaoshan (of Zhejiang Province), a physician of the Yuan and Ming Dynasties.

243. 甄权(公元 540—643),许州(属河南)人,隋唐针灸学家)。
　　　Zhen Quan (540—643), a native of Xuzhou (of today's Henan Province), an acupuncturologist in the Sui and Tang Dynasties.

244. 浦湘澄 (1899—1962),四川射洪人,近代针灸家。
　　　Pu Xiangcheng (1899—1962), a native of Shehong, Sichuan Province, an acupuncturologist of the Modern times.

245. 雷丰,亦名雷少逸,衢州(属浙江)人,清代灸法专家。
Lei Feng, also named Lei Shaoyi, a native of Quzhou (of today's Zhejiang Province), an expert in moxibustion of the Qing Dynasty.

246. 鲍同仁,亦名鲍国良,歙县(属安徽)人,元代针灸家。
Bao Tongren, also named Bao Guoliang, coming from Shexian (of Anhui Province), an acupuncturist of the Ming Dynasty.

247. 鲍姑,亦名潜光,丹阳句容(属江苏)人,东晋女针灸家。
Bao Gu, also named Bao Qianguang, a native of Jurong, Danyang (of today's Jiangsu Province), a woman acupuncturist of the Eastern Jin Dynasty.

248. 窦汉卿(1196—1280),亦名窦杰、窦汉卿、窦默、窦子声、窦太师、窦文贞公,广平肥乡(属河北)人,金元著名针灸学家。
Dou Hanqing (1196—1280), also named Dou Jie, Dou Mo, Dou Zisheng, Dou Taishi, Dou Wenzhengong, a native of Feixiang, Guangping (of today's Hebei Province), a distinguished acupuncturologist in the Jin and Yuan Dynasties.

249. 窦材(公元1100—?),真定(属河北)人,南宋医家。
Gou Cai(1100—?) a native of Zhending (of today's Hebei Province), a physician in the Southern Song Dynasty.

250. 窦桂芳,亦名窦静斋,建安(属福建)人,元代针灸家。
Dou Guifang, also named Dou Jingzhai, a native of Jianan (of today's Fujian Province), an acupuncturologist in the Yuan Dynasty.

十四画以上 (more over 14 strokes)

251. 僧坦然,太平箬村(属安徽)人,明代针灸家。
Seng Tanran, a native of Youcun, Taiping (of today's Anhui Province), an acupuncturist in the Ming Dynasty.

252. 廖润鸿,亦名逵宾,绿江(属湖南)人,清代著名针灸家。
Liao Runhong, also named Liao Kuibin, a native of Lüjiang (of Hunan Province), a famous acupuncturologist in the Qing Dynasty.

253. 潭志光(1852—1930),亦名容国,湖南长沙人,近代针灸家。
Tan Zhiguang (1852—1930), also named Tan Rongguo, a native of Changsha, Hunan Province, an acupuncturologist of the modern times.

254. 熊宗立,亦名熊道轩,建阳(属福建)人,明代医学家。
Xiong Zongli, also named Xiong Daoxuan, a native of Jianyang (of Fujian Province), a physician in the Ming Dynasty.

255. 樊阿,彭城(属江苏)人,三国时针灸家。
Fan E, a native Pongcheng (of today's Jiangsu Province), an acupuncturist in the Three Kingdoms Period.

256. 薛己(1488—1558),亦名薛新甫,薛立斋,吴县(属江苏)人,明代外科针灸家。
Xue Ji (1488—1558), also named Xue Xinfu, Xue Lizhai, a native of Wuxian (of today's Jiansu Province), a surgical acupuncturist of the Ming Dynasty.

257. 潘韫辉。常州(属江苏)人,明代针灸家。
Pan Yunhui, a native of Changzhou (of Jiangsu Province), an acupuncturist of the Ming Dynasty.

258. 翟良,亦名玉华,益都(属山东)人,明清经络专家。
Zhai Liang, also named Zhai Yuhua, a native of Yidu (of today Shandong Province), an expert in Jingluology in the Ming Dynasty.

附录二
APPENDIX 2

穴 名 索 引
POINTS INDEX

B

Bāfēng 八风(EX-LE 10) ……………… (4)
Bāxié 八邪(EX-UE 9) ………………… (8)
Báihuánshū 白环俞(BL 30) …………… (10)
Bǎichóngwō 百虫窝(EX-LE 3) ………… (11)
Bǎihuì 百会(DU 20) …………………… (11)
Bāohuāng 胞肓(BL 53) ………………… (13)
Běnshén 本神(GB 13) ………………… (18)
Bìnào 臂臑(LI 14) …………………… (21)
Bìguān 髀关(ST 31) …………………… (22)
Bǐngfēng 秉风(SI 12) ………………… (25)
Bùróng 不容(ST 19) …………………… (28)
Bùláng 步廊(KI 22) …………………… (29)

C

Chángqiáng 长强(DU 1) ……………… (39)
Chéngfú 承扶(BL 36) ………………… (42)
Chéngguāng 承光(BL 6) ……………… (43)
Chéngjiāng 承浆(RN 24) ……………… (43)
Chéngjīn 承筋(BL 56) ………………… (43)
Chénglíng 承灵(GB 18) ……………… (44)
Chéngmǎn 承满(ST 20) ……………… (44)
Chéngqì 承泣(ST 1) …………………… (44)
Chéngshān 承山(BL 57) ……………… (45)
Chǐzé 尺泽(LU 5) ……………………… (46)
Chìmài 瘈脉(SJ 18) …………………… (48)
Chōngmén 冲门(SP 12) ……………… (48)
Chōngyáng 冲阳(ST 42) ……………… (49)
Cìliáo 次髎(BL 32) …………………… (53)
Cuánzhú 攒竹(BL 2) ………………… (58)

D

Dàbāo 大包(SP 21) …………………… (59)
Dàchángshū 大肠俞(BL 25) ………… (61)
Dàdū 大都(SP 2) ……………………… (61)
Dàdùn 大敦(LR 1) …………………… (62)
Dàgǔkōng 大骨空(EX-UE 5) ………… (62)
Dàhè 大赫(KI 12) ……………………… (62)
Dàhéng 大横(SP 15) ………………… (63)
Dàjù 大巨(ST 27) ……………………… (64)
Dàlíng 大陵(PC 7) …………………… (64)
Dàyíng 大迎(ST 5) …………………… (65)
Dàzhōng 大钟(KI 4) ………………… (66)
Dàzhù 大杼(BL 11) …………………… (68)
Dàzhuī 大椎(DU 14) ………………… (69)
Dàimài 带脉(GB 26) ………………… (70)
Dǎnnáng 胆囊(EX-LE 6) …………… (74)
Dǎnshū 胆俞(BL 19) ………………… (75)
Dànzhōng 膻中(RN 17) ……………… (75)
Dāngyáng 当阳(EX-HN 2) …………… (76)
Dìcāng 地仓(ST 4) …………………… (78)
Dìjī 地机(SP 8) ……………………… (78)
Dìwǔhuì 地五会(GB 42) ……………… (79)
Dìngchuǎn 定喘(EX-B 1) …………… (84)
Dūshū 督俞(BL 16) …………………… (87)
Dúyīn 独阴(EX-LE 11) ……………… (88)
Dúbí 犊鼻(ST 35) …………………… (88)
Duìduān 兑端(DU 27) ………………… (89)

E

Ěrhéliáo 耳和髎(SJ 22) ……………… (94)

Ěrjiān 耳尖(EX-HN 6) ……………… (95)
Ěrmén 耳门(SJ 21) ……………… (96)
Èrbái 二白(EX-UE 2) ……………… (100)
Èrjiān 二间(LI 2) ……………… (101)

F

Fēiyáng 飞扬(BL 58) ……………… (106)
Fèishū 肺俞(BL 13) ……………… (108)
Fēnglóng 丰隆(ST 40) ……………… (109)
Fēngchí 风池(GB 20) ……………… (110)
Fēngfǔ 风府(DU 16) ……………… (111)
Fēngmén 风门(BL 12) ……………… (113)
Fēngshì 风市(GB 31) ……………… (115)
Fūyáng 跗阳(BL 59) ……………… (116)
Fútù 伏兔(ST 32) ……………… (117)
Fútū 扶突(LI 18) ……………… (118)
Fúbái 浮白(GB 10) ……………… (118)
Fúxì 浮郄(BL 38) ……………… (118)
Fǔshè 府舍(SP 13) ……………… (119)
Fùfēn 附分(BL 41) ……………… (120)
Fùliù 复溜(KI 7) ……………… (121)
Fù'āi 腹哀(SP 16) ……………… (121)
Fùjié 腹结(SP 14) ……………… (121)
Fùtōnggǔ 腹通谷(KI 20) ……………… (122)

G

Gānshū 肝俞(BL 18) ……………… (127)
Gāohuāng 膏肓(BL 43) ……………… (132)
Géguān 膈关(BL 46) ……………… (139)
Géshū 膈俞(BL 17) ……………… (139)
Gōngsūn 公孙(SP 4) ……………… (142)
Guānchōng 关冲(SJ 1) ……………… (146)
Guānmén 关门(ST 22) ……………… (147)
Guānyuán 关元(RN 4) ……………… (148)
Guānyuánshū 关元俞(BL 26) ……………… (149)
Guāngmíng 光明(GB 37) ……………… (149)
Guīlái 归来(ST 29) ……………… (150)

H

Hǎiquán 海泉(EX－HN 11) ……………… (154)
Hányàn 颔厌(GB 4) ……………… (158)
Hégǔ 合谷(LI 4) ……………… (160)
Héyáng 合阳(BL 55) ……………… (161)
Hèdǐng 鹤顶(EX－LE 2) ……………… (162)
Hénggǔ 横骨(KI 11) ……………… (163)
Hòudǐng 后顶(DU 19) ……………… (165)
Hòuxī 后溪(SI 13) ……………… (166)
Huágài 华盖(RN 20) ……………… (168)
Huáròumén 滑肉门(ST 24) ……………… (169)
Huántiào 环跳(GB 30) ……………… (170)
Huāngmén 肓门(BL 51) ……………… (172)
Huāngshū 肓俞(KI 16) ……………… (173)
Huìyáng 会阳(BL 35) ……………… (178)
Huìyīn 会阴(RN 1) ……………… (178)
Huìzōng 会宗(SJ 7) ……………… (178)
Húnmén 魂门(BL 47) ……………… (179)

J

Jīmén 箕门(SP 11) ……………… (182)
Jíquán 极泉(HT 1) ……………… (183)
Jímài 急脉(LR 12) ……………… (184)
Jǐzhōng 脊中(DL 6) ……………… (185)
Jiājǐ 夹脊(EX－B 2) ……………… (186)
Jiáchē 颊车(ST 6) ……………… (187)
Jiānshǐ 间使(PC 5) ……………… (188)
Jiānjǐng 肩井(GB 21) ……………… (189)
Jiānliáo 肩髎(SJ 14) ……………… (189)
Jiānwàishū 肩外俞(SI 14) ……………… (190)
Jiānyú 肩髃(LI 15) ……………… (191)
Jiānzhēn 肩贞(SI 9) ……………… (191)
Jiānzhōngshū 肩中俞(SI 15) ……………… (191)
Jiànlǐ 建里(RN 11) ……………… (192)
Jiāoxìn 交信(KI 8) ……………… (198)
Jiǎosūn 角孙(SJ 20) ……………… (199)

17

Jiěxī 解溪(ST 41) ……………… (202)

Jīnjīn,Yùyè 金津、玉液(EX－HN 12,13)
……………… (202)

Jīnmén 金门(BL 63) ……………… (203)

Jīnsuō 筋缩(DU 8) ……………… (204)

Jīnggǔ 京骨(BL 64) ……………… (207)

Jīngmén 京门(GB 25) ……………… (207)

Jīngqú 经渠(LU 8) ……………… (213)

Jīngmíng 睛明(BL 1) ……………… (217)

Jìngbǎiláo 颈百劳(EX－HN 15) …… (218)

Jiūwěi 鸠尾(RN 15) ……………… (219)

Jūliáo 居髎(GB 29) ……………… (225)

Jùgǔ 巨骨(LI 16) ……………… (226)

Jùliáo 巨髎(ST 3) ……………… (226)

Jùquè 巨阙(RN 14) ……………… (226)

Jùquán 聚泉(EX－HN 10) ……………… (228)

Juéyīnshū 厥阴俞(BL 14) ……………… (230)

K

Kǒngzuì 孔最(LU 6) ……………… (232)

Kǒuhéliáo 口禾髎(LI 19) ……………… (232)

Kùfáng 库房(ST 14) ……………… (234)

Kuāngǔ 髋骨(EX－LE 1) ……………… (235)

Kūnlún 昆仑(BL 60) ……………… (236)

L

Lánwěi 阑尾(EX－LE 7) ……………… (237)

Láogōng 劳宫(PC 8) ……………… (237)

Lígōu 蠡沟(LR 5) ……………… (242)

Lìduì 厉兑(ST 45) ……………… (243)

Liánquán 廉泉(RN 23) ……………… (244)

Liángmén 梁门(ST 21) ……………… (245)

Liángqiū 梁丘(ST 34) ……………… (246)

Lièquē 列缺(LU 7) ……………… (246)

Língdào 灵道(HT 4) ……………… (247)

Língtái 灵台(DU 10) ……………… (249)

Língxū 灵墟(KI 24) ……………… (250)

Lòugǔ 漏谷(SP 7) ……………… (256)

Lúxī 颅息(SJ 19) ……………… (257)

Luòquè 络却(BL 8) ……………… (259)

M

Méichōng 眉冲(BL 3) ……………… (265)

Mìngmén 命门(DU 4) ……………… (270)

Mùchuāng 目窗(GB 16) ……………… (272)

N

Nǎohù 脑户(DU 17) ……………… (276)

Nǎokōng 脑空(GB 19) ……………… (277)

Nàohuì 臑会(SJ 13) ……………… (277)

Nàoshū 臑俞(SI 10) ……………… (277)

Nèiguān 内关(PC 6) ……………… (278)

Nèihuáijiān 内踝尖(EX－LE 8) …… (279)

Nèitíng 内庭(ST 44) ……………… (280)

Nèixīyǎn 内膝眼(EX－LE 4) …… (281)

Nèiyíngxiāng 内迎香(EX－HN 9) …… (281)

P

Pángguāngshū 膀胱俞(BL 28) …… (290)

Píshū 脾俞(BL 20) ……………… (293)

Pǐgēn 痞根(EX－B 4) ……………… (296)

Piānlì 偏历(LI 6) ……………… (297)

Pòhù 魄户(BL 42) ……………… (298)

Púcān 仆参(BL 61) ……………… (299)

Q

Qīmén 期门(LR 14) ……………… (300)

Qìchōng 气冲(ST 30) ……………… (303)

Qìduān 气端(EX－LE 12) ……………… (304)

Qìhǎi 气海(RN 6) ……………… (305)

Qìhǎishū 气海俞(BL 24) ……………… (305)

Qìhù 气户(ST 13) ……………… (307)

Qìshè 气舍(ST 11) ……………… (309)
Qìxué 气穴(KI 13) ……………… (311)
Qiándǐng 前顶(DU 21) ………… (316)
Qiángǔ 前谷(SI 2) ……………… (317)
Qiángjiān 强间(DU 18) ………… (318)
Qīnglíng 青灵(HT 2) …………… (320)
Qīnglěngyuān 清冷渊(SJ 11) … (321)
Qiūxū 丘墟(GB 40) …………… (322)
Qiúhòu 球后(EX-HN 7) ……… (322)
Qūbìn 曲鬓(GB 7) ……………… (323)
Qūchā 曲差(BL 4) ……………… (323)
Qūchí 曲池(LI 11) ……………… (323)
Qūgǔ 曲骨(RN 2) ……………… (324)
Qūquán 曲泉(LR 8) …………… (325)
Qūyuán 曲垣(SI 13) …………… (325)
Qūzé 曲泽(PC 3) ……………… (326)
Quánliáo 颧髎(SI 18) ………… (327)
Quēpén 缺盆(ST 12) ………… (328)

R

Rángǔ 然谷(KI 2) ……………… (329)
Rényíng 人迎(ST 9) …………… (333)
Rìyuè 日月(GB 24) …………… (337)
Rǔgēn 乳根(ST 18) …………… (338)
Rǔzhōng 乳中(ST 17) ………… (339)

S

Sānjiān 三间(LI 3) …………… (341)
Sānjiāoshū 三焦俞(BL 22) …… (343)
Sānyángluò 三阳络(SJ 8) …… (345)
Sānyīnjiāo 三阴交(SP 6) …… (346)
Shāngqiū 商丘(SP 5) ………… (350)
Shāngqū 商曲(KI 17) ………… (350)
Shāngyáng 商阳(LI 1) ………… (350)
Shàngguān 上关(GB 3) ……… (352)
Shàngjùxū 上巨虚(ST 37) …… (352)
Shànglián 上廉(LI 9) ………… (352)

Shàngliáo 上髎(BL 31) ……… (353)
Shàngwǎn 上脘(RN 13) ……… (353)
Shàngxīng 上星(DU 23) …… (354)
Shàngyíngxiāng 上迎香(EX-HN 8) ……… (355)
Shàochōng 少冲(HT 9) ……… (356)
Shàofǔ 少府(HT 8) ………… (356)
Shàohǎi 少海(HT 3) ………… (357)
Shàoshāng 少商(LU 11) …… (357)
Shàozé 少泽(SI 1) …………… (358)
Shēnmài 申脉(BL 62) ……… (359)
Shēnzhù 身柱(DU 12) ……… (360)
Shéncáng 神藏(KI 25) ……… (360)
Shéndào 神道(DU 11) ……… (360)
Shénfēng 神封(KI 23) ……… (361)
Shénmén 神门(HT 7) ……… (362)
Shénquè 神阙(RN 8) ……… (363)
Shéntáng 神堂(BL 44) …… (363)
Shéntíng 神庭(DU 24) …… (363)
Shénshū 肾俞(DL 23) ……… (365)
Shíqīzhuī 十七椎(EX-B 8) … (379)
Shíxuān 十宣(EX-UE 11) …… (383)
Shíguān 石关(KI 18) ……… (384)
Shímén 石门(RN 5) ………… (385)
Shídòu 食窦(SP 17) ……… (386)
Shǒusānlǐ 手三里(LI 10) …… (390)
Shǒuwǔlǐ 手五里(LI 13) …… (401)
Shūfǔ 俞府(KI 27) ………… (405)
Shùgǔ 束骨(BL 65) ………… (407)
Shuàigǔ 率谷(GB 8) ……… (408)
Shuǐdào 水道(ST 28) ……… (408)
Shuǐfēn 水分(RN 9) ……… (409)
Shuǐgōu 水沟(DU 26) …… (409)
Shuǐquán 水泉(KI 5) ……… (410)
Shuǐtū 水突(ST 10) ……… (411)
Sīzhúkōng 丝竹空(SJ 23) … (412)
Sìbái 四白(ST 2) …………… (412)
Sìdú 四渎(SJ 9) …………… (412)
Sìfèng 四缝(EX-UE 10) …… (413)

19

Sìmǎn 四满(KI 14) …………… (414)
Sìshéncōng 四神聪(EX—HN 1)……… (415)
Sùliáo 素髎(DU 25) …………… (416)

T

Tàibái 太白(SP 3) …………… (419)
Tàichōng 太冲(LR 3) …………… (419)
Tàixī 太溪(KI 3) …………… (420)
Tàiyáng 太阳(EX—HN 5)……… (420)
Tàiyǐ 太乙(ST 23) …………… (421)
Tàiyuān 太渊(LU 9) …………… (423)
Táodào 陶道(DU 13) …………… (426)
Tiānchí 天池(PC 1) …………… (429)
Tiānchōng 天冲(GB 9) …………… (430)
Tiānchuāng 天窗(SI 16) …………… (430)
Tiāndǐng 天鼎(LI 17) …………… (431)
Tiānfǔ 天府(LU 3) …………… (431)
Tiānjǐng 天井(SJ 10) …………… (431)
Tiānliáo 天髎(SJ 15) …………… (432)
Tiānquán 天泉(PC 2) …………… (433)
Tiānróng 天容(SI 17) …………… (433)
Tiānshū 天枢(ST 25) …………… (434)
Tiāntū 天突(RN 22) …………… (434)
Tiānxī 天溪(SP 18) …………… (435)
Tiānyǒu 天牖(SJ 16) …………… (436)
Tiānzhù 天柱(BL 10) …………… (437)
Tiānzōng 天宗(SI 11) …………… (437)
Tiáokǒu 条口(ST 38) …………… (437)
Tīnggōng 听宫(SI 19) …………… (439)
Tīnghuì 听会(GB 2) …………… (439)
Tōnglǐ 通里(HT 5) …………… (440)
Tōngtiān 通天(BL 7) …………… (441)
Tóngzǐliáo 瞳子髎(GB 1) …………… (443)
Tóulínqì 头临泣(GB 15) …………… (444)
Tóuqiàoyīn 头窍阴(GB 11) …………… (444)
Tóuwéi 头维(ST 8) …………… (445)

W

Wàiguān 外关(SJ 5) …………… (453)
Wàihuáijiān 外踝尖(EX—LE 9)……… (454)
Wàiláogōng 外劳宫(EX—UE 8)……… (455)
Wàilíng 外陵(ST 26) …………… (455)
Wàiqiū 外丘(GB 36) …………… (455)
Wángǔ 完骨(GB 12) …………… (456)
Wàngǔ 腕骨(SI 4) …………… (457)
Wéidào 维道(GB 28) …………… (460)
Wěiyáng 委阳(BL 39) …………… (461)
Wěizhōng 委中(BL 40) …………… (461)
Wèicāng 胃仓(BL 50) …………… (462)
Wèishū 胃俞(BL 21) …………… (467)
Wèiwǎnxiàshū 胃脘下俞(EX—B 3)
………………… (468)
Wēnliū 温溜(LI 7) …………… (470)
Wūyì 屋翳(ST 15) …………… (472)
Wǔchù 五处(BL 5) …………… (475)
Wǔshū 五枢(GB 27) …………… (478)

X

Xīguān 膝关(LR 7) …………… (482)
Xīyǎn 膝眼(EX—LE 5) …………… (483)
Xīyángguān 膝阳关(GB 33) ……… (484)
Xìmén 郄门(PC 4) …………… (484)
Xiábái 侠白(LU 4) …………… (485)
Xiáxī 侠溪(GB 43) …………… (486)
Xiàguān 下关(ST 7) …………… (487)
Xiàjíshū 下极俞(EX—B 5) ……… (488)
Xiàjùxū 下巨虚(ST 39) …………… (489)
Xiàlián 下廉(LI 8) …………… (489)
Xiàliáo 下髎(BL 34) …………… (489)
Xiàwǎn 下脘(RN 10) …………… (490)
Xiàngǔ 陷谷(ST 43) …………… (492)
Xiāoluò 消泺(SJ 12) …………… (494)
Xiǎochángshū 小肠俞(BL 27) ……… (496)

Xiǎogǔkōng 小骨空(EX—UE 6) …… (503)
Xiǎohǎi 小海(SI 8)……………… (503)
Xīnshū 心俞(BL 15) ……………… (509)
Xìnhuì 囟会(DU 22) ……………… (510)
Xíngjiān 行间(LR 2) ……………… (511)
Xiōngxiāng 胸乡(SP 9) …………… (513)
Xuánlí 悬厘(GB 6) ………………… (518)
Xuánlú 悬颅(GB 5) ………………… (519)
Xuánshū 悬枢(DU 5) ……………… (519)
Xuánzhōng 悬钟(GB 39) ………… (519)
Xuánjī 璇玑(RN 21) ……………… (520)
Xuèhǎi 血海(SP 10) ……………… (524)

Y

Yǎmén 哑门(DU 15) ……………… (533)
Yángbái 阳白(GB 14) …………… (536)
Yángchí 阳池(SJ 4) ……………… (536)
Yángfǔ 阳辅(GB 38) ……………… (536)
Yánggāng 阳纲(BL 48) …………… (537)
Yánggǔ 阳谷(SI 5) ………………… (537)
Yángjiāo 阳交(GB 35) …………… (538)
Yánglíngquán 阳陵泉(GB 34) …… (538)
Yángxī 阳溪(LI 5) ………………… (541)
Yǎnglǎo 养老(SI 6) ……………… (544)
Yāoqí 腰奇(EX—B 9) …………… (545)
Yāoshū 腰俞(DU 2) ……………… (545)
Yāotòngdiǎn 腰痛点(EX—UE 7) … (546)
Yāoyǎn 腰眼(EX—B 7) …………… (546)
Yāoyángguān 腰阳关(DU 3) …… (546)
Yāoyí 腰宜(EX—B 6) …………… (547)
Yèmén 液门(SJ 2) ………………… (549)
Yìshè 意舍(BL 49) ………………… (553)
Yìxǐ 譩譆(BL 45) ………………… (553)
Yìfēng 翳风(SJ 17) ……………… (553)
Yìmíng 翳明(EX—HN 14) ……… (554)
Yīnbāo 阴包(LR 9) ……………… (554)
Yīndū 阴都(KI 19) ……………… (554)
Yīngǔ 阴谷(KI 10) ……………… (555)

Yīnjiāo 阴交(RN 7) ……………… (556)
Yīnlián 阴廉(LR 11) ……………… (556)
Yīnlíngquán 阴陵泉(SP 9) ……… (557)
Yīnshì 阴市(ST 33) ……………… (558)
Yīnxī 阴郄(HT 6) ………………… (559)
Yīnmén 殷门(BL 37) ……………… (563)
Yínjiāo 龈交(DU 28) ……………… (564)
Yǐnbái 隐白(SP 1) ………………… (565)
Yìntáng 印堂(EX—HN 3) ……… (565)
Yíngchuāng 膺窗(ST 16) ………… (566)
Yíngxiāng 迎香(LI 20) …………… (567)
Yǒngquán 涌泉(KI 1) …………… (568)
Yōumén 幽门(KI 21) ……………… (569)
Yújì 鱼际(LU 10) ………………… (571)
Yúyāo 鱼腰(EX—HN 4) ………… (572)
Yùtáng 玉堂(RN 18) ……………… (573)
Yùzhěn 玉枕(BL 9) ……………… (574)
Yùzhōng 彧中(KI 26) …………… (575)
Yuānyè 渊液(GB 22) ……………… (575)
Yúnmén 云门(LU 2) ……………… (580)

Z

Zhāngmén 章门(LR 13) …………… (585)
Zhàohǎi 照海(KI 6) ……………… (586)
Zhéjīn 辄筋(GB 23) ……………… (587)
Zhèngyíng 正营(GB 17) ………… (600)
Zhīgōu 支沟(SJ 6) ……………… (600)
Zhīzhèng 支正(SJ 7) …………… (601)
Zhìyáng 至阳(DU 9) ……………… (605)
Zhìyīn 至阴(BL 67) ……………… (605)
Zhìshì 志室(BL 52) ……………… (605)
Zhìbiān 秩边(BL 54) …………… (606)
Zhōngchōng 中冲(PC 9) ………… (608)
Zhōngdū 中都(LR 6) …………… (608)
Zhōngdú 中渎(GB 32) …………… (609)
Zhōngfēng 中封(LR 4) …………… (609)
Zhōngfǔ 中府(LU 1) …………… (609)
Zhōngjí 中极(RN 3) ……………… (611)

Zhōngkuí 中魁(EX—UE 4) ……… (611)
Zhōngliáo 中髎(BL 33) ……… (612)
Zhōnglǚshū 中膂俞(BL 29) ……… (612)
Zhōngquán 中泉(EX—UE 3) ……… (613)
Zhōngshū 中枢(DU 7) ……… (613)
Zhōngtíng 中庭(RN 16) ……… (614)
Zhōngwǎn 中脘(RN 12) ……… (614)
Zhōngzhǔ 中渚(SJ 3) ……… (615)
Zhōngzhù 中注(KI 15) ……… (616)
Zhōuróng 周荣(SP 20) ……… (618)

Zhǒujiān 肘尖(EX—UE 1) ……… (619)
Zhǒuliáo 肘髎(LI 12) ……… (620)
Zhùbīn 筑宾(KI 9) ……… (622)
Zǐgōng 子宫(EX—CA 1) ……… (624)
Zǐgōng 紫宫(RN 19) ……… (628)
Zúlínqì 足临泣(GB 41) ……… (631)
Zúqiàoyīn 足窍阴(GB 44) ……… (631)
Zúsānlǐ 足三里(ST 36) ……… (632)
Zútōnggǔ 足通谷(BL 66) ……… (644)
Zúwǔlǐ 足五里(LR 10) ……… (644)

附录三
Appendix 3

插 图 索 引
Index of Figures

Ancient Nine Needles, the	27(222)
Acupuncture drills	30(245)
Bafeng and Qiduan points	3(5)
Bladder Meridian of Foot-Taiyang	84(641)
Bone proportional cun(B-cun)(Anterior view)	19.1(142)
Bone proportional cun(B-cun)(Posterior view)	19.2(143)
Changqiang & Huiyin points	4(39)
Chengqi and other point of head(Anterior view)	5(45)
Circulation of the 14 meridians	47(381)
Dazhu and other points of back	7(68)
Dannang point	9(75)
Dangyang point	10(76)
Dermal needles	36(292)
Dingchuan and Jiaji points	11(83)
Direct moxibustion	74(602)
Du Meridian, the	12.1(86)
Duyin Point	13(88)
Erbai point	15(101)
Filiform needles, round-sharp needle, and three-edged needle	21(159)
Finger-breadth measurement	22(164)
Gallbladder Meridian of Foot-Shaoyang, the	82(634)
Haiquan, Jinjin and Yuye points	20(154)
Heart Meridian of Hand-Shaoyin	51(396)
Huantiao and other points of chest and abdomen	23(171)
Indirect moxibustion	25(192)
Intradermal needles	38(292)
Jiache, Xiaguan and Touwei points	24(187)
Kidney Meridian of Foot-Shaoyin, the	83(639)
Kouheliao and other points of head and face	28(234)
Lanwei point	29(237)
Large Intestine Meridian of Hand-Yangming, the	53(402)
Lifting and thrusting	57(427)
Liver Meridian of Foot-Jueyin, the	80(629)
Lung Meridian of Hand-Taiyin, the	52(399)
Luoque and other points of occiput	31(259)
Manipulation of a dermal needle	37(292)
Methods of Needle Insertion	26(205)

Entry	Reference
Middle finger cun	77(615)
Mild warm moxibustion	62(469)
Moxa stick	1(2)
Moxa cones	2(3)
Moxibustion with a warm needle	63(471)
Neixiyan and Neihuaijian points	33(281)
Neiyingxiang point	34(281)
Points of Bladder Meridian (Leg)	35.1(289)
Points of Bladder Meridian (Foot)	35.2(289)
Points of Bladder Meridian (Lower limb)	35.3(290)
Points of Du Meridian (Back)	12.2(86)
Points of Du Meridian	12.3(87)
Points of Gallbladder Meridian (Lower limbs)	8.1(73)
Points of Gallbladder Meridian (Foot)	8.2(74)
Points of Gallbladder Meridian (Thigh)	8.3(74)
Points of Gallbladder Meridian (Leg)	8.4(74)
Points of Heart Meridian	67(508)
Points of Kidney Meridian (Foot & leg)	46(364)
Points of Large Intestine Meridian (Forearm)	6.1(60)
Points of Large Intestine Meridian (Arm)	6.2(60)
Points of Large Intestine Meridian (Hand)	6.3(60)
Points of Large Intestine Meridian & Stomch Meridian (Neck)	6.4(61)
Points of Liver Meridian (Leg)	17.1(125)
Points of Liver Meridian (Foot)	17.2(125)
Points of Lung Meridian	16(107)
Points of Pericardium Meridian	66(508)
Points of Ren Meridian	43.2(335)
Points of Sanjiao Meridian (Shoulder)	44.1(342)
Points of Sanjiao Meridian (Arm)	44.2(342)
Points of Sanjiao Meridian (Forearm)	44.3(343)
Points of Sanjiao Meridian (Hand)	44.4(343)
Points of Small Intestine Meridian (Shoulder)	65.1(495)
Points of Small Intestine Meridian (Hand)	65.2(496)
Points of Spleen Meridian (Foot)	39.1(293)
Points of Spleen Meridian (Abdomen)	39.2(294)
Points of Spleen Meridian (Chest)	39.3(294)
Points of Spleen Meridian (Leg)	39.4(294)
Points of Stomach Meridian (Leg)	60.1(464)
Points of Stomach Meridian (Thigh)	60.2(464)
Points of Stomach Meridian (Foot)	60.3(465)
Points of Stomach Meridian (Abdomen)	60.4(465)
Points of Stomach Meridian (Lower limb)	60.5(466)
Points of the three yang meridians of hand	48(391)

Points of the three yin meridians of foot	81(633)
Points of the three yin meridians of hand	49(392)
Qihu and other points of chest and abdomen	40(307)
Ququan and Yinbao points	41(325)
Ren Meridian, the	43.1(334)
Salt-separated moxibustion	18(138)
Sanjiao Meridian of hand-Shaoyang	50(394)
Scalp acupuncture lines(Anteior view)	59.1(446)
Scalp acupuncture lines(Vertex view)	59.2(446)
Scalp acupuncture lines(Lateral view)	59.3.1(447)
Scalp acupuncture lines(Lateral view)	59.3.2(447)
Scalp acupuncture lines(Posterior view)	59.4(448)
Shaofu, Shaochong, Laogong and Zhongchong points	45(356)
Sifeng point	54(413)
Sishencong point	55(415)
Sparrow-pecking moxibustion	42(328)
Spleen Meridian of Foot-Taiyin, the	85(643)
Standard international chart of auricular points, the	14(99)
Stomch Meridian of Foot-Yangming, the	87(647)
Taiyang, Erjian, and Yiming points	56(420)
Three Yin Meridians of Foot	81(633)
Thumb cun	32(271)
Tiantu, Lianquan and Chengjing points	58(435)
Weiwanxiashu and other extra points(Back view)	61(468)
Wushu, Weidao and Juliao points	64(478)
Xuehai point	68(524)
Yaotongdian and Wailaogong points	69(545)
Yinjiao point	70(564)
Yongquan point	71(569)
Yuanye, Zhejin and Daimai points	72(575)
Zhangmen and Qimen points	73(585)
Zhongfu and Yunmen points	75(610)
Zhongquan and other extra points(Dorsum of hand)	76(613)
Zhoujian point	78(620)
Zigong point	79(624)
Zuwuli, Yinlian and Jimai points	86(645)

Index

A

Ashi Point 1
  Natural reactive point 436
  Non-fixed Point 28
  Ouch Point 532
Abdomen 121
Abdomen (MA)121
Abdomen below hypochondrium 268
Abdominal pain 122
    ∼ due to pathogenic cold 157
    ∼ due to retention of food 387
    ∼ due to stagnation of liver-qi 127
    ∼ due to Yang deficiency 542
  Abdominal pain during pregnancy 335
    Lower abdominal pain during pregnancy 336
      Embarrassment of the fetus 15
      Pain due to fetus 626
Abnormal position of fetus 13
  Malposition of fetus 418
Acromion scapulae 572
Acupoint electrometry 215
Acupoint magnetotherapy 522
Acupoint selection along the affected meridian 18
Acupoints 407
  Applicable places for Stone needling and moxibustion 22
  Bone holes 143
  Gathering sites 177
  Holes 232
  Locus 521
  Point 521
  Point channel 521
  Transmission 406
Acupuncture and moxibustion 54
  ∼ therapy 592
  Moxibustion and acupuncture 223
Acupuncture and moxibustion in the dog-days 117
Acupuncture anesthesia 588
  A. A. 596
Acupuncture diagram and model 268
Acupuncture drills 244
Acupuncture manipulation 589
Acupuncture operator 590
Acupuncture needle 587
Acupuncture with filiform needle 160
Acupuncture zone of meridians 211
Acupuncturist 596
Acute appendicitis 41
  ∼ with legs flinching 418
Acute infantile convulsion 183
Acute mastitis 52, 339
  ∼ due to external blowing 452
  ∼ due to stagnation of liver-qi 129
  ∼ due to stomach-heat 466
  Galactostitis 88
  Mammary abscess 52
  Ru chui(Breast blowing) 338
Adhesive plaster substitute for moxibustion 429
Adjacent puncture 13
Age moxa cones 416
Aijiu Tongshuo 1
Alopecia areata 12
  ∼due to pathogenic wind 569
    Haircut by ghost 151
Alumen-separated moxibustion 135
Amenorrhea 208
  ∼due to blood stasis caused by accumulation of pathogenic cold 155
  ∼ due to deficiency of blood 525

~due to deficiency of the liver
　　and kidney 126
~ due to menstrual disorder 208
~ due to phlegm-dampness 425
~due to stagnancy of qi and blood
　　stasis 315
~due to weakness of the spleen and
　　stomach 295
Blockage of menstruation 579
Blood stoppage 524
Closing of menstruation 578
Disappearances of menses 579
Menopause 505
Irregular monthly coming 578
No arrival of Menstrual flow 579
No flow of menses 208
Mo flow of menstrual blood 211
No menses 29
No menstrual flow 213
No menstruation 579
No mensual blood 29
No-coming of monthly envoy 579
Obstruction of menstrual flow 213,580
Obstruction of menstruation 578,579
Obstruction of menstrual blood 211
Anal itching in children 496
Anatomical landmarks on body surface
　　428
　　Landmarks on body surface 428
　　Location according to ~ 428
Ancient book copied on silk
　　discovered in the tomb of Han Dynasty
　　at Mawangdui 261
Angle of Cymba Conchae(MA) 440
　　Prostate(MA) 318
Angle of needle insertion 588
Angulus mandibulae 324
Ankle 170,458
Ankle(MA-AH 2) 170

Anonymous finger, the 472
Anterior ear lobe 52
　　Neurasthenia point 362
Antihelix 89
Antitragic apex 89
　　Parotid Gland (MA) 340
　　Relieving Asthma 297
Antitragus 89
　　Posterior groove of ~ 89
Anus(MA) 131
　　Hemorrhoid Nucleus 607
Apoplexy 617
　　~ in pregnancy 336
　　~involving the meridians and
　　　　collaterals 617
　　~involving zang and fu 618
　　　　Excess-syndrome of ~ 618
　　　　Collapse-syndrome of ~ 618
　　Wind-stroke 57
　　　　Sudden stroke 58
　　　　Sudden wind-stroke 57
　　Zhongfenbuyuxue 616
　　Zhongfengqixue 616
Appendix(MA) 237
Appliance for needle insertion 206
Areas for stimulation 54
Arrival of qi 77
Arrival of qi at the affected area
　　314
Arteries of the Twelve Meridians 376
Arthralgia syndrome 20
　　Arthralgia aggravated by pathogenic
　　　　cold 443
　　Fixed arthralgia 623
　　Heat arthralgia 330
　　Lingering arthralgia(damp arthralgia) 623
　　Migratory arthralgia 511
　　Pain arthralgia(cold arthralgia) 443
Ascariasis of biliary tract 72

Epigastric pain due to enterositosis 50
　Epigastric pain due to bite by parasites 49
　Epigastric pain due to snap by parasites 50
　Colic caused by ascariasis 157
Assembled Meridians 628
Asthma 495
　~ due to deficiency of lung 109
　~ due to phlegm-heat 424
　~ due to retention of cold fluid
　　158
Auxiliary manipulations 120
　Scraping 146

B

Ba Dou(Semen Crotonis)-separated moxibustion 133
Back-Shu Meridian 406
　Meridian of Back-Shu 406
Back-shu points 16
Bafeng 4
　Bachong 4
　Yindubaxue 555
Bahua 5
　Liuhua 253
Bai Fu Zi(Rhizoma Typhonii)-separated moxibustion 10
Bai Zheng Fu(A verse on 100 diseases) 12
Bai Jie Zi(Semen Sinapis Albae) moxibustion 10
Baichongwo 1, 11
　Xuexi 528
Baifa magic needling 11
Baihuanshu 10
　Yuhuanshu 573
　Yufangshu 572
Baihui 11
　Dianshang 79
　Niwangong 282
　Sanyang 345

Sanyangwuhui 345
Tianman 433
Weihui 460
Wuhui 475
Bailao 12
Balsam pear moxibustion 234
Bamboo needle 622
Ban Xia(Rhizoma pinelliac) moxibustion 13
Baohuang（胞肓）13
　Baohuang（包肓）13
Baomen and Zihu 14
　Zihu 625
Basic joints of extremities 17
Baxie 8
　Baguan 5
　Big puncture at Baguan 5
　Dadu 2, 61
　Shangdu 351
　Xiadu 487
Bazhuixia 8
Beiji Jiufa (Moxibustion Method for Emergency) 16
Beijiazhongjian 16
Below belt 71
　Leukorrhea disease 71
　　Leukorrhea due to noxious dampness 370
　　Leukorrhea due to the deficiency of the kidney 366
　　Leukorrhea due to the deficiency of the spleen 295
　　Multicolored vaginal mucoid discharge 477
　　　Leukorrhea with multicolored discharge 71
　　　Vaginal mucoid discharge of five colors 71
　　　Bloody leukorrhea 47
　　　　Leukorrhea with bloody discharge 71

Blackish leukorrhea 163
　　　　Leukorrhea with blackish discharge
　　　　71
　　　Greenish leukorrhea 320
　　　　Leukorrhea with greenish discharge
　　　　71
　　　Yellowish leukorrhea 173
　　　　Leukorrhea with yellowish dicharge
　　　　71
Benshen 18
　Zhier 602
Beriberi 200
　Cardiac ～ 200
　　Beriberi attacking the heart 200
　　Beriberi entering the heart 200
　Dry beriberi 123
　Foot-asthenia 200
　Moxibustion at eight points for ～ 200
　Slow wind 172
　Wet beriberi 370
Bian Que 23
Bian Que Shenying Zhenjiu Yulong Jing
　(Bian Que's Dragon Classics of
　Accupuncture and Moxibustion) 23
Bian Que Xin Shu(Bian Que's Medical
　Experiences) 23
Bian Que Zhen Chuan(Bian Que's
　Bequeathed Acupuncture Techniques) 23
Biandu 24
Big granary 419
Big valley 62
Biguan 22
Bihuan 19
Bijiaoezhong 19
　Bijiao 19
Biliu 19
Binao (臂臑) 21
　Binao (臂脑) 21
　Jingchong 219

　Jingzhong 219
　Touchong 444
Bingfeng 25
Bird-pecking moxibustion 328
Bird-pecking needling 328
Bishizitou 21
Biwuli 21
　Wuli1 426
Bleeding of post-moxibustion sores 103
Bleeding with cupping 55
　Blood-letting cuping 56
Blepharoptosis 535
　Dysfunction of eyelid 192
　Ptosis of the eyelid 82
Blood-letting therapy 56,105
　Collateral pricking therapy 55
Blood-reflowing to Pericardium
　Meridian 526
Blurred vision 273
　Fat deposition opacity 285
　Interstitial keratitis 179
　Hypopyon 176
　Thin nebula 25
　Trachomatous pannus 52
Bo Shu Jingmai(Meridians of the Silk
　Book) 25
　Eleven meridians,the 384
Body acupuncture 429
Boiling the needle 621
Bolt-door-pivot 147

Bolt-pivot 148
Bone end 228
Bone needle 145
Bone of the thigh 22
Bone proportional measurement 143
　Bone measurement 142
　Bone-length movement 143
Border of white skin 10

29

Bowl moxibustion 457
  Bowl-separated moxibustion 138
Breaking of the inserted needle 587
Breast nodules 338
  ~ due to phlegm turbidity 425
  ~ due to yin deficiency 561
Bright hall 268
Brow origin 265
Brow source 265
Bronze Statue 342
Bu Xie Xue Xin Ge(Verse for Clear Understanding of Reinforcing and Reducing) 27
Bulang(步廊) 29
  Bulang(步郎) 29
Bulging muscles 230
Burning moxibustion 356
  Blistering moxibustion 103
  Festering moxibustion 169
Burong 28
Buttock 231
Buttock (MA-AH 5) 450
Buzhu Tongren Shuxue Zhenjiu Tujing (Supplementary Annotation for the Illustrated Mannual of Points of Acupuncture and Moxibustion on a Bronze Status with Acupoints) 27

C

Caiai Bian(A Book on Adoption of Moxibution) 30
Caiai Bian Yi(Supplement to the book on Adoption of Moxibustion) 30
Calf 623
Cang Zhu(Rhizoma Atractylodis) moxibution 30
  Cang Zhu(Rhizoma **Atractylodis**)-separated moxibustion 134
Cardiac Orifice(MA-IC 7) 291

Cardialgia 510
Catgut embedding 262
  Catgut embedding at acupoints 523
Cauda helicis 96
  Back of ~ ,the 96
Cauterisation with Folium Cannabis 261
Cavity cocha 95
Central forehead 535
Central jaw 552
Central Rim (MA) 577
  Brain point(MA) 276
Chahua 31
Changgu 39
  Changping2,39
  Xunji(循脊)2,532
  Xunji(循际)2,532
  Xunyuan 532
Changqiang 39
  Jiuwei 219
  Juegu 228
  Qizhiyinxi 283
  Weilǔ 461
  Xiajizhishu 488
  Xiongzhiyinshu 514
Changrao 41
Changsang Jun 40
Changyang meridian 38
Changyi 41
  Changdao 40
Cheek 187
Cheek(MA) 187
Chen Hui 42
Chen Tingquan 42
Chen Yan 42
Chenjue 41
  Jujiao 226
  Jujue 226
Cheng Gao 45
Cheng Jie 46

Cheng Tianzuo 46
Cheng Yue 46
Chengfu 42
  Fucheng 118
  Rouxi 338
  Yinguan 555
Chenggu 42
Chengguang 43
Chengjiang 43
  Chuijiang 52
  Guishi 151
  Tianchi 429
  Xuanjiang 518
Chengjin 43
  Zhenchang 598
  Zhichang 601
  Zhuanchang 623
Chengling 44
Chengman 44
Chengming 44
Chengqi 44
  Mianjiao 266
  Xixue 482,484
Chengshan 45
  Changshan 41
  Rouzhu 338
  Yuchang 571
  Yufu 571
  Yuyao(鱼腰2) 572
  Yuzhu 574
Chest 512
Chest (MA) 512
Chi Wu Shen Zhen Jing(Classic on Red-Black Miraculous Acupuncture) 47
Chicken claw acupuncture 181
Chimai 47
  Zimai 624
  Chinao 46
Chinese-Chives-separated moxibustion 136

Chize 46
  Guishou 151
  Guitang 151
Cholera morbus 331
  ~due to cold 138
  ~ due to cold-qi 139
  Summer ~ 330
Chonggu 50
  Taizu 423
  Zhuiding 623
Chongmen 48
  Cigong1,52
  Shangcigong 351
Chongyang 49
  Huiyuan 178
Chorea-trembling controlled area, the 481
Chuan Jiao(Pericarpium Zanthexyli)-separated moxibustion 134
Chuanshijiu 51
Chunli 52
Chunyu Yi 52
Cigong2, 52
Cijiu Xinfa Yaojue(Essentials of Acupuncture and Moxibustion in Verse) 55
Ciliao 53
Clavicle(MA-F5) 418
Clay coin 282
Clay moxibustion 282
Climacterium 228
  Menopausal sundromes 208
Cold limbs 155
  Chilly limbs 241
Cold limbs in children 497
  ~ due to excess of heat 498
  ~ due to yang trouble 502
  ~ due to yin trouble 502
Cold moxibustion 241
Cold needle 241

Cold needling 241
Cold-application at accupoints 523
Collateral branch of the large
　　meridian 259
Collateral of the same yin 442
Collateral pricking 55,259
Collateral qi 259
Collaterals 259
Collaterals located at the thenar
　　eminence 571
Color blindness 347
　　Monochromation 388
　　Seeing red as if seeing white 388
Column bone 622
Coma in children 497
Combination of local points, the 206
　　Local selection 207
　　Point selection near the affected
　　　region 206
Combination of points on meridians
　　with the same name 395
Combination of points on yin meridian
　　with those lon yang meridian, the 562
Combination of the Back-Shu and the
　　Front-Mu points 405
Combination of the lift-right points,
　　the 648
Combination of the superior-inferior
　　points 354
Combined selection of the Yuan
　　(Primary) point and the Luo(Connect-
　　ing) point 576
Common cold 131
　　~ due to summer-heat and dampness 407
　　~ due to wind-cold pathogen 111
　　~ due to wind-heat patogen 113
Comprehensive manipulations 628
Connecting 259
Constipation 24

~of cold type 241
　　Cold accumulation 155
　~ due to heat 329
　~of insufficient type 514
　　Yin-accumulation 556
Dyschesia 59
Difficult bowel movement 59
Dry stool 59
Continuous lifting-thrusting technique 77
　　Bird-pecking needling 328
Contraindications of needling 54
　　Five contraindications 476
　　Five deteriorating cases 477
　　Five excesses 475
　　Needling for five kinds of exhaustions
　　　forbidden 475
　　Twelve contraindications 374
Contralateral needling 225
Contralateral prick 270
Convulsive syndrome 219
　　Convulsion 219
　　~due to impairment of yin caused
　　　by high fever 132
Corresponding point selection 89
Cough 231
　~ due to cold-wind pathogen 112
　~ due to dry heat pethogen 583
　~ due to liver fire 124
　~ due to phlegm-dampness 424
　~ due to wind-heat pathogen 114
　~ due to yin deficiency 561
Cough in children 497
Crossing needling 198
Crossing point 193
Cuan 58
Cuanzhu 58
　　Guangming 149
　　Meiben 265
　　Meitou 265

Mingguang 268
Shiguang(始光) 388
Yeguang 549
Yuanzai 576
Yuanzhu 576
Cunzhen Tu(Pictures of Reserving the True) 58
Cunping 58
Cupping 9
　～ bu extracting air 50
　～ by pushing the cup 449
　～ with boiled cup 410
　～ with glasses in alignment 288
　Bamboo cupping 9
　Fire cupping 180
　　Cups with heated air 180
　Flash-fire cupping 348
　Quick cupping 348
　　Successive flash cupping 348
　Horn cupping 199
　　Horn 199
　Moving cupping 628
　Pulling cupping 236
　Sucking cup 482
　Sucking tube 482
Cutaneous regions 291
Cutaneous regions of the six meridians 253
　Bolt-dormancy 149
　Firm hinge 405
　Gentlle hinge 405
　Haifei 154
Cutting therapy 133
Cymba auriculae 85

D

Dabao 59
Dachangshu 61
Dachui 61
Dadu1, 61
Dadun 62
　Shuiquan 410
　Zudazhicongmao 628
Dagukong(大骨空) 62
　Dagukong(大骨孔) 62
Dahe 62
　Yinguan 555
　Yinwei(阴维穴2②) 559
Daheng 63
　Hengwen 164
　Renheng 332
　Shenqi 365
Daju 564
　Yemen(液门2) 549
Daling 64
　Guixin 151
　Tailing 420
　Xinzhu 510
Damen 64
Damuzhitou 64
Daying 65
　Suikong 417
Dazhijiehengwen 66
　Dazhijieli 66
Dazhijumao 66
Dazhong 66
　Taizhong 423
Dazhu 68
　Dashu 65
Dazhui 69
　Bailao 12
Dan Jie (Double-singular acupoint selection) 72
Dannang 74
Danshu 75
Danzhong(膻中) 75
　Danzhong 75
　Shangqihai 353

Xiongtang 513
Yuaner 576
Yuanjian 576
Daquan2, 65
Dangrong 76
Dangyang 76
Dan Medicine for health preservation 574
Day-prescription of extra meridians
　302
Deafness 95
　Bi syndrome of the ear 94
　Loss of listening ability 255
Deep-sited Chong Meridian 117
　Deep-sited meridian in the spine 117
Delayed menstruation 214
　～due to blood-cold 525
　　Delayed menses due to blood-cold 524
　～ due to blood deficiency 528
　～ due to qi stagnation 314
　Backward menstruation 579
　Delayed menstrual period 154
　Later menstruation than usual 208
　Postponed menstrual cycle 213
Depletive heat 493
Dermal needle 292
　Casing-type ～ 427
　Plum-blossom needle 266
　Seven-star needle 300
Deterioration due to fire 180
Determination of heat sensitivity 601
Di fu zi(Fructus kochiae) steaming
　moxibustion 78
Dicang 78
　Huiwei 177
　Weiwei 469
Dihe 78
Diji（地机）78
　Diji（地箕）79
　Pishe 293

Dishen 79
Diwuhui 79
　Diwu 79
Diabetes 494
　～ involving the lower jiao 491
　～ involving the middle-jiao 615
　～ of the upper jiao 354
　Thirst due to consumptive heat 495
Diagnosis by Examining the meridians
　and points 215
Diarrhea 507
　～ due to improper diet 349
　～ due to stagnation of liver-qi 129
　Cold-damp ～ 157
　Damp-heat ～ 335
　Diarrhea before dawn 329,475
　　Early morning diarrhea 42
　Diarrhea in children due to pathogenic heat 499
　Diarrhea in children due to phlegm 499
Ding Deyong 82
Ding Yi 82
Dingchuan 84
　Chuanxixue 51
　Zhichuan 606
Dingshanghuimao 84
Direct moxibustion 602
　Male-female thunderbolt fire 53
　Moxibustion on muscle 624
　Moxibustion on skin 624
　Visible moxibustion 268
Directing-qi method 581
Dispersing 507
Distal segment point selection 577
Distal-proximal point association 578
Distant poin selection 577
　Distal point selection 577
　Distant selection 518
Distention(胀1) 585

Disease of Distention 586
　　Tympanites 146
　　Single abdominal distention 72
Dizziness 520
　　Deficiency syndrome of ～ 521
　　Excess syndrome of ～ 520
　　Faintness 345
Dongyi Baojian (A Treasured Mirror of Oriental Medicine) 84
Dou Cai 85
Dou Chi (Semen sojae praeparatum)-cake-separated moxibustion 134
　　Dou Chi (Semen sojae praeparatum) moxibustion 85
Dou Guifang 85
Dou Hanqing 85
Douzhou 85
　　Xiaozhoujian 505
Dragon-tiger ascending and prancing 254
　　Dragon-tiger ascending and descending 254
Dragon-tiger alternate prance 254
Dragon-tiger alternate fight 254
Drainage needling 65
Dredging the meridians by connecting meridian qi 201
Dripping with sweat after delivery 34
Drought of moxibustio
i 8 Win 5Dj 8
mi6Duhu7
Gaga 11 agga 3
Dyin 88
Duiduan 89
Duodenum(MA-SC 1) 379
Duoming 91
　　Dushu 87
　　Gaogai 131
　　Hama 154

　　Xingxing 511
Dysentery 244
　　～ due to cold-dampness 156
　　～ due to damp-heat pathogen 371
　　Chang Pi 40
　　Chronic dysentery with frequent relapse 514
　　Fasting ～ 207
　　Frequent bowel motions 489
　　Fulminant ～ 552
　　Prolonged defecation with difficulty 607
Dysentery 244
Dysmenorrhea 444
　　～ due to blood stasis 531
　　～ due to cold-dampness 156
　　～due to impaired liver and kidney 126
　　～ due to qi stagnation 314
　　Abdominal pain after menstruation 209
　　Abdominal pain during menstruation 214
　　Abdominal pain in menstrual period 579
　　Lower abdominal pain before menstruation 212
Dyspepsia during pregnancy 302
Dysphagia 548
　　Choke 548
　　Difficult deglutition 140

E

Ear acupuncture 100
　　～ anesthesia 100
　　Ear poin acupuncture therapy 100
Ear Center(MA-H 1) 100
　　Diaphragm(MA) 139
Ear lobe 94

Back side of the ~ 94
Eclampsia gravidarum 627
　Convulsion due to wind pathogen 113
　Convulsion during pregnancy 335
　Epilepsy during pregnancy 336
　Epilepsy in a pregnant womwn 93
　Epileptiform Dizziness in a pregnant woman 94
　Epileptiform Spasm in a pregnant woman 93
　Spasm due to fetus 418
　Wind-type convulsion during pregnancy 335
Eczema 373
　~ due to blood deficiency 529
　~ due to damp-heat pathogen 372
　~ of the ear 518
　Infantile eczema 276
　Eczema of breast 339
　Fetus eczema 418
　Scrotal eczema 365,514
Edema 411
　Yang ~ 539
　Yin ~ 558
　Egen 91
Egg moxibustion 181
Eight Confluence Points 7
　Bamai Jiaohui Baxue Ge (Verses on the Eight Confluence Points) 7
　Combination of Eight Confluence Points, the 6
　Dou's Eight Points 85
　Eight ebb-flow points 251
　Eight crossing points 198
　Eight points of the eight meridians 5
Eight Directions 8
Eight evading-items of puncturing 337
　Eight Extra Meridians 301
　Eight Meridians 5

Chong Meridian, the 48
　Great Chong Vessel 420
　Diseases of the Chong Meridian 48
Dai Meridian 70
　Diseases of the Dai Meridian 71
Du Meridian, the 85
　Diseases of the Du Merdian 85
Ren Meridian, the 334
　Diseases of the Ren Meridian 334
Yangqiao Meridian 539
　Diseases of the Yangqiao Meridian 539
　Yangqiao 539
Yangwei Meridian, the 540
　Diseases of the Yangwei Meridian 540
　Yangwei points 540
Yinqiao Meridian 558
　Diseases of the Yinqiao Meridian 558
Yinwei Meridian 59
　Diseases of the Yinwei Meridian 559
Eight Influential Points 5
　Bahui 5
Eight Methods 4
　Eight methods for needling manipualtion 491
　Eight methods of intelligent Turtle 248
　　Soaring of the intelligent turtle 225
　Eight methods of Soaring 105
Eight winds 5
Eight-wood fires 8
Elbow 619
Electric stimulator 81
Electrical acupuncture anesthesia 81
Electric-heating moxibustion 80
Electroacupuncture therapy 80
Eleven heavenly-star points 436
　Twelve heavenly-star points 436
Eleven meridians, the 384
　Bo Shu Jingmai(Meridians of the Silk Book) 25

Elongated needle 263
   Therapy with ∼ 264
Elu 91
Empirical selection of points 2116
Emission 552
   Leaking of the seminal fluid 552
Enuresis in children 502
Epigastric pain 510
Epiphora induced by wind 567
   Epiphora with cold tear induced by
     wind 566
   Epiphora with warm tear induced by
     wind 567
Epilepsy disease 491
   Deficiency type of ∼ 492
   Depressive psychosis(癫证2) 80
   Excess type of ∼ 492
   Feng xuan 115
Epistaxis 19
   ∼ due to liver fire 124
   ∼ due to lung-heat 108
   ∼ due to stomach-heat 464
   Bleeding from inside the nose 20
   Serious case of ∼ 19
   Nasal bleeding 19
Erbai 100
Erchui 94
Erheliao 94
   Heliao 162
Erhoufaji 95
Erjian（耳尖）95
   Eryong 100
Erjian（二间）101
   Jiangu 188
   Zhougu 618
Erkongzhong 95
Ermen 96
Ermenqianmai 96
Ershang 97

Ershangfaji 100
   Ershang 97
Erzhishang 102
Erzhong 100
Erzhuixia 102
   Wuming 472
Erysipelas 71
   ∼ due to damp-heat pathogens 371
   ∼ due to wind-heat pathogens 113
   ∼ overhead 15
   Burning sores along belt 160
   Fire ∼ 180
     Heavenly fire 431
     Red fire 71
     Unfixed red ∼ 48
   Running fire 251
Esophagus(MA-IC 6) 386
Exterior-interior point selection 24
External Ear(MA) 452
   Ear 94
External Genitalia(MA-H) 406
External meridians 454
External moxibustion adhesive plaster
   454
External Nose (MA-T 1) 452
Extra points 214
   Extraordinary points 214
   Peculiar points 302
   Peculiar transmissive points 302
Eye outline 272
Eye source 271
Eye1 (MA) 273
   Eye(MA-L 11) 535
Eye2 (MA) 272
Eyebrow-like knife 504
   Sha knife 347
Eyebrow-occiput line 265

F

Face acupuncture 267
Facial Pain 267
Facial paralysis 266
  Deviation of the eye and mouth 234
Fainting during acupuncture 581
Fainting during moxibustion 581
Faji 103
Fan E 103
Fan Jiusi 105
Fan Peixian 105
Fan Yuyi 105
Feimu 108
Feishu 108
Feiyang（飞扬）106
  Feiyang（飞阳）106
  Jueyang 229
Feiyang Meridian 106
Femur 193
Feng Qu 116
Feng Zhuohuai 116
Fengchi 110
Fengchitong 110
Fengfeixue 110
Fengfu 111
  Caoxi 31
  Guizhen 152
  Guixue 152
  Sheben 358
  Xingxing 511
Fengguan 111
Fenglong 109
Fengmen 113
  Fengmenrefu 113
  Refu 330
Fengshi 115
  Chuishou 52
Fengxi（MA）115

Allergic Area(MA) 153
  Urticaria Point (MA) 318
Fengyan(风岩) 115
Fengyan(风眼) 115
Fermented soyabean-cake-separated moxibustion 134
  Fermented soyabean-cake moxibustion 47
Festering moxibustion 169
  Scarring moxibustion 12
Fifteen Main Colleterals 382
  Fifteen collaterals 382
  Fifteen separating collaterals 382
  Collateral of the Du Meridian, the 87
    Branch of the Du Meridian 87
  Collateral of the Ren Meridian, the 335
    Branch of the Ren Meridian 335
    Diseases of the the collateral of the Ren Meridian 335
  Collateral of Foot-Jueyin 630
    Branch of Foot-Jueyin 631
    Diseases of ~ 631
  Collateral of Foot-Shaoyang 636
    Branch of Foot-Shaoyang, the 636
    Diseases of ~ 636
  Collateral of Foot-Shaoyin 638
    Branch of Foot-Shaoyin, the 638
    Diseases of ~ 638
  Collateral of Foot-Taiyang 640
    Branch of Foot-Taiyang 640
    Diseases of ~s640
  Collateral of Foot-Taiyin, the 643
    Branch of Foot-Taiyin 644
    Diseases of ~ 643
  Collateral of Foot-Yangming, the 646
    Branch of Foot-Yangming, the 646
    Diseases of ~ 646
  Collateral of Hand-Jueyin, the 389
    Diseases of ~ 390

Collateral of Hand-Shaoyang, the 393
   3
      Disease of ~ 393
   Collateral of Hand-Shaoyin, the 395
      Branch of Hand-Shaoyin, the 395
      Diseases of ~ 395
   Collateral of Hand-Taiyang, the 397
      Branch of Hand-Taiyang, the 398
      Diseases of ~ 397
   Collateral of Hand-Taiyin, the 400
      Branch of Hand-Taiyin, the 401
      Diseases of ~ 400
   Collateral of Hand-Yangming, the 403
      Branch of Hand-Yangming 404
      Diseases of ~ 404
   Large Collateral of the Spleen, the 296
      Diseases of ~ 296
15th Vertebra, the 383
Fifty-nine acupoints for febrile
   diseases 330
Fifty-nine needlings 478
Filiform needle 159
   ~ acupuncture 160
Finger pressing 604
Finger(MA-Sf 1) 603
Finger(Toe) Next to the Little One
   504
Finger reinforcing and reducing 404
Finger-breadth measurement 164, 550
   Finger cun 442
   Hand measurement 389
Finger-nail pressing 315
Fire needle 180
   Heated needle 104
   Red-hot needle 58
Fire needling 180
   Puncturing with heated needle 355
Five ancient needling techniques 475
   Needling methods for five zang-

      organ
      Extremely shallow puncture 12
      Hegu puncture 161
      Joint puncture 146
      Leopard-spot puncture 15
      Shu needling2, 406
   Five acupuncture techniques 476
      Dispelling of perplexity 201
      Hydrops discharge by the stiletto
         needle 326
      Rousing the blind and awakening the
         deaf 103
      Shaking Off Dust 598
      Taking off clothes 41
   Five changes 474
   Five elements 480
   Five gates 476
   Five-change acupuncture 474
   Five-Shu points 479
      He(Sea) points 143
         ~ are used to treat disorders of
         the fu organs 162
      Jing(River) points 218
      Shu(Stream) points 406
   Fixed marks 146
   Flaccidity syndrome 462
      ~due to lung-heat damaging
         body fluid 108
      ~due to the invasion of damp-heat
         pathogen 371
      ~due to deficiency of liver-
         kidney yin 126
   Flaccidity syndrome in children 500
      Infantile paralysis 498
   Flat bone 23
   Flat wart 23
   Flour-cake-separated moxibustion 136
   Flour Sauce-separated moxibustion 136
   Flying method 105

Foot motor sensory area 648
Foot-Jueyin Vessel, the 631
Foot-Shaoyang Vessel 636
Foot-Yangming Vessel 647
Forearm bones 20
Forehead 91
Four confluences 414
Four meridians 414
Four Seas, the 414
  Sea of blood, the 524
    Sea of the Twelve Meridians 340
    Sea of five zang-organs and six fu-organs, the1, 378
  Sea of marrow, the 417
Four sources and three tubers 413
Fourteen meridians, the 380
Fourteen needling methods 341
  Fourteen methods for needling manipulation 491
  Assisting 359
  Circling 288
  Flicking 423
  Massage along the meridian 531
  Method of insertion 206
  Moving 85
  Nail-pressing 586
  Palpation method 266
  Pressing 3
  Pressure method 319
  Rotating 547
    Handle-rotating manipulation 547
  Twirling 283
  Twisting 59
  Withdrawing 450
Fresh gingesh ginger moxibustion 368
Front-Mu points 274
Fu Weng 119
Fu Xi 117
Fu Zi(Monk´shood) cake 120

Fu Zi(Aconium Carmichaeli)-separated Moxibustion 135
  Fu Zi (Monkshood) moxibustion 120
Fu´ai 121
Fufen 120
Fugu 120
Fujie 121
  Changjie 40
  Changku 40
Fuliu（复溜）120
  Changyang 38
  Fubai 117
  Fuliu（伏溜）117
  Fuliu（复留）117
  Fuqu 120
Fullness（胀2）585
Fumigating moxibustion 531
Fumigating the umbilicus 531
Fundamental manipulation 182
Furuncle 82
  ～complicated by septicemia 73
    Spread of furuncle 176
  ～ on the lower lip 487
  Boil on philtrum 33
    Boil on dragon stream 255
  Felon 603
  Furunculosis 83
  Red-streaked infection 164
    Blood-streaked infection 528
  Red-thread infection 165
  Snake's head-like Furuncle 359
Furuncle of nose 19
  Cichuang 52
  Fire bead-like furuncle 181
  Naked-sword-like furuncle 10
Fushe 119
Futonggu 122
  Tonggu 440
Futu（伏兔）117

Waigou 453
Fuyang 116
Futu(扶突) 118
Shuixue 411
Fuxi 117

G

Gangrene of finger or toe 451
　～due to deficiency of both qi and yin 312
　～ due to qi and blood stasis 315
　Bone-dropping boil 451
　Bone-dropping cellulitis 451
　Dropping carbuncle 451
Ganshu 127
Gansui (Radix Euphorbiae Kabnsui) moxibustion 123
Gao Huang 132
Gao Wu 132
Gaogu 131
Gaohuang 132
　Gaohuangshu 133
Gaohuangshuxue Jiufa (Moxibustion on Gaohuangshu Point) 133
Garlic-separated moxibustion 137
Gastric area, the 463
Ge Hong 140
Ge Kejiu 140
Geguan 139
Gemen 133
Geshu 139
Ghost points 152
　Thirteen ghost points, the 379
　Guicang 150
　Guichen 150
　Guichuang 150
　Guifeng 150
　Guigong 150
　Guiku(鬼窟) 151

Guilei 151
Guilu(鬼路) 151
Guishi 151
Guitang 151
Guixin(鬼心) 151
Guixin(鬼信2) 151
Guizhen 152
Giant needle 227
Ginger-separated moxibustion 136
Glabella(印堂2) 565
Glass statue with meridians and acupoints 210
Globus hyertericus 265
Gold needle(金针1) 203
Gongsun 142
Goiter 568
　Big neck 59
　Qi goiter 313
Great stomach collateral, the 469
　Xuli 515
Great yang 227
Green dragon wagging its tail 320
　Blue dragon wagging its tail 30
Green turtle probing its cave 30
Groove on the Back of Auricle(MA4) 94
Growing and grown numbers 368
Grub-separated moxibustion 137
　Grub moxibustion 303
Guzheng Bing Jiufang(Moxibustion Methods for Concumptive Diseases) 145
Guanchong 146
Guanmen 147
Guanming 148
Guanyi 148
Guanyuan 148
　Cimen 53
　Dantian 72
　Dazhongji 67
　Sanjiejiao 343

Xiaji（下纪）434
Guanyuanshu 149
Guangming 149
Guidang 150
Guilai 150
　　Xixue 482
Guixin（鬼信1）152
Guiyan（鬼眼1）152
　　Shouzudazhizhaojia 405
Guiyan（鬼眼2）152
　　Guiku（鬼哭）150
　　Yaoyan 546
Guiding yang from yin 57
Guiding yin from yang 57
Guo Yu 152
Guo Zhong 152
Guoliangzhen 136

H

Haiquan 154
Haircut by ghost 151
Hairline 103
Han Lian Cao（Herb Eclipta）moxibustion 158
Hanyan 158
Hand acupuncture 404
Hand fish 404
Hand pressing 533
Hand separating and pressing 406
He Ruoyu 162
Heding1，162
　　Xiding 482
Heding2，162
Hegu（合谷）160
　　Hegu（合骨）161
　　Hukou1，167
Heyang 161
Head needle 446
　　Scalp needle 444

Headache 445
　　~ due to cold-wind pathogen 112
　　~ due to blood deficiency 529
　　~ due to blood stasis 570
　　~ due to phlegm turbidity 425
　　~ due to wind-damp pathogen 115
　　~ due to wind-heat pathogen 114
　　Liver yang ~ 127
　　Pain in the head 445
Heart（MA）507
Heart system 510
Heart dominator1 510
Heat needling（燔针1）104
Heat-needling（Red-hot needling）58
Heated needle（燔针2）104
Heatstroke 617
　　Mild ~ 617
　　Serious ~ 617
　　Sunstroke 618
Heaven portion 384
　　Heaven-cai 384
Heavenly treatment 390
Heel 616
Heel（MA-AH 1）141
Helix 96
　　~ tubercle 96
　　Crus of ~ 96
　　Posterior sulcus to the ~ 96
　　Upper and lower branches of
　　　　Posterior sulcus to the ~ 96
　　Spine of ~ 96
Helix 1-6（MA）258
Hemafecia 24
　　~ before menstruation 212
　　~ due to damp-heat 371
　　~ due to deficiency of the spleen 295
　　Loosing the bowels with blood 491
Hematuria（尿血1）284

~ due to flaring heart-fire 509
~due to yin deficiency and hyper
   activity 561
Urine with blood 284
Bloody urine 416
Hemiplegia in children 496
Hemoptysis 232
~due to attack of liver fire on the
   lung 124
~due to yin deficiency and hyper-
   activity of fire 560
Cough with blood 231
Hemorrhoid 606
~ due to damp-heat pathogen 373
~ due to qi-deficiency 311
~-pricking 438
External ~ 456
Internal ~ 282
Internal-external ~ 280
Mixed hemorrhoid 179
Henggu 163
Xiaheng 488
Xiaji（下极）488
Hernia 348
Hernial qi 348
~ due to invasion of cold 156
~ due to heat 331
Inguinal hernia 167
Pathogenic qi of the small intestine
   495
Scrotal ~ 555
Hiccough in children 502
Hiccup in children 496
Hiccup 92
~ due to qi stagnation 313
~ due to stomach cold 463
~ due to stomach heat 464
~ due to yang deficiency 542
~ due to yin deficiency 560

~ while eating 46
Hiccough 578
Hidden bone 20
Xiphoid 20
High fever 131
Hill foot 348
Hip bone 235
Hip(MA-AH 4) 235
Holy medicinal cake 369
Horn needle 199
Host and guest 621
Host-guest combination of acupoints,
   the 621
Host-guest combination of Yuan(Primary)
   and Luo(Connecting) points 621
Hot moxibustion 330
Houding 165
Jiaochong 193
Houshencong 166
Houxi 166
Houyexia 148
Houye 166
House of tendons 204
Hukou2, 167
Hua Tuo 169
Hua Shou 169
Huagai 168
Huaroumen 169
Huanmen 172
Huantiao 170
Biyan 22
Bingu 25
Fenzhong 109
Kuangu 235
Huandiao 170
Huantiao needle 172
Huanzhong 172
Huang Shiping 176
Huang Shizhen 176

43

Huang Zhongzi 176
Huangdi (The Yellow Emperor) 174
Huangdi Jiu Xu Neijing (The Yellow Emperor's Canon of Internal Medicine in Nine Parts) 174
Huangdi Mingtang Jiujing (The Yellow Emperor's Classic of Mingtang Chart and Moxibustion 174
Huangdi Mingtang Yan Ce Rentu (The Yellow Emperor's Mingtang chart of Anterior and Lateral View) 174
Huangdi Neijing (The Yellow Emperor's Canon of Internal Medicine) 174
  Neijing (Internal Classic) 279
Huangdi Neijing Mingtang (The Yellow Emperor's Inner Classic Acupoints) 175
Huangdi Neijing Mingtang Leicheng (Classification of Acupoints of the Yellow Emperor's Canon of Internal Medicine) 175
Huangdi Qi Bo Lun Zhenjiu Yaojue (Essentials of Acupuncture and Moxibustion Expounded in Verse by the Yellow Emperor and Qi Bo) 175
Huangdi Shier Jingmai Mingtang Wu Zang Ren Tu (The Yellow Emperor's Chart of Twelve Meridians, Acupoins and Five Zang-Organs as Shown on Human Figure) 175
Huangdi Zhenjiu Hama Ji (Frog Contraindications of the Yellow Emperor's Acupuncture and Moxibustion) 175
Huangfu Mi 173
Huangmen 172
Huangmu 172
Huangshu 173
Huge bone(巨骨2) 226

Huifawuchu 177
Huiqi(回气) 177
  Huiqi(迴气) 177
Huitu Jingluo Tushuo (Illustrated Manual of Meridians and Collaterals) 179
Huiyang 178
  Liji 243
Huiyin 178
  Haidi 154
  Pinyi 298
  Xiaji 488
  Xiajizhishu 488
Huizong 178
Human portion 332
  Human-cai 332
Human tunnels 213
Hungry horse ringing a bell 93
Hunmen 179
Hunshe 179
Huoren Miaofa Zhenjing (Acupuncture Canon of Magical Methods for Saving Life) 180
Hypochondriac pain 505
  ~ due to blood stasis 570
  ~ due to damp-heat 372
  ~ due to stagnation of liver-qi 129
  ~ due to yin deficiency 562
Hypochondrium 505
  ~ (季胁2) 186
Hypogalactia 339
  ~due to deficiency of qi and blood 312
  ~ due to stagnation of liver-qi 128
  Lack of lactation 328
Hysteria 582

I

Illness of deficiency type should be

treated by tonifying method 516
Impairment of qi 370
Impotence 540
　Deficiency syndrome of ∼541
　Excess syndrome of ∼ 541
　Flaccidness of penis 559
Index finger 387
Inapplicable points 186
Induced period of acupuncture anesthesia 596
Indirect moxibustion 192
　Separated moxibustion 192
　Tablet moxibustion 547
Inducing fire method 645
Inducing qi 76
Infantile convulsion 217
　Acute ∼ 183
　Chronic ∼ 263
　Convulsion due to fright 217
Infantile diarrhea 501
Infantile headache 500
Infantile malnutrition sickness 130
　Infantile malnutrition 130
　Infantile malnutrition disease 130
　Infantile mslnutrition syndrome 130
Infantile needle 503
Infantile vomiting 498
　∼ due to cold 140
　∼due to fright 157
　　Vomiting due to fright 217
　　Vomiting in infancy due to fright 187
　∼due to heat 332
　　Vomiting due to stomach-heat 466
　∼ due to improper diet 349
　∼ due to intestinal parasitosis 49
　∼ due to retained food 182
　Milk vomiting in infants 349
Infantile vomiting with diarrhea

and fever 499
Inferior crus of antihelix 89
Inflammation of the throat 165
　Sore throat 165
Infrared radiation 165
　Infrared moxibustion 164
Ingot-shaped tablet moxibustion 547
Inner canthus 272
Inserting the needle as if injecting it 621
　Quick needle insertion 235
Inserting the needle by twirling 284
Inserting the needle through a pipe 427
Inserting the needle while pinching the skin 285,428
Inserting the needle while unfolding the skin 42
　Hand separating and pressing 406
Insertion 204
Insomnia 28,370
　∼due to yin deficiency and hyperactivity of fire 560
　∼ due to deficiency of the heart and spleen 509
　∼due to derangement of the stomach 463
　　∼due to upward disturbance of liver fire 124
　Difficult sleep 28
　Inability to Sleep 27
Instep 116
Intermuscular needling 109
Internal cauterization 279
Internal Ear (MA) 278
Internal Genitalia (MA) 254
　Seminal Palace(MA)(精宫3) 280
　Tiangui (MA) 413
　Uterus (MA) (子宫3) 624

Internal meridians 279
Internal Nose (MA) 278
Intradermal needle 292
　Granular ～ 231
　Thumb-back ～ 319
Iron needle 438
Invasion by cold after delivery 35
Invaluable experience in verse 369
Invasion by wind after delivery 34
Irregular menstruation 578
　Abnormal menstruation 208
　Disorder of menstral flow 213
　Disorder of menstruation 208
　Irregular menses 579
　Irregular menstrual flow 208,579
　Irregular menstrual qi 212
　Irregular menstrual vessel 211
　Irregular monthly envoy 579
　Unfixed amount of menstrual flow 213

J

Jaundice 173
　Huan Dan 174
　　Yang ～ 538
　　Yin ～ 555
Jaw (MA) 162
Jibeiwuxue 185
Jigujiezhong 185
Jijupikuaixue 182
Jimai 184
Jimen 182
Jiquan 183
Jisanxue 185
Jizhong 185
Jishu 185
　Shenzong 364
Jiache 187
　Chiya 47
　Guichuang 150

Jiguan 181
　Quya 325
Jiafeng 188
Jiagen 188
Jiaji 186
　Huatuojiaji 170
　Huatuoxue 170
Jianjing 189
　Bojing 26
Jianju 192
Jianli 192
Jianliao（肩髎）189
Jianliao（肩聊）189
Jianneishu 190
Jianneiyu 190
Jianshi 188
　Guilu（鬼路）151
　Guiying 152
Jianshu 190
Jiantou 190
Jianwaishu 190
Jianjian 189
Jianyu 191
　Biangu（扁骨1）23
　Jianjian 168
　Jianjing 168
　Piangu 296
　Pianjian 297
　Shanggu 355
　Zhongjianjing 611
Jianzhen 191
Jianzhongshu 191
Jianzhugu 192
Jianzhu 192
Jiangwei 193
Jiao Yunwen 199
Jiaosun 199
Jiaoxin 198
　Neijin 279

Jie 201
Jieji 200
　Jiegu 200
Jiemai 202
Jienüe 201
Jiexi 202
Jin Kongxian 203
　Caoxiedaixue 31
Jin Yetian 203
Jinjin, Yuye 202
　Jinjin 202
　Youyuye 570
　Yuye 574
Jinlan Xunjing(Gold Orchid Book on Meridians) 203
Jinlan Xunjing Quxue Tujie(Gold Orchid boolk with Illustrations for Selecting Points along Meridians) 203
Jinmen 203
　Guanliang 147
　Liangguan 245
Jinsuo 204
　Jinshu 204
Jinteng Yugui Zhenjin(Acupuncture Canon of the Gold Bag and Jade Chamber) 203
Jingbailao 218
Jingbi 219
Jinzhen Fu(Ode to Gold Needle) 203
Jinggu(京骨2), 207
Jinggu(京骨1), 207
　Dagu 62
Jingluo Huibian(A Collection of Meridians and Collaterals) 210
Jingluo Jianzhu(Notes and Commentary on Meridians and Collaterals) 210
Jingluo Kao(Study on Meridians and Collaterals) 210
Jingluo Quanshu(A Complete Work on Meridians and Collaterals) 210
Jingluo Shuyao(The Pivot of Meridians and Collaterals) 210
Jingmai Fentu(Illustrated book on Meridian) 211
Jingmai Fenye(Seperate Exposition on Meridians) 211
Jingmen 207
　Qifu 304
　Qishu 310
Jingming（睛明）217
Jingming（精明）218
Leikong（泪空）240
Leikong（泪孔）240
Muneizi 272
Jingqu 213
Jingxue Faming(Invention on Meridian Points) 215
Jingxue Huijie(Collective Exposition on meridian points) 215
Jingxue Zuanyao(Essentials of Meridian Points) 216
Jingzhong(睛中) 218
Jingzhong（经中）217
　Yindu(阴都2), 554
Jiu Bu Zhenjing(A Collection of Nine Acupuncture Classics) 220
Jiu Juan(Nine Volumes) 221
Jiu Ling 221
Jiudianfeng 223
Jiufa Michuan(Secretly Bequeathed Method of Moxibustion) 223
Jiulao 224
Jiuquzhongfu 221
Jiuqu 221
Jiuwei 219
　Weiyi 461
Jiuweiguduan 220
Jiuxiao 224

Jiuxuebing 225
Juchu 225
Jugu 226
Juliao（巨髎）226
Juliao（居髎）225
　Jujiao（巨節）226
Juquan 228
Juque 226
Jueshu 227
Jueyunxue 229
Jueyinshu 230
　Queshu 229
Junction of the red and white skin 47

K

Kao vitality in nine palaces 220
　Human vitality 231
Kaozheng Zhoushen Xuefa Ge（Verse on Methods of Textual Research on Points of the Whole Body）2131
Keeping the needling qi 405
Kidney qi 365
Kidney（MA）364
Knee（MA-AH 3）482
Knife with an eye-shaped edge 504
Knife-shaped stone 598
Kong Guangpei 232
Kongzui 232
Kouheliao 232
　Changhui 39
　Changjia 39
　Changliao 39
　Changping 39
　Heliao 162
Ku Hu（Lagenaria Sicerarria）moxibustion 234
　Ku Hu（Lagenaria Sicerarria）-separated moxibustion 136
Kufang 234

Kuangu 235
Kunlun 236
　Shangkunlun 352
　Xiakunlun 489

L

Lama 236
Lan Jiang Fu（Intercepting-River Fu）237
Lanmen 236
Lanwei 237
Laogong 237
　Guiku（鬼窟）151
　Guiying 152
　Wuli 476
　Zhangzhong 585
Laozhen 239
　Xiangqiangxue 493
Large collaterals（络2）259
Large Intestine（MA）60
　Tooth Meridian 47
Laser acupuncture 183
Laser irradiation of acupoints 182
Laser therapy on the acupoint 522
Lateral aspect 452
Lateral canthus 272
　Outer canthus 273
Lateral malleolus 454
Lateral recumbent position 31
Layer of kidney and liver 364
Left to li and south to you 241
Left and right twirling 649
Lei Feng 239
Leihuo Zhenfa（Moxibustion with Thunder-Fire Herbal Moxa Stick）239
Leijing（Classified Canon）240
Leijing Fyyi（An Addition to Supplements to Illustrated Classified

Canon of Internal Medicine of the
Yellow Emperor) 240
Leijing Tuyi(Illustrated Supplements
to Classified Canon of Internal
Medicine of the Yellow Emperor) 240
Leitou 240
Leixia 240
Li Hao 242
Li Mengzhuo 242
Li Shoudao 242
Li Shouxian 242
Li Xuechuan 242
Li Yu 243
Li Yuan 243
Lidui 243
Ligou 242
   Jiaoyi 199
Lineiting 243
Liyue Pianwen(A Rhymed Discourse on
External Therapies) 243
Lianquan(廉泉1) 244
   Benchi 17
   Sheben 358
Lianquan(廉泉2) 244
Liangmen 245
Liangqiu 246
Liaoliao 246
Lieque 246
   Tongxuan 443
   Wanlao 457
Life door(命门3) 270
Life gate(命门4) 270
Life pass(命关3) 269
Lifting 428,450
Lifting-pushing method 50
Lifting and thrusting 428
Lifting while twirling the needle 84
Limbs and joints 600
Linqi 247

Linquan 247
Ling Shu(Miraculous Pivot) 249
   Jiu Xu(Nine Mysteries) 221
   Jiu Ling 221
Ling Shu Jingmai Yi(Supplement to the
Meridians of the Miraculous Pivot) 249
Lingdao 247
Lingguang Fu(Ode to the Brilliance of
Gods) 248
Linghou 250
Lingtai 249
   Feidi 107
Lingxu 250
Liu Zhu moxibustion 252
   Xiang Sha(Moschus Chinnabaris) moxi-
bustion 493
Liu Dang 250
Liu Jin 250
Liu Wansu 250
Liu Yuanbin 251
Liufeng 252
Liuhe 253
Liuzhu Zhiwei Fu(Lyrics of Flow) 251
Liver (MA) 123
Liver (MA-SC 5) 123
Liver yang 127
Liver-Yang(MA) 127
Local point selection 225
Locating points by finger-cun measure-
ment 603
Lochiorrhea 92
   Persistent lochia 92
Lochiostasis 92
Loess-cake-separated moxibustion 176
Long needle 40
   Huantiao needle 172
Long retention of the needle for cold
sundromes 158
Long snake moxibustion 40

Extending moxibustion 299
Long Xiansu 255
Longhan 253
Loss of qi 370
Lou Ying 256
Lougu 256
  Dayinluo 65
  Taiyinluo 422
  Zutaiyinluo 642
Louyin 257
Lower auricle root 487
Lower Auricle Root (MA) 487
Lower cofluent points 487
  ∼ of the six fu organs 252
Lower end, the (下极1) 488
Lower Portion of Rectum (MA) 602
Luxi 257
  Luxin 257
Luo (Connecting) points 260
Luoque 259
  Luoxi 260
  Naogai 276
  Qiangyang 319
Lu Guang 257
Lu Kui 258
Lushang 258
Lumbar pain 545
  ∼ due to cold and dampness 157
  ∼ due to internal injury caused by overstrain 238
  ∼ due to kidney deficiency 367
  Pain along the spinal column 544
Lumbosacral Vertebrae (MA) 544
Lung (MA) 107
Lung (MA-IC 1) 107

M

Ma Danyang 261
Ma Danyang's twelve points 261

Ma Siming 261
Magical fire-needle 364
  Peach-twig cauterisation 426
Magical light illumination 361
  Magicala lilght fire 361
Malaria 200, 287
  ∼ disease 286
  ∼ illness 286
  ∼ with general debility 238
  Algid ∼ 156
  Pyrexial ∼ 470
  Typical ∼ 600
Malignant Malaria 586
  ∼ due to heat 332
  Cold ∼ 241
Malleolus 170
Mangchangxue 264
Mao Gen (Herba Ranunculi Japonici) vesiculation 264
Mass-disintegrating miraculous-fire needle 494
Match-head moxibustion 180
Measurement of the meridian qi flow by respiration 368
  Dredging the meridians by connecting meridian qi 201
  Resperation times for measuring the meridian qi flow 84
Measurement of meridians 263
Medical needle 550
Medicated-stick moxibustion 547
Medicinal blister-causing moxibustion 548
Medicinal vesiculation 432
  Juice vesiculation 410
Medial Malleolus 279
Medial side 278
Meeting-once-again period, the 50
  Meetin-once-again of the Heavenly

Stems 337
Megnetic needle 53
Meichong 265
    Xiaozhu 505
Melancholia 574
Menic-depressive psychosis 79
    Depressive psychosis(癫证1) 80
    Mania 235
Menorrhagia 579
    ~ due to qi deficiency 310
    ~with internal injury caused by overstrain 238
    Hypermenorrhea 578
    Profuse Menstruation 217
Menstruation in an unfixed(either preceded of delayed) period 214
    ~ due to kidney deficiency 366
    ~ due to stagnation of liver-qi 127
    Disorder of menstrual flow（经水无常2） 213
    Either preceded or delayed menstruation 214
    Menstruation irregularity 209
    Unfixed menstrual period 216
Meridian diseases and primary diseases of zang and fu organs 348
    Meridian diseases 388
    Meridian diseases due to related organs 418
Meridian of Arm-Juyin 21
Meridian of Arm-Shaoyang 21
Meridian of Arm-Shaoyin 21
Meridian of Arm-Taiyang 21
Meridian of Arm-Taiyin 21
Meridian of Arm-Yangming 22
Meridian in muscle 337
Meridian points 215
Meridian proper,the(正经2) 599
Meridian qi 212

Meridian transmission phenomenon 209
    Meridian phenomenon 211
    Meridian sensation phenomenon 210
    Phenomenon of acupuncture and moxibustion response 592
Meridian waters 213
Meridians 211,(脉1)262,(血脉1)526
Meridians and collaterals 209
Metal needle(金针2) 203
Method of connecting meridians 63
Method of leading the needling sensation 590
Method of needle insertion 206
Methods of accelerating qi-flow over the meridians 105
    Dragon-tiger-turtle-phoenix 254
    Dredging the meridians to promote the qi-circulation 440
Methods of point selection 326
Metrorrhagia and metrostaxis 18
    ~ due to blood deficiency 530
    ~ due to blood-heat 527
    ~ due to qi deficiency 310
    ~ due to qi stagnation 313
    ~ due to yang deficiency 541
    ~ due to yin deficiency 560
    ~ due to damp-heat 371
    Bursting and leaking 18
Mianyan 267
Middle Cymba Conchae (MA) 440
    Around Umbilicus (MA) 303
Middle finger cun 615
Middle Ear(MA-H1) 100
    Diaphragm(MA) 139
Middle Triangular Fossa(MA) 199
Mild moxibustion 469
    Warming moxibustion 469
Mild moxibustioner 470
    Moxibustion apparatus 224

Mingguan 269
Mingjia Jiuxuan(Moxibustion Collection by Famous Experts) 268
Mingmen(命门1) 270
    Jinggong 218
    Shulei 407
Mingtang Jingluo Tuce(Illustrated Manual of Meridians and Collateral of
Mingtang Jingtu(Mingtang classic with Illustration) 268
Mingtang Kongxue(An Acupoint Atlas) 268
Mingtang Kongxue Tu(An Atlas of Points for Acupuncture and Moxibustion) 268
Mingtang Kongxue Zhnju Ziao MntagPoins a Esenal of cuntue an Moxibustion Treatlment) 269
Mingtang Renxing Tu(Chart of Acupoints as Shown on a Human Figure) 269
Mingtang Tu(Mingtang Charts of Acupoints) 269
Mingtang Xuanzhen Jingjue(Mingtang Miraculous and Essential Classic in Verse) 269
Mingtang ZhenjiuTu(Charts for Acupuncture and Moxibustion) 269
Minute collaterals 417
    Minute vessels 417
Minute needle 460
    Small needle 504
Moderate stimulation 608
Monthly forbidding 578
Morbid condition, a(泄4) 507
Morning sickness 93
    ~ due to liver heat 125
    ~ due to phlegm stagnation 425
    ~ due to stomach cold 463

    ~ due to stomach deficiency 469
Affected diaphragm causing sickness 25
Aversion to fetus 481
Aversion to food 481
Choosing food 520
Disease due to fetus 624
Sickness due to gravidity 25
Sickness in pregnancy 25
Vomiting and nausea during pregnancy 648
Vomiting during pregnancy 336
Wuzi 481
Mother-child reinforcing-reducing method 625
    Combination of reinforcing mother point and reducing son point, the 26
    Reducing son according to mother 507
Motor Area, the 580
Mouse manure cauterization 407
Mouth(MA-ICS) 232
Mouth-width measurement 232
Moving landmarks 179
Moxa ball 3
Moxa cone 3
    ~ moxibustion 3
Moxa down 2
Moxa roll 2
    ~ moxibustion 2
Moxa rolls with medicinal powder 548
Moxa sphere 3
Moxa stick 2
    ~moxibustion 2
        Revolving moxibustion 177
Moxa wool 2
    ~ moxibustion 1
Moxibustion 223
Moxibustion by steaming with herbal medicine 548
Moxibustion cauterisation 224

Moxibustion cover 225
Moxibustion dipper 1
　Moxibustion plate 225
Moxibustion doctor 224
Moxibustion for health protection 15
Moxibustion on skin 624
Moxibustion sensation 223
Moxibustion with a warm tube 471
Moxibustion with apparatus 224
Moxibustion with Ba Dou Shuang(Pulvis Croton Tiglium) 9
Moxibustion with Bai Fu Zi(Rhizoma Tyghonii) 10
Moxibustion with electric warming needles 81
Moxibustion with garlic and coin 416
Moxibustion with salt 387
Moxibustion with scallion stalk 56
Moxibustion with scallion stalk and fermented soyabean 56
Moxibustion with thunder-fire herbal moxa stick 239
Moxibustion with vapor from the Ba Dou(Croton Tiglium) spirit 9
Moxibustion with wheat-grain-like moxa-cone 62
Moxibustion with Xiao Hui Xiang (Fructus Foennniculi) 503
Moxibustion wood 224
Moxibustion-acupuncture 223
Moxibustionist 224
Mu SHu Jing (Classic of Front-Mu and Back-Shu Points) 274
Mu Xiang(Radix Aucklandiao) cake 271
Mu Xiang(Radix Aucklandiae)-cake-separated moxibustion 137
Muchuang 272
　Zhigong 605
　Zhirong 605
　Zhiying 605
Mulberry Moxibustion 347
Mulberry twig moxibustion 347
Mumps 583
　Epidemic parotiditis 583
　Pyogenic inflammation of cheeks 154
　Sore inside cheek 155
Muscle(分肉1) 109
Multiple cupping 91
Muzhilihengwen 271

N

Ncil-like furuncle in tiger's mouth 168
　Carbuncle of hand 388
　Clapping-crab poison 288
　Deep-rooted carbunc;e om toger's mouth 168
　Fore-legs of a diseased crab 25
　Nail-like boil around tiger's mouth 532
　Nail-like boil in Hegu area 161
　Poison in the area of tiger's mouth 168
　Pustule in tiger's mouth 168
　Pyogenic infection in the area of tiger's mouth 168
　Thumb-crab poison 26
　Y-shaped finger 532
Nail pressing insertion 586
　Finger pressing insertion 604
Nail-pressing technique 586
Nanyinfeng 276
Nangdi 276
Naohu 276
　Helu 161
　Huie 177
　Zafeng 582

Naohui 277
　Naojiao（臑交）277
　Naojiao（臑窌）277
Naokong 277
　Nieru 285
Naoshu 277
Nasal acupuncture 20
Natural reactive points 436
Navel Center(MA)（脐中2）303
Navel-steaming therapy 599
　Fumigating umbilicus method 531
　Steaming the navel 598
Near sighted disease 282
　Short-sightedness 207
Nearby point selection 247
　All-round point selection 415
Neck(MA-AH) 218
Needle and stone 596
Needle box 590
Needle transmission 512
　Needle conveying 581
Needle-embedding 262
Needle-holding hand 55
Needle-like finger pressing 604
Needle-moxa 588
Needling for five kinds of exhaustions forbidden 475
　Contraindications of needling 54
Needling forward three times and lifting backward once 344
Needling Method 589
　Acupuncture technique 53
Needling methods of midnight-noon ebb-flow 626
Needle container 30
Needling Sensation 590
　Needling response 588
Needling stone 596
Needling treating five pathogenic factors 480
Nei Wai Er Jing Tu(Two Illustrations on Interior and Exterior of the Body) 280
Neiguan 278
　Yinweixue（阴维穴2①）559
Neihuaijian 279
　Huaijian 170
　Lǔxi 258
Neihuaiqianxia 279
Neijingming 279
Neitaichong 280
Neiting 280
Neixiyan 281
　Neilongyan 280
Neiyangchi 281
Neiyingxiang 281
Neizhiyin 282
Neurodermatitis 285
　~due to blood deficiency and wind-dryness 528
　~due to heat transformation of wind-damp pathogen 114
　Sores around the nape 359
Nian Ying medicinal moxa roll 284
Niaoxue 284
Nie Ying 285
Nieru 285
Nine compatibilities 221
Nine needles 221
　Big needle 66
　Lance needle 116
　Shear needle 31
　　Arrow-head needle 193
　Stiletto needle 291
　　Flying needle 106
　　Sword-shaped needle 193
Nine needlings 220
Nine-six number 221

Nine-six reinforcing and reducing 221
Nipple-moth(Tonsillitis) 338
　Moth 91
　Moth-like throat 165
　Nipple-goose 338
Nocturnal emission 266
　Loss of essence in dream 266
Nodules of breast 338
　∼ due to stagnation of liver-qi 129
　Lump in breast 276
　Mass in breast 276
Non-scarring moxibustion 472
　Non-festering moxibustion 106
Non-warming moxibustion 472
Notch between the tragus and the antihelix 298
Nu(努法2) 286
Nuxi 286
　Nüxu 286

O

Oblique insertion 505
Obstruction of qi in the chest 513
　∼ due to blood stasis 571
　∼ due to cold of insufficiency 515
　∼ due to phlegm turbidity 426
Obvious part(明堂3) 268
Occiput (MA) 598
Occipialt node 598
Ocular system 273
　Eye system 535
Oil wick moxibustion 569
Omalgia 257
　Frozen shoulder 190
One insertion and three liftings 550
　Three liftings and one insertion 344
One yang 550
One-cun distance with three cones side by side 164

Onion-separated moxibustion 134
Opening of the external auditory meatus 453
Opening-closing-pivot 231
Opposite qi 304
Optic Area, the 388
Ordinary needling 11
　Cold needling 241
　Warm needling 471
Otitis media suppurative 439
　∼ due to wind 110
　Chronic suppurative otitis media 94
　Ear cyst 276
　Deficiency syndrome of ∼ 440
　Excess syndrome of ∼ 439
　Troublesome ear 31
Outer canthus 273
Outer net of the eye 273

P

Pain below the umbilicus before menstruation 212
Painful locality taken as acupoint 552
Palmar cross striation of the wrist 458
Palpebral cyst 271
Palpitation 509
　∼ due to blood deficiency 529
　∼ due to blood stasis 570
　∼ due to fright 217
　∼ due to phlegm-fire 423
　∼ due to qi deficiency 310
　Severe ∼ 598
Pancreas, Gallbaldder (MA-SC 6) 551
Pangguangshu 290
Pangting 288
　Zhushi 621
Paper-separated moxibustion 139
Paravertebral musculature of back 258

Paroxymal cough 90
  Chicken cough 181
  Egret cough 257
  Epidemic ~ 386
  Epidemic cough with asthma 435
  Epidemic cough with dyspnea 436
  Epidemic severe cough 553
  Epidemic whooping cough 386
  Pressed cough 298
  Wooping cough 12
Pass of thigh 22
Pass of tibia 154
Pause 505
Pearl-like projection 620
Pectoral muscle 566
Penetrating needling 448
Penis(宗筋3) 628
Penis and testis(宗筋2) 628
Peng Jiusi 291
Peng Yongguang 291
Penglai fire 291
People of five kinds 479
Pepper cake-separated moxibustion 135
  Pepper-cake moxibustion 167,199
Pericarpium zanthoxili-cake-separated moxibustion 134
  Pericarpium zanthoxyli-cake moxibustion 51
Perineum(会阴2) 178
Perineum Meridian 178
Pharynx-larynx (MA-T 3)534
Pigen 296
Piheng 293
Pipa 292
Pishu 293
Pianli 297
Pinching needle method 186
Pinching technique 186
Plate for moxibustion 222

Pleurdiaphragmatic interspace 274
  Pleurdiaphragmatic field 270
Pohu 298
  Hunhu 179
Point aspirator 523
Point injection therapy 523
  Acupoint block therapy 522
Point prescription 290
Point prescription of the five shu 478
Point selection according to the affected area 231
Point selection in accordance with differentiation of syndrome 24
Point selection on disparate meridians 552
  Selection of points on other meridians 418
Poin selection on mated meridians 288
Point-radiation therapy 523
Point-ultrasonic stimulation therapy 521
Points on the fourteen meridians 380
Pokeberry Root-cake moxibustion 350
  Pokeberry Root separated moxibustion 137
Popliteal fossa 153
Post-decoction cupping 621
  Decocting the cupping tube 621
  Medicinal cupping 547
Post-moxibustion pox 224
Post-moxibustion scar 222
Post-moxibustion sore 222
  Adhesive plaster for ~ 223
Posterior eminence of inferior concha 95
Posterior fossa of the intertragic notch 298
Posterior groove of antihelix 89

Postpartum abdominal pain 33
  Abdominal pain after delivery 94
Postpartum aphasia 32
Postpartum constipation 32
Postpartum convulsion 32
  Postpartum spasm 33
Postpartum deafness 32
Postpartum dyspepsia 35
Postpartum diarrhea 36
  Postpartum dysentry 34
Postpartum dizziness due to blood problems 37
  Oppressive feeling and dizziness 574
  Postpartum dizziness 37
Postpartum edema 35
Postpartum fever 33
Postpartum frequency of urination 36
Postpartum headache 35
  ~ due to blood deficiency 528
  ~ due to blood stasis 530
Postpartum heat-stroke 38
Postpartum hypochondriac pain 37
Postpartum ophthalmodynia 34
Postpartum paralysis 35
Postpartum prolapse of genital structure 38
  Postpartum prolapse of uterus 38
  Postpartum relaxation of uterus 38
Postpartum retention of urine 36
Postures for acupuncture and moxibustion 594
  Postures 383
  Lying posture 471
    Prone position 120
    Supine posture 544
  Posture for cupping chin in hands 450
  Sitting postures 580
    Sitting in flexion 119
    Sitting position like a winnowing pan 182
    Sitting with back and head on a lazy back 544
    Sitting with head bending aside 31
Pottery and porcelain needles 426
  Pottery needle 426
Preceded menstrual cycle 214
  ~ due to blood-heat 527
  ~ due to qi deficiency 310
  ~ due to stagnation of liver-qi 128
  Earlier-than-usual menstruation 216
    Earlier-than-usual menstruation due to bloodheat 527
  Forward menstruation 579
  Menstruation twice a month 550
  Preceded menstrual flow 213
Pressing for diagnosis 4
Pressing moxibustion 386
Pressing pain point 475
  Diagnosis by pressing 532
  Pressing for diagnosis 532
Pricking 80,438
Pricking therapy 438
  Pricking out grass seed 438
  Root-cutting therapy 201
Professor of Acupuncture 596
Projecting bones bilateral to the occipital bone 574
Prolapse of uterus and vagina 559
  Appearing of the uterus 487
  Cockscomb sore 181
  Contraction failure of uterus 624
  Egg-plant-like prolapse 319
  Fall-off of uterus and vagina 559
  Falling of uterus 559
  Hysteroptosis 625
    ~ due to qi deficiency 311
    ~ due to kidney deficiency 368
  Prolapse of uterus 624,558

Prolapse of rectum 451
　~ of deficiency type 451
　~ of excess type 451
　Blockage of rectum 201
Prolapse of rectum in children 500
Prolonged defecation with difficulty 607
　Dysentery 244
Primary infertility 238
Prominence of pectoral muscle(膺中1) 566
Prone needling 471
Prostate(MA) 318
Prostration syndrome 452
Protracted labor 607
　Delivery with difficulty 38
　Difficult labor 276
Protuberant bones(高骨2) 117
Pruritus vulvae 562
　Itching of vaginal orifice 557
　Pruritus in female pudindum 554
　Pruritus of vaginal orifice 557
Pucan 299
　Anxie 2
Puji Fang(Prescriptions for Universal Relief 299
Pulling out the needle 9
Pulmonary system 109
Pulmonary tuberculosis 107
　Corpse-walking tuberculosis 51
　Ghost tuberculosis 152
　Tuberculosis of a corpse 369
　Walking corpse 51
Pulse condition 263
Puncturing along or against the direction of meridians 567
Puncturing with needles in alignment (排针2) 288
Purgative prescription(泄3) 507

Pushing and pulling 449
Pylorus(幽门1) 569

Q

Qi Bo 301
Qi Bo Jiujing(Qi Bo's Acupuncture Classic) 301
Qi entering sanjiao 309
Qi needle 314
Qi-lifting method 428
　Needle-lifting method 428
Qi-moving method 251
　Qi-flowing method 251
Qi-receiving method 275
　Qi-intaking method 613
Qi-regulating method 438
　Qi-promoting method 512
Qi-street(气街1) 308
　Four qi-streets 415
　Four streets 414
Qibojiu 301
　Qixialiuyi 303
Qichong(气冲1) 303
　Qijie(气街3) 278
Qiduan 304
Qihai 305
　Boyang 26
　Dantian 72
　Xiahuang 488
　Xiaqihai 490
Qihaishu 305
Qihu 307
Qijing Ba Mai Kao (A Study on the Eight Extra Meridians) 302
Qijing Najia Fa(Day-Prescription of Acupoints of Extra Meridians) 302
Qimen (期门) 300
Qimen (气门) 309
Qishangxiawufenxue 302

Qishe 309
Qitang 310
  Qichong(气冲2) 303
Qixue 311
  Baomen 14
  Zihu 625
Qizhong(脐中) 303
Qizhongsibianxue 303
Qizhong(气中) 315
  Qichong(气冲3) 303
Qizhuma Points 303
Qian Jinghu 318
Qianding 316
Qianfaji(前发际穴1)，317
Qiangu 317
Qianjin Fang(Prescriptions Worth a Thousand Gold) 315
Qianjin Shi Xue Ge(A Verse of Ten Acupoints Worth a Gold) 315
Qianjin Yaofang(Essential Prescriptions Worth a Thousand Gold) 316
Qianjin Yifan(Supplement to Essential Prescriptions Worth a Thousand Gold) 316
Qianshencong 318
Qianzheng 316
Qiangjian 318
Qiaoyin 319
Qin Chengzu 319
Qin Yueren 319
Qinglengyuan 321
  Qinghao 320
  Qinglengquan 321
Qingling 320
  Qinglingquan 320
Qiong Yao Faming Shenshu(Miraculous Book of the Pretty Jade's Invention) 321
Qiongyaozhenren Ba Fa Shenzhen (Miraculous Book of the Pretty Jade's Inventions) 322
Qiu Jingli 322
Qiu Jue 322
Qiuxu(丘墟) 322
  Qiuxu(丘虚) 322
Qu 326
Qubin 323
  Qufa 324
Qucha 323
  Bichong 18
Quchi 323
  Guichen 150
  Guitui 151
  Yangze 542
Qugu(曲骨) 324
  Ergu 94
  Huigu 177
  Qugu(屈骨) 326
Quguduan 326
  Henggu 163
  Niaobao 284
Qujia 324
Qujiao 324
Ququan 325
Quya 325
Quyuan 325
Quze 326
Quan Xunyi 327
Quanjianxue 327
Quanliao(颧髎) 327
  Duigu 90
  Quanliao(权髎) 327
Quanmen 327
Quanyin 327
Quantification of acupuncture anesthesia 596
Quepen1，328
Quepen2，328

Tiangai 431
Quick needling for heat 332

R

Rangu(然谷) 329
    Longquan 255
    Longyuan 255
    Rangu（然骨）329
Ranhou 329
Rapid-yet-slow needling weakens evil-qi 184
Reaching 59
Rectum(MA-H 2)(直肠1) 601
Red Pheonix Encountering the source 47
    Pheonix spreading the wings 116
Redness, swelling and pain of the eye 271
    Red eye 165
    Epidemic red eye 436
    Epidemic red-hot eye 436
    Eye disease due to wind-heat pathogen 114
    Fiery eye 180
    Wind-fire eyes 113
Reducing by puncturing against the direction of meridian qi 566
    Reducing by puncturing adversely to meridian-qi 282
Reducing round and reinforcing square 507
Reducing south and reinforcing north 506
Reducing square and reinforcing round 506
Regulating qi according to pathogenic changes 416
Regurgitation of food from the stomach 104
    Reversing movement of food from the stomach 463
    Upside-down stomach 103
Regular meridians(正经1) 599
Regulating qi 438
Reinforcement can be acheived by slow-yet-rapid needling 516
Reinforcing and reducing achieved by keeping the hole open or closed 230
Reinforcing and reducing by lifting and thrusting the needle 427
Reinforcing and reducing by means of respiration 167
Reinforcing and reducing by puncturing along and against the direction of the meridians respectively 567
Reinforcing and reducing manipulations in acupuncture therapy 588
Reinforcing and reducing method at Zi-Wu portions 626
Reinforcing and reducing manipulation 27
Reinforcing and reducing of moxibustion 1
Reinforcing and reducing with needle tip 597
Reinforcing by puncturing a point following its meridian course 416
Reinforcing the growing and reducing the grown 27
Removing the needle 262
    Withdrawing the needle 51
Removing the stagnation of blood, qi and other pathogenic factors in the xue stage 574
Renjing Jing(Classic of Mirror for Human Being) 332
Renshen(The vitality) 333
Renying 333
    Tianwuhui 435
    Wuhui 475
Repeated moxibustion 15

Reproduction area 369
Retained fluid(水气2) 410
Retching 110
　Noisy nausea without food 550
Retention of the needle 251
　Retaining the needle 607
　Retention 251
Retention of placenta 14
　Delayed delivery of pacenta 482
　Lingering fetus 419
　Lingering placenta 14
　Resting placenta 482
　Retained placenta 15
　Retardative delivery of afterbirth 94
　Retardative fetus 419
Retroauricular upper groove 95
Returning ben and yuan 104
Reverse moxibustion 282
Reverse acupuncture and moxibustion 283
Rhinorrhea 19
　~due to heat resulting from wind-cold 111
　~due to fire in the liver and gall-bladder 124
　Serious sinusitis with purulent discharge 232
　Brain coldness 276
　Brain collapse 276
　Brain leakage 277
　Oozing of brain 277
　Tingling in the roof of the nose and rhinorrhea 510
Riyue 337
　Shenguang 362
Roller needle 152
Root and branch 140
Root of Ear Vagus(MA) 97

Root of the tongue(舌本3) 358
Round needle (员针,圆针) 576
Rubella 116
　~ due to exopathogen 453
　~ due to stomach-heat 466
　Urticaria 318,565
　Wheal 116
Rugen 338
　Bixi 20
　　Xiongbi 513
Rushang 338
Ruxia 339
Ruzhong 339
Rush-fire cauterization 77
　Burning rush moxibustion 77
　Rush moxibustion 77

S

Sacrum end 70
Salt-separated moxibustion 138
Sancai points(三才2) 341
Sanchi 306
Sanguan 341
Sanjian 341
　Shaogu 357
　Xiaogu 503
Sanjiao 307
Sanjiaoshu 342
　Solitary fu 42
Sanqi Liuyi Zhen Yaojing("Three- Six" Canon of Essentials of Acupuncture) 344
Sanshang 344
Sanshui 344
Sanxiao 345
Sanyangluo 345
　Guomen 153
　Tongjian 440
　Tongmen 441

Sanyinjiao 345
　Taiyin 422
Sanyinsanyang 346
Scalp acupuncture 446
Scapha 100
　Posterior eminence of ∽ 100
Scapula 188
Scanty menstruation 217, 579
　∽ due to blood-cold 525
　∽ due to blood deficiency 530
　∽ due to blood stasis 531
　∽ due to phlegm-dampness 424
　∽ due to kidney deficiency 367
　Difficult and scanty menstruation 213
　Hard menstrual flow 213
　Infrequent menstruation 579
　Oligomenorrhea 579
Scarf needle 202
Scattered pulse(散脉2) 347
Scattered vessel(散脉1) 347
Scattering needling 347
Sciatie nerve(MA-AH 6) 649
Science of acupuncture and moxibustion 594
Scraping manipulation 370
Scrofula 258
　∽ due to stagnation of liver-qi 128
　∽ due to wind-heat pathogen 114
　∽ due to yin deficiency 561
　Mouse sore 239
　Mouse-like scorufa 407
　Scrofulous neck 244
Sea of meridians 212
Second digit from the thumb(big toe) 66
Second Speech Area, the 534
Selecting points on only the
　Yangming Meridians for the treat-
　ment of flaccidity syndromes 544

Selecting points on the affected
　meridian where a neither-excess-nor-
　deficiency syndrome lies 28
Selecting related He(Sea) points to
　treat diseases of fu organs 602
Selecting related Shu(Stream) points
　to treat diseases of zang organs 602
Selecting side points to treat
　diseases in the middle 608
Selecting Taiyang meridians for
　fulminating diseases 15
Selecting Ying(Spring) and Shu(Stream)
　points for treating meridian disorder 567
Selecting Yuan(Primary) points for
　diseases of zang organs 582
Selection of contralateral points 193
　Selection of points on the opposite side 89
Selection of lower points for upper diseases 351
　Selection of lower points 490
Selection of points according to muscle groups 3
Selection of points according to the distribution of nerves 4
Selection of points on connected meridians 201
　Selectng points on the meridians with the same name 442
Selection of Shaoyang points for bone convulsion and shakes 145
Selection of upper points for lower diseases 487
　Selection of upper points 353
Selection of Yuan(Primary) Points 9
Seng Tanran 347
Sensation transmission along the meridians 532

Sensory Area, the 131
Separative vessel 507
Setting the mountain on fire 355
Seven-line points 300
Shan Zhi(Capejasmine) and fresh ginger
  separated moxibustion 348
Shanqixue 349
  Qipangxue 302
  Sanjiaojiu 343
Shantiao Zhenjiu Jing(Shantiao Classic
  of Acupuncture and Moxibustion) 348
Shang Lu(Radix Phytolaccae)-cake
  moxibustion 350
  Shang Lu(Radix Phytolaccae)-separated
    moxibustion 137
Shang'exue 351
Shangguan(上关) 352
  Kezhuren 232
Shangjuxu 352
  Juxu 227
  Shanglin 353
  Juxushanglian 227
  Zushanglian 632
Shanglian 352
  Shoushanglian 391
Shangliao 353
Shangqu 350
  Gaoqu 131
Shangwan 353
  Shangguan(上管) 352
  Shangji 352
Shangxing 354
  Guitang 151
  Mingtang 268
  Shentang 363
Shangyang 350
  Jueyang 229
Shangyinli 354
Shangyingxiang 355

Bichuan 18
Bitong 19
Chuanbi 51
Shaochong 356
  Jingshi 213
Shaofu 356
Shaohai 357
  Qujie 325
Shaoshang 357
Shaoyang vessel 357
Shaoyangwei 358
Shaoyin vessel 358
Shaoze 358
Shaoji 357
  Xiaoji 504
Sharp stone 22
  Sagital stone 31
Shexiaxue 358
Shear needle 31
  Arrow-head needle 193
  Sharp needle 339
Shen Haowen 364
  Shen Nong Jing(Shen Nong Classic) 362
Shen Ying Jing(Classic of God Merit)
  364
Shendao 360
  Chongdao 48
  Zangshu(藏俞) 583
  Zhuangshu 623
Shenfeng 361
Shenfu 361
Shenjiao 360
Shenjiu Jinglun(Principles of Magic
  Moxibustion) 362
Shenmai 359
  Guilu(鬼路) 151
  Juyang 227
Shenmen(神门1) 362
  Duichong 89

Duigu 90
Ruizhong 340
Zhongdu2 608
Shenmen (MA)(神门2) 362
Shenque 363
　Huangu 170
　Qihe 307
　Qizhong 315
　Weihui 460
Shenshu 365
　Shaoyinshu 358
Shentang 363
Shenting 363
　Faji 103
Shenxi 365
Shenzhu 360
Shengji Zonglu(Imperial Medical Ency-
　clopaedia) 369
　　Zhenghe Shengji Zonglu (Zhenghe
　　ImperialMeil Enycopeda60Si BinTeChanes
　　73Sion Ru(Rancuius) 385
Shi Sengkuang 388
Shi Sengkuang Zhenjiu Jing(Shi
　Sengkuang's Classic of Acupuncture
　and Moxibustion 388
Shi Zangyong 386
Shi Zhanchi 388
Shidou 386
　Mingguan 269
Shier Jing Zimu Bu Xie Ge(Verses of
　the Child-Mother Reinforcing-Reducing
　Method of the Twelve Meridians) 340
Shier Jingmai Ge(A Verse of the
　Twelve Meridians) 378
Shier Ren Tu(The Twelve Pictures of
　Man) 378
Shiguan(石关1) 384
　Shique 385
　Youguan 570

Shiguan(石关2) 384
Shiguan(食关) 387
Shimen 385
　Dantian 72
　Jinglu 218
　Liji 243
　Mingmen 270
Shimianxue 370
Shiqizhui 379
Shisi Jing Fahui(An Elaboration of
　the Fourteen Meridians) 380
Shisu 388
Shiwang 382
Shiwuzhui 383
Shixuan 383
　Guicheng（鬼城）150
Shiyi Mai Jiujing(Moxibustion Classic
　Classsic of the Eleven Meridians) 384
　Bo Shu Jingmai(Meridians of the Silk
　Book) 25
Shoudazhijiahou 389
Shouhuai 389
Shoulder(肩1) 188
Shoulder (MA-SF 4)(肩2) 168
Shoulder Meridian 190
Shounizhu 390
Shousanli 390
　Guixie 151
　Sanli 344
　Shangsanli 353
Shouwuli 401
　Biwuli 21
　Chizhiwuli 47
Shouxin 401
Shouzhanghoubairoujixue 404
Shouzhanghoubijianxue 404
Shouzusuikong 405
　Shousuikong 396
Shu-point needling 406

Shuaigu 408
  Erjian 95
Shufu 405
Shugu 407
Shuwei 407
Shuxue Zhezhong(Acupoint Compromise) 408
Shuidao 408
Shuifen 409
  Zhongshou 613
Shuigou 409
  Guigong 150
  Guishi 151
  Renzhong 333
Shuiquan 410
  Shuiyuan 411
Shuitu 411
  Shuimen 410
Si Wan Feng(Atopic Eczema) 415
Si Zongxue Ge(A Vere about the Four General Acupoints) 415
Sibai 412
Sidu 412
Sifeng 413
Sihengwen 414
  Xiasifeng 490
  Zhigen 604
Sihua（四花）414
  Sihua（四华）414
  Jin Men Sihua 212
Silver needle 564
Siman（四满2）414
Siman（四满1）414
  Suifu 417
  Suizhong 417
Sishencong 415
  Shencong 360
Sizhukong 412
  Jujiao 226

Mujiao 272
Sizhu 412
Six meridians 253
Six pairs of combinations 253
Sixteen Collaterals, the 379
Sleep sage powder 412
Slow-rapid reinforcing-reducing method 517
Slurry pill palace(泥丸宫2) 282
Small Intestine (MA-SC) 495
Small moxa cone moxibustion 505
  Cone Moxibustion 505
Snake-like herpes zoster 359
  ∼ due to damp-heat pathogen 372
  ∼ due to wind-fire pathogen 112
  Heavenly fire 431
  Herpes zoster 31
    Snake-like blisters 359
Snapping of the inserted needle 88
Specifications of filiform needles 160
Sole(足心3) 645
Solution-injected moxibustion 411
Source, flow, pour and entry 141
South to mao and north to mao 264
South to mao and north to you 265
Spading 228
Specific points 427
Spermatorrhoea 168
  Incontinence of seminal fluid 218
Spitting blood 449
  ∼ due to deficiency of the spleen 295
  ∼ due to liver fire 125
  ∼ due to stomach-heat 467
  Cough with blood 416
  Hematemesis 287
Spleen(MA) 292
Spoon needle 77
  Pushing needle 450
Sprain 286

Stainless steel needle 29
Steaming with a decoction of ginger
  and chili 193
Stem-Prescription of acupoints 275
  Day-prescription of acupoints 275
Sterility 29
  ~due to blood deficiency 528
    Sterility due to insufficiency of
      blood 528
  ~ due to blood stasis 530
  ~ due to phlegm-dampness 424
  ~ due to kidney deficiency 365
  ~due to retention of cold in uterus
    13
    Sterility due to ice-cold lower abdomen
      487
    Childlessness due to cold in the
      uterus 14
    Infertility due to cold uterus 628
  Childlessness 472
  No delivery 228
  No offspring 229
  No posterity 88
Stiffneck(落枕1) 239
  Torticollis 376
Stimulation parameter 53
Stimulation point 53
Stimulation intensity 54
Stimulation therapy with warm needle
  340
Stomach(MA) 462
Stomachache 467
  ~ due to accumulaion of cold 155
  ~ due to blood stasis 570
  ~ due to cold of insufficiency 515
  ~ due to qi stagnation 313
  ~ due to retention of food 387
  ~ due to yin deficiency 562
  Epigastric pain 468

Stomach-heart pain 469
Stone needle 386
Stone needling 22
  Stone needling therapy 22
  Flying needle 106
Strabismus 506
  due to wind pathogen 113
  Cross-eye 408
Stranguria 247
  ~caused by the disorder of qi 308
    Dysuria due to the disorder of qi 385
  Dysuria with milky urine 133
  ~caused by the passage of
    Urine Stone 385
  ~ complicated by hematuria 526
  ~ due to heat 331
  ~ induced by overstrain 238
  Internal ~ 280
  Sand ~ 348
    Sand-stone ~ 348
Streams and valleys 482
  Small streams 504
Stretch skin to open the striae 158
Strong stimulation 318
Stuck needle 607
Stye 597
  Bail of eye 444
  Disorder of earth-orbiculus 449
  Wheat grain-like swelling 238
Su Wen(Plain Questions) 416
Subcortex(MA) 292
Subcutaneous needling 535
  Transverse insertion 163
Sublingual gland(廉泉3) 244
Submental region 158
Sudden collapse 16
Sudden loss of vision 16
Sulfur cauteriztion 252
Sulfur-Cinnabaris cauterization 252

Sulfur-made lozenge moxibustion 540
Suliao 416
  Bizhun(鼻准2) 20
  Mianwang 267
  Mianyu 2667
  Mianzheng 267
Sun Dingyi 417
Sun Simiao 417
Sun Simiao Zhenjing (Sun Simiao's Classic of Acupuncture) 418
Sun Zhuosan 418
Sunlight moxibustion 337
Superficial collaterals 118
Superficial venules 526
Superficialities and origins of the Twelve meridians 375
  Superficialities and origins of the six meridians 253
  Superficiality and origin of Foot-Jueyin, the 629
  Superficiality and origin of Foot-Shaoyang, the 632
  Superficiality and origin of Foot-Shaoyin, the 637
  Superficiality and origin of Foot-Taiyang, the 639
  Superficiality and origin of Foot-Taiyin, the 642
  Superficiality and origin of Foot-Yangming, the 645
  Superficiality and origin of Hand-Jueyin, the 389
  Superficiality and origin of Hand-Shaoyang, the 392
  Superficiality and origin of Hand-Shaoyin, the 394
  Superficiality and origin of Hand-Taiyang, the 396
  Superficiality and origin of Hand-Taiyin, the 398
Superior crus of antihelix 89
Superior Triangular Fossa (MA) 199
  Point for Lowering Blood Pressure (MA) 193
Suprapubic hair margin 264
Suspended moxibustion 519
Sweling and pain of the throat 534
  ∼ due to excessive heat 386
  ∼due to heat of deficiency type 515
  ∼ due to wind-heat pathogen 114
Swift insertion and slow lifting 204
Swift lifting and slow insertion 204
Sympathetic(MA-AH 7) 193
Symptomatologic point selection 417
  Point selection in accordance with the symptoms 89
Syncope syndrome 230
  Syncope 229
    ∼ due to excess of heat 331
    ∼ due to excessive loss of blood 525
    ∼ due to phlegm 424
    ∼resulting from disorder of qi 308
  Cold limbs 155

T

Tachea(MA-IC 2) 305
Taibai 419
Taichong 419
  Dachong 61
Taixi 420
  Daxi 65
  Luxi 257
  Neikunlun 280
Taiyang(太阳1) 420
Taiyang(太阳2) 420
  Dangyang(当阳2) 76

Qianguan 317
Taiyang（MA）（太阳4）420
Taiyang（太阳5）376
Taiyi（太乙）421
　　Taiyi（太一）421
Taiyi Miraculous moxa roll 421
Taiyi Shen Zhen(Magic Moxibustion with Great Monad Herbal Stick) 421
Taiyi Shenzhen Fang(Recipes of Great Monad Herbal Moxa Stick) 422
Taiyi Shenzhen Jijie(Exposition on Methods of Moxibustion with Great Monad Herbal Stick) 422
Taiyi Shenzhen Xinfa(Experiences in Moxibustion with Great Monad Herbal Stick) 422
Taiyin 422
Taiyin Meridians 422
Taiyin vessel 422
Taiyuan 423
　　Daquan1，65
　　Guixin 151
　　Taiquan 420
Taking qi from rong 56
Taking qi from wei 56
Taodao 426
Techniques of acupuncture and moxibustion 54
Techniques of filiform needle acupuncture 160
　　Filiform needle acupuncture 160
Temple(MA) 285
Tendons 209
Tetanus 298
　　～ due to injury 349
　　Convulsion due to wound by a metalic tool 202
Thenar eminence 571
Thigh pivot 22

Epiglottis of thigh 22
Third Speech Area, the 534
Thirteen ghost points, the 379
　　Thirteen points 379
　　Guicang 150
　　　Huiyin 178
　　　Yumentou 573
　　Guichen 150
　　Guitui 151
　　　Quchi 323
　　Guichuang 150
　　　Jiache 187
　　Guifeng 150
　　　Haiquan 154
　　Guigong 150
　　　Shuigou 409
　　Guiku 151
　　　Laogong 237
　　Guilei 151
　　　Yinbai 565
　　Guilu（鬼路）151
　　　Guiying 152
　　　Laogong 237
　　　Shenmai 359
　　Guishi 151
　　　Chengjiang 43
　　Guitang 151
　　　Shangxing 354
　　Guixin（鬼心）151
　　　Daling 64
　　Guixin（鬼信）151
　　　Shaoshang 357
　　Guizhen 152
　　　Fengfu 111
Thorocic Cavity Area 513
Thorough heavenly cool 448
Thoracic Vertebrae (MA) 514
Thready collateral 412
Three cai´s 341

Three hundred and sixty-five hui 340
Three hundred and sixty-five section 340
Three hundred and sixty- five collacterals 340
Three hundred and sixty-five acupoints 340
Three portions 341
Thre types of diabetes 345
Three yang meridians of foot, the 632
Three yang meridians of hand, the 391
Three yang´s 345
Three yang´s and three yin´s 345
Three yin meridians of foot, the 632
Three yin meridians of hand, the 391
Three yin´s 346
Three yin´s and three yang´s 346
Three-edged needle 344
Thrusting while pushing the needle 449
Thumb cun 270
Thunder-like miraculous needle 239
Tianchi 429
    Tianhui 431
Tianchong 430
    Tianqu 433
Tianchuang 430
    Chuanglong2, 51
    Tianlong 433
Tiancong 430
Tianding（天鼎）431
    Tianding（天顶）430
Tianfu 431
Tianjing（天井）431
Tianliao 432
Tianquan 433
    Tianjing（天泾）431
    Tianshi 434
    Tianwen 435

Tianrong 433
    Darong 65
Tiansheng Zhenjing(Imperial Holy Classic of Acupuncture 433
Tianshu 434
    Buyuan 27
    Changxi 40
    Gumen 142
    Xunji 532
    Xunyuan 532
Tiantu 434
    Yuhu 572
Tianqu 433
Tianxi 435
Tianyou 436
Tianyuan Taiyi Ge(Verse of Taiyi in Nature) 436
Tianzhu 437
Tianzhu bone 437
Tianzong 437
Tiaokou 437
Tiger´s mouth 167
Ting Li Zi (Lipidium Seed)-cake- separated moxibustion 123
    Cake-moxibustion of Tingli (Semen Lepidi Seu Desocurainiae) 439
Tinggong 439
    Duosuowen 91
Tinghui 439
    Houguan 166
    Tinghe（听呵）438
    Tinghe（听河）438
Tinnitus 97
    ~ during pregnancy 335
    Chip of cicada in the ear 100
    Deficiency-type of ~ and deafness 97
    Excess-type ~ and deafness 97
Tinplate needle 262

Tiny collaterals 484
Toad(虾蟆2) 154
Toad-separated moxibustion 134
Toe(MA) 604
Tongli（通里）440
   Tongli（通理）441
Tongli（通理）441
Tongren (A Bronze Statue) 442
Tongren Shuxue Zhenjiu Tujing
(Illustrated Manual of Points for
Acupoints and Moxibustion on a Bronze
with Acupoints) 442
Tongren Zhenjiu Fang (Prescription
for acupuncture and Moxibustion on a
Bronze Statue) 443
Tongren Zhiyao Fu (A Prose on the
Essentials of a Bronze Statue) 443
Tongtian 441
   Tianjiu 432
Tongue(MA) 321
Tongxuan Zhiyao Fu (Ode to the appre-
hension of Abstruse Essentials of
Acupuncture 441
Tongziliao 443
   Houqu 166
   Qianguan 317
   Taiyang 420
   Yuwei 572
Tonsil(MA) 22
Top of shoulder(肩髃2) 191
Tooth (MA) 533
Toothache 533
   ~ due to deficiency fire 515
   ~ due to excess-heat 386
   ~ due to wind-fire pathogen 112
Top 79
Touchong 444
Toulinqi 444
   Lingqi 247

Mulinqi 272
Touqiaoyin 444
   Shouqiaoyin 405
   Zhengu 598
Touwei 445
   Sangda 347
   Toufeng 444
Tragic apex (MA) 298
   Zhuding 620
Tragus 97
   Ear pearl 100
Training-navel method 245
Transmission 406
Transverse bone(横骨2) 163
Transverse bone of head 444
Transverse crease(横纹1) 164
Transverse Meridian 164
Treating edema by selecting the Jing
(River) points 119
Treating excess with reducing
methods 369
Treating subsidence with moxibustion
493
Trembling method 98
Triangular fossa 343
Tubercle posterior to the triangular
fossa 343
Tuangang 449
   Huangang 170
Tube for needle insertion 206
Tube moxibustion 443
Twelve contraindications 374
Twelve Cutaneous Regions, the 378
   Cutaneous regions 291
   Cutaneous regions of the six
      meridians 253
Twelve Divergent Meridians 376
   Divergent meridians 208
   Divergent Meridian of Foot- Jueyin,

the 630
Divergence of Foot-Jusyin, the 631
Divergent Meridian of Foot-Shaoyang, the 635
Divergence of Foot-Shaoyang, the 647
Divergent Meridian of Foot-Shaoyin, the 637
Divergence of Foot-Shaoyin, the 639
Divergent Meridian of Foot-Taiyang, the 639
Divergence of Foot-Taiyang, the 642
Divergent Meridian of Foot-Taiyin, the 642
Divergence of Foot-Taiyin, the 644
Divergent Meridian of Foot-Yangming, the 645
Divergence of Foot-Yangming, the 648
Divergent Meridian of Hand-Jueyin, the 389
Divergence of Hand-Jueyin, the 401
Divergent Meridian of Hand-Shaoyang, the 392
Divergence of Hand-Shaoyang, the 394
Dvergent Meridian of Hand-Shaoyin, the 394
Divergence of Hand-Shaoyin, the 396
Divergent Meridian of Hand-Taiyang, te 396
Divergence of Hand-Taiyang, the 398
Divergent Meridian of Hand-Taiyin, the 400
Divergence of Hand-Taiyin, the 401
Divergent Meridian of Hand-Yangming, the 403
Divergence of Hand-Yangming, the 404
Divergent Meridians of Hand-Yangming and Hand-Taiyin 404
Divergent Meridians of Foot-Shaoyang and Foot-Jueyin, the 637
Divergent Meridians of Foot-Taiyang and Foot-Shaoyin, the 642
Divergent Meridians of Foot-Yangming and Foot-Taiyin, the 648
Divergent Meridians of Hand- Shaoyang and Hand-Jueyin, the 393
Divergent Meridians of Hand-Taiyang and Hand-Shoyin, the 397
Twelve Meridians, the 377
Twelve Regular Meridians, the 379
Bladder Meridian of Foot-Taiyang, the 640
Bladder Meridian, the 289
Diseases of ∼ 641
Bladder Vessel of Foot-Taiyang 290
Gallbladder Meridian of Foot-Shaoyang 633
Gallbldder Meridian, the 74
Diseases of ∼ 635
Gallbadder Vessel of Foot-Shaoyang, the 75
Heart Meridian of Hand-Shaoyin, the 395
Heart Meridian, the 509
Diseases of ∼ 396
Vessel of the Heart Hand-Shaoyin, the 509
Kidney Meridian of Foot-Shaoyin, the 638
Kidney Meridian, the 364
Diseases of ∼ 639
Foot-shaoyin Vessel of the Kidney 368
Large Intestine Meridian of Hand-Yangming, the 401
Large Intestine Meridian 60
Diseases of ∼ 403
Hand-Yangming Vessel of Large Intestine 61
Liver Meridian of Foot-Jueyin, the 629

Liver Meridian, the 125
　Diseases of ∼ 630
　Foot-Jueyin Vessel of the Liver 130
Lung Meridian of Hand-Taiyin 398
　Lung Meridian, the 107
　Diseases of ∼ 399
　Lung Vessel of Hand-Taiyin 108
Pericardium Meridian of Hand-Jueyin, the 390
　Pericardium Meridian 510
　Diseases of ∼ 390
　Pericardium Vessel of Hand-Jueyin 510
Sanjiao Meridian of Hand-Shaoyang, the 393
　Sanjiao Meridian, the 342
　Diseases of ∼ 393
　Sanjiao Vessel of Hand-Shaoyan, 342
Small Intestine Meridian of Hand-Taiyang, the 398
　Small Intestine Meridian 495
　Diseses of ∼ 398
　Small Intestine Vessel of Hand-Taiyang 495
Spleen Meridian of Foot-Taiyin, the 643
　Spleen Meridian, the 293
　Diseases of ∼ 644
　Spleen Vessel of Foot-Taiyin, the 296
Stomach Meridian of Foot-Yangming, the 647
　Stomach Meridian, the 463
　Diseases of ∼ 648
　Stomach Meridian in Neck, the 566
　Stomach Vessel of Foot-Yangming 469
　Yangming Vessel, the 481
Twelve methods of acupuncture 374
　Twelve puncturing methods 373
　　Twelve needlings(十二节1) 374

Adjacent puncture 13
Assembling puncture 300
　Gathering puncture 185
Centro-square needling 542
　Yang puncture 536
Lateral puncture 176
Mated puncture 287
Repeated shallow puncture 582
Short-thrust needling 88
Shu needling 406
Straight puncture 602
Superficial puncture 118
Trigger puncture 15
Yin puncture 554
Twelve muscle regions 377
　Muscle Region of Foot-Jueyin, the 630
　　Diseases of ∼ 630
　Muscle Region of Foot-Shaoyang, the 635
　　Diseases of ∼ 636
　Muscle Region of Foot-Shaoyin, the 637
　　Diseases of ∼ 638
　Muscle region of Foot-Taiyang, the 640
　　Diseases of ∼ 640
　Muscle region of Foot-Taiyin, the 642
　　Diseases of ∼ 642
　Muscle region of Foot-Yangming, the 645
　　Diseases of ∼ 646
　Muscle Regions of Hand-Jueyin 389
　　Diseases of ∼ 389
　Muscle Region of Hand-Shaoyang, the 392
　　Diseases of ∼ 392
　Muscle Region of Hand-Shaoyin, the 395
　　Diseases of ∼ 395
　Muscle Region of Hand-Taiyang, the 397
　　Diseases of ∼ 397
　Muscle Region of Hand-Taiyin, the 400

Diseases of ~ 400
  Muscle Region of Hand-Yangming, the 403
    Diseases of ~ 403
Twelve needling methods 378
  Orderly needling methods with 12
    words 379
  1. Nail pressing(爪切) 586
  2. Finger holding 603
  3. Mouth warming 234
  4. Method of insertion 206
  5. Finer pressing 604
  6. Nail scratching 586
  7. Needle lifting 597
  8. Finger rotating 603
  9. Finger twirling 604
  10. Finger retaining 604
  11. Needle shaking 597
  12. Finger pulling 603
Twelve pictures of man 378
Twelve sections(十二节2) 336
Twelve successions 373
Twenty-seven kinds of qi 102
Twining collaterals 31
Twirling reinforcing and reducing 283
Twirling the acupuncture needle 283
Twisting 257
Two fires 101
Two yang´s, the 102
Two yin´s, the 102
Tympanites 146
  ~due to blood stasis 524
    Abdominal distention due to
      accumulated blood 518
  ~ due to fluid retention 407
  ~ due to the stagnation of qi 305
  Bulge 146
  Disease of Distention 586
  Distention(胀1) 585
  Single abdominal distention 72

Spider-like distention 540
Single meteorism 72

U

Umbilical warming 470
Uniform reinforcing-reducing 297
Unripeness and ripness 368
Upper arm 277
Upper bone 351
Upper ear root(上耳根1) 351
Upper eye outline 272
  Upper eye net 273
Upper Root of Auricle (MA)(上耳根2) 315
  Middle Stasis (MA) 575
  Spinal Cord 1(MA) 185
Upper tragic notch 298
Ureter(MA-SC 7) 406
Urethra(MA) 284
Urogenitial region(宗筋1) 628
Uroschesis 255
  Deficiency syndrome of ~ 256
  Excess syndrome of ~ 256
  Retention of urine 255
  Dysuria 20
Urticaria 318
Urticaria Point (MA) 318
Usage area, the 581

V

Verse-fu on acupuncture and moxibustion 592
Vessel of Foot-Juyang 629
Vessel of Foot-Juanyang 629
Vessel of Foot-Jueyin 631
Vessel of Foot-Shaoyang 636
Vessel of Foot-Shaoyin 638
Vessel of Foot-Taiyang 644
Vessel of Foot-Taiyin 644
Vessel qi 263
Vigorous reduction 65
Vigorous reinforcing and reducing method 59

Penetrating heaven coolness 448
Setting the mountain on fire 355
Vomiting 287
～ due to cold of insufficiency 514
～ due to exopathogen 453
～ due to improper diet 349
～ due to liver qi 125
～ due to retention of phlegm 425
～ due to yin deficiency 561

W

Waiguan 453
   Yangweixue 540
Waihuaijian 454
Waihuaiqianjiaomai 454
Waihuaishang 454
Waijinjinyuye 454
Waike Jiufa Luncui Xinshu (A New Book on Essentials of Moxibustion for External Diseases) 455
Wailaogong 455
   Xiangqiangxue 493
Waiqiu 455
Waitai Miyao (Clandestine Essentials from the Imperial Library) 456
Waixiyan 456
Waiting for qi 166
Waiting for the proper time 167
Walnut-like bone 162
Walnut-separated moxibustion 162
Wangu (完骨) 456
Wangu (腕骨) 457
Wang Bing 458
Wang Chuming 458
Wang Guorui 458
Wang Haogu 458
Wang Huaiyin 458
Wang Kai 458
Wang Keming 458

Wan Tao 459
Wang Weiyi 459
Wang Yu 459
Wang Zhizhong 459
Wang Zongquan 459
Wang Zuan 459
Warm needle moxibustion 471
   Needle-handle moxibustion 588
   Heat-conducting moxibustion 51
   Heating the needle end 355
   Warm needling 471
Water 408
Water-ditch 409
Wter-flow of the Twelve Meridians, 378
Watery disease 408
Wei Shijie 462
Weibao 460
Weicang 462
Weicui 460
   Xiaoerganli 496
   Xiaoerganshou 496
Weidao 460
Waishu 456
Weigong 460
Weiqionggu 461
Weisheng Zhenjiu Xuanji Miyao (Mysterious Clandestine Essentials of Acupuncture and Moxibustion for Health Protection) 462
Weishu 467
Weiwanxiashu 468
   Yishu 493
Weiyang 461
   Xiyang 485
Weizhong 461
   Weizhongyang 462
   Xizhong 485
   Xuexi 528

Zhongxi 614
Wenliu 470
　Chitou 46
　Nizhu 283
　Shetou 359
Wenren Qinian 471
White pepper moxibustion 10
White tiger shaking it's head 10
Wind gate 113
Withdraw 450
Withdrawing the needle 51
　Pulling away the needle 564
　Pulling out the needle 103
　Removing the needle(排针1) 288
Wrinkle, the 578
Wrist(腕2) 457
Wrist-ankle needling 457
Wrist(MA-SF 2)(腕1) 457
Wu Bei Zi(Galla Chinesis) moxibustion 474
Wu Bei Zi(Galla Chinensis) steaming moxibustion 474
Wu Fugui 472
Wu Jiayan 473
Wu Kun 473
Wu Qian 473
Wu Wenbing 473
Wu Yiding 473
Wu Zhiying 474
Wuchu 475
Wuhu 475
Wumei (Fructus Mune steam moxibustion 419
　Wushu 478
Wuyi 472

X

Xi Fang Zi Mingtang Jiujing (Xi Fang Zi Classic of Moxibustion) 482

Xi Hong 484
Xi Hong Fu (Ode to Xi Hong) 484
Xi Xin(Herba Asari) vesiculation 485
Xi(Cleft) points 485
Xiguan 482
Ximen 484
Xipang 483
Xishang 483
Xiwai 483
Xixia 483
Xiyan 483
　Guiyan 152
　Ximu 483
Xiyangguan 484
　Guanling 147
　Guanyang 148
　Hanfu 155
　Yangling 538
Xia Ying 491
Xiabai 485
　Jiabai 186
Xiachengjiang 486
Xiaguan(下关) 487
Xiajishu 488
　Xiajizhishu 488
Xiajuxu 489
　Juxu 227
　Juxuxialian 227
Xialian 489
Xialin 490
　Zuxialian 645
Xiakunlun 489
　Neikunlun 280
Xialian 489
　Shouxialian 401
Xialiao 489
Xiashangxing 486
Xiawan 490
　Xiaguan(下管) 487

75

Youmen 569
　Xiangu（陷谷）492
　Xiangu（陷骨）493
Xiaxi 486
Xiayao 491
Xiang Fu（Rhizoma Cyperi）cake 493
Xiang Fu(Cyperustuber)-cake-separated moxibustion 138
Xiang Liu(Moschussulfur) cake 493
Xiangqiangxue 493
Xiaochangshu 496
Xiaoerjixiongxue 497
　Xiaoerguixiongxue 497
Xiaoershixian 499
Xiaoershuijing 499
Xiaogukong（小骨空）503
　Xiaogukong（小骨孔）503
Xiaohai 503
Xiaoli 494
Xiaoluo 494
Xiaotianxin 504
Xiaozhijian（小指尖）504
　Shoutaiyangxue 398
　Xiaozhitou 504
　Yanxiao 535
Xiaozhijian（小趾尖）504
Xiaozhizhaowen 504
Xie Ye(Bulbus Allii Macrostemi)-separated moxibustion 138
Xietamg 505
Xin Ji Mingtang Jiufa (Mew Collection of Mingtang Moxibustion) 510
Xinhui 510
　Dingmen 83
Xinjian 510
Xinshe 510
Xinshu 509
Xinzhong 511
Xingjian 511

Xinglong 511
Xinzhen Zhiyao Fu (Ode to the Essentials of Acupuncture) 512
Xingzhen Zongyao Ge (A Verse on Generals of Acupuncture) 512
Xiongtang 513
Xiongtonggu 513
Xiongxiang 513
Xu Chunfu 516
Xu Feng 517
Xu Tingzhang 517
Xu Wenzhong 517
Xu Yue 517
Xu Xi 517
Xu Yuqing 517
Xu-needle 461
Xuanji 璇玑 518
　Xuanji（旋机）518
　Xuanji（旋玑）518
Xuanli 518
Xuanlu 519
Xuanming 519
　Guilu(鬼禄) 151
Xuanshu 519
　Xuanzhu 520
Xuanwu Huiyao Zhenjing (Canon for Understanding the Essentials of Acupuncture 518
Xuanwu Sishen Zhenfa (Comprehension of Four-Spirit Methods of Acupuncture) 518
Xuanzhong 519
　Juegu 228
Xue Ji 521
　Xue Lizhai 521
Xuehai 524
　Baichongwo(百虫窝2) 11
Xuemen 526
Xunjing Kaoxue Bian (Studies on

Acupoints along Meridians) 532

Y

Yamen 533
    Hengshe 164
    Sheheng 358
    Sheyan 359
    Yinmen（瘖门）563
Yan Zhen 477
Yankou 534
Yanzi 535
    Liangshouyanzigu 246
Yang collaterals 539
Yang occluded in yin 563
Yang Jizhou 543
Yang Jie 543
Yang Jingzhai Zhenjiu Quanshu (Yang Jingzhai's Complete Book of Acupuncture and Moxibustion) 543
Yang needling 536
Yang Shangshan 543
Yang Xun 543
Yang Yanqi 544
Yangbai 536
Yangchi 536
    Bieyang（别阳1）25
Yangfu 536
    Fenrou 109
    Juegu 207
Yanggang（阳刚）537
Yanggang（阳纲）537
    Changfeng 40
    Yanggang（阳刚）537
Yanggu 537
Yangguan 537
    Beiyangguan 17
    Yangling（阳陵2）538
Yangjiao 538
    Bieyang（别阳2）25

Yanglao 544
Yanglingquan 538
    Yangling（阳陵1）538
    Yangzhilingquan 542
Yangweixue 540
Yangxi 541
    Zhongkui 611
Yaomu 545
Yaoqi 545
Yaoshu 545
    Beijie 16
    Suikong 417
    Suishu 417
    Yaohu 544
    Yaizhu（腰注）547
    Yaizhu（腰柱）547
Yaotongdian 546
Yaotongxue 546
Yaoyan 546
    Guiyan 152
    Yaomujiao 549
Yaoyangguan 546
    Beiyangguan 17
Yaoyi 547
Ye Chashan 548
Ye Guangzuo 549
Yemen（液门）549
    Yemen（腋门1）549
    Yemen（掖门2）549
    Yemen（掖门1）549
    Yejian（掖间）549
    Yemen（腋门3）549
Yexiaxue 550
Yellow wax moxibustion 176
Yi Huan 550
Yidao 552
Yifeng 553
Yijing Xiaoxue (Collection of Elementary Medical Classics) 551

Yiming 554
Yishe 553
Yixi 553
   Wuqushu 477
Yixue Gangmu (An Outline of Medicine) 511
Yixue Rumen (An Introduction to Medicine) 551
Yizong Jinjian (Gold Mirror of Orthodox Medical Lineage) 551
Yin collaterals 557
Yin occluded in yang 542
Yin Ju 563
Yin knotted pulse(阴结2) 556
Yinbai 565
   Guilei 151
Yinbao（阴包）554
   Yinbao（阴胞）554
Yindu 554
   Shigong(食宫) 387
   Shigong(石宫) 384
   Tongguan 440
Yingu 555
Yinjiao（阴交）556
   Henghu 163
   Shaoguan 357
Yinjiao（龈交）564
   Yinjiao（断交）564
Yinjingxue 556
   Shitou 388
Yinlian 556
Yinlingquan 557
   Yinling 557
   Yinzhilingquan 563
Yinmen（殷门）563
Yinmen（寅门）564
Yinnangfeng 557
   Nangxiafeng 276
Yinnangxiahengwen 557

Yinshi 558
   Yinding 554
Yintang（印堂1）565
Yinwei points(阴维穴1) 559
Yinxi(阴郄) 559
   Shaoyinxi 321
   Shoushaoyinxi 354
Yinxi（饮郄）565
Yinyangxue（阴阳穴1）562
Ying(Spring) points 568
Yingchi 568
   Yinyangxue（阴阳穴2）562
Yingchuang 566
Yingtu 565
Yingxiang 567
   Chongyang 49
Yongju Shenmi Jiujing (Mysterious Canon of Moxibustion for Carbuncle) 568
Yongju Shenmiao Jiujing (Wonderful Canon of Moxibustion for Carbuncle) 68
Yongquan（涌泉）568
   Diwei 79
   Dichong 78
   Yongquan（勇泉）568
   Zuxin 645
Youmen 569
   Shangmen 353
Yu Fakai 571
Yugui Zhenjing (Canon of Acupuncture of the Jade Chamber) 572
Yuji 571
Yulong Fu (Jade Dragon Ode) 573
Yumentou 573
   Guicang 150
   Nuyinfeng 286
Yuquan(玉泉2, 3) 573
Yutang 573
   Yuying 574

Yutian 573
Yuwei 572
Yuyao(鱼腰)1, 572
Yuzhen 574
Yuzhong（彧中）575
  Huozhong 181
  Yuzhong（域中）575
Yuan(Primary) point 577
Yuanye（渊腋）575
  Quanye 327
  Yuanye（渊液）575
Yun Qizi 580
Yunmen 580

Z

Zabing Shiyi Zheng Ge (Eleven Verses for Miscellaneous Diseases) 582
Zang organ points(藏俞2) 583
Zangshu(藏俞1) 583
Zhang Di 585
Zhang Jiebin 584
Zhang Quan 584
Zhang Yuansu 584
Zhang Zhicong 584
Zhang Zhongjing 584
Zhangmen 585
  Changping(长平1) 369
  Jixie 186
  Xiejiao 505
Zhaohai 586
  Taiyiqiao 423
  Yinqiaoxue 558
Zhejin 587
Zhen Quan 598
Zhenfang (Acupuncture Prescriptions) 589
Zhenfang Liuji (Six Collections of Acupuncture Prescription) 589
Zhenjing (Canon of Acupuncture) 590
Zhenjing Jieyao (Essentials of Acupuncture Classics) 590
Zhenjing Zhaiying Ji (A Collection of Gems from Acupuncture Classics) 591
Zhenjing Zhinan (Guide to the Classics of Acupuncture) 591
Zhenjiu Dacheng (A Great Compendium of Acupunture and Moxibustion) 591
Zhenjiu Daquan (A Complete Work of Acupuncture and Moxibustion) 591
Zhenjiu Jicheng (A Collection of Acupucture and Moxibustion) 592
Zhenjiu Jia-Yi Jing (A-B Classic of Acupuncture and Moxibustion) 592
Zhenjiu Jingxue Tukao (Study on Acupoints Illustrations of Acupuncture and Moxibustion) 593
Zhenjiu Juying (Essentials of Acupuncture and Moxibustion) 593
Zhenjiu Juying Fahui (An Elaboration of Essentials of Acupuncture and Moxibustion) 593
Zhenjiu Quansheng (A Book on Acupuncture and Moxibustion for Saving Life) 593
Zhenjiu Si Shu (Four Books on Acupuncture and Moxibustion) 593
Zhenjiu Su Nan Yaozhi(The Essentials of Acupuncture and Moxibustion in Plain Questions and The Classic of Questions) 593
Zhenjiu Tu Yaojue (Essentials of the Diagrams of Acupunture and Moxibustion) 594
Zhenjiu Tujing (Illustrated Canon of Ackupunture and Moxibustion) 594
Zhenjiu Wen Da (Questions and Answers on Acupuncture and Moxibustion) 594
Zhenjiu Wen Dui (Catechism of Acupunc-

ture and Moxibustion) 594
Zhenjiu Yaozhi (Essentials of Acupuncture and Moxibustion) 595
Zhenjiu Yi Xue (Acupuncture and Moxibustion Are Easy to Learn) 595
Zhenjiu Zashuo (Miscellaneous Remarks on Acupuncture and Moxibustion) 595
Zhenjiu Zeri Bianjiu (A Collection of Acupunture and Moxibustion Selected Days 595
Zhenjiu Zisheng Jing (Acupuncture-Moxibustion Classic for Saving life) 595
Zhenjiu Zuanyao (A Compilation of Essentials of Acupuncture and Moxibustion) 596
Zhenjiuxue (Science of Acupuncture and Moxibustion) 594
Zhengying 600
Zhi Lugu 602
Zhi Mi Fu (Ode for Dispelling Confusions) 604
Zhibian 606
Zhigen 604
   Xiasifeng 490
Zhigou 600
   Feichu 105
   Feihu 105
Zhigu 602
Zhishi 605
   Jinggong 218
Zhiyang 605
Zhiyin 605
Zhizheng 601
Zhongchong 608
Zhongdu (中都1) 608
Zhongdu (中渎) 608
   Xiadu 487

Zhongdu(中犊) 609
Zhongfeng 609
   Xuanquan 519
Zhongfengbuyuxue 616
Zhongfengqixue 616
Zhongfu 609
   Feimu 108
   Fuzhongshu 119
   Longhan 253
   Yingshu 566
   Yingzhong 566
   Yingzhongshu 566
Zhonggao Kongxue Tujing(Zhong Gao Canon of Acupoints with Illustrations) 610
Zhongguo Zhenjiu Zhiliaoxue(Therapeutics of Chinese Acupuncture and Moxibustion) 610
Zhongguo Zhenjiuxue(Chinese Acupuncture and Moxibustion) 610
Zhonghua Zhenjiuxue (Acupuncture and Moxibustiuon of China) 610
Zhongji 611
   Qiyuan 314
   Yuquan(玉泉1) 573
Zhongju 611
   Chuiju 52
Zhongliao 612
Zhongkong 611
Zhonglüshu 612
   Jineishu 185
   Zhonglü 612
   Zhonglüneishu 612
   Zhonglüshu(中膂输) 612
Zhongkui2, 611
Zhongping 612
Zhongquan 613
Zhongshu 613
   Zhongzhu(中柱) 616

Zhongting 614
Zhongwan 614
  Dacang 59
  Shangji 352
  Taicang 419
  Weiguan 463
  Zhongguan 610
Zhongwu 614
Zhongxi 614
Zhongzhijie 615
  Shouzhongzhidiyijiexue 361
Zhongzhu（中渚）615
  Xiadu 487
Zhongzhu（中注）616
Zhou Hanqing 618
Zhouhou Beiji Fang（A Handbook of Prescriptions for Emergencies）619
Zhouhou Ge（A Verse for Convenience of Acupuncture and Moxibustion）619
Zhoujian 619
Zhouliao（肘髎）620
  Zhouliao（肘聊）620
Zhourong 618
  Zhouying 619
Zhoushu 620
Zhouzhui 620
Zhubin（筑宾）622
Zhubin（筑滨）622
Zhubu 622
Zhushi 621
Zhuxia 622
Zhuan 623
Zhuang 623
Zhuangshu 623
Zi Bao 624

Zigong（子宫2）624
  Xiayuquan 486
Zigong（紫宫）628
Zi-wu dao jiu needling 626
Zi-Wu Jing（Classic on Midnight-Noon）626
Zi-Wu Liuzhu（Midnight-Noon Ebb-Flow）626
Zi-Wu Liuzhu Zhen Fa（Needling Methods of Midnight-Noon Ebb-Flow）626
Zi-Wu Liuzhu Zhenjing（Acupuncture Classic on Midnight-Noon Ebb-Flow）627
Zi-Wu Liuzhu Zhu Ri An Shi Ding Xue Ge（Rhymes for Selecting Points in Terms of Heavenly Stems and Time of Each Day of Midnight Noon Ebb-Flow）627
Zi-wu（midnight noon）methods 626
Zudierzhishang 628
Zujiao 629
Zulinqi 631
Zuqiaoyin 631
Zusanli 632
  Guixie 151
  Sanli 344
  Xialing 489
  Xialingsanli 490
  Xiasanli 490
Zushaoyangxue 636
Zutaiyangxue 641
Zutonggu 644
  Tonggu 440
Zuwuli 644
  Wuli 476
Zuxin 645
Zuan 648
Zygomatic region 327

图书在版编目(CIP)数据

汉英双解针灸大辞典/石学敏,张孟辰主编. — 北京:华夏出版社,1998.1
ISBN7—5080—1377—8
Ⅰ.汉… Ⅱ.①石…②张… Ⅲ.针灸学—词典—汉、英 Ⅳ.R245-61
中国版本图书馆 CIP 数据核字(97)第 23180 号

华 夏 出 版 社 出 版 发 行
(北京东直门外香河园北里4号 邮编:100028)
新 华 书 店 经 销
北京房山先锋印刷厂印刷
787×1092 1/16开本 49.5印张 1640千字
1998年1月北京第1版 1998年1月北京第1次印刷
定价:160.00元

(本版图书凡印刷、装订错误,可及时向我社发行部调换)